Jean-Claude Givel (Ed.)

Surgery of the Thymus

Pathology, Associated Disorders and Surgical Technique

Co-editors:
Marco Merlini David B. Clarke Michael Dusmet

With 239 Figures and 45 Tables

Springer-Verlag Berlin Heidelberg New York
London Paris Tokyo Hong Kong

Editor

PD Dr. Jean-Claude Givel

Centre Hospitalier Universitaire Vaudois
1011 Lausanne, Switzerland

Co-editors

Dr. Marco Merlini
Dr. Michael Dusmet

Service de Chirurgie A, Centre Hospitalier
Universitaire Vaudois, 1011 Lausanne
Switzerland

David B. Clarke MB FRCS

The Queen Elizabeth Hospital, Queen Elizabeth
Medical Centre, Edgbaston, Birmingham B15 2TH
United Kingdom

ISBN-13:978-3-642-71078-0 e-ISBN-13:978-3-642-71076-6
DOI: 10.1007/978-3-642-71076-6

Library of Congress Cataloging-in-Publication Data.
Surgery of the thymus : pathology, associated disorders and surgical technique / Jean-Claude Givel (ed.) ; co-editors, Marco Merlini, David B. Clarke, Michael Dusmet. p. cm. Includes bibliographical references.
ISBN-13:978-3-642-71078-0 (U. S. : alk. paper)
1. Thymus-Surgery. 2. Thymus-Diseases. 3. Thymus-Pathophysiology. I. Givel, J.-Cl. (Jean-Cl.). 1946- [DNLM: 1. Thymus Gland-pathology. 2. Thymus Gland-physiopathology. 3. Thymus Gland-surgery. WK 400 S961]
RD598.8.S87 1990 617.5'46-dc20 DNLM/DLC 89-26267

Softcover reprint of the hardcover 1st edition 1990

2124/3140/543210 - Printed on acid-free paper

Preface

The thymus gland has always fascinated me and, despite the ever-growing abundance of medical books, this subject seemed to be a bit of a "poor relation." As a surgeon, the lack of information was particularly frustrating, and this is why I decided to edit a text covering the different aspects of thymic pathology, surgery, and prognosis.

It is always difficult to strike a balance between what is to be included and left out of a book about a subject intended for readers of different specialities. This one was written primarily to provide valuable information to surgeons on most aspects related to thymic surgery and to other specialists who are often confronted with thymic diseases. Written by leaders in their respective fields, I hope it will provide an excellent reference for those interested in an up-to-date synthesis of general knowledge of such highly specialized areas as immunology, pathology, and neuroscience.

The opening chapters on clinical management provide a historical review and descriptions of the normal thymus and surgical pathology. Later chapters review the various diseases related to the surgical pathology of the thymus. Investigations, surgical procedures, and other therapeutic modalities are also extensively covered. The book closes with chapters on the postoperative evolution of myasthenia gravis and thymic tumors, as well as on the effect of thymectomy in human oncogenesis.

A book of such a wide spectrum takes time to be edited. As new developments take place so rapidly in some fields (particularly immunology and neurophysiology), it is inevitable that some chapters may not cite the very latest references. Nevertheless, it should not be forgotten that the aim of this book is rather to offer the nonspecialist a synthesis which will not go out of date too quickly, even in these highly specialized areas.

I would like to pay special tribute to all the authors who have collaborated by submitting outstanding contributions. A book of this scope would not have been possible without their cooperation. I asked researchers and clinicians with a special interest in the thymus to give overviews of their respective fields in light of recent findings. I am sure that their texts will not only prove of value as a current review of surgical aspects of thymic pathology, but will also act as a stimulus to those interested in further study of the many unresolved problems. The delays encountered in the preparation of this book have been a great nuisance to those authors who submitted their manuscripts according to my original schedule and who have had to revise their chapters. I am grateful for their cooperation.

I would also like to thank my coeditors Marco Merlini, David Clarke, and Michael Dusmet for their excellent help in the tremendous job of editing these 32 chapters.

Lausanne, 1990 JEAN-CLAUDE GIVEL

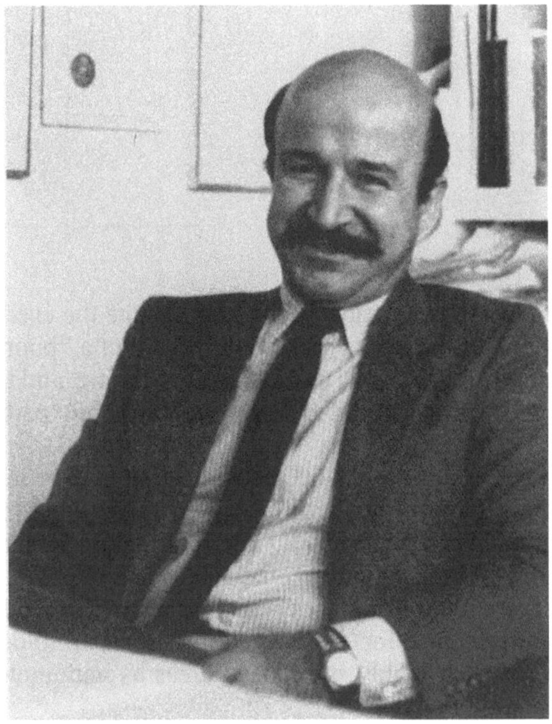

This book is dedicated to the memory of Professor ANGELOS E. PAPATESTAS (1939–1989). His outstanding contribution to the surgery of the thymus and to our understanding of the importance of thymectomy in myasthenia gravis is even more remarkable in view of the fact that his career was tragically short and his interests were manifold. We regret his untimely death all the more deeply because he was one of the more enthusiastic authors of our book from the outset, believing that there was a true need for a volume dedicated to the surgery of the thymus. This was both a great honor and an encouragement for us all.

Table of Contents

List of Contributors

BACH, JEAN-FRANÇOIS, Prof.; Unité de Recherches Immunopathologiques et Néphrologiques de l'INSERM U 25, Laboratoire Associé du CNRS 122, Immunologie Clinique, Hôpital Necker, 161, rue de Sèvres, 75743 Paris Cedex 15, France

BERGMANS, JOSEPH A. M., M. D.; Laboratory of Clinical Neurophysiology, Faculty of Medicine, Catholic University of Louvain, Avenue Hippocrate 54, 1200 Brussels, Belgium

BHARDWAJ, SUSHIL, M. B. B. S.; Dept. of Neoplastic Diseases, Mount Sinai School of Medicine, One Gustave L. Levy Place, New York, NY 10029, USA

BOUMGHAR, MOHAMED, M. D.; Service de Chirurgie A, Centre Hospitalier Universitaire Vaudois, 1011 Lausanne, Switzerland

CHAHINIAN, A. PHILIPPE, M. D.; Dept. of Neoplastic Diseases, Mount Sinai School of Medicine, One Gustave Levy Place, New York, NY 10029, USA

CLARKE, DAVID B., MB FRCS; Cardiothoracic Surgery Unit, Queen Elizabeth Hospital, Edgbaston, Birmingham 15, United Kingdom

DARDENNE, MIREILLE; Unité de Recherches Immunopathologiques et Néphrologiques de l'INSERM U 25, Laboratoire Associé du CNRS 122, Immunologie Clinique, Hôpital Necker, 161, rue de Sèvres, 75743 Paris Cedex 15, France

DUSMET, MICHAEL, M. D., Service de Chirurgie A, Centre Hospitalier Universitaire Vaudois, 1011 Lausanne, Switzerland

FULPIUS, BERNARD W., Prof., M. D. Ph. D.; Dept. of Biochemistry, University of Geneva, Faculty of Sciences, 30, quai Ernest-Ansermet, 1211 Genève, Switzerland

GAMSU, GORDON, M. D.; Dept. of Radiology, University of California Medical Center, San Francisco, CA 94143, USA

GIVEL, JEAN-CLAUDE, M. D. Privat-Docent; Service der Chirurgie A, Centre Hospitalier Universitaire Vaudois, 1011 Lausanne, Switzerland

GRAY, STEPHEN W., Ph. D.; Center for Surgical Anatomy and Technique, Emory University School of Medicine, 1440 Clifton Road, 105 WHSCAB, Atlanta, GA 30322, USA

HESS, MAX W., M. D.; Institute of Pathology, University of Bern, Freiburgstraße 30, 3010 Bern, Switzerland

HOFMANN, WALTER J., Dr.; Institute of Pathology, University of Heidelberg, Im Neuenheimer Feld 220/221, 6900 Heidelberg, Federal Republic of Germany

HONG, RICHARD, M. D.; Dept. of Pediatrics, University of Wisconsin, Clinical Science Center, 600 Highland Avenue, Madison, WI 53792, USA

HOWELLS, T. HILARY, M. D.; Dept. of Anaesthesia, Royal Free Hospital, Pond Street, London NW3 2QG, United Kingdom

KATER, LOUIS, M. D.; Division of Immunopathology, Dept. of Internal Medicine and Institute of Pathology, University Hospital, 101 Catharijnesingel, 3511 GV Utrecht, The Netherlands

KENDALL, MARION D., Prof. M. D.; Division of Anatomy, United Medical and Dental Schools, Guy's and St. Thomas's Hospitals Medical School, Lambeth Palace Road, London SE1 7EH, United Kingdom

thyroid and parathyroids, "thymic asthma" and operations for tumors and cysts arising in the thymus. Reciprocally, surgery has made important contributions to a better understanding of the pathology, if not the physiology, of this organ.

Early Thymic Surgery

Myasthenia Gravis

That thymectomy can influence myasthenia gravis was first demonstrated by the German thoracic surgeon Ernst Ferdinand Sauerbruch (1875-1951) in 1911 when he was Professor of Surgery at the University of Zürich, Switzerland. The case was reported in detail by Schumacher and Roth in 1912. The patient, a 20-year-old woman, had clinical manifestations of both hyperthyroidism and myasthenia, a hypervascular and symmetrically enlarged thyroid and roentgenologically visible enlargement of the thymus. After ligation of the right superior thyroid artery and vein the myasthenia was worse and the thyroid condition unchanged. Aware from Laquer and Weigert's findings of a connection between myasthenia and thymus hyperplasia, Sauerbruch decided that thymectomy was justifiable, and in March 1911 he removed through a cervical incision an enlarged thymus weighing 49 g. Examination of the specimen showed thymic hypertrophy (but no tumour) and numerous Hassall's corpuscles. The operation was followed by marked improvement in the myasthenia, but not in the hyperthyroidism. Subtotal thyroidectomy was done 18 months after the thymectomy. At that time the myasthenia was still improving.

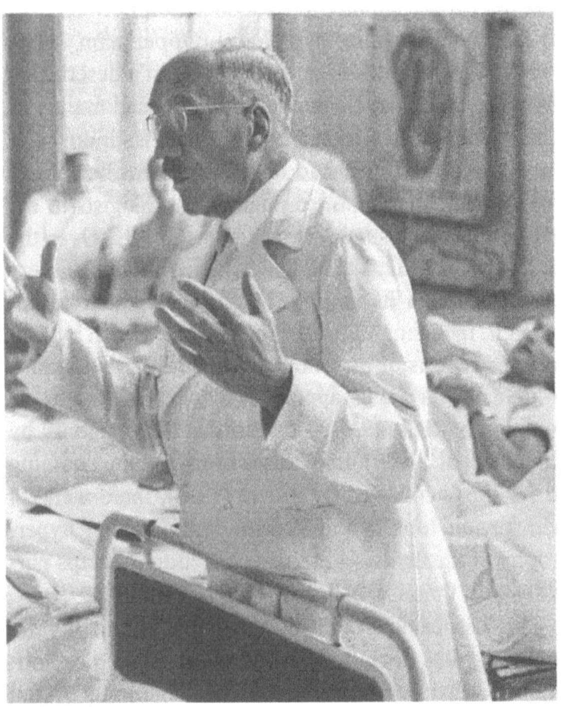

Fig. 1. Ernst Ferdinand Sauerbruch (1875-1951)

As a result of Sauerbruch's experience, several thymectomies were done during the First World War. Von Haberer (1917), reviewing operations on the thymus for a variety of conditions, reported a partial transcervical thymectomy in a 27-year-old man with myasthenia gravis, but no evidence of thymic enlargement, the gland being "in involution"; improvement was noted when the patient was seen 3 years later.

Sauerbruch himself performed two other thymus operations, both consisting in removal of thymic tumors in myasthenic subjects. Both patients died; one (reported by Adler 1937), despite initial improvement, from mediastinitis, the other (Obiditsch 1937) from a streptococcal infection, 8 and 5 days respectively after operation.

The resection of thymomas in myasthenic subjects at this time was attended by a heavy mortality. Lièvre (1936) knew of no published report of the successful removal of a thymoma. Reporting successful excision of an "essentially non-malignant" thymic tumor unaccompanied by myasthenia gravis in a boy of 13, Andrus and Foot (1937) stated: "No case that we can find has survived operative removal of a thymoma more than a few days, which makes our case unique." (They could not know of the survival of Blalock's patient operated on in the previous year, as we shall describe later.)

Hyperthyroidism

That thymic hyperplasia complicating simple or exophthalmic goitre may cause death from suffocation or from "thymic intoxication" leading to hyperthymism or acidosis, was pointed out in 1918 by Crotti, a surgeon who trained in Switzerland, with Stilling in Lausanne and Kocher in Berne. Crotti's practice in such cases, as indeed in all cases of goitre on which he operated, was to follow up thyroidectomy by thymectomy. On completion of thyroidectomy he explored the mediastinum systematically and whenever he found thymus removed it. This procedure, he claimed, had the advantages of eliminating a possible mechanical cause of death, diminishing the postoperative reactions that often follow operations for goitre, especially toxic goitre, and giving better long-term results. In cases of thymic hyperplasia in children, if the mechanical symptoms, i. e. attacks of choking, were alarming he operated at once, but otherwise he regarded roentgen irradiation as the method of choice (Crotti 1918). The thymic hyperplasia associated with hyperthyroidism, noted by Sauerbruch and by Crotti, is an occasional finding, the cause of which is not known. It is discussed further in Chap. 7.

"Thymic Asthma"

At the beginning of the twentieth century the thymus was thought to be responsible for a condition in children known as "thymic asthma", characterized by recurrent difficulty in breathing associated with stridor and cyanosis. One of the principal exponents of surgical treatment of this condition was a French surgeon, Victor Veau, who removed thymuses from young children on the assumption that the glands were enlarged and causing respiratory symptoms by compression.

In 1910 Veau described the three surgical procedures that had been tried up to that time for the relief of supposed thymic pressure: (1) exothymopexy, or fixation of the gland to the substernal fascia; (2) resection of the manubrium sterni to relieve pressure; and (3) thymectomy. Veau advised against (1) and (2), but claimed substantial success for subtotal, subcapsular, transcervical thymectomy. Through a vertical incision made above the sternum he dissected the soft tissue down to the thymus, seized the gland at its upper pole, freed it from its capsule, drew it up through the opening, and resected it. Thymectomy was always partial, as the lower pole could not be reached through the suprasternal incision (Veau 1910).

Some 13 years later, at the Sixth Congress of the International Surgical Society in 1923, Veau reviewed the experience of the intervening period. He was by then acquainted with 50 thymectomies performed for "thymic asthma" in children, 14 by himself. There had been only one postoperative death, but 30% of the patients had died within 1 month of operation from infections or pneumonia. Chronic dyspnoea was relieved in some 65% of the patients, attacks of suffocation in 80%, and stridor in 35%. Despite these favourable results, however, and after referring somewhat nostalgically to 1910 as *"l'âge d'or de la chirurgie thymique"*, Veau predicted, correctly, that thymectomy for this condition would soon be abandoned, as roentgen therapy of the gland produced the same results without effusion of blood (Veau 1924).

As to whether the thymus is in fact the cause of "thymic asthma" opinion has varied. The relevant literature was reviewed by Boyd (1932). Certainly "status lymphaticus", or "status thymolymphaticus", said by Paltauf (1889, 1890) to be a cause of sudden death, can no longer be accepted as an entity (Boyd 1932). Another reason for the decline of surgery in conditions allegedly of thymic origin was that (as Veau had noted) an elarged thymus, which consists largely of lymphoid cells, shrinks rapidly under roentgen irradiation.

Cysts

Surgery of the thymus has included removal of cysts. Partial excision of a congenital polycystic cervical thymic tumour in an 18-month-old boy, who died on the day of the operation, was reported by Pollosson and Piéry in 1901. Pezcoller (1929) set out to remove a cervical thymic cyst, with a stalk apparently arising in the mediastinum, in a 5-year-old boy, but gave up the attempt because of haemorrhage. Histologic examination of a fragment of cyst wall showed typical thymic tissue. The first complete and successful removal of a cervical thymic cyst was reported by Hyde et al. (1944), and of mediastinal thymic cysts by Bradford et al. (1947) and Smart (1947). Cases have been reported subsequently by Schillhammer and Tyson (1962), Al-Shihabi and Jackson (1982) and Baroudi et al. (1982).

Modern Thymic Surgery

Alfred Blalock

Twenty-five years after Sauerbruch's excision of an enlarged thymus without tumor in a patient with both myasthenia and hyperthyroidism, followed by improvement in the myasthenia but not in the hyperthyroidism, and 19 years after von Haberer's partial excision of a thymus showing neither enlargement nor tumour in a patient with myasthenia, likewise followed by improvement, an American surgeon, Alfred Blalock (1899-1964), removed a benign cystic tumour from the thymic region of a patient with myasthenia.

The operation took place at the Vanderbilt University School of Medicine, Nashville, Tennessee, in May 1936. The patient was a 19-year-old girl suffering from severe generalized myasthenia. The disease had run a 4-year course with partial remissions and relapses, but myasthenic crises were becoming progressively more severe. Roentgenography had shown a dense shadow in the mediastinum and the presumed thymic tumor had been treated by roentgen therapy, but a new series of crises had occurred. Blalock observed the patient carefully so as to operate during a mild remission. This cautious procedure underlines the fact that thymectomy should never be an emergency operation, but should be timed to coincide with an optimal phase of the disorder. The myasthenia improved greatly, and the improvement was still present many years later.

torical eponym which has not been adopted by the anatomists (Keynes 1981).

Keynes acquainted himself with the best use of antimyasthenic drugs in the perioperative phase of thymectomy. His collaboration with a pharmacologist, Andrew Wilson of the University of Liverpool, England, in the early 1950s led to the discovery of a rational basis for thymectomy in myasthenia gravis. Wilson prepared an extract of thymus glands which Keynes had removed from myasthenic subjects. He found that the extract exerted a neuromuscular blocking action in rat nerve-muscle preparations and that it could paralyse small animals. The activity of the extracts correlated with the clinical results of the operation, the most potent extracts being obtained from the patients who had benefited most from thymectomy (Keynes 1953, 1954; Wilson et al. 1953). When he retired from active surgery in 1956 Keynes had performed 281 thymectomies in myasthenic patients, the largest series then on record (Keynes 1961), thus establishing a definitive advance in the treatment of myasthenia gravis.

Tribute must be paid, not only to Keynes' meticulous operating technique, but also to his courage. The myasthenic subjects on whom he operated were usually desperately ill. The operation itself was more hazardous than today; for example, there was at that time no positive pressure ventilation (Harmer 1982). The patients who had undergone thymectomy joined to form the British Association of Myasthenics, whose letterhead carries the slogan: "Help conquer myasthenia gravis 'the disease nobody knows'". At the end of his life Keynes received a well-deserved tribute from this Association. They recorded their "total and sincere appreciation" of his life's work, and their gratitude for his "dedication and services in the treatment of all those who suffer from the disease of myasthenia gravis" (Keynes 1981).

The Thymectomy Controversy

During the 40 years following Blalock's pioneer operation in 1936 the evaluation of thymectomy as treatment for myasthenia gravis had the features of a seesaw, with the "for-and-against" fluctuation of Mayo Clinic opinion as the plank, and Keynes' unwavering confidence in the soundness of his own judgment as the fulcrum.

Initially, the consensus of American surgical opinion was favourable to thymectomy. In 1942 two resections of thymomas in myasthenic patients, successful in one, were reported from Albany, New York by Campbell et al., and a successful resection of a thymoma by Clagett at the Mayo Clinic was reported by Eaton. In 1945 Viets (who in 1935 had established the world's first special clinic for myasthenia gravis at the Massachusetts General Hospital, Boston), reported on thymectomy in 15 patients with this disease, 4 with thymomas. There were 4 operative deaths, 8 of the 11 survivors were considered to be improved, and 3 were awaiting assessment. Viets reported again in 1950, this time on 36 patients with myasthenia gravis treated by thymectomy - 7 with thymomas, of whom 3 improved and 29 with no thymoma, of whom 14 improved (Viets 1945, 1950). In contrast to Keynes, Viets stressed that he had been conservative in patient selection, and had operated only on patients with longstanding disease, i.e. the group that fared worst in Keynes' series.

In 1948 Harvey, of Johns Hopkins Hospital, Baltimore, studied 125 myasthenic subjects, of whom 32, including 7 with thymomas, underwent thymectomy. (These 32 included the 20 reported by Blalock in 1944.) Of 26 patients followed for at least 6 months since operation, 20 were improved. Among those who did not have thymectomy, Harvey found that if lasting clinical remissions occurred they did so early in the disease, but were unusual in patients who had received neostigmine for over 6 months (Harvey 1948). Further favourable results with thymectomy were reported from the Massachusetts General Hospital by Schwab and Passouant in 1952. They recommended early resection of thymomas to avoid the risk of malignancy developing, and considered that in nonthymomatous myasthenia gravis the best results were obtained in young patients, especially females.

Meantime, at the Mayo Clinic at Rochester, Minnesota, the downward movement of the seesaw had begun. In 1947 Clagett and Eaton, reporting on thymectomy in 32 patients with myasthenia gravis, 15 with and 17 without thymic tumor, had opined that "thymectomy has been of value in the treatment of myasthenia gravis", but in 1949 Eaton et al., although reporting that 60% of the same 32 patients showed improvement 6 months to 4½ years after operation, declared that these results "must not be looked on as conclusive evidence that thymectomy is of value in the treatment of myasthenia gravis".

In the following year (1950) Eaton and Clagett compared 72 patients with myasthenia gravis who had thymectomy with 142 control patients not treated surgically. Although the results in the thymectomy group were better than in the control group they were not attributed to the thymectomy, but to factors connected with patient selection. The recommendation was that thymectomy should be performed only for the removal of thymic tumors on account of their potential malignancy, and not because of expected improvement in the myasthenia gravis. This was at variance with the policy adopted by Keynes who, in assessing results, had placed patients with thymomatous myasthenia gravis in a category apart (Keynes 1949, 1953, 1954, 1961, 1981).

The adverse view of thymectomy for myasthenia gravis, emanating from so authoritative a source as the Mayo Clinic and published in the *Journal of the American Medical Association,* was soon universally known and placed Keynes in a difficult position (Keynes 1961). But it did not cause him to alter his views, and he continued to perform thymectomies in myasthenic subjects from all over the world: "I felt I could ignore the criticism and pursue my own path" (Keynes 1981).

It was not long, however (3 years, to be exact), before the Mayo workers were influenced by Keynes' results to revise the conclusions given in Eaton and Clagett's paper of 1950. They perceived that the group operated on in that study had been heavily loaded with patients who had thymomas. Elimination of these patients revealed that the series had indeed provided evidence supporting the value of thymectomy in myasthenia gravis. Unfortunately this new report (Eaton et al. 1953) appeared in a specialized journal of relatively restricted circulation.

In 1954 Keynes, delivering the Annual Oration before the Medical Society of London, clarified his position with regard to the by then much criticized operation for myasthenia gravis (Keynes 1954). He pointed out that the results obtained by the Mayo group were not comparable to his because of differences in operative technique, in postoperative patient management and, most important of all, in patients classification and selection. In selecting patients for operation the Mayo group had given preference to those with thymomas, but had pooled all the results, so that the results of simple thymectomies had been lost among the poor results obtained in the numerically superior thymomectomies. Keynes was also able to tell his hearers of the 1953 report by Eaton et al., in which the Mayo Clinic had reversed its stand in regard to the value of thymectomy in myasthenia gravis. The affair, Keynes said, was an interesting study in the formation of medical opinion. It showed how truth may become overlaid by confused thinking, and how harm can be done by misuse of statistics and by paying exaggerated deference to views simply because they originate in a large and well-known centre.

A fuller and more widely read recantation was published by Eaton and Clagett in 1955. It is evident, they then declared, that thymectomy is of value in the treatment of female myasthenic patients under the age of 50 and who do not have thymomas. The harm had, however, been done and much time was to pass before Keynes' views achieved general acceptance.

That thymectomy had been underrated in the United States as a therapeutic approach to myasthenia gravis and in consequence insufficiently used was the opinion expressed to Keynes, in a conversation in 1960, by Kermit Osserman of the Mount Sinai Hospital, New York, a leading American authority on myasthenia (Keynes 1961).

While agreement on the role of thymectomy in myasthenia gravis was thus gradually being reached at the four major centres with extensive experience of the procedure and its results - Baltimore (Johns Hopkins Hospital), Boston (Massachusetts General Hospital), Rochester (Mayo Clinic), and London (St. Bartholomew's, New End and National Hospitals) - pleas for medical versus surgical treatment of the disease were being made by Ferguson, a neurologist at Manchester, England, who reported good results in 70% of 145 patients treated medically and observed over periods ranging from 2 to 28 years (Ferguson et al. 1955; Ferguson 1962). However, the 70% included cases of ocular myasthenia gravis which is known to run a benign course and is not considered for thymectomy (Eaton et al. 1953; Osserman and Genkins 1971).

In 1976 the Mayo Clinic announced its full and final conversion to Keynes' views in a paper published in the prestigious journal *Annals of Surgery* (Buckingham et al. 1976). The authors referred to Keynes' report *The surgery of the thymus gland* published 30 years earlier (Keynes 1946) and pronounced an identical opinion: "Until more effective treatment is available for myasthenia gravis, thymectomy deserves consideration for both sexes." This contrasted with Eaton and Clagett's restricted recantation of 1955, approving of thymectomy in female patients "particularly if they are young", but with strict reservations as regards male patients.

On the European continent thymectomy gained favour as treatment for myasthenia gravis after respiratory assistance became available and drug therapy improved during the 1950s, and since then it has been performed with increasing frequency. Because of limitations of space only some of the principal series can be mentioned here. The following list is by no means exhaustive, but the papers are useful as sources of reference and points of departure for further studies: Finland (Mattila et al. 1976); France (Gamondes et al. 1981) (Lyon); (Le Brigand 1982; Le Brigand et al. 1972, 1980) (Paris); (Ribet et al. 1982) (Lille); Italy (Maggi and Paletto 1982); Poland (Rzepecki et al. 1981); Switzerland (Givel et al. 1982, 1986; Givel 1983). In Japan Masaoka and Monden (1981) have reported interesting comparisons of different surgical approaches to the gland.

Part I

Normal Thymus

2 Embryology and Congenital Anomalies

Stephen W. Gray and John E. Skandalakis

Comparative Anatomy

The thymus has claimed more attention from embryologists than have many other organs. After the publication of Haeckel's *Generelle Morphologie*, which was influenced by Darwin, in 1866, the pharyngeal region of the embryo was seen as an outstanding example of embryonic recapitulation of the phylogeny of the organism: "The development of the embryo is an abstract of the history of the genus" (Haeckel 1866).

The branchial clefts and pouches become functional gills in the lower vertebrates only, but the early stages of gill development are present in mammals, including humans. Throughout the vertebrates certain epithelial structures associated with the embryonic clefts and pouches will become the thyroid, parathyroids, thymus, and ultimobranchial bodies. Their formation and their homologies from one organism to another occupied much of the literature of embryology in the last quarter of the nineteenth century and the first quarter of the twentieth.

Although thymus bodies may be recognized as far down the scale as elasmobranch fishes, the thymus and parathyroid glands become transposed in mammals. In submammalian vertebrates the thymus arises from the dorsal portion of the pharyngeal pouch and the parathyroid from the ventral portion. Godwin (1939) has reviewed the literature on the comparative anatomy of these structures.

When the search for homologies was complete, or at least was less zealously pursued, it was realized that the thymus, alone of the pharyngeal derivatives, had no demonstrated function. To consider this large lymphoid structure merely as a part of Waldeyer's ring of lymphoid tissue (Shier 1963) seemed inadequate.

Because the endocrine function of the thyroid and parathyroid glands was well known, it was widely assumed that the thymus also produced a hormone. Many reports of thymic hormones appeared in the early literature, but they were equivocal or could not be confirmed. It was not until 1961, when Archer and Pierce removed the thymus in newborn animals, that the resulting reduction of immunologic capacity revealed the gland's humoral action. The hormone thymopoietin probably arises in the epithelial reticulum cells (Basch and Goldstein 1975).

Embryology

The definitive studies of the development of the pharyngeal pouch derivatives are those of Weller (1933) and Norris (1937). Although their concept of the ultimobranchial body as "lateral thyroid" has been modified, their description of thymus development has not been surpassed.

In mammals the thymus gland develops from the ventral portion of the third branchial pouch, with an inconstant contribution from the fourth pouch (Gilmour 1941). At about the 6th gestational week (g. w.) (10 mm) the third pouch separates from the pharynx and is in contact with the fourth cleft, which has itself lost its connection with the surface ectoderm (Figs. 1 and 2). From the dorsal portion of the pouch, parathyroid III (inferior parathyroid) has begun to differentiate. Unlike the parathyroids, which are solid from their first appearance, the thymus primordium retains a lumen, the thymopharyngeal duct, pinched off from the third branchial pouch (Figs. 2 and 3). The epithelium of this duct is endodermal, and there is possibly an ectodermal contribution from the fourth cleft.

During the 7th and 8th g. w., the thymuses elongate caudally and anteromedially. By the end of the 8th

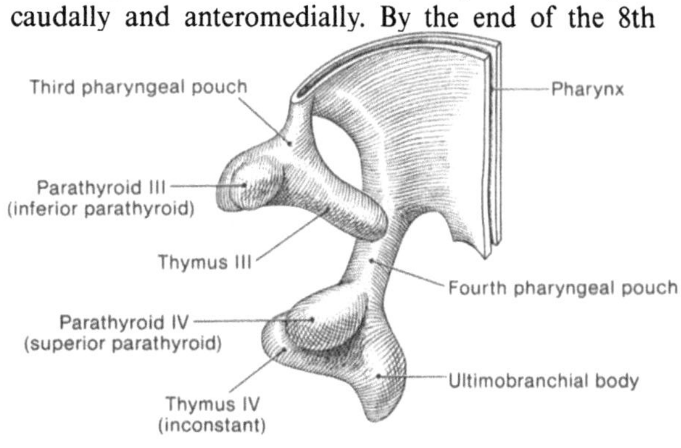

Fig. 1. Pharynx with right third and fourth branchial pouches at 6th gestational week. From Arey 1959

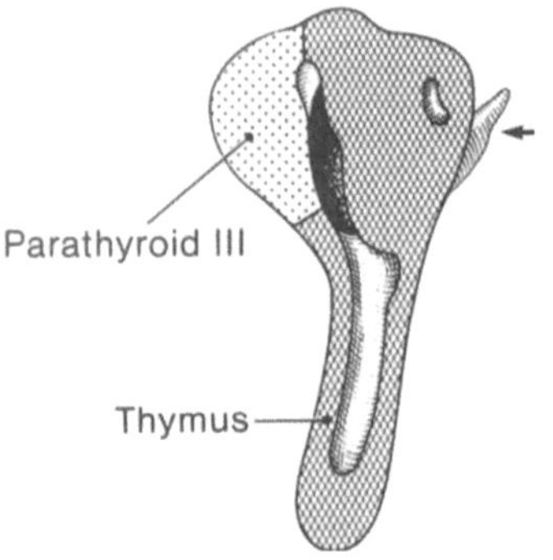

Fig. 2. Long section through the derivatives of the third branchial pouch. The ventral (thymic) portion retains a lumen. The *arrow* indicates the point of detachment from the pharynx. From Arey 1959

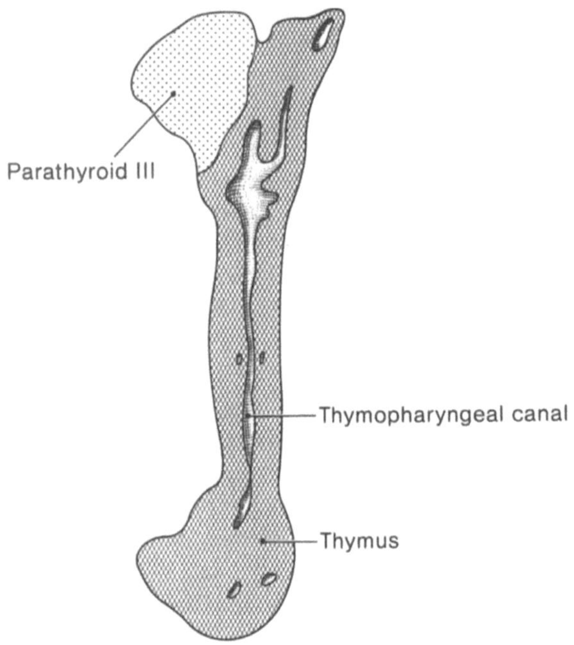

Fig. 3. Elongation of the thymic portion of the third pouch derivative. The thymopharyngeal canal is disappearing. From Arey 1959

g. w., the advancing distal ends of the primordia meet and fuse at the level of the superior margin of the aortic arch (Fig. 4; Weller 1933). This midline fusion affects only the connective tissue; the parenchyma does not fuse (Siegler 1969). After fusion, the distal ends of the thymuses enlarge. The cephalic portions lose their connection with the pharynx and disappear during the 8th g. w., leaving the definitive thymus in the mediastinum. Cervical thymic cysts may form from persistent remnants of the tubular upper end of the primitive organ.

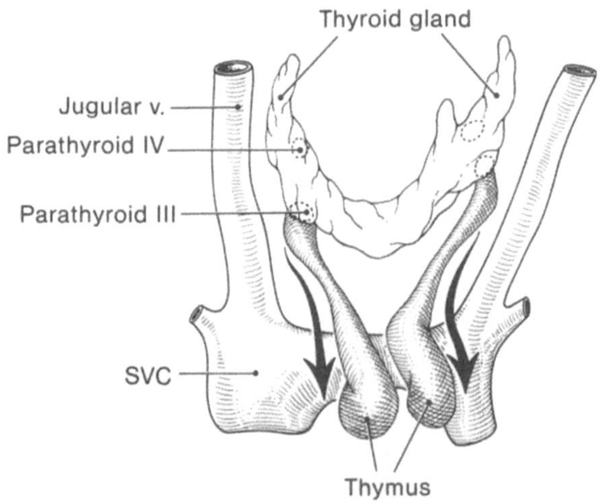

Fig. 4. The descent of the thymus at the end of the second month. The cranial ends of the thymus will disappear; the descending caudal ends will form the definitive thymus. Note that parathyroid III, attached to the thymus, has descended to a site below that of parathyroid IV. *SCV* superior vena cava. From Arey 1959

The thymus is the first of the lymphoid organs to develop. It appears essentially mature by the 15th g. w. (Haynes 1984) or the 20th g. w. (Papiernik 1972). Normal peripheral lymph nodes depend on seeding by small lymphocytes from the thymus. In patients with the DiGeorge syndrome (thymic aplasia), lymph nodes with germinal centers are found, but few lymphocytes. In severe combined immunodeficiency disease, lymph nodes contain reticulum cells only.

Until the 7th g. w., only undifferentiated epithelial cells are present. This cell mass becomes invaded by mesenchyme containing the lymphocytic stem cells. During the 8th to 10th g. w., precursors of hemopoietic cells reach the thymus from the bone marrow and the liver (Moore and Metcalf 1970; Haynes 1984). There is evidence from chick embryos that the neural crest may act as an organizer of an interaction between the epithelial primordium and the invading mesenchyme (Bockman and Kirby 1984). Thymus lobes appear in the 9th g. w. and Hassall's corpuscles are present by the 11th g. w. Between the 12th and 14th g. w., the cortex and medulla are defined and presumptive T-lymphocytes (rosette-forming cells) are present (Raitsina and Kalinina 1984).

That reticulum cells may have a dual origin has been suggested by von Gaudecker and Müller-Hermelink (1980), the reticulum cells of the cortex differentiating from epithelial cells of the thymus primordium, and other cells, resembling the reticulum cells of peripheral lymph nodes, entering the medulla with the mesenchymal septa between the 10th and 12th g. w. The difference in the stroma, according to these investigators, may be correlated with differences between cortical and medullary lymphocytes.

The means by which precursor T-lymphocytes reach the thymus is obscure. Owen and Jenkinson (1981) point out that embryonic chick thymus is not vascularized at the stage at which cell migration takes place. Stem cells must leave the blood vessels and pass through mesenchyme to reach the primitive epithelial thymus.

The origin and significance of Hassall's corpuscles are not clear. They are not present in the early stage of thymic development. Shier (1963) considered them to be of endodermal origin, remnants of epithelial cords around which the mesenchymal portion develops. Similarities between Hassal's corpuscles and epidermal keratinocytes have been pointed out by von Gaudekker and Schmale (1974), using electron microscopic and histochemical methods. More recently, Bonnefoy et al. (1984) showed that epithelial cells from the thymic medulla and Hassall's corpuscles share an antigenic specificity common to epidermal granulosa cells.

The thymus reaches its greatest size at puberty and then undergoes slow involution, although nonatrophic portions may continue to function normally for many years. There is a loss of total lymphoid mass, and both cortical lymphocytes and T-lymphocytes in peripheral blood are reduced. Much of the thymus is replaced by fat. Table 1 recapitulates the development of the thymus.

Table 1. Chronology of the developing thymus

Developmental event	Gestational week
Pouch III formed	5th
Elongation of epithelial primordia	7th-8th
Invasion of mesenchyme (stem cells)	7th
Disappearance of cephalic portion, descent of thymus	8th
Stem cell in thymus	8th-10th
Lobes visible	9th
Hassall's corpuscles present	11th
Cortex and medulla defined	12th-14th
Maturity of thymus	15th-20th
Greatest size of thymus	Puberty

Anomalies of the Thymus

Undescended Thymus and Accessory Thymus Bodies

The thymus occasionally fails to descend into the mediastinum. Failure of descent may be bilateral, but is usually unilateral and on the left side. If affects about twice as many females as males. Most cases are diagnosed in infancy or childhood.

Usually, the main body of the thymus descends, leaving a strip of thymus tissue or a fibrous remnant along the line of embryonic descent (Harman 1901). The persistent strip may separate into nodules of accessory thymus. Accessory thymus bodies may also originate from the fourth pharyngeal pouch (Van Dyke 1941). They may be attached to the superior parathyroid glands, or be embedded in the thyroid, or lie on its posterior surface (Gilmour 1937, 1941). Both thymus and parathyroid tissue at the site of the tonsil (second pouch) have been reported (Robinson et al. 1959). None of these accessory thymus bodies is of clinical significance.

Although a swelling in the neck is usually the only symptom of cervical thymus, a pedunculated thymic tumor reported by Epstein and Loeb in 1955 in a 3-week-old infant presented as a mass in the mouth. It was diagnosed as a hamartoma and removed surgically without sequelae. A single case of hyperdescent of the thymus - an anomalous lobe of thymus growing into the left posterior mediastinum and blocking expansion of the left lung - has been reported (Terribile 1967).

Cysts of the Third Branchial Pouch (Thymic Cysts)

Cervical cysts of the thymus large enough to attract the attention of the patient or physician are extremely rare. Up to 1982, a total of 38 cases had been reported, 35 by Al-Shihabi and Jackson (1982), and 3 others by Baroudi et al. (1982). About twice as many males were affected as females, and over half the sufferers were under 10 years of age. In two older patients, the cyst was found incidentally to a surgical operation on the thyroid, and in one patient aged 74 years it was revealed at necropsy. In one case, the cyst was present at birth; in most of the others, it had been evident for between a few days and a few weeks.

The cervical thymic cysts reported were firm, immobile, and rarely tender to palpation. Their diameters ranged from 2 to 17 cm, and they were usually lined with simple squamous epithelium, although cuboidal or even pseudostratified linings were reported. Their fluid contents were clear to brow, and they usually contained cholesterol crystals.

It would be easy to assign thymic cysts an origin from the third pharyngeal pouch, but evidence for such an assignment is frequently lacking. Thymus tissue in the wall of the cyst is the exception. Crawford et al. (1957) found it in the wall of a thymic cyst they removed from the neck of a 6-year-old boy. Rarely, thymic cysts have been formed in the mediastinum (Schillhammer and Tyson 1962). Most mediastinal cysts are of pericardial, bronchogenic, or esophageal origin.

Table 2. Thymic agenesis, aplasia, and hypoplasia

Syndrome	Thymus	Lymphocytes	Associated anomalies	Etiology	Possible effective treatment	Prognosis (untreated)
Thymic aplasia (DiGeorge syndrome)	Total or partial absence; lymph nodes with germinal centers, but few lymphocytes	Decreased, normal, or increased B-lymphocytes	Absence of parathyroids; characteristic facies; cardiac defects	Possible autosomal recessive	Thymus and parathyroid transplants	Early death from infection or cardiac defect
Metaphyseal chondrodysplasia with thymolymphopenia	Absence of thymus, tonsils, and lymph nodes	Decreased T- and B-lymphocytes	Dwarfism with skeletal defects	Autosomal recessive	None	Early death from infection
Severe combined immune deficiency (Swiss-type agammaglobulinemia, autosomal)	1. Thymus small but partially normal; deficient ADA 2. Thymus vestigial; no lymphocyts or Hassall's bodies; no germinal centers in lymph nodes; normal ADA	Decreased T-lymphocytes	None	Autosomal[a] recessive; stem cell defect	Thymus and liver transplants	Early death from infection

ADA = Adenosine deaminase

[a] An X-linked form of this syndrome exists in males only.

Thymic Agenesis, Aplasia, and Hypoplasia

Any classification of thymus deficiency diseases is difficult and must be considered tentative. Bergsma's (1982) arrangement into three main syndromes is perhaps the most convenient at the present time (Table 2). Most cases appear to be familial with autosomal recessive genes. The sexes are equally affected.

Total thymic agenesis is often associated with agenesis of parathyroid glands (the DiGeorge syndrome), suggesting failure of development of the entire third pouch. In other cases, the parathyroids are normal. A rare variety of severe combined immunodeficiency is X-linked and occurs only in male infants (Gatti and O'Reilly 1979). All of these syndromes result in early death from opportunistic infections.

Haynes (1984) suggested that the DiGeorge syndrome is the result of an early failure of stem cells to enter the epithelial primordium (1-7 weeks), and that the severe combined immunodeficiency syndrome arises from failure of T-lymphocytes to induce epithelial proliferation.

The aplastic thymus is small; reticular cells and large thymocytes are usually present, but small lymphocytes and Hassall's bodies are usually absent. Other lymphoid organs have few lymphocytes, and may themselves be aplastic. Reconstitution of the T-cell function by thymus implants, and of B- and T-cell function by fetal liver implants has met with some success. Patients with the DiGeorge syndrome have survived with thymus and parathyroid implants (Lapointe and Pahwa 1979).

References

Al-Shihabi BM, Jackson JMcG (1982) Cervical thymic cyst: case report. J Laryngol Otol 96: 181-189

Archer O, Pierce JC (1961) Role of thymus in development of the immune response. Fed Proc 20: 26

Arey LB (ed) (1959) Dev Anat, 6th edn. Saunders Philadelphia

Baroudi IF, Lewis E, Paletta FX (1982) Thymic cyst of the neck. Plast Reconstr Surg 70: 230-232

Basch RS, Goldstein G (1975) Thymopoietin-induced acquisition of responsiveness to T cell mitogen. Cell Immunol 20: 218-228

Bergsma D (1979) (ed) Birth defects compendium, 2nd edn. The National Foundation-March of Dimes. Liss, New York

Bockman DE, Kirby ML (1984) Dependence of thymus development on derivatives of the neural crest. Science 223: 498-500

Bonnefoy JY, Reano A, Schmitt D, Thivolet J (1984) Thymic Hassall's corpuscles-epidermis antigenic relations defined by a common glycoprotein in man (GP 37). Thymus 6: 387-394

Crawford AS, Evans PV, Thompson W (1957) Thymic cyst in the neck: case report. J Indiana State Med Assoc 50: 715-719

Epstein HC, Loeb WJ (1955) Thymic tumor of the pharynx. J Pediatr 47: 105-108

Gatti RA, O'Reilly RJ (1979) Immunodeficiency, X-linked severe combined. In: Bergsma D (ed) Birth defects compendium, 2nd edn. The National Foundation-March of Dimes. Liss, New York, pp 578-579

Gilmour JR (1937) The embryology of the parathyroid glands, the thymus and certain associated rudiments. J Pathol Bacteriol 45: 507-522

Gilmour JR (1941) Some developmental abnormalities of the thymus and parathyroids. J Pathol Bacteriol 52: 213-218

Godwin MC (1939) The mammalian thymus IV: the development in the dog. Am J Anat 64: 165-201

Haeckel EHPA (1866) Generelle Morphologie der Organismen, 2 vols. Reimer, Berlin

Harman NB (1901) "Socia thymi cervicalis", and thymus accessorius. J Anat Physiol 36: 47-53

Haynes BF (1984) Phenotypic characterization and ontogeny of components of the human thymic microenvironment. Clin Res 32 (5): 500-507

Lapointe N, Pahwa S (1979) Thymic agenesis. In: Bergsma D (ed) Birth defects compendium, 2nd edn. The National Foundation-March of Dimes. Liss, New York, pp 1018-1019

Moore MAS, Metcalf D (1970) Ontogeny of the haemopoietic system: Yolk sac origin of in vivo and in vitro colony forming cells in the developing mouse embryo. Br J Haematol 18: 279-296

Norris EH (1937) The parathyroid glands and the lateral thyroid in man: their morphogenesis, histogenesis, topographic anatomy and prenatal growth. Contrib Embryol (Carnegi Inst Washington DC) 26 (no 159): 247-294

Owen JJT, Jenkinson EJ (1981) Embryology of the lymphoid system. Prog Allergy 29: 1-34

Papiernik M (1972) Ontogeny of the human lymphoid system: study of the cytological maturation and the incorporation of tritiated thymidine and uridine in the foetal thymus and lymph node and in the infantile thymus. J Cell Physiol 80: 235-242

Raitsina SS, Kalinina II (1984) Differentiation of thymic lymphoid cells during human embryogenesis. Dev Comp Immunol 8: 225-230

Robinson M, Ferguson C, Flake CG (1959) Aberrant parathyroid and thymus in the pharynx. Arch Otolaryngol 69: 312-314

Schillhammer WR Jr, Tyson MD (1962) Mediastinal thymic cysts. Arch Surg 85: 410-417

Shier KJ (1963) The morphology of the epithelial thymus: observations on lymphocyte-depleted and fetal thymus. Lab Invest 12: 316-326

Siegler R (1969) The thymus and the unicorn - two great myths of gross anatomy. Anat Rec 163: 264

Terribile V (1967) Su di un caso di pancreatite fetale associata ad anomalia timica. Boll Soc Ital Patol 10: 46-48

Van Dyke JH (1941) On the origin of accessory thymus tissue, thymus IV: the occurrence in man. Anat Rec 79: 179-209

Von Gaudecker B, Müller-Hermelink HK (1980) Ontogeny and organization of the stationary non-lymphoid cells in the human thymus. Cell Tissue Res 207: 287-306

Von Gaudecker B, Schmale EM (1974) Similarities between Hassall's corpuscles of the human thymus and the epidermis: an investigation by electron microscopy and histochemistry. Cell Tissue Res 151: 347-368

Weller GL Jr (1933) Development of the thyroid, parathyroid and thymus glands in man. Contrib Enbryol (no 141): 93-139

3 Anatomy

Marion D. Kendall

Morphology and Topography

The thymus gland in the adult is an elongated, lobulated, pinkish yellow structure comprising thymic tissue and fat (Fig. 1), situated in the midline in the anterior and superior mediastina. It extends from the level of the fourth costal cartilage below to the level of the inferior border of the thyroid gland above, but occasionally its cranial limit extends over the thyroid. Anteriorly it is related to the sternum, the adjacent parts of the upper four costal cartilages and the sternothyroid and sternohyoid muscles. Posteriorly it is related to the pericardium, the aortic arch and its branches, the left brachiocephalic (left innominate) vein, the trachea and sometimes the thyroid gland.

Although referred to and appearing as a single organ, the thymus is composed of two distinct elements, termed the right and left lobes of the thymus. Each lobe is surrounded by a collagenous capsule and the lobes are joined in the midline by loose connective tissue. The lobes are further divided into lobules (often confusingly called lobes). Since the septa, extending from the capsule, reach only to the corticomedullary junction, the medulla is confluent throughout.

In infants and children the thymus has little fat (Fig. 1). It may appear pale with pinkish red areas, or be pale to deep red. Its bilobed structure is more obvious than in adults, as are the cervical horns (Fig. 2), which account for its greater extent in children.

As the thymus descends caudally after its bilateral derivation from the ventral part of the pharyngeal pouches III (Norris 1938) and in some cases IV (van Dyke 1941), nodules or strands of thymic tissue may be found in relation to the thyroid gland (often posteriorly and laterally), the parathyroid glands and the thyroid cartilage. Ectopic thymic tissue is in fact common in humans; Goldstein and Mackay (1969) estimated that it may be found in 25% of the population.

Derivation

Studies in lower animals on the anatomy and relations of the thymus that may be of significance in cardiothoracic surgery concern the derivatives of the neural crest (Le Douarin and Jotereau 1975; Bockman and Kirby 1984; Le Douarin et al. 1984). Whereas the neural crest cells themselves contribute only to the development of the connective tissues of the thymic septa and blood vessels, neural crest mesectoderm contributes to thymus formation, via interaction with endoderm from pharyngeal pouches III and IV, to give tis-

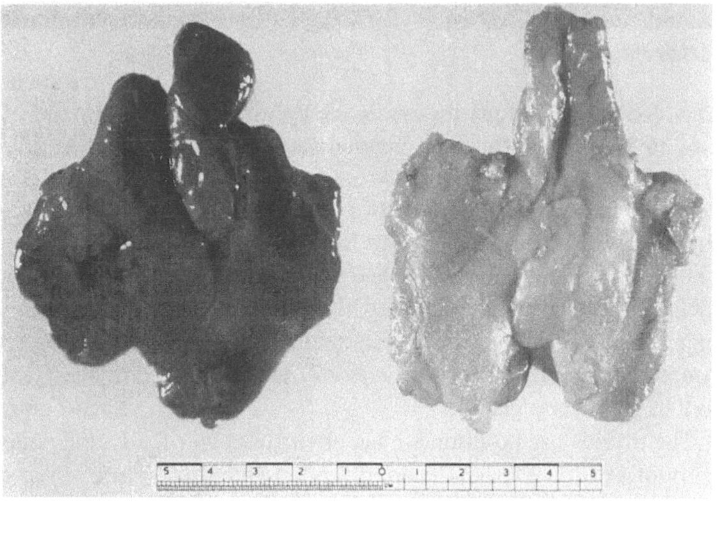

Fig. 1. Thymus glands from a 9-year-old girl (left) and an 80-year-old man (right). Despite the fatty infiltration that usually accompanies ageing the gland's characteristic shape is retained. (Kendall et al. 1980)

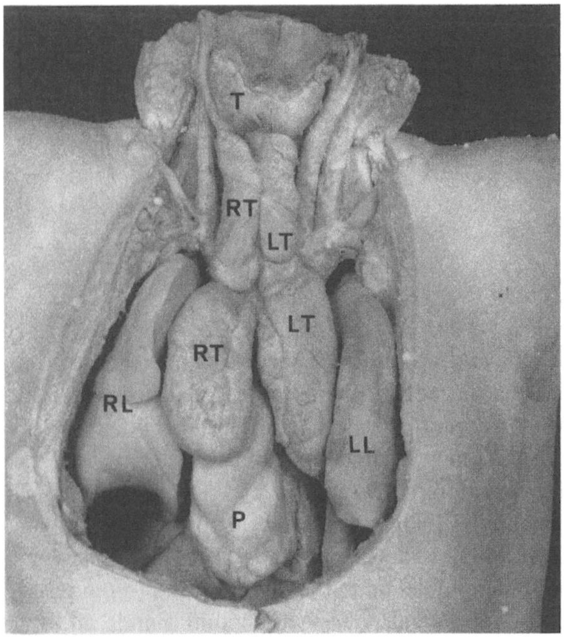

Fig. 2. Museum specimen of the left *(LT)* and right *(RT)* lobes of the thymus gland in a child, showing the great size of the gland relative to other organs. *LL*, Left lung; *RL*, right lung; *P*, pericardium; *T*, thyroid gland. Note the cervical extensions (horns) of the thymus

sues that subsequently differentiate to support thymopoiesis. The mesenchyme of the aortic arches is derived from neural crest, and the truncal septum also contains neural crest cells. The significance of this is that developmental abnormalities of neural crest derivatives affect the formation of the heart, the thymus and the peripheral ganglia. Couly et al. (1983) have proposed this explanation for the DiGeorge and Pierre Robin syndromes, where there is absence or hypoplasia of the thymus with cardiac malformations.

Arteries

The blood supply to the thymus probably varies. It is said to be derived from the internal thoracic artery (Deaver 1903) and the inferior thyroid artery (Williams and Warwick 1980), from these two plus the superior thyroid artery (Dawson 1966) and from all three plus branches of the subclavian and carotid arteries (Schäfer and Symington 1898). These mediastinal branches are small and supply fat, areolar tissue and lymphatics in the superior and anterior mediastina as well as the thymus gland.

The thymus has no distinct hilus or single point of entry or exit for vessels. The arteries often enter dorsally through the capsule and course along the connective tissue septa to the corticomedullary junction where they turn and run as arterioles between cortex and medulla. Siegler (1964) reports that they branch after passing through the capsule and enter the cortex directly. Capillaries run radially into the cortex and return to the corticomedullary junction. The medulla receives irregular branches. According to Williams and Warwick (1980), the thymus contains high-walled postcapillary venules similar to those of the lymph nodes, but they are not commonly seen and few accounts mention them. Blanc and Koritké (1970) using Indian ink injection methods have described in detail the angioarchitecture of the perinatal human thymus.

Veins

The interlobar septa carry large veins from the corticomedullary junction to the capsule, and in addition small veins leave the cortex to form a venous plexus on the posterior surface of the capsule. As a result of the fusion of smaller veins a single vein frequently leaves the medial side of each lobe and the two join to form a short wide vein (the great vein of Keynes) which drains into the anteroinferior surface of the left brachiocephalic vein just proximal to the entry of the superior intercostal vein (Goldstein and Mackay 1969; Last 1984). A lateral vein drains from each side of the gland, that from the right side to the superior vena cava and that from the left side to the left brachiocephalic vein. Additional veins may drain to the inferior thyroid vein, the thyreoidea ima vein and the internal thoracic (internal mammary) vein (Goldstein and Mackay 1969; Hollinshead 1971; Williams and Warwick 1980).

Lymphatics

There are no afferent lymphatics to the thymus (Goldstein and Mackay 1969; Bloodworth et al. 1975). The perivascular spaces probably form the first channels for the conduction of thymocytes from the gland. Hwang et al. (1974), however, assign this function to the postcapillary venules. Small lymph capillaries form within the gland and join to form larger lymphatic vessels that run with the blood vessels to reach the capsule (Arya et al. 1982). The lymph vessels of the thymus end in the brachiocephalic (innominate), tracheobronchial and parasternal (internal mammary) lymph nodes (Goldstein and Mackay 1969). The efferent vessels from the brachiocephalic nodes unite with efferents from the tracheobronchial nodes to form the left and right bronchomediastinal lymph trunks. These most frequently open independently into the internal jugular and subclavian veins of their own side. Sometimes, however, the left bronchomediastinal trunk may join the thoracic duct, and the right trunk the right lymphatic duct (Williams and Warwick 1980).

Nerves

The vagus nerve, the phrenic nerve, the cervicothoracic (stellate, inferior cervical) ganglion and the ansa cervicalis (ansa hypoglossi) have all been described as contributing to the innervation of the thymus. The vagus nerve contains both special visceral (branchial) efferent fibres originating in the nucleus ambiguus and serving striated (skeletal) muscle, and general visceral (parasympathetic) efferent fibres originating in the dorsal motor vagus nucleus (DMV) and serving smooth and cardiac muscle. Although there are smooth muscles in the vascular supply of the thymus, the myoid cells (Chap. 4) resemble cardiac muscle in having centrally located nuclei with sometimes clearly defined sarcomeres.

Hammar (1935) studied the innervation of the thymus in 18 foetuses ranging in length from 12.9 to 81.1 mm. He found that the central part of the thymus anlage, when still in the neck (middle of the second month), receives branches from the vagus on each side. These branches enter from the dorsal, lateral or medial aspect and result in the formation of a rich plexus (rete) in the medulla. After the organ has descended it receives a sympathetic innervation from ganglia positioned near the thoracic inlet. These fibres enter from several points, usually along the interlobular blood vessels, pass radially without much branching, and then turn centrally. The vagal and sympathetic fibres meet, after the differentiation of cortex and medulla, at the corticomedullary border. The innervation is complete by the time Hassall's corpuscles have developed and the gland is functional.

The role of the vagal innervation of the thymus has not been fully established. When labelled horseradish peroxidase was injected directly into the thymus of rats and mice (Bulloch and Moore 1981) there was no labelling of neurones in the DMV, although a few neurones were consistently labelled in the dorsal medullary tegmentum adjacent to the DMV. The largest population of labelled neurones was in the retrofacial nucleus and labelled neurones were seen throughout the rostrocaudal length of the nucleus ambiguus.

In addition to the vagal supply, there is also some innervation from the cervical spinal nerves. Schäfer and Symington (1898) quote previous work suggesting that the nerves of the thymus are minute and that they are partly derived from the phrenic nerve. They also quote Cooper's view that filaments from the vagus (pneumogastric) and sympathetic nerves descend on the thyroid to the upper part of the thymus, and add that sympathetic nerves are found along the arteries of the thymus. Bulloch and Moore (1981) recorded that spinal cord neurones in segments C2–4 labelled with horseradish peroxidase in two distinct columns in the ventral horn, one lying laterally and the other medially. A third group of neurones also labelled in the medial part of the ventral horn of C-1.

The sympathetic nerve supply to the thymus is from the cervicothoracic ganglion or from the ansa subclavia. Sergeeva (1974) demonstrated a rich sympathetic innervation not restricted to the thymus vasculature, but distributed widely through the parenchyma of the gland including the Hassall's corpuscles. Williams and Felten (1981) used fluorescence microscopy of thymus and spleen from mice to identify noradrenergic fibres in perivascular and parenchymal regions of both organs. Thymic innervation was mainly perivascular, but isolated islands and strings of free noradrenergic fibres were noted among thymic parenchymal cells. Felten and Felten (1989) have reviewed current knowledge on the innervation of the thymus gland, and this is further considered in Chapter 4.

Now that the innervation of the thymus is being established in animal models, further work is required in man. The human thymus becomes fatty with age, and in rodents the ageing thymus does not appear to loose its adrenergic innervation (Felten and Felten, 1989). If this should be so in man too, would it mean that the ageing thymus could be reawakened in man as in rats (Fitzpatrick et al. 1985; Fitzpatrick et al. 1986; Kendall et al. submitted)?

Brain-Thymus Connections

The neural connections between the thymus and the brain have been studied by Cross et al. (1980, 1982) in rodents. Whereas lesions in the preoptic-anterior hypothalamus result in thymic involution, lesions in the hippocampus increase thymic (and splenic) mitogenic responsiveness and cellularity. Since hypothalamic neurones are known to project to the nucleus ambiguus, there may be a hypothalamic-thymic pathway. In addition, Renoux et al. (1980) showed that ablation of the left cerebral cortex abrogates the production of thymic hormones, reduces the number of splenic T cells, and impairs immunization with sheep erythrocytes.

Recently, there has been increased interest in the relationships between the central nervous system and the immune system particularly with regard to the effects of neuropeptides and cytokines, some of which are considered in Chapter 4. Part of this is enacted through the hypothalamic-hypophyseal-gonadal axis, but all the other endocrines glands are involved, especially the adrenal. The channels of communication are bidirectional, with hormones and cytokines being the mediators of the message. Now that many lymphocytes have been shown to contain neuropeptides (see Chapter 4) the complexities of the system appear enormous. Work in this are may now begin to explain the numerous social, psychological, and environmental factors that have been shown to influence the immune system (Ader, 1981; Ader et al. 1987).

Size

The size of the thymus in humans and most animals studied increases with age until about puberty, when the gland is said to involute and be largely replaced by fat. Much of this information dates from between 1900 and 1930, when studies were conducted to investigate status thymicolymphaticus, a condition which is no longer recognized. The thymus was weighed at necropsy and sometimes prepared for histological examination. Although some authors included figures for sudden death in apparently normal patients, many of the values were obtained after chronic illness in children and adults or after unexplained death in infants. Since it is now well established that the thymus atrophies under stress and chronic disease (Boyd 1927, 1932; Goldstein and Mackay 1969; Watts 1969) these data do not help to establish normal adult thymus weights in health. Hammar (1905, 1906, 1914, 1921) was fully aware of this problem. In addition, great variability in the size of normal adult thymus glands has been reported (Anderson and Cameron 1927; Young and Turnbull 1931; Boyd 1932; Sloan 1943; Kreel 1969; Kendall et al. 1980), and many authors have stated that the thymus is present and active throughout life in normal healthy adults (Bratton 1925; Young and Turnbull 1931; Keynes 1954; Kendall 1984). Studies on thymic hormone levels (Dardenne and Bach 1981), on ageing (Walford 1980), and on immunology (Steinmann and Müller-Hermelink 1984) now support this view, and the thymus should be regarded as of value throughout life despite normal age-related fatty involution.

Weight

Thymic weight in the foetus was studied by Scammon (1927). He found great variability, but in 1043 foetuses he demonstrated a linear relation between thymic weight and body weight. Schulz et al. (1962) reported mean thymus weights of 0.9 g for five male foetuses and 1.5 g for four female foetuses at 5 months gestational age. They recorded a steady increase in weight until birth, when male values were 8.6 ± 5.5 g ($n=91$) and female values 7.2 ± 3.6 g ($n=55$), although thymuses from stillborn infants weighed more (12 ± 5 g in 64 males and 10 ± 5 g in 72 females). Similar figures were given by Anderson and Cameron (1927).

Thymic weight in children is well documented. Bratton (1925) studied 337 thymuses from previously healthy subjects under 16 years of age who had died within 12 h of the onset of acute medical or surgical conditions, or within 1 day of accidents, and compared the findings with those of previous workers. In newborn infants, Bratton found a mean thymic weight of 11.18 g in his own material ($n=58$), and in the earlier literature a range of 9-14.4 g, i.e. values slightly higher than those found by Schulz et al. (1962). In contrast, Young and Turnbull (1931) (Fig. 3) recorded thymus weights of 24.8 ± 12.8 g at birth, but in the 11- to 16-year-old group their values were similar to those of Bratton. Young and Turnbull's study, and the studies of Greenwood and Woods (1927) and of Schulz et al. (1962) reported higher mean thymic birth weights for males than females, but by 1-6 years the differences had disappeared. All authors have shown an increase in thymus weight to about 15 years of age (mean values 25-37.52 g).

The data for thymic weight in adults are more sketchy and difficult to interpret because of the difficulty, outlined previously, of knowing what is normal when information is culled from necropsies. Within these limitations, the data given by Young and Turnbull (1931) which included Hammar's values of 1906 and 1929, are useful. Both studies showed a gradual fall in weight from the period of puberty to over 66 years of age. They provided no evidence of sex differences during adult life.

In a more representative sample of necropsy thymus weights (wet, lipid and lean dry weights), Kendall et al. (1980) found a wide range in the different age groups, and higher mean values (Fig. 3) than previously recorded. Mean wet weight decreased with age, but mean thymic weight in the over-80-year-old group was only 23.7% less than in the 0- to 20-year-old group. The marked scatter of values showed that at all ages there were thymus weights as great as or greater than those found around puberty (when thymus weight is

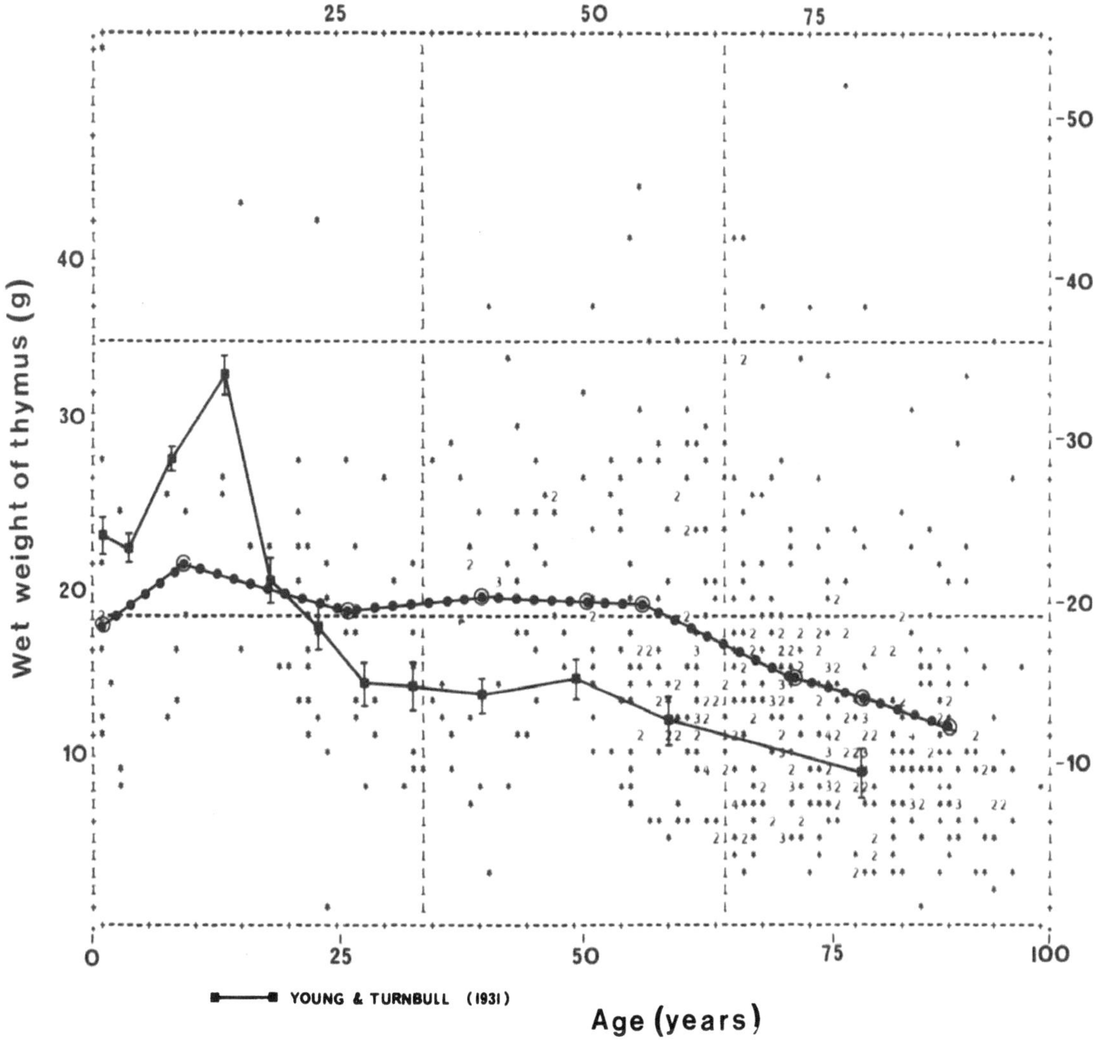

Fig. 3. Age changes in the weight of normal human thymus. *Circles* wet weights of human thymus glands from 574 coroners' necropsies. Means superimposed. The standard deviations ranged from 6.4 to 9.9 g. *Squares*, thymus weights in 464 persons in "normal" health at the time of death (values taken from Young and Turnbull 1931). (Modified from Kendall et al. 1980)

supposed to be at its maximum). Body weight did not help much in explaining the range in thymic weights. The lipid weight of the thymus increased rapidly and linearly ($p < 0.001$) up to the age of 50 years then levelled off (with a wide range of values at any given age) and showed a very slight decrease in the older groups (over 70 years of age). The lean dry material (protein and carbohydrate) decreased significantly with age ($p < 0.001$), being greatest in the under-30-year-old group. A small percentage of thymuses from the over-80-year-old group had as high a lean dry weight as those from the under-50-year-old group.

Age-Related Changes

Since both the mass of thymus tissue and the degree of fatty infiltration are variable, attempts have been made at further evaluation of the age-related changes. Labrecque et al. (1972) showed that thymic tissue could be found and evaluated in 91% of a series of necropsies in the age range 18-92 years, and that reliable quantitative work could be done on any sections of thymus taken from the anterior mediastinum. Biopsies of the gland from 89 patients immediately before thyroidectomy for nontoxic nodular goitre (Simpson et al. 1975) showed that the cortex atrophied slightly faster than the medulla in young people (age group "17" years), but not later (age group "57" years). Although the numbers in any category were low and standard deviations high, there was evidence for a biphasic pattern of age involution in the cortex (but not the medulla) in women, with atrophy taking place faster up to and including the third decade of life, and thereafter linearly as in the male thymuses examined.

In 25 of 26 thymic biopsies from male patients undergoing open-heart surgery, Singh and Singh (1979) noted that the distinction between cortex and medulla was clear and that the parenchyma remained lymphoid, although the cortex involuted 2.5 times faster than the medulla. They recorded an age-related decline in E-rosette-forming (T) cells in males and females from about 95% (0-20 years of age) to about 60% (60-70 years of age).

In an electron microscope study of material from five boys (4-11 years) and two adults undergoing heart surgery, von Gaudecker (1978) concluded that the age-involuted adult human thymus, though greatly reduced quantitatively, contains a remnant of lymphoid tissue unchanged in cellular composition and presumably able to serve its function in cell-mediated immunological responses by providing new T cells, even in the aged. Studying the duration of thymic function, Stutman and Good (1974) found that significant numbers of aged subjects can develop vigorous responses to new antigens. That adult thymectomy reduces this ability was shown by Björkholm et al. (1975). In 31 of 146 patients who underwent thymectomy on account of thymomas, extrathymic malignancies developed 10-15 years after the operation (Souadjian et al. 1968). More subtle changes in T-helper and suppressor cell populations in peripheral blood are now becoming evident (Berrih et al. 1983; Björkholm et al. 1975). (Earlier work on T-cell changes after adult thymectomy has been reviewed by Newsom-Davis and Vincent 1982.)

Recent work on ageing rats (18 months old) in which the thymus gland was greatly reduced and virtually nonexistent, has shown that 30 days after orchidectomy or implants of the stable analogue of luteinizing hormone-releasing hormone, the thymus reappears as a large bilobed (or even four-lobed) organ and the peripheral blood lymphocyte counts are raised (Fitzpatrick et al. 1985; Adcock et al. 1986; Greenstein et al. 1986). Further work has demonstrated that this is preventable by giving the animals subcutaneous implants of testosterone (Fitzpatrick et al. 1986). If the human thymus is affected in a similar manner this finding is of great potential in the search for methods of boosting the body's immune responses.

Thus, although it is true that in general the thymus involutes with age, this does not necessarily mean that it becomes nonfunctional. Some individuals appear to have a large, lymphoid thymus well into old age.

References

Adcock IM, Fitzpatrick FTA, Greenstein BD (1986) Regeneration of thymus in ageing rats after orchidectomy: effects of testosterone. J Physiol 372: 66
Ader R (1981) Psychoneuroimmunology. Academic Press, New York
Ader R, Cohen N, Felten DL (1987) Brain, behaviour and immunity. Brain Behav Immun 1: 1-6
Anderson J, Cameron JAM (1927) Status lymphaticus and sudden death. Glasgow Med J 108: 129-147
Arya S, Gilbert EF, Hong R, Bloodworth JMB Jr (1982) The thymus. In: Bloodworth JMB Jr (ed) Endocrine pathology. General and surgical, 2nd edn. Williams and Wilkins, Baltimore, pp 767-832
Berrih S, Le Brigand H, Levasseur P, Gaud C, Bach JF (1983) Depletion of helper/inducer T cells after thymectomy in myasthenic patients. Clin Immunol Immunopathol 28: 272-281
Besedovsky HO, del Rey AE, Sorkin E (1983) What do the immune system and the brain know about each other? Immunology Today 4: 342-346
Björkholm M, Holm G, Johansson B, Mellstedt H (1975) T-lymphocyte deficiency following adult thymectomy in man. Scand J Haematol 14: 210-215
Blalock JE (1984) The immune system as a sensory organ. J Immunol 132: 1067-1070
Blanc F, Koritké JG (1970) Considérations sur l'angioarchitectonie du thymus humain dans la période périnatale. CR Assoc Anat 55: 665-673
Bloodworth JMB Jr, Hiratsuka H, Hickey RC, Wu J (1975) Ultrastructure of the human thymus, thymic tumors, and myasthenia gravis. In: Sommers SC (ed) Pathology annual, vol 10. Appleton-Century-Crofts, New York, pp 329-391
Bockman DE, Kirby ML (1984) Dependence of thymus development on derivatives of the neural crest. Science 223: 498-500
Boyd E (1927) Growth of the thymus: its relation to status thymicolymphaticus and thymic symptoms. Am J Dis Child 33: 867-879
Boyd E (1932) The weight of the thymus gland in health and in disease. Am J Dis Child 43: 1162-1214
Bratton AB (1925) The normal weight of the human thymus. J Pathol Bacteriol 28: 609-620
Bulloch K, Moore RY (1981) Innervation of the thymus gland by brain stem and spinal cord in mouse and rat. Am J Anat 162: 157-166
Couly G, Lagrue A, Griscelli C (1983) Le syndrome de Di-George, neurocristopathie rhombencéphalique exemplaire. Rev Stomatol Chir Maxillofac 84: 103-108
Cross RJ, Markesbery WR, Brooks WH, Roszman TL (1980) The acute effect of hypothalamic lesions on the immune response. Fed Proc 39: 1162 (4711)
Cross RJ, Brooks WH, Roszman TL, Markesbery WR (1982) Hypothalamic-immune interactions: effect of hypophysectomy on neuroimmunomodulation. J Neurol Sci 53: 557-566

Dardenne M, Bach JF (1981) Thymic hormones. In: Kendall MD (ed) The thymus gland. Academic, London, pp 113-131

Dawson HL (1966) Basic human anatomy. Appleton-Century-Crofts, New York, pp 148-149

Deaver JB (1903) Surgical anatomy III. Rebman, London, p 425

Felten DL, Felten SY (1989) Innervation of the thymus. Thymus Update 2: 73-88

Fitzpatrick FTA, Kendall MD, Wheeler MJ, Adcock IM, Greenstein BD (1985) Reappearance of thymus of ageing rats after orchidectomy. J Endocrinol 106: R17-R19

Fitzpatrick FTA, Kendall MD, Wheeler MJ, Adcock IM, Greenstein BD (1986) Reappearance of thymus in ageing male rats treated for one month with a stable analogue of luteinizing hormone-releasing hormone. J Endocrinol 108 (Supplement: abstract 32)

Goldstein G, Mackay IR (1969) The human thymus. Heinemann, London, p 3

Greenstein BD, Fitzpatrick FTA, Adcock IM, Kendall MD, Wheeler MJ (1986) Reappearance of the thymus in old rats after orchidectomy: inhibition of regeneration by testosterone. J Endocrinol 110: 417-422

Greenwood M, Woods HM (1927) "Status thymico-lymphaticus" considered in the light of recent work on the thymus. J Hyg (Lond) 26: 305-326

Hall NR, McGillis JP, Spangelo B, Palaszynski E, Moody T, Goldstein AL (1982) Evidence for a neuroendocrine-thymus axis mediated by thymosin polypeptides. In: Serrou B et al. (eds) Current concepts in human immunology and cancer immunomodulation. Elsevier, Amsterdam, pp 653-660

Hammar JA (1905) Zur Histogenese und Involution der Thymusdrüse. Anat Anz 27: 23-30; 41-89

Hammar JA (1906) Über Gewicht, Involution und Persistenz der Thymus im Postfötalleben des Menschen. Arch Anat Phys Anat Abt [Suppl]: 91-182

Hammar JA (1914) Methode, die Menge der Rinde und des Marks der Thymus, sowie die Anzahl und Größe der Hassallschen Körper zahlenmäßig festzustellen. Z Angew Anat Konstitutionslehre 1: 311-396

Hammar JA (1921) The new views as to the morphology of the thymus gland and their bearing on the problem of the function of the thymus. Endocrinology 5: 543-573; 731-760

Hammar JA (1935) Konstitutionsanatomische Studien über die Neurotisierung des Menschenembryos. IV. Über die Innervationsverhältnisse der Inkretorgane und der Thymus bis in den 4. Fötalmonat. Z Mikrosk Anat Forsch 38: 253-293

Hollinshead WH (1971) Anatomy for surgeons, 2nd edn, vol 2. Harper and Row, New York, p 37

Hwang WS, Ho TY, Luk SC, Simon GT (1974) Ultrastructure of the rat thymus. A transmission, scanning electron microscope, and morphometric study. Lab Invest 31: 473-487

Kendall MD (1984) Have we underestimated the importance of the thymus in man? Experientia 40: 1181-1185

Kendall MD, Johnson HRM, Singh J (1980) The weight of the human thymus gland at necropsy. J Anat 131: 485-499

Kendall MD, Fitzpatrick FTA, Greenstein BD, Khoylou F, Safieh B, Hamblin A (submitted) The histology of the ageing rat thymus after treatment with a stable analogue of luteinizing hormone-releasing hormone

Keynes G (1954) The physiology of the thymus gland. Br Med J 2: 659-663

Kreel L (1969) The radiology in diagnosis. In: Greene R (ed) Myasthenia gravis. Heinemann, London, p 57

Labrecque PG, Souadjian JV, Titus JL (1972) Etude morphologique quantitative du thymus humain dans une série d'autopsies. Union Med Can 101: 695-697

Last RJ (1984) Anatomy regional and applied, 7th edn. Churchill Livingstone, Edinburgh, p 228

Le Douarin NM, Jotereau FV (1975) Tracing of cells of the avian thymus through embryonic life in interspecific chimeras. J Exp Med 142: 17-40

Le Douarin NM, Jotereau FV, Houssaint E, Thiery JP (1984) Primary lymphoid organ ontogeny in birds. In: Le Douarin NM, McLaren A (eds) Chimeras in developmental biology. Academic, New York, pp 179-216

Newsom-Davis J, Vincent A (1982) Myasthenia gravis. In: Lachmann PJ, Peters DK (eds) Clinical aspects of immunology, 4th edn, vol 2. Blackwell, Oxford, pp 1011-1068

Norris EH (1938) The morphogenesis and histogenesis of the thymus gland in man: in which the origin of the Hassall's corpuscles of the human thymus is discovered. Contrib Embryol (Carnegie Inst Washington DC 27) (no 166): 193-209

Rebar RW, Miyake A, Low TLK, Goldstein AL (1981) Thymosin stimulates secretion of luteinizing hormone-releasing factor. Science 214: 669-671

Renoux G, Bizière K, Renoux M, Guillaumin JM (1980) Le cortex cérébral règle les réponses immunes des souris. CR Acad Sci [III]: 719-722

Scammon RE (1927) The prenatal growth of the human thymus. Proc Soc Exp Biol Med 24: 906-909

Schäfer EA, Symington J (1898) In: Schäfer EA, Thane GD (eds) Quain's elements of anatomy, 10th edn: vol 3 (N), Splanchnology. Longmans, London, pp 307-310

Schulz DM, Giordano DA, Schulz DH (1962) Weights of organs of fetuses and infants. Arch Pathol Lab Med 74: 244-250

Sergeeva VE (1974) Histotopography of catecholamines in the mammalian thymus. Bull Exp Biol Med 77 (4): 115-118

Siegler R (1964) The morphology of the thymuses and their relation to leukemia. In: Good RA, Gabrielsen AE (eds) The thymus in immunobiology: structure, function, and role in disease. Hoeber, Harper and Row, New York, pp 623-655

Simpson JG, Gray ES, Beck JS (1975) Age involution in the normal human adult thymus. Clin Exp Immunol 19: 261-265

Singh J, Singh AK (1979) Age-related changes in human thymus. Clin Exp Immunol 37: 507-511

Sloan HE Jr (1943) The thymus in myasthenia gravis: with observations on the normal anatomy and histology of the thymus. Surgery 13: 154-174

Souadjian JV, Silverstein MN, Titus JL (1968) Thymoma and cancer. Cancer 22: 1221-1225

Steinmann GG, Müller-Hermelink HK (1984) Lymphocyte differentiation and its microenvironment in the human thymus during aging. Monogr Dev Biol 17: 142-155

Stutman O, Good RA (1974) Duration of thymic function. Ser Haematol 7: 505-523

Van Dyke JH (1941) On the origin of accessory thymus tissue, thymus IV: the occurrence in man. Anat Res 79: 179-209

Von Gaudecker B (1978) Ultrastructure of the age-involuted adult human thymus. Cell Tissue Res 186: 507-525

Walford RL (1980) Immunology and aging. Am J Clin Pathol 74: 247-253

Watts T (1969) Thymus weights in malnourished children. J Trop Pediatr 15: 155-158

Williams JM, Felten DL (1981) Sympathetic innervation of murine thymus and spleen: a comparative histofluorescence study. Anat Rec 199: 531-542

Williams PL, Warwick R (1980) (eds) Gray's anatomy, 36th edn. Churchill Livingstone, Edinburgh, pp 770; 782; 800

Young M, Turnbull HM (1931) An analysis of the data collected by the status lymphaticus investigation committee. J Pathol Bacteriol 34: 213-258

4 Histology

Marion D. Kendall

Introduction

The two encapsulated lobes that together comprise the thymus gland contain three main populations of cells. A supporting stroma of *epithelial cells* is a fairly constant component, in which cell turnover appears relatively slow and which forms an integrated framework for rapidly mitosing populations of *haemopoietic cells* and motile *accessory cells.*

The collagenous capsule constitutes a discrete boundary, even when the gland is very fatty and embedded in mediastinal adipose tissue. Inside the main capsule each lobule of cortex is bounded by collagen, fibroblasts, mast cells and a connective tissue matrix that extends into the gland at least to the corticomedullary junction, ensheathing neurovascular bundles and lymphatics. The thymic septa of neonates contain adipose cells which, with increasing age, invade the subcapsular region, gradually replacing it and the cortex, and eventually reaching the medulla. The cortex appears capable of regrowing within this fatty infiltration, since small spherical areas of densely packed and mitosing cortical thymocytes, superficially resembling germinal centres, but without the characteristic cells or organization, are commonly observed in the fat in adults. Typical germinal centres have been recorded in "normal" thymus glands (Henry 1981; Kendall 1981), but they are unusual as thymus tissue normally contains less than 2% of plasma cells (Singh 1980 and personal communication).

The perivascular spaces in the septa may contain many different cell types, often of the myeloid series (such as eosinophils), in which case it is difficult to identify lymphatics in these spaces. The perivascular space of the interlobular septa is completely surrounded by type-1 epithelial cells (see later), but once the blood vessels have entered the stroma of the gland they may lack the epithelial surround. If the sheath is deficient the gap is usually filled by a macrophage. Some capillaries within the gland are fenestrated (Singh 1979).

Epithelial Cells

The supporting stroma of the thymus is composed of epithelial cells (sometimes called epithelial reticular cells) characterized by intracellular tonofilaments and desmosomes, and staining with keratin-specific antibodies (de Maagd et al. 1985). The thymus anlage of the 8th gestational week (g. w.) contains almost exclusively immature epithelial cells (sometimes with cilia), regularly arranged at the periphery and randomly distributed at the centre (von Gaudecker and Müller-Hermelink 1979). At about 9 weeks haemocytoblasts enter the gland, and medulla gradually develops as the central cells become more spindle-shaped and the first Hassall's corpuscles appear (9th g. w.). Interdigitating reticulum cells (see later) are seen at about 12 weeks, after mesenchymal septa have begun to invade the cortex. Characteristic differences between cortical and medullary epithelial cells are established by the 15th g. w. There are differences in electron density and the medullary cells are associated with basement membrane material whereas those within the cortex are not. The detailed use of monoclonal antibodies to antigens of the major histocompatibility complex, such as cytokeratins and thymulin *(facteur thymique sérique),* has shown that the adult organization of epithelial cells occurs between the 16th and 20th g. w. (Müller-Hermelink and Steinmann 1984).

Recent work on the epithelial cells of the cortex and medulla in thymuses from children and young adults categorizes these cells into six types with intermediate gradations (van de Wijngaert et al. 1984; Kendall et al. 1985). Previous descriptions of the ultrastructure of epithelial cells in humans (Arya et al. 1982; Bearman et al. 1978; Haar 1974; Hirokawa 1969; Kameya and Watanabe 1965; Savino and Santa-Rosa 1982; Singh 1981) did not recognize so much variation in cell types. In these studies the epithelial cells were often referred to as "pale" and "dark", as in other animal studies, "pale" cells being said to occur in the cortex, both types in the medulla. The features of epithelial cells suggesting a secretory function were often mentioned, and since Gelfand et al. (1980) pointed out that T cells need contact with epithelial cells and their

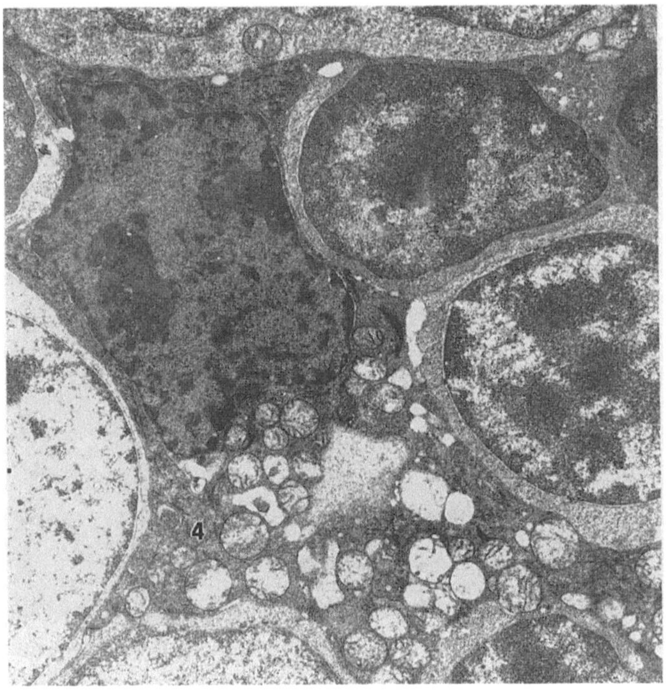

Fig. 3. A type-4 epithelial cell (4) from the deep cortex of a man aged 46 years. × 15000

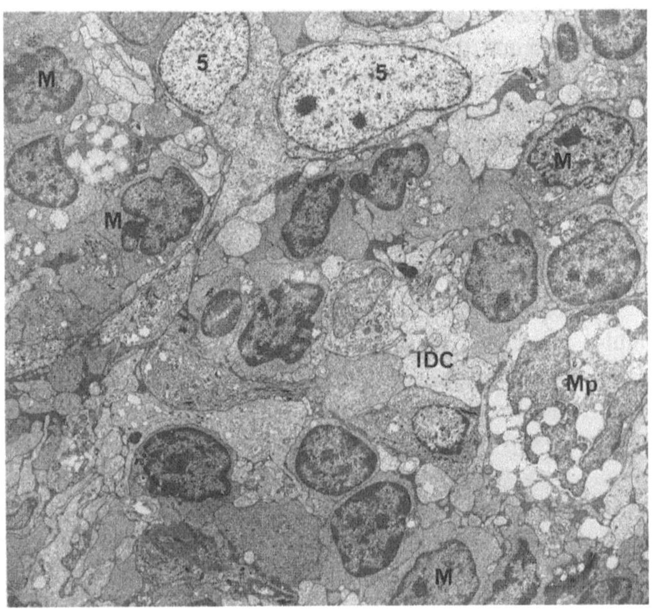

Fig. 4. Type-5 epithelial cells (5) in the thymic medulla of a man aged 19 years. *Mp* macrophage; *IDC* interdigitating cell cytoplasm. The medullary thymocytes *(M)* differ from those of the cortex (see text and Figs. 2 and 6). × 4000

epithelial cells show many of the features of keratinizing skin (Mandel 1968; von Gaudecker and Schmale 1974) and contain a variety of cell types (other epithelial cells, eosinophils, macrophages and occasionally mast cells and plasma cells). Thus Blau (1967) suggested that they were "graveyards" for dead thymocytes and other cell types. Marshall and White (1961) showed that Hassall's corpuscles can accumulate antigen and this theory has been taken up by others, especially by Kater, who showed in 1973 that antigenic stimulation can cause an increase in the number and size of these structures, although it is recognized that age, thymic atrophy and certain diseases can also do so.

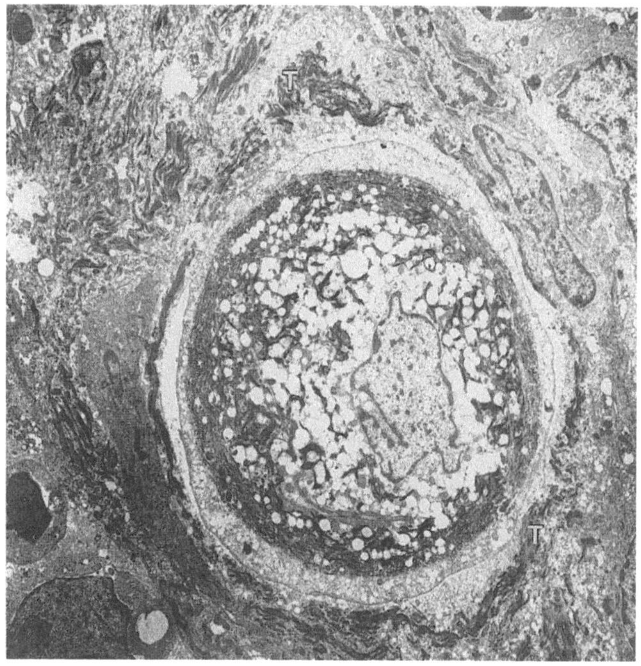

Fig. 5. A small Hassall's corpuscle from the thymus of a man aged 46 years. *T* tonofilaments. ×6000

Haemopoietic Cells

The lymphoid cells of the adult human thymus are in general small cells with a pachychromatic nucleus and few cytoplasmic organelles. However, detailed ultrastructural studies (Bloodworth et al. 1975; Haar 1974; Jones et al. 1975; von Gaudecker 1978; Singh 1980) show a surprising range of cellular morphology amongst thymocytes, the functional implications of which (Bhan et al. 1980; Janossy et al. 1986) will be dealt with in Chap. 6. For a full and recent summary of thymocyte maturation and differentiation the reader is referred to review articles in Kendall and Ritter (1989).

The lymphoid cells under the capsule in the subcapsular zone are often larger (see Fig. 1) than those in the cortex, ranging in size from 6-8 μm (medium thymocytes) to 9-14 μm (large thymocytes). The larger the cell the more leptochromatic the nucleus. The many cells that contain numerous monoribosomes or polyribosomes in the comparatively extensive cytoplasm are normally regarded as prothymocytes. Some of them could equally well be multipotential stem cells (Yoffey 1981). Mitotic figures are common in this region, and the progeny are presumed to be the small thymocytes (diameter 4-6 μm) seen slightly deeper in the gland (see Fig. 1). The outer cortical zone contains many of these small thymocytes with a pachychromatic nucleus, a small rim of cytoplasm, and few organelles. The range of morphology observed in cells of this zone (see Fig. 2) mainly reflects the changes that take place as cells pass through the mitotic cycle. These cells are commonly located within or between type-2 and type-3 epithelial reticular cells (see Fig. 2). In the deep cortex there are subtle changes in cellular morphology: in sections, some cells have a wide rim of electron-lucent cytoplasm whereas others are typical small cortical thymocytes (Fig. 6). Mitosis occurs here too, so it is possible that this zone is a region of clonal expansion. The epithelial cells are now mainly of types 3 and 4, so that islands of cells are seen with strands of electron-dense epithelial reticular cell processes around and between them (Fig. 6).

The thymocytes of the medulla (see Fig. 4) are larger (4-7 μm diameter) than small cortical thymocytes. The nuclear size is similar, but they contain more cytoplasm, sometimes with small dense granules, and the cells and nuclei are often irregular in outline with small projections that indent adjacent cells. Larger thymocytes also occur within lymphatics in the septa in humans (Singh 1980 and personal observations).

If correlation between structure and function is sought, the three main morphologically distinct types of thymocytes (subcapsular, cortical and medullary) do seem to correspond to the three subsets of thymocytes recognized by the identification of clusters of differentiation antigens, i. e. classes I, II, and III of Reinherz et al. (1980). Moreover, the sporadic occurrence of class-II thymocytes in the medulla and of class-III thymocytes in the cortex has morphological correlates.

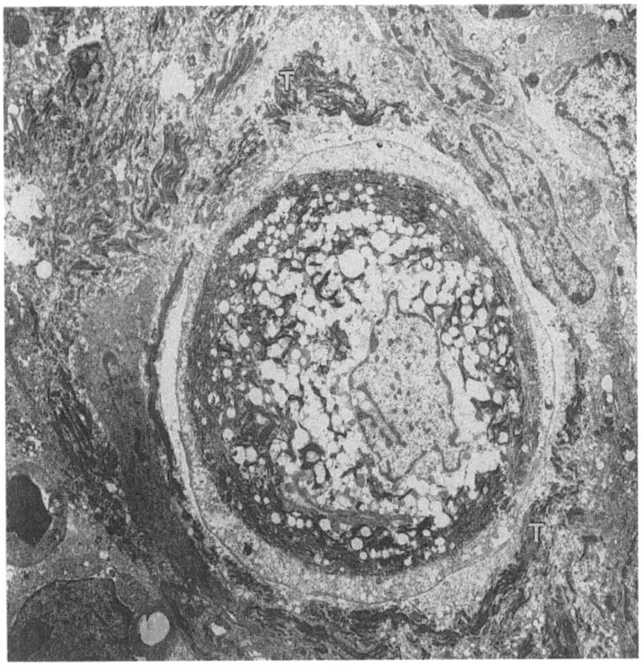

Fig. 6. The deep cortex of the thymus in a man aged 19 years with small cortical thymocytes *(T)* and larger thymocytes with medullary thymocyte *(M)* features. A type-4 epithelial cell (4) and a macrophage *(Mp)* are also present. (Singh 1981) ×6000

A greater degree of equivalence is probably demonstrable only by specialized techniques.

Other reasons make the correspondence difficult to achieve. The motile mononuclear cells in the thymus are not all thymocytes. The human thymus (like that of most animals), especially in the foetus, supports erythropoiesis (Albert et al. 1966; Taylor and Skinner 1976; Kendall and Singh 1980) and granulopoiesis (Harris 1958; Bhathal and Campbell 1965; Burnet 1965; Sin and Sainte-Marie 1965a, b; van Haelst 1967; Singh 1980; Kendall 1981). Taylor and Skinner (1976) found that 30% of small round cells in the foetal and neonatal thymus contained haemoglobin, and Kendall and Singh (1980) reported that approximately 80% of the adult thymus glands examined contained erythroblasts (Fig. 7), if only a few. In addition, mast cells are formed in the thymus throughout life. Many of these cell lines have progenitors that could be confused morphologically with thymocytes. Although ontogenetic studies are beginning to elucidate the developmental pathways and factors influencing T-cell production, there remain many unanswered questions about thymic haemopoiesis in general.

It was established many years ago that the first thymic rudiment in the embryo of all animals studied is epithelial, and that large basophilic cells enter the thymus before the blood vessels develop (Moore and Owen 1967; Owen and Ritter 1969; Le Douarin and Jotereau 1981). These early cells are thought to be derived from the yolk sac and are thus termed haemocytoblasts. Avian studies have shown that they enter in waves during periods when the gland is receptive, and possibly under the influence of chemoattractants (Le Douarin and Joterau 1981). Do some progeny of these cells remain within the thymus, perhaps throughout life as stem cells? Is the developing thymus receptive to later waves of infiltrating cells, and if so are these from the foetal liver, developing bone marrow or possibly the foetal spleen? How committed are these infiltrating cells? Later in adult life in animals, prethymic T-restricted cells derived from bone marrow enter the thymus and give rise to thymocytes (Jordan and Robinson 1981). Immature T-cell precursors are present in the human thymus to the end of life (Steinmann and Müller-Hermelink 1984). Does this mean a continual influx of prethymic T-restricted cells or can these cells divide to maintain a reserve pool within the thymus? Can these prethymic T-restricted cells enter other organs? Can they develop in, for example, the spleen, the bone marrow or other as yet undefined sites, to give rise to extrathymically produced T cells? And if they do so, must the thymus remain active? Athymic (nude) mice develop host cells with T-cell features after thymic grafting (Loor and Kindred 1973). Thus, extrathymic T-cell production may well depend on circulating thymic factors and so still rely upon an active thymus.

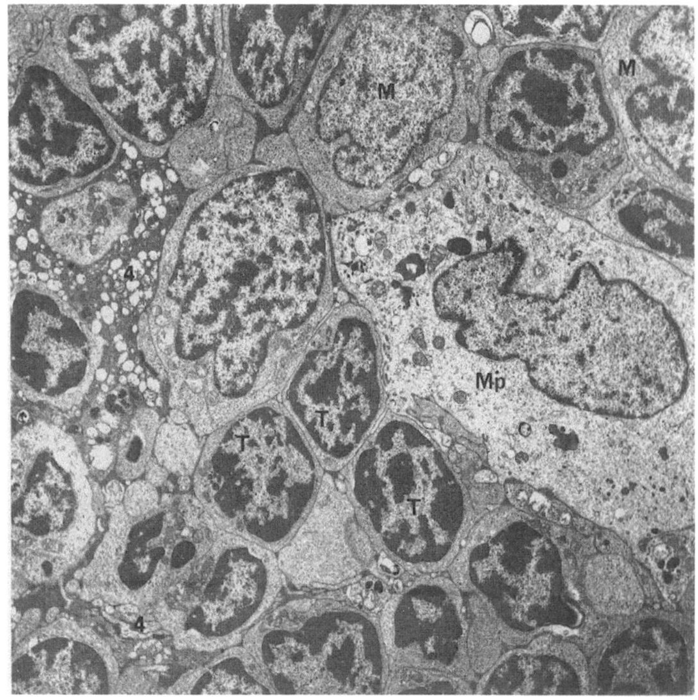

Fig. 7. Normoblasts *(N)* in the thymus of a man aged 48 years. Type-1 epithelial cells (1) separate the normoblasts from the perivascular space *(PVS)*. (Kendall and Singh 1980) ×6000

Accessory and Other Cells

Both macrophages and interdigitating cells occur in the thymus (Klug and Mager 1979; von Gaudecker and Müller-Hermelink 1980; Duijvestijn and Hoefsmit 1981) and are considered to play a specific role in T-cell maturation (Beller and Unanue 1980; Wong et al. 1982). Macrophages secrete a thymocyte-differentiating factor (Beller and Unanue 1977) which is mitogenic for thymocytes. It induces the functional maturation of thymocytes in vitro and may also do so in vivo (Beller et al. 1978). In studies in rats, Duijvestijn (1983) formed the opinion that the thymic macrophages in the cortex were scavengers and that cells from the macrophage line that reside in the medulla become interdigitating reticulum cells. It is here that the more mature thymocytes are found with most of the characteristics of immunocompetent T cells (Stobo and Paul 1972; Weissman 1973; Weissman et al. 1975).

Macrophages have been identified throughout the thymus and in the connective tissues of its capsule and septa. The greatest numbers are said to be around the corticomedullary junction, although numbers appear to vary extensively in different glands and probably increase with age. These very large cells (15-35 μm diameter) display all the features of macrophages found elsewhere in the body. A useful identifying feature is that many macrophages have short regions of electron-dense plasma membrane (Fig. 8) that can be seen in the electron microscope at relatively low magnifications (Henry, personal communication). They generally have an indented and irregular nucleus with marginally arranged heterochromatin, but the nature and extent of their inclusions vary. In foetal and neonatal glands macrophages may contain pyknotic nuclei, and this can become an important and obvious activity of macrophages if there is sudden involution of the thymus. In general, however, the gland macrophages do not contain many pyknotic nuclei. This is at variance with the assertion that most thymocytes die within the thymus because of the lethally high intracellular levels of deoxynucleosides (Ma et al. 1983) and never leave the gland (Scollay 1983). Study of the mitosis rates of thymocytes shows that cell cycle times (9-12 h in mice) are almost certainly shorter than the time taken for a macrophage to destroy an engulfed pyknotic cell completely (2-3 days) (Kendall 1984a). Furthermore, it is possible that at least some pyknotic cells are extruded erythrocyte nuclei, especially during foetal development (Kendall 1984b).

Cells known as foamy macrophages (Bloodworth et al. 1975), lipid-laden foamy cells (Loewenthal and Smith 1952), periodic acid-Schiff (PAS)-positive reticulum cells (Metcalf and Ishidate 1962) and autofluorescent cells (Sainte-Marie 1968) have been described, and they are probably all macrophages.

The interdigitating reticulum cells are characterized by an extensive electron-lucent cytoplasm with a much

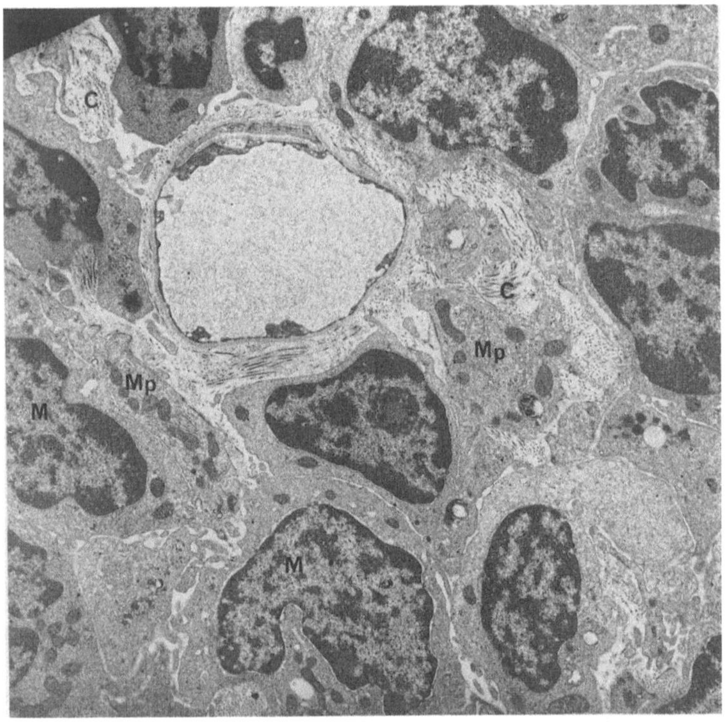

Fig. 8. From the thymus of a man aged 23 years. Macrophages *(Mp)* and "medullary" thymocytes *(M)* in a wide perivascular space that contains a fenestrated capillary. *C* collagen. × 10000

invaginated cell membrane. The leptochromatic, eccentrically placed and lobulated nucleus has a thin margin of heterochromatin under the nuclear membrane. Most of the organelles are in the central area where there are abundant stacks of Golgi membranes, small vesicles, coated vesicles, mitochondria and a few strands of RER. Many dense bodies are situated in the central area and appear to be secondary lysosomes. Characteristically they contain Birbeck granules, i.e. curious "tennis-racquet-shaped" inclusions first described by Birbeck et al. (1961) in the Langerhans cells of the skin. They are not particularly numerous in human interdigitating cells. Langerhans cells are Ia-positive (Stingl et al. 1978), and the Ia-positive antigen-presenting dendritic thymic macrophages described in vitro (Beller and Unanue 1980) are probably the same cell line. Kaiserling et al. (1974) first described these cells in the human thymus, although Oláh et al. (1968) described a "special cell" which although not phagocytic was probably an interdigitating cell. Interdigitating reticulum cells are especially prominent in the medulla and at the corticomedullary junction. They occur in T-dependent areas of lymph nodes and spleen (Heusermann et al. 1974; van Ewijk et al. 1974; Veerman 1974) where they are believed to be responsible for the T microenvironment. Zinkernagel et al. (1978) working with mice concluded that they had a role in determining which T precursors are activated to become effector, helper or killer cells during an immunological challenge.

Myoid cells are large single cells, with centrally located indented nuclei and irregularly arranged sarcomeres in the cytoplasm, which may be joined by desmosomes to other (notably epithelial) cells. Their histology in humans has been described by Bockman (1968), Bockman and Winborn (1969), Ito et al. (1969), Henry (1972) (who also reviews earlier work) and Puchtler et al. (1975). They are a regular feature of human thymuses, occurring in particular at the corticomedullary junction and extending into the medulla and close to the capsule. Henry (1981) considers that they may have a role in expelling thymocytes from the gland, but their chief interest has been their possible role in myasthenia gravis, especially since Kao and Drachman (1977) demonstrated acetylcholine receptors on myoid (and epithelial) cells. The thymus is a production site (although not the only one) of antibody to acetylcholine receptor substance (Vincent et al. 1978), but the significance of this in myasthenia gravis is not known.

Nerves, Neurotransmitters, Neuroendocrine Cells and Hormone Producing Cells

One of the greatest areas of advance in examining the function of the thymus *in vivo* since this chapter was first written (1985) is current work in progress on the innervation of the gland, neurotransmitters in nerves and in lymphocytes, and thymic hormones. The field is moving fast as information accumulates. Although many peptides have been reported from the thymus, it is not always clear which are synthesised in the gland, and which can be taken up by cells such as epithelial cells and thymocytes. Many peripheral blood lymphocytes are now known to contain neuropeptides (Blalock, 1984; Ottaway and Greenberg, 1984; Weigent and Blalock, 1987; Dion and Blalock, 1988; Weigent et al. 1988) and the interactions between the immune and neuroendocrine systems is an important area of current research activity (Smith and Blalock, 1988).

A useful review of the noradrenergic innervation of the thymus can be found in Felten and Felten (1989). This paper also discusses the problems with establishing a cholinergic innervation and briefly mentions the presence of other peptides such as neuropeptide Y and Vasoactive Intestinal Peptide (VIP) both of which form plexuses in the subcapsular zone and cortex. The VIP innervation appears to be independent of the noradrenergic network (Al-Shawaf et al., submitted). High levels of the neuropeptides, oxytocin and vasopressin are found in the gland and the activity has been localised to the subcapsular type 1 cells, medullary epithelial cells and Hassall's corpuscles (Geenen 1986 a, 1986 b). These cells are also immunoreactive with monoclonal antibodies raised to thymulin, thymopoeitin and thymosin alpha 1 (Savino and Dardenne, 1984; Auger et al., 1987), and A2B5 (a marker for neurones, neural crest cells and neuropeptide-secreting endocrine cells) (Haynes, Shimizu and Eisenbarth, 1983). Substance P is also present in human thymus glands, perhaps in the sensory innervation (Geppetti et al. 1987), but preprotachykinin mRNA detection in the thymus raises the possibility of intrathymic synthesis (Geenen, personal communication). Calcitonin related gene product reactivity in the rat thymus has recently been observed in our laboratory.

Work on acetylcholinesterase activity in the thymus (Bulloch and Moore, 1981; Bulloch and Pomerantz, 1984; Bulloch, 1985, 1988; Bulloch et al. 1987) demonstrated fibres that indicated a cholinergic innervation. This was also confirmed by Kendall et al. (1989) who also found large AChE positive cells in the medulla that were not myoid cells. Similar cells are enolase positive. However, the work of Bulloch and Moore (1981) has been repeated but not confirmed by Nance, Hopkins and Biegler (1987). More recently Bulloch and Lucito (1988) describe the effects of cortisone on acetylcholinesterase activity in the mouse thymus, and discuss the forms of acetylcholinesterase present showing that much more work needs to be conducted on the area of the cholinergic innervation of the gland.

Microenvironment

The thymus is a rapidly mitosing primary lymphoid organ with an ability to maintain defined microenvironments. The cellular content of the medulla differs from that of the cortex, and not all regions of the cortex contain cells in the same state. The subcapsular region also differs from the main part of the cortex and from the deep cortex adjacent to the medulla. Some of the microenvironmental differences are created by morphologically distinct epithelial cells types and cells of the monocyte/macrophage line that appear to have different functions in the various regions, but also the innervation could create locally distinct microenvironments.

The cortical microenvironment was considered to be a distinct 'antigenically pure' region as antigen injected directly into the thymus evoked histological changes that could not be elicited by antigen in the circulation. Marshall and White's blood-thymus barrier concept of 1961, proposed to account for these findings gained support from Raviola and Karnovsky (1972) who studied the permeability of the blood vessels of the thymus with electron-opaque tracers. The cortical capillaries have a specialised structure: being surrounded by a ring of type 1 epithelial cells that enclose the connective tissue of the perivascular spaces as well as various migrating cells (Kendall, in press). However the blood vessels of the corticomedullary region and the medulla may be deficient in this sheath of epithelial cells and the efficiency of the thymus-blood barrier has been questioned.

Recent work however has presented a completely different view of the 'antigenically protected' nature of the thymus which completely questions the validity of the blood-thymus barrier concept (Nieuwenhuis et al. 1988). Antigens were shown to enter the thymus by a transcapsular route and it is proposed that the free, differentiating, and maturing thymocytes may be constantly bathed by circulating self-antigens (Nieuwenhuis, in press). This is of fundamental importance for our understanding of thymocyte education in the gland and the learning of self recognition. Also, thymocytes contained within epithelial cells by emperiopoleisis could however be temporarily removed from this bathing medium, creating yet another form of microenvironment.

From this knowledge it can be seen that the microenvironments of the gland are dynamic concepts that vary with physiological conditions such as ageing, and could change rapidly with a variety of events such as stress, viral infection and chemical toxicity - sometimes resulting in irreparable damage from which the gland cannot fully recover. The constantly changing cellular dynamics of the thymus need to be carefully appraised throughout life to understand the impact of a fully functional thymus on immune function.

References

Albert S, Wolf PL, Pryjma I, Vazquez J (1966) Erythropoiesis in the human thymus. Am J Clin Pathol 45: 460-464

Al-Shawaf A, Cowen T, Kendall MD (submitted) Neural profiles in the normal and chemically sympathectomised rat thymus

Arya S, Gilbert EF, Hong R, Bloodworth JMB Jr (1982) The thymus. In: Bloodworth JMB Jr (ed) Endocrine pathology. General and surgical, 2nd edn. Williams and Wilkins, Baltimore, pp 767-832

Auger C, Stahli C, Fabien N, Monier JC (1987) Intracellular localization of thymosin alpha 1 by immunoelectron microscopy using a monoclonal antibody. J Histochem Cytochem 35: 181-187

Bearman RM, Levine GD, Bensch KG (1978) The ultrastructure of the normal human thymus: a study of 36 cases. Anat Rec 190: 755-782

Beller DI, Unanue ER (1977) Thymic maturation in vitro by a secretory product from macrophages. J Immunol 118: 1780-1787

Beller DI, Unanue ER (1980) IA antigens and antigen-presenting function of thymic macrophages. J Immunol 124: 1433-1440

Beller DI, Farr AG, Unanue ER (1978) Regulation of lymphocyte proliferation and differentiation by macrophages. Fed Proc 37: 91-96

Berczi I (1986) Pituitary function and immunity. CRC, Florida

Bhan AK, REinherz EL, Poppema S, McCluskey RT, Schlossman SF (1980) Location of T cell and major histocompatibility complex antigens in the human thymus. J Exp Med 152: 771-782

Bhathal PS, Campbell PE (1965) Eosinophil leucocytes in the child's thymus. Aust Ann Med 14: 210-213

Birbeck MS, Breathnach AS, Everall JD (1961) An electron microscope study of basal melanocytes and high-level clear cells (Langerhans cells) in vitiligo. J Invest Dermatol 37: 51-64

Blalock JE (1984) The immune system as a sensory organ. J Immunol 132: 1067-1070

Blau JN (1967) The dynamic behaviour of Hassall's corpuscles and the transport of particulate matter in the thymus of the guinea-pig. Immunology 13: 281-292

Bloodworth JMB Jr, Hiratsuka H, Hickey RC, Wu J (1975) Ultrastructure of the human thymus, thymic tumors, and myasthenia gravis. In: Sommers SC (ed) Pathology annual, vol 10. Appleton-Century-Crofts, New York, pp 329-391

Bockman DE (1968) Myoid cells in adult human thymus. Nature 218: 286-287

Bockman DE, Winborn WB (1969) Ultrastructure of thymic myoid cells. J Morphol 129: 201-210

Bulloch K (1985) Neuroanatomy of lymphoid tissue: a review. Neural Modulation of immunity. Raven Press, New York, pp 111-141

Bulloch K (1988) A comparative study of the autonomic nervous system innervation of the thymus in the mouse and chicken. Intern J Neuroscience 40: 129-140

Bulloch K, Cullen MR, Schwartz RH, Longo DL (1987) Development of innervation within syngeneic thymus tissue transplanted under the kidney capsule of the nude mouse: a light and ultrastructural microscopic study. J Neurosci Res 18: 16-27

Bulloch K, Lucito R (1988) The effects of cortisone on acetylcholinesterase (AChE) in the neonatal and aged thymus. Ann NY Acad Sci 521: 59-71

Bulloch K, Moore RY (1981) Innervation of the thymus gland by brain stem and spinal cord in mouse and rat. Am J Anat 162: 157-166

Bulloch K, Pomerantz W (1984) Autonomic nervous system innervation of thymic-related lymphoid tissue in wildtype and nude mice. J Comp Neurol 228: 57-68

Burnet FM (1965) Mast cells in the thymus of NZB mice. J Pathol Bacteriol 89: 271-284

De Maagd RA, Mackenzie WA, Schuurman HJ, Ritter MA, Price KM, Broekhuizen R, Kater L (1985) The human thymus microenvironment: heterogeneity detected by monoclonal anti-epithelial cell antibodies. Immunology 54: 745-754

Dion LD, Blalock JE (1988) Neuroendocrine properties of the immune system. Adv Biochem Psychopharmacol 44: 15-20

Duijvestijn AM (1983) The rat thymus: non-lymphoid cells in the microenvironment of T-cell differentiation. PhD Thesis, Krips Repro Meppel

Duijvestijn AM, Hoefsmit ECM (1981) Ultrastructure of the rat thymus: the micro-environment of T-lymphocyte maturation. Cell Tissue Res 218: 279-292

Felten DL, Felten SY (1989) Innervation of the thymus. Thymus Update 2: 73-88

Felten DL, Felten SY, Bellinger DL, Carlson SL, Ackermann KD, Madden KS et al. (1987) Noradrenergic sympathetic neural interactions with the immune system structure and function. Immunol Rev 100: 225-260

Geenen V, Legros JJ, Franchimont P, Baudrihaye M, Defresne MP, Boniver J (1986) The neuroendocrine thymus: coexistence of oxytocin and neurophysin in the human thymus. Science 232: 508-511

Geenen V, Legros JJ, Franchimont P, Defresne MP, Boniver J, Ivell R, Richter D (in press) The thymus as a neurosecretory organ: synthesis of vasopressin and oxytocin in human thymic epithelium. Ann NY Acad Sci

Gelfand EW, Dosch HM, Shore A, Limatibul S, Lee JWW (1980) Role of the thymus in human T cell differentiation. In: Gelfand EW, Dosch HM (eds) Biological basis of immunodeficiency. Raven, New York, pp 39-56

Geppetti P, Maggi CA, Zecchi-Orlandini S, Santicioli P, Meli A, Frilli S, Spillantini MG, Amenta F (1987) Substance P-like immunoreactivity in capsaicin-sensitive structures of the rat thymus. Regul Pept 18: 321-329

Haar JL (1974) Light and electron microscopy of the human fetal thymus. Anat Rec 179: 463-476

Harris PF (1958) Changes in thymus and lymph node activity, and alterations in bone marrow lymphocyte levels during recovery of the guinea-pig from whole body gamma irradiation. Br J Exp Pathol 39: 557-573

Hay ED, Revel JP (1963) Autoradiographic studies of the origin of the basement lamella in *Ambystoma*. Dev Biol 7: 152-168

Haynes BF, Shimizu K, Eisenbarth GS (1983) Identification of human and rodent thymic epithelium using tetanus toxin and monoclonal antibody A2B5. J Clin Invest 71: 9-14

Henry K (1972) An unusual thymic tumour with a striated muscle (myoid) component (with a brief review of the literature on myoid cells). Br J Dis Chest 66: 291-299

Henry K (1981) The human thymus in disease with particular

emphasis on thymitis and thymoma. In: Kendall MD (ed) The thymus gland. Academic, London, pp 85-111
Heusermann U, Stutte HJ, Müller-Hermelink HK (1974) Interdigitating cells in the white pulp of the human spleen. Cell Tissue Res 153: 415-417
Hirokawa K (1969) Electron microscopic observation of the human thymus of the fetus and the newborn. Acta Pathol Jpn 19: 1-13
Hirokawa K, McClure JE, Goldstein AL (1982) Age-related changes in localization of thymosin in the human thymus. Thymus 4: 19-29
Ito T, Hoshino T, Abe K (1969) The fine structure of myoid cells in the human thymus. Arch Histol Jpn 30: 207-215
Jambon B, Montagne P, Bene MC, Brayer MP, Fascere G, Duheille J (1981) Immunohistologic localization of facteur thymique sérique (FTS) in human thymic epithelium. J Immunol 127: 2055-2059
Janossy G, Bofill M, Trejdosiewicz LK, Willcox HNA, Chilosi M (1986) Cellular differentiation of lymphoid subpopulations and their microenvironments in the human thymus. In: Müller-Hermelink HK (ed) The human thymus: histophysiology and pathology. Curr Top Pathol 75: 89-125
Jones DL, Thomas K, Williams WJ, (1975) A fine structure study of human thymus. Beitr Pathol 156: 387-400
Jordan RK, Robinson JH (1981) T lymphocyte differentiation. In: Kendall MD (ed) The thymus gland. Academic, London, pp 151-177
Kaiserling E, Stein H, Müller-Hermelink HK (1974) Interdigitating reticulum cells in the human thymus. Cell Tissue Res 155: 47-55
Kameya T, Watanabe Y (1965) Electron microscopic observations on human thymus and thymoma. Acta Pathol Jpn 15: 223-246
Kao I, Drachman DB (1977) Thymic muscle cells bear acetylcholine receptors: possible relation to myasthenia gravis. Science 195: 74-75
Kater L (1973) A note on Hassall's corpuscles. In: Davies AJS, Carter RL (eds) Contemporary topics in immunobiology, vol 2. Thymus dependency. Plenum, London, pp 101-109
Kendall MD (1981) Introduction. In: Kendall MD (ed) The thymus gland. Academic, London, pp 1-6
Kendall MD (1984a) Have we underestimated the importance of the thymus in man? Experientia 40: 1181-1185
Kendall MD (1984b) More pieces of the jigsaw puzzle. Immunology Today 5: 286-287
Kendall MD (1985) The outer and inner thymus cortex is a functional syncytium. Cell Biol Int Rep 9: 3
Kendall MD (1986) The syncytial nature of epithelial cells in the thymic cortex. J Anat 147: 3-12
Kendall MD (in press) The morphology of the perivascular spaces in the thymus. Thymus
Kendall MD, Singh J (1980) The presence of erythroid cells in the thymus gland of man. J Anat 130: 183-189
Kendall MD, van de Wijngaert FP, Schuurman HJ, Rademakers LHPM, Kater L (1985) Heterogeneity of the human thymus epithelial microenvironment at the ultrastructural level. In: Klaus GGB (ed) Microenvironments in the lymphoid system. Adv Exp Med Biol 186: 289-297
Kendall MD, Al-Shawaf A, Zaidi SAA (1989) The cholinergic and adrenergic innervation of the rat thymus. Adv Exp Med Biol 237: 255-261
Kendall MD, Ritter MA (1989) T lymphocyte differentiation in the human thymus. In: Thymus update, vol 2. Harwood Academic Publishers, London
Klug H, Mager B (1979) Ultrastructure and function of interdigitating cells in the guinea pig thymus. Acta Morphol Acad Sci Hung 27: 11-19
Le Douarin NM, Jotereau FV (1981) The ontogeny of the thymus. In: Kendall MD (ed) The thymus gland. Academic, London, pp 37-62
Loewenthal LA, Smith C (1952) Studies on the thymus of the mammal. IV. Lipid-laden foamy cells in the involuting thymus of the mouse. Anat Rec 112: 1-15
Loor F, Kindred B (1973) Differentiation of T-cell precursors in nude mice demonstrated by immunofluorescence of T-cell membrane markers. J Exp Med 138: 1044-1055
Ma DDF, Sylwestrowicz T, Janossy G, Hoffbrand V (1983) The role of purine metabolic enzymes and terminal deoxynucleotidyl transferase in intrathymic T-cell differentiation. In: Inglis JR (ed) T lymphocytes today. Elsevier, Amsterdam, pp 62-65
Mandel T (1968) The development and structure of Hassall's corpuscles in the guinea pig: a light and electron microscopic study. Z Zellforsch Mikrosk Anat 89: 180-192
Marshall AHE, White RG (1961) The immunological reactivity of the thymus. Br J Exp Pathol 42: 379-385
Metcalf D, Ishidate M (1962) PAS-positive reticulum cells in the thymus cortex of high and low leukaemia strains of mice. Aust J Exp Biol Med Sci 40: 57-71
Monier JC, Dardenne M, Pleau JM, Schmitt D, Descheaux P, Bach JF (1980) Characterization of facteur thymique sérique (FTS) in the thymus. I. Fixation of anti-FTS antibodies on thymic reticuloepithelial cells. Clin Exp Immunol 42: 470-476
Moore MAS, Owen JJT (1967) Experimental studies on the development of the thymus. J Exp Med 126: 715-726
Müller-Hermelink HK, Steinmann GG (1984) Age-related alterations of intrathymic micro-environments. In: de Weck AL (ed) Lymphoid cell functions in aging. Topics in aging research in Europe, vol 3. Eurage, The Netherlands, pp 75-82
Nance DM, Hopkins DA, Biegler D (1987) Re-investigation of the innervation of the thymus gland in mice and rats. Brain Behav Immunol 1: 134-147
Nieuwenhuis P (in press) Self tolerance induction and the blood-thymus barrier. Thymus Update 3
Nieuwenhuis P, Stet RJM, Wagenaar JPA, Wubbena AS, Kampinga J, Karrenbeld A (1988) The transcapsular route: a new way for (self-)antigens to by-pass the blood-thymus barrier? Immunol Today 9: 372-375
Oláh I, Dunay C, Röhlich P, Toro I (1968) A special type of cells in the medulla of the rat thymus. Acta Biol Acad Sci Hung 19: 97-113
Ottaway CA, Greenberg GR (1984) Interaction of vasoactive intestinal peptide with mouse lymphocytes: specific binding and the modulation of mitogen responses. J Immunol 132: 417-423
Owen JJT, Ritter MA (1969) Tissue interaction in the development of thymus lymphocytes. J Exp Med 129: 431-442
Potworowski EF, Pyke KW, Brodniewkz-Proba I, Zelechowska M (1985) TMF, a thymic epithelial glycoprotein: chemotaxis of hematopoietic precursor cells. In: Klaus GGB (ed) Microenvironments in the lymphoid system. Adv Exp Med Biol 186: 683-691
Puchtler H, Meloan SN, Branch BW, Gropp S (1975) Myoepithelial cells in human thymus: staining, polarization and fluorescence microscopic studies. Histochemistry 45: 163-176
Raviola E, Karnovsky MJ (1972) Evidence for a blood-thymus barrier using electron-opaque tracers. J Exp Med 136: 466-497

Reinherz EL, Kung PC, Goldstein G, Levey RH, Schlossman SF (1980) Discrete stages of human intrathymic differentiation: analysis of normal thymocytes and leukemic lymphoblasts of T-cell lineage. Proc Natl Acad Sci USA 77: 1588-1592

Sainte-Marie G (1968) The autofluorescent cells of the lymphocytic tissues of the rat. Anat Rec 151: 133-150

Savino W, Dardenne M (1984) Thymic hormone containing cells: VI. Immunohistologic evidence for the simultaneous presence of thymulin, thymopoietin and thymosin alpha 1 in normal and pathological human thymuses. Eur J Immunol 14: 987-991

Savino W, Santa-Rosa GL (1982) Histophysiology of thymic epithelial reticular cells. Arch Histol Japan 45: 139-144

Schuurman HJ, Kater L (1985) Relevance of "nurse cells" in histophysiology of lymphoid tissues. Thymus 7: 317-322

Schuurman HJ, van de Wijngaert FP, Delvoye L, Broekhuizen R, McClure JE, Goldstein AL, Kater L (1985) Heterogeneity and age dependency of human thymus reticulo-epithelium in production of thymosin components. Thymus 7: 13-23

Scollay R (1983) Intrathymic events in the differentiation of T-lymphocytes: a continuing saga. In: Inglis JR (ed) T lymphocytes today. Elsevier, Amsterdam, pp 52-56

Scollay R, Andrews P, Boyd R, Shortman K (1985) The role of the thymic cortex and medulla in T cell differentiation. In: Klaus GGB (ed) Microenvironments in the lymphoid system. Adv Exp Med Biol 186: 229-234

Sin YM, Sainte-Marie G (1965a) Granulocytopoiesis in the rat thymus. I. Description of the cells of the neutrophilic and eosinophilic series. Br J Haematol 11: 613-623

Sin YM, Sainte-Marie G (1965b) Granulocytopoiesis in the rat thymus. II. Pattern for granulocyte formation based on cell counts in granulocytopoietic islands. Br J Haematol 11: 624-632

Singh J (1979) Observations on the capillaries and perivascular spaces in the human thymus. J Anat 128: 424-425

Singh J (1980) Studies on the human thymus with particular reference to age changes. PhD thesis, University of London, pp 369-370

Singh J (1981) The ultrastructure of epithelial reticular cells. In: Kendall MD (ed) The thymus gland. Academic, London, pp 133-150

Smith ME, Blalock JE (1988) A molecular basis for interactions between the immune and neuroendocrine systems. Int J Neurosci 38: 455-464

Steinmann GG, Müller-Hermelink HK (1984) Lymphocyte differentiation and its microenvironment in the human thymus during aging. Monogr Dev Biol 17: 142-155

Stingl G, Katz SI, Shevach EM, Wolff-Schreiner E, Green I (1978) Detection of Ia antigens on Langerhans cells in guinea pig skin. J Immunol 120: 570-578

Stobo JD, Paul WE (1972) Functional heterogeneity of murine lymphoid cells. II. Acquisition of mitogen responsiveness and of theta antigen during the ontogeny of thymocytes and "T" lymphocytes. Cell Immunol 4: 367-380

Taylor CR, Skinner JM (1976) Evidence for significant hematopoiesis in the human thymus. Blood 47: 305-313

Trowell OA (1949) Intracellular lymphocytes in thymus reticular cells and in fibroblasts cultured in vitro. J Physiol (Lond) 110: 5P

Van Ewijk W, Verzijden JHM, van der Kwast TH, Luijex-Meijer SWM (1974) Reconstitution of the thymus dependent area in the spleen of lethally irradiated mice: a light and electron microscopical study of the T-cell microenvironment. Cell Tissue Res 149: 43-60

Van Haelst U (1967) Light and electron microscopic study of the normal and pathological thymus of the rat. I. The normal thymus. Z Zellforsch Mikrosk Anat 77: 534-553

Van de Wijngaert FP, Rademakers LHPM, Schuurman HJ, de Weger RA, Kater L (1983) Identification and in situ localization of the "thymic nurse cell" in man. J Immunol 130: 2348-2351

Van de Wijngaert FP, Kendall MD, Schuurman HJ, Rademakers LHPM, Kater L (1984) Heterogeneity of epithelial cells in the human thymus: an ultrastructural study. Cell Tissue Res 237: 227-237

Veerman AJP (1974) On the interdigitating cells in the thymus-dependent area of the rat spleen: a relation between the mononuclear phagocyte system and T-lymphocytes. Cell Tissue Res 148: 247-257

Vincent A, Scadding GK, Thomas HC, Newsom-Davis J (1978) In-vitro synthesis of anti-acetylcholine-receptor antibody by thymic lymphocytes in myastenia gravis. Lancet 1: 305-307

Von Gaudecker B (1978) Ultrastructure of the age-involuted adult human thymus. Cell Tissue Res 186: 507-525

Von Gaudecker B, Müller-Hermelink HK (1979) Ontogenetic differentiation of epithelial and non-epithelial cells in the human thymus. Adv Exp Med Biol 114: 19-23

Von Gaudecker B, Müller-Hermelink HK (1980) Ontogeny and organization of the stationary non-lymphoid cells in the human thymus. Cell Tissue Res 207: 287-306

Von Gaudecker B, Schmale EM (1974) Similarities between Hassall's corpuscles of the human thymus and the epidermis: an investigation by electron microscopy and histochemistry. Cell Tissue Res 151: 347-368

Weigent DA, Baxter JB, Wear WE, Smith LR, Bost KL, Blalock JE (1988) Production of immunoreactive growth hormone by mononuclear leukocytes. FASEB J 2: 2812-2818

Weigent DA, Blalock JE (1987) Interactions between the neuroendocrine and immune systems: common hormones and receptors. Immunol Rev 100: 79-108

Weissman IL (1973) Thymus cell maturation: studies on the origin of cortisone-resistant thymic lymphocytes. J Exp Med 137: 504-510

Weissman IL, Small M, Fathman CG, Herzenberg LA (1975) Differentiation of thymus cells. Fed Proc 34: 141-144

Wekerle H, Ketelsen UP (1980) Thymic nurse cells: Ia-bearing epithelium involved in T-lymphocyte differentiation? Nature 283: 402-404

Wong TW, Klinkert WEF, Bowers WE (1982) Immunological properties of thymus cell subpopulations: rat thymic dendritic cells are potent accessory cells and stimulators in a mixed leukocyte culture. Immunobiology 160: 413-423

Yoffey JM (1981) Stem cells and the thymus with special reference to cellular migration streams. In: Kendall MD (ed) The thymus gland. Academic, London, pp 185-202

Zinkernagel RM, Callahan GN, Althage A, Cooper S, Klein PA, Klein J (1978) On the thymus in the differentiation of "H-2 self-recognition" by T cells: evidence for dual recognition? J Exp Med 147: 882-896

5 Physiology

Jean-François Bach and Mireille Dardenne

Introduction

The thymus gland plays a major role in immunity by producing T cells whose effector and regulatory subsets are major components of the immune system. It may also have other functions, as is suggested by thymoma-associated erythroblastopenia (which is cured by thymectomy) and by the sterility that is usual in thymus-deprived nude mice. These nonimmune functions, however, are still questionable and are not fully substantiated. In fact, all the effects of thymectomy, whether in adults or newborns, seem explicable on the basis of the action of the thymus on the immune system (Table 1).

The intrathymic differentiation and immunological functions of T cells are described in another section of this volume. Here we shall concentrate on the physiology of the nonlymphoid compartment of the thymus, which essentially includes two cell types: epithelial cells and phagocytic cells (macrophages and interdigitating dendritic cells). The epithelium is the original element of the thymus. Grafted into a thymus-deprived animal it can achieve reconstitution of a normal thymus. Neither lymphocytes nor macrophages, both of which arise from haematopoietic stem cells, can do this. The lymphocytes, perhaps the macrophages too, are attracted by a chemotactic factor, after which they colonize the epithelium. The thymic epithelium has a fundamental role in the maturation of T cells. It provides the principal signals of differentiation, both by direct cell contact - presentation of major histocompatibility complex (MHC) antigens - and through the intermediary of multiple polypeptidic hormones, whose chemical nature we shall describe, together with the properties and secretion physiology of one of them, thymulin.

Table 1. Effects of thymectomy in the mouse

Neonatal thymectomy (before 24 h)	Thymectomy at weaning (3 weeks)	Adult thymectomy[a] (2 months)
Loss of circulating thymic hormone	Loss of circulating thymic hormone	Loss of circulating thymic hormone
↓ Thy-1$^+$, Lyt-1$^+$, Lyt-2$^+$, Lyt-1.2$^+$ cells		Lyt-1.2$^+$ cells ↓ Thy-1$^+$ rosette-forming cells ↑ Autologous rosette-forming cells
↓ PHA, ConA responses ↓ MLC, CML, allograft rejection and GvH reaction	PHA, ConA responses	
↓ Antibody formation to thymus-dependent antigens		↑ Response to thymus-independent antigens and to some thymus-dependent antigens (IgE)
↑ Incidence of viral infections and non-induced tumours		
Variable effect on autoimmune responses	↑ Spontaneous antinuclear antibody formation	↑ Some autoimmune responses (e.g. rat erythrocyte-induced haemolytic anaemia) ↑ Syngeneic GvH reaction

Thy- and Lyt-designate cell surface differentiation antigens for mouse T cells.
PHA phytohaemagglutinin, ConA concanavalin A: MLC mixed lymphocyte culture, CML cell-mediated lympholysis, GvH = graft-versus-host; IgE immunoglobulin E
[a] In addition, adult thymectomy accelerates the age-associated decline in immune responses.

Signals of T-Cell Differentiation

General

Intrathymic T-cell differentiation occurs in discrete stages that have been demonstrated by the study of antigenic phenotypes using anti-TL or anti-Lyt alloantibodies in mice and anti-T-cell xenogeneic monoclonal antibodies in humans. Thymic lymphocytes acquire immunocompetence progressively, and concomitantly with the variations of antigenic phenotype. All these major intrinsic changes, conferred upon pre-T cells by the thymus, depend on cellular and humoral signals emanating from the gland's various cell types (Bach and Papiernik 1981).

It has been known for over a decade that direct contact between pre-T cells and the thymic epithelium is essential for the onset of differentiation. This direct contact, which probably accounts for the simultaneous presence in the thymus of the differentiating tissue (epithelial cells) and its target cells (marrow or liver-derived lymphoid progenitor cells), may relate primarily to the now well-documented intrathymic T-cell education of the receptor repertoire. It is not known, however, whether the educator cells (which are radioresistant) are epithelial cells or macrophages also present in the thymic reticulum.

Several humoral signals are probably instrumental at different maturation stages. Epithelial cells produce polypeptides that have been fully characterized, some of which may act as chemoattractants, others as lymphocyte-differentiating agents. Macrophages, particularly the recently described interdigitating cells, give rise to interleukin 1 (IL-1) (Papiernik and Homo-Delarche 1983) and probably to prostaglandins (Homo et al. 1981). Lymphocytes, notably those of the medulla with the Lyt-1 phenotype, generate interleukin 2 (IL-2), probably under the stimulation of IL-1 or autologous stimulation. Other lymphokines, such as IL-3 whose role in colony-forming unit in S phase (CFU-S) proliferation has recently been outlined (Garland 1984), may also be concerned. All these mediators have been shown to induce some aspects of T-cell differentiation in vitro and in vivo (Bach and Papiernik 1981). Evaluation of the physiological significance of thymus-generated interleukins and prostaglandins is still difficult. Only the peptidic hormones produced by epithelial cells will be studied here.

Migration of T-Cell Precursors to the Thymus: Role of Chemotactic Factors

The intervention of a chemotactic factor produced by the thymic epithelium in the colonization of the gland by pre-T cells is suggested by two findings derived from in vivo and in vitro experiments respectively.

In vivo, in the chicken, Le Douarin and Joterau (1981) showed that colonization of the embryonic thymic anlage occurs in successive waves of cells which, although present in the circulation, can penetrate into the interior of the thymus only during those periods in which the gland is "receptive". This migration is an active phenomenon during which stem cells are sensitive to a concentration gradient of a chemotactic factor of epithelial origin whose secretion is associated with a specific stage of epithelial maturation.

In an in vitro system of cellular migration under agar Pyke and Bach (1979) showed that 14-day-old foetal murine liver cells were attracted by explants of thymic epithelium. The migration, induced by a soluble factor produced by the thymic epithelium, is active and directed. It can be inhibited by the presence of thymic tissue among the pre-T cells contained in the foetal liver cell preparation. These experiments were reinvestigated and further developed by Slimane et al. (1983) in a different in vitro experimental system which enable them to characterize the chemical nature of the factor, shown to be a peptide with a molecular weight close to 1000.

Presentation of Major Histocompatibility Complex Products

The fact that lymphocytes remain in the thymus for several days undergoing the early phases of their differentiation suggests that if the thymus acts by secreting humoral factors the effect of these factors is not exclusive, and must be associated with or completed by direct contact between pre-T cells and the epithelium. In fact, a thymus graft in a Millipore chamber placed in a 45-day-old mouse thymectomized at birth does not lead to reconstitution of the animal's immune competence, which only the grafting of free thymus, into which the pre-T cells can penetrate, will achieve.

The nature of the cell contact in question remained obscure until Zinkernagel's experiments showed recognition of the MHC antigens by the pre-T cells to be responsible. If an irradiated $(A \times B)F_1$ mouse, reconstituted with $(A \times B)F_1$ bone marrow, is transplanted with an irradiated thymus of A origin, the T cells generated at the periphery can recognize only antigens associated with strain A MHC products (Zinkernagel et al. 1978). The interpretation of these experiments is not as easy as was first thought. Thus, partial maturation of T cells can be obtained in nude mice by treating their cells with IL-2, independently of all contact with the thymic epithelium (Gillis et al. 1979). However, the recognition of autologous MHC antigens, both classes of which are expressed on the thymic epithelium, is probably concerned in the education of the specificities of T-cell recognition. This autorecognition, for which the syngeneic mixed lymphocyte reaction is a good in vitro model, may be the source of the intense proliferation of lymphoid cells observed in the thymic cortex, during which the selection of T-cell clones and the rearrangements of the T-cell receptor genes characteristic of each clone probably occur.

Lymphocyte Differentiation Peptides

The thymus exerts some of its differentiating activities by secreting hormones acting both within the organ and at the periphery. Thus, the immune competence of mice thymectomized at birth can be restored by thymic grafts in Millipore chambers or by thymic extracts. Many attempts have been made to characterize the active factors contained in the biologically functional extracts. Several peptides have been described and analysed biologically and biochemically. If we exclude the thymic humoral factor described by Trainin et al. (1975) (well documented biologically, but not definitively characterized chemically), and if we abide strictly by the known criteria, namely, amino acid sequence, proof of thymic origin and in vivo and in vitro demonstration of biological activities in humans and experimental animals, we are left with three peptides: thymopoietin, thymosin α_1 and thymulin (previously called *facteur thymique sérique*, FTS).

Thymopoietin is a peptide composed of 49 amino acids (molecular weight 5562), initially isolated by its unexpected capacity to depress neuromuscular transmission (Goldstein and Manganaro 1971). It or one of its active fragments, a pentapeptide (TP5) (Goldstein et al. 1979), binds to specific receptors and has many immunopharmacological properties both in vitro (induction of T-cell markers) and in vivo (generation of cytotoxic T cells, prevention of autoimmunity) (Audhya et al. 1984).

Thymulin was isolated from porcine serum, and is produced exclusively by the thymic epithelium. It is a nonapeptide (molecular weight 847) which binds to zinc and thus obtains its biologically active conformation (and modifies its antigenicity). Its biological activities show wide diversity. It can stimulate most T-cell functions provided the cells are not too immature, in which case they would need concomitant direct contact with the thymic epithelium. In particular, thymulin induces auxiliary and cytotoxic T-cell functions, and at high doses can stimulate suppressor T-cell function. It binds to high affinity receptors characterized on lymphoblastoid cell lines. The nature of the second messenger is unknown (cyclic AMP or, more probably, prostaglandins) (Goldstein and Lau 1980).

Thymosin α_1 is a polypeptide composed of 28 amino acids (molecular weight 3108) (Bach 1983). Although it was isolated from the thymus an exclusive thymic origin has not been demonstrated. In contrast, recent studies suggest that it could also be produced by the brain, and even by T-lymphocytes (which are usually considered to be its target) (Goldstein et al. 1977). Several biological activities have been described, without providing specific information concerning its possible intervention in the physiological maturation of T cells (Goldstein et al. 1983).

The other factors described remain secondary. This may be because their chemical natures have not been definitively elucidated, as in the case of the thymic humoral factor (THF) described by Trainin et al. (1975), or because they are ubiquitous, i. e. produced by many categories of cells other than thymus cells, such as thymosin β_4 or the aptly named ubiquitin. Finally, it may be because they have not been defined biochemically, or attributed thymic origins or biological activities.

There is no indication of any interrelation between these peptides. No homology exists between the known amino acid sequences, and there is no evidence of cross-reactivity with antibodies raised against any of them or with the thymulin receptor. It is possible, however, that a chemical relation will be found when the sequence of THF is known. It may also be that some of these peptides are cleavage by-products of a larger precursor molecule. DNA recombinant studies currently in progress should cast light on this possibility.

Undoubtedly several distinct peptides exist. Before the actual number of thymic hormones can be determined, evidence is needed as to whether all these peptides are truly physiological lymphocyte-differentiating hormones, exclusively produced by the thymic epithelium (lymphokines can also be isolated from whole thymic extracts). Some of them may be original and significant substances; others, although pharmacologically active, may have no physiological role or may be related to already known substances (such as polymers or carrier proteins) (Dardenne et al. 1980). Perhaps there exist other thymic factors that we do not know about. Although definitive conclusions are not yet possible, a plausible minimal hypothesis postulates two to four different thymic hormones, perhaps originating in part from the same precursor, and acting at different stages of T-cell differentiation.

Physiology of the Thymic Epithelium as Studied by Thymulin Production

Site of Hormone Production

That the thymus is the only source of thymic hormones has been shown chiefly in studies of thymulin, at first by indirect evidence, namely, the absence of thymulin from the sera of thymus-deprived animals such as the nude mouse and of thymectomized animals and humans (Goldstein and Lau 1980). Direct evidence that thymulin is produced only by thymic epithelial cells was obtained later by immunohistochemical methods depending on polyclonal and monoclonal antibodies directed against the synthetic or the natural hormone. These techniques established the exclusive presence of thymulin in certain thymic epithelial cells in situ, and in cultured cells in vitro (Savino et al. 1982; Berrih et al. 1984).

Thymulin has been demonstrated within epithelial cell cytoplasmic vacuoles in electron microscopic studies (Schmitt et al. 1980). In fact, the same epithelial cells contain the three thymic peptides, thymopoietin, thymosin α_1 and thymulin, indicating that these cells can generate different thymic hormones simultaneously (Savino and Dardenne 1984). Using primary cultures of thymic epithelial cells as a model, Cohen et al. (1983) have found the biologically active hormone in these culture supernatants.

Ontogeny and the Relation Between Thymulin Secretion and Ageing

The fact that thymulin can be detected in the serum of pregnant thymectomized mice as early as the 14th day of gestation by indirect immunofluorescence studies on thymic epithelial cells (Goldstein and Lau 1980) suggests that its production is probably associated with activity of the foetal thymus.

In humans, the maximal normal serum thymulin activity can be measured at birth. This level is maintained unchanged until adulthood is reached, after which it gradually falls, in parallel with the involution of the thymus. Thymulin is undetectable in the serum after the age of 60. Although the appearance of hormone inhibitory factors has been reported in mice as well as humans (Dardenne et al. 1984), the fall in thymulin level can be attributed to the reduced secretion during ageing that results from a significant decrease, as evaluated by immunofluorescence, in the number of thymus cells synthesizing it.

Regulation of Thymulin Production

Regulation of thymulin secretion has been demonstrated both in vivo and in vitro, but its mechanism has not been elucidated. Hormone depletion in vivo, produced for example by injections of monoclonal thymulin-specific antibodies or by immunization against the hormone, induces a significant increase in the number of cells synthesizing the hormone in normal mouse thymuses (Savino et al. 1983). On the other hand, repeated injections of thymulin lead to a moderate but significant reduction in the number of these cells. These observations suggest that secretion of thymulin, like secretion of other hormones, is subject to a feedback regulation. The existence of this regulatory mechanism has been confirmed by in vitro studies of thymulin secretion by cultured thymic epithelial cells (Cohen et al. 1983). The number of cells synthesizing the hormone, minimal at the onset of the culture, increased in a highly significant manner during the culture, because of the lack of inhibitory serum factors. Addition of the synthetic hormone to the culture prevented the increase, a fact which suggests that the hormone itself can regulate its own production by these epithelial cells (Cohen et al. 1983). Nevertheless, other hormones, in particular glucocorticoids and the sex steroids, are concerned in the regulation of thymic hormone secretion, and receptors for these hormones are present in thymic epithelial cells.

Conclusion

The fact that the thymus is both a lymphocyte-differentiating gland and an endocrine gland is well documented. The thymic epithelial cells have the principal role. They influence the different stages of intrathymic maturation and present the products of the MHC to lymphocytes. They also produce chemotactic factors, which enable the gland to be colonized by pre-T cells, and thymic hormones, whose biological activities have been demonstrated in vivo and in vitro at the different stages of T-cell differentiation.

References

Audhya T, Talle MA, Goldstein G (1984) Thymopoietin radioreceptor assay utilizing lectin-purified glycoprotein from a biologically responsive T cell line. Arch Biochem Biophys 234: 167-177

Bach JF (1983) Thymulin (FTS-Zn). Clinics in Immunology and Allergy, vol 3. Saunders, London, pp 133-156

Bach JF, Papiernik M (1981) Cellular and molecular signals in T cell differentiation. In: Microenvironments in haemopoietic and lymphoid differentiation. Ciba Found Symp 84: 215-235

Berrih S, Savino W, Azoulay M, Dardenne M, Bach JF (1984) Production of anti-thymulin (FTS) monoclonal antibodies by immunization against human thymic epithelial cells. J Histochem Cytochem 32: 432-438

Cohen S, Berrih S, Dardenne M, Bach JF (1983) Régulation in vitro de la sécrétion de thymuline (FTS) par les cellules épithéliales thymiques humaines. CR Séances Acad Sci (III) 297: 63-65

Dardenne M, Pléau JM, Bach JF (1980) Evidence of the presence in normal serum of a carrier of the serum thymic factor (FTS). Eur J Immunol 10: 83-86
Dardenne M, Savino W, Gastinel LN, Bach JF (1984) Thymulin, zinc and aging. In: de Weck AL (ed) Lymphoid cell functions in aging. Topics in aging research in Europe, vol 3. Eurage Ryswyk, pp 187-199
Garland JM (1984) Involvement of interleukin 3 in lymphocyte biology and leukemogenesis. In: Pick E (ed) Lymphokines. A forum for immunoregulatory cell products, vol 9. Academic, London, pp 201-256
Gillis S, Union NA, Baker PE, Smith KA (1979) The in vitro generation and sustained culture of nude mouse cytolytic T-lymphocytes. J Exp Med 149: 1460-1476
Goldstein G, Lau C (1980) Thymopoietin and immunoregulation. In: Beers RF Jr, Basset EG (eds) Polypeptide hormones. Raven, New York, pp 459-465
Goldstein G, Manganaro A (1971) Thymin: a thymic polypeptide causing the neuromuscular block of myasthenia gravis. Ann NY Acad Sci 183: 230-240
Goldstein AL, Low TLK, McAdoo M, McClure J, Thurman GB, Rossio J, Lai CY, Chang D, Wang S, Harvey C, Ramel AH, Meienhofer J (1977) Thymosin α_1: isolation and sequence analysis of an immunologically active thymic polypeptide. Proc Natl Acad Sci USA 74: 725-729
Goldstein G, Scheid MP, Boyse EA, Schlesinger DH, Van Wauwe J (1979) A synthetic pentapeptide with biological activity characteristic of the thymic hormone thymopoietin. Science 204: 1309-1310
Goldstein AL, Low TLK, Latz MM, Hall NR, Naylor PH (1983) Thymosins. Clinics in Immunology and Allergy, vol 3. Saunders, London, pp 119-132
Homo F, Russo-Marie F, Papiernik M (1981) Steroid modulation of in vitro prostaglandin secretion by human thymic epithelium. Prostaglandins 22: 377-385
Le Douarin NM, Jotereau FV (1981) The ontogeny of the thymus. In: Kendall MD (ed) The thymus gland. Academic, London, pp 37-62
Papiernik M, Homo-Delarche F (1983) Thymic reticulum in mice. III. Phagocytic cells of the thymic reticulum in culture secrete both prostaglandin E_2 and interleukin 1 which regulate thymocyte proliferation. Eur J Immunol 13: 689-692
Pyke KW, Bach JF (1979) The in vitro migration of murine fetal liver cells to thymic rudiments. Eur J Immunol 9: 317-323
Savino W, Dardenne M (1984) Thymic hormone-containing cells. VI. Immunohistologic evidence for the simultaneous presence of thymulin, thymopoietin and thymosin α_1 in normal and pathological human thymuses. Eur J Immunol 14: 987-991
Savino W, Dardenne M, Papiernik M, Bach JF (1982) Thymic hormone-containing cells. Characterization and localization of serum thymic factor in young mouse thymus studied by monoclonal antibodies. J Exp Med 156: 628-633
Savino W, Dardenne M, Bach JF (1983) Thymic hormone-containing cells. III. Evidence for a feedback regulation of the secretion of the serum thymic factor (FTS) by thymic epithelial cells. Clin Exp Immunol 52: 7-12
Schmitt D, Monier JC, Dardenne M, Pléau JM, Deschaux P, Bach JF (1980) Cytoplasmic localization of FTS (facteur thymique sérique) in thymic epithelial cells. An immunoelectron-microscopical study. Thymus 2: 177-186
Slimane SB, Houllier F, Tucker G, Thiery JP (1983) In vitro migration of avian hemopoietic cells to the thymus: preliminary characterization of a chemotactic mechanism. Cell Differ 13: 1-24
Trainin N, Small M, Zipori D, Umiel T, Kook AL, Rotter V (1975) Characteristics of THF, a thymic hormone. In: Van Bekkum DW (ed) The biological activity of thymic hormones. Kooyker, Rotterdam, pp 117-132
Zinkernagel RM, Callahan GN, Althage A, Cooper S, Klein PA, Klein J (1978) On the thymus in the differentiation of "H-2 self-recognition" by T cells: evidence for dual recognition? J Exp Med 147: 882-896

6 Immunology

Henk-Jan Schuurman and Louis Kater

Introduction

Over the last 25 years studies of the role of the thymus in the generation of cellular immune competence have been stimulated and facilitated after the classical thymectomy experiments of Metcalf (1960) and Miller (1961), by the recognition of defects of cellular immunity in children with congenital aplasia of the thymus (DiGeorge 1965; Huber et al. 1967) and by the development of cardiac surgery with attendant removal of thymus tissue.

Despite substantial progress in thymology, however, Scollay stated in 1983 that "a careful analysis of available data shows how poorly we understand the role of the thymic cortex and medulla and how little we know of the exact processes which give rise to thymus-dependent peripheral T cells".

The thymus occupies a unique position among lymphoid organs in that most of its lymphoid elements are immature thymus-derived (T)-lymphocytes and that it has a microenvironment consisting mainly of epithelial cells. Its reticuloepithelial meshwork is in fact generally held to be responsible for its two principal functions, namely: processing immature T-precursor lymphocytes to become mature T cells and synthesizing humoral factors that are biologically active in T-cell maturation. This review of the role of the thymus gland in the immune system will begin with a description of the lymphoid compartment of the thymus, as a logical preliminary to examining the functions of its microenvironment inT-lymphocyte maturation. It concerns the state of knowledge in June 1985 and has been updated for some details in 1986 and finally in November 1987. For a review including more recent data on the biological functions of the thymus microenvironment, the reader is referred to Schuurman (1988). Apart from the final section on the adult thymus, all remarks refer to the human thymus in childhood.

T-Cell Subpopulations in the Thymus

Cytological Heterogeneity

The cytological features of lymphocytes differ in different parts of the thymus. In the subcapsular zone the principal lymphoid elements are large lymphoblastoid cells with abundant cytoplasm, prominent nucleoli, and frequent mitotic figures. The cortex is normally heavily populated by small lymphocytes with little or no cytoplasm. The medulla is less densely populated, mainly by medium-sized cells having little cytoplasm and resembling the lymphocytes in T-dependent areas of peripheral lymphoid organs. In cell suspensions of thymus tissue the ratio lymphoblasts: intermediate cells: small cells is about 5:20:75. This cytological heterogeneity of lymphocytes at various locations in the thymus is matched by heterogeneity of the cells' immunological characteristics, such as the expression of cell markers or functional capacity.

Relation Between Cell Markers, Function and Tissue Location

The first application of monoclonal antibody technology to leucocytes was in the characterization of T-lymphocyte (sub)populations. The monoclonal antibodies that recognize antigens on the surface of T cells have been compared and grouped at international workshops on leucocyte differentiation antigens. There are now eight so-called clusters of differentiation (CD) of antigens on cells of the T-cell lineage (International Union of Immunological Societies, IUIS, World Health Organization, WHO, Nomenclature Subcommittee 1984; McMichael and Gotch 1987), and an additional two on activated T cells (Table 1). The expression of CD antigens on the cell membrane is associated with the maturation and differentiation stages of the cell.

To denote the three main cell subsets, each with a distinct CD phenotype composition, that exist in the thymus, Reinherz et al. (1980) have proposed stages I, II and III (Table 2). These subsets correlate with the

Table 1. Clusters of differentiation for T-lymphocytes[a]

CD no. (cell, MW)	Leucocyte subset	Examples of well-known antibodies
1 (Thy, gp45,12)	Corticothymocytes	OKT6, NA1/34
2 (T, gp50)	T with sheep erythrocyte receptor	OKT11, anti-Leu-5
3 (T, gp19-29)	Mature T	OKT3, anti-Leu-4
4 (T, gp56-62)	T-helper, inducer	OKT4, anti-Leu-3
5 (T, gp67)	Pan-T, subset B	OKT1, anti-Leu-1
6 (T, gp120)	Mature T, subset B	Tü 33
7 (T, gp41)	Pan-T	Anti-Leu-9, WT1, 3A1
8 (T, gp32-33)	T-cytotoxic, suppressor	OKT8, anti-Leu-2
25 (T, B, p55)	T- and B-activated	Tac, anti-IL-2 receptor
w26 (T, p120, 200)	T-activated	

CD cluster of differentiation; MW molecular weight; gp glycoprotein; p protein; w workshop
[a] CD 1-8 are described in IUIS-WHO Nomenclature Subcommittee (1984). Additional data on certain antibodies are presented in Reinherz et al. (1980), Ledbetter et al. (1981), Reinherz et al. (1983) and Tax et al. (1984).

cytological heterogeneity described. Stage I are the large lymphoblasts of the subcapsular zone, stage II are the small thymocytes of the cortex and stage III are the medium-sized thymocytes of the medulla. The stage III thymocytes comprise two segregated subsets, two-thirds of them expressing the CD4 phenotype and one-third the CD8 phenotype. Stage I thymocytes are the most immature and stage III thymocytes the most mature among the T-cell subpopulations. The phenotype of stage I cells is similar to that of the so-called prothymocytes, which are precursor cells in the bone marrow destined to go to the thymus to become immunocompetent (van Dongen et al. 1985; Janossy et al. 1986). The phenotype of stage III cells corresponds to that of T-lymphocytes in peripheral blood and peripheral lymphoid organs.

Other markers, in addition to antigens of the CD series, that distinguish T-cell subsets in the thymus include the T9 (transferrin receptor) antigens, the CD38 antigen, human leucocyte antigen (HLA) class I, peanut agglutinin binding capacity and the nuclear en-

Table 2. Markers for human thymocyte subpopulations

Marker	Prothymocytes (bone marrow)	Stage I blasts (subcapsule)	Stage II small cells (cortex)	Stage III medium-sized (medulla)		Peripheral T cells	
				1/3	2/3	1/3	2/3
Antigens							
CD1	–	–	+	–	–	–	–
CD2	+	+	+	+	+	+	+
CD3	–	–	±	+	+	+	+
CD4	–	–	+	–	+	–	+
CD5	–	–	±	+	+	+	+
CD6	–	–	–	+	+	+	+
CD7	+	+	+	+	+	+	+
CD8	–	–	+	+	–	+	–
CD25	?	±	–	–	–	–	–
T9	?	±	–	–	–	–	–
CD38	+	+	+	–	–	–	–
HLA class I	–	–	–	+	+	+	+
Peanut agglutinin binding capacity	–	–	+	–	–	–	–
TdT	+	+	+	–	–	–	–
Enzymes of purine nucleotide metabolism							
ADA		480	300	130		45	74
PNP		85	27	120		75	99
ADA/PNP		5.6	11	1.1		0.6	0.8
ecto-5′-NT		8.3	4.1	25		33	10
dCK		1.2	0.5	0.3		0.1	0.3
ecto-5′-NT/dCK		6.9	8.2	81		330	32

HLA human leucocyte antigen; TdT terminal deoxynucleotidyl transferase; ADA adenosine deaminase; PNP purine nucleoside phosphorylase; ecto-5′-NT ecto-5′-nucleotidase; dCK deoxycytidine kinase
[a] The data for markers are derived from Reinherz et al. (1980), Schuurman et al. (1981), Schuurman, van Laarhoven, Broekhuizen et al. (1983), IUIS-WHO Nomenclature Subcommittee (1984), Tax et al. (1984), Ceredig et al. (1985), van Dongen et al. (1985), Janossy et al. (1986). Data on purine enzymes (nmol per 10^6 cells per hour) are from Ma et al. (1982) and Schuurman, van Laarhoven, Broekhuizen et al. (1983).

zyme, terminal deoxynucleotidyl transferase (TdT) (Table 2). In the mouse Scollay et al. (1984) have described the marker B2A2, present in high density on stage II lymphocytes and in lower density on stage III lymphocytes. B2A2 is present on only a minor proportion of T cells in peripheral lymphoid organs and is the only known marker that distinguishes mature thymic T cells from peripheral T cells.

A relation between cell phenotype and cell function has been established for thymocyte subpopulations in suspension, separated according to size and density or according to marker expression. It has been thus shown that thymocytes of stage III, but not thymocytes of stage II, respond to stimulation with mitogens or alloantigens (Schuurman et al. 1981; Ma et al. 1982; Umiel et al. 1982; de Vries et al. 1983; Schuurman, Brekelmans, Daemen et al. 1983; Schuurman, van Laarhoven, Broekhuizen et al. 1983). Studies on thymocytes in suspension have also thrown light on the occurrence of relatively small lymphocyte subsets with maturation between stages I, II or III. Some 25% of peanut agglutinin binding thymocytes are CD3-positive and 10%-20% are strongly CD5-positive; unlike the peanut agglutinin binding CD5-negative population, these cells respond to mitogen and alloantigen stimulation like stage III thymocytes (Umiel et al. 1982).

Tissue location by immunohistochemical methods using monoclonal antibodies on frozen tissue sections have extended the phenotypic characteristics of thymocytes (Bhan et al. 1980; Janossy et al. 1986). Cytomorphological studies have revealed phenotype expression of stage II thymocytes in the thymus cortex and of stage III thymocytes in the medulla. Immunohistochemistry enables single-cell analysis to be performed on tissue sections, by which technique stage II thymocytes have been identified in the medulla and stage III thymocytes in the cortex (Bhan et al. 1980; Umiel et al. 1982). In mice, cells with receptors for interleukin 2 (IL-2), equivalent to CD25 in humans), being about half of stage I thymocytes, occur at scattered locations throughout the cortex and medulla (Ceredig et al. 1985), a finding which indicates that stage I thymocytes may be dispersed throughout the organ, morphologically mainly in the subcapsular area. On the other hand, a small subset of stage III lymphocytes that have been located in the cortex, but not in the medulla of mice bear a receptor for high endothelial venules in T-dependent areas in peripheral lymphoid tissues (Fink et al. 1985). These observations influence the concepts, to be discussed later, of thymocyte migration through the thymus in relation to the microenvironment of the organ.

Significance of Cell Marker Molecules in Cell Function

Apart from their association with differentiation or maturation stages, cell surface markers may have specific functions. For example, a receptor function in cell activation or proliferation has been demonstrated in peripheral mature T-cell subsets with immunoregulatory functions. The CD4-bearing cell population comprises lymphocytes with helper-inducer function in immune reactions and the CD8-bearing population includes cells with suppressor-cytotoxic function (Ballieux and Heijnen 1982). This relation between cell marker expression and cell function apparently does not apply to stage II thymocytes which coexpress CD4 and CD8. Reinherz et al. (1983) have established a functional significance for these antigens. The CD4 antigen functions as a receptor for a nonpolymorphic determinant of the HLA class II molecule, which is concerned in cell-cell interactions of helper cells in the initiation of immune reactions. Similarly, the CD8 antigen acts as a receptor for HLA class I molecules, concerned in cell-cell interaction during T-cell-mediated cytotoxicity.

The CD3 antigen has a peculiar relevance, as it forms part of the antigen recognition structure on T cells (Reinherz et al. 1983). This consists of a heterodimer comprising a CD3 molecule and a so-called Ti antigen receptor. The CD3 molecule consists of three polypeptide chains and Ti is a disulphide-linked dimer composed of one α- and one β-chain (Acuto and Reinherz 1985). The Ti molecule recognizes the antigen in association with a polymorphic determinant of the major histocompatibility complex (MHC) (Reinherz et al. 1983), an interaction which results in cell activation. One of the features of T-cell activation is the synthesis of IL-2 and IL-2 receptor molecules (CD25). The interaction between IL-2 receptor on the cell surface and secreted IL-2 is necessary for subsequent proliferation and expansion of the cell. The close association between CD3 and Ti has been confirmed using antibodies to either CD3 or the variable part of Ti; at present there are no indications for a segregated occurrence of both molecules on the cell membrane. Before being expressed on the cell membrane, the CD3 molecule occurs in the cytoplasm during a more immature stage of the cell (Campana et al. 1987; Allison and Lanier 1987; Van Dongen 1987). We therefore assume that in the thymus Ti occurs only on CD3-positive cells, i.e. stage III and part of stage II thymocytes.

This assumption has been confirmed in studies on the molecular genetics of the antigen receptor. Apart from CD3 genome, three genes are concerned, one for the α- and one for the β-chain, and in addition a γ-

chain gene. For transcription, rearrangements are required to form a combination between gene segments coding for variable, diversity, joining and constant parts of the chain. These arrangements are generally assessed by detection of mRNA molecules (the transcription product). At the DNA level, γ-gene rearrangements occur early in differentiation, before prothymocytes enter the thymus. The rearrangement of α- and β-genes occurs in the thymus (Van Dongen 1987; Allison and Lanier 1987). mRNA for β-chain is abundant in stage II and III cells (Acuto and Reinherz 1985; Collins et al. 1985) in which it exceeds that in peripheral mature T cells 10- to 20-fold (Yoshikai et al. 1984). Whereas mRNA for α-chain is detected only in stage III thymocytes, γ-chain gene transcripts have been found in stage II and to a less extent in stage III thymocytes (Raulet et al. 1985). These data support the view that the antigen recognition repertoire of T cells is acquired during maturation in the thymus, and that functional antigen receptors become expressed on stage III thymocytes.

The marker TdT may have a function in the process of gene rearrangements. This enzyme functions as a DNA polymerase catalysing the coupling of dNTP to the free 3′-OH end of DNA, and may thus participate in somatic mutations during gene rearrangements (Gearhart 1982). As TdT is present in stage I and II thymocytes, its putative function in gene rearrangements concerns especially the β-chain of Ti.

A function for the CD2 antigen in lymphocyte activation has recently been hypothesized (Reinherz 1985). CD2 is the first marker established for human T-lymphocytes, viz. the receptor for sheep erythrocytes. Interaction with the molecule on the cell surface (by means of CD2-specific antibodies) results in suppression of IL-2 synthesis by mature T cells (Tadmori et al. 1985). For thymocytes this interaction leads to suppression of IL-2 receptor expression (Reed et al. 1985). Further, O'Flynn et al. (1985) have claimed that interaction with the CD2 molecule on the cell surface plays a part in activation of T cells by phytohaemagglutinin. Reinherz (1985) suggested that stage I and II thymocytes, which are CD2-positive but CD3- (hence Ti)-negative, can be activated by "natural ligands" in the microenvironment binding to CD2, with resultant IL-2-independent maturation or expansion of the cell. This ligand has been identified as the LFA-3 (leukocyte function associated) molecule (Selvaraj et al. 1987; Vollger et al. 1987).

Enzymes of Purine Nucleotide Metabolism

Interest in purine metabolism in lymphoid cells arose from studies of the causal relation between certain forms of immunodeficiency on the one hand and deficiency of purine nucleotide metabolizing enzymes on the other. Purine enzyme composition is different in stage I, II and III thymocytes (Table 2). Determination of these enzymes helps to assess maturation stage; for example, the enzyme activity ratio of adenosine deaminase (ADA) to purine nucleoside phosphorylase (PNP) is higher in stage I and II thymocytes than in stage III thymocytes, and the reverse applies to the ratio of ecto-5′-nucleotidase (ecto-5′-NT) to deoxycytidine kinase (dCK). The purine enzyme profile also gives information on the capacity of the cell to synthesize DNA, hence on its capacity to proliferate. In this respect the enzyme profile of stage I and II thymocytes seems suicidal. When compared with stage III thymocytes, for example, the low ratio of ecto-5′-NT to dCK indicates that (deoxy)nucleosides are more easily converted into toxic (deoxy)nucleotide triphosphates, a suggestion that has been confirmed in functional analyses as follows. In vitro proliferative responses of T cells are inhibited by addition of deoxynucleosides to the culture. The responses of immature (cortical) thymocytes are inhibited by lower concentrations than are the responses of more mature (medullary) thymocytes or peripheral T-lymphocytes (Cohen et al. 1980; Schuurman, van Laarhoven, Broekhuizen et al. 1983). Ma et al. (1983) have put forward the hypothesis that this "suicide" of stage I and stage II thymocytes is prevented in situ by "metabolic cooperation" in intimate contacts between the cells and the thymus microenvironment. This hypothesis is discussed in the next section.

The Thymus Nonlymphoid Microenvironment

Composition of the Microenvironment

The principal constituents of the nonlymphoid microenvironment of the thymus are epithelial cells, macrophages and interdigitating cells. In addition there are, of course, blood vessels, lymph vessels and connective tissue.

The morphology of the epithelial reticulum, which constitutes the major component, is heterogeneous, as ultrastructural studies by van de Wijngaert et al. (1984) have shown. Different subtypes have also been observed in antigen expression detected by monoclonal epithelial cell-specific antibodies, both in humans (McFarland et al. 1984; Bofill et al. 1985; de Maagd et al. 1985; Janossy et al. 1986; Ritter and Haynes 1987; Schuurman et al. 1987a) and mice (van Vliet et al. 1984a). Epithelial cells in the cortex differ in phenotype from epithelial cells in the medulla, and the medulla itself contains subtypes with different phenotype expression. It is remarkable that epithelial cells in the subcapsular zone show a phenotype expression similar to that of a subtype of cells in the medulla (de Maagd et al. 1985; Janossy et al. 1986). Expression of HLA class II antigens in epithelial cells varies with the location, cells in the subcapsular zone and medulla being negative or showing a low epression, whereas cells in the cortex are strongly HLA class II-positive (Bofill et al. 1985; Schuurman, van de Wijngaert, Huber et al. 1985). The epithelium is also heterogeneous in expression of thymic humoral factors.

Using an intracellular dye injection technique, Kendall (1985, 1986) has demonstrated that there is communication between thymic cortical epithelial cells in mice and in humans. The epithelial cells of the thymus cortex may therefore be regarded as a functional syncytium. Preliminary quantitative X-ray microanalysis studies, also by Kendall (personal communication), show that in the rat the concentrations of biologically important elements such as sodium and potassium are similar in the cortical epithelial cells and lymphocytes, but different in those of the subcapsular zone and the medulla.

As regards the other constituents of the thymic nonlymphoid microenvironment, the macrophages occur scattered throughout the cortex and medulla. The interdigitating cells are found chiefly in the medulla; they are rich in HLA class II expression, and this may influence lymphocyte differentiation in the thymus.

The macrophage-derived factor interleukin 1 (IL-1) enhances the proliferative response of immature thymocytes, presumably by induction of IL-2 receptors necessary for cell proliferation and expansion (Oppenheim and Gery 1982). IL-1-induced changes in the phenotype of stage II thymocytes compatible with a transition to stage III thymocytes have been noted by de Vries et al. (1983).

An insoluble thymic stromal fraction originating in the perivascular basement membranes of the thymic medulla and mediating the homing of bone marrow precursor cells to the thymus has been described by Fournier and Potworowski (1979).

Processing of Thymocytes by the Microenvironment

That the thymus has an important role in the production of leucocytes was first demonstrated by Kölliker (1879). Kölliker's researches ware taken further by Beard (1899), who believed that all the leucocytes in the body originate from epithelial cells in the thymus: "... the original leucocytes, starting from their birthplace and home in the thymus, have penetrated into almost every part of the body and have there created new centres for growth, for increase, and for useful work for themselves and for the body" (Beard 1899). We now know that Beard's postulate holds only for lymphocytes of the thymus-dependent T-cell lineage, which originate in the bone marrow and have to pass through the thymus to become mature T cells, competent for their function in immune reactions (Ford et al. 1966). Induction of this maturation apparently requires intimate contact between lymphoid cells and cells of the matrix of the organ.

In the mouse thymus, the daily immigration of prothymocytes accounts for about 0.001% of the total thymocyte population. The newly generated thymocytes account for about 30% and the emigrant population for only 1%. Some 29% of the total thymocyte pool dies each day (Scollay et al. 1984).

The migration pathways of lymphocytes through the thymus during generation of immunocompetence, and the fate of dead thymocytes, are still controversial subjects. The fact that migration concerns only a small percentage of the total thymocyte pool does not facilitate clarification. The immigrant population is immature, whereas the emigrant population has almost all the characteristics of the immunocompetent lymphocytes present in the peripheral blood and in the T-dependent areas of peripheral lymphoid organs. The tissue location of T-cell subpopulations suggests that the main migration pathway is immigration into the subcapsular zone, then via the cortex to the medulla for export. There is evidence, some of it based on single-cell analysis of tissue sections, that other pathways, such as direct migration of immigrants to the medulla, or direct export of emigrants from the cortex, may also exist (Scollay 1983). The presence in both cortex and medulla of cell clusters that are the progeny of one immigrant cell, and of cells bearing the IL-2 receptor (representing recently immigrated stage I cells) has been reported by Ezine et al. (1984) and Ceredig et al. (1985) respectively. The fact that cells with a receptor for high endothelial venules (which form a subset of immunocompetent stage III thymocytes) occur scattered throughout the cortex may reflect the presence of emigrant cells at this location (Fink et al. 1985).

In vitro and in vivo assays, including the use of neonatally thymectomized or congenitally athymic (nude) animals, have helped to determine the functions of the thymic microenvironment. For example, after transplantation of cultured thymic fragments, depleted of lymphocytes and consisting of epithelial cells only, into nude animals, thymus-dependent immunocompetence develops to a level comparable to that prevailing in immunocompetent animals. The transplanted graft becomes populated with lymphoid elements and its histology comes to resemble that of the normal thymus. This observation supports the concept that the function of the graft (e. g. thymus epithelium) is the induction of immune competence during passage of immature T cells through the epithelial microenvironment (Hong et al. 1979; Schuurman et al. 1982; Jenski and Hong 1985; Jordan et al. 1985; Schuurman, Vos, Broekhuizen et al. 1985; Schuurman, Vaessen, Vos et al. 1986; Schuurman et al. 1987 b).

Interactions Between Thymocytes and the Epithelial Reticulum

In both human and murine thymus cell suspensions, lymphocyte-epithelial cell complexes consisting of epithelial cells with lymphocytes in their cytoplasm have been described and designated "thymic nurse cells" (Wekerle et al. 1980; Ritter et al. 1981; Kyewski and Kaplan 1982; van de Wijngaert et al. 1983). Electron microscopy of tissue sections has revealed the presence in the cortex of epithelial cells with elongated processes that surround or even completely enclose thymocytes (van de Wijngaert et al. 1983, 1984). In the case of thymic nurse cells in suspension, the phenotype of the enveloped lymphocytes and of the epithelial cells supports the cortex tissue location (Ritter et al. 1981; Kyewski and Kaplan 1982; van Vliet et al. 1984 b). The only difference between enveloped lymphocytes and "common" stage II thymocytes seems to be the higher response to allogeneic stimulation of lymphocytes isolated from thymic nurse cells in vitro (Vakharia 1983). The biological significance of the internalization of lymphocytes within the epithelial cell is not known (Schuurman and Kater 1985).

These close interactions between precursor T cells and epithelial cells can be mimicked in vitro by incubation of cell suspensions containing precursor T-lymphocytes (e. g. bone marrow from normal individuals or bone marrow and peripheral blood of patients with various forms of immunodeficiency) on monolayers of cultured thymic epithelial cells. Such incubation results in induction of T-lymphocyte markers on the precursor T-lymphocytes (Willis-Carr et al. 1978; Gelfand and Dosch 1982). The relevance of this observation can, however, be disputed. Rubenfeld et al. (1981) have demonstrated a similar biological effect of cultured epidermal cells and cultured thymic epithelium in induction of TdT in bone marrow cells. Furthermore, the induction of T-cell markers concerns mainly the induction of CD2, but this marker is already present on prothymocytes entering the thymus (Table 2). We have been unable to detect markers of cortical epithelium on cultured epithelial monolayers, but have observed markers of medullary epithelium on some of these cells (Schuurman, Hendriks, Lange et al. 1986; Schuurman et al. 1987 a). We therefore suggest that the in vitro incubation of precursor T cells with epithelial monolayers has no relevance to T-cell maturation processes that are believed to occur in the cortex.

The close interaction between thymocytes and the epithelial reticulum in the cortex thus remains a subject for hypothetical models. One such model proposed by Ma et al. (1983) is based on the purine enzyme profile of the cortical thymocyte population (Table 2) which, as mentioned already, is rather unsuitable for cell proliferation and DNA synthesis. Cell death may be prevented during close contact with the microenvironment either by temporary metabolic cooperation with transfer of toxic nucleotides or enzyme molecules, or by rapid induction of maturation associated with changes into a less suicidal purine enzyme composition, such as change from stage II to stage III thymocytes.

Shore et al. (1981) studied the in vitro induction of T-cell markers during incubation on thymic epithelial monolayers. Using monolayers from normal subjects, they found induction for bone marrow cells from patients with immunodeficiency associated with ADA deficiency. If ADA activity in the monolayer was blocked there was no induction. Observing the in vivo induction of immune competence in nude mice by transplantation of cultured thymic fragments, Hong et al. (1982) reported that fragments cultured under conditions of blocked ADA activity were devoid of biological effect in vivo. These experimental data indicate the relevance of the ADA-mediated metabolic pathway in the interaction between thymocytes and epithelium.

Restriction Specificity in Recognition of Major Histocompatibility Complex Antigens

The thymus was originally assumed to be a privileged site for restriction or expansion of precursor T-cell clones which recognize nonpolymorphic self-major histocompatibility complex (MHC) antigens (Zinkernagel and Doherty 1979; Wagner et al. 1981). This recognition is a property of the complex of CD3 and Ti on the cell surface and is "learned" during the transition from stage II to stage III thymocytes. Data from murine experiments, however, indicate that precursor T cells in the bone marrow can already recognize class I antigens (Morrissey et al. 1982) and class II antigens (Bradley et al. 1982), and that cells in this prothymic stage of maturation can already be tolerized for effector reactivity to self-MHC structures. Studying self-MHC recognition during the development of virus-specific cytotoxic responses in mice, Kast et al. (1984) found that the thymus dictates class II specificity, but not class I specificity. Von Boehmer and Schubiger (1984) have claimed that cytotoxic T-lymphocytes that recognize class I antigens develop independently of the class I genotype of the thymus. Thus, the restriction specificity function of the thymus apparently applies only to class II MHC antigens. It appears not to include the generation of new structures recognizing antigen, but rather the expansion or selection of self-recognizing cells in the immigrant population. This restriction specificity has been documented for helper T-lymphocyte development, which requires class II antigen recognition (Singer et al. 1982), a process in which expression of class II antigens on the thymus microenvironment is required (Kruisbeek et al. 1983).

A strong expression of class II antigens has been observed on the epithelial reticulum of the cortex and on interdigitating cells in the medulla (Janossy et al. 1986). Interdigitating cells originate in the bone marrow (Longo and Schwartz 1980; Barclay and Mayrhofer 1981; Oliver and Le Douarin 1984). In a study of "chimeric" thymuses in which the epithelium and interdigitating cells differ in MHC haplotype, Longo and Schwartz (1980) found evidence that the interdigitating cells mediate the restriction specificity. Using the model of cultured thymic fragment implantation in athymic nude rats, Schuurman, Vaessen, Vos et al. (1986) found similar phenomena in allogeneic combinations, suggesting a role for interdigitating cells in intrathymic T-cell competence induction. This observation is supported by in vitro experiments in which thymocyte populations containing precursors with different haplotype-recognizing ability were cocultured with accessory cells from the spleen expressing a single haplotype; only thymocytes recognizing the haplotype of the accessory population developed (Rock et al. 1984). A role of the epithelial cells expressing MHC antigens cannot be excluded, but it appears to be related more to the induction of tolerance than to the clonal expansion of self-MHC recognizing T-cell precursors (Jordan et al. 1985).

The thymus medulla, where interdigitating cells are located, may therefore be the site of expansion of self-MHC recognizing T cells. This expansion follows the rearrangement of antigen receptor (Ti) genes which occurs predominantly in the immature thymocyte population in the cortex. Such function by interdigitating cells is not peculiar to the thymus. Interdigitating cells also occur in thymus-dependent areas of peripheral lymphoid organs, where they function by presentation of antigens to adjacent CD4-positive T-lymphocytes. There are indications that interdigitating cells in the thymus medulla also function in antigen presentation. They can stimulate T cells in syngeneic sensitization, which is related to the antigen presentation process (Papiernik et al. 1983). Further, the blood-thymus barrier apparently exists only for the thymus cortex, as soluble protein antigens can enter the thymus medulla (Kater 1973; Kyewski et al. 1984). As a site of initiation of immune responses the medullary compartment of the thymus resembles thymus-dependent areas of peripheral lymphoid organs and functions as a secondary lymphoid organ.

A similar situation may exist in humans. In thymus biopsy specimens from two patients with the so-called bare lymphocyte syndrome - a condition characterized by defective expression of HLA class I and in some cases also of class II molecules on blood mononuclear cells - Schuurman, van de Wijngaert, Huber et al. (1985) found that the (immuno) histology, including the expression of T-cell markers, was normal except for the absence of HLA expression on cortical epithelial cells. In two of the thymuses class II-positive interdigitating cells were observed in the medulla, whereas one of them was negative for HLA class II antigen expression at this location. These results suggest that the expression of HLA class I and class II antigens on epithelial cells in the normal thymus cortex has no role in T-cell maturation as judged by changes in T-cell phenotypes (including CD3).

Thymic Humoral Factors

The synthesis of humoral factors significant in T-cell maturation both within the thymus and elsewhere in the body is an important function of the thymic microenvironment. There are many thymic humoral factors, differing in chemical structure and in biological activity. They include extracts of the thymus and purified products from these extracts (Goldstein et al. 1981, 1983; Trainin et al. 1983, 1985), supernatants of cultured thymic stromal cells (Kruisbeek 1979; Oosterom et al. 1979; Gelfand and Dosch 1982), and substances present in the blood. The purified products are peptides, some of which have been sequenced and subsequently prepared synthetically. The best-documented preparations are thymosin and thymosin components, thymulin (formerly denoted *facteur thymique sérique*), thymic humoral factor, thymostimulin and thymopoietin.

The thymic humoral factors differ in biological activity with regard to in vitro and in vivo T-lymphocyte maturation (Ahmed et al. 1979; Kruisbeek 1979; Goldstein et al. 1981, 1983; Trainin et al. 1983). That they differ as regards both the target cells sensitive to their action and their effects on target cell populations suggests that the soluble products of the thymic microenvironment have a broad biological activity on T-lymphocytes in different stages of maturation (Bach and Goldstein 1980). This conclusion is illustrated by the following studies on thymosin. The crude thymosin extracted from calf thymus has been separated into peptides of which thymosin α_1, α_7, β_3 and β_4 are biologically active, each in its own way. Thymosin α_1 induces TdT expression in prothymocytes in the mouse bone marrow (Goldschneider et al. 1981), but reduces the TdT content of TdT-positive thymocytes on incubation with them (Hu et al. 1981), thus indicating that its biological effects differ with the maturation stage of the target cell. Thymosin α_1 induces T-helper cell function and thymosin α_7 induces T-suppressor cell function, in both cases in the more mature thymocytes. Thymosin β_3 and β_4, in contrast, exert their biological effects mainly on prothymocytes and presumably also on stage I thymocytes (Ahmed et al. 1979; Goldstein et al. 1981).

The major site of synthesis of thymic humoral factors appears to be the thymus medulla, but cortical epithelial cells also contain these factors (Kater et al. 1979; Hirokawa, McClure, Goldstein 1982; Savino and Dardenne 1984; Schuurman, van de Wijngaert, Delvoye et al. 1985). The thymosin components are synthesized by different cells in the epithelial microenvironment. Epithelial cells in the subcapsular zone are positive for thymosin α_1, β_3 and β_4; epithelial cells in the medulla are in part positive for thymosin α_1 and in part for thymosin α_7 (Hirokawa, McClure, Goldstein 1982; Schuurman, van de Wijngaert, Delvoye et al. 1985).

Humoral factors might be expected to exert their biological effects primarily in the immediate neighbourhood of the site of synthesis. In the case of thymosin components this would imply that the subcapsular zone where thymosin β_3 and β_4 are synthesized is the site of first maturation of immature thymocytes on their arrival in the thymus, the final maturation mediated by thymosin α_1 and α_7 occurring in the medulla. The site of synthesis of the different thymosin components is compatible with the tissue location of T-lymphocyte subsets which need these factors to mature.

Thymic factors are secreted into the bloodstream and may therefore also function at other body locations. The induction of TdT expression mediated by factors such as thymosin α_1, β_3 and β_4 appears to occur in the bone marrow, as prothymocytes entering the thymus are already TdT-positive (Table 2). This also applies to induction of CD2 on human precursor T cells. In mice, on the other hand, thymic emigrants contain a marker (B2A2) present on few peripheral T cells, a fact which is suggestive of the occurrence of T-cell maturation in peripheral lymphoid organs (Scollay et al. 1984). The presence of a small subset of peanut agglutinin binding T cells which reveal low mitogen responsiveness in the human tonsil (Schuurman, Brekelmans, Daemen et al. 1983) supports this suggestion. We have already seen how, apart from thymic humoral factors, products of other nonlymphoid components of the thymus may influence T-cell maturation.

The Adult Thymus

As regards thymus function in adulthood, Friedleben (1858) was the first to show that adult animals can be thymectomized without harm. The involution of the organ after puberty (Kendall et al. 1980) is associated with a decrease in intrinsic function of the epithelial cells (Oosterom and Kater 1981; Hirokawa, McClure, Goldstein 1982; Hirokawa, Sato, Makinodan 1982; Small et al. 1984; Schuurman, van de Wijngaert, Delvoye et al. 1985). Although it seems logical to assume that the thymus no longer functions in adulthood, all its components are present in the involuted organ till old age in the normal subject (Steinmann and Müller-Hermelink 1984). When the body has a demand, the thymus can generate immunocompetent T cells at other periods of life than during ontogeny. Such demand may occur especially in pathological situations (Kendall 1984), and an example is now appearing in centres practising bone marrow transplantation. The reconstitution of the T-cell system after transplantation is mediated chiefly by immunocompetent T cells present in the graft (de Gast et al. 1985). To avoid graft-versus-host reactions in allogeneic transplantation, grafting of bone marrow depleted of immunocompetent T cells has been introduced, in the belief that the T-cell system will be rebuilt by precursor cells in the graft which have to pass through the thymus. Scanty data from animal experiments point to a pivotal role for the thymus in T-cell reconstitution under these conditions (Müller-Hermelink et al. 1984). The "true function of the thymus" in T-cell generation, other than during ontogeny, may become an important subject of clinical research during the coming years.

References

Acuto O, Reinherz EL (1985) The human T-cell receptor; structure and function. N Engl J Med 312: 1100-1111
Ahmed A, Wong DM, Thurman GB, Low TLK, Goldstein AL, Sharkis SJ, Goldschneider I (1979) T-lymphocyte mat-

uration: cell surface markers and immune function induced by T-lymphocyte cell-free products and thymosin polypeptides. Ann NY Acad Sci 332: 81-94
Allison JP, Lanier LL (1987) The T-cell antigen receptor gamma chain: rearrangement and cell lineages. Immunol Today 8: 293-296
Bach J-F, Goldstein G (1980) Newer concepts of thymic hormones. Thymus 2: 1-4
Ballieux RE, Heijnen CJ (1982) Antigen-specific helper and suppressor T cell factors in man. Clin Haematol 11: 711-718
Barclay AN, Mayrhofer G (1981) Bone marrow origin of Ia-positive cells in the medulla of rat thymus. J Exp Med 153: 1666-1671
Beard J (1899) The true function of the thymus. Lancet 1: 144-146
Bhan AK, Reinherz EL, Poppema S, McCluskey RT, Schlossman SF (1980) Location of T cell and major histocompatibility complex antigens in the human thymus. J Exp Med 152: 771-782
Bofill M, Janossy G, Willcox N, Chilosi M, Trejdosiewicz LK, Newsom Davis J (1985) Microenvironments in the normal thymus and the thymus in myasthenia gravis. Am J Pathol 119: 462-473
Bradley SM, Morrissey PJ, Sharrow SO, Singer A (1982) Tolerance of thymocytes to allogeneic I region determinants encountered prethymically. Evidence for expression of anti-Ia receptors by T cell precursors before their entry into the thymus. J Exp Med 155: 1638-1652
Campana D, Thompson JS, Amlot P, Brown S, Janossy G (1987) The cytoplasmic expression of CD3 antigens in normal and malignant cells of the T lymphoid lineage. J Immunol 138: 648-655
Ceredig R, Lowenthal JW, Nabholz M, MacDonald HR (1985) Expression of interleukin-2 receptors as a differentiation marker on intrathymic stem cells. Nature 314: 98-100
Cohen A, Lee JWW, Dosch H-M, Gelfand EW (1980) The expression of deoxyguanosine toxicity in T lymphocytes at different stages of maturation. J Immunol 125: 1578-1582
Collins MKL, Tanigawa G, Kissonerghis A-M, Ritter M, Price KM, Tonegawa S, Owen MJ (1985) Regulation of T-cell receptor gene expression in human T-cell development. Proc Natl Acad Sci USA 82: 4503-4507
De Gast GC, Verdonck LF, Middeldorp JM, The TH, Hekker A, v d Linden JA, Kreeft HAJG, Bast BJEG (1985) Recovery of T cell subsets after autologous bone marrow transplantation is mainly due to proliferation of mature T cells in the graft. Blood 66: 428-431
De Maagd RA, MacKenzie WA, Schuurman H-J, Ritter MA, Price KM, Broekhuizen R, Kater L (1985) The human thymus microenvironment: heterogeneity detected by monoclonal anti-epithelial cell antibodies. Immunology 54: 745-754
De Vries JE, Vyth-Dreese FA, Figdor CG, Spits H, Leemans JM, Bont WS (1983) Induction of phenotypic differentiation, interleukin 2 production, and PHA responsiveness of "immature" human thymocytes by interleukin 1 and phorbol ester. J Immunol 131: 201-206
DiGeorge AM (1965) Discussion. In: Cooper MD, Peterson RDA, Good RA. A new concept of the cellular basis of immunity. J Pediatr 67: 907-908
Ezine S, Weissman IL, Rouse RV (1984) Bone marrow cells give rise to distinct cell clones within the thymus. Nature 309: 629-631
Fink PJ, Gallatin WM, Reichert RA, Butcher EC, Weissman IL (1985) Homing receptor-bearing thymocytes, an immunocompetent cortical subpopulation. Nature 313: 233-235
Ford CE, Micklem HS, Evans EP, Gray JG, Ogden DA (1966) The inflow of bone marrow cells to the thymus: studies with part-body irradiated mice injected with chromosome-marked bone marrow and subjected to antigenic stimulation. Ann NY Acad Sci 129: 283-296
Fournier M, Potworowski EF (1979) Role of a thymic stromal fraction in the homing of bone marrow precursor cells to the thymus. J Reticuloend Soc 25: 463-467
Friedleben A (1858) Die Physiologie der Thymusdrüse in Gesundheit und Krankheit, vom Standpunkte experimenteller Forschung und klinischer Erfahrung. Literarische Anstalt, Frankfurt
Gearhart PJ (1982) Generation of immunoglobulin variable gene diversity. Immunol Today 3: 107-112
Gelfand EW, Dosch H-M (1982) Differentiation of precursor T lymphocytes in man and delineation of the selective abnormalities in severe combined immune deficiency disease. Clin Immunol Immunopathol 25: 303-315
Goldschneider I, Ahmed A, Bollum FJ, Goldstein AL (1981) Induction of terminal deoxynucleotidyl transferase and Lyt antigens with thymosin: identification of multiple subsets of prothymocytes in mouse bone marrow and spleen. Proc Natl Acad Sci USA 78: 2469-2473
Goldstein AL, Low TLK, Thurman GB, Zatz MM, Hall N, Chen J, Hu S-K, Naylor PB, McClure JE (1981) Current status of thymosin and other hormones of the thymus gland. Recent Prog Horm Res 37: 369-415
Goldstein AL, Low TLK, Zatz MM, Hall NR, Naylor PH (1983) Thymosins. Clinics Immunol Allergy 3: 119-132
Hirokawa K, McClure JE, Goldstein AL (1982) Age-related changes in localization of thymosin in the human thymus. Thymus 4: 19-29
Hirokawa K, Sato K, Makinodan T (1982) Influence of age of thymic grafts on the differentiation of T cells in nude mice. Clin Immunol Immunopathol 24: 251-262
Hong R, Horowitz SD, Fortman C, Martin DW Jr (1982) Effect of ADA deficiency on cultured murine thymus transplantation. Clin Immunol Immunopathol 23: 448-458
Hong R, Schulte-Wissermann H, Jarrett-Toth E, Horowitz SD, Manning DD (1979) Transplantation of cultured thymic fragments. II. Results in nude mice. J Exp Med 149: 398-415
Hu S-K, Low TLK, Goldstein AL (1981) Modulation of terminal deoxynucleotidyl transferase activity by thymosin. Mol Cell Biochem 41: 49-58
Huber J, Cholnoky P, Zoethout HE (1967) Congenital aplasia of parathyroid glands and thymus. Arch Dis Child 42: 190-192
IUIS-WHO Nomenclature Subcommittee (1984) Nomenclature for clusters of differentiation (CD) of antigens defined on human leukocyte populations. Bull WHO 62: 809-811
Janossy G, Bofill M, Trejdosiewicz LK, Willcox HNA, Chilosi M (1986) Cellular differentiation of lymphoid subpopulations and their microenvironments in the human thymus. In: Müller-Hermelink HK (ed) The human thymus: histophysiology and pathology. Springer, Berlin Heidelberg New York Tokyo, pp 89-125 (Current topics in pathology, vol 75)
Jenski LJ, Hong R (1985) Transplantation of cultured thymic fragments. VI. *H-2* recombinant donors. J Immunol 135: 947-953
Jordan RK, Robinson JH, Hopkinson NA, House KC, Bentley AL (1985) Thymic epithelium and the induction of

transplantation tolerance in nude mice. Nature 314: 454-456
Kast WM, de Waal LP, Melief CJM (1984) Thymus dictates major histocompatibility complex (MHC) specificity and immune response gene phenotype of class II MHC-restricted T cells but not of class I MHC-restricted T cells. J Exp Med 160: 1752-1766
Kater L (1973) A note on Hassall's corpuscles. Contemp Top Immunobiol 2: 101-109
Kater L, Oosterom R, McClure J, Goldstein AL (1979) Presence of thymosin-like factors in human thymic epithelium conditioned medium. Int J Immunopharmacol 1: 273-284
Kendall MD (1984) Have we underestimated the importance of the thymus in man? Experientia 40: 1181-1185
Kendall MD (1985) The outer and inner thymus cortex is a functional syncytium. Cell Biol Int Rep 9: 3
Kendall MD (1986) The syncytial nature of epithelial cells in the thymic cortex. J Anat 147: 3-12
Kendall MD, Johnson HRM, Singh J (1980) The weight of the human thymus gland at necropsy. J Anat 131: 485-497
Kölliker A (1879) Entwicklungsgeschichte des Menschen und der höheren Tiere, 2nd edn. Engelmann, Leipzig, pp 875-880
Kruisbeek AM (1979) Thymic factors and T cell maturation in vitro: a comparison of the effects of thymic epithelial cultures with thymic extracts and thymus dependent serum factors. Thymus 1: 163-185
Kruisbeek AM, Fultz MJ, Sharrow SO, Singer A, Mond JJ (1983) Early development of the T cell repertoire. In vivo treatment of neonatal mice with anti-Ia antibodies interferes with differentiation of I-restricted T cells but not K/D restricted T cells. J Exp Med 157: 1932-1946
Kyewski BA, Kaplan HS (1982) Lymphoepithelial interactions in the mouse thymus: phenotypic and kinetic studies on thymic nurse cells. J Immunol 128: 2287-2294
Kyewski BA, Fathman CG, Kaplan HS (1984) Intrathymic presentation of circulating non-major histocompatibility complex antigens. Nature 308: 196-199
Ledbetter JA, Evans RL, Lipinsky M, Cunningham-Rundles C, Good RA, Herzenberg LA (1981) Evolutionary conservation of surface molecules that distinguish T lymphocyte helper/inducer and cytotoxic/suppressor subpopulations in mouse and man. J Exp Med 153: 310-323
Ling NR, MacLennan ICM, Mason DY (1987) B-cell and plasma cell antigens: new and previously defined clusters. In: McMichael AJ and thirteen others (eds) Leucocyte typing III. White cell differentiation antigens. Oxford University Press, Oxford, pp 302-335
Longo DL, Schwartz RH (1980) T-cell specificity for H-2 and Ir gene phenotype correlates with the phenotype of thymic antigen-presenting cells. Nature 287: 44-46
Ma DDF, Sylwestrowicz TA, Granger S, Massaia M, Franks R, Janossy G, Hoffbrand AV (1982) Distribution of terminal deoxynucleotidyl transferase and purine degradative and synthetic enzymes in subpopulations of human thymocytes. J Immunol 129: 1430-1435
Ma DDF, Sylwestrowicz T, Janossy G, Hoffbrand AV (1983) The role of purine metabolic enzymes and terminal deoxynucleotidyl transferase in intrathymic T-cell differentiation. Immunol Today 4: 65-68
McFarland EJ, Scearce RM, Haynes BF (1984) The human thymic microenvironment: cortical thymic epithelium is an antigenically distinct region of the thymic microenvironment. J Immunol 133: 1241-1249
McMichael AJ, Gotch FM (1987) T-cell antigens: new and previously defined clusters. In: McMichael AJ and thirteen others (eds) Leucocyte typing III. White cell differentiation antigens. Oxford University Press, Oxford, pp 31-62
Metcalf D (1960) The effect of thymectomy on the lymphoid tissues of the mouse. Br J Haematol 6: 324-333
Miller JFAP (1961) Immunological function of the thymus. Lancet 2: 748-749
Morrissey PJ, Kruisbeek AM, Sharrow SO, Singer A (1982) Tolerance of thymic cytotoxic T lymphocytes to allogeneic H-2 determinants encountered prethymically: evidence for expression of anti-H-2 receptors prior to entry into the thymus. Proc Natl Acad Sci USA 79: 2002-2007
Müller-Hermelink HK, Gülden M, Bathmann R (1984) Restitution of the thymus in lethally irradiated mice after transplantation of syngeneic or allogeneic bone marrow. Immunobiology 167: 462-482
O'Flynn K, Krensky AM, Beverley PCL, Burakoff SJ, Linch DC (1985) Phytohaemagglutinin activation of T cells through the sheep red blood cell receptor. Nature 313: 686-687
Oliver PD, Le Douarin NM (1984) Avian thymic accessory cells. J Immunol 132: 1748-1755
Oosterom R, Kater L (1981) The thymus in the aging individual. II. Thymic epithelial function in vitro in aging and in thymus pathology. Clin Immunol Immunopathol 18: 195-202
Oosterom R, Kater L, Oosterom J (1979) Effects of human thymic epithelial-conditioned medium on mitogen responsiveness of human and mouse lymphocytes. Clin Immunol Immunopathol 12: 460-470
Oppenheim JJ, Gery I (1982) Interleukin 1 is more than an interleukin. Immunol Today 3: 113-119
Papiernik M, Nabarra B, Savino W, Pontoux C, Barbey S (1983) Thymic reticulum in mice. II. Culture and characterization of nonepithelial phagocytic cells of the thymic reticulum: their role in the syngeneic stimulation of thymic medullary lymphocytes. Eur J Immunol 13: 147-155
Raulet DH, Garman RD, Saito H, Tonegawa S (1985) Developmental regulation of T-cell receptor gene expression. Nature 314: 103-107
Reed JC, Tadmori W, Kamoun M, Koretzky G, Nowell PC (1985) Suppression of interleukin 2 receptor acquisition by monoclonal antibodies recognizing the 50 KD protein associated with the sheep erythrocyte receptor on human T lymphocytes. J Immunol 134: 1631-1639
Reinherz EL (1985) A molecular basis for thymic selection: regulation of T11 induced thymocyte expansion by the T3-Ti antigen/MHC receptor pathway. Immunol Today 6: 75-79
Reinherz EL, Kung PC, Goldstein G, Levey RH, Schlossman SF (1980) Discrete stages of human intrathymic differentiation: analysis of normal thymocytes and leukemic lymphoblasts of T-cell lineage. Proc Natl Acad Sci USA 77: 1588-1592
Reinherz EL, Meuer SC, Schlossman SF (1983) The delineation of antigen receptors on human T lymphocytes. Immunol Today 4: 5-8
Ritter MA, Sauvage CA, Cotmore SF (1981) The human thymus microenvironment: in vivo identification of thymic nurse cells and other antigenically-distinct subpopulations of epithelial cells. Immunology 44: 439-446
Ritter MA, Haynes BF (1987) Summary of thymic epithelium workshop. In: McMichael AJ, et al. (eds) Leucocyte typing III. White cell differentiation antigens. Oxford University Press, Oxford, p 247
Rock KL, Yeh ETH, Benacerraf B (1984) Selection of thymo-

cyte MHC restriction specificity in vitro. J Mol Cell Immunol 1: 311-320
Rubenfeld MR, Silverstone AE, Knowles DM, Harper JP, de Sostoa A, Fenoglio CM, Edelson RL (1981) Induction of lymphocyte differentiation by epidermal cultures. J Invest Dermatol 77: 221-224
Savino W, Dardenne M (1984) Thymic hormone-containing cells. VI. Immunohistologic evidence for the simultaneous presence of thymulin, thymopoietin and thymosin α_1 in normal and pathological human thymuses. Eur J Immunol 14: 987-991
Schuurman HJ, Kater L (1985) Relevance of "nurse cells" in histophysiology of lymphoid tissues. Thymus 7: 317-322
Schuurman HJ, Klerx JPAM, van den Brink E,Figdor CG, Kater L (1981) Lymphocyte differentiation in the human thymus: characteristics and function of human thymocyte subpopulations. Hum Lymph Differ 1: 263-278
Schuurman HJ, Vos JG, van de Brink E, Kater L (1982) Culture of thymic epithelium for transplantation purposes: morphological characterization and in vivo biological effect on thymus-dependent immunity in athymic (nude) rats. Clin Immunol Immunopathol 24: 418-431
Schuurman HJ, Brekelmans P, Daemen T, Broekhuizen R, Kater L (1983) T-cell maturation in the human thymus and tonsil: peanut agglutinin binding T lymphocytes in thymus and tonsil differ in maturation stage. Clin Immunol Immunopathol 29: 271-281
Schuurman HJ, van Laarhoven JPRM, Broekhuizen R, Spierenburg GT, Brekelmans P, Figdor CG, de Bruyn CHMM, Kater L (1983) Lymphocyte maturation in the human thymus. Relevance of purine nucleotide metabolism for intrathymic T cell function. Scand J Immunol 18: 539-549
Schuurman HJ, van de Wijngaert FP, Delvoye L, Broekhuizen R, McClure JE, Goldstein AL, Kater L (1985 a) Heterogeneity and age dependency of human thymus reticulo-epithelium in production of thymosin components. Thymus 7: 13-23
Schuurman HJ, van de Wijngaert FP, Huber J, Schuurman RKB, Zegers BJM, Roord JJ, Kater L (1985 b) The thymus in "bare lymphocyte" syndrome. Significance of expression of major histocompatibility complex antigens on thymic epithelial cells in intrathymic T-cell maturation. Hum Immunol 13: 69-82
Schuurman HJ, Vos JG, Broekhuizen R, Brandt CJWM, Kater L (1985 c) In vivo biological effect of allogeneic cultured thymic epithelium on thymus-dependent immunity in athymic nude rats. Scand J Immunol 21: 21-30
Schuurman HJ, Hendriks RW, Lange JMA, van der Linden JA, Gmelig Meyling FHJ, Danner SA, Kater L (1986) Cultured human thymus epithelial monolayer cells induce CD4 expression on mononuclear cells of AIDS patients in vitro. Clin Exp Immunol 64: 348-355
Schuurman HJ, Vaessen LMB, Vos JG, Hertogh A, Geertzema JGN, Brandt CJWM, Rozing J (1986) Implantation of cultured thymic fragments in congenitally athymic nude rats: ignorance of thymic epithelial haplotype in generation of alloreactivity. J Immunol 137: 2440-2447
Schuurman HJ, Ritter MA, Broekhuizen R, Ladyman H, Larché M (1987 a) The thymic epithelium panel of antibodies: immunohistologic analysis of human tissues. In: McMichael AJ and thirteen others (eds) Leucocyte typing III. White cell differentiation antigens. Oxford University Press, Oxford, pp 259-262
Schuurman HJ, Vaessen LMB, Broekhuizen R, Brandt CJWM, Holewijn MC, Vos JG, Rozing J (1987 b) Implantation of cultured thymic fragments in congenitally athymic (nude) rats. Influx of lymphocytes and dendritic cells. Scand J Immunol 26: 129-139
Schuurman HJ (1988) Biological functions of the thymic microenvironment. In: Thymus Update 1: 67-99. Harwood Academic Publishers, London
Scollay R (1983) Intrathymic events in the differentiation of T lymphocytes: a continuing enigma. Immunol Today 4: 282-286
Scollay R, Bartlett P, Shortman K (1984) T cell development in the adult murine thymus: changes in the expression of the surface antigens Ly2, L3T4 and B2A2 during development from early precursor cells to emigrants. Immunol Rev 82: 79-103
Selvaraj P, Plunkett ML, Dustin M, Sanders ME, Shaw S, Singer TA (1987) The lymphocyte glycoprotein CD2 binds the cell surface ligand LFA-3. Nature 326: 400-402
Shore A, Dosch H-M, Gelfand EW (1981) Role of adenosine deaminase in the early stages of precursor T cell maturation. Clin Exp Immunol 44: 152-155
Singer A, Hathcock KS, Hodes RJ (1982) Self recognition in allogeneic thymic chimeras. Self recognition by T helper cells from thymus-engrafted nude mice is restricted to the thymic H-2 haplotype. J Exp Med 155: 339-344
Small M, Barr-Nea L, Aronson M (1984) Culture of thymic epithelial cells from mice and age-related studies on the growing cells. Eur J Immunol 14: 936-942
Steinmann GG, Müller-Hermelink H-K (1984) Lymphocyte differentiation and its microenvironment in the human thymus during aging. Monogr Dev Biol 17: 142-155
Tadmori W, Reed JC, Nowell PC, Kamoun M (1985) Functional properties of the 50 kd protein associated with the E-receptor on human T lymphocytes: suppression of IL2 production by anti-p50 monoclonal antibodies. J Immunol 134: 1709-1716
Tax WJM, Tidman N, Janossy G, Trejdosiewicz L, Willems R, Leeuwenberg J, de Witte TJM, Capel PJA, Koene RAP (1984) Monoclonal antibody (WT 1) directed against a T cell surface glycoprotein: characteristics and immunosuppressive activity. Clin Exp Immunol 55: 427-436
Trainin N, Pecht M, Handzel ZT (1983) Thymic hormones: inducers and regulators of the T-cell system. Immunol Today 4: 16-21
Trainin N, Handzel ZT, Pecht M (1985) Biological and clinical properties of THF. Thymus 7: 137-150
Umiel T, Daley JF, Bhan AK, Levey RH, Schlossman SF, Reinherz EL (1982) Acquisition of immune competence by a subset of human cortical thymocytes expressing mature T cell antigens. J Immunol 129: 1054-1060
Vakharia DD (1983) Demonstration of keratin filaments in thymic nurse cells (TNC) and alloreactivity of TNC-T cell population. Thymus 5: 43-52
Van de Wijngaert FP, Rademakers LHPM, Schuurman H-J, De Weger RA, Kater L (1983) Identification and in situ localization of the "thymic nurse cell" in man. J Immunol 130: 2348-2351
Van de Wijngaert FP, Kendall MD, Schuurman H-J, Rademakers LHPM, Kater L (1984) Heterogeneity of epithelial cells in the human thymus. An ultrastructural study. Cell Tissue Res 237: 227-237
Van Dongen JJM (1987) Analysis of immunoglobulin genes and T cell receptor genes as a diagnostic tool for the detection of lymphoid malignancies. Neth J Med 31: 201-209
Van Dongen JJM, Hooijkaas H, Comans-Bitter M, Hählen K, de Klein A, van Zanen GE, Van't Veer MB, Abels J, Benner R (1985) Human bone marrow cells positive for terminal deoxynucleotidyl transferase (TdT), HLA-DR,

and a T cell marker may represent prothymocytes. J Immunol 135: 3144-3150
Van Vliet E, Melis M, van Ewijk W (1984a) Monoclonal antibodies to stromal cell types of the mouse thymus. Eur J Immunol 14: 524-529
Van Vliet E, Melis M, van Ewijk W (1984b) Immunohistology of thymic nurse cells. Cell Immunol 87: 101-109
Vollger LW, Tuck DT, Springer TA, Haynes BF, Singer KH (1987) Thymocyte binding to human thymic epithelial cells is inhibited by monoclonal antibodies to CD-2 and LFA-3 antigens. J Immunol 138: 358-363
Von Boehmer H, Schubiger K (1984) Thymocytes appear to ignore class I major histocompatibility complex antigens expressed on thymus epithelial cells. Eur J Immunol 14: 1048-1052
Wagner H, Hardt C, Stockinger H, Pfizenmaier K, Bartlett R, Röllinghoff M (1981) Impact of thymus on the generation of immunocompetence and diversity of antigen-specific MHC-restricted cytotoxic T-lymphocyte precursors. Immunol Rev 58: 95-129
Wekerle H, Ketelsen U-P, Ernst M (1980) Thymic nurse cells. Lymphoepithelial cell complexes in murine thymuses: morphological and serological characterization. J Exp Med 151: 925-944
Willis-Carr JI, Ochs HD, Wedgwood RJ (1978) Induction of T-lymphocyte differentiation by thymic epithelial cell monolayers. Clin Immunol Immunopathol 10: 315-324
Yoshikai Y, Yanagi Y, Suciu-Foca N, Mak TW (1984) Presence of T-cell receptor mRNA in functionally distinct T cells and elevation during intrathymic differentiation. Nature 310: 506-508
Zinkernagel RM, Doherty PC (1979) MHC-restricted cytotoxic T cells: studies on the biological role of polymorphic major transplantation antigens determining T-cell restriction-specificity, function, and responsiveness. Adv Immunol 27: 51-177

Part II

Surgical Pathology

7 Hyperplasia

Walter J. Hofmann, Peter Möller and Herwart F. Otto

Introduction

It was in 1614 that Platter described the condition "mors thymica" (mors subita = "sudden infant death") caused by pressure of an enlarged (hyperplastic) thymus ("thymus magnum") on the trachea. "Thymus ingens" was also described by Morgagni (1761) in the *Epistola de morbis thoracis* of his epochal work *"De sedibus, et causis morborum per anatomen indagatis*.

The concept of thymic hyperplasia has been the subject of controversy since A. Paltauf of Vienna proposed his concept of "status thymicolymphaticus" in 1889 and 1890: "A lymphatic constitution distinguished by a persistent thymus gland, active Hassall's corpuscles, hypoplasia of the arterial system and abundant (hyperplastic) lymphatic tissue". "Status thymicolymphaticus" was also described by Osler (1914) who defined it as "a condition in childhood of hyperplasia of lymphatic tissue and of the thymus in association with a flabby fat overgrowth of the body and hypoplasia of the heart and blood vessels".

An elaborate study of status thymicolymphaticus was published in 1945 by Carr. He reviewed the historical background and the spectrum of normal thymic weight (Bratton 1925; Greenwood and Woods 1927; Young and Turnbull 1931; Boyd 1936), experimental and clinical findings of status thymicolymphaticus and causes of death in "Lymphatism". By establishing the normal thymic weight range, several studies disproved the concept that thymic enlargement was associated with sudden infant death (Hammar 1926, 1936; Kendall et al. 1980). The findings of Hammar on the normal age-dependent weight range of the thymus are shown in Fig. 1.

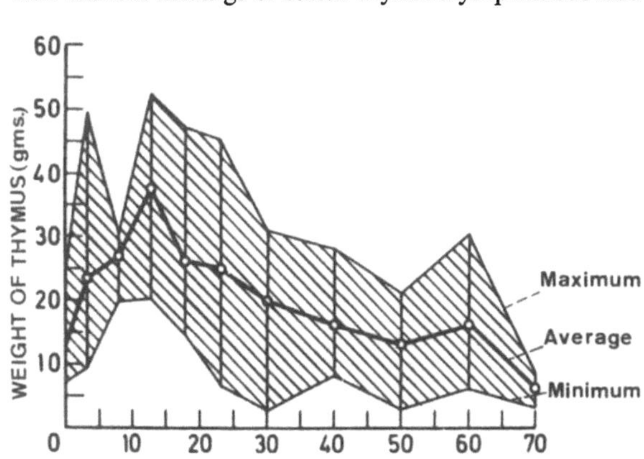

Fig. 1. Normal weight range of the human thymus during life, according to the findings of Hammar (1926). (Otto 1984, p 38; Castleman and Norris 1949)

Hyperplasia is an increase in volume in a tissue or organ by formation of new cellular elements in a normal microscopic arrangement. Thymic hyperplasia is one of numerous conditions which present themselves clinically and/or roentgenologically as mediastinal masses. Therefore, the diagnosis of a mediastinal mass represents a challenging diagnostic and management problem (Haller et al. 1969; Saegesser and Zoupanos 1970; Wychulis et al. 1971; Bower and Kiesewetter 1977; Blasimann et al. 1977; Filler et al. 1979; Barcia and Nelson 1979; Silverman and Sabiston 1980). Currently, on the basis of morphological criteria, two types of thymic hyperplasia are recognized (Levine and Rosai 1978; Otto 1984): (a) true hyperplasia; and (b) lymphofollicular hyperplasia, defined by the presence of lymph follicles with germinal centres, regardless of the size or weight of the thymus (Castleman and Norris 1949). This is the type classically associated with myasthenia gravis (Sloan 1943).

True Thymic Hyperplasia

True hyperplasia is characterized by an increase in both size and weight of the thymus gland with a normal microscopic appearance appropriate for the patient's age. True thymic hyperplasia is rare. The three clinicopathological subtypes of this form of hyperplasia are:

1. Thymic hyperplasia with massive enlargement of the gland (massive thymic hyperplasia);
2. Thymic rebound in childhood and adolescence;
3. Rare instances of thymic hyperplasia which are associated with other diseases, endocrinopathies being of major importance here.

Thymic Hyperplasia with Massive Enlargement of the Gland

There are very few well-documented examples of thymic hyperplasia with massive enlargement, and these are summarized in Table 1. In our review of the literature we found only eleven cases of this condition. The cause and functional significance of giant thymic hyperplasia (thymomegaly) are unclear.

"Enlargement of the thymus" is a common observation in infancy. Haller et al. (1969) reported a series of 80 children who were seen for "mediastinal masses" at

Table 1. Clinicopathological features of thymic hyperplasia with massive enlargement, but normal, age-related histology. Summary of eleven published cases

Case	Age, sex	Clinical and laboratory findings	Treatment	Weight and size of thymus	Reference
1	7 months, m	Hepatomegaly. Peripheral blood and bone marrow lymphocytosis. "Large soft tissue density in the right hemithorax." 2 years after thymectomy: reduced serum IgG	Thymectomy	224 g 9 × 8 × 6 cm	Katz et al. 1977
2	12 months, m	Respiratory distress. "Large anterior mediastinal mass ... (decreased in size after steroid therapy, but quickly enlarged again)." Peripheral blood lymphocytosis, 92% T-lymphocytes[a]	Corticosteroids, thymectomy	420 g	O'Shea et al. 1978
3	4 years, f	Asymptomatic. Moderate peripheral lymphocytosis[b]. Median opacity occupying both lung fields almost entirely	Thymectomy	800 g	Rasore-Quartino et al. 1979
4	14 years, m	"Anterior mediastinal mass ... (discovered on routine chest roentgenogram)"	Thymectomy	490 g	Lack 1981[c]
5	11 years, m	"Right anterior mediastinal mass ... (discovered on routine chest roentgenogram)"	Thymectomy	324 g 15.2 cm diameter	Lack 1981[c]
6	7 months, f	Large liver cyst. Respiratory distress syndrome ("by displacement and compression of the bronchopulmonary system"). "Huge" mediastinal mass	Corticosteroids (for 3 weeks)[d], thymectomy	230 g 18 × 11 × 8.5 cm	Lamesch 1983
7	10 years, f	Cough. A regularly outlined X-ray shadow in the anterior mediastinum	Thymectomy	93 g	Nezelof and Normand 1986
8	5 years, f	Slightly asthenic. Moderate and disseminated lymphadenopathy. Leucocytosis without lymphocytosis[e]. Abnormal mediastinal shadow	Biopsy		Nezelof and Normand 1986
9	11 years, f	Mild, nonproductive cough, localized bonchitis, bronchopneumonia. Homogeneous mass occupying the thymic region	Biopsy		Nezelof and Normand 1986
10	12 years, m	Respiratory distress, dysphagia. Large anterior mediastinal mass	Thymectomy	245 g 13 × 8 × 3.5 cm	Judd RL 1987
11	15 years, m	Multiple childhood viral infections, chronic persistant hepatitis 2 years before the detection of a large anterior mediastinal mass	Thymectomy	680 g 17 × 16 × 6 cm	Arliss et al. 1988

[a] Lymphocytosis disappeared after total thymectomy. Phytohaemagglutinin blastogenesis was normal in peripheral blood lymphocytes, but diminished in the thymic cells. The aetiology of lymphocytosis is unknown. The authors postulated that a disorder in T-suppressor activity may have been a factor in their case. [b] Disappeared after thymectomy. [c] In both instances the hyperplasia was demonstrated by morphometric studies using the point-counting method. [d] Steroid therapy without effect on the mediastinal mass. [e] Normal number of peripheral T-lymphocytes and normal lymphocyte proliferation assays.

the Johns Hopkins Hospital, Baltimore, between July 1933 and July 1968; there were 8 "hyperplastic thymus glands" in 4 newborn infants and 4 children 3 months to 5 years old. In a review of 16 cases of thymic hyperplasia by Blasimann et al. (1977), 9 were found in infants in their first year of life. Barcia and Nelson (1979) reported a series of 11 children, 1-13 years of age, who underwent thymectomy for an undiagnosed thymic enlargement. The weight of the resected masses was 47-92 g. On histological examination, one proved to be an anaplastic thymic malignancy, the other ten were shown to be histologically normal thymuses without germinal centre formation.

Clinical symptoms in this type of thymic hyperplasia range from none at all to respiratory distress (Table 1). Four of the cases in Table 1 (cases 3, 4, 5, 11) were asymptomatic and mediastinal widening was discovered by chance on a routine chest radiograph. If the mediastinal mass is symptomatic most of the symptoms are local ones and due to the irritation of mediastinal structures. Respiratory symptoms, i.e. mild dyspnoea, nonproductive cough, bronchopneumonia or acute respiratory distress, occurred in four of the eleven cases (cases 2, 6, 7, 9). However, some of them might have also been unrelated to the mediastinal mass which was then detected during the routine diagnostic procedure of an upper respiratory infection, for example. Other, nonlocal symptoms which have been reported are a moderate and disseminated lymphadenopathy in one of the eleven cases (case 8) and hepatomegaly with a questionable splenomegaly which disappeared 6 months after thymectomy in another case (case 1). It is tempting to correlate the lymphadenopathy with the thymic hyperplasia although there was only a peripheral leucocytosis, but without lymphocytosis. The hepatomegaly, on the other hand, might be correlated with the thymic hyperplasia since the patient also had an increase in the number of peripheral T cells and a disturbance of the architecture of a mediastinal lymph node, owing to an expansion of the thymus-dependent lymph node area.

Pathological laboratory findings may also be absent, but, if present, they mostly concern the peripheral leucocyte blood count. Seven of the eleven cases in Table 1 (cases 4, 5, 6, 7, 9, 10, 11) did not reveal any abnormal results of routine laboratory test. The remaining four cases presented with leucocytosis (case 8) or lymphocytosis (cases 1, 2, 3) with (cases 1, 2) or without (case 3) an increase in the number or ratio of peripheral T-lymphocytes. Hypogammaglobulinaemia was detected in one case (case 1) 6 months after thymectomy. The authors postulate that the thymic hyperplasia might have induced hypogammaglobulinaemia through an imbalance of the T-B-cell ratio in the peripheral lymphoid organs (a mediastinal lymph node with an expanded T-cell zone was examined) and blood. This hypothesis, however, could not be proven and congenital or acquired hypogammaglobulinaemia could not be ruled out.

The morphology in many instances is not well illustrated or defined and it is conceivable that many cases of "thymic hyperplasia" (borderline enlargement) are examples of lymphofollicular hyperplasia (see later in this chapter). This might be true not only for those cases without histological examination, but also for those in which only a small biopsy obtained through mediastinoscopy or only one random section of the thymectomy specimen is examined. The number of lymph follicles in lymphofollicular hyperplasia of the thymus varies considerably from case to case and between different histological slides from the same specimen (Grody et al. 1986). Therefore, if only one random section of the specimen is examined the correct diagnosis of lymphofollicular hyperplasia might be overlooked (see later in this chapter).

Thymectomy specimens of very well documented cases are macroscopically encapsulated. Histological examination reveals a normal, lobular thymic architecture with a clear demarcation of the dark cortical and the lighter medullary areas. As usual the cortex contains many more lymphocytes than the medulla where Hassall's corpuscles, normal in distribution and number, can be found. No lymph follicles with germinal centres occur within the specimen.

Aetiology and pathogenesis of this rare lesion still remain to be elucidated. The most convenient explanation for its formation is thymic hyperfunction or dysfunction, which might be related to the endocrine activity of the thymic epithelial cells. This was suggested by Lack (1981), Katz et al. (1977) and more recently by Nezelof and Normand (1986). The findings of lymphocytosis with high numbers of peripheral T cells in some of the reported cases, and the expansion of the thymus-dependent area in a lymph node near the resected thymus in another case, would argue for thymic hyperfunction with an effect on the peripheral lymphoid organs. Thymic dysfunction, on the other hand, with an arrest in T-cell differentiation and an accumulation of immature T cells could be postulated on the basis of the findings of Nezelof and Normand (1986). They found that the number of mature T-lymphocytes, estimated by the intracellular dot-like α-naphthyl acetate esterase activity, was markedly reduced in three cases of massive thymic hyperplasia in comparison with a normal control thymus. Lastly, besides the functional disturbances a mechanical one has been discussed by Lack (1981) who found an increase of perivascular collagen in one of his two reported cases.

Since the perivascular spaces are believed to be the pathway of lymphocyte emigration from the thymus, an increase of the perivascular collagen might inhibit the normal migration and lead to a local accumulation of T cells.

The fact that thymic hyperplasia with massive enlargement can simulate malignant mediastinal tumours and tumour-like lesions, however, is of greater practical concern. Tumours of the anterior mediastinum to be considered in the differential diagnosis of thymic hyperplasia with massive enlargement are thymoma, carcinoid tumours of the thymus, thymolipoma, Hodgkin's disease or non-Hodgkin's lymphomas, neoplasms of germ cell origin, Castleman's disease, and cysts of various histogenesis. If a child with a newly recognized mass is thriving and if most of the alternative possibilities have been ruled out by appropriate clinical and laboratory evaluation, the patient can just be observed carefully. A trial of corticosteroid therapy, as proposed by Caffey and Silbey (1960), should only be done if a corticosteroid-sensitive tumour can be ruled out. A brief course of corticosteroids will often shrink the hyperplastic thymus within a few days. However, this measure is not conclusive in all cases and also failed to be effective in one of two cases in Table 1. Therefore, diagnostic mediastinoscopy or, in the case of severe respiratory symptoms, a thoracotomy with resection of the mediastinal mass may be necessary. Thymic hyperplasia can then easily be diagnosed because it is histologically different from all the tumours mentioned here.

Thymic Rebound in Childhood and Adolescence

The phenomenon of *rebound* or *regeneration* of thymic tissue in children has been described in a number of conditions, including recovery from severe thermal burns (Gelfand et al. 1972; Lee et al. 1979), cardiac surgery (Rizk et al. 1972), and after ending oral administration of steroids (Caffey and Silbey 1960), as well as following recovery from tuberculosis (Bertoye et al. 1956).

This phenomenon of thymic rebound has also been reported after treatment for Hodgkin's disease (Grissom et al. 1983; Shin and Ho 1983; Tartas et al. 1985; Carmosino et al. 1985). Furthermore, it has been described after treatment for other malignancies such as lymphoblastic leukemia, malignant lymphoma, poorly differentiated lymphocytic lymphoma, Wilms' tumour, osteosarcoma of the left distal femur, malignant abdominal teratoma (Hill and Dodd 1970; Cohen et al. 1980) and embryonal rhabdomyosarcoma of the left testicle (Bell et al. 1984).

One group of six cases of thymic rebound hyperplasia has been reported in children after severe thermal burns (Table 2). In three of them true thymic hyperplasia was proven by histological examination of the thymectomy specimen or a biopsy. The age range of the patients was 22 months to 12 years, the thymic hyperplasia was detected 1-9 months after the burn. None of the patients had any clinical symptoms or pathological laboratory findings and the mediastinal widening was detected on a routine chest radiographs.

Table 2. Clinicopathological features of thymic rebound hyperplasia in children recovering from severe thermal burns. Summary of six published cases

Case	Age, sex	Degree of burn	Time between burning and thymic hyperplasia	Treatment	Weight and size of thymus	Reference
1	10 years, f	32%, mostly 2nd degree	5 months	Thymectomy	130 g	Gelfand et al. 1972
2	8 years, m	55%, 3rd degree	8 months	Biopsy[a]	Roughly 3 times normal	Gelfand et al. 1972
3	5 years, f	47%, 2nd and 3rd degree	9 months	None[b]	–	Gelfand et al. 1972
4	6.5 years, f	48%, 2nd and 3rd degree	7 months	None[c]	–	Gelfand et al. 1972
5	12 years, m	15%, 3rd degree	8.5 months	None[d]	–	Gelfand et al. 1972
6	20 months, f	~ 25%, 2nd degree	1 month	Corticosteroids[e], thymectomy	550 g 19 × 12 × 4.5 cm	Lee et al. 1979

[a] Size of thymus, on serial radiographs did not change over the next 2 years.
[b] Mediastinal mass disappeared gradually over the next 10 months.
[c] Mediastinal mass decreased in size over the next 7 months.
[d] Mediastinal mass decreased in size for 3 months; the child has been asymptomatic for 1 year.
[e] Prednisone 1.5 mg per kilogram body weight for 5 days without effect on the mediastinal mass.

Table 3. Clinicopathological features of thymic rebound hyperplasia after treatment for malignancies. Summary of fourteen published cases

Case	Age, sex	Malignancy	Treatment of malignancy	Time from treatment to thymic hyperplasia	Clinical and laboratory findings	Treatment of thymic hyperplasia	Reference
1	19 years, f	Hodgkin's disease IIsB	Chemotherapy, including corticosteroids[a]	← 10 months 8 months → 3 months →	Interstitial lung disease Herpes zoster, nonproductive cough, definite left hilar mass	Partial resection (6 × 4 cm)	Grissom et al. 1983
2	4.5 years, m	Wilms' tumour	Nephrectomy, Radiotherapy Vincristine	← 12 months ← 11 months ← 8 months	Widening of the mediastinum	Thymectomy	Hill and Dodd 1970
3	3 years, m	Wilms' tumour	Nephrectomy, Radiotherapy Vincristine	 ← 12 months ← 9 months	Lobulated mass in a widened mediastinum	Thymectomy	Cohen et al. 1980
4	32 months, f	Lymphoblastic leukemia	Chemotherapy	← Several months	Definite widening of the anterior mediastinum	Biopsy	Cohen et al. 1980
5	9 years, m	Osteosarcoma of the distal femur	Amputation Chemotherapy	← 17 months ← 1 month	Anterior mediastinal mass	None[b]	Cohen et al. 1980
6	5 years, f	Malignant teratoma	Resection Chemotherapy	 ← 5 months	Widened anterior mediastinum	None[c]	Cohen et al. 1980
7	4 years, m	Malignant lymphoma	Radiotherapy Chemotherapy	 ← During	Mediastinal widening	None[d]	Cohen et al. 1980
8	4 years, f	Poorly differentiated, lymphocytic lymphoma (convoluted type)	Chemotherapy	← 10 months	Polyarthritis[e], widening of the mediastinum	Corticosteroids[f]	Cohen et al. 1980
9	23 months, f	Wilms' tumour	Nephrectomy Radiotherapy Chemotherapy	 ← 10 months	Large left mediastinal mass	Corticosteroids[g]	Cohen et al. 1980
10	2.5 years, m	Embryonal rhabdomyosarcoma left testicle	Orchiectomy, chemotherapy	← 12 months	Enlargement of the superior mediastinum	Resection of the right thymic lobe (28 g)	Bell et al. 1984
11	33 years, f	Hodgkin's disease IIB	Chemotherapy Radiotherapy	← 22 months	Anterior mediastinal soft tissue mass seemed to be of thymus origin. Laboratory findings normal	Partial resection[h]	Tartas et al. 1985
12	23 years, m	Hodgkin's disease III_2A	Chemotherapy	← during	Persistant anterior mediastinal mass	Thymectomy 10 × 6 × 2 cm	Carmosino et al. 1985
13	23 years, f	Endodermal sinus tumour left ovary	Hysterectomy with bilateral salpingo-oophorectomy, chemotherapy	← 10 months	Widened mediastinum, anterior mediastinal mass	Thymectomy 75 g 10 × 9 × 2 cm	Carmosino et al. 1985

Table 3. (continued)

Case	Age, sex	Malignancy	Treatment of malignancy	Time from treatment to thymic hyperplasia	Clinical and laboratory findings	Treatment of thymic hyperplasia	Reference
14	16 years, m	Mixed germ cell tumour with elevated tumour markers (α-FP, β-HCG)	Orchiectomy Chemotherapy	← 6 months	Anterior mediastinal mass 3 cm in diameter; tumor markers negativ	Thymectomy 58 g 120 × 80 × 20 cm	Düe et al. 1988

[a] Corticosteroids were given as part of therapy for Hodgkin's disease and to treat drug-induced interstitial lung disease.
[b] The mediastinal contour returned to normal after 1 year.
[c] No significant change in the mediastinal silhouette.
[d] Observation (no change).
[e] Therapy with corticosteroids.
[f] Prednisone (60 mg/m^2); 24 h after the first dose a definite shrinking of the mediastinal mass was evident; the mediastinal shadow was entirely normal by 48 h.
[g] Striking reduction of the mass after 7 days oral prednisone therapy.
[h] The mediastinal mass disappeared in two months.

Another group of patients with thymic rebound hyperplasia consists of children and four young adults treated for different malignant tumours (Table 3). In most of these cases, however, there was no histological examination of the mediastinal mass, but the diagnosis was based on routine chest radiographs and the clinical exclusion of other causes for the mediastinal widening. In two cases, shrinkage of the mediastinal mass was achieved by corticosteroid administration.

The histological appearance of this type of thymic hyperplasia is the same as that of true thymic hyperplasia with massive enlargement of the gland as discussed in the previous section. It is merely the circumstances and the possible pathogenetic explanations of this type of thymic hyperplasia that differentiate the two. The microtopography and cellular composition of the enlarged thymi are the same as in normal thymus as could be shown by immunohistological examination of a thymic rebound hyperplasia (Düe et al., 1988). After treatment of a malignant tumour, this form of thymic hyperplasia may simulate radiologically a recurrence or a metastasis.

Pathogenetically, different factors can be implicated as the cause of thymic hyperplasia in these patients. The reversal of greatly elevated endogenous corticosteroid levels in patients with severe thermal burns (Gelfand et al. 1972), the withdrawal of exogenous corticosteroids and antimitotic drugs in patients with malignancies (Hill and Dodd 1970; Shin and Ho 1983) or the stimulatory effects of the cellular mediated immunity by viral infections (Grissom et al. 1983) might, alone or in combination, cause thymic hyperplasia under certain conditions. However, to be operative, these factors can only cause thymic hyperplasia in a susceptible thymus. The age-dependent size of the thymus with thymic atrophy during ageing indicates a functionally active thymus in childhood and adolescence which might be susceptible to such effects. Indeed, most of the reported cases were 20-month- to 12-year-old children; only four patients were between 19 and 33 years old. The occurrence of thymic rebound hyperplasia in patients with malignant tumours has recently been reported to represent an immunological rebound phenomenon that can be used clinically as a good prognostic indicator of successful control of Hodgkin's disease and other malignancies (Cohen et al. 1980).

True Thymic Hyperplasia in Association with Other Diseases

Rare instances of non-neoplastic enlargement of the thymus gland have also been described in patients with endocrine abnormalities, sarcoidosis (Oh et al. 1971; Pardo-Mindan et al. 1980) and the Beckwith-Wiedemann syndrome (Balcom et al. 1985). This enlargement is due to a true thymic hyperplasia which again, on histological grounds, cannot be distinguished from true thymic hyperplasia with massive enlargement or thymic rebound hyperplasia as discussed in the two previous sections. For instance, it has been found that in cases of thyrotoxicosis (the so-called thymic form of Graves' disease) and in children treated for hypothyroidism (Nicholson 1978; Yulish and Owens 1980; Rose and Lam 1982) an enlargement of the thymus gland occurred.

Scheiff et al. (1977) studied the influence of thyroid hormones on the size of the thymus in their experimental work on thymic hyperplasia. To our knowledge, this is the only experimental study on this subject. In their murine model of thymic hyperplasia induced by triiodothyronine administration they demonstrated a 2-fold increase in the total number of epithelial cells in both the cortex and medulla. However, whereas the number of epithelial cells per unit volume also increased in the medulla this value decreased in the cortex, indicating that the volume of the thymic cortex was mainly increased by the nonepithelial component, i. e. the lymphocytes.

Thus, thymic hyperplasia induced by triiodothyronine administration is caused by multiplication and proliferation of epithelial cells in both the cortex and medulla on the one hand and by invasion or proliferation of lymphocytes in the cortex on the other hand. Thereby the cortical volume is increased 2-fold and the medullary volume about 1.6-fold. Since these data were obtained by delicate morphometric studies using semithin and ultrathin sections of the tissue it is doubtful whether these criteria can be used in the differential diagnosis of thymic hyperplasia in normal histological tissue sections.

Other conditions in which true thymic hyperplasia occurs include Addison's disease, acromegaly, congenital absence of pituitary gland and anencephaly (Potter and Craig 1975; Goldstein and Mackay 1969).

Lymphofollicular Hyperplasia of the Thymus*

Lymphofollicular hyperplasia of the thymus has been described in autoimmune diseases such as myasthenia gravis, systemic lupus erythematosus, scleroderma, rheumatoid arthritis, periarteritis nodosa, Hashimoto's thyroiditis, autoimmune anemia, Behçet's disease and Sjögren's syndrome (Rosai and Levine 1976; Levine and Rosai 1978; Otto 1984; Tridente 1985). The characteristic non-neoplastic lesion of the thymus gland in myasthenia gravis, for example, is lymphofollicular hyperplasia. Between 60% and 90% of myasthenic patients show such thymic changes (Sloan 1943; Castleman and Norris 1949; Kirchner et al. 1986). Further thymic abnormalities include an increased number of B-lymphocytes, T-helper cells, myoid cells and epithelial cells containing detectable intracytoplasmatic thymosin (Dalakas et al. 1981; Scadding et al. 1981; Thomas et al. 1982; Kornstein et al. 1984).

Lymphofollicular hyperplasia of the thymus can also be observed in patients with ulcerative colitis, multiple sclerosis, hepatic cirrhosis and other liver diseases, in some endocrinopathies (Addison's disease, thyrotoxicosis, acromegaly, gonadal hypofunction, diabetes) and in chronic disseminated infections (toxoplasmosis). Lymphofollicular hyperplasia has also been found in epithelial thymic tumours and in the uninvolved portion of a thymus with a thymoma.

The size of the thymus in lymphofollicular hyperplasia lies within the normal range (Fig. 1; Castleman and Norris 1949; Rosai and Levine 1976; Levine and Rosai 1978). Lymphofollicular hyperplasia of the thymus is defined by its histological appearance (Castleman and Norris 1949; Rosai and Levine 1976).

Histologically lymph follicles with germinal centres are found in the thymic medulla (Fig. 2). Their number, however, varies considerably from case to case and even within one case (Grody et al. 1986). Thus, if lymphofollicular hyperplasia of the thymus is suspected, sections from different regions of the organ should be examined in order to rule out the presence or absence of lymph follicles. The medullary area seems to be blown up by the presence of lymph follicles and the thymic cortex is arranged in the form of a cap covering this region (Figs. 2 and 4). Thymuses with lymphofollicular hyperplasia may also present with fatty involution, depending on the patient's age (Fig. 4).

The configuration, microtopography, cellular composition, ultrastructure and immunohistological findings of thymic germinal centres in lymphofollicular hyperplasia associated with myasthenia gravis are essentially the same as in those occurring in lymph nodes and in other lymphatic tissue. Ultrastructurally and immunohistologically the cellular population is composed of long branching dendritic reticulum cells, lymphocytes in various stages of transformation, "starry-sky" macrophages and the marginal zone is populated by small lymphocytes (Fig. 3 a–e; Tamaoki et al. 1971; Staber et al. 1975; Levine and Bearman 1980; Löning et al. 1980; Wiersbowsky-Schmeel et al. 1984). Our findings are summarized in Table 4 (Hofmann et al. 1987, 1988 a). Furthermore labelling with *Ulex europaeus* lectin-I (UEA-I) reveals hyperplasia of capillary blood vessels and the appearance of epithelial venules in the parafollicular zone (Fig. 3 f).

Immunohistology with monoclonal antibodies against B-cell differentiation antigens is a useful tool in those cases where the lymph follicles are rare or difficult to detect morphologically. Aggregates of the B-

* Synonyms of this term frequently used in the literature are lymphoid hyperplasia and follicular hyperplasia. We, however, prefer the term lymphofollicular hyperplasia as we and others (Kornstein et al. 1984) were able to show that the follicular structures correspond to lymph follicles in the peripheral lymphatic tissue (see later discussion).

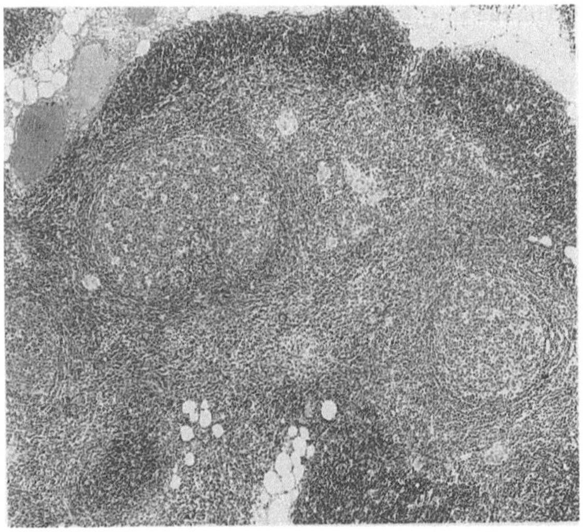

Fig. 2. Lymphofollicular hyperplasia of the thymus with active germinal centres (female, 31 years, myasthenia gravis without thymoma, thymectomy specimen 30 g). Three lymph follicles seemingly situated within thymic medulla. Atrophic thymic cortex. Epithelial cells and Hassall's corpuscles are seen in the intervening zone (Otto 1984, p 110, H & E × 80)

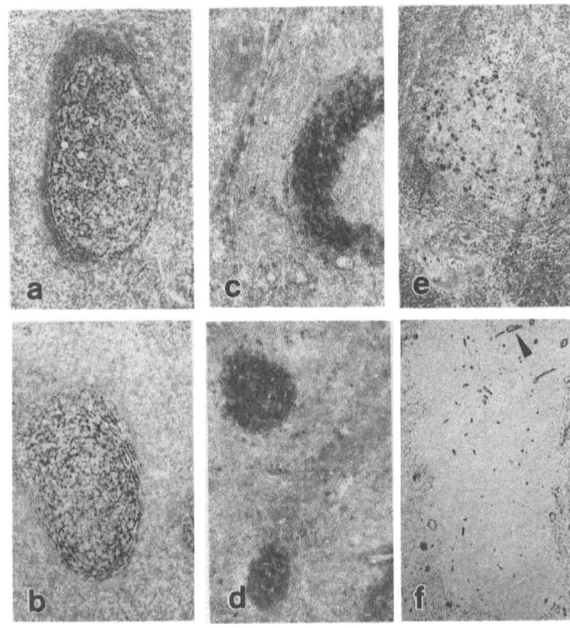

Fig. 3 a–f. Lymph follicles and surroundings in lymphofollicular hyperplasia of the thymus (**a** male, 19 years, osteosarcoma; **b–f** female, 23 years, myasthenia gravis without thymoma). **a** C3bR antibody detects the dendritic reticulum cells of the germinal centre and the marginal zone. × 70, **b** only the dendritic reticulum cells of the follicle centre are DRC1-positive. × 70, **c** positive staining of the lymphocytes of the marginal zone by anti-IgD. Note a few positively labelled cells in the parafollicular area representing plasma cells. × 67, **d** germinal centre cells express surface IgM. Again the few positively labelled cells in the parafollicular area represent plasma cells. × 54, **e** natural killer cells within the germinal centre of a lymph follicle detected by the antibody Leu-7; a pattern typical of activated germinal centres. × 70, **f** UEA-I stains the epithelial network of the thymic medulla (left, bottom, right border), and also the blood vessel endothelium, thus revealing an extension of the regional pre-existing capillary tree and formation of epitheloid venules *(arrowhead)* in the parafollicular area. × 45

cell population are clearly visible by the reaction of the cells with such antibodies. Furthermore, the relation of the lymph follicles in lymphofollicular hyperplasia to the different compartments of the thymus becomes evident when using immunohistological methods.

In agreement with Levine and Rosai (1978) and Levine and Bearman (1980) we propose that the thymus is divided into three major compartments, as illustrated in Fig. 5 (Hofmann et al. 1984, 1988). The cortex and the medulla constitute the *true* thymic parenchyma (i. e. intraparenchymal zone), the third compartment, the so-called extraparenchymal zone, being located within the perivascular (paraseptal) spaces of the thymus.

Staining with anti-keratin serum quite clearly reveals the borders between thymic and extrathymic compartments (Figs. 6 and 7). Thus, two statements about the localization of the lymph follicles in the lymphofollicular hyperplastic thymus can be made: (a) there is a very clear demarcation line between the lymph follicles and the thymic medulla, consisting of a continuous row of epithelial cells; and (b) the lymphofollicular hyperplastic tissue is connected with the surrounding fat and connective tissue of the interlobular septa.

These two facts suggest that the lymphofollicular hyperplastic tissue originates from the interlobular fibrous septa; as the connection to the fibrous septa has the shape of a stalk (Fig. 7, *arrow*), it depends very much on the section level whether this connection is visible or not. Thus, for geometrical reasons the most frequent picture to be seen is that of lymph follicles seeming to be imbedded in the thymic medulla (see Fig. 5).

During further development of the lesion this border between the extraparenchymal zone with the lymph follicles and the thymic medulla may be interrupted (Bofill et al. 1985; Kirchner et al. 1986) thus facilitating the B-lymphocytes infiltrating the thymic medulla, a situation which is also called "thymitis" (Otto 1984; Kirchner et al. 1986). This infiltration of the thymic medulla by B-lymphocytes in the course of lymphofollicular hyperplasia and myasthenia gravis, however, has to be distinguished from the previously

Table 4. Immunohistological characteristics[a] of the lymph follicles and their surroundings in lymphofollicular hyperplasia of the thymus

Antibody	Reactivity	Germinal centre			Mantle zone		Parafollicular
		DRC	CBCC	Lympho	DRC	Lympho	Lympho
Dako-DRC1	DRC	+++	–	–	–	–	–
CD35(To5)	Receptor for C3b	+++	–	–	+++	–	–
ISCR3	HLA-DR	+++	++	–	++	–	+ (IDC)
CD20(B1)	B-cell specific	++	–	++	–	+++	–
CD21(B2)	B-cell specific	+++	–	–	+++	+++	–
CD22(HD6, HD39)[b]	B-cell specific	+++	–	+	–	+++	–
CD37(HD28)[c]	B-cell associated	+++	–	+	–	+++	–
Dako-IgM	μ-chain of the IgM molecule	–	+++	–	–	+	+ (PC)
Dako-IgD	δ-chain of the IgD molecule	–	–	–	–	+++	+ (PC)
HNK1(Leu-7)	Natural killer cells	–	–	+	–	–	–
CD3(OKT3)	Medullary thymocytes + peripheral T cells	–	–	+	–	+	++
CD1(OKT6)	Cortical thymocytes	–	–	–	–	–	+ (IDC)
CD4(Leu-3a)	Thymocytes + helper T cells	–	–	+	–	+	++
CD8(OKT8)	Suppressor, cytotoxic T cells	–	–	–	–	–	+

+++ all; ++ many; + few; – no cells stained by the respective antibody
DRC dendritic reticulum cells; IDC interdigitating reticulum cells; CBCC centrocytes and centroblasts of the follicle centre; PC plasma cells
[a] For antibody sources, references, and methods used see Hofmann et al. (1988)
[b, c] Monoclonal antibodies directed against B-cell-specific differentiation antigens 130, 140 Kdalton[b] auc 39-52 Kdalton, respectively, presented at the 2nd International Conference on Leucocyte Typing (Boston, 1984), were a kind gift of the producer, Dr. B. Dörken, Haematological Department of the Medizinische Poliklinik of the University of Heidelberg

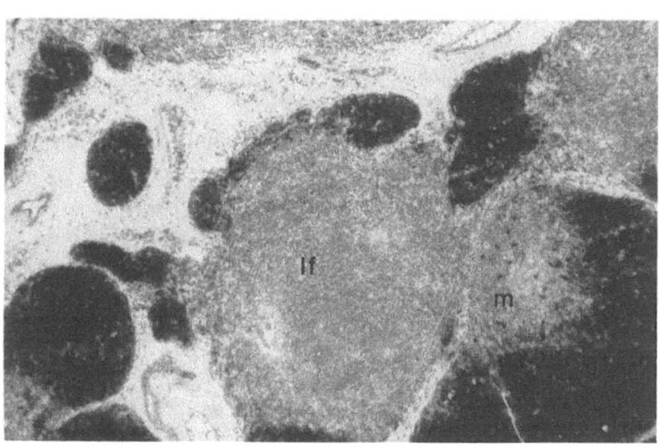

Fig. 4. Lymphofollicular hyperplasia of the thymus (same patient as Fig. 3 b–f). Labelling with anti-T6 reveals atrophy of the thymic cortex in the area displaced by lymph follicles and surroundings. lf lymph follicle; m medulla with some positively stained interdigitating reticulum cells. ×53

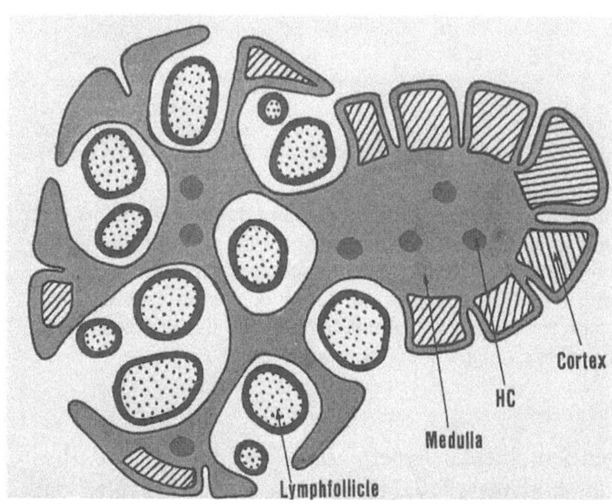

Fig. 5. Diagram summarizing our results: Normal thymus (right) and lymphofollicular hyperplasia of the thymus (left). The complex histological pattern of lymphofollicular hyperplasia is the result of expansion of the septal space in which the lymph follicles emerge, displace the thymic medulla, and lead to atrophy of the cortical area

reported occurrence of B-lymphocytes within the thymic medulla (Hofmann et al. 1988a and b).

Diagnosis of lymphofollicular hyperplasia of the thymus should not be difficult in those cases where a thymectomy is performed for myasthenia gravis when a thymus of normal weight is removed, showing the typical histological picture of lymphofollicular hyperplasia. However, if a biopsy of an anterior mediastinal tumour shows thymic tissue with lymphofollicular hyperplasia this is most probably not the cause of the mediastinal widening, since a thymus with lymphofollicular hyperplasia is not greatly enlarged and its weight lies within normal limits. Thus, tumours of the anterior mediastinum which can be associated with

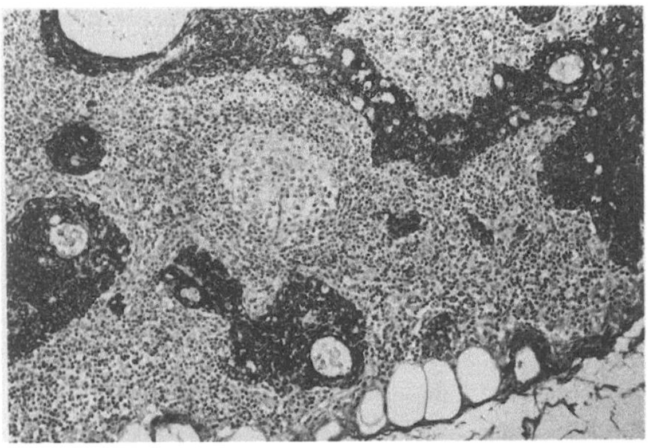

Fig. 6. Lymphofollicular hyperplasia of the thymus (female, 28 years, myasthenia gravis without thymoma, thymectomy specimen 80 g). Lymph follicle and surroundings clearly demarcated from the medullary epithelial cells positively labelled by a pan-keratin antibody. Hassall's corpuscles with cystic degeneration. × 132

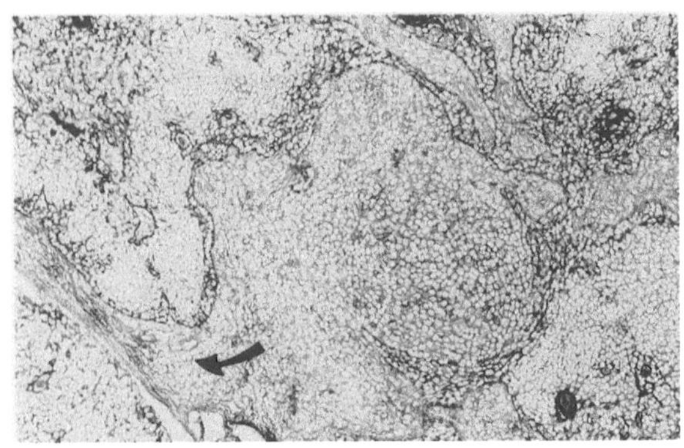

Fig. 7. Lymphofollicular hyperplasia of the thymus (same patient as Fig. 3). Clear demarcation of the lymph follicle from the medullary epithelial cells positively stained by a pan-keratin antibody. There is no structural barrier between the lymph follicle and the septal and adipose tissue surrounding the thymic compartment *(arrow)* × 132

lymphofollicular hyperplasia of the thymus, i. e. thymoma or metastasizing tumours, should be ruled out by a second biopsy.

Lesions which might be confused with lymphofollicular hyperplasia of the thymus because of their microscopic appearance are angiofollicular lymph node hyperplasia (giant lymph node hyperplasia, Castleman's disease) of the anterior mediastinum and follicular lymphomas. Both lesions, however, clinically present themselves as mediastinal masses, a feature uncommon for lymphofollicular hyperplasia of the thymus. On histological examination, the absence of thymic tissue, the hyalinization of the centres of lymphoid follicles in the hyaline-vascular type of giant lymph node hyperplasia and the numerous plasma cells in the plasma cell typ of giant lymph node hyperplasia help to distinguish this lesion from lymphofollicular hyperplasia of the thymus.

References

Arliss J, Scholes J, Dickson PR, Messina JJ (1988) Massive thymic hyperplasia in an adolescent. Ann Thorac Surg 45: 220-222

Balcom RJ, Hakanson DO, Werner A, Gordon LP (1985) Massive thymic hyperplasia in an infant with Beckwith-Wiedemann syndrome. Arch Pathol Lab Med 109: 153-155

Barcia PJ, Nelson TG (1979) Hyperplasia of the thymus and thymic neoplasms in children. Milit Med 144: 799-801

Bell BA, Esseltine DW, Azouz EM (1984) Rebound thymic hyperplasia in a child with cancer. Med Pediatr Oncol 12: 144-147

Bertoye A, Beraud C, Depierre A, Duc H, Beraud A (1956) Hypertrophie thymique et primo-infection du nourrisson. Pediatrie 11: 545-549

Blasimann B, Kuffer F, Bettex M (1977) Chirurgische Betrachtungen über die Thymushyperplasie. Z Kinderchir 21: 214-230

Bofill M, Janossy G, Willcox N, Chilosi M, Trejdosiewicz LK, Bagott M, Newsom-Davis J (1985) Microenvironments in the normal and myasthenia gravis thymus. Am J Pathol 119: 462-473

Bower RJ, Kiesewetter WB (1977) Mediastinal masses in infants and children. Arch Surg 112: 1003-1009

Boyd E (1936) Weight of the thymus and its component parts and number of Hassall corpuscles in health and in disease. Am J Dis Child 51: 313-335

Bratton AB (1925) The normal weight of the human thymus. J Pathol Bacteriol 28: 609-620

Caffey J, Silbey R (1960) Regrowth and overgrowth of the thymus after atrophy induced by the oral administration of adrenocorticosteroids to human infants. Pediatrics 26: 762-770

Carmosino L, DiBenedetto A, Feffer S (1985) Thymic hyperplasia following successful chemotherapy. A report of two cases and review of the literature. Cancer 56: 1526-1528

Carr JL (1945) Status thymico-lymphaticus. J Pediatrics 27: 1-43

Castleman B, Norris EH (1949) The pathology of the thymus in myasthenia gravis. Medicine (Baltimore) 28: 27-58

Cohen M, Hill CA, Cangir A, Sullivan MP (1980) Thymic rebound after treatment of childhood tumors. AJR 135: 151-156

Dalakas MC, Engel WK, McClure JE, Goldstein AL, Askanas V (1981) Immunocytochemical localization of thymosin-α_1 in thymic epithelial cells of normal and myasthenia gravis patients and in thymic cultures. J Neurol Sci 50: 239-247

Düe W, Dieckmann K-P, Stein H (1988) Thymic hyperplasia following chemotherapy of a testicular germ cell tumor. Cancer 63: 446-449

Filler RM, Simpson JS, Ein SH (1979) Mediastinal masses in infants and children. Pediatr Clin North Am 26: 677-690

Gelfand DW, Goldman AS, Law EJ, MacMillan BG, Larson D, Abston S, Schreiber JT (1972) Thymic hyperplasia in children recovering from thermal burns. J Trauma 12: 813-817

Goldstein G, Mackay IR (1969) The human thymus. Heinemann, London, pp 13, 134-135, 242-245, 290-291
Greenwood M, Woods HM (1927) "Status thymico-lymphaticus" considered in the light of recent work on the thymus. J Hyg (Lond) 26: 305-326
Grissom JR, Durant JR, Whitley RJ, Flint A (1983) Thymic hyperplasia in a case of Hodgkin's disease. South Med J 76: 1189-1192
Grody WW, Jobst S, Keesey J, Herrmann C, Maeim F (1986) Pathologic evaluation of thymic hyperplasia in myasthenia gravis and Lambert-Eaton syndrome. Arch Pathol Lab Med 110: 843-846
Haller JA Jr, Mazur DO, Morgan WW Jr (1969) Diagnosis and management of mediastinal masses in children. J Thorac Cardiovasc Surg 58: 385-393
Hammar JA (1926) Die Menschenthymus in Gesundheit und Krankheit. Ergebnisse der numerischen Analyse von mehr als tausend menschlichen Thymusdrüsen. Teil I: Das normale Organ. Zugleich eine kritische Beleuchtung der Lehre des "Status thymicus". Z Mikrosk Anat Forsch 6 [Suppl]: 11-73, 459-489, 502
Hammar JA (1936) Die normal-morphologische Thymusforschung im letzten Vierteljahrhundert. Analyse und Synthese nebst einigen Worten zu der Funktionsfrage. Barth, Leipzig, pp 297-301
Hill CA, Dodd GD (1970) Thymic hyperplasia simulating mediastinal metastasis. Tex Med 66: 78-81
Hofmann WJ, Möller P, Momburg F, Moldenbauer G, Otto HF (1984) Struktur des normalen Thymus, der lymphofollikulären Thymushyperplasie und der Thymome, dargestellt mit Lectinen, S-100-Protein und Keratin-Antiseren und monoklonalen (epitheliotropen) Antikörpern. Verh Dtsch Ges Pathol 68: 504
Hofmann WJ, Möller P, Otto HF (1987) Thymic hyperplasia. II. Lymphofollicular hyperplasia of the thymus. An immunohistologic study. Klin Wochenschr 65: 53-60
Hofmann WJ, Momburg F, Möller P, Otto HF (1988a) Intra- und extrathymic B cells in physiological and pathological conditions. Immunohistochemical study on normal thymus and lymphofollicular hyperplasia of the thymus. Virchows Arch A 412: 431-442
Hofmann WJ, Momburg F, Möller P (1988b) Thymic medullary cells expressing B-lymphocyte antigens. Hum Pathol 19: 1280-1287
Judd RL (1987) Massive thymic hyperplasia with myoid cell differentiation. Hum Pathol 18: 1180-1183
Katz SM, Chatten J, Bishop HC, Rosenblum H (1977) Massive thymic enlargement. Am J Clin Pathol 68: 786-790
Kendall MD, Johnson HRM, Singh J (1980) The weight of the human thymus gland at necropsy. J Anat 131: 485-499
Kirchner T, Schalke B, Melms A, von Kügelen T, Müller-Hermelink HK (1986) Immunohistological patterns of non-neoplastic changes in the thymus in myasthenia gravis. Virchows Arch B (Cell Pathol) 52: 237-257
Kornstein MJ, Brooks JJ, Anderson AO, Levinson AI, Lisak RP, Zweiman B (1984) The immunohistology of the thymus in myasthenia gravis. Am J Pathol 117: 184-194
Lack EE (1981) Thymic hyperplasia with massive enlargement. J Thorac Cardiovasc Surg 81: 741-746
Lamesch AJ (1983) Massive thymic hyperplasia in infants. Z Kinderchir 38: 16-18
Lee Y, Moallem S, Clauss RH (1979) Massive hyperplastic thymus in a 22-month-old infant. Ann Thorac Surg 27: 356-358
Levine GD, Rosai J (1978) Thymic hyperplasia and neoplasia: a review of current concepts. Hum Pathol 9: 495-515
Levine GD, Bearman RM (1980) The thymus. In: Johannessen JV (ed) Electron microscopy in human medicine, vol 5. McGraw-Hill, New York, pp 214-254
Löning T, Caselitz J, Otto HF (1981) The epithelial framework of the thymus in normal and pathological conditions: immunohistochemical demonstration of an autopsy series. Virchows Arch (Pathol Anat) 392: 7-20
Morgagni GB (1761) De sedibus, et causis morborum per anatomen indagatis, vol 1, book 2 (De morbis thoracis). Venetiis, Typographia Remondiniana, pp 129-298
Nezelof C, Normand C (1986) Tumor-like massive thymic hyperplasia in childhood: a possible defect of T-cell maturation, histological and cytoenzymatic studies of three cases. Thymus 8: 177-186
Nicholson RL (1978) Thymic hyperplasia in thyrotoxicosis. J Can Assoc Radiol 29: 264-265
Oh KS, Weber AL, Borden S (1971) Normal mediastinal mass in late childhood. Radiology 101: 625-628
O'Shea PA, Pansatiankul B, Farnes P (1978) Giant thymic hyperplasia in infancy: immunologic, histologic, and ultrastructural observations. Lab Invest 38: 391 (abstr.)
Osler W (1914) Principles and practice of medicine. Appleton, New York
Otto HF (1984) Pathologie des Thymus. Springer, Berlin Heidelberg New York, pp 106-115, 186-188 (Spezielle pathologische Anatomie, vol 17)
Paltauf A (1889) Über die Beziehungen der Thymus zum plötzlichen Tod. Wien Klin Wochenschr 2: 877-881
Paltauf A (1890) Über die Beziehungen der Thymus zum plötzlichen Tod. Wien Klin Wochenschr 3: 172-175
Pardo-Mindan FJ, Crisci CD, Serrano M, Arcas R (1980) Immunological aspects of sarcoidosis associated with true thymic hyperplasia. Allergol Immunopathol (Madr) 8: 91-96
Platter F (1614) Observationum in hominis affectibus plerisque.... L König, Bask, Book I p 172
Potter EL, Craig JM (1975) Pathology of the fetus and infant, 3rd edn. Year Book Medical Publishers, Chicago, p 321-322
Rasore-Quartino A, Rebizzo F, Romagnoli G (1979) Iperplasia gigante del timo nell'infanzia. Pathologica 71: 711-715
Rizk G, Cueto L, Amplatz K (1972) Rebound enlargement of the thymus after successful corrective surgery for transposition of the great vessels. AJR 116: 528-530
Rosai J, Levine GD (1976) Tumors of the thymus. In: Atlas of tumor pathology, sec ser, fasc 13. Armed Forces Institute of Pathology, Washington DC, pp 26-33, 133-137
Rose JS, Lam C (1982) Thymic enlargement in association with hyperthyroidism. Pediatr Radiol 12: 37-38
Saegesser F, Zoupanos G (1970) Thymomas, tumors of the thymic site, and the para-neoplastic immunological syndromes associated with them. In: Saegesser F, Pettavee J (eds) Surgical oncology. Huber, Bern, pp 447-488
Scadding GK, Vincent A, Newsom-Davis J, Henry K (1981) Acetylcholine receptor antibody synthesis by thymic lymphocytes: correlation with thymic histology. Neurology 31: 935-943
Scheiff JM, Cordier AC, Haumont S (1977) Epithelial cell proliferation in thymic hyperplasia induced by triiodothyronine. Clin Exp Immunol 27: 516-521
Shin MS, Ho KJ (1983) Diffuse thymic hyperplasia following chemotherapy for nodular sclerosing Hodgkin's disease. Cancer 51: 30-33
Silverman NA, Sabiston DC Jr (1980) Mediastinal masses. Surg Clin North Am 60: 757-777

Sloan HE Jr (1943) The thymus in myasthenia gravis. Surgery 13: 154-174

Staber FG, Fink U, Sack W (1975) B lymphocytes in the thymus of patients with myasthenia gravis. N Engl J Med 292: 1032-1033

Tamaoki N, Habu S, Kameya T (1971) Thymic lymphoid follicles in autoimmune disease. II. Histological, histochemical and electron microscopic studies. Keio J Med 20: 57-68

Tartas NE, Korin J, Dengra CS, Barazutti LM, Blasetti A, Avalos JCS (1985) Diffuse thymic enlargement in Hodgkin's disease. J Amer Med Association 19: 406

Thomas JA, Willcox HNA, Newsom-Davis J (1982) Immunohistological studies of the thymus in myasthenia gravis: correlation with clinical state and thymocyte culture responses. J Neuroimmunol 3: 319-335

Tridente G (1985) Immunopathology of the human thymus. Semin Hematol 22: 56-57

Wiersbowsky-Schmeel A, Helpap B, Totovic V, Grouls V (1984) Thymus in myasthenia gravis: a light and electron microscopic study of a case with thymic follicular hyperplasia. Pathol Res Pract 178: 323-331

Wychulis AR, Payne WS, Clagett OT, Woolner LB (1971) Surgical treatment of mediastinal tumors. J Thorac Cardiovasc Surg 62: 379-392

Young M, Turnbull HM (1931) An analysis of the data collected by the status lymphaticus investigation committee. J Pathol 34: 213-258

Yulish BS, Owens RP (1980) Thymic enlargement in a child during therapy for primary hypothyroidism. AJR 135: 157-158

8 Thymic Cysts

Anthony S.Y. Leong

Introduction

Although cysts of thymic origin are rare, their recognition dates back to the early nineteenth century. In 1832, at necropsy of two young syphilitic men, Lieutaud found suppurative changes in the thymuses, and related them to the concomitant necropsy finding of caseous pulmonary tuberculosis (Lieutaud 1832, cited by Dubois 1850). Dubois, in 1850, attributed cystic changes in the thymuses of three newborn infants who died from congenital syphilis to syphilitic suppuration and suggested that this, not tuberculous suppuration, had been the lesion in Lieutaud's patients. Cystic changes in the thymus were described subsequently by Chiari (1894), Pollosson and Piéry (1901), Erdheim (1904), Hammar (1905), Pappenheimer (1910) and Klose (1914). All of those early studies were made on necropsy material and the cysts were either ascribed to syphilis or regarded as being of congenital origin. The thymuses were generally multicystic, with individual cysts varying from a few millimetres in diameter to "almost walnut size".

Embryology

Thymic cysts may be found anywhere along a line extending medially from the angle of the mandible to the manubrium sterni, often adjacent to or within the anterior cervical triangle, and in the anterior mediastinum down to the diaphragm. To understand the location of these cysts the embryogenesis of the thymus must be discussed.

The thymus is derived from the third pair of pharyngeal pouches, with a minor and inconstant contribution from the fourth pair (Weller 1933; Norris 1937; Gilmour 1941). During the 6th week of foetal life sacculations of thymic ectoderm appear on the ventrolateral surfaces of the third pharyngeal pouch. These diverticular buds elongate into hollow thymopharyngeal ducts which eventually pinch off from the pharynx to form paired primordia or anlage. With proliferation and elongation of the lining entoderm the ducts become solid stalks which migrate caudally and approximate in the midline. The thymic anlage passes behind the developing thyroid gland, becomes adherent to the pericardium and descends with the pericardium into the anterior mediastinum as a paired organ by about the 13th week of development. In the 8th week, the proximal portions of the elongated thymic stalks usually atrophy and disappear. If the upper end of the thymopharyngeal stalk fails to regress its remnants may be found in any position along the line of thymic descent. Wenglowski (1912) reported necropsies in which he found small thymic cysts and rests in the necks of 2 of 10 adults and 21 of 65 infants. Gilmour (1941) reported 13 cases showing thymic tissue in unusual positions, and Kind (1949) found thymic cysts in the neck at necropsy in 8 cases. Thymic cysts have also been described as coincidental findings on histological examination of surgically excised thyroid gland (Indeglia et al. 1967).

Derivation

Speer (1938) hypothesized that thymic cysts may be derived: (1) from embryonal remnants of the thymopharyngeal ducts, the branchial clefts or the thymic tubules; (2) from sequestration products in pathological involution of the thymus; (3) from neoplastic processes in lymphoid, "cytoreticular" or connective tissue; (4) from degenerating Hassall's corpuscles; or (5) from vascular or connective tissue elements during various stages of thymic development, involution or hyperplasia.

Krech et al. (1954) divided thymic cysts into three groups: (1) congenital; (2) inflammatory; and (3) neoplastic. So-called Dubois' abscesses or inflammatory cysts appeared invariably to be due to syphilis and cysts occurring in thymic neoplasm could probably be attributed to degeneration and necrosis of the tumour. These authors suggested that non-neoplastic and non-inflammatory cysts were probably of congenital origin in that persistent congenital defects in the form of patent thymic or thymopharyngeal ducts would predispose to cyst formation after haemorrhage or accumulation of fluid from unknown causes. Fielding et al.

(1963), however, revived an older theory that cysts arose from degenerated Hassall's corpuscles. They maintained that degenerative changes, if extensive enough, caused cystic dilatation of Hassall's bodies, and accounted for the variety of appearances of the cyst lining and even the granulomatous changes consequent upon rupture of the cyst.

The fact that Hassall's corpuscles are connected together as part of the complex epithelial network of branching cords and tubules derived from the thymopharyngeal tract (Shier 1963), has given rise to the suggestion that degenerative changes within this system could explain the development of a multilocular or multicystic mass within the thymus. Willis (1962) described a case in which the cysts developed in later life, and Schlumberger (1946) referred to work on the thymuses of dogs and cats in which cysts developed after birth. Multiple small epithelial-lined cysts appeared in the thymuses of rats injected with oestrogens, and it is likely that these cysts originated in Hassall's corpuscles (Ross and Korenchevsky 1941).

Cystic degeneration in Hassall's corpuscles is not, however, a constant finding in thymic cysts (Krech et al. 1954). When such degeneration is in the cyst wall it may well be a secondary phenomenon resulting from local distortion of the normal gland structure. Most thymic cysts, moreover, occur in the first decade of life when degenerative changes are unlikely; indeed, they have not been demonstrated in the normally developing child (Shier 1963). In view of the evidence that Hassall's corpuscles derive from the thymopharyngeal duct which is subsequently incorporated in the lymphoreticular component of the organ, unincorporated remnants of the duct may be expected to persist, either outside the thymus or within its septal tissue (Bieger and McAdams 1966), and that such is in fact the case has been demonstrated by Gilmour (1937) and by Shier (1963). All the clinical and pathological features of thymic cysts can thus be explained by persistence of the thymopharyngeal duct system. Further evidence of congenital origin is the relatively frequent association of cervical thymic cysts with other endocrine gland inclusions. Inclusions of normal parathyroid tissue, less often of normal thyroid tissue, were found by Guba et al. (1978). Cystic parathyroid adenomas with mixtures of thymic elements (Schlumberger 1946; Bradford et al. 1947) and an unusual cystic choristoma of the mediastinal thymus containing a mixture of normal thymic, parathyroid and salivary gland tissue (Breckler and Johnson 1956) have been reported. The frequent connection between cervical thymic cysts and the normal mediastinal thymus also points to a congenital aetiology. Thus, the development of thymic cysts may logically be attributed to the presence of sequestered remnants of the thymopharyngeal duct within and adjacent to the gland. Subsequent degenerative changes such as haemorrhage and the accumulation of fluid may be responsible for the clinical manifestations of these congenital structures.

Histopathology

Thymic cysts are loculated and have diameters ranging from 2 to 15 cm. The fluid they contain may be clear, or it may be turbid because of cholesterol crystals or haemorrhage (Fig. 1). The cyst lining may consist of flattened, cuboidal, columnar, ciliated-columnar or squamous epithelium (Fig. 2). Although the squamous epithelium is usually regarded as being derived from Hassall's corpuscles, metaplastic change may also account for its presence. The lining is often degenerated and replaced by granulation tissue, inflammatory cellular infiltrate and foamy macrophages (Fig. 3). Cholesterol-type granulomas or clefting are usually seen and foreign body giant cells and haemosiderin-laden macrophages may occur in the fibrous cyst wall. Thymic epithelial elements in intimate relation to the cyst lining are essential to the diagnosis of thymic cysts (Fig. 4). In the absence of Hassall's corpuscles or diffuse thymic epithelial elements thymic cysts cannot be distinguished histologically from branchial cleft cysts (Willis 1962). Because of the atrophic condition of the thymic remnant, extensive sampling and careful microscopic examination are often necessary. Multiple minute cysts sometimes detected in the walls indicate that one cyst has enlarged at the expense of the others (Dyer 1967). The histological appearance of cervical and medistinal thymic cysts are identical.

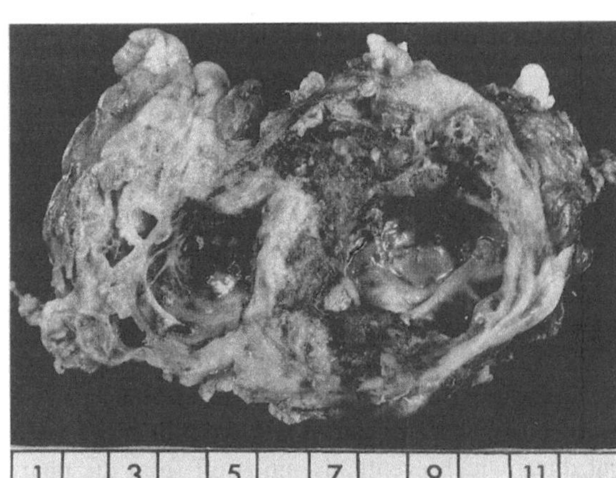

Fig. 1. Bisected 7-cm diameter multiloculated cyst showing areas of shaggy fibrin and granulation tissue on the cyst wall

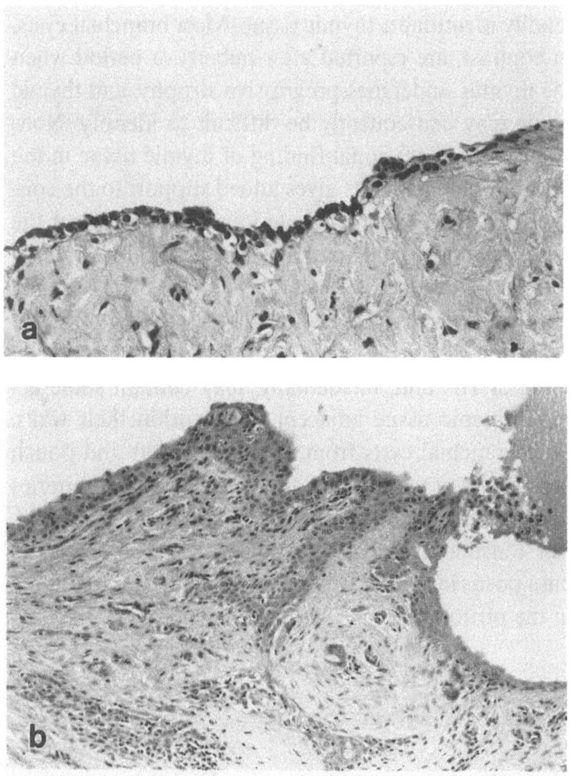

Fig. 2a, b. The lining epithelium of thymic cysts. **a** Low cuboidal epithelium on fibrous stroma. ×125 **b** Stratified squamous lining connected to underlying Hassall's corpuscles and tubules of the thymus. ×125

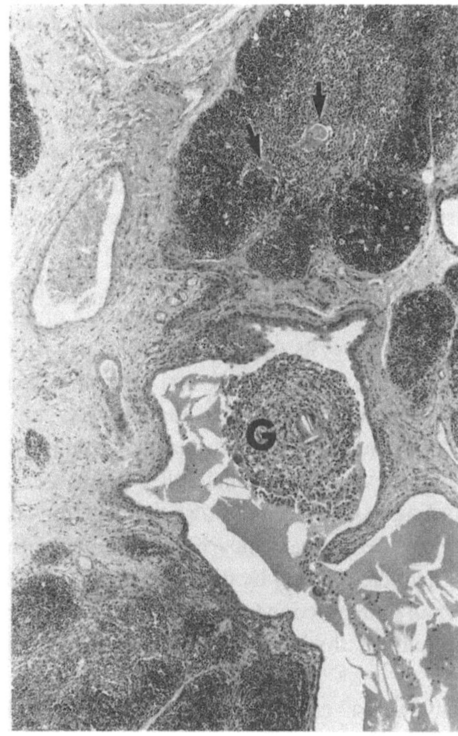

Fig. 4. A prominent and characteristic granuloma *(G)* projects into the cyst. Thymic lymphocytes and epithelial nests *(arrows)* are present (Courtesy of Dr. G. E. Phillips) ×60

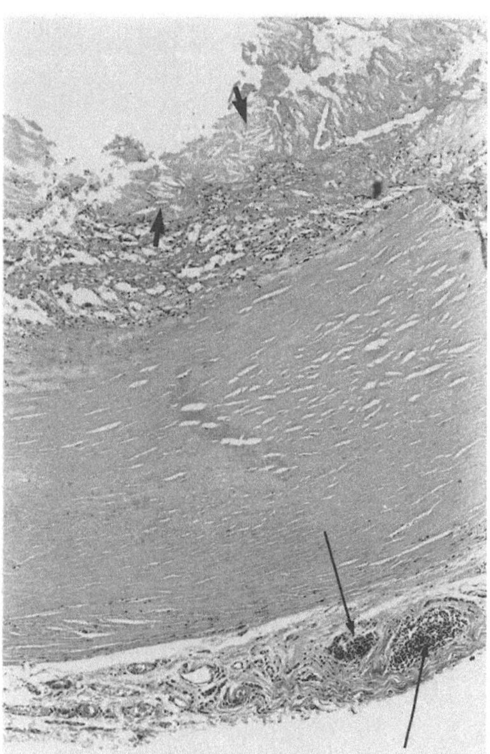

Congenital Thymic Cysts

The ratio of mediastinal thymic cysts to cervical thymic cysts has been estimated as 2.5:1, with an approximately equal sex distribution (Indeglis et al. 1967).

Cervical Thymic Cysts

Cervical thymic cysts were studied extensively by Guba et al. (1978), who reviewed reports of 56 histologically confirmed cases. The lesions were left-sided in 70% of the patients, right-sided in 23% and midline or pharyngeal in 7%. In 90% the presenting symptom was a painless swelling, and in the remainder it was dysphagia, dyspnoea, hoarseness or, rarely, pain. In 16 additional cases of their own, these workers occasionally noted fluctuation in cyst size, presumably owing to in-

Fig. 3. Anterior mediastinal cyst with denuded epithelial lining. The thick fibrous cyst wall is covered with necrotic debris and foamy macrophages. Cholesterol clefts are present *(short arrows)* and small nests of epithelial cells and lymphocytes *(long arrows)* identify its thymic origin. ×60

fection or haemorrhage. As was to be expected from the fact that the thymus gland reaches its greatest relative size at 2-4 years of age and its greatest absolute size at puberty, the incidence of cervical thymic cyst was highest in the paediatric age group. In the group of 56 cases the average age was 12 years and the median age at presentation 7 years. Over 75% of all patients were under 20 years. These lesions have, nevertheless, occasionally been observed in older patients. Indeglia et al. (1967) reported three patients over the age of 60, two with mediastinal cysts (one of them a 75-year-old woman) and one with a cervical cyst. Behring and Bergman (1963) found that cervical thymic cysts may be unilocular or multilocular, and that they appeared to occur almost exclusively unilaterally. It has been stated, according to Guba et al. (1978), that as many as 50% of cervical thymic cysts may be continuous with mediastinal thymus, possibly by direct extension of the cyst substernally, or by connection to a solid cord or vestigial remnant of thymic tissue extending into the thorax.

In an analysis of 47 cases of cervical cysts by Mikal (1974), 25 were branchial, 12 thyroglossal, 8 thyroid, 1 thymic and 1 parathyroid. The relation of cervical thymic cysts to branchial cysts remains controversial. Fahmy (1974) has argued that branchial cysts also originate from the thymopharyngeal tract of the third pharyngeal pouch. The location of the classical branchial cyst along the line of descent of the thymopharyngeal tract, and the similarity of its epithelial lining to that of the thymic cyst, support the contention that they both derive from the same vestigial structure. Most cervical thymic cysts are recognized before puberty. As thymic size and activity are maximal at this period, it is not surprising that the cyst wall contains readily identifiable thymic tissue. Most branchial cysts, in contrast, are reported after puberty, a period when the thymus undergoes progressive atrophy, and thymic tissue may consequently be difficult to identify. Nonetheless, the occasional finding of thymic tissue in the wall of branchial cysts gives added support to the concept that both these cystic lesions are variants of the same developmental anomaly. The classical view, however, is that branchial cysts are derived from vestigial branchial pouch-cleft complexes. According to Mikal (1974) they arise from the second cleft or the cervical sinus of His and, incidentally, may contain some ectopic thymic tissue adjacent to or within their walls. True branchial cysts from the second cleft and pouch pass between the internal and external carotid arteries just above the carotid bifurcation and end in the superior tonsillar fossa, unlike thymic cysts whose tracts pass posterior to the carotid bifurcation and terminate in the piriform fossa.

Mediastinal Thymic Cysts

Mediastinal thymic cysts are rare. Of 1064 mediastinal tumours described by Wychulis et al. (1971), 196 were benign cysts, of which only 19 were of thymic origin and only 2 were in patients under the age of 30 years.

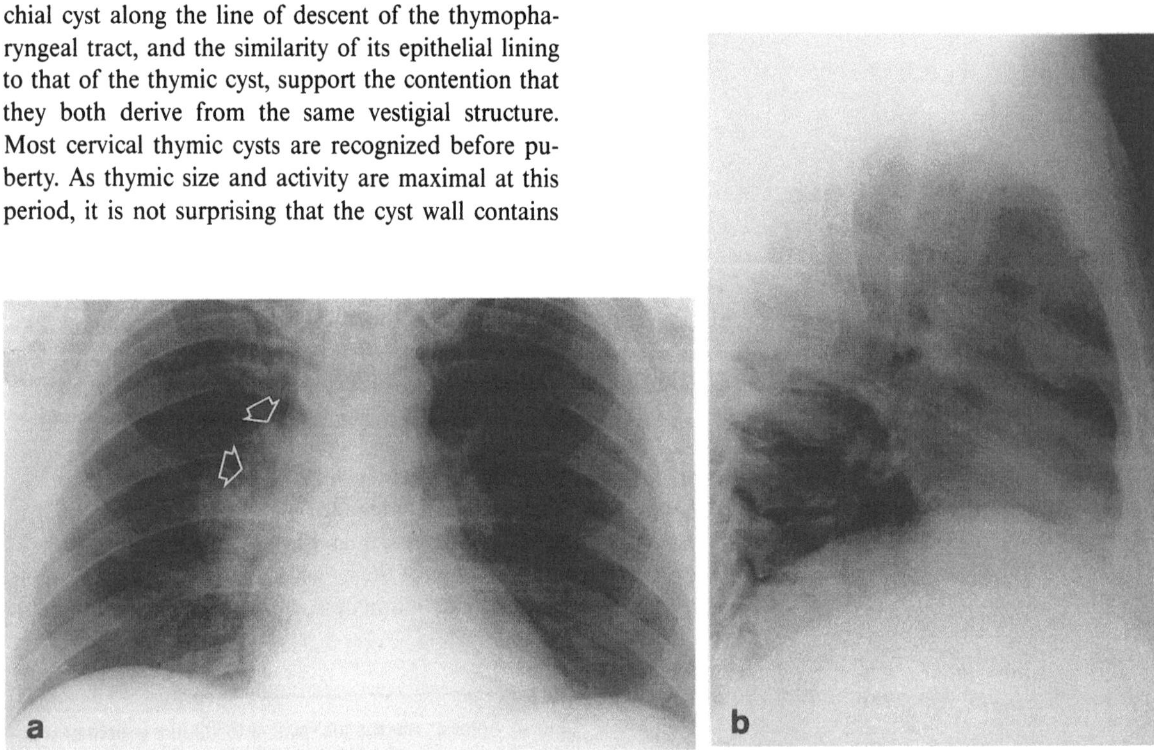

Fig. 5. Benign cyst presenting as an asymptomatic anterior mediastinal mass on chest roentgenogram. A thin rim of peripheral calcification is apparent *(arrows)*. (Courtesy of Dr. J. H. Brown)

Silverman and Sabiston (1977) have provided a composite analysis from several reported series on the frequency of mediastinal tumours and cysts in adults and in children.

Mediastinal thymic cysts are often asymptomatic, being discovered incidentally on chest roentgenograms done for unrelated reasons. There are no specific diagnostic measures that would indicate clinically that an anterior mediastinal mass is a thymic cyst. Other cystic structures that may occur in the anterior mediastinum include bronchogenic, oesophageal, gastroenteric, mesothelial, neoplastic, parasitic, pericardial, thoracic duct and tracheo-oesophageal cysts, and cystic hematomas (see Chap. 11). Hydatid disease, which can affect practically any organ, has been reported as a cystic mass in the thymus (Giraud et al. 1963). Some mediastinal cysts are labelled "nonspecific" because they defy diagnosis even after histological examination (Dyer 1967). It is likely that many of these "nonspecific" mediastinal cysts may represent thymic cysts in which the epithelial lining is destroyed by degenerative changes and replaced by granulation tissue.

Investigating a group of 138 patients with thymic tumours, Bernatz et al. (1961) found that when roentgenologically demonstrable peripheral linear calcification was present it was invariably in the wall of a noninvasive cystic thymoma or in the fibrous capsule of a well-demarcated tumour. An example of such peripheral calcification in a benign thymic cyst is shown in Fig. 5. Rim calcification may, however, occur in other mediastinal lesions, such as dermoids and hydatids (Harper and Guyer 1965). In fact, the separation of mediastinal cysts from solid tumours is rarely achieved and a precise diagnosis is seldom made before operation (Krech et al. 1954; Dyer 1967). The role of computer-assisted tomographic scanning in the diagnosis of thymic cysts is discussed in Chap. 17.

Acquired Thymic Cysts

The commonest cause of acquired thymic cysts is infection. Although this type of thymic cyst was the subject of many of the earlier reports, it seems to have vanished from the literature in recent years. "Dubois' abscesses" were almost always reported at necropsy as multicystic glands of variable size filled with pus, and were thought to be due to congenital syphilis. Ribbert (1912) described some of these cysts as being formed of markedly enlarged Hassall's corpuscles filled with keratin and necrotic debris, thus raising doubts as to the causative role of syphilis (Rosai and Levine 1976).

Mediastinal thymic cysts have been observed after roentgen therapy for Hodgkin's disease (Katz et al. 1977; Baron et al. 1981; Murray and Parker 1984). They present as persistent mediastinal masses and have to be distinguished from recurrence of Hodgkin's disease. It has been suggested that such cysts relate solely to the effects of roentgen therapy (Katz et al. 1977), but a case has been described in which only chemotherapy had been given (Scully et al. 1982).

Cystic Thymic Neoplasms

Yamakawa et al. (1961) suggested that neoplastic change may occur in a simple thymic cyst. However, they described a cyst with areas of thymoma in the cyst wall, was probably a thymoma undergoing characteristic cystic degeneration with cholesterol clefts and lymphocytic foci. Foci of germinoma (seminoma) have been described in the walls of cystic thymuses (Iverson 1956; Indeglia et al. 1967). True malignant transformation in a thymic cyst has, however, been reported only once, by Leong and Brown in 1984. The patient was a 64-year-old male in whom they excised an asymptomatic cystic mediastinal tumour measuring $11 \times 7 \times 4$ cm. Areas of well-differentiated papillary squamous cell carcinoma were found in the squamous epithelium lining the cyst (Fig. 6). Follow-up 7 years

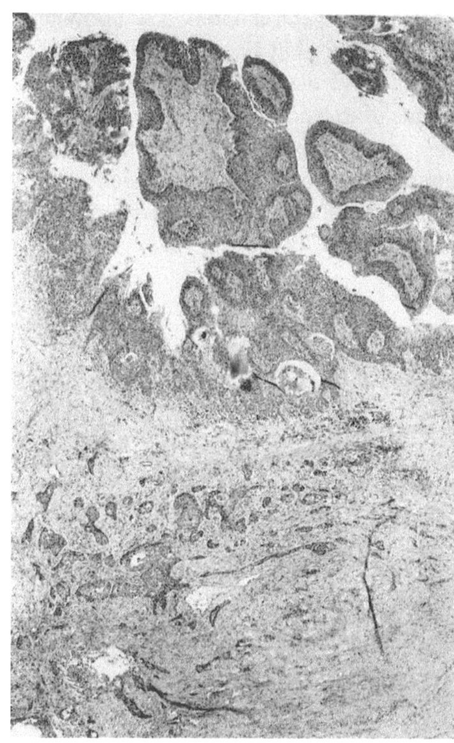

Fig. 6. Well-differentiated papillary squamous cell carcinoma arising in the lining of a thymic cyst. Note the invasion of the cyst wall. Definite epithelial and lymphoid elements of the thymus were identified elsewhere in the cyst wall. ×60

after complete excision showed no evidence of metastasis.

Cysts are encountered in 40% of thymomas, more frequently in the larger tumours than in the smaller ones (Rosai and Levine 1976). They vary from inconspicuous spaces containing clear fluid to large cavities containing blood or thick yellow-brown material rich in cholesterol and other breakdown products of blood. Cystic tumours are particularly prone to calcification. Cystic degeneration is sometimes so extensive that identifiable thymoma tissue is reduced to small nodules attached to the capsule, and may be difficult to find, a fact which reemphasizes the need for careful gross examination and extensive microscopic sampling. Some thymomas may be associated with true cystic change in the non-neoplastic thymus surrounding the tumour (Rosai and Levine 1976). Microscopic cystic change may also occur in other thymic neoplasms such as germinomas and teratomas. Lymphangiomas and lymphatic cysts may also rarely occur in the thymus (Videbaek and Thomsen 1959; Bernatz et al. 1961).

Treatment

Most authors agree that excision is the only method of treatment of thymic cysts (Dyer 1967). It not only provides a positive diagnosis, but also removes any malignant or locally invasive tissue. Frozen section examination at the time of excision helps in determining the extent of the procedure necessary for removal. The surgical treatment of thymic cysts dates back to 1901 (Pollosson and Piéry 1901), and its subsequent history is outlined in Chap. 1.

References

Baron RL, Sagel SS, Baglan RJ (1981) Thymic cysts following radiation therapy for Hodgkin disease. Radiology 141: 593-597

Behring C, Bergman F (1963) Thymic cyst of the neck: report of a case. Acta Pathol Microbiol Scand 59: 45-50

Bernatz PE, Harrison EG, Clagett OT (1961) Thymoma: a clinicopathologic study. J Thorac Cardiovasc Surg 42: 424-444

Bieger RC, McAdams AJ (1966) Thymic cysts. Arch Pathol 82: 535-541

Bradford ML, Mahon HW, Grow JB (1947) Mediastinal cysts and tumors. Surg Gynecol Obstet 85: 467-491

Breckler IA, Johnston DG (1956) Choristoma of the thymus. Am J Dis Child 92: 175-178

Chiari H (1894) Über Cystenbildung in der menschlichen Thymus, zugleich ein Beitrag zur Lehre von den "Dubois'schen Abscessen". Z Heilkd 15: 403-425

Dubois P (1850) Du diagnostic de la syphilis considérée comme une des causes possibles de la mort du foetus. Gaz Méd de Paris 21: 392-395

Dyer NH (1967) Cystic thymomas and thymic cysts: a review. Thorax 22: 408-421

Erdheim J (1904) Befunde von Cysten und Drüsenbläschen neben und in branchiogenen Organen. Beitr pathol Anat allg Pathol (Jena) 35: 412-433

Fahmy S (1974) Cervical thymic cysts: their pathogenesis and relationship to branchial cysts. J Laryngol Otol 88: 47-60

Fielding JF, Farmer AW, Lindsay WK, Conen PE (1963) Cystic degeneration in persistent cervical thymus: a report of four cases in children. Can J Surg 6: 178-186

Gilmour JR (1937) The embryology of the parathyroid glands, the thymus and certain associated rudiments. J Pathol Bacteriol 45: 507-522

Gilmour JR (1941) Some developmental abnormalities of the thymus and parathyroids. J Pathol Bacteriol 52: 213-218

Giraud G, Nègre E, Thevenet A, Beraud P (1963) Kyste hydatique du thymus. Presse Méd 71: 1375-1376

Guba AM Jr, Adam AE, Jaques DA, Chambers RG (1978) Cervical presentation of thymic cysts. Am J Surg 136: 430-436

Hammar JA (1905) Zur Histogenese und Involution der Thymusdrüse. Anat Anz 27: 23-30

Harper RAK, Guyer PB (1965) The radiological features of thymic tumours: a review of sixty-five cases. Clin Radiol 16: 97-105

Indeglia RA, Shea MA, Grage TB (1967) Congenital cysts of the thymus gland. Arch Surg 94: 149-152

Iverson L (1956) Thymoma: a review and reclassification. Am J Pathol 32: 695-719

Katz M, Piekarski JD, Bayle-Weisgerber C, Laval-Jeantet M, Teillet F (1977) Masses médiastinales résiduelles post-radiothérapiques au cours de la maladie de Hodgkin. Ann Radiol (Paris) 20: 667-672

King ESJ (1949) The lateral lympho-epithelial cyst of the neck ("branchial" cyst). Aust NZ J Surg 19: 109-121

Klose H (1914) Chirurgie der Thymusdrüse. Ergeb Chir Orthop Berl 8: 274-423

Krech WG, Storey CF, Umiker WC (1954) Thymic cysts: a review of the literature and report of two cases. J Thorac Surg 27: 477-493

Leong AS-Y, Brown JH (1984) Malignant transformation in a thymic cyst. Am J Surg Pathol 8: 471-475

Lieutaud E (1832) Mémoires d'Haugsted. (In part published in Arch Med, T III, Second Series, 1833)

Mikal S (1974) Cervical thymic cyst: case report and review of the literature. Arch Surg 109: 558-562

Murray JA, Parker AC (1984) Mediastinal Hodgkin's disease and thymic cysts. Acta Haematol (Basel) 71: 282-284

Norris EH (1937) The parathyroid glands and the lateral thyroid in man: their morphogenesis, histogenesis, topographic anatomy and prenatal growth. Contrib Embryol (Carnegie Inst Wash Publ) 26 (no 159): 247-294

Pappenheimer AM (1910) A contribution to the normal and pathological histology of the thymus gland. J Med Research Bost 22: 1-73

Pollosson A, Piéry M (1901) Un cas d'épithélioma primitif du thymus. Province Méd (Lyon) 16: 1-4

Ribbert H (1912) Die Entwicklungsstörung der Thymusdrüse bei kongenitaler Lues. Frankfurt Z Pathol 11: 209-218

Rosai J, Levine GD (1976) Tumors of the thymus. In: Atlas of tumor pathology, sec ser, fasc 13. Armed Forces Institute of Pathology, Washington DC, pp 48-49, 207-211

Ross MA, Korenchevsky V (1941) The thymus of the rat and sex hormones. J Pathol Bacteriol 52: 349-360

Schlumberger HG (1946) Teratoma of the anterior mediastinum in the group of military age: a study of sixteen cases,

and a review of theories of genesis. Arch Pathol 41: 398-444
Scully RE, Mark EJ, McNeely BU (1982) Case records of the Massachusetts General Hospital (case 47). N Engl J Med 307: 1391-1397
Shier KJ (1963) The morphology of the epithelial thymus: observations on lymphocyte-depleted and fetal thymus. Lab Invest 12: 316-326
Silverman NA, Sabiston DC Jr (1977) Primary tumors and cysts of the mediastinum. Curr Probl Cancer 2: 1-55
Speer FD (1938) Thymic cysts: report of a thymus presenting cysts of three types. NY Med Coll Flower Hosp Bull 1: 142-150
Videbaek A, Thomsen G (1959) Tumours of the thymic region: follow-up on 36 operated cases. Acta Radiol [Diagn] (Stockh) [Suppl 188]: 261-275
Weller GL Jr (1933) Development of the thyroid, parathyroid and thymus glands in man. Contrib Embryol (Carnegie Inst Wash Publ) 24 (no 141): 93-139
Wenglowski R (1912) Über die Halsfisteln und Cysten. Langenbecks Arch Klin Chir 100: 789-892
Willis RA (1962) The borderland of embryology and pathology, 2nd edn. Butterworths, London, pp 283-287
Wychulis AR, Payne WS, Clagett OT, Woolner LB (1971) Surgical treatment of mediastinal tumors: a 40 year experience. J Thorac Cardiovasc Surg 62: 379-392
Yamakawa K, Tsuchiya Y, Naito S, Kawaguchi JS (1961) A case report of thymic cyst. Am J Dis Chest 39: 542-545

9 Epithelial Tumors

Mark R. Wick and Juan Rosai

Introduction

Over the past 25 years, the definition, diagnosis, and treatment of thymic epithelial tumors has been refined continually. The group of neoplasms formerly designated generically as "thymomas" has now been divided into several distinct clinicopathologic entities (Bernatz et al. 1961; Lattes 1962; Katz and Lattes 1969; Rosai and Higa 1972; Levine 1973; Sterchi and Cordell 1975; Rosai and Levine 1976; Levine and Rosai 1978; Gray and Gutowski 1979, Snover et al. 1982; Wick et al. 1982; Lewis et al. 1987). The true spectrum of the morphological appearance and behavior of thymomas (i. e., cytologically bland tumors of the thymic epithelium) has thus been better characterized.

The pathologic features of both cytologically bland and cytologically malignant thymic epithelial tumors are the subject of this chapter. Whenever appropriate, the relationship between histopathology and biology will be outlined. In addition, microscopic differential diagnostic considerations will be described, along with appropriate methods for separating one from another.

Accordingly, we shall only use the term "thymoma" in conjunction with neoplasms consisting of cytologically bland thymic epithelial cells. Modified expressions of this concept, such as "malignant thymoma," will be considered subsequently.

Thymoma

Clinical Features

Thymomas usually present as anterior-superior mediastinal masses which may be discovered incidentally by chest X-ray during routine medical examinations (Fig. 1), or they may produce symptoms of thoracic structural displacement, such as cough, dyspnea, palpitations, and substernal or interscapular aching pain. A variety of paraneoplastic syndromes (myasthenia gravis, pure erythroid aplasia, acquired hypogammaglobulinemia, etc.) may herald the presence of a thymoma (Gafni et al. 1960; Hirst and Robertson 1967; Rogers et al. 1968; Souadjian et al. 1974; Slater et al. 1978). These syndromes will be discussed in Chaps. 12-15.

Rarely, thymomas may occur in ectopic locations, such as the posterior mediastinum (Cooper and Narodick 1972), the pulmonary parenchyma (McBurney et al. 1951), and the base of the neck (Rosai et al. 1984). These phenomena relate to flaws in the embryologic development of the thymus gland (Chap. 2). Among the examples just mentioned, the posterior mediastinal mass caused chest pain, the pulmonary lesion was associated with myasthenia gravis, and the neck masses were asymptomatic.

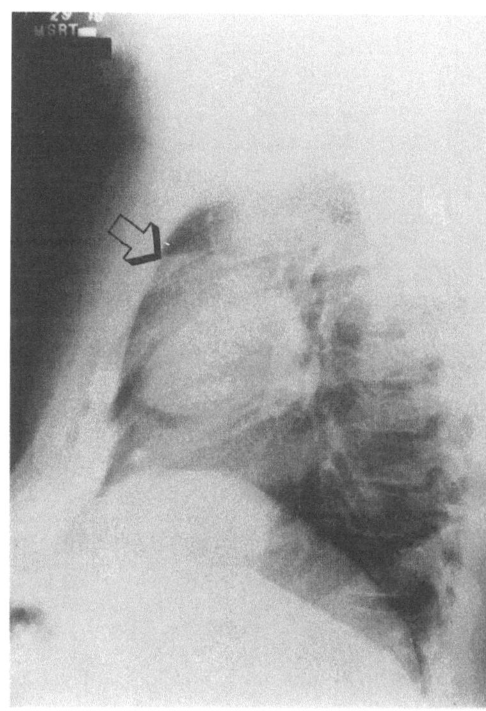

Fig. 1. Anterior mediastinal mass *(arrow)* found at routine chest roentgenography, which proved to be a thymoma

Gross Characteristics

Classically, thymomas are encapsulated, circumscribed, lobulated neoplasms. Their cut surfaces are typically firm, tan-pink, and homogeneous, and they are divided into macroscopic lobules by thick fibrous internal bands (Fig. 2). The capsule is also characteristically thick and fibrous. Up to 50% of thymomas may contain gross internal cysts (Fig. 3) which are usually filled with fluid or with grumous cellular debris. Limited foci of necrosis may be present, but extensive necrotic changes, with or without hemorrhage, are unusual and should alert one to the possibility of an alternative diagnosis.

Occasional thymomas may display gross internal foci of calcification or an incomplete peripheral rim of calcification (or even ossification). Others (particularly lymphocyte-predominant thymomas) sometimes lack obvious fibrous capsules and internal fibrous septa, and take on a tan-gray, homogeneous appearance, like that of "fish flesh." Rarely, small, nodular thymomas may be seen within a single lobe of an otherwise normal thymus; this is commonest in glands which have been removed for the treatment of myasthenia gravis. Thymomatous nodules have also been seen in the walls of thymic cysts (Rosai and Levine 1976).

An important feature of the gross assessment of thymomas is the surgeon's detailed description of the tumor in situ. Thymomas which are totally encapsulated and therefore easily resectable differ in behavior from those that invade contiguous mediastinal structures (Bernatz et al. 1973). The prognostic significance of these gross features will be discussed subsequently. Tumor size is extremely variable, and logically correlates with the presence or absence of clinical symptoms. Rosai and Levine (1976) have reported a thymoma of merely 1 mm diameter; on the other hand, Smith et al. (1970) described one which weighed 5700 g and measured 34 cm in its greatest dimension. Two-thirds of all thymomas are between 5 and 10 cm in diameter, excluding those composed exclusively of spindle cells which tend to be larger in size.

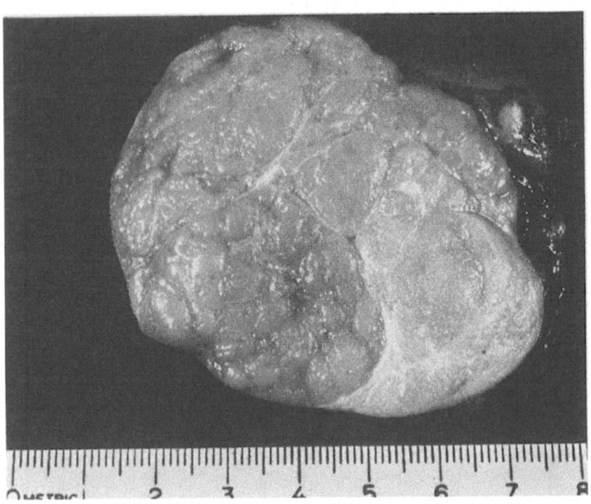

Fig. 2. Typical gross appearance of thymoma. The tumor is encapsulated, and subdivided by fibrous bands

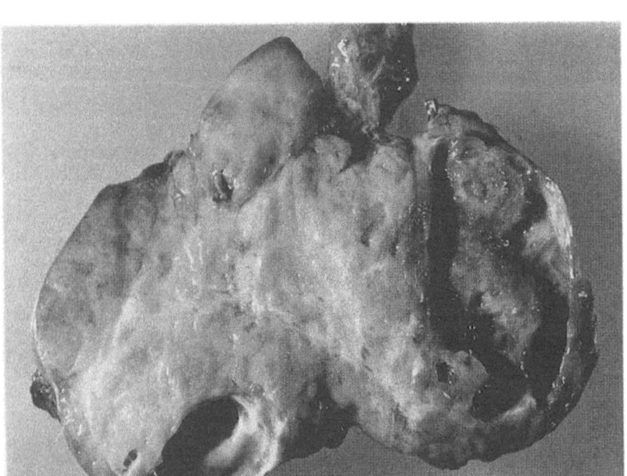

Fig. 3. Multifocal cystic change in an otherwise typical thymoma. This appearance is seen in a minority of these neoplasms

Microscopic Characteristics

Thymomas are composed of varying proportions of epithelial cells and lymphocytes. However, the thymic epithelial cells are the only neoplastic cells in these tumors. These are at least three times the size of mature lymphocytes, and have a moderate amount of amphophilic cytoplasm (Fig. 4). Their nuclear membranes are slightly indented, and chromatin is evenly dispersed, with inconspicuous nucleoli. Mitotic activity is usually scanty in the epithelial cells of thymomas, and atypical mitoses are absent.

Throughout this chapter, we shall employ the terms "predominantly lymphocytic," "mixed lymphoepithelial," and "predominantly epithelial" to describe types of thymoma. These are arbitrarily defined as neoplasms in which lymphocytes comprise respectively two-thirds or more, one-third to two-thirds, and less than one-third of the intratumoral cell population (Figs. 5-7). Spindle cell thymomas are regarded as a special variant of the last of these three groups.

A salient microscopic feature of most thymomas is their gross fibrous septation. Histologically, these tumors are composed of lobules, which are divided by intersecting bands of paucicellular fibrous tissue (Fig. 8) which often form acute angles at points of

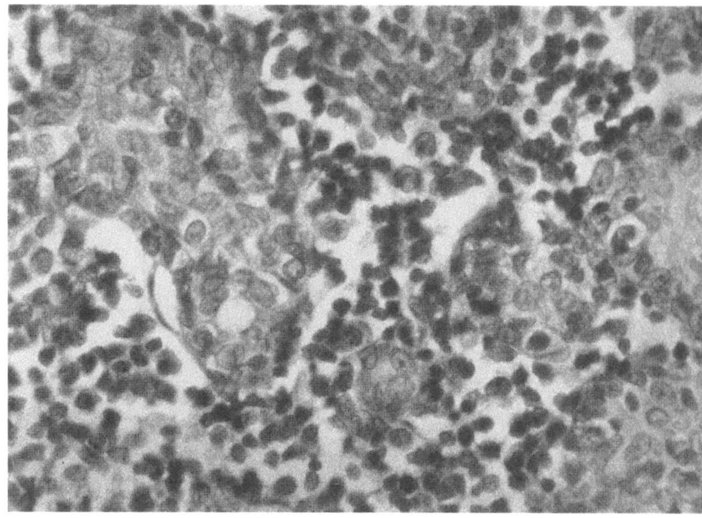

Fig. 4. Thymic epithelial cells are cohesive, and from one-and-a-half times to twice the size of reactive lymphocytes in this thymoma

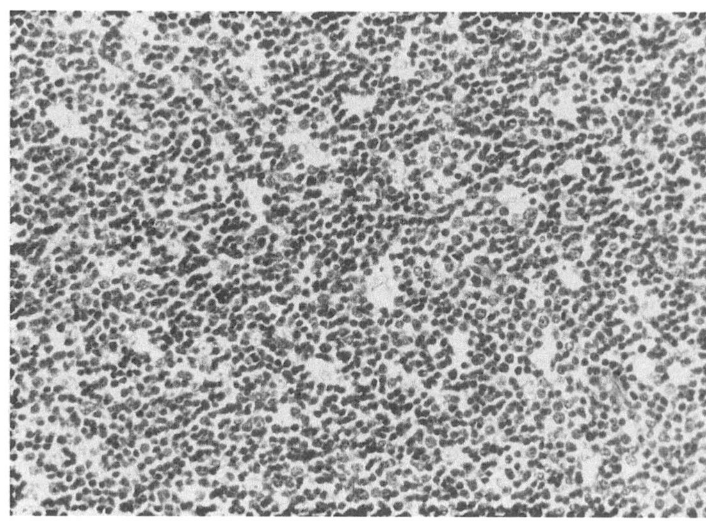

Fig. 5. Predominantly lymphocytic thymoma. Sheets of relatively mature lymphocytes are plunctuated randomly by sparse thymic epithelial cells

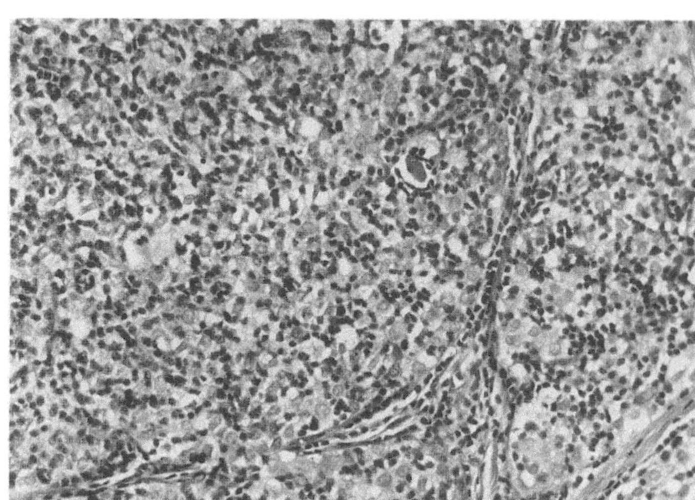

Fig. 6. Mixed lymphoepithelial thymoma. Thymic epithelial cells and reactive lymphocytes are admixed in roughly equal proportions

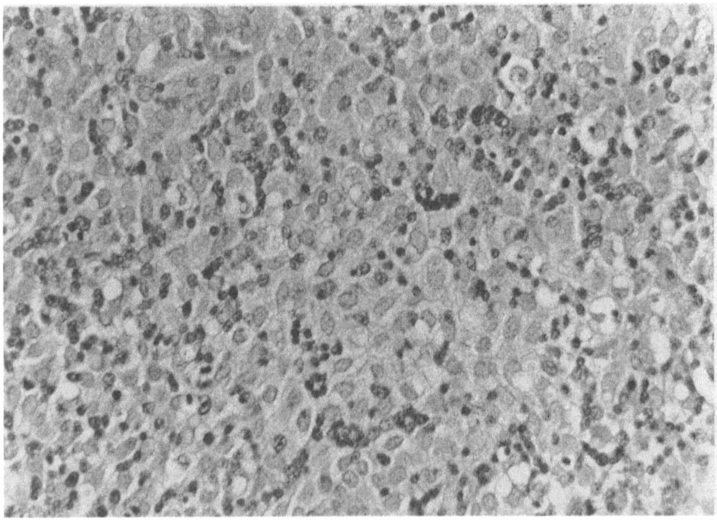

Fig. 7. Predominantly epithelial thymoma. The tumor is almost entirely composed of thymic epithelial cells

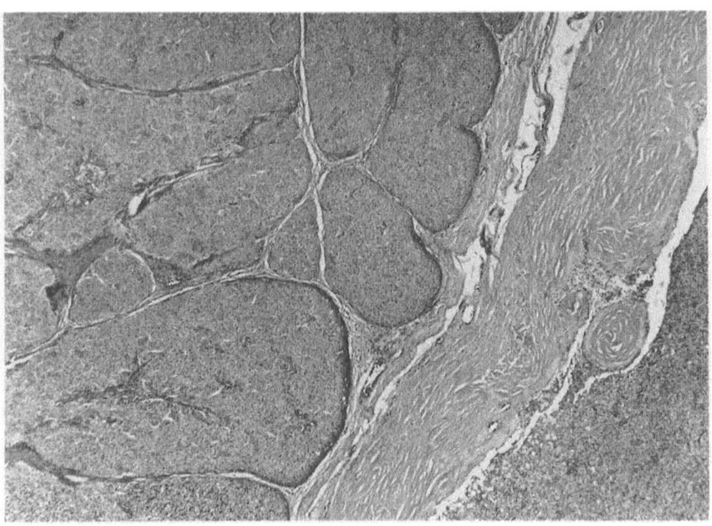

Fig. 8. Typical low power microscopic appearance of thymoma. This neoplasm is comprised of cellular lobules, which fit together in an angular jigsaw fashion. They are separated by fibrous stromal bands

junction. Peripherally, a fibrous capsule is usually also apparent. Remnants of non-neoplastic thymus gland may be included in operative specimens of thymoma. These may be distinguished from tumor tissue by their normal corticomedullary relationship (Fig. 9), which is not seen in the thymoma.

Intratumoral lymphocytes are generally small and mature, but may occasionally take on an "activated" appearance. In this case, their nuclei are enlarged, with slightly folded membranes and increased mitotic activity (Fig. 10). However, they never attain the "convoluted" nuclear appearance of lymphoblasts, nor do they manifest increased nucleocytoplasmic ratios.

Occasional thymomas of the predominantly lymphocytic variety contain numerous, scattered, "tingible body" macrophages. As a result, a "starry sky" pattern is seen on low power microscopy (Fig. 11). However, the intervening lymphoid cells are cytologically mature, unlike those of small cell noncleaved follicular center cell (Burkitt's) lymphoma, which is associated with a similar histologic appearance (Banks et al. 1975). Furthermore, epithelial cells are usually obvious in the variant of thymoma with a "starry sky" pattern.

Other focal or subtle microscopic features of predominantly lymphocytic thymomas are helpful in distinguishing them from lymphomas. One such change has been called "medullary differentiation" (MD) (Rosai and Levine 1976) because it is reminiscent of the appearance of the normal thymic medulla. Thymomas with MD show rounded, low density areas within the lymphocytic population on low magnification (Fig. 12). These may be confused with germinal centers, or

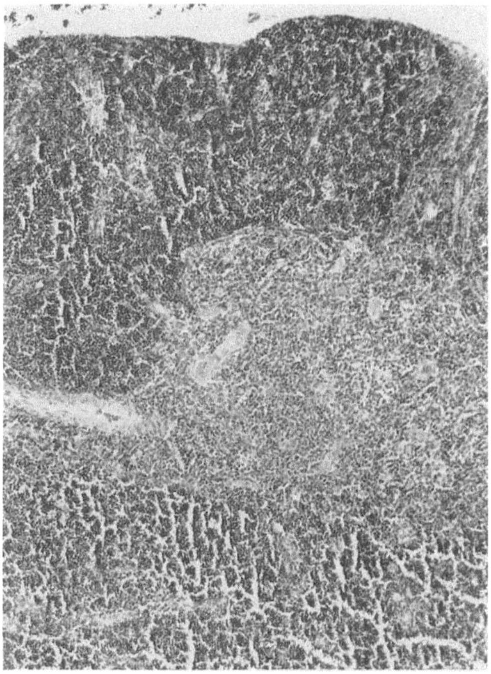

Fig. 9. Remnant of normal thymus, found adjacent to a thymoma. This gland shows a well-defined cortex and medulla

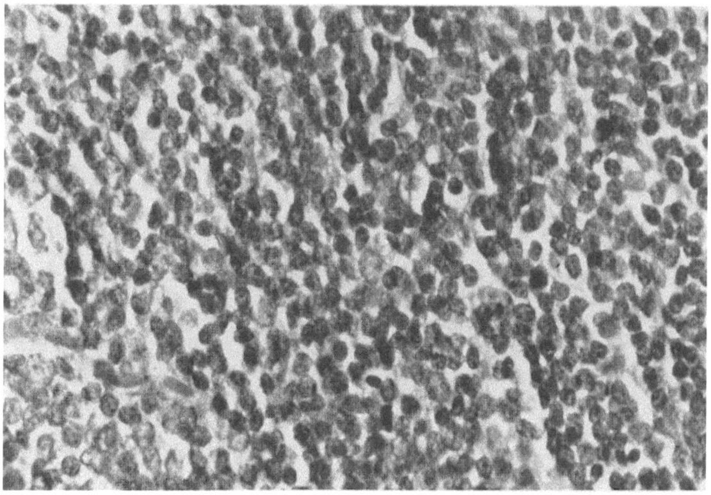

Fig. 10. Some predominantly lymphocytic thymomas contain "activated" lymphocytes, which are slightly larger than normal, with somewhat folded nuclear membranes

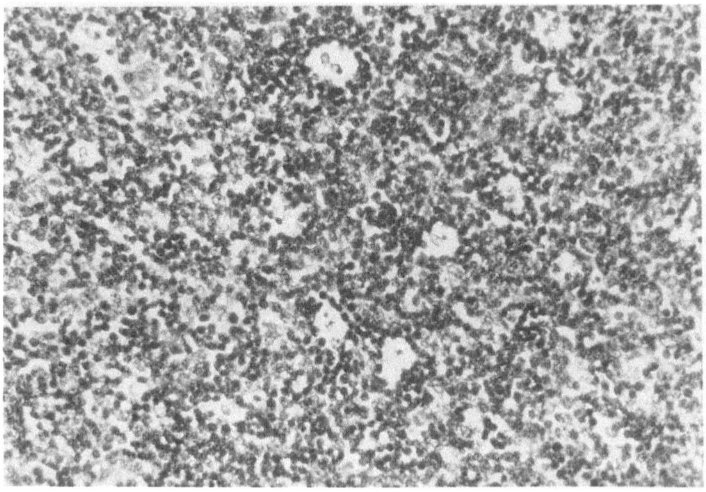

Fig. 11. Predominantly lymphocytic thymoma containing reactive histiocytes. This feature results in a "starry sky" appearance, and may lead to confusion with small cell noncleaved follicular center cell lymphoma

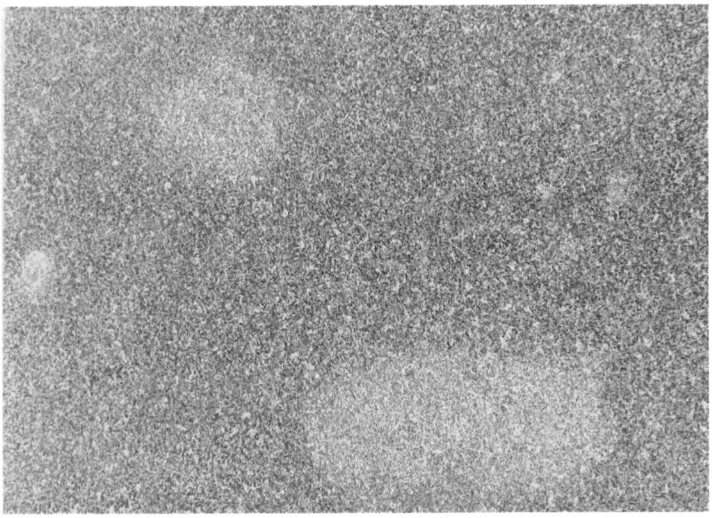

Fig. 12. Predominantly lymphocytic thymoma with medullary differentiation. The medullary differentiation is represented by areas of loose cellular aggregation, and is not seen in lymphomas of the thymus

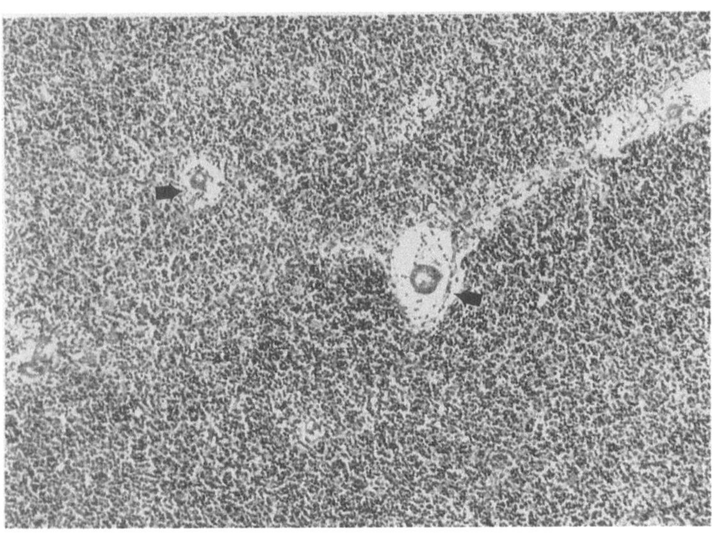

Fig. 13. Perivascular "clearing" by serum lakes *(arrows)* in a predominantly lymphocytic thymoma, a finding which helps to distinguish thymomas from small cell malignant lymphomas

with the neoplastic follicles of nodular lymphoma. However, unlike germinal centers, immunoblasts and tingible body macrophages are not present. In contrast to the follicular structures of nodular lymphoma which are composed of small, closely apposed "cleaved" follicular center cells, areas of MD in thymoma show only loosely aggregated, small, mature lymphocytes. Furthermore, small Hassall's corpuscle-like structures may also be evident within foci of MD. Another feature which differentiates predominantly lymphocytic thymomas from thymic small cell lymphomas is the presence of perivascular spaces ("lakes") and microcystic changes in the epithelial tumors.

Perivascular spaces surround centrally located, intratumoral, capillary or venule-sized blood vessels. The area between these vessels and the basement membrane of bordering epithelial cells is filled with a proteinaceous material, giving it slightly eosinophilic staining characteristics. Lymphocytes, scattered red cells, or foamy macrophages may be suspended within the serous contents (Fig. 13). Occasionally, the perivascular spaces may be replaced with hyaline-like material. Microcysts, on the other hand, are admixed with lymphocytes within the neoplasm itself. They appear as small, sometimes clustered areas of lucency, which may contain occasional degenerating epithelial cells or lymphocytes.

True germinal centers are seen in roughly 10% of all thymomas, again usually of the predominantly lymphocytic type. The germinal center content of thymomas has been reported to be closely related to clinical

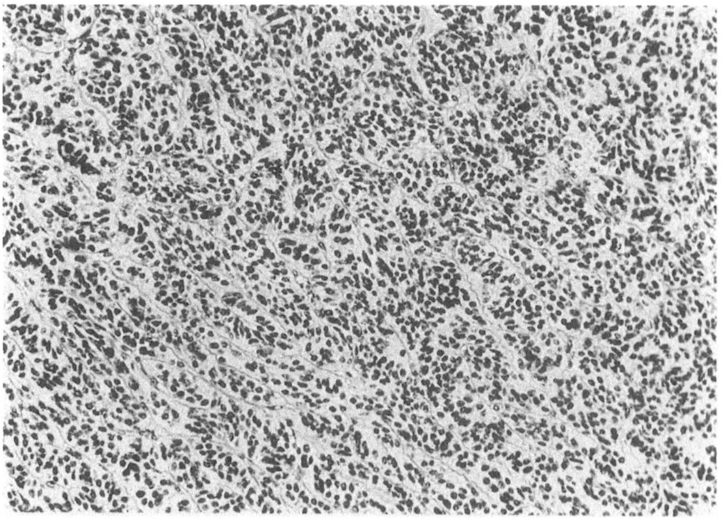

Fig. 14. Organoid growth pattern in a predominantly epithelial thymoma, simulating the appearance of an endocrine tumor

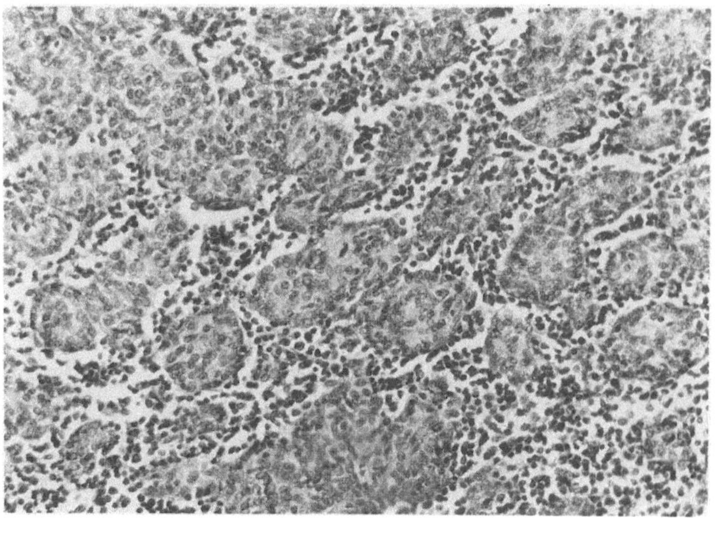

Fig. 15. Pseudorosettes in a mixed lymphoepithelial thymoma. Thymic epithelial cells are clustered around small central blood vessels

myasthenia gravis (Rosai and Levine 1976). The primary alternative to a diagnosis of thymoma in such cases is one of angiofollicular lymph node hyperplasia (Castleman's disease) (Keller et al. 1972). However, thymomas do not show the "onion skin" configuration of plasma cells and lymphocytes around germinal center-like structures, nor the intercellular, eosinophilic material within them, as are seen in angiofollicular lymph node hyperplasia.

At the opposite end of the spectrum, the predominantly epithelial thymomas may express histologic variations which could cause diagnostic confusion with other neoplasms. Neuroendocrine tumors of the thymus (thymic carcinoids) often contain true rosettes (in which the spherically arranged cells enclose open spaces) or pseudorosettes (in which tumor cells surround small blood vessels) (Rosai et al. 1976). Since epithelial thymomas may also assume a vaguely organoid growth pattern as well as displaying rosette or pseudorosette formation (Figs. 14 and 15), in some cases the similarity to thymic carcinoids may be great. Indeed, one of us has seen five tumors with these characteristics in which specialized studies (electron microscopy, histochemistry, and immunohistochemistry) were required to reach a conclusive diagnosis of epithelial thymoma (Wick et al. 1980). A useful stain for the solution of this problem is the chloroacetate esterase (CAE) method (which may be employed with paraffin-embedded tissue). Thymomas tend to show scattered mast cells throughout (Rosai and Levine 1976), as highlighted by the CAE stain, whereas carcinoid tumors do not.

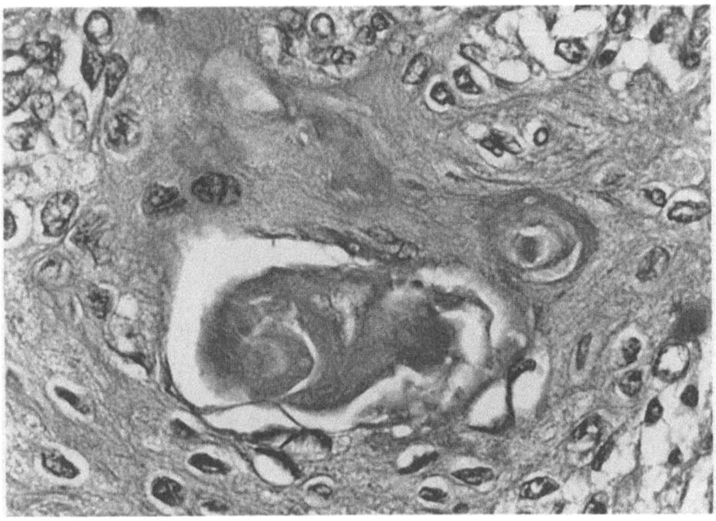

Fig. 16. Keratin "pearl" in a predominantly epithelial thymoma

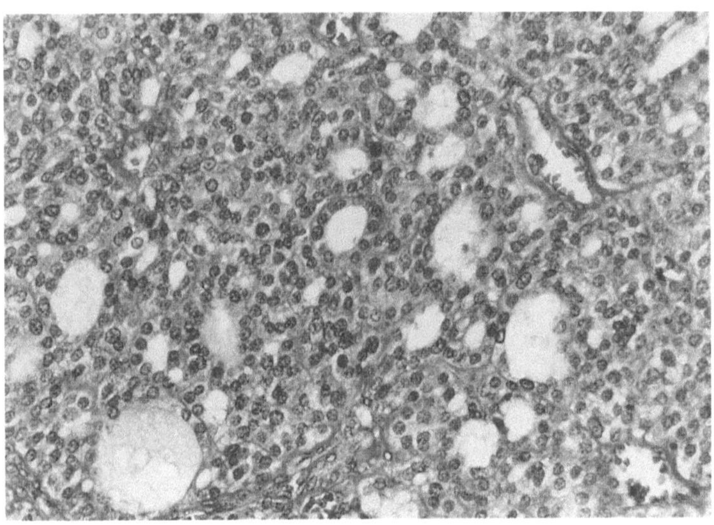

Fig. 17. True glandular spaces in a predominantly epithelial thymoma. These structures, seen in up to 20% of thymomas, may lead to confusion with metastatic adenocarcinoma

Squamous metaplasia is common in thymoma (Fig. 16), with the acquisition of acidophilic, glassy cytoplasm by tumor cells, and a tendency for them to be arranged in incipient keratin "pearls." However, unless care is taken to ensure that the nuclei of the squamoid cells are bland, cases of squamous carcinoma of the thymus will be missed (Wick et al. 1982).

Gland-like spaces are present in up to one-fifth of epithelial thymomas. They are lined by low columnar or cuboidal epithelial cells, and are similar in appearance to thyroid follicles without colloid (Fig. 17). Papillary epithelial formations may sometimes be present within these inclusions. These spaces represent true epithelial structures made up of thymic epithelium, and may cause confusion with metastases of adenocarcinoma to the thymus. This possibility is excluded by the overall appearance and cellular content of the tumor, which is in general typical of thymoma, as outlined already.

A distinctive variant of epithelial thymoma is that in which the tumor cells assume a spindled appearance, causing a resemblance to mesenchymal neoplasms. If a prominent vascular stroma (Fig. 18) or a storiform growth pattern (Fig. 19) accompanies the spindle-cell change, diagnoses of hemangiopericytoma or fibrous histiocytoma may alternatively be considered. However, experience with this spectrum of neoplasms indicates that most spindle cell tumors of the anterosuperior mediastinum are of thymic epithelial origin (Lowenhaupt 1948; Rosai and Levine 1976). In such cases, short, blunt, spindle cells are grouped cohesively into an organoid pattern. Cells at the periphery of epithelial nests are often oriented in parallel with one another, giving a palisaded appearance (Fig. 20). The intervening tumor stroma is densely fibrous.

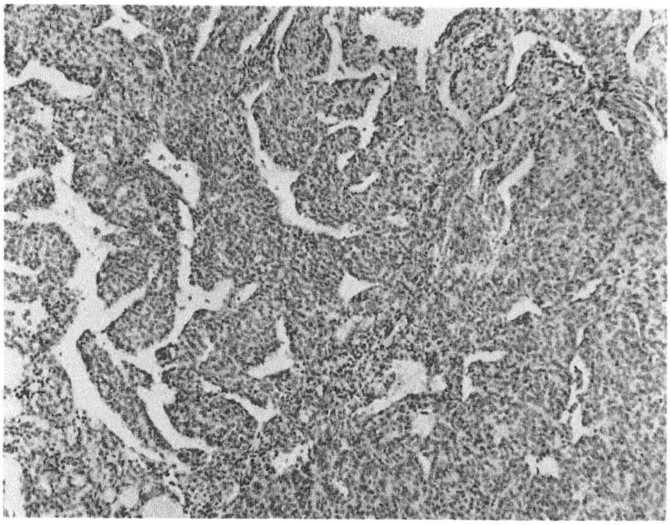

Fig. 18. Hemangiopericytoma-like vascular pattern in a thymoma. Most, if not all, neoplasms of the anterior mediastinum with this appearance are of thymic epithelial, rather than mesenchymal, origin

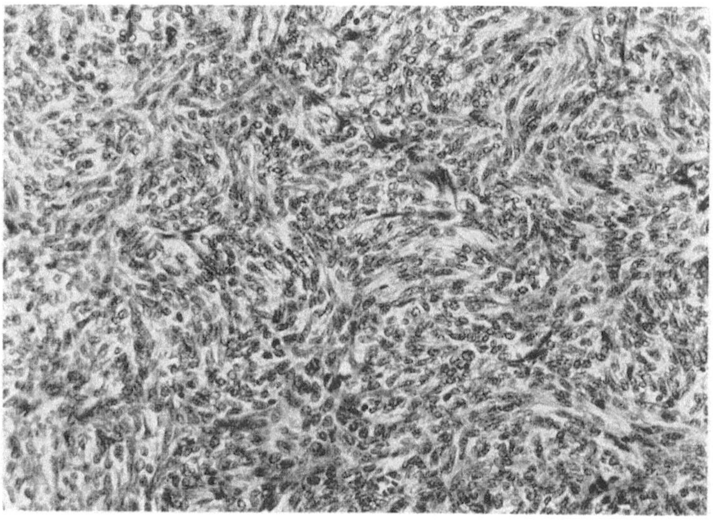

Fig. 19. Storiform arrangement of tumor cells in a spindle cell thymoma, a finding which may lead to confusion with fibrous histiocytomas

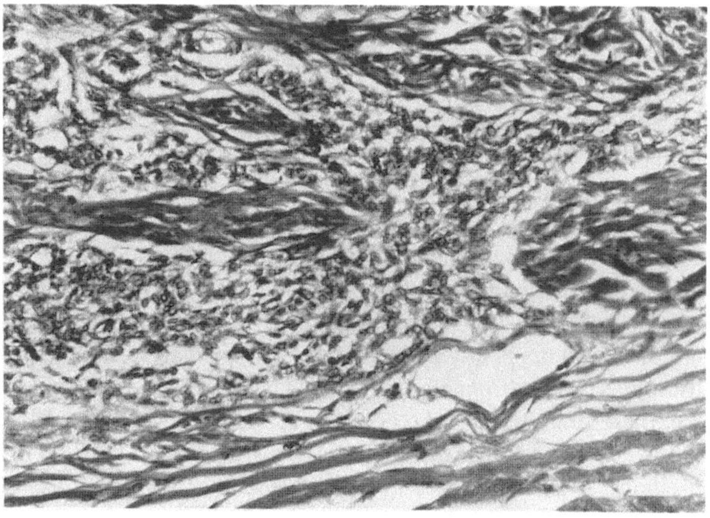

Fig. 20. "Adamantinoma-like" epithelial thymoma, in which nests of blunt spindle cells are separated by broad bands of stromal collagen. Nuclear palisading is sometimes seen at the periphery of tumor cell clusters

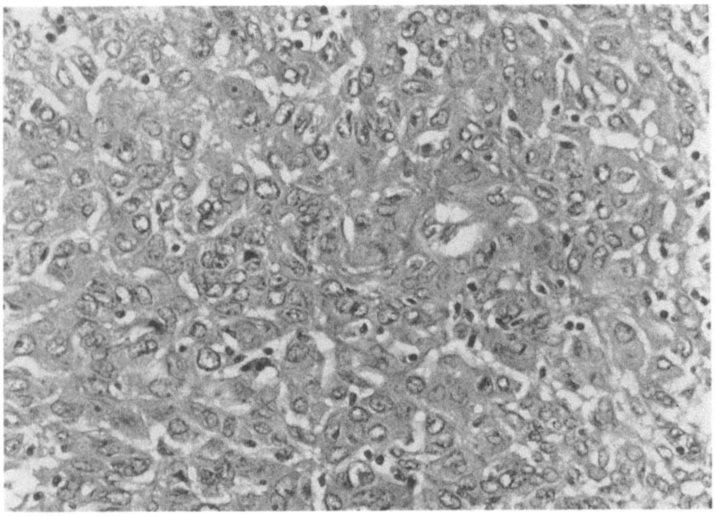

Fig. 21. Cellular atypia in a predominantly epithelial thymoma. Moderate nuclear pleomorphism, vesicular chromatin, and occasional nucleoli may raise the possibility of thymic carcinoma

Nuclear Atypia

A spectrum of cytologic atypia may be seen in the epithelial cells of thymomas, e. g., nuclear pleomorphism, hyperchromasia, and nucleolar prominence (Fig. 21). These changes may be either focal or diffuse. In some cases, it can be quite difficult to determine whether an atypical thymic epithelial neoplasm should be called a thymoma or a thymic carcinoma. However, as will be discussed later in this chapter, thymic carcinomas usually display nucleolar prominence, abundant mitotic activity, markedly increased nuclear: cytoplasmic ratios, and multifocal spontaneous necrosis, in addition to the nuclear changes just described. The distinction between thymoma and thymic carcinoma is an important one because of the marked difference in their clinical behavior.

Electron Microscopy

The ultrastructural features of thymomas bear a striking similarity to those of the normal gland (Levine and Bensch 1972; Levine and al. 1975; Pascoe and Miner 1976; Rosai and Levin 1976; Shier 1981). Since the proliferating element in these tumors is the thymic epithelial cell, the electron microscopic diagnosis of thymoma rests on the identification of this cell's characteristics. Epithelial cells of the thymus and of thymomas have oval or slightly irregular nuclei, with evenly distributed heterochromatin and small nucleoli (Fig. 22). These features are in accord with corresponding histologic attributes. The cytoplasm contains the usual metabolic organelles, as well as broad, electron-dense skeins of cytokeratin-containing intermediate filaments (tonofilaments) (Fig. 23). Long, overlapping cytoplasmic extensions, which may traverse relatively long distances before joining to one another (Fig. 24), are typical. Junctions between the epithelial cells are well formed and desmosomal in nature (see Fig. 23) and, not uncommonly, tonofilaments may be seen inserting into them. Basal lamina is regularly present

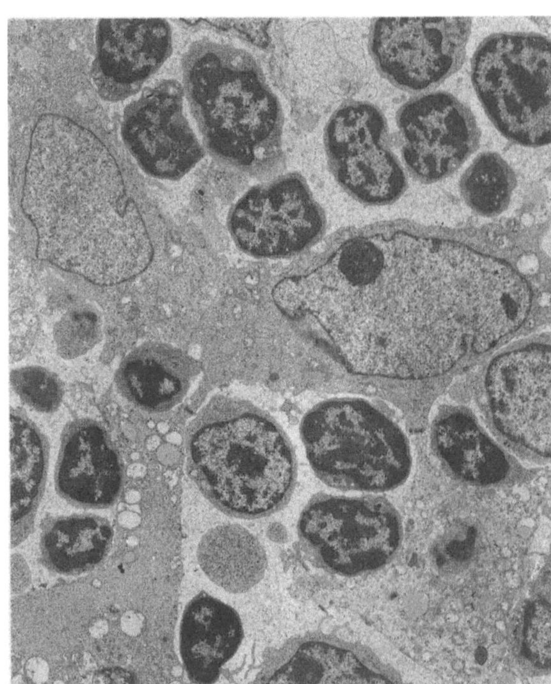

Fig. 22. Electron micrograph of a mixed lymphoepithelial thymoma. Epithelial cells are large, with evenly distributed chromatin, and are attached to one another through desmosomal junctions. Reactive lymphocytes are numerous

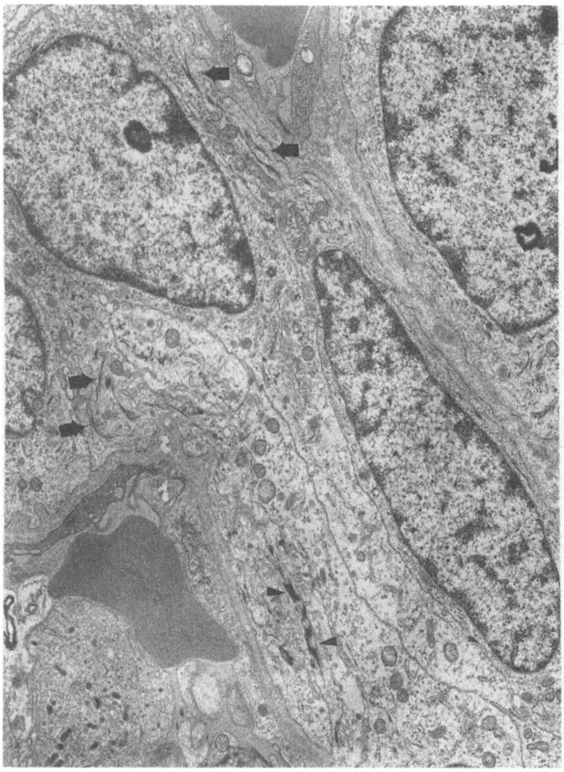

Fig. 23. Ultrastructural study of a thymoma showing, typically, cytoplasmic tonofilaments *(arrows)*, and intercellular desmosomes *(arrowheads)*, into which such filaments insert

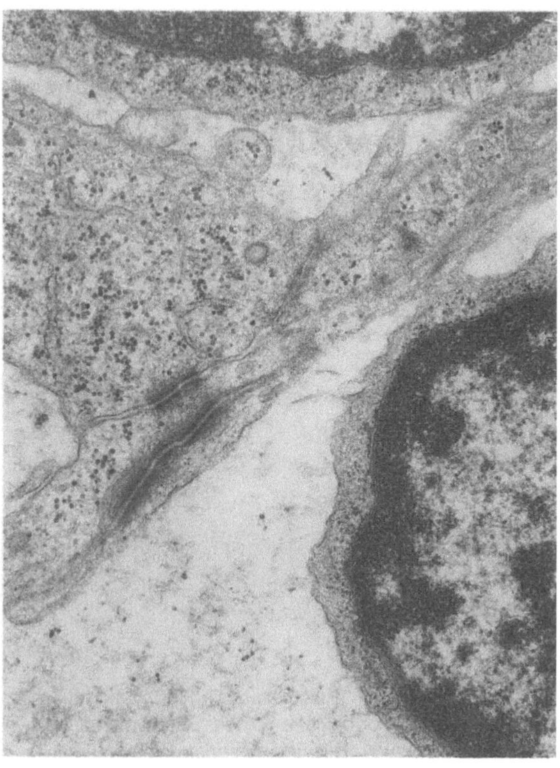

along the plasma membranes of cytoplasmic extensions.

In predominantly lymphocytic or lymphoepithelial thymomas, the reactive lymphoid population is composed of cells with smooth borders, compact nuclei, and few organelles. This is consistent with immunologic and immunohistochemical data (Griffin et al. 1978; Wick et al. 1981; Reddick and Jennette 1983; Chan et al. 1984; Sato et al. 1986) showing that intratumoral lymphocytes in thymomas are T cells. Careful study may be necessary to find epithelial cells or their extensions in order to make a definite diagnosis of predominantly lymphocytic thymoma.

Immunohistochemistry

Immunocytochemical studies, using either the peroxidase-antiperoxidase (PAP) or avidin-biotin-peroxidase complex (ABC) methods, may be of value in selected cases in confirming the thymomatous nature of a mediastinal mass. The epithelial cells of thymomas express keratin proteins (Battifora et al. 1980) and epithelial membrane antigen (EMA) (Figs. 25 and 26; Lewis et al. 1987) in contrast to the large lymphoid cells and histiocytes with which they may be confused in predominantly lymphocytic lesions. Conversely, common leukocyte antigen (CLA) is lacking in thymic epithelial cells, but this determinant is expressed by virtually all lymphoid cells (Kurtin and Pinkus 1985; Kodama et al. 1986). Hence, a panel of anti-cytokeratin, anti-EMA, and anti-CLA antibodies will usually suffice to distinguish between predominantly lymphocytic or mixed lymphoepithelial thymoma and small cell or mixed large-small cell lymphoma. This differential diagnosis is one which is typically problematic for the histopathologist, especially in needle biopsy or aspiration cytology specimens.

Anti-cytokeratin and anti-EMA are also quite useful in differentiating pure spindle cell thymomas, which are cytokeratin- and EMA-reactive (Fig. 27; Lewis et al. 1987; Wick, unpublished observations), from mesenchymal tumors, which are not. Furthermore, anti-vimentin will bind to the latter of these groups of neoplasms (Osborn and Weber 1983), whereas in our experience thymomas are vimentin-negative (unpublished observations).

Fig. 24. Long cytoplasmic extensions in a thymoma, joined to each other by desmosomes. The nuclei are those of surrounding reactive lymphocytes

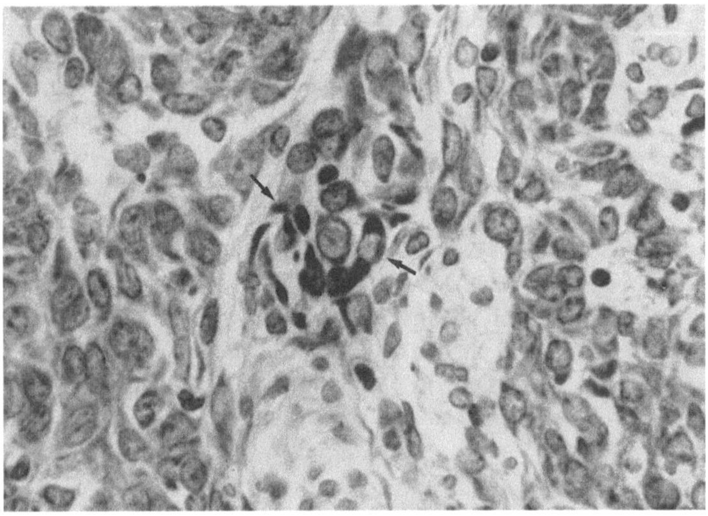

Fig. 25. Immunoreactivity for cytokeratin *(arrows)* in a thymoma

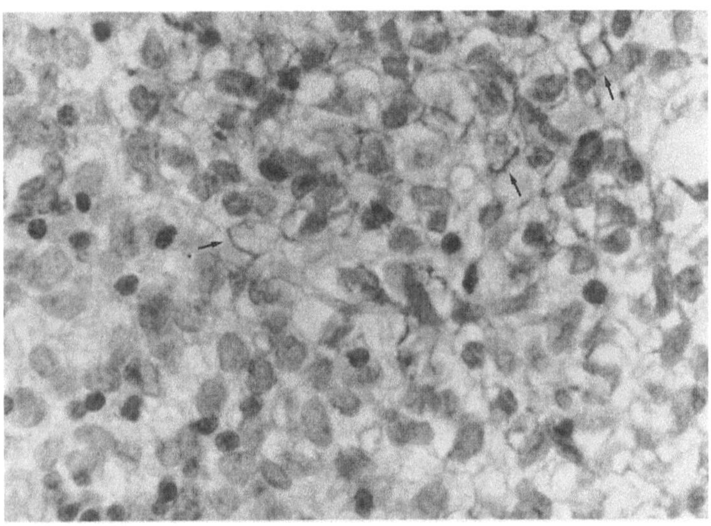

Fig. 26. Delicate labeling of epithelial membrane antigen in tumor cells of a thymoma *(arrows)* by the immunoperoxidase technique

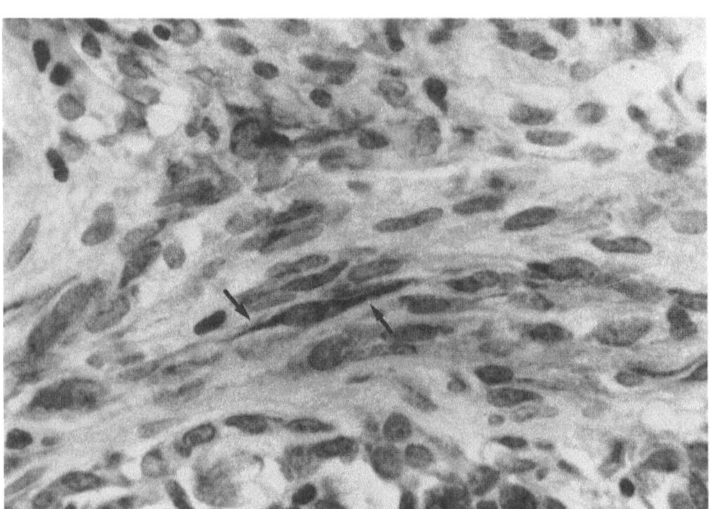

Fig. 27. Positive staining for cytokeratin in a tumor cell of a spindle cell thymoma *(arrows)*. This finding separates spindle cell thymomas from mesenchymal neoplasms

Recent studies have utilized monoclonal antibodies against specific lymphoid differentiation antigens to study the lymphocyte population of predominantly lymphocytic thymomas. These have shown a preponderance of OKT6-positive and terminal deoxynucleotidyl transferase (TdT)-positive cells, with an almost complete absence of OKT3-reactive lymphocytes (mature thymic lymphocytes) (Chan et al. 1984). A variable number of cells with the OKT8 (suppressor) phenotype have been observed, with the tentative conclusion that this subpopulation is reduced within thymomas associated with myasthenia gravis (Chan et al. 1984). Both the reactive lymphocytes and epithelial cells of predominantly lymphocytic thymomas have been shown to express the Leu-7 and HLA-DR antigens. The former of these markers is usually detected focally on epithelial cells bordering perivascular serum lakes (Chan et al. 1984).

These data on OKT, Leu, and HLA-DR immunoreactivity could cause diagnostic misadventures if employed alone in the evaluation of mediastinal tumors. Lymphoblastic lymphoma and well-differentiated lymphocytic lymphoma are characterized respectively by OKT6 and TdT positivity, and HLA-DR reactivity (Knowles 1985). This emphasizes the need for inclusion of epithelial cell markers in the immunocytochemical assessment of thymomas. Immunoreactivity for such thymic "hormones" as thymosin and serum thymic factor in normal thymic epithelium has been reported (Bach 1979; Wara 1981). However, no convincing reports are available on the presence of these hormones in thymomas. Thus, their use as specific markers for thymic epithelial neoplasms remains to be determined.

Needle Biopsy and Aspiration Cytology

Needle biopsies and aspiration cytologic studies have been performed increasingly often in the last 10 years to obtain a histologic diagnosis of mediastinal masses (Rosenberger and Adler 1978; Haaga 1979; Sajjad et al. 1982; Sterett et al. 1983). These techniques may provide surgeons with useful information for planning definitive treatment procedures. As experience with such specimens has grown, the diagnostic confidence of pathologists dealing with them has improved commensurately.

Nevertheless, certain well-defined problems continue to apply to the needle biopsy diagnosis of thymomas. Particularly in predominantly lymphocytic and spindle cell epithelial neoplasms, it may be impossible to exclude the possibilities of small cell malignant lymphoma and mesenchymal lesions, respectively, by conventional microscopic study. It is in these circumstances that such special techniques as immunocytochemistry make a valuable diagnostic contribution.

In addition, there is no way that needle biopsies or aspiration cytologic procedures can predict the potential invasiveness of thymoma, as seen at ensuing thoracotomy. This, however, is not a major issue, as surgery is recommended for both encapsulated and invasive thymomas (with debulking in the latter instance) (Chahinian et al. 1981).

Encapsulated and Invasive Thymomas

The most important factor in predicting the behavior of a thymoma is the encapsulation of the tumor, or the lack of it. Neoplasms which have intact fibrous capsules and are not densely adherent to mediastinal structures are curable by surgical excision alone in 85%–90% of cases. Conversely, those which invade contiguous soft tissues, the lung, the adventitia of the great vessels, or the pericardium are likely to recur if adjuvant therapy is not administered postoperatively. Hence, it is obvious that careful gross inspection of tumors submitted to the pathology laboratory, and multiple microscopic sections of their capsules, are indicated in all cases. In addition, excellent communication between the surgeon and pathologist concerning the in situ characteristics of thymomas is essential. Four clinical stages have been described with respect to these tumors (Masaoka et al. 1981). Stage I includes completely encapsulated thymomas without microscopic invasion of the calpsule; stage II denotes macroscopic invasion of the mediastinal fat or pleura, or microscopic invasion of the capsule; stage III corresponds to macroscopic invasion of neighboring organs (i.e., pericardium, great vessels, lungs); and stage IV implies pleural or pericardial seeding or distant metastasis.

Somewhat surprisingly, there is a definite risk of recurrence for totally encapsulated neoplasms, although it is small. Fechner (1969) has reported several examples of this phenomenon, and 15% of encapsulated thymomas seen at the Mayo Clinic showed subsequent recurrence. In such cases, reoperation and radiotherapy are suggested.

"Invasive thymoma" is the preferred term for tumors showing infiltrative growth, yet retaining a typically bland cytologic appearance. These lesions have often been referred to as "malignant thymoma" in the past; however, this term can cause confusion with thymic *carcinoma*, and thus should be discarded. Invasive thymomas require postoperative radiotherapy for adequate control (Penn and Hope-Stone 1972; Marks et al. 1978; Arriagada et al. 1981) and the combination of radiotherapy and chemotherapy has also been employed with good results (Boston 1976; Shellito et al. 1978; Evans et al. 1980; Needles et al. 1981). However, the 10-year survival rate for patients with invasive thymoma is inferior to that for encapsulated tumors, in spite of radiotherapy (Bernatz et al. 1973; Masaqka et al. 1981). Newer treatment regimens may equalize survival in these two groups, but this remains to be proven.

Metastasizing Thymoma

Thymomas may demonstrate implantation on pleural surfaces (either visceral or parietal) at surgery, or subsequent to it (Fig. 28). As expected, invasive tumors are most likely to show such behavior. Whether this phenomenon represents true metastasis or pleural fluid-mediated implantation is a matter of controversy; however, the incidence of *embolic* spread of thymoma to *extrathoracic* sites is extremely low (<5%) (Rachmaninoff and Fentress 1964; Gravanis 1968; Nickels and Franssila 1976; MacDonald et al. 1978; Baud et al. 1981; Needles et al. 1981). In the Mayo Clinic's experience, 8 of 283 neoplasms displayed true metastasis to cervical lymph nodes, bones, liver, brain, or peripheral soft tissues. One remarkable case showed selective involvement of cranial and peripheral nerves (Wick et al. 1981). Osseous implants tended to be blastic radiographically (Fig. 29) and occurred most often with predominantly epithelial tumors; a minority of them manifested nuclear atypia, but the other criteria required for a diagnosis of thymic carcinoma were not fulfilled.

We agree with Lattes (1962), Gravanis (1968), Salyer and Eggleston (1976), and LeGolvan and Abell (1977) that there are no reliable histologic features which predict potential metastatic behavior in thymomas, while emphasizing that this statement specifically excludes cytologically malignant tumors from consideration. An appropriate diagnostic term for these thymomas is the simply descriptive "metastasizing thymoma." Recent case reports have documented the efficacy of chemotherapy for thymomas which have spread outside the thorax (Needles et al. 1981).

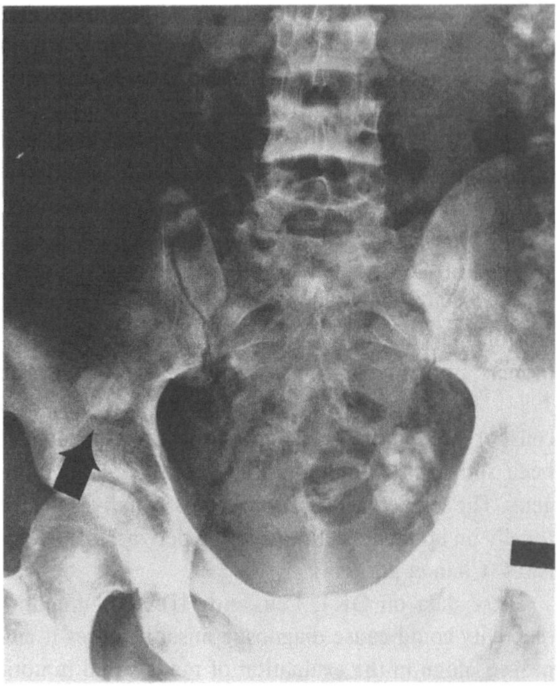

Fig. 29. Metastasizing thymoma with secondary implant in the pelvic bones. The implant is blastic roentgenographically *(arrow)*. This neoplasm was predominantly lymphocytic, and lacked cytologic evidence of malignancy

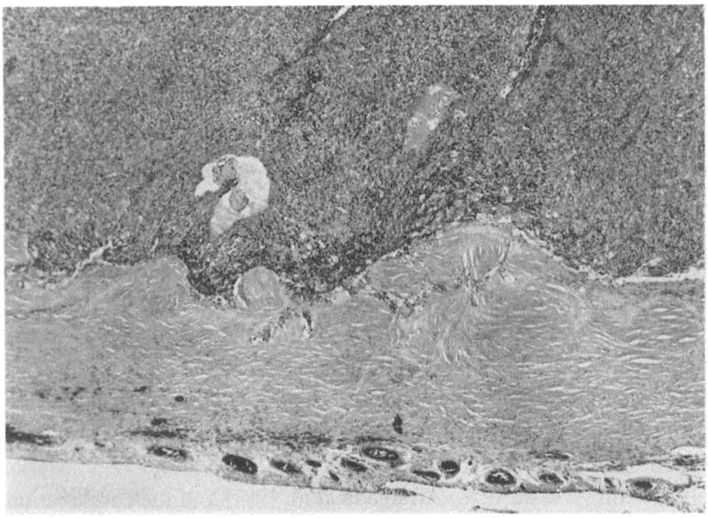

Fig. 28. Tumor implant of thymoma in the parietal pleura, which contains dilated blood vessels

Relationship Between Histologic Features and Clinical Behavior

A substantial amount of conflicting information has been offered on the relationship between microscopic types of thymoma and their clinical behavior. Topics included under this heading concern the relative incidence of paraneoplastic syndromes, the risk of recurrence and extrathoracic metastasis, and overall survival, as related to different microscopic patterns.

Previous publications have stated that subcategorization of thymomas into predominantly lymphocytic, mixed lymphoepithelial, and predominantly epithelial types had little practical application (Rosai and Levine 1976). However, in a recent review of 283 cases of thymoma seen at the Mayo Clinic, Lewis et al. (1985) found that overall death rates were 44 per 1000 patient years for predominantly lymphocytic thymomas, 76 for mixed lymphoepithelial tumors, and 93 for predominantly epithelial neoplasms (excluding spindle cell lesions). These data approach statistical significance ($P < 0.1$) and are similar to the results obtained by Masaoka et al. (1981). Maggi et al. (1986) found that survival was significantly diminished in the lymphoepithelial group in a study of 169 cases of thymoma (76% 5-year survival compared with 88% for predominantly lymphocytic and predominantly epithelial types, respectively; $P < 0.05$). Admittedly, multiple sections of each neoplasm must be studied in order to assign an accurate microscopic classification of this type, and the influence of the latter on prognosis remains controversial.

In the past, the significance of nuclear atypia in predominantly epithelial tumors had been reported to be unrelated to the clinical outcome in the absence of overt cytologic malignancy, and there were no microscopic features which reliably correlated with the clinical course of thymomas (Gravanis 1968; Levine 1973; Salyer and Eggleston 1976; LeGolvan and Abell 1977; Gray and Gutowski 1979). However, in the group of 283 Mayo cases referred to, nuclear atypia (without other features of overt carcinoma) was linked to a higher rate of local recurrence and extrathoracic metastasis ($P < 0.004$). This finding is not totally unexpected, in view of the concept that thymoma and thymic carcinoma show similar cellular differentiation; thus, it is likely that intermediate forms between the two will show occasionally aggressive behavior. Indeed, we have seen several cases in which some microscopic sections would have yielded a diagnosis of atypical thymoma, while others demonstrated overt carcinoma.

At present, the therapeutic implications of finding nuclear atypia in any given thymoma are unclear, since the behavioral propensities just discussed are statistical, and as such are applicable to a *group* of tumors, rather than to individual neoplasms. Close monitoring of all patients with atypical thymomas with regular (e.g., twice yearly) physical and radiographic examinations, seems advisable. However, there appears no justification at present for advocating adjuvant radiation treatment or chemotherapy in such cases, in the absence of macroscopic invasion or metastasis at initial surgery.

With respect to microscopic subtypes of thymoma and their relationship to paraneoplastic syndromes, it would seem that only two statements can be made with any degree of confidence (Rosai and Levine 1976): (1) myasthenia gravis is usually associated with histologic types of thymoma *other* than spindle cell tumors; and (2) acquired erythroid hypoplasia or hypogammaglobulinemia are typically found *in conjunction with* spindle cell thymomas.

Differential Diagnosis

Throughout this section, we have pointed out the differential diagnostic considerations of thymomas. Simply put, if one excludes obviously cytologically malignant lesions, the possibilities include small cell and mixed malignant lymphoma of the thymic region, carcinoid tumor of the thymus, spindle cell mesenchymal neoplasms, angiofollicular lymphoid hyperplasia, and thymic cysts (Rosai and Levine, 1976). The last of these lesions are distinguished from cystic thymoma on conventional gross and microscopic examination; they contain only a simple squamous or low columnar lining, without evidence of discrete foci of neoplastic epithelial proliferation (Fig. 30). Tables 1-3 summarize the findings of special studies which may be required to reach a final diagnosis of thymoma or another of these tumors.

Prognostic Factors

Patients presenting at age 60 or older were found to have a higher actuarial fatality rate due to tumor growth in the Mayo Clinic study, as were patients with tumors 10 cm in diameter or greater. Conversely, no neoplasm under 5 cm recurred or led to death. The presence of symptoms of mediastinal structural displacement was also a poor prognostic indicator in this study.

Earlier reports had documented a negative influence on survival by tumor-related myasthenia gravis (Bernatz et al. 1973; Rosai and Levine 1976). However,

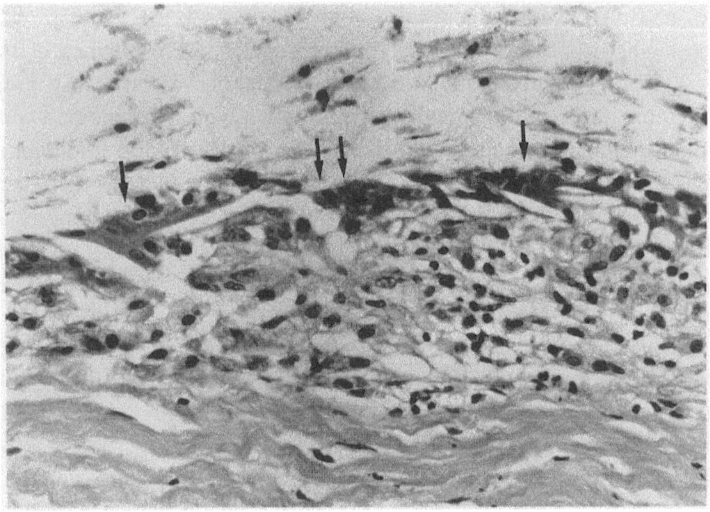

Fig. 30. Lining of a simple thymic cyst, composed of flattened and cuboidal epithelial cells *(arrows)*

Table 1. Light microscopic findings in thymoma and its differential diagnostic alternatives

Tumor	Lobulation	MD	PSL	Micro-cysts	Lymphoid cells	Rosettes/pseudo-rosettes	Organoid growth	Stromal hemorrhage/cholesterol
Predominantly lymphocytic thymoma	++-+++	++	+	±	+++	0	0	0
Epithelial thymoma	++-+++	0	++	±	±-+	±-+	0-±	0-++
Spindle cell thymoma	++-+++	0	±	±	±	0	0	0
Angiofollicular lymphoid hyperplasia	0	0	0	0	+++	0	0	0
Small or mixed small-large cell lymphomas	0	0	0	0	+++	0	0	0
Hemangiopericytoma	0	0	0	0	0	0	0	0
Fibrous histiocytoma	0	0	0	0	0	0	0	0
Thymic cysts	0	0	0	0[a]	+-++	0	0	++-+++
Carcinoid of thymus	0	0	0	0	±	++-+++	++-+++	0

MD medullary differentiation; PSL perivascular serum lakes; 0 absent; + focally present or observed in less than all cases; ± variably present; ++ uniformly present; +++ uniformly present and prominent

[a] Thymic cysts may show small outpouchings of main cyst wall microscopically.

Table 2. Electron microscopic features of thymoma and its differential diagnostic alternatives

Tumor	ECP	PBM	Tonofil	CIF	ICJ	PCL	Pinocytosis	CDB	NSG
Thymoma (all variants)	++	++	++	±	++(D)	0	0	0	0
Malignant lymphoma	0	0	0	±	0	±	0	0	0
Thymic carcinoid	0	+	±	+[a]	+(MA)	0	0	0	++-+++
Hemangiopericytoma	±	+	0	+	+(AP)	0	+-++	++	0
Fibrous histiocytoma	±	0	0	±	±(AP)	+-++	0	0	0

ECP elongated cellular processes; PBM pericellular basement membrane; Tonofil cytoplasmic tonofilaments; CIF cytoplasmic intermediate filaments; ICJ intercellular junctions; D desmosomes; MA maculae adherentes; AP appositional plaques; PCL prominent cytoplasmic lysosomes; CDB cytoplasmic dense bodies; NSG neurosecretory granules; 0 absent; ± variably present; + present focally; ++ uniformly present; +++ uniformly present and prominent

[a] Intermediate filaments in thymic carcinoid are often localized to perinuclear cytoplasm, and whorled.

Table 3. Immunohistologic findings in thymoma and its differential diagnostic alternatives

Tumor	EMA	CKER	NSE	VIM	ACT	AACT	CLA	Chromogranin
Thymoma (all variants)	+	+	±	0	0	0	+[a]	0
Malignant lymphoma	0	0	0	±[b]	0	±[b]	+	0
Thymic carcinoid	±	±	+	0	0	0	0	+
Hemangiopericytoma	0	0	0	+	±	0	0	0
Fibrous histiocytoma	0	0	0	+	±	+	0	0
Angiofollicular lymphoid hyperplasia	0	0	0	±[c]	+[c]	0	+[a]	0

EMA epithelial membrane antigen; CKER cytokeratin; NSE neuron-specific enolase; VIM vimentin; ACT actin; AACT α-1-antichymotrypsin; CLA common leukocyte antigen; 0 absent; ± variably, present; + present
[a] Reactivity is confined to reactive lymphoid cells.
[b] Reactivity is confined to large cells of mixed small-large cell lymphomas.
[c] Reactivity is confined to proliferating vascular elements.

most recent series have not shown a statistically significant association between this syndrome and heightened mortality (Verley and Hollmann 1985; Maggi et al. 1986). Others with acquired erythroid hypoplasia or hypogammaglobulinemia did manifest diminished survival, but this was of borderline significance statistically.

Pure spindle cell epithelial neoplasms seem to behave in a relatively innocuous fashion, rarely causing fatality, and should not be included with *type ordinaire* epithelial thymomas for prognostic purposes. Nevertheless, as pointed out by Masaoka et al. (1981) and Bergh et al. (1978) high tumor stage at diagnosis (invasion of mediastinal structures, pleural implants, distant metastases) again has an adverse effect on survival.

Thymic Carcinoma

Thymic carcinoma is the best designation for tumors derived from thymic epithelium which are cytologically malignant. Thus, an adequate distinction is made from the invasive (and thus biologically malignant) but cytologically bland neoplasms (i.e., thymomas). These two groups of tumors differ significantly in their clinical behavior, making such a separation both justifiable and desirable.

Relatively little has been written on the clinicopathologic features of thymic carcinomas. There are three reasons for this:

1. Many tumors in early reports on "carcinomas of the thymus" were later recognized to have been in reality malignant lymphomas, germ cell tumors, or carcinomas metastatic to the thymus (Ewing 1916; Jacobsen 1923; Lemann and Smith 1926; Bedford 1930; Symmers 1932; Lowenhaupt and Brown 1951). This discredited the concept of primary thymic carcinoma for many years;
2. Thymic carcinomas are rare - only 16 cytologically malignant neoplasms of the thymic epithelium were found in a review of Mayo Clinic cases seen over a 75-year period (Wick et al. 1982);
3. Even today, there are few specific pathologic findings which can be relied on to distinguish primary thymic carcinomas from metastatic neoplasms to which they are histologically similar.

Clinical Features

The clinical presentation of thymic carcinomas is similar to that of thymomas, with the exception that symptoms of mediastinal structural displacement are more frequent and may evolve more rapidly (Wick et al. 1982); radiographic or clinical evidence of extrathoracic metastasis is also more likely to be present at diagnosis. Myasthenia gravis, acquired erythroid hypoplasia, or hypogammaglobulinemia have not been reported in association with thymic carcinoma.

Gross Characteristics

In general, thymic carcinomas lack the well-defined fibrous encapsulation and internal septation of thymomas, although occasional specimens may appear to be totally encapsulated at initial presentation. The cut surfaces of thymic carcinomas are typically rubbery or gritty and gray-white; areas of necrosis and hemorrhage are common (Fig. 31). Cystic change has been reported only rarely as discussed later. Snover et al. (1982) have described a mucoepidermoid carcinoma of the thymus which had a gelatinous or "slimy" cut

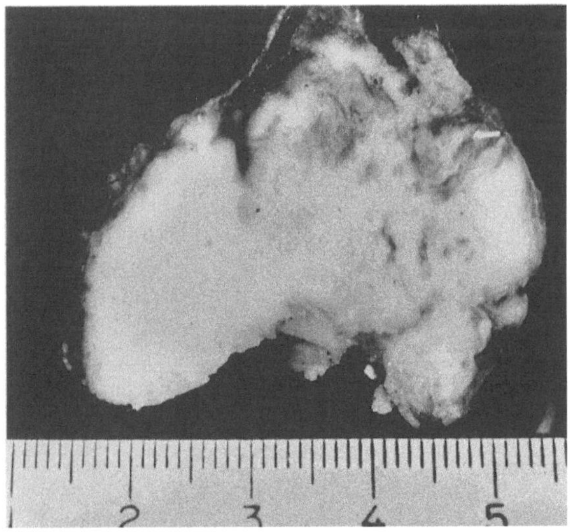

Fig. 31. Characteristic macroscopic appearance of thymic carcinoma. The tumor lacks obvious fibrous septation and encapsulation, and contains foci of necrosis and hemorrhage

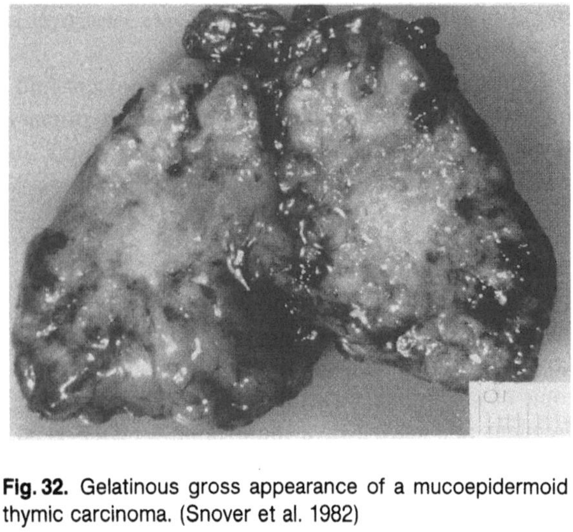

Fig. 32. Gelatinous gross appearance of a mucoepidermoid thymic carcinoma. (Snover et al. 1982)

surface (Fig. 32), as well as a case of a grossly cystic thymic basaloid carcinoma. Leong and Brown (1984) documented a cystic squamous carcinoma.

Microscopic Characteristics

Although thymic carcinomas are extremely rare, several distinctive microscopic variants are currently recognized. These will be discussed in order of their relative frequency.

Lymphoepithelioma-like squamous carcinoma (Levine and Rosai 1978; Rosai 1981; Wick et al. 1982; Marino and Müller-Hermelink 1985) is composed of sheets or nests of oval or round cells, with large, vesicular nuclei and prominent eosinophilic nucleoli. Nucleocytoplasmic ratios are high, the cytoplasm is amphophilic with indistinct cell borders, and mitoses are numerous (Figs. 33 and 34). Areas of spontaneous intratumoral necrosis are commonly seen. As this description is virtually identical to that of "lymphoepithelioma" of the nasopharynx (poorly differentiated squamous carcinoma) (Easton et al. 1980), the term "lymphoepithelioma-like thymic carcinoma" is appropriate for diagnostic use.

Keratinizing squamous carcinoma (Thomson and Thackray 1957; Shimosato et al. 1977; Easton et al. 1980; Rosai 1981; Wick et al. 1982; Swinborne-Sheldrake et al. 1985) is composed of tumor cells with large, hyperchromatic nuclei and a moderate amount of acidophilic, occasionally "glassy" cytoplasm. Nucleocytoplasmic ratios are again high, and mitoses are easily found. The distinctive feature of these neoplasms is the formation of keratin pearls, which are concentric arrangements of tumor cells in association with extracellular keratin (Fig. 35). Either a sheet-like or an organoid growth pattern may be seen; occasionally there is a predominantly spindle cell, yet obviously clustered, epithelial appearance (Fig. 36; Wick et al. 1982). Leong and Brown (1984) have described a keratinizing squamous thymic carcinoma which was a mural nodule in an otherwise typical thymic cyst, lined by variably dysplastic squamous epithelium.

Basaloid squamous carcinoma (Snover et al. 1982) is composed of small, uniform, polygonal cells with scanty amphophilic cytoplasm. Nuclei are oval, with equally distributed chromatin, indistinct nucleoli, and high nucleocytoplasmic ratios (Fig. 37). Mitoses are abundant, and small foci of metaplastic-type keratinizing squamous cells may be interspersed throughout these neoplasms. Tumor cells ar arranged in nests or trabeculae, with a palisaded nuclear configuration at their periphery (Fig. 38). Gland-like spaces may also be observed, the contents of which contain weakly periodic acid-Schiff (PAS)- and mucicarmine-positive material. The two examples of basaloid thymic carcinoma described by Snover et al. (1982) appeared to be intimately related to thymic cyst-like structures which were lined by squamoid, focally dysplastic cells, and were associated with contiguous cholesterol clefts and hemorrhage.

Clear cell thymic carcinoma. Two cases have been reported by Snover et al. (1982) and by Wolfe et al. (1983). Both consisted of sheets of polygonal cells with

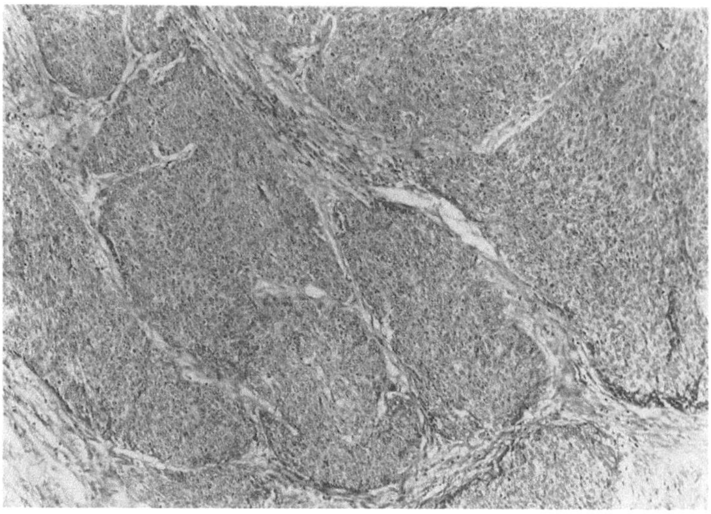

Fig. 33. Lymphoepithelioma-like variant of thymic carcinoma. Clusters of neoplastic cells are separated by a fine fibrovascular stroma, and may superficially recall the appearance of conventional thymomas on low power microscopy

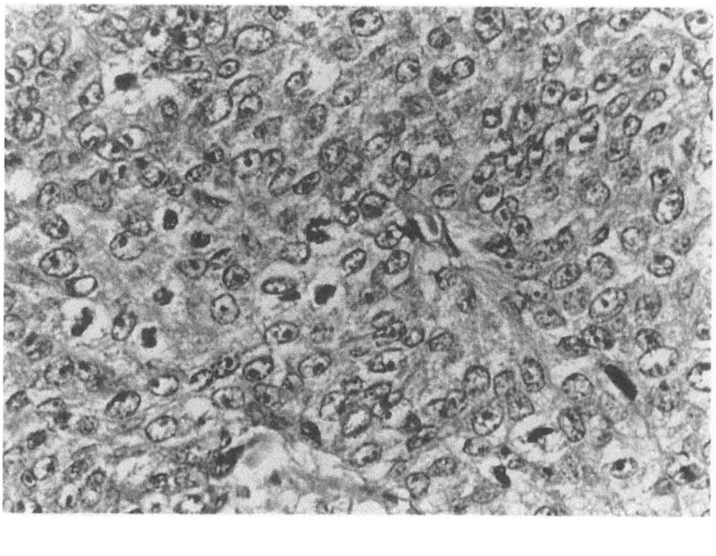

Fig. 34. High power view of the neoplasm shown in Fig. 33. Tumor cells have large vesicular nuclei with prominent nucleoli. Mitoses are evident

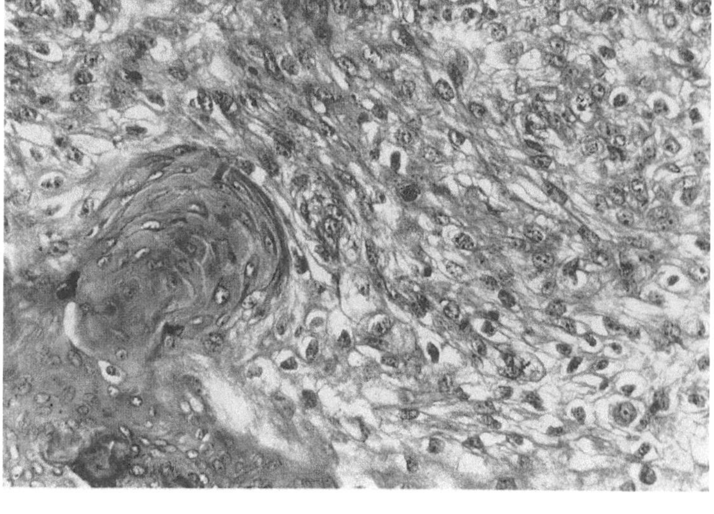

Fig. 35. Keratinizing squamous carcinoma of the thymus. A keratin "pearl" is present at the left of the photograph; the cytologic aspects of the tumor cells point to a diagnosis of malignancy

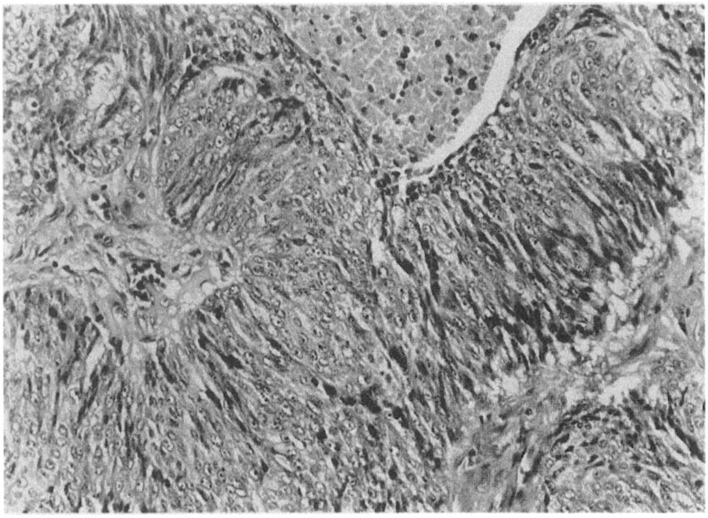

Fig. 36. Lymphoepithelioma-like thymic carcinoma with spindle cell change. This pattern is also seen in histologically similar neoplasms of the nasopharynx

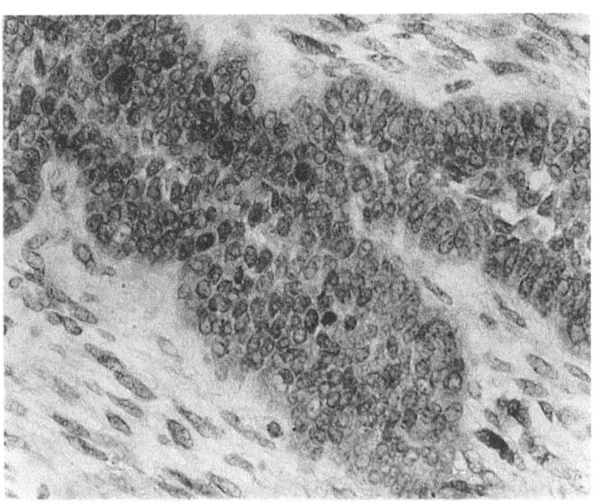

Fig. 37. Basaloid carcinoma of the thymus. Small tumor cells with high nuclear: cytoplasmic ratios are clustered in trabeculae, with a suggestion of peripheral nuclear palisading

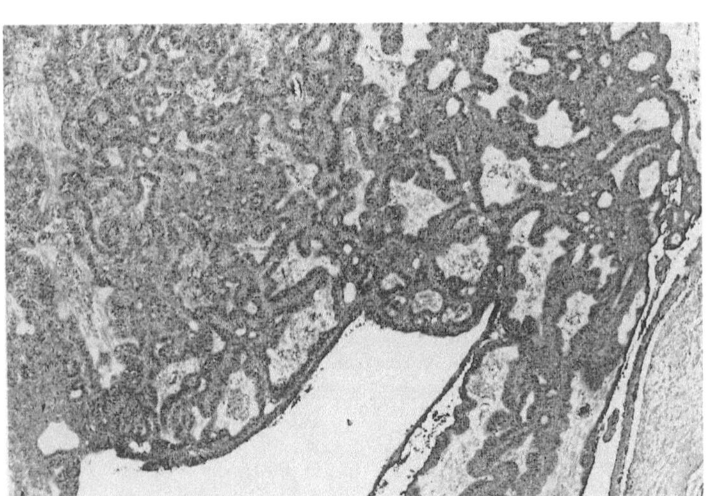

Fig. 38. Partially cystic basaloid thymic carcinoma. Nuclear palisading is apparent within cords of neoplastic cells. (Snover et al. 1982)

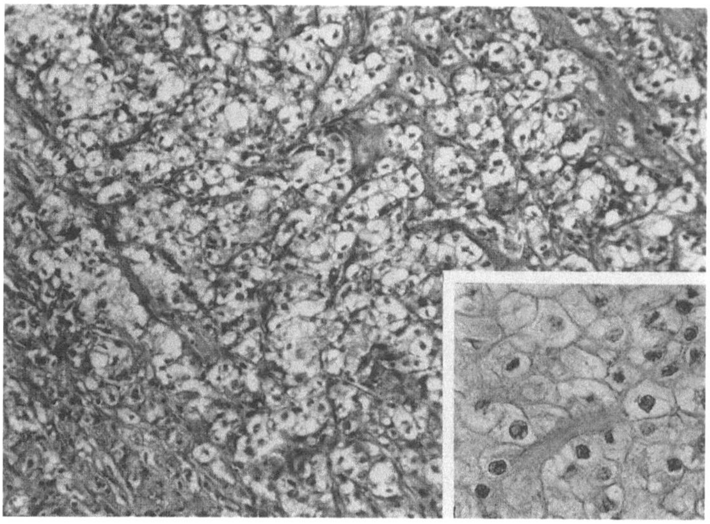

Fig. 39. Clear cell carcinoma of the thymus. This rare variant is characterized by nests of tumor cells with optically clear cytoplasm, separated by fine fibrous stroma. *Inset* demonstrates moderate nuclear atypia and relatively abundant clear cytoplasm. A similarity to renal cell carcinoma is striking

an abundant, optically clear cytoplasm which were occasionally subdivided by fibrovascular septa (Fig. 39). The nuclei were oval with evenly dispersed chromatin in some areas, whereas in others they were more vesicular and contained prominent eosinophilic nucleoli. Mitoses were rare. A striking similarity to renal cell carcinoma was obvious in both cases. The cytoplasm of the tumor cells described by Snover et al. (1982) contained PAS-stainable glycogen, while the other tumor showed only scant PAS reactivity. Stains for mucin were negative.

Sarcomatoid carcinoma has also been described twice (Snover et al. 1982; Wick et al. 1982). In both instances, foci of cytologically malignant squamous growth, as described already, were admixed with spindle cell areas. In one tumor, these assumed a storiform pattern with focal cytoplasmic cross-striations and acidophilia (Fig. 40; Snover et al. 1982). In the case reported by Wick et al. (1982) fascicles of spindle cells regularly punctuated a background population of epithelial elements. The nuclei of spindle cells in both tumors were hyperchromatic, with occasionally prominent nucleoli and high nucleocytoplasmic ratios. We have seen a third case of sarcomatoid carcinoma which was composed almost exclusively of spindle cells in a storiform arrangement (Fig. 41); only occasional small nests of squamoid epithelial cells were apparent in this tumor and cross-striations were not observed in the spindle cell component.

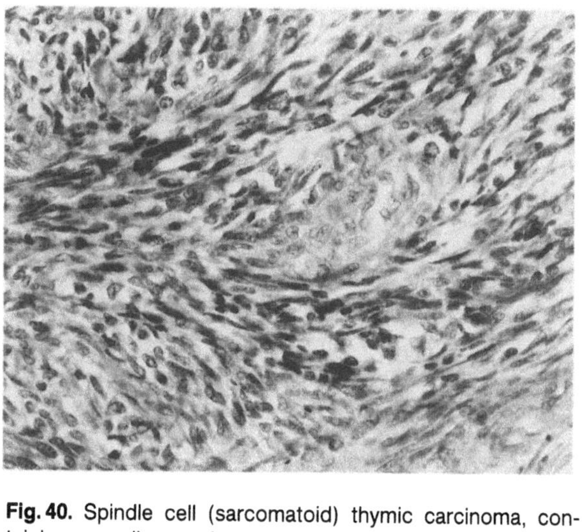

Fig. 40. Spindle cell (sarcomatoid) thymic carcinoma, containing a small nest of overtly epithelial (polygonal) cells. Cytoplasmic cross-striations were evident in other areas of this neoplasm

Mucoepidermoid carcinoma: An example of thymic carcinoma reported by Snover et al. (1982) was essentially identical microscopically to mucoepidermoid carcinomas of salivary gland origin. It was composed of three cell types: one was polygonal with moderate eosinophilic cytoplasm; another contained slightly basophilic, PAS-positive (diastase-resistant) cytoplasmic vacuoles which compressed nuclei; and the third was squamoid, with intercellular "bridges," nuclear hyperchromasia and enlargement, and mitotic activity (Figs. 42 and 43). Occasional dyskeratotic cells were scattered throughout the mass. The tumor documented by Tanaka et al. (1982) was microscopically similar. In both cases the tumor cells were arranged in partially cystic, partially necrotic nests which were separated by fibrous bands; the microcysts contained mucinous material.

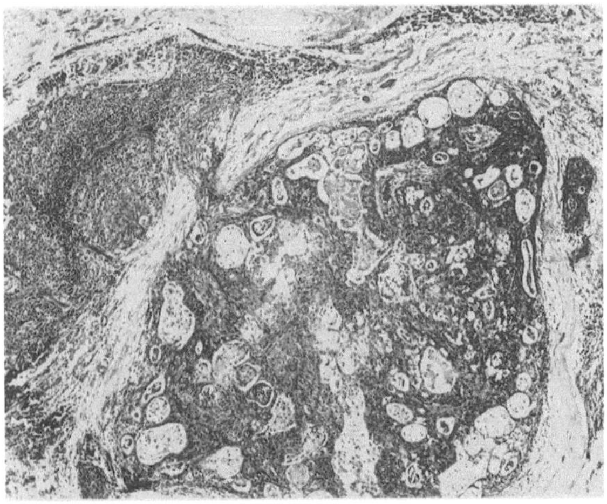

Fig. 41. Sarcomatoid thymic carcinoma, with marked resemblance to a fibrohistiocytic tumor

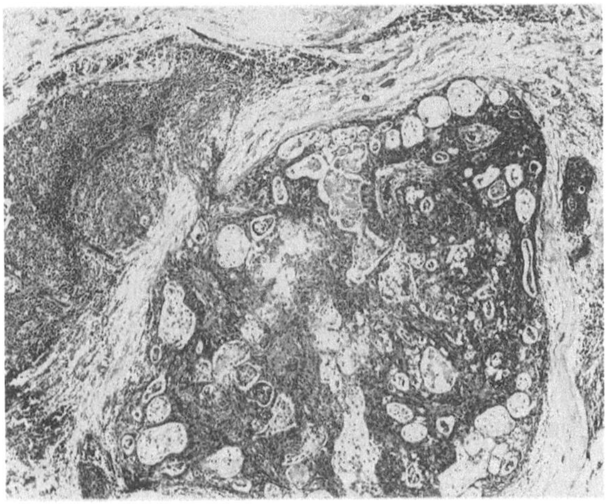

Fig. 42. Mucoepidermoid carcinoma of the thymus. Mucin-filled microcysts punctuate the central cellular lobule. (Snover et al. 1982)

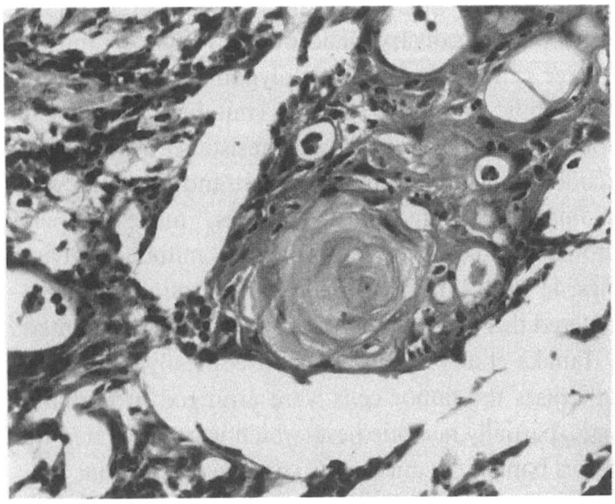

Fig. 43. Keratinized cell nest in mucoepidermoid thymic carcinoma, surrounded by microcysts. (Snover et al. 1982)

Electron Microscopy

Lymphoepithelioma-like, keratinizing squamous, basaloid, and clear cell thymic carcinomas have similar ultrastructural features (Snover et al. 1982; Wick et al. 1982; Wolfe et al. 1983). They all display high nucleocytoplasmic ratios, coarsely distributed heterochromatin, and complex nucleoli. The cytoplasm of the tumor cells contains the usual metabolic organelles and some glycogen, as well as variable numbers of tonofilaments (Figs. 44 and 45) which insert into numerous well-formed desmosomes, as in thymomas. Indeed, reliance must be placed solely on nuclear characteristics and the relative cell volume which they occupy in distinguishing between thymomas and thymic carcinoma.

We have seen two carcinomas of the thymus which had the light microscopic appearance of lymphoepithelioma-like thymic carcinoma, but which contained a moderate number of cytoplasmic granules ultrastructurally (Fig. 46; Wick et al. 1982). Otherwise, these neoplasms showed the electron microscopic features described already, including tonofilaments and prominent desmosomes. Current opinion may favor the classification of such lesions as "large cell neuroendocrine carcinoma," in analogy to certain tumors of the lung (Mills et al. 1987).

Snover et al. (1982) demonstrated cytoplasmic sarcomeric development, correlating with the cross-striations which were observed by light microscopy (Fig. 47) in a case of sarcomatoid thymic carcinoma. No epithelial features such as intercellular junctional complexes were observed, but this was attributed to sampling limitations. To date, mucoepidermoid thymic carcinoma has not been studied ultrastructurally.

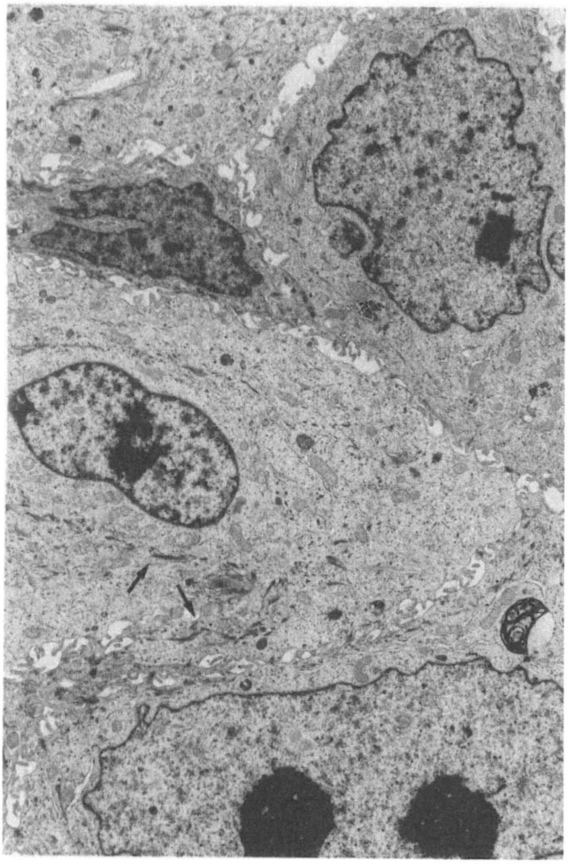

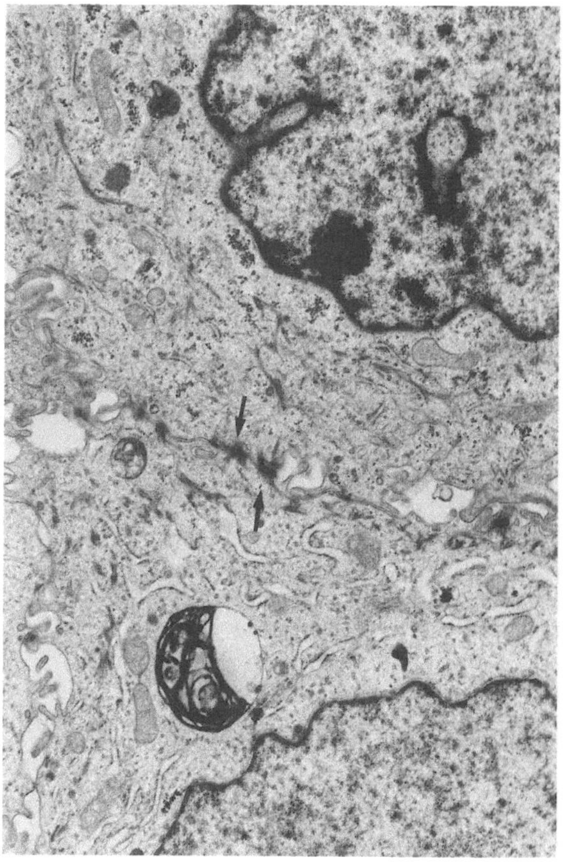

Fig. 44. Electron micrograph of lymphoepithelioma-like thymic carcinoma, showing cytoplasmic tonofilaments within tumor cells *(arrows)*. The ultrastructural characteristics of this tumor are virtually identical to those of conventional thymoma

Fig. 45

Fig. 45. Higher power view of tumor shown in Fig. 44. Tumor cells are joined by desmosomes *(arrows)*, into which tonofilaments insert

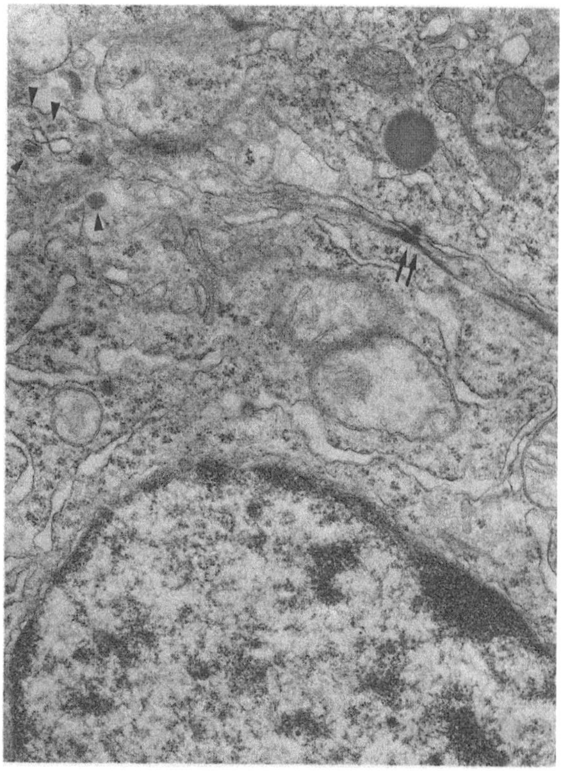

Fig. 46. Lymphoepithelioma-like thymic carcinoma, showing ultrastructural evidence of combined squamous and endocrine differentiation. Tonofilament-desmosomal complexes *(double arrow)* are accompanied by cytoplasmic neurosecretory granules *(arrowheads)*

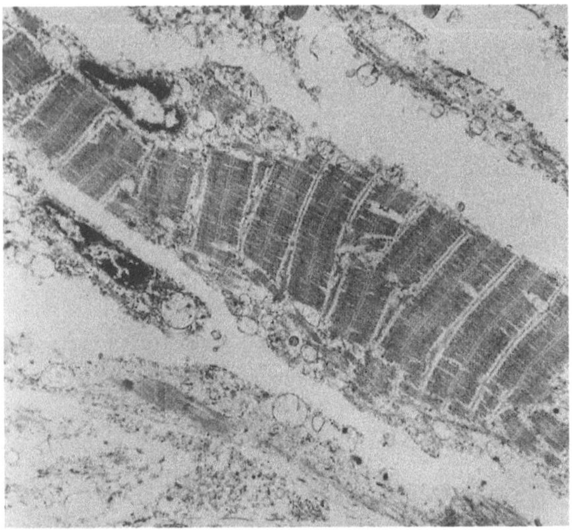

Fig. 47. Myogenous differentiation in a tumor cell of sarcomatoid thymic carcinoma. Well-oriented sarcomeres are present in the cytoplasm. (Snover et al. 1982)

Immunohistochemistry and Serologic Studies

Immunohistochemistry provides perhaps the most useful method for distinguishing thymic carcinoma from many of its differential diagnostic alternatives. All forms of thymic carcinoma are immunoreactive for epithelial membrane antigen and cytokeratin (Figs. 48 and 49), but not for α-fetoprotein (AFP), β-human chorionic gonadotropin, placental alkaline phosphatase, or common leukocyte antigen (Wick et al. 1982 and unpublished work). Myoglobin reactivity has been reported in an example of sarcomatoid thymic carcinoma, with the PAP technique (Fig. 50) (Snover et al. 1982). This neoplasm also expressed cytokeratin positivity. Leyvraz et al. (1985) have reported a case of lymphoepithelioma-like thymic carcinoma with positive serologic studies for Epstein-Barr virus (EBV) infection. This finding suggests that EBV may play an etiologic role for such tumors, as it does in a proportion of "lymphoepitheliomas" of the nasopharynx (Klein 1979; Ringborg et al. 1983). It is possible that immunohistochemical methods may reveal EBV antigens in additional examples of thymic carcinoma in the future.

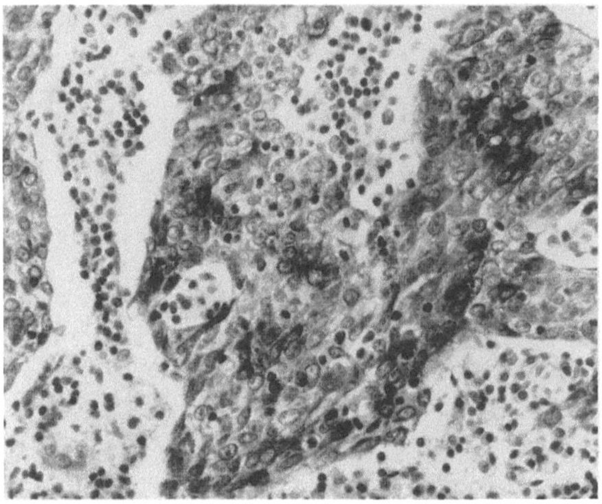

Fig. 49. Darkly staining cytoplasmic reactivity for cytokeratin in lymphoepithelioma-like thymic carcinoma

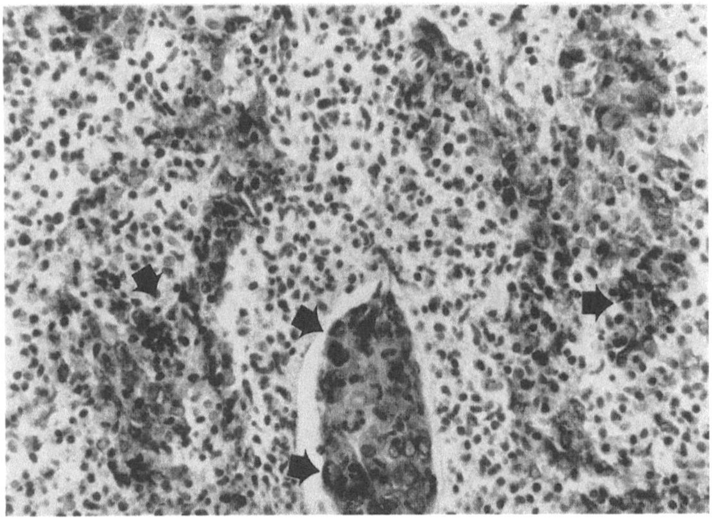

Fig. 48. Darkly staining cells are immunoreactive for epithelial membrane antigen *(arrows)* in this lymphoepithelioma-like thymic carcinoma. Intervening lymphocytes fail to stain

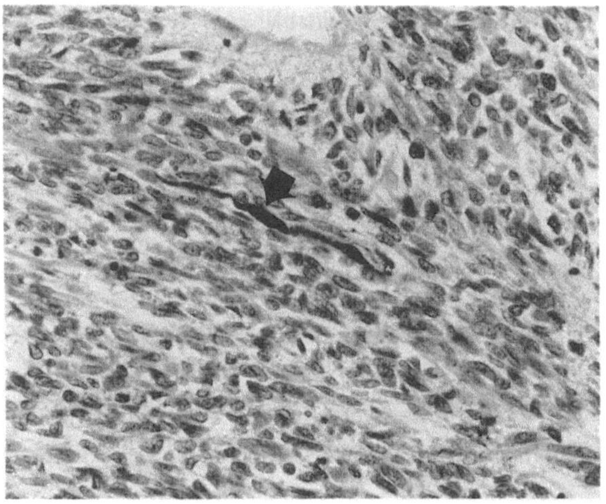

Fig. 50. A single cell is reactive for the presence of myoglobin, in this sarcomatoid thymic carcinoma. (Snover et al. 1982)

Differential Diagnosis

The differential diagnostic considerations in cases of thymic carcinoma are summarized in Tables 4-6. The most important one, because of the close similarity of variants of thymic carcinoma to nasopharyngeal, pulmonary, renal, salivary glandular, genital, and anorectal carcinomas, is a metastasis to the anterior mediastinum from an occult tumor in one of these sites. Electron microscopy and immunohistochemistry are of limited value in differentiating primary from secondary tumors. The only form of thymic carcinoma which is dissimilar ultrastructurally to its extrathymic "mimic" is clear cell carcinoma of the thymus; unlike clear cell carcinomas of the kidney and female urogenital tract, it contains abundant cytoplasmic tonofilaments and well-formed desmosomes, and lacks microvillous development and copious amounts of glycogen (Wolfe et al. 1983). However, in any case where thymic carcinoma is considered to be the diagnosis, exhaustive clinical investigation to rule out a primary extrathymic neoplasm should be considered mandatory.

Another major problem in the differential diagnosis of thymic carcinoma lies in the similarity between lymphoepithelioma-like squamous carcinoma and large cell lymphoma of the thymic region (van Heerden et al. 1970; Lichtenstein et al. 1980). This is the commonest problem referred to us for evaluation in our consultation practices. Fortunately, the availability of antibodies directed at cytokeratin, EMA, and CLA provides a satisfactory solution to this dilemma in most cases. Thymic carcinoma is immunoreactive for cytokeratin and EMA, but not for CLA (unpublished observations); the converse of these findings typifies large cell lymphomas (Sloane and Ormerod 1981; Wood et al. 1984).

Extragonadal germ cell tumors of the mediastinum such as seminoma and embryonal carcinoma may also be confused with thymic carcinoma (Levine 1973; Cox 1975; Luna and Valenzuela-Tamariz 1976; Fox et al. 1979; Wick and Siegal 1980). Detailed histopathologic examination will usually resolve this uncertainty (Table 4), but occasional cases require the use of electron microscopy (Table 5) and immunocytochemistry (Table 6). Seminomas do not contain cytoplasmic tonofilaments or fully formed desmosomes (Levine 1973; Battifora et al. 1984), as do thymic carcinomas; on the other hand, seminomas demonstrate abundant cytoplasmic glycogen and complex nucleolar forms. Embryonal carcinoma commonly contains cytoplasmic AFP globules ultrastructurally, and lacks true tonofilaments (Wick and Siegal 1980; Battifora et al. 1984). Immunohistochemically, seminoma is positive for placental alkaline phosphatase (PLAP) (Aguirre et al. 1985; Wick et al. 1987), but is nonreactive for EMA (Sloane and Ormerod 1981) and cytokeratin (Battifora

Table 4. Points of histologic distinction between thymic carcinoma and other primary mediastinal neoplasms

Tumor	Nesting growth	Round/oval nuclei	Complex nucleoli	Rudimentary glands	Lymphoid infiltrate	Prominent angioinvasion	PAS positivity
Thymic carcinoma (polygonal cell)	+-++	++	0	0	±	0	±
Thymic carcinoma (sarcomatoid)	± (focal)	±	0	0	±	0	±[a]
Large cell lymphoma	0[b]	0	0	0	++	++	0
Seminoma	+	+	++	0	+	0	+-++
Embryonal carcinoma	+-++	+	±	+-++	±	0	+
True sarcomas	0	0	0	0	0	0	0

0 absent; ± variably present; + present; ++ present and prominent

[a] Isolated cells with densely eosinophilic cytoplasm may be strongly PAS-positive and show cross-striations.

[b] Some examples of large cell lymphoma with sclerotic stroma may have a clustered growth pattern.

Levine GD (1973) Primary thymic seminoma: a neoplasm ultrastructurally similar to testicular seminoma and distinct from epithelial thymoma. Cancer 31: 729-741

Levine GD, Bensch KG (1972) Epithelial nature of spindle-cell thymoma: an ultrastructural study. Cancer 30: 500-511

Levine GD, Rosai J (1978) Thymic hyperplasia and neoplasia: a review of current concepts. Hum Pathol 9: 495-515

Levine GD, Rosai J, Bearman RM, Polliack A (1975) The fine structure of thymoma, with emphasis on its differential diagnosis: a study of ten cases. Am J Pathol 81: 49-86

Leyvraz S, Henle W, Chahinian AP, Perlmann C, Klein G, Gordon RE, Rosenblum M, Holland JF (1985) Association of Epstein-Barr virus with thymic carcinoma. N Engl J Med 312: 1296-1299

Lewis JE, Wick MR, Scheithauer BW, Bernatz PE, Unni KK, Taylor WF (1987) Thymoma: a clinicopathologic review. Cancer 60: 2727-2743

Lichtenstein AK, Levine A, Taylor CR, Boswell W, Rossman S, Feinstein DI, Lukes RJ (1980) Primary mediastinal lymphoma in adults. Am J Med 68: 509-514

Lowenhaupt E (1948) Tumors of the thymus in relation to the thymic epithelial anlage. Cancer 1: 547-563

Lowenhaupt E, Brown R (1951) Carcinoma of the thymus of granulomatous type: a clinical and pathological study. Cancer 4: 1193-1209

Luna MA, Valenzuela-Tamariz J (1976) Germ-cell tumors of the mediastinum: postmortem findings. Am J Clin Pathol 65: 450-454

MacDonald J, Parker JC Jr, Brown S, Page LK, Wolfe DE (1978) Cerebral metastasis from a malignant thymoma. Surg Neurol 9: 58-60

Maggi G, Giaccone G, Donadio M, Ciuffreda L, Dalesio O, Leria G, Trifiletti G, Casadio C, Palestro G, Mancuso M, Calciati A (1986) Thymomas: a review of 169 cases, with particular reference to results of surgical treatment. Cancer 58: 765-776

McBurney RP, Clagett OT, McDonald JR (1951) Primary intrapulmonary neoplasm (thymoma?) associated with myasthenia gravis: report of a case. Mayo Clin Proc 26: 345-353

Marino M, Müller-Hermelink HK (1985) Thymoma and thymic carcinoma. Virchows Arch A 407: 119-149

Marks RD Jr, Wallace KM, Pettit HS (1978) Radiation therapy control of nine patients with malignant thymoma. Cancer 41: 117-119

Masaoka A, Monden Y, Nakahara K, Tanioka T (1981) Follow-up study of thymomas with special reference to their clinical stages. Cancer 48: 2485-2492

Mills SE, Cooper PH, Walker AN, Swanson PE, Wick MR (1987) Large-cell neuroendocrine carcinoma of the lung (abstract). Lab Invest 56: 52A

Needles B, Kemeny N, Urmacher C (1981) Malignant thymoma: renal metastases responding to cis-platinum. Cancer 48: 223-226

Nickels J, Franssila K (1976) Thymoma metastasizing to extrathoracic sites: a case report. Acta Pathol Microbiol Immunol Scand [A] 84: 331-334

Osborn M, Weber K (1983) Tumor diagnosis by intermediate filament typing: a novel tool for surgical pathology. Lab Invest 48: 372-394

Pascoe HR, Miner MS (1976) An ultrastructuralstudy of nine thymomas. Cancer 37: 317-326

Penn CRH, Hope-Stone HF (1972) The role of radiotherapy in the management of malignant thymoma. Br J Surg 59: 533-539

Rachmaninoff N, Fentress V (1964) Thymoma with metastasis to the brain. Am J Clin Pathol 41: 618-625

Reddick RL, Jennette JC (1983) Immunologic and ultrastructural characterization of the small cell population in malignant thymoma. Hum Pathol 14: 377-380

Ringborg U, Henle W, Henle G, Ingimarsson S, Klein G, Silfversward C, Strander H (1983) Epstein-Barr virus-specific serodiagnostic tests in carcinomas of the head and neck. Cancer 52: 1237-1243

Rogers BHG, Manaligod JR, Blazek WV (1968) Thymoma associated with pancytopenia and hypogammaglobulinemia: report of a case and review of the literature. Am J Med 44: 154-164

Rosai J (1981) Mediastinum. In: Rosai J (ed) Ackerman's surgical pathology, vol 1, 6th edn. Mosby, St. Louis, pp 306-311

Rosai J, Higa E (1972) Mediastinal endocrine neoplasm, of probable thymic origin, related to carcinoid tumor: clinicopathologic study of 8 cases. Cancer 29: 1061-1074

Rosai J, Levine GD (1976) Tumors of the thymus. In: Atlas of tumor pathology, sec ser, fasc 13. Armed Forces Institute of Pathology, Washington, DC

Rosai J, Levine G, Weber WR, Higa E (1976) Carcinoid tumors and oat cell carcinomas of the thymus. Pathol Annu 11: 201-226

Rosai J, Limas C, Husband EM (1984) Ectopic hamartomatous thymoma: a distinctive benign lesion of lower neck. Am J Surg Pathol 8: 501-513

Rosenberger A, Adler O (1978) Fine needle aspiration biopsy in the diagnosis of mediastinal lesions. AJR 131: 239-242

Sajjad SM, Lukeman JM, Llamas L, Fernandez T (1982) Needle biopsy diagnosis of thymoma: a case report. Acta Cytol (Baltimore) 26: 503-506

Salyer WR, Eggleston JC (1976) Thymoma: a clinical and pathological study of 65 cases. Cancer 37: 229-249

Sato Y, Watanabe S, Mukai K, Kodama T, Upton M, Goto M and Shimosato Y (1986) An immunohistochemical study of thymic epithelial tumors. II. Lymphoid component. Am J Surg Pathol 10: 862-870

Shellito J, Khandekar JD, McKeever WP, Vick NA (1978) Invasive thymoma responsive to oral corticosteroids. Cancer Treat Rep 62: 1397-1400

Shier KJ (1981) The thymus according to Schambacher: medullary ducts and reticular epithelium of thymus and thymomas. Cancer 48: 1183-1199

Shimosato Y, Kameya T, Nagai K, Suemasu K (1977) Squamous cell carcinoma of the thymus: an analysis of eight cases. Am J Surg Pathol 1: 109-121

Slater G, Papatestas AE, Genkins G, Kornfeld P, Horowitz SH, Bender A (1978) Thymomas in patients with myasthenia gravis. An Surg 188: 171-174

Sloane JP, Ormerod MG (1981) Distribution of epithelial membrane antigen in normal and neoplastic tissues and its value in diagnostic tumor pathology. Cancer 47: 1786-1795

Smith WF, DeWall RA, Krumholz RA (1970) Giant thymoma. Chest 58: 383-385

Snover DC, Levine GD, Rosai J (1982) Thymic carcinoma: five distinctive histological variants. Am J Surg Pathol 6: 451-470

Souadjian JV, Enriquez P, Silverstein MN, Pépin JM (1974) The spectrum of diseases associated with thymoma: coincidence or syndrome? Arch Intern Med 134: 374-379

Sterchi M, Cordell AR (1975) Seminoma of the anterior mediastinum. Ann Thorac Surg 19: 371-377

Sterrett G, Whitaker D, Shilkin KB, Walters MN-I (1983) The fine needle aspiration cytology of mediastinal lesions. Cancer 51: 127-135

Swinborne-Sheldrake K, Gray GF, Glick AD (1985) Thymic epithelial neoplasms. Southern Med J 78: 790-800

Symmers D (1932) Malignant tumors and tumor-like growths of the thymic region. Ann Surg 95: 544-572

Tanaka M, Shimokawa R, Matsubara O, Aoki N, Kamiyama R, Kasuga T, Hatakeyama S (1982) Mucoepidermoid carcinoma of the thymic region. Acta Pathol Jpn 32: 703-712

Thomson AD, Thackray AC (1957) The histology of tumours of the thymus. Br J Cancer 11: 348-364

Van Heerden JA, Harrison EG Jr, Bernatz PE, Kiely JM (1970) Mediastinal malignant lymphoma. Chest 57: 518-529

Verley JM, Hollmann KH (1985) Thymoma: a comparative study of clinical stages, histological features and survival in 200 cases. Cancer 55: 1074-1086

Wara DW (1981) Thymic hormones and the immune system. Adv Pediatr 28: 229-270

Wick MR, Siegal GP (1980) Primary mediastinal embryonal carcinoma. Minn Med 63: 723-726

Wick MR, Scott RE, Li C-Y, Carney JA (1980) Carcinoid tumor of the thymus: a clinicopathologic report of seven cases with a review of the literature. Mayo Clin Proc 55: 246-254

Wick MR, Nichols WC, Ingle JN, Bruckman JE, Okazaki H (1981) Malignant, predominantly lymphocytic thymoma with central and peripheral nervous system metastases. Cancer 47: 2036-2043

Wick MR, Weiland LH, Scheithauer BW, Bernatz PE (1982) Primary thymic carcinomas. Am J Surg Pathol 6: 613-630

Wick MR, Swanson PE, Manivel TC (1987) Placental-like alkaline phosphatase reactivity in human tumors. Hum Pathol 18: 946-954

Wolfe JT III, Wick MR, Banks PM, Scheithauer BW (1983) Clear cell carcinoma of the thymus. Mayo Clin Proc 58: 365-370

Wood GS, Link M, Warnke RA, Dilley J, Levy R (1984) Panleukocyte monoclonal antibody L3B12: characterization and application to research and diagnostic problems. Am J Clin Pathol 81: 176-183

10 Neuroendocrine, Germ Cell, and Nonepithelial Tumors

Mark R. Wick and Juan Rosai

Introduction

As mentioned in Chap. 9, many neoplasms of the thymic region which were formerly classified as thymomas are now known to be primary neuroendocrine, germ cell, lymphoid, and mesenchymal lesions (Rosai and Levine 1976). This chapter summarizes the clinicopathologic features of these thymic neoplasms, with emphasis on their differential diagnosis.

Neuroendocrine Thymic Tumors (Carcinoids and Oat Cell Carcinomas)

Historical Aspects

Although it had been known for many years that some thymic neoplasms were associated with clinical endocrinopathies such as Cushing's syndrome (Leyton et al. 1931; Scholz and Bahn 1959; Cohen et al. 1960; Azzopardi and Williams 1968; Kay and Wilson 1970), these tumors were not distinguished from thymomas until 1972. At that time, Rosai and Higa remarked on their morphological similarity to neuroendocrine tumors of other sites, and suggested that they be called "thymic carcinoids."

Similarly, Duguid and Kennedy reported the existence of primary mediastinal "oat cell" carcinoma in 1930. However, this rare lesion went unstudied for nearly 50 years, because of skepticism owing to the well-known phenomenon of metastasis to the mediastinum from occult oat cell carcinomas of the bronchi.

Clinical Features

Roughly 30% of carcinoid tumors of the thymus are associated clinically with Cushing's syndrome (Wick et al. 1980). In addition, inappropriate ectopic production of antidiuretic hormone (Levine and Rosai 1976), hypertrophic osteoarthropathy (Lowenthal et al. 1974), and the Eaton-Lambert syndrome (Wick and Rosai, in press) have been occasionally seen in patients with these neoplasms. Extremely high serum levels of adrenocorticotropic hormone (ACTH) (greater than 1000 pg/ml) are often recorded in patients with Cushing's syndrome along with cutaneous hyperpigmentation (Brown et al. 1982). The latter is enhanced after misdirected adrenalectomy; this situation has been designated as "pseudo-Nelson's sydrome" (Wick and Rosai, in press).

The vast majority of thymic carcinoids and all reported oat cell carcinomas have presented with symptoms and signs of thoracic structural displacement, such as dyspnea, cough, chest pain, the superior vena cava syndrome, or are found incidentially on chest roentgenograms (Fig. 1, Wick et al. 1980, 1982a). Rarely, metastasis to the cervical lymph nodes, bones, or skin may be the first manifestation of thymic carcinoids (Wick et al. 1980).

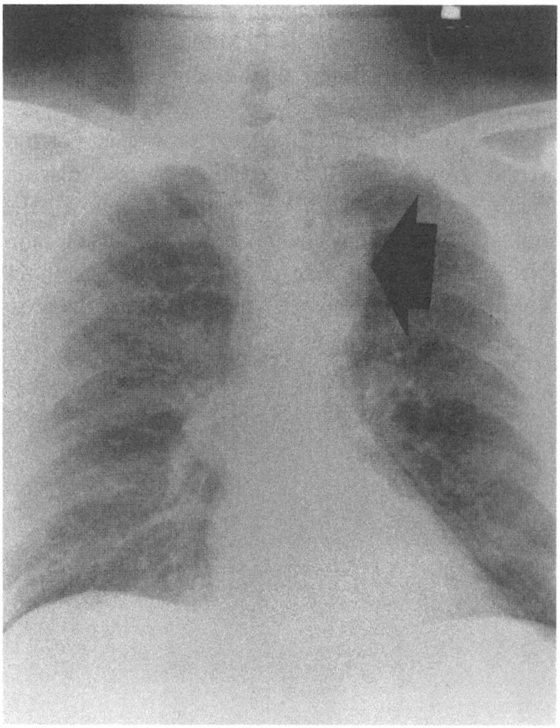

Fig. 1. Anterosuperior mediastinal mass *(arrow)* found on routine chest roentgenogram. This tumor proved to be a thymic carcinoid

Pathology

Gross Characteristics

Thymic carcinoids and oat cell carcinomas are virtually identical macroscopically, and differ in appearance from thymomas. The majority are unencapsulated and average 8-10 cm in their greatest dimension (Fig. 2; Rosai et al. 1976). They are gray-white and firm on cut section, often have a gritty consistency, and lack internal fibrous septation. Foci of hemorrhage and necrosis are apparent in approximately 70% of cases. When associated with Cushing's syndrome, carcinoid tumors of the thymus tend to be smaller at diagnosis (3-5 cm diameter), and may be totally confined within the capsule of one thymic lobe (Brown et al. 1982).

Light Microscopy

Thymic Carcinoid

Most thymic carcinoids display an "organoid" growth pattern, characterized by nests of relatively uniform tumor cells separated by a fine fibrovascular stroma (Fig. 3). Individual cell borders are indistinct, cytoplasm is slightly eosinophilic and granular, and nuclei are round to oval with evenly distributed chromatin and indistinct nucleoli (Fig. 4). Mitotic activity is variable, but is usually found; abnormally shaped division figures may be apparent.

Over 50% of thymic carcinoids show areas of trabecular growth and the formation of true rosettes (Fig. 5, Rosai et al. 1976; Wick et al. 1980, 1982a). The lumina of rosettes may contain material which is stainable with the alcian blue or colloidal iron methods (Rosai et al. 1976). Another typical feature is the presence of central necrosis within tumor cell nests (Fig. 6) which manifest dystrophic calcification (Rosai and Higa 1972; Wick et al. 1980); this is the histological basis for the gritty consistency that may be observed in gross examination of carcinoid tumors of the thymus.

Application of argyrophilic techniques such as the Churukian-Schenk or Sevier-Munger stains yields positive results in virtually all cases (Rosai et al. 1976; Wick et al. 1980), whereas argentaffin methods such as the Fontana-Masson stain give uniformly negative results. These findings are consistent with those obtained in other neuroendocrine neoplasms of foregut derivation (Williams and Sandler 1963).

Ancillary microscopic features typical of thymomas, such as a significant lymphoid cell population, microcyst formation, perivascular serum lakes, medullary differentiation, and a hemangiopericytoma-like vascular pattern, are not seen in thymic carcinoids (Rosai et al. 1976; Rosai and Levine 1976; Wick et al. 1980). However, these do share a capacity for spindle cell growth with thymoma (Fig. 7; Levine and Rosai 1976), and occasional cases of either tumor type may require extensive special study to make a definitive diagnosis. Nonetheless, attention to the nuclear chromatin pattern in spindle cell carcinoid of the thymus usually allows this distinction to be made with conventional microscopy, since it is like that of "classic" carcinoid cells. The use of touch preparations made from resected tumor tissue facilitates this facet of pathologic evaluation.

Stromal amyloid, demonstrated by the Congo red or crystal violet stains, has been reported in rare examples of thymic carcinoid with a spindle cell growth pattern (Fig. 8; Rosai et al. 1976; Wick and Rosai, in press). The similarity of these neoplasms to medullary carcinoma of the thyroid was striking (Chong et al.

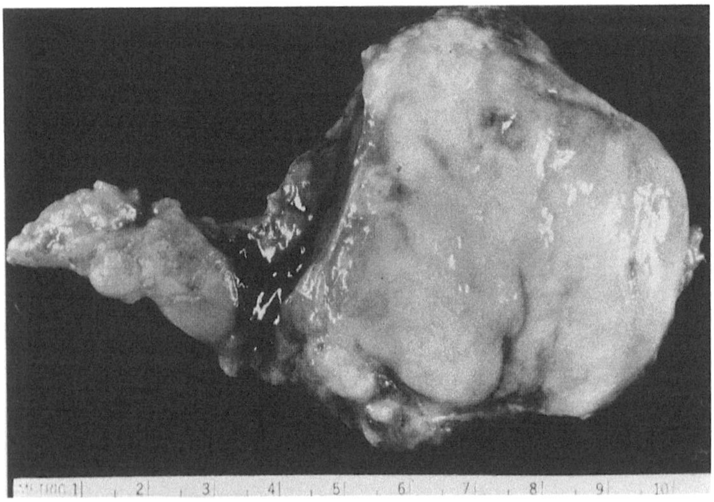

Fig. 2. Gross appearance of thymic carcinoid. The tumor is pseudoencapsulated, but lacks internal fibrous septation. Small foci of necrosis are visible

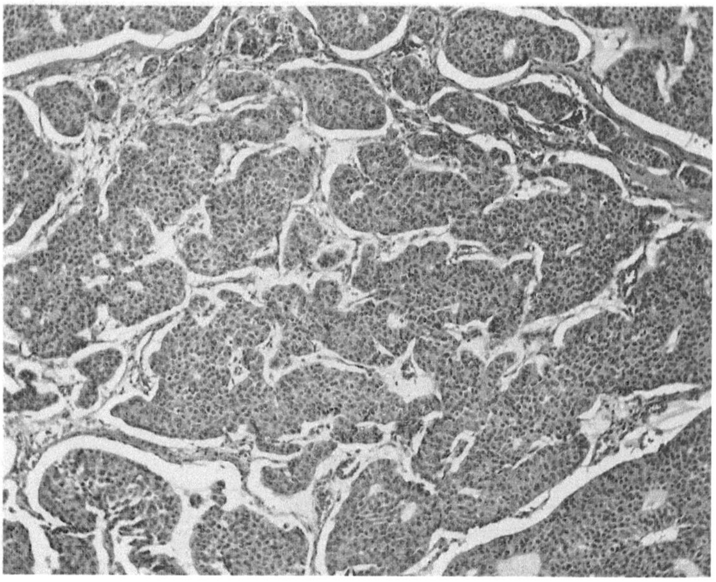

Fig. 3. Complex, organoid growth pattern in a thymic carcinoid

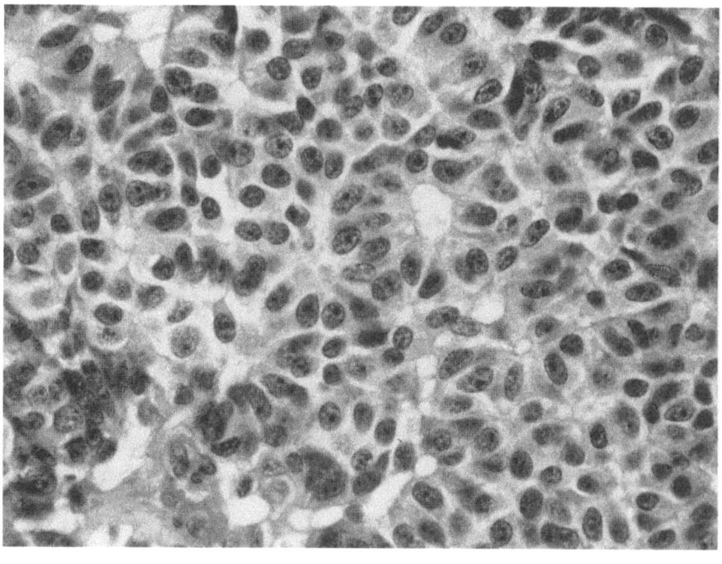

Fig. 4. Cytologic detail of carcinoid tumor of the thymus. The tumor cells have regular, oval nuclei, with evenly distributed chromatin and inconspicuous nucleoli. The cytoplasm is finely granular

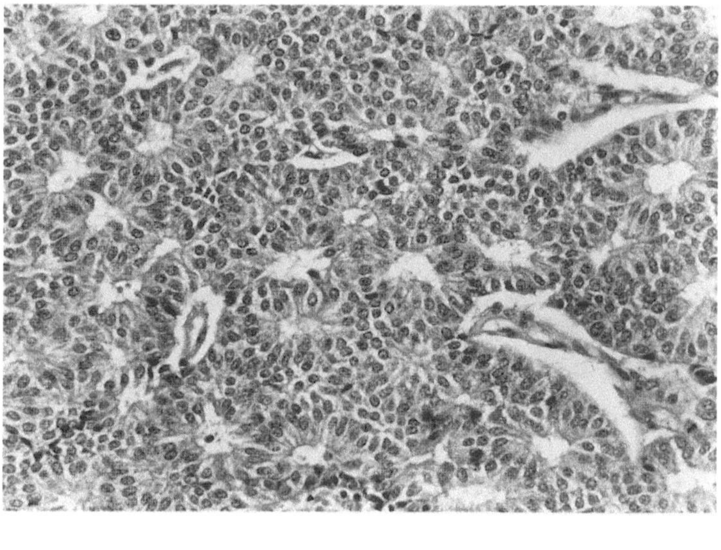

Fig. 5. Formation of numerous true rosettes in a thymic carcinoid

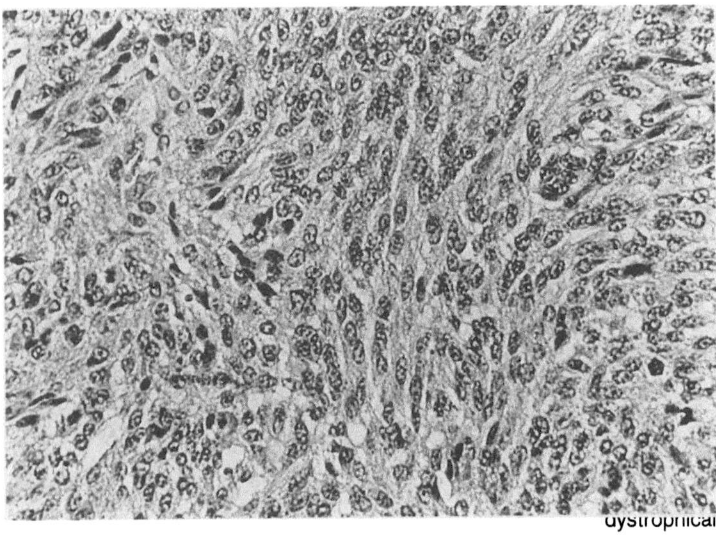

...al necrosis within an artifactually detached "ball" ...ls, in a thymic carcinoid. Such foci may become ...y calcified

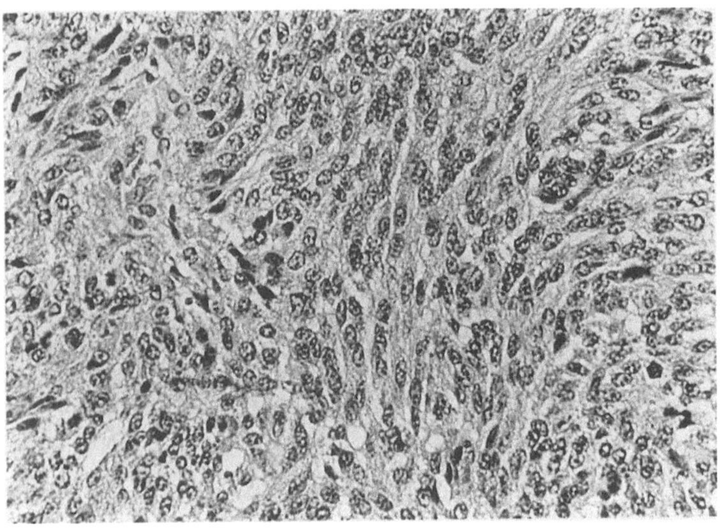

Fig. 7. Spindle cell growth in a thymic carcinoid tumor. This appearance may lead to confusion with spindle cell thymoma

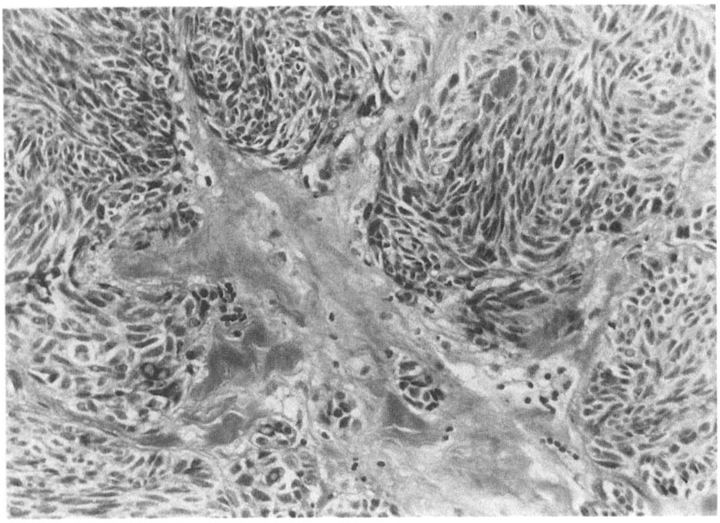

Fig. 8. A spindle cell growth pattern is associated with stromal amyloid matrix in this medullary thyroid carcinoma-like thymic carcinoid

1975). However, the thyroid glands in the affected patients were entirely normal in both location and structure.

Other microscopic variants of thymic carcinoid have been described: some have intracytoplasmic lipofuscin-like or melanin pigment (Fig. 9; Ho and Ho 1977; Wick et al. 1982a; Wick and Scheithauer 1984); others have an extensively fibrous "scirrhous" stroma (Fig. 10), as well as examples with focally cribriform or diffuse growth patterns (Fig. 11; Wick et al. 1982a). The significance of these histologic subtypes lies in their potential confusion with metastatic carcinomas or malignant lymphoma, as will be discussed subsequently.

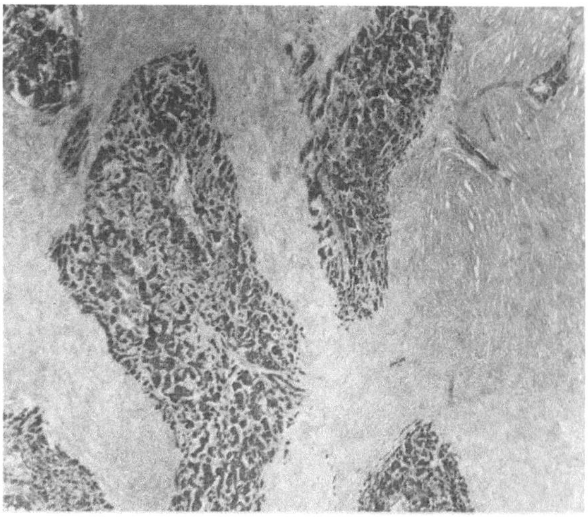

Fig. 10. Sclerotic stroma in this thymic carcinoid is reminiscent of that seen in desmoplastic carcinomas

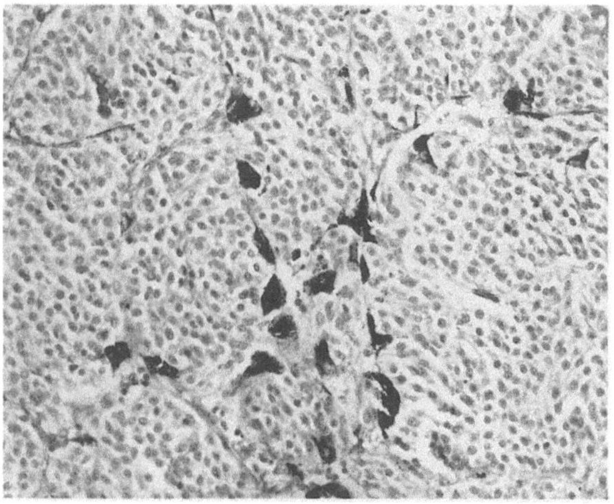

Fig. 9. Pigmented variant of thymic carcinoid. Grimelius stain highlights lipofuscinoid material within several tumor cells

Oat Cell Carcinoma

There are less than 20 reported examples of primary thymic neoplasms with the histologic appearance of bronchogenic oat cell (small cell) carcinoma (Duguid and Kennedy 1930; Rosai et al. 1976; Rosai and Levine 1976; Wick and Scheithauer 1982; Wick et al. 1982b). These differ from carcinoid tumors in that their cytoplasm is extremely scanty, mitoses are more numerous, and organoid growth is less apparent (Fig. 12). Tumors with an intermediate form of cytologic morphology may also be encountered, making it difficult to decide whether they should be classified as "carcinoids" or "oat cell carcinomas" (Fig. 13; Wick and Rosai, in press). In such cases, the terms "atypical

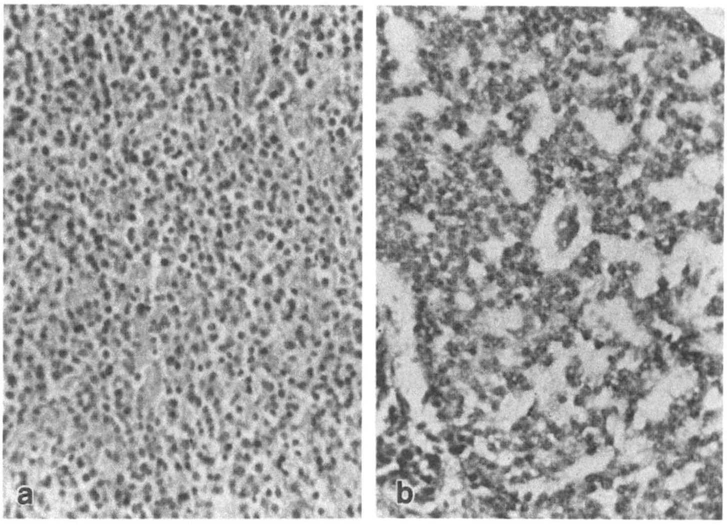

Fig. 11 a, b. Diffuse (**a**) and cribriform (**b**) growth patterns in carcinoid tumors of the thymus. These appearances may lead to confusion with lymphoma or germinoma, and with metastatic carcinoma

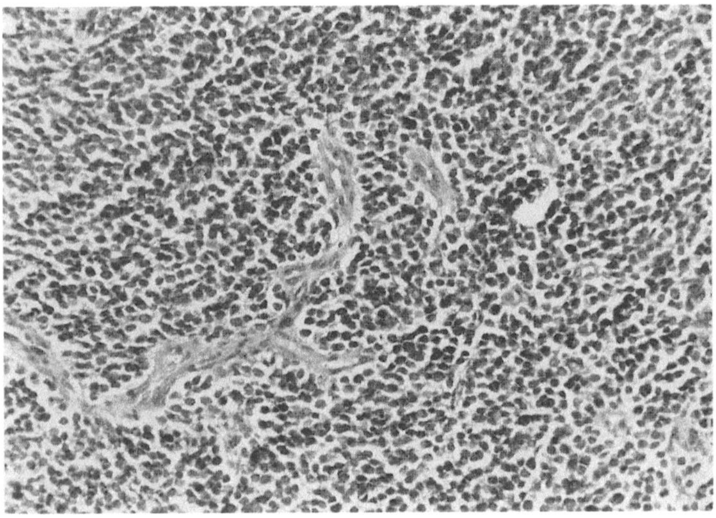

Fig. 12. Small cell neuroendocrine (oat cell) carcinoma of the thymus. Lymphocyte-like cells are arranged in an only vaguely organoid fashion, and are separated by delicate fibrovascular stroma

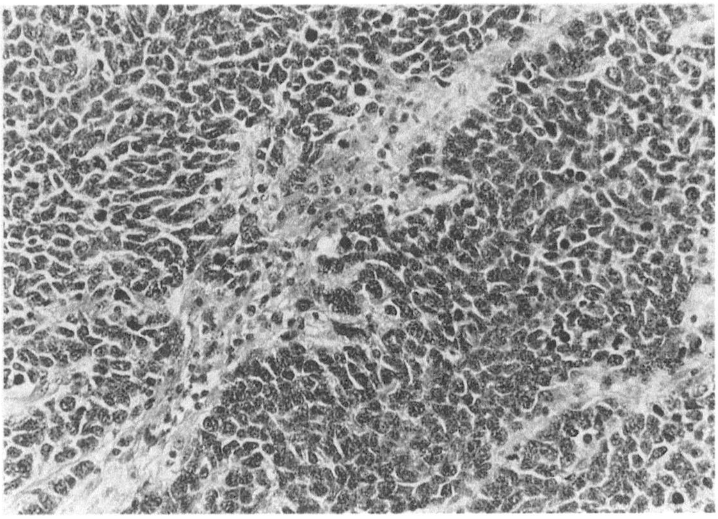

Fig. 13. Neuroendocrine carcinoma (atypical caracinoid) of the thymus. The cells are intermediate in size between those of conventional carcinoid and those of oat cell carcinoma, and mitotic activity is easily seen

carcinoid" or "neuroendocrine carcinoma" have been employed. These neoplasms have not been discussed under the heading of "thymic carcinoma" in Chap. 9, because they do not show differentiation toward thymic epithelium, but are thought to be ultrastructurally and immunohistochemically similar to Kulchitsky-type neuroendocrine cells (Rosai et al. 1976). However, this is a fine point and in practical terms oat cell carcinoma is indeed a form of primary thymic carcinoma in the sense that it arises within the thymus.

We cannot stress too strongly the fact that most apparent oat cell carcinomas of the thymic region are actually metastases from occult bronchial neoplasms. There are no reliable pathologic points of distinction between primary thymic and primary pulmonary oat cell carcinoma, making exhaustive clinical exclusion of the latter mandatory before accepting a definitive diagnosis of the former.

Snover et al. (1982) have described three cases of primary, combined oat cell carcinoma squamous carcinoma of the thymus (Fig. 14). Squamous elements in these tumors were confined to small, randomly distributed cell nests amid the oat cell population; the boundary between the two was sharp microscopically. Again, because similar mixed differentiation has been observed in primary bronchogenic neoplasms, the exclusion of metastasis to the mediastinum is necessary in such cases.

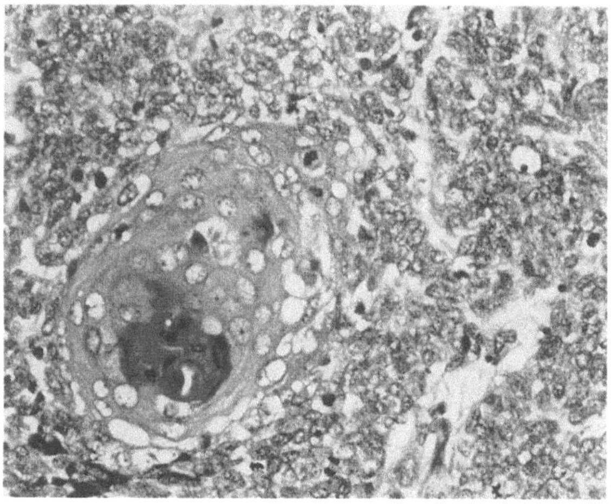

Fig. 14. Combined squamous/small cell neuroendocrine carcinoma of the thymus. A keratin "pearl" is formed by cytologically malignant squamous cells at the left of the photograph, and is sharply separated from surrounding lymphocyte-like tumor cells

Electron Microscopy

Ultrastructurally, thymic carcinoids are composed of closely apposed, polygonal cells (Fig. 15; Rosai et al. 1976; Wick and Scheithauer 1984). Adjacent cells may display blunt, interdigitating cytoplasmic processes, and are incompletely invested by basement membrane material. The interstitium consists of a mixture of collagen and flocculogranular matrix. Rarely, pseudoacini, formed by individual cell necrosis within cellular nests, may be evident. Intercellular junctions are invariably present, but are not abundant, and are of the maculae adherentes type. Nuclei are ovoid, or only slightly irregular in shape, with evenly districuted chromatin. Cytoplasmic invaginations within the nuclear contours may produce "pseudoinclusions." Nucleoli are characteristically inconspicuous.

Typical membrane-bound dense-core neurosecretory granules are usually abundant in the cytoplasm of tumor cells. These measure between 140 and 500 nm diameter (Fig. 16), although the size of such inclusions is usually rather uniform in any given neoplasm. "Misplaced" exocytosis, similar to that seen in pituitary prolactinomas, may be observed occasionally (Wick and Scheithauer 1984).

Other cytoplasmic organelles are rather nondescript, with three exceptions. Rough endoplasmic reticulum may be abundant and arranged in parallel arrays or concentric formations, particularly in hormonally active tumors. In these neoplasms, Golgi bodies are also numerous and prominent. Finally, thymic carcinoids which synthesize ACTH also appear to show an abun-

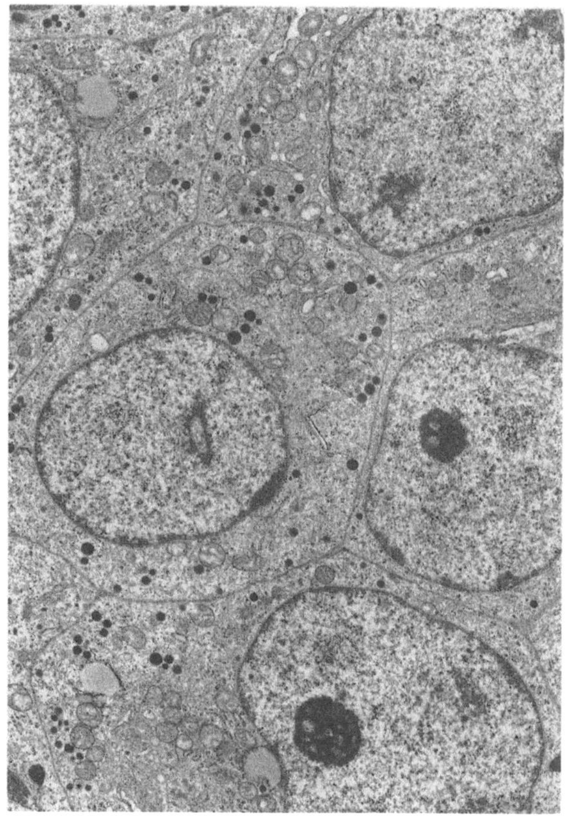

Fig. 15. Electron photomicrograph of a thymic carcinoid. Polygonal tumor cells contain round nuclei with evenly distributed chromatin, and numerous cytoplasmic neurosecretory granules. Inconspicuous macula adherens-like junctions are evident between apposed cell membranes

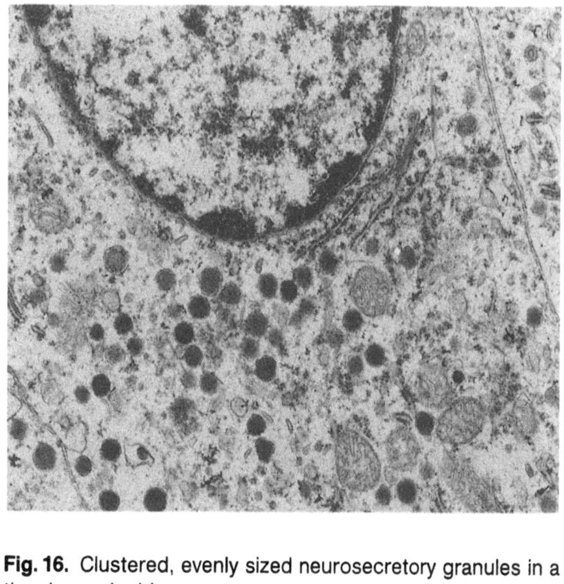

Fig. 16. Clustered, evenly sized neurosecretory granules in a thymic carcinoid

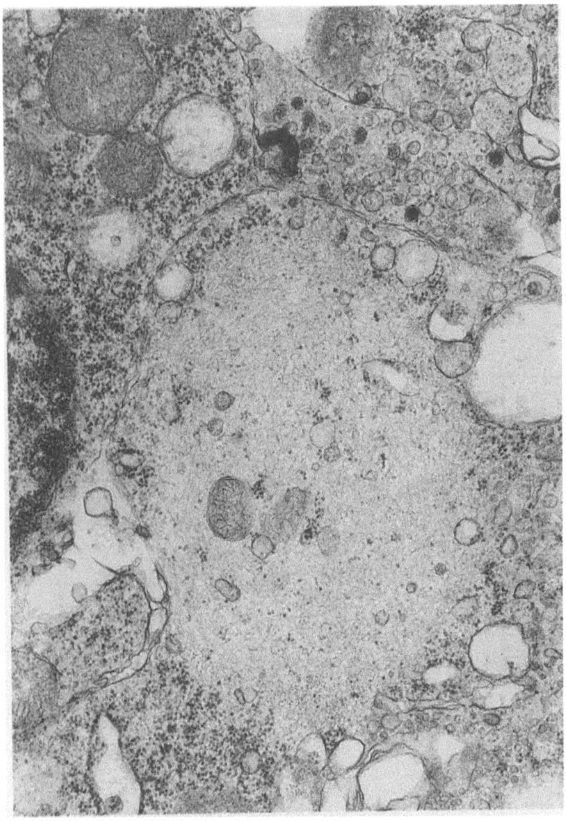

Fig. 17. A cytoplasmic whorl of "intermediate" filaments is present in this thymic carcinoid

dance of smooth endoplasmic reticulum (Wick and Scheithauer 1984).

Cytoplasmic filaments of the "intermediate" type are often present in thymic carcinoids, and not uncommonly assume a whorled, perinuclear configuration, in which dense-core granules may be enmeshed (Fig. 17; Fetissof et al. 1982; Wick and Scheithauer 1984). Short, scanty tonofilaments may also be evident in thymic carcinoids (Wick and Scheithauer 1984), although they never assume the prominence seen in thymomas.

The elecron microscopic features of thymic oat cell carcinoma are generally similar to those of carcinoid tumors, except that their cytoplasm is more scanty, and neurosecretory granules are much less numerous (Wick and Scheithauer 1982; Wick et al. 1982b) and may indeed require diligent searching. Somewhat unexpectedly, intercellular junctional complexes may be more prominent in thymic oat cell carcinoma than in carcinoid tumors. Tumors showing focal squamous differentiation by light microscopy manifest an abundance of cytoplasmic tonofilaments in such areas ultrastructurally (Snover et al. 1982, Wick et al. 1982). It should be noted that dense-core granules may also be seen within the squamoid cells.

Immunohistochemistry

Immunohistochemically, there are similarities and important differences between thymic carcinoids and true thymomas, with which they are most commonly confused. Both display reactivity for low molecular weight cytokeratin (Fig. 18; Wick et al., unpublished work), although this class of intermediate filament is much more abundant in thymomas than in thymic carcinoids or oat cell carcinomas. Some oat cell carcinomas, like thymomas, express epithelial membrane antigen (EMA), and this determinant is seen in 50% of thymic carcinoids as well (Sloane and Ormerod 1981; Wick, unpublished work).

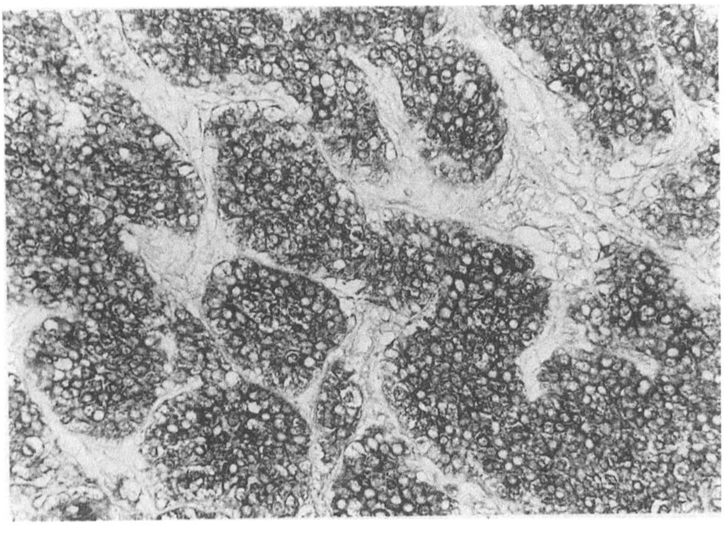

Fig. 18. Cytoplasmic immunoreactivity for low molecular weight cytokeratin in a carcinoid tumor of the thymus

Two antisera are particularly valuable in differentiating epithelial thymoma from thymic carcinoid or oat cell carcinoma: those directed at neuron-specific enolase (NSE) (Tapia et al. 1981; Wick et al. 1983b) and chromogranin (Wilson and Lloyd 1984). The first of these substances is an isoenzyme of 2-D-phosphoglycerate hydrolase, which is found in neurons and the diffuse neuroendocrine cellular system (Hullin et al. 1980). The second is a protein which is seemingly an integral part of the membrane of neurosecretory granules. In our experience, both have been consistently present in thymic neuroendocrine neoplasms, regardless of their degree of differentiation; however, NSE may be seen in thymomas as well (Wick et al., unpublished work). Accordingly, specificity testing of these two antisera has shown anti-chromogranin to be the more reliable in the definition of neuroendocrine neoplasms as a group, making it the probe of choice in the circumstances just described (Fig. 19).

In keeping with their line of differentiation, thymic carcinoids and oat cell carcinomas may exhibit immunoreactivity for any of the neuropeptide hormones or for serotonin (Wick et al. 1982a; Wick and Scheithauer 1982; Wick et al. 1982b; Wick and Scheithauer 1984); ACTH, somatostatin, and calcitonin have been the neuropeptides most frequently observed (DeLellis and Wolfe 1976); Wick and Scheithauer 1984). Thymomas do not manifest synthesis of any of these peptides, and we are of the firm opinion that all previous reports of "thymomas" showing ACTH production were, in fact, examples of thymic carcinoids (Wick et al. 1983a).

Confusion with malignant lymphoma may arise in the rare cases of carcinoid tumor of the thymus with a diffuse growth pattern (Wick et al. 1982a). However, thymic carcinoid fails to show immunoreactivity for common leukocyte antigen (Kurtin and Pinkus 1985), like the former lesion.

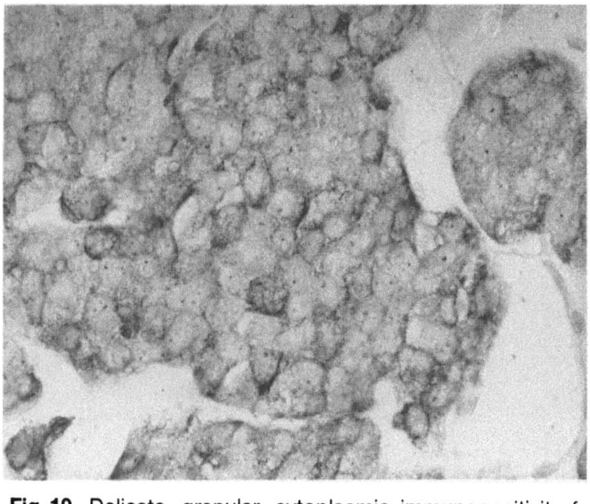

Fig. 19. Delicate, granular, cytoplasmic immunopositivity for chromogranin in a thymic carcinoid

Positive immunohistochemical staining results for neuropeptides are clinically valuable not only to confirm the origin of obivous endocrinopathies, but also to provide useful data on "silent" tumors. In both circumstances, the serum may be assayed for the hormone concerned (e.g., somatostatin) as a potential marker of tumor progression or recurrence.

Behavior and Prognosis

The primary reason for emphasizing the distinction between thymic carcinoid and oat cell carcinoma on the one hand, and true thymoma on the other, is the disparity in their respective biologic behaviors. Whereas at least 30%-40% of thymic neuroendocrine neoplasms present with extrahoracic metastases to bones, skin, lymph nodes, and liver (Wick et al. 1982), which are usually refractory to adjuvant chemotherapy or radiotherapy, thymomas exhibit such behavior in less than 5% of all cases.

The mortality rate for carcinoid tumor of the thymus is higher in patients with the multiple endocrine neoplasia (MEN) syndrome, type I (pituitary adenoma, parathyroid adenoma or hyperplasia, and pancreatic islet cell tumor; Rosai et al. 1972; Manes and Taylor 1973; Dry et al. 1976; Lokich and Li 1978: Wick et al. 1980). Individuals with ectopic Cushing's syndrome due to tumoral synthesis of ACTH also fare more poorly than those without clinical endocrinopathy (Wick et al. 1980).

Thymic carcinoid has the potential to act aggressively, even if encapsulated at initial diagnosis, as does oat cell carcinoma of the thymus (Wick et al. 1980; 1982a). Thus, this macroscopic feature does not have the same prognostic significance that it does in cases of true thymoma. Since metastasis of thymic carcinoid and oat cell carcinoma may occur as late as 10 years after initial presentation (Wick et al. 1982a; Wick and Rosai, in press), long-term clinical follow-up is necessary. The few cases of oat cell carcinoma of the thymus which have been reported have not shown the rapidly fatal behavior of histologically identical pulmonary tumors, with an average survival in one series of 36 months (Wick et al. 1982b). A possible exception to this statement concerns examples of these lesions with focal squamous differentiation. Among three cases reported by Snover et al. in 1982, widespread metastases occurred within 2 years after diagnosis.

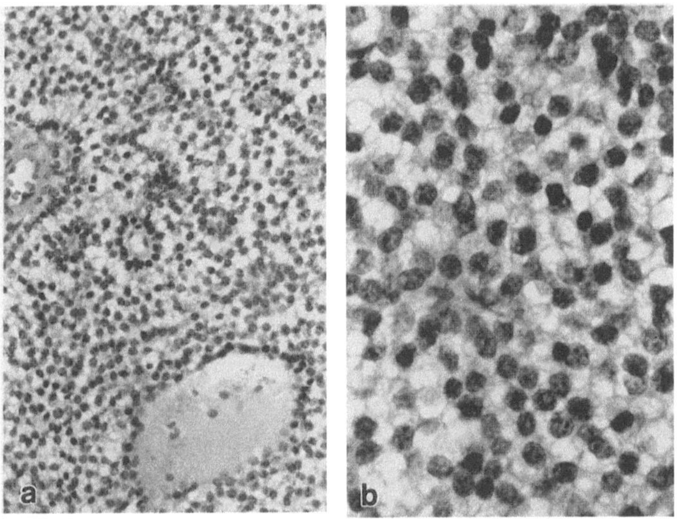

Fig. 20 a, b. Intrathymic parathyroid adenoma. Tumor cells have more abundant clear cytoplasm (a) and more compact nuclei (b) than those of thymic carcinoid

Differential Diagnosis

Several other pathologic entities enter into the differential diagnosis with thymic carcinoid and oat cell carcinoma. *Epithelial thymoma* has been extensively discussed in Chap. 9 as well as in the preceding sections. To recapitulate, thymoma does not display the uniformity of nuclear chromatin seen in thymic carcinoids, and commonly shows lobulation by internal fibrous bands. Thymic carcinoids are immunoreactive for chromogranin, in contrast to thymomas.

Intrathymic parathyroid adenoma usually has a clinical course with hypercalcemia, which betrays the nature of this endocrine lesion (Russell et al. 1981; Roslyn et al. 1983). However, occasional cases may be hormonally silent, thereby causing possible confusion with thymic carcinoid. Several points of distinction between these lesions are evident microscopically. Most notably, parathyroid adenomas do not contain the focal necrosis, organoid growth pattern, or rosette formation which typify thymic carcinoids (Fig. 20), and they are usually strongly periodic acid-Schiff (PAS)-positive (Woolner et al. 1952; Wick and Rosai, in press). Electron microscopy shows far fewer neurosecretory granules in parathyroid adenoma than in thymic carcinoid. Parathyroid hormone may be demonstrated immunohistochemically in the former, but not the latter of these lesions (Wick, unpublished work).

Paraganglioma of the mediastinum is also morphologically similar to thymic carcinoid; however, it does not characteristically occur in the thymic bed, but rather is seen in association with large blood vessels because of its presumed origin from the aorticopulmonary bodies or intravascular paraganglia (Glenner and Grimley 1974; Olson and Salyer 1978). A more tightly clustered cellular growth pattern (*Zellballen* formation) typifies paragangliomas (Fig. 21), as compared with the larger organoid cell nests of thymic carcinoids. Furthermore, whereas paragangliomas are usually devoid of mitotic activity, division figures are readily visible in thymic carcinoids. Argentaffin reactions are likely to yield positive results in paragangliomas, but not in thymic carcinoids. Finally, both neoplasms may be immunoreactive for Met- and Leuenkephalin (Baker et al. 1982; DeLellis et al. 1983), although this is much more frequent in paragangliomas (DeLellis et al. 1983).

Metastases to the thymus pose a difficult diagnostic problem in some cases, as they can mimic thymic car-

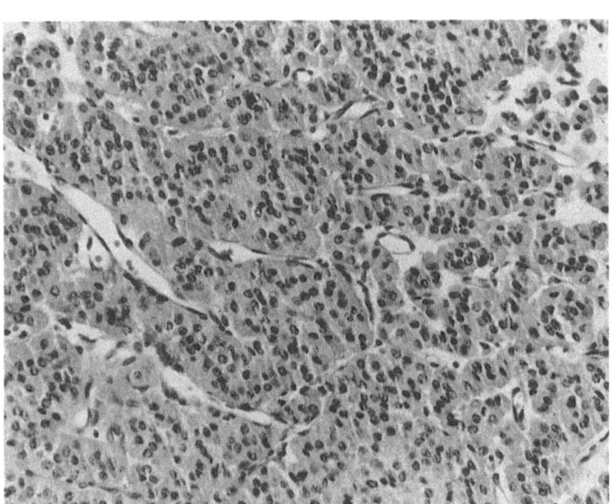

Fig. 21. Anterior mediastinal paraganglioma. Tumor cells have more abundant cytoplasm and are more obviously clustered into *Zellballen* than in thymic carcinoids

cinoid tumors. Conversely, the variant of thymic carcinoid which displays a cribriform growth pattern may suggest the presence of a secondary tumor, rather than a primary thymic lesion (Wick et al. 1982a). It is extremely unusual for carcinoids of the lung or intestine to metastasize selectively to the mediastinum, in the absence of overt disease at the primary site. Nevertheless, bronchoscopy and radiologic evaluation of the alimentary tract should be performed before making a definitive diagnosis of thymic carcinoid. The problems in differentiating primary and secondary oat cell carcinomas in the thymus, as well as the necessity to do so, have already been discussed.

Immunocytochemical stains have limited utility in the solution of these problems. NSE, chromogranin, and the neuropeptide hormones may be observed in primary or metastatic neuroendocrine neoplasms, and thus have little differential diagnostic application in this setting.

Lastly, rare examples of *malignant lymphoma* or *mediastinal germ cell tumor* may be confused with thymic carcinoid. In these circumstances, immunohistologic evaluation *is* helpful diagnostically. Lymphomas display the presence of common leukocyte antigen (Kurtin and Pinkus 1985) and germinomas contain placental alkaline phosphatase (Beckstead 1983) both of which are absent in carcinoid tumors of the thymus.

Germ Cell Tumors of the Thymus

It is not surprising that neoplasms showing germinal cell differentiation should arise in the thymus in view of the embryologic development of the gonads, which are the most frequent sites for such tumors. In early fetal life, the germinal ridges are paired midline structures, which extend virtually throughout the axial dimension of the developing human (Gillman 1948). With time, the cells in these ridges migrate caudally, to reach an eventual destination in the gonadal anlage. However, if they are arrested in this process, the surviving germinal cells may serve as a focus for subsequent neoplasia; this most typically evolves in the cranial sellar region (Bjornsson et al. 1985), thymic bed (Friedman 1951; Oberman and Libcke 1963; Cox 1975; Bergh et al. 1978b; Recondo and Libshitz 1978), and retroperitoneum (Abell et al. 1965; Engel et al. 1968; Buskirk et al. 1982).

The terminology of germ cell neoplasia is potentially confusing, as it has gone through several permutations and changes over the years. Throughout this chapter, we shall use the following nosologic system, which has been chosen because of its simplicity and general acceptance:

1. Mature teratomas: tumors composed of mature tissues showing differentation representative of at least two of the three embryonal germinal layers.
2. Immature teratomas: tumors containing primitive, embryonic neuroepithelial tissues as well as mature elements, as just described, but without undifferentiated components.
3. Seminomas: tumors composed of cells showing monodifferentation into spermatogonia-like elements.
4. Embryonal carcinomas: tumors comprised of undifferentiated cellular elements, showing a tendency to form primitive glands or ducts. The germinal origin of such neoplasms must be substantiated by the use of special techniques, and may not be obvious on conventional microscopy.
5. Yolk sac tumors (endodermal sinus tumors): neoplasms in which morphogenesis recapitulates such extraembryonic structures as the yolk sac endoderm and extra embryonic mesoblasts, in the absence of other lines of differentiation.
6. Teratocarcinomas: mature or immature teratomas combined with embryonal carcinoma, yolk sac tumor, or choriocarcinoma (with or without a seminomatous component).
7. Choriocarcinomas: tumors showing sole differentiation into placental tissues, including the cytotrophoblast and syncitiotrophoblast.

A well-known feature of germ cell neoplasms in their tendency to display more than one of these patterns. In a review of 56 cases of mediastinal germ cell tumors seen at the Mayo Clinic, Knapp et al. (1985) found mixed tumors in 34% of their cases. Hence, it is not rare for the pathologist to render such diagnoses as "mixed germ cell tumor, containing embryonal carcinoma and choriocarcinoma." This practice is preferable to attemps at "forcing" tumors into the strict nosologic categories described here, and is of use to clinicians in planning therapeutic interventions and determining accurate prognoses. With this caveat in mind, we shall nonetheless provide more detailed descriptions of each form of germ cell neoplasia, in the following sections. The premise that they represent tumors of the thymus, in a topographic sense, is substantiated by the observations that they may be totally confined within the capsule of this gland (Rosai and Levine 1976), or that thymic elements are intermingled within the tumor (Burns and McCaughey 1986).

Mature Teratoma

Mature teratomas are the commonest germ cell tumors of the mediastinum, accounting for 9%-20% of all tu-

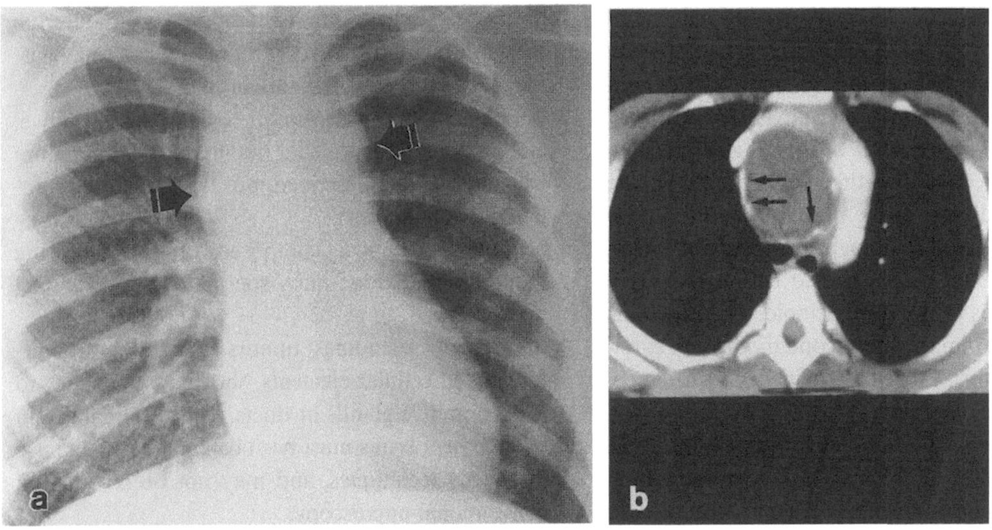

Fig. 22 a, b. Anterosuperior mediastinal teratoma (**a**) shows "eggshell" calcification on corresponding computed tomogram (**b**). (Courtesy of Dr. Bradley Lewis, Mayo Clinic, Rochester, Minnesota, USA)

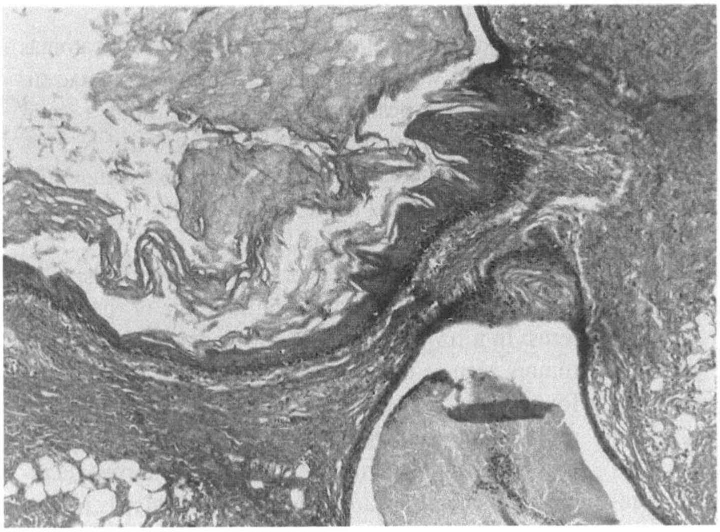

Fig. 23. Keratinizing squamous epithelium in mature thymic teratoma

mors in this location (Ringertz and Lidholm 1956; Lewis et al. 1983). They occur with equal frequency in men and women, with a peak during the third decade of life (Lewis et al. 1983). However, an increased incidence has been reported in men with Klinefelter's syndrome (Lachman et al. 1986). Roughly one-third are asymptomatic, and are found during routine chest radiography. The remainder present with chest, back, or shoulder pain, dyspnea, the superior vena cava syndrome, or cough. Rupture of such neoplasms into the bronchi may produce the dramatic symptom of trichoptysis, if hair is contained within the mass, and lipid pneumonia may also ensue. Foci of calcification are evident on roentgenograms of mediastinal teratomas in roughly 25% of all cases (Fig. 22; Lewis et al. 1983).

Grossly, mature teratomas are encapsulated, internally cystic masses averaging 10–11 cm in their greatest dimension. The cyst cavities often contain keratinous debris, with or without hair; cartilage or bone may also be macroscopically obvious (Adebonojo and Nicola 1976). Histologically, the predominant elements are usually integumentary, including keratinizing squamous epithelium with pilosebaceous and sudoriferous adnexa (Fig. 23). Respiratory and gut epithelium and pancreatic tissue are also frequently observed, along with fibroblastic or smooth muscular

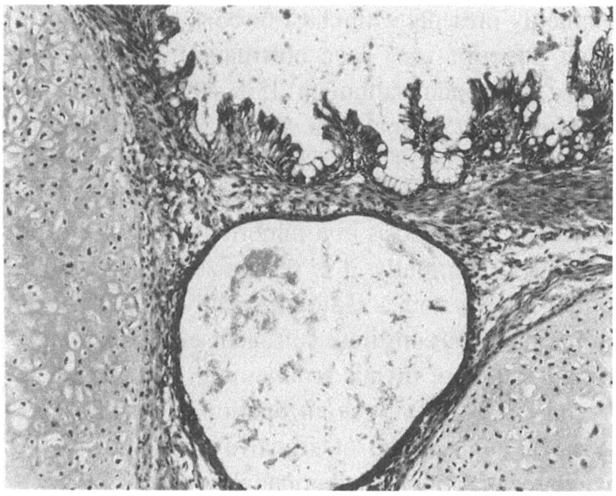

Fig. 24. Bronchial epithelium-lined cyst (top), squamous cyst (bottom), and well-formed cartilage (left and right) in a mature thymic teratoma

mesenchymal tissue, or cartilage and bone, as mentioned already (Fig. 24). Less than 10% of mature teratomas contain teeth, choroid plexus, nervous tissue, bone marrow, striated muscle, renal tissue, or retinal tissue (Lewis et al. 1983).

Care must be taken to sample these tumors thoroughly for microscopic exmination, since the finding of foci of seminoma or other germ cell tumors changes not only their classification, but their prognosis. In addition, rare examples of mature mediastinal teratomas harboring squamous cell carcinoma, adenocarcinoma, or sarcoma have been reported (Ulbright et al. 1984). In the absence of these complicating elements, surgery is curative, and the prognosis is therefore excellent.

Immature Teratoma

Immature teratomas, again defined as showing embryonic neuroepithelial, mesenchymal, and epithelial elements in varying combinations, account for only 1% of mediastinal teratomas (Carter et al. 1982). In other locations, particularly in the gonads and the sacrococcygeal region, the quantity of primitive neuroectodermal tissue in immature teratomas has been determined to be an important prognostic feature (Norris et al. 1976; Gonzalez-Crussi et al. 1978). The microscopic appearance of this element will be described later. In the mediastinum, however, it would appear that the patient's age is the most important prognostic factor (Carter et al. 1982). The immature teratomas occurring after age 15 have tended to behave aggressively (Ringertz and Lidholm 1956; Hodge et al. 1959; Daniel et al. 1960; Oberman and Libcke 1964; Canty and Siemens 1978), while all those in younger individuals have pursued an innocuous course after surgery alone (Berry et al. 1969; Carney et al. 1972; Carter et al. 1982). This point is an interesting one, since it correlates with the behavior of gonadal germ cell tumors such as yolk sac tumors, which are less aggressive in infants and children than in adults (Donaldson et al. 1973; Dehner 1975).

Grossly, there are no significant differences between mature and immature teratomas. Microscopically, the latter contain foci of fetal-appearing cartilage or primitive neuroectodermal tissue (Carter et al. 1982) which is represented by clusters of basaloid cells with high nucleocytoplasmic ratios, and mitotic activity (Fig. 25). These may show a tendency toward the formation of rudimentary neural tube-like structures, and may be embedded in a fibrillar, neuroglial-like stroma. The presence of overt embryonal carcinoma, choriocarci-

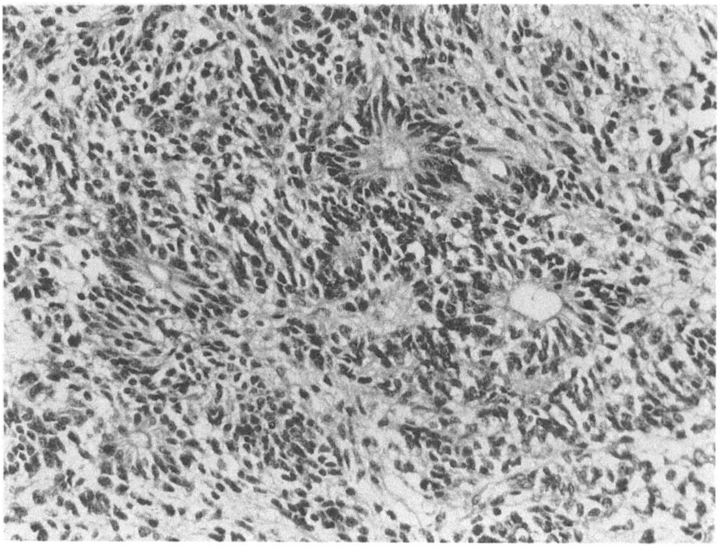

Fig. 25. Aggregates of small neuroepithelial cells with formation of primitive neural tube-like rosettes, in immature thymic teratoma

noma, yolk sac tumor, seminoma, or somatic carcinoma/sarcoma in an otherwise typical teratoma mandates its exclusion from this group.

Seminoma

Seminoma of the thymus is the commonest pure germ cell tumor of the mediastinum, and has been confused in the past with true thymoma (seminomatous thymoma) (Schantz et al. 1972; Levine 1973; Martini et al. 1974; Rosai and Levine 1976; Burt and Javadpour 1981). However, compelling evidence has accrued which both dispels any notion that this neoplasm is of thymic epithelial origin and demonstrates its pathologic identity with seminoma of the testis and dysgerminoma of the ovary (Levine 1973).

This neoplasm occurs almost exclusively in males, mostly in the third and fourth decades of life. Like other space-occupying lesions of the mediastinum, it commonly presents with chest or back pain, dyspnea, cough, superior vena cava obstruction, fever, weight loss or bone pain, although 15%-40% of cases are asymptomatic (Schantz et al. 1972; Cox 1975; Recondo and Libschitz 1978; Knapp et al. 1985). Cervical and supraclavicular lymph nodes may be involved by metastases at diagnosis in a minority of cases (Knapp et al. 1985). Currently, it is recognized that palpably normal gonads and a radiographically unremarkable retroperitoneum constitute sufficient evidence for the primary nature of thymic seminoma in any given case (Aygun et al. 1984). Such an opinion is based on the statistical unlikelihood of selective metastasis to the thymic region of an occult gonadal tumor of this type.

Grossly, thymic seminoma is usually unencapsulated, and freely invades mediastinal great vessels, pleura, or pericardium (Fig. 26; Rosai and Levine 1976). On cut section, it is solid, rubbery, and gray-white, without the internal lobulation which characterizes true thymoma. Foci of necrosis and hemorrhage are

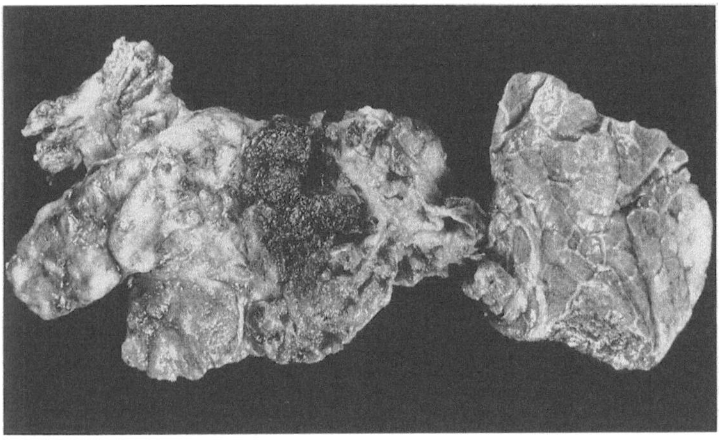

Fig. 26. Thymic seminoma (left) showing nonencapsulation, hemorrhage, and necrosis. A fragment of residual thymus borders the mass (right)

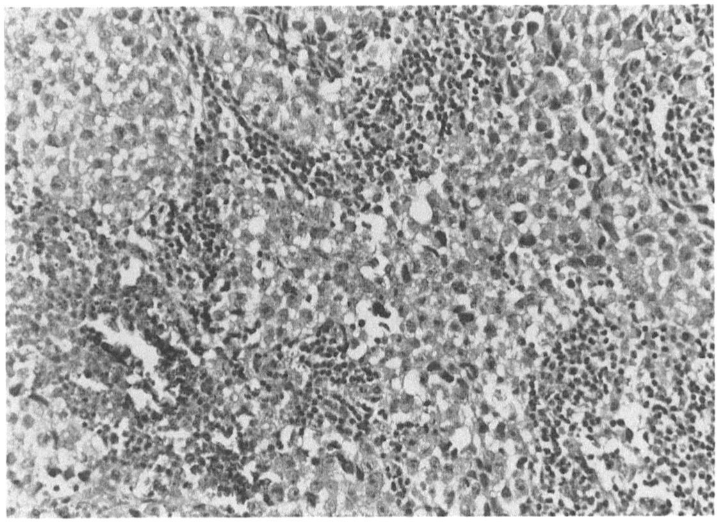

Fig. 27. Sheets of lossely cohesive tumor cells are surrounded by reactive lymphocytes in this thymic seminoma

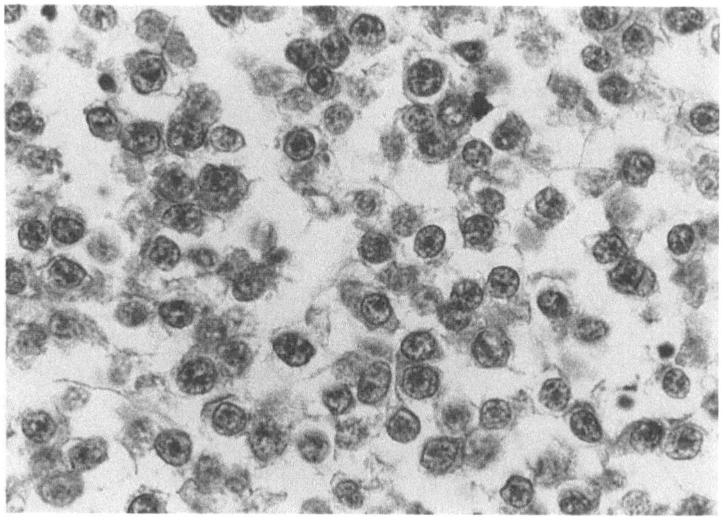

Fig. 28. Cytologic detail of seminoma of the thymus. Tumor cels have indistinct cytoplasmic borders, coarse, distinct nuclear membranes, and prominent nucleoli

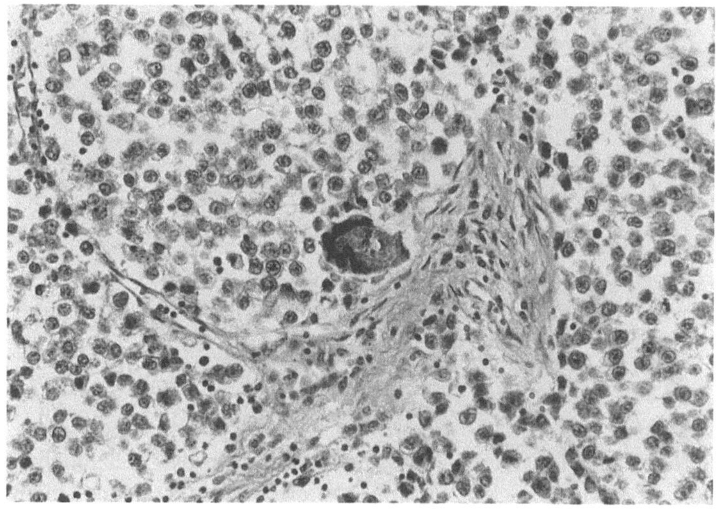

Fig. 29. Syncytial trophoblastic cell in thymic seminoma (center). The presence of such elements in isolation does not affect the classification or prognosis of this tumor

common, and cysts can occasionally be seen (Burns and McCaughey 1986).

Histologically, sheets of uniform tumor cells are subdivided by fine fibrovascular septa, which are typically heavily invested by reactive lymphocytes (Fig. 27). The cells of seminoma contain abundant, clear or slightly eosinophilic cytoplasm, which is PAS-positive and labile to diastase digestion. Nuclei are round or oval, with thick membranes, coarse chromatin, and complex nucleoli (Fig. 28). Mitotic activity is variable. A peculiar feature, which, like the lymphoid infiltrates of such neoplasms is thought to reflect a host immune response, is the admixture of noncaseating epithelioid granulomas throughout some thymic seminomas. These may be prominent enough to obscure the tumor proper, and may result in erroneous diagnoses of granulomatous inflammatory processes such as sarcoidosis (Burns and McCaughy 1986; Dusmet, personal communication). Occasional cases contain syncytiotrophoblastic cells, scattered randomly among the typical seminomatous cells (Fig. 29). If unassociated with cytotrophoblastic elements, this finding does not alter diagnosis or prognosis (Rosai 1981). However, it should be noted in pathologic reports, since production of human chorionic gonadotropin (HCG) by the syncytiotrophoblastic cells may account for elevated serum levels of this hormone.

On ultrastructural examination, seminoma does not display the overt features of epithelial differentiation (tonofilaments and desmosomes) which are seen in true thymomas (Levine 1973; Rosai and Levine 1976). Only primitive "appositional plaques" serve to join adjacent tumor cells, and basal lamina is absent (Fig. 30). The cytoplasm contains few metabolic organelles, and

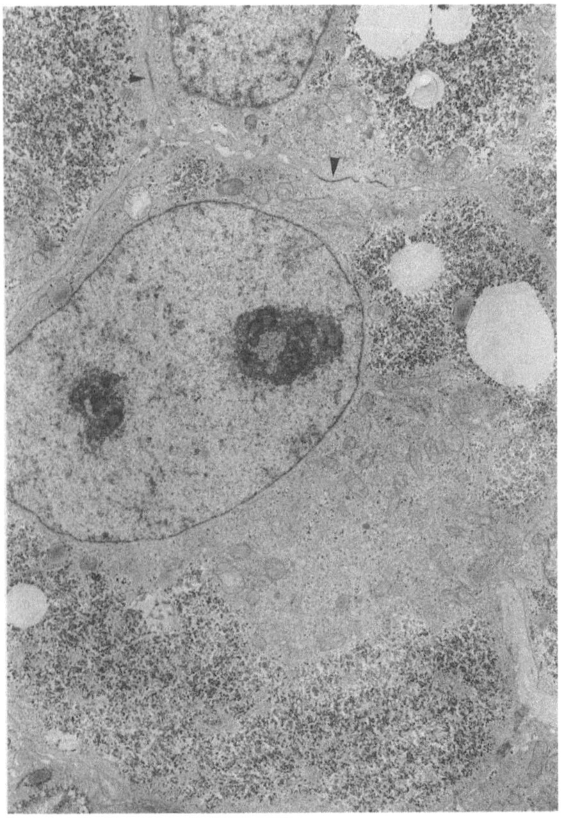

Fig. 30. Electron micrograph of thymic seminoma. Tumor cells contain cytoplasmic glycogen "pools," and are joined by "appositional plaques" *(arrowheads)*

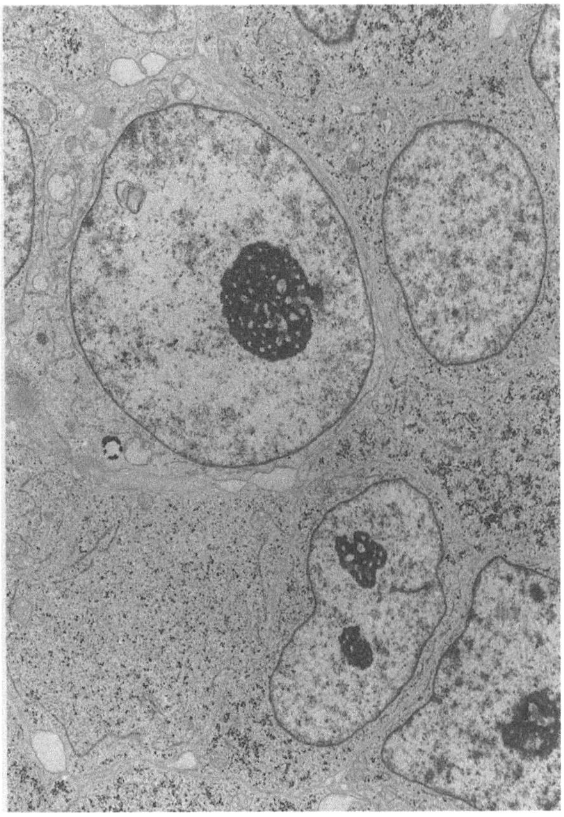

Fig. 31. Complex nucleolonemas, in nucleoli of thymic seminoma cells

lacks neurosecretory granules, but "lakes" of glycogen particles may be abundant. The most distinctive feature of seminomas on electron microscopy is the aspect of the nucleoli in this tumor - they are complex, with dispersed nucleolonema, and are present in nearly all neoplastic cells (Fig. 31).

Immunohistochemically, seminoma is again typified by a relative lack of positive findings. It does not express EMA (Sloane and Ormerod 1981) or cytokeratin (Battifora et al. 1984), nor does it contain α-fetoprotein (AFP), α_1-antitrypsin (AAP), neuropeptides, chromogranin, or common leukocyte antigen (Jacobsen et al. 1981; Wick, unpublished work). Indeed, aside from the aforementioned presence of HCG immunoreactivity in rare cases, the only determinant exhibited by seminoma is placental alkaline phosphatase (PLAP) (Fig. 32; Beckstead 1983; Manivel et al. 1987). Nonetheless, this isoenzyme is present in virtually all such tumors, a feature which is invaluable in defining their germinal nature, and which aids in excluding the differential diagnostic alternatives of *malignant lymphoma, thymoma,* and *thymic carcinoma,* in which PLAP reactivity is absent (Beckstead 1983; Wick, unpublished work). Keratin-specific antibodies, however, can highlight a meshwork of thymic epithelial cells which are intimately intermingled with the seminoma cells (Burns and McCaughey 1986).

Aygun et al. (1984) have recently reviewed the clinical features of mediastinal seminoma, with particular attention to prognosis and response to treatment. As with gonadal tumors of this type, radiation therapy is recommended as the primary modality. Although seminoma is thought to be equally sensitive to radiation regardless of its site of origin, a greater proportion (approximately 11%) of primary mediastinal tumors fail to respond to this treatment, and metastasize to bones, liver, brain, and soft tissue. Salvage chemotherapy regimens including cisplatin and etoposide have yielded encouraging results (Einhorn 1986). This observation may relate to the larger size of thymic seminoma at diagnosis, and consequently greater incidence of vascular invasion, compared with that of more accessible gonadal lesions. In any event, the 5-year survival of mediastinal seminoma is currently 75%, while that of testicular and ovarian germinoma is 85%-90% (Aygun et al. 1984).

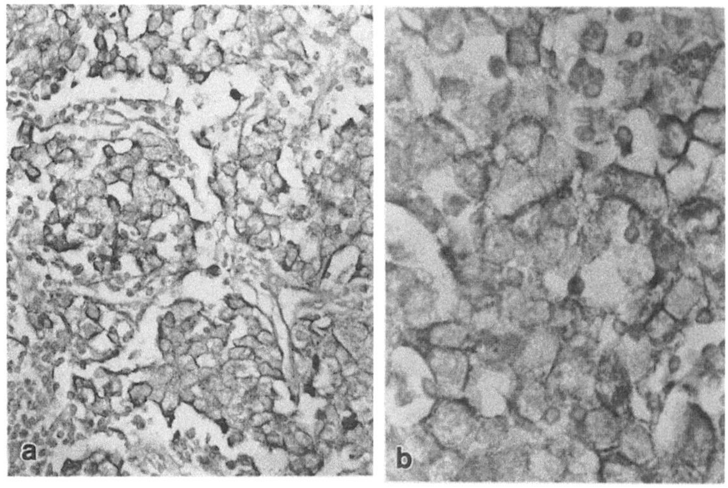

Fig. 32 a, b. Immunoreactivity for placental alkaline phosphatase is evident in this thymic seminoma, taking the form of membranous and cytoplasmic staining

Embryonal Carcinoma (MEC)

Pure embryonal carcinoma arising in the thymus is relatively rare, and this neoplasm is most commonly encountered in combination with seminoma, yolk sac tumor, choriocarcinoma, or teratomatous elements (Knapp et al. 1982). Like seminoma, mediastinal embryonal carcinoma (MEC) is commoner in male patients, and has a peak incidence in early adulthood. Males with Klinefelter's syndrome may have a higher risk of developing this neoplasm (McNeil et al. 1981). Symptoms and signs of MEC are similar to those of thymic seminoma, but may evolve more rapidly; however, serum levels of AFP are often elevated in cases of embryonal carcinoma (Javadpour 1979; Wick and Siegal 1980), as can be serum HCG levels (Knapp et al. 1985).

Grossly, MEC presents a similar appearance to that of seminoma, except that intratumoral necrosis and hemorrhage are somewhat commoner findings. Invasion of other mediastinal structures is frequently observed at surgery (Oberman and Libcke 1964; Cox 1975; Recondo and Libshitz 1978). Microscopically, this neoplasm is composed of nests, sheets, or cords of undifferentiated cells with large vesicular nuclei, scanty amphophilic cytoplasm, and abundant mitotic activity (Figs. 33 and 34; Oberman and Libcke 1964; Cox 1975; Rosai and Levine 1976; Wick and Siegal 1980; Knapp et al. 1982). Papillary structures may also be apparent. This description is generally quite similar to that of thymic carcinoma (Wick et al. 1982), and therefore the two tumors may be easily confused. Nevertheless, careful sampling of MEC will almost always reveal foci of primitive glandular or ductal differentiation (Fig. 35), features which are not present in thymic carcinoma.

Ultrastructural findings in cases of embryonal carcinoma are generally nondescript, and may lead to an

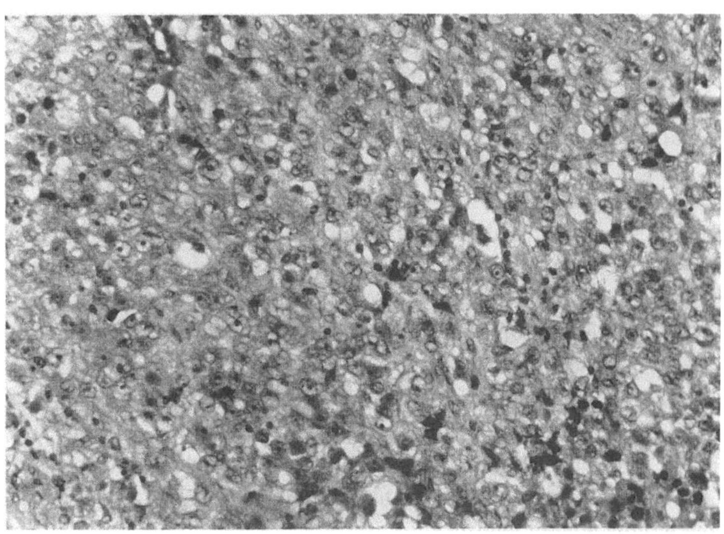

Fig. 33. Embryonal carcinoma of the thymus, composed of sheets of tumor cells with indistinct cytoplasmic borders, and large vesicular nuclei with prominent nucleoli. A resemblance to lymphoepithelioma-like thymic carcinoma is marked

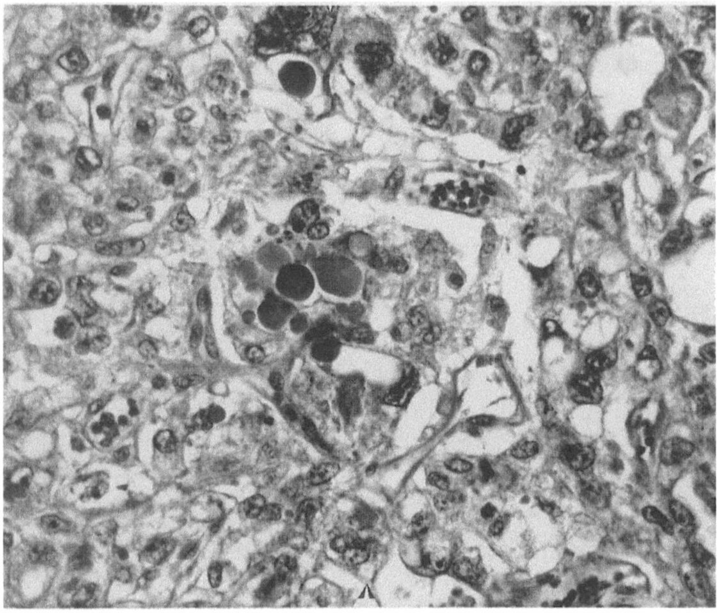

Fig. 34. Higher power view of tumor shown in Fig. 33 demonstrates cytologic detail to better advantage. In addition, several extracellular globules of refractile material are present (center). The latter are characteristic of embryonal carcinoma, and are not seen in thymic carcinoma

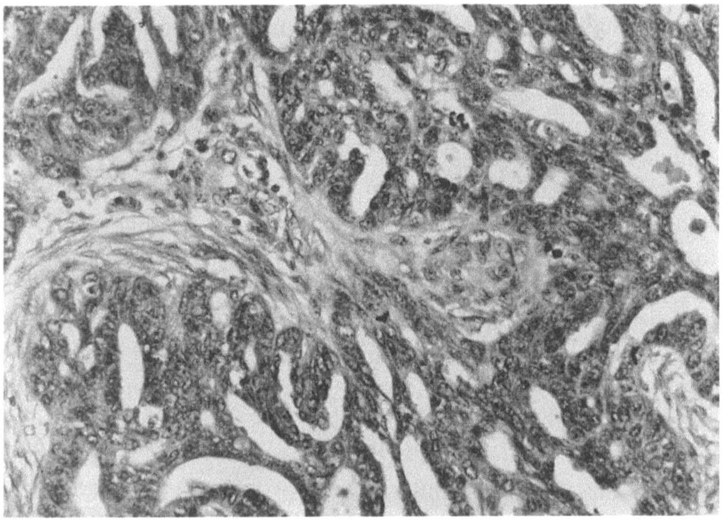

Fig. 35. Primitive glandular and ductal differentiation in thymic embryonal carcinoma

erroneous diagnosis of "undifferentiated carcinoma, not otherwise specified" (Mc Neil et al. 1981). Desmosomal intercellular junctions are more prominent than in cases of thymic seminoma, but cytoplasmic tonofilaments and pericellular basal lamina are again lacking (Fig. 36; Battifora et al. 1984). Occasional nuclei may display focally complex nucleoli. The most distinct feature of MEC on electron microscopy is probably the presence of cytoplasmic AFP globules. These are moderately electron-dense, and relatively large (500-900 nm), and often found in close association with rough endoplasmic reticulum (Fig. 37; Saas et al. 1983). Rare cases of MEC may demonstrate microvillous plasmalemmal differentiation, but intracytoplasmic lumina are not evident.

Immunocytochemical study reveals a typical antigenic profile in cases of MEC, and is therefore the pathologic investigation most likely to yield an accurate diagnosis. Embryonal carcinoma is EMA-negative (Sloane and Ormerod 1981), but cytokeratin-positive (Battifora et al. 1984), and shows immunoreactivity for PLAP, like seminoma (Beckstead 1983; Manivel et al. 1987). AFP is also detectable in 50%-75% of all cases immunohistochemically (Kurman et al. 1977), as is AAT (Wick, unpublished work). These results are unlike those obtained in *primary thymic carcinoma* or *metastatic carcinomas* from other sites, which represent the major differential diagnostic alternatives to MEC.

The clinical course of thymic embryonal carcinoma is highly malignant (Cox 1975; Martini et al. 1974;

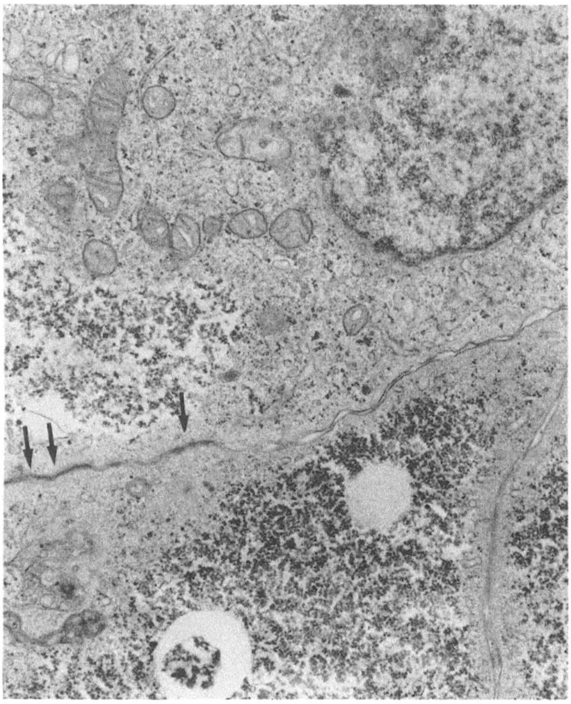

Fig. 36. Electron photomicrograph of embryonal carcinoma of the thymus, showing intercellular junctional complexes *(arrows)* and cytoplasmic glycogen. This neoplasm is similar in appearance to the seminoma in Fig. 30

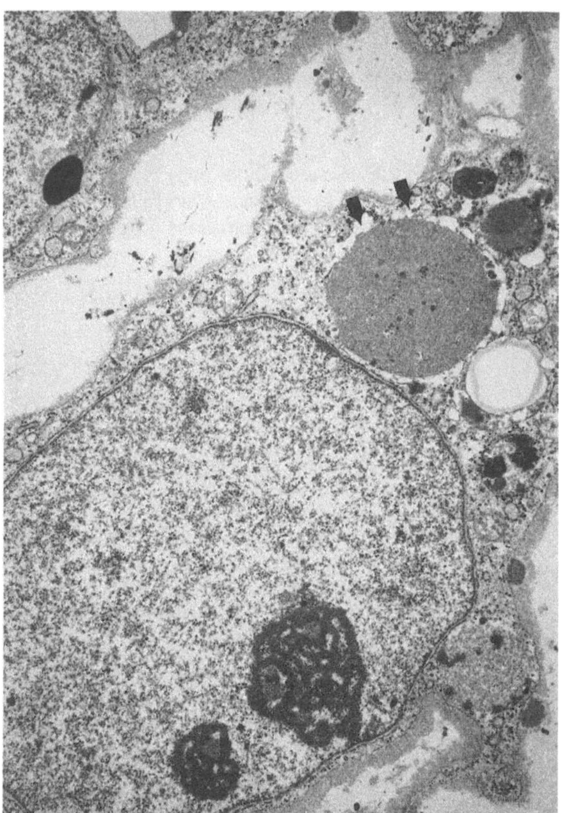

Vogelzang et al. 1982). It is often refractory to surgical resection, radiotherapy, and aggressive combination chemotherapy, and proves fatal through massive intrathoracic growth and/or metastasis to the lungs, bones, liver, and brain. Median survival for patients with MEC is less than 12 months (Burt and Javadpour 1981; Knapp et al. 1985). Once again, this pattern of behavior is worse than that of histologically identical gonadal tumors, perhaps for the same reasons cited in connection with thymic seminoma. As with testicular embryonal carcinoma, the response to therapy of MEC may be followed clinically by monitoring serum AFP levels (Javadpour 1979; Burt and Javadpour 1981).

Yolk Sac Tumor (Endodermal Sinus Tumor)

The clinical and gross pathologic features of yolk sac tumor (YST) of the mediastinum are virtually identical to those of embryonal carcinoma; indeed, the two tumors are commonly admixed with one another within the same mass (Teilmann et al. 1967; Huntington and Bullock 1970; Roth and Panganiban 1976; DeSmet et al. 1977; Mukai and Adams 1979). Pure thymic YST is exceedingly rare, and less than 20 cases have been documented (Fox and Vix 1980), only 2 in females (Gooneratne et al. 1985; Knapp et al. 1985).

Microscopically, this neoplasm is characterized by thin anastomosing cords composed of cuboidal cells with oval, hyperchromatic nuclei. Reticular or microcystic patterns may be evident (Fig. 38). A distinctive structure in YST, for which the neoplasm is named, is the Schiller-Duval body, which resembles the embryonic yolk sac (Fig. 39). It is composed of one or two layers of tumor cells mantling a central fibrovascular core, with an overall papillary configuration (Teilum 1959). Another characteristic feature is the formation of embryoid bodies (Fig. 40; Mostofi and Price 1973), composed of small groups of flattened tumor cells within microcystic spaces, and reminiscent of the embryonic growth plate. Extracellular, eosinophilic basement membrane material is sometimes abundant in YST, and is PAS-positive (Mukai and Adams 1979). In addition, PAS-positive, diastase-resistant globules are commonly evident within the cytoplasm of the tumor cells.

Fig. 37. A globule of α-fetoprotein is present within a dilated profile of endoplasmic reticulum *(arrows)*, in this thymic embryonal carcinoma

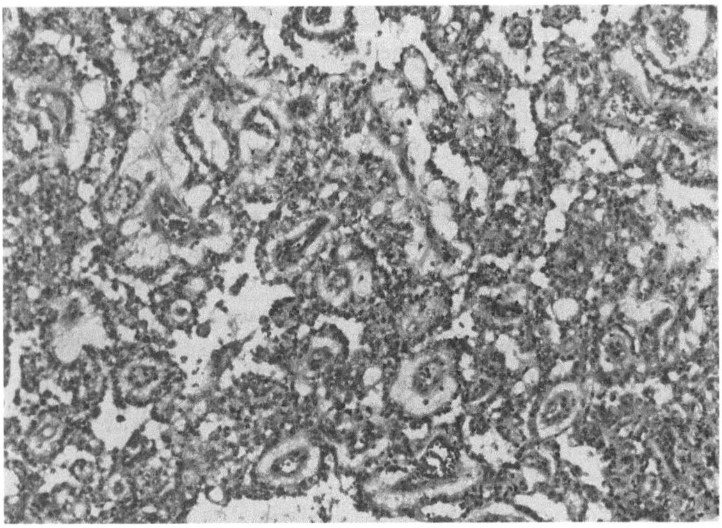

Fig. 38. Microcystic or "reticular" variant of endodermal sinus tumor (yolk sac carcinoma) of the thymic region

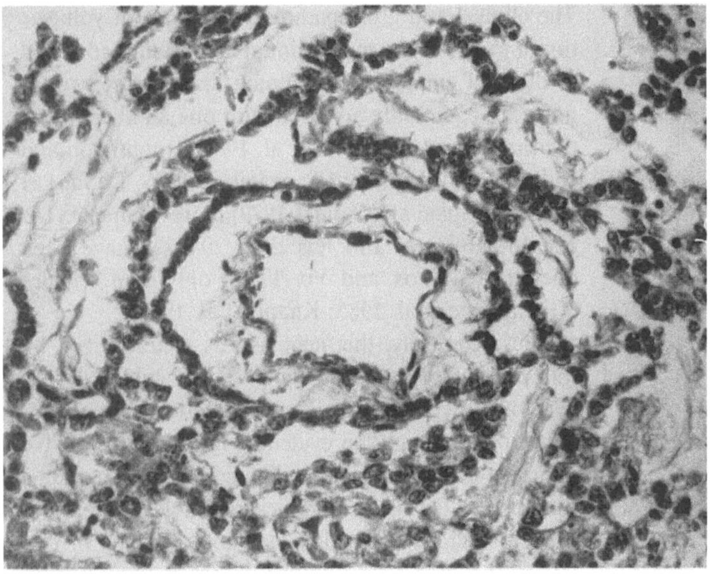

Fig. 39. Schiller-Duval body in thymic endodermal sinus tumor. A single layer of flattened tumor cells surrounds a central blood vessel

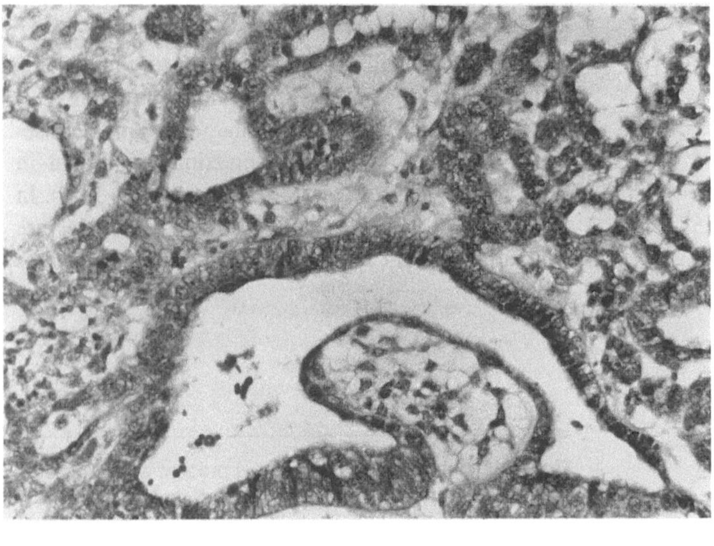

Fig. 40. An embryoid body is evident in this endodermal sinus tumor of the thymus (bottom of figure). It is represented by a bud-like protrusion of tumor cells into a central cavity, and rsembles the primitive embryonic growth plate

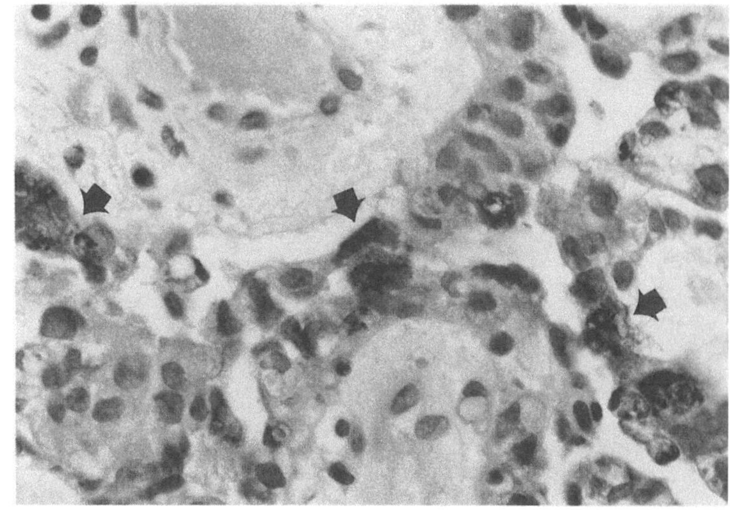

Fig. 41. Immunoreactivity for α-fetoprotein *(arrows)*, in endodermal sinus tumor of the thymus

Ultrastructurally, YST is nearly identical to MEC, except that extracellular basement membrane material is much more prominent (Nogales-Fernandez et al. 1977; Vuletin et al. 1977; Mukai and Adams 1979). Cytoplasmic globules of AFP are also more numerous than in the latter neoplasm (Javadpour 1979). Immunocytochemical features parallel those of MEC qualitatively, but AFP and AAT positivity is stronger and more uniform in YST (Fig. 41; Kurman et al. 1977; Mukai and Adams 1979; Sass et al. 1983; Wick, unpublished work). The AAT reactivity corresponds to the PAS-positive intracytoplasmic material seen on conventional microscopy (Mukai and Adams 1979).

The prognosis of thymic YST is generally poor. It is commonly unresectable at diagnosis, and the majority of documented cases have shown metastases to the lungs, liver, brain, lymph nodes, and bones (Mukai and Adams 1979; Fox and Vix 1980). Response to radiotherapy and chemotherapy is uncommon, and patients with residual mediastinal or metastatic disease have a median survival of 10 months (Kuzur et al. 1982). However, after reviewing the literature, Mukai and Adams (1979) proposed clinicopathologic criteria which may correlate with a better prognosis in YST. These include an asymptomatic status at diagnosis, surgical resectability of the neoplasm, and the absence of metastatic spread at presentation. Serum levels of AFP are again useful monitors of therapeutic efficacy in cases of YST of the mediastinum (Talermann et al. 1977).

Teratocarcinoma

As might be expected, the clinical and macroscopic features of mediastinal teratocarcinoma resemble those of either mature or immature teratoma, embryonal carcinoma, yolk sac tumor, or seminoma, depending on the relative proportions of these elements in any given case (Figs. 42 and 43; Pugsley and Carleton 1953; Pachter and Lattes 1964; Cox 1975; Bergh et al. 1978b). Similarly, the histologic aspects of teratocarcinoma represent an amalgam of the aforementioned tumor types.

Recent attention has been given to the development of non-germ cell malignancies (NGCM) within mediastinal teratocarcinomas. Ulbright et al. (1984) have described four cases in which rhabdomyosarcoma, liposarcoma, fibrosarcoma, angiosarcoma, or glioblastoma multiforme occurred in this setting. We have observed seven such examples, all of which featured rhabdomysarcoma or angiosarcoma in conjunction

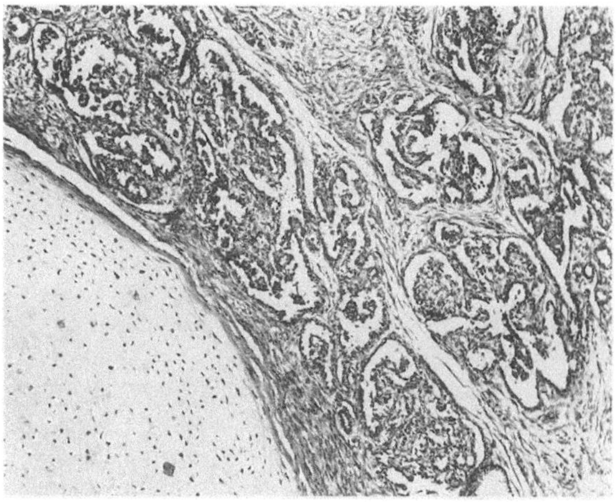

Fig. 42. Teratocarcinoma of the anterior mediastinum, composed of chondroid tissue (lower left) and juxtaposed embryonal carcinoma/endodermal sinur tumor

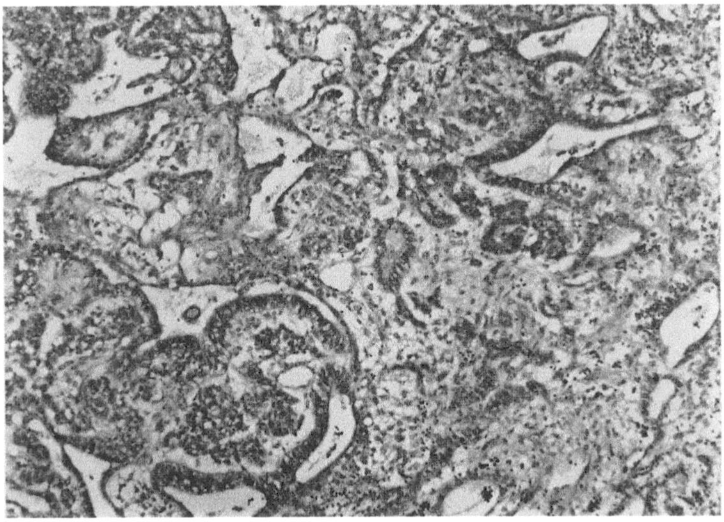

Fig. 43. Higher power view of the germ cell component of tumor shown in Fig. 42

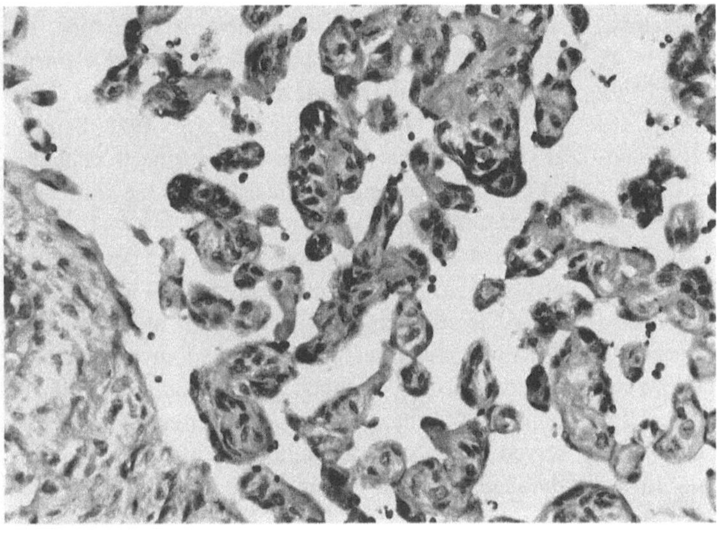

Fig. 44. Angiosarcomatous differentiation in a teratomatous tumor of the thymus. Papillary stromal projections are covered by cytologically malignant endothelial cells

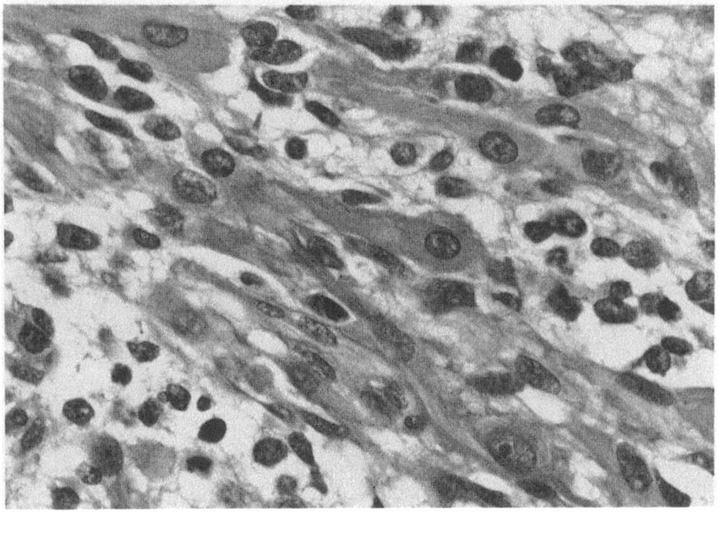

Fig. 45. Rhabdomyosarcomatous focus in a thymic germ cell tumor. Strap-like cells contain refractile eosinophilic cytoplasm; some of these elements showed cross-striations

with malignant germ cell elements (Fig. 44; Manivel et al. 1986). One of these cases contained areas of both rhabdomyosarcomatous and angiosarcomatous differentiation (Fig. 45). Whether or not these tumor tissues arise as a reflection of differentiation induced by the therapy of teratocarcinoma, or are present de novo, they do not respond to standard germ cell tumor treatment protocols, as shown in the high rate of therapeutic failure and mortality in such cases. Similar comments apply to the equally rare circumstance of squamous cell carcinoma or adenocarcinoma arising in a teratocarcinoma of the mediastinum (Wick et al. 1982b).

Until recently, the outlook for uncomplicated thymic teratocarcinoma was said to be dismal. However, a report by Parker et al. (1983) has documented the efficacy of aggressive surgical intervention after cyclic chemotherapy. Surgery was performed after serum AFP levels had fallen, indicating the cytolysis of MEC or YST components of the tumors. Five of six patients treated with this regimen were apparently cured; notably, another two patients who died had undergone chemotherapy alone, without subsequent surgical resections of their neoplasms.

Choriocarcinoma

Choriocarcinoma as a pure thymic germ cell neoplasm is vanishingly rare, and this tumor type is almost invariably admixed with MEC, YST, or both (Wenger et al. 1968, Sickels et al. 1974; Sandhaus et al. 1981; Knapp et al. 1982). It only exceptionally occurs within teratocarcinomas of the mediastinum. Nevertheless, any focus of choriocarcinoma, no matter how small, in a thymic germ cell neoplasm assumes major prognostic importance. Patients with such lesions are nearly all males, in their 30s or 40s, who may present with rapidly enlarging mediastinal masses and superior vena cava obstruction if the choriocarcinoma component of their tumors is sizable (Wenger et al. 1968). Erosion into bronchi by the mass may produce hemoptysis, and the synthesis of HCG by choriocarcinomas produces gynecomastia, decreased libido, and testicular atrophy (Greenwood et al. 1971). The rare tumors which occur in females cause menstrual irregularities.

Grossly, choriocarcinoma is a friable, reddish-gray, largely necrotic invasive neoplasm. Hence, any areas resembling this description in mediastinal germ cell tumors should be sampled thoroughly. Microscopically, choriocarcinoma is defined by the presence of cytotrophoblast, represented by sheets and nests of polygonal cells with single, large, vesicular nuclei and a moderate amount of amphophilic cytoplasm (Fig. 46), and by syncytiotrophoblast, which is composed of multinucleated cellular elements occurring in apposition to the cytotrophoblastic elements (Fig. 47; Golding et al. 1968). Spontaneous necrosis and hemorrhage are common, and cytotrophoblastic mitotic activity is typically brisk. As mentioned previously, occasional seminomas of the thymus may contain syncytiotrophoblastic cells; however, unless unequivocal cytotrophoblast is also present, such neoplasms should not be labeled as choriocarcinomas.

In contrast to thymic seminoma, MEC, and YST, the absence of palpable gonadal mass does not confirm the primary nature of a mediastinal choriocarcinoma (Knapp et al. 1982), for choriocarcinomas have a well-known tendency to form early, distant metastases, while only a miniscule primary tumor is present in the ovary or testis. This issue is currently of little prognostic importance (Reynolds et al. 1979), but may influ-

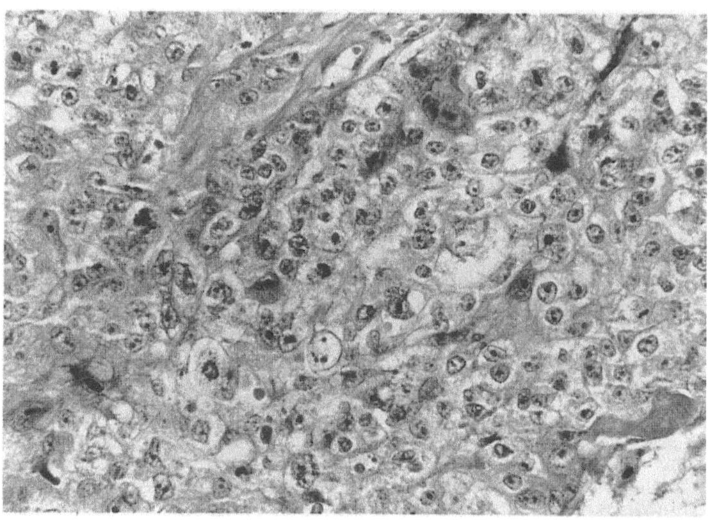

Fig. 46. Cytotrophoblastic component of thymic choriocarcinoma, represented by relatively uniform polygonal cells with clear cytoplasm

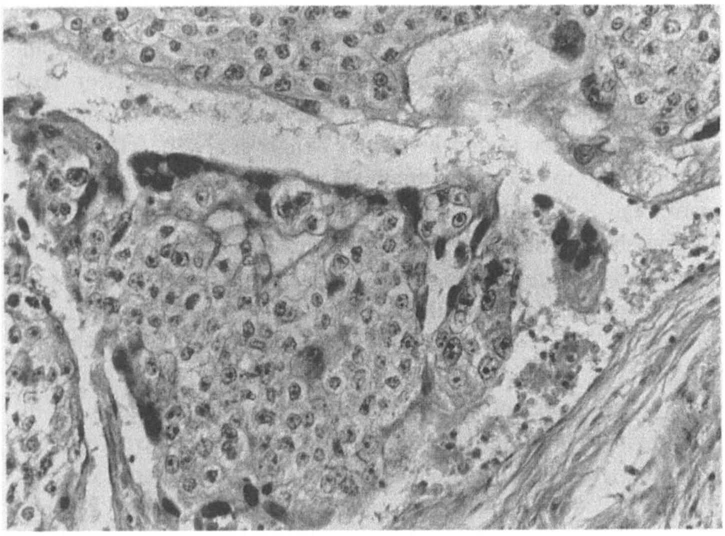

Fig. 47. Syncytiotrophoblastic cells, containing multiple nuclei, cover nests of cytotrophoblasts in this thymic choriocarcinoma

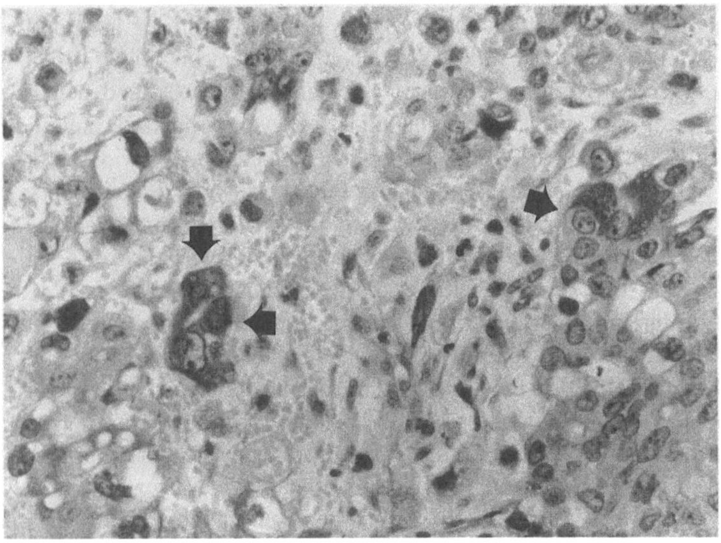

Fig. 48. Darkly staining cytoplasmic immunoreactivity for β-human chorionic gonadotropin *(arrows)* in syncytiotrophoblastic cells of thymic choriocarcinoma

ence the decision of the thoracic surgeon as to whether or not a therapeutic thoracotomy is warranted.

Ultrastructural study is of little benefit in the pathologic identification of thymic choriocarinoma. However, immunocytochemistry may be invaluable in confirming the presence of syncytiotrophoblastic elements. As one would expect, antisera to HCG are employed for this purpose (Fig. 48; Sandhaus et al. 1981; Knapp et al. 1982).

Other immunohistologic markers may be useful to exclude a limited number of differential diagnostic alternatives. *Metastases* of anaplastic, pleomorphic carcinomas to the thymic region, which may mimic choriocarcinoma, are EMA-positive, but nearly always PLAP-negative (Sloane and Ormerod 1981; Beckstead 1983; Nagle et al. 1983; Wick, unpublished work). Choriocarcinomas exhibit the converse of these findings (Beckstead 1983). Rare examples of *pleomorphic sarcomas* of the mediastinum, which may contain syncytiotrophoblast-like giant cells, would be expected to show vimentin immunoreactivity (Altmannsberger et al. 1981; Miettenen et al. 1983), whereas choriocarcinomas instead express cytokeratin.

As stated previously, the diagnosis of choriocarcinoma of the mediastinum has grave prognostic implications, even if the size of this neoplastic element is small. Thymic choriocarcinoma is invariably refractory to even the most heroic treatment regimens, and rapidly metastasizes to the lungs, liver, bones, and brain. Indeed, pulmonary metastases are commonly present at initial diagnosis. The median survival in reported cases of this entity has been no longer than 7 months after presentation (Reynolds et al. 1979; Knapp et al. 1985).

Malignant Lymphomas of the Thymic Region

The thymus is not uncommonly involved in Hodgkin's or non-Hodgkin's malignant lymphoma. This gland may be invaded secondarily from disease in mediastinal lymph nodes, or may be the primary (and only) focus of involvement (Rosai and Levine 1976). Inasmuch as clinical and pathologic findings differ significantly in thymic Hodgkin's disease (HD) and non-Hodgkin's lymphoma (NHL), these two classes of malignant lymphoma will be discussed separately.

Hodgkin's Disease of the Thymus (HD)

HD is the form of malignant lymphoma which is most likely to arise in the thymus and mediastinum (Marshall and Wood 1957; Fechner 1969; Bergh et al. 1978a). In the thymus, the nodular sclerosing type (NSHD) is by far the commonest of the four currently accepted variants of HD (lymphocyte-predominant, nodular sclerosing, mixed cellularity, and lymphocyte-depleted) (Fechner 1969).

For many years, NSHD of the thymus was considered to be a form of thymoma (granulomatous thymoma) (Lowenhaupt and Brown 1951) rather than a lymphoreticular malignancy, because of the gross and microscopic aspects of NSHD, which show certain similarities to those of thymomoa. These include gross and microscopic nodularity (interpreted as lobulation by thymoma proponents), and internal septation by broad fibrous bands. However, over the past two decades, several authors have considered this point in detail (Katz and Lattes 1969; Keller and Castleman 1974; Null et al. 1977), and there is now universal agreement that "granulomatous thymoma" is a misnomer.

Clinical Features

NSHD usually affects young individuals (under the age of 40), with an equal sex distribution. Patients may occasionally present with symptoms and signs of thoracic structural displacement, as outlined repeatedly throughout this chapter, or, more frequently, with nonlocalizing systemic complaints. The latter include fever, weight loss, fatigue, and sweating. Anemia or eosinophilia may be present (Colby et al. 1982). Rare cases associated with paraneoplastic sydromes such as those seen with thymoma have been reported (Remigio 1971; Null et al. 1977; Peck 1977). This is not evidence that "granulomatous thymoma" exists as an entity distinct from HD of the thymus, since pure red cell aplasia and hypogammaglobulinemia have also been seen in conjunction with lymphoreticular malignancies in other locations (Nagasawa et al. 1981).

Pathologic Features

Grossly, NSHD presents as a multinodular, firm, pink gray mass, which may or may not be confined within the thymic capsule (Fig. 49). Cystic degeneration and necrosis may be present internally. Microscopically, the low power view of NSHD is distinctive, and differs from that of true thymoma. The cellular nodules of NSHD have a rounded configuration (Fig. 50), as opposed to the angular outlines of cell nests in thymoma, owing to the configuration of the intersecting stromal fibrous bands which are present in both. In addition, the cellular composition of NSHD is much more heterogeneous than that of thymoma, and in-

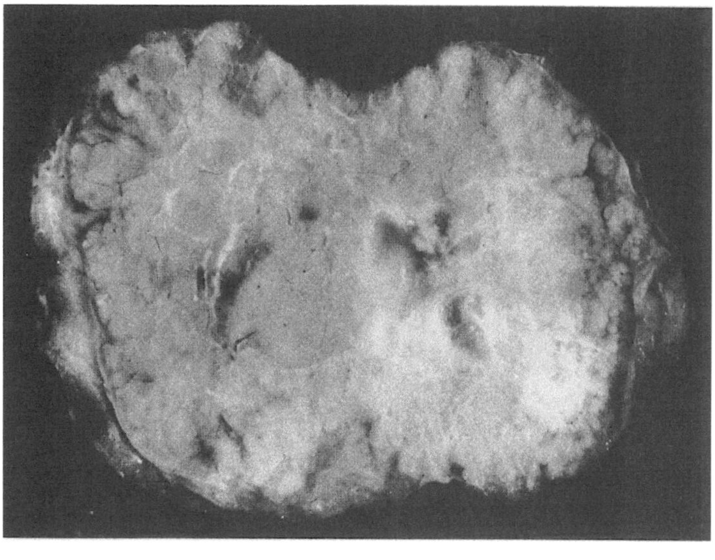

Fig. 49. Gross photograph of anterior mediastinal mass, which proved to represent nodular sclerosing Hodgkin's lymphoma. The tumor displays numerous internal fibrous bands, and may be confused with thymoma because of this feature

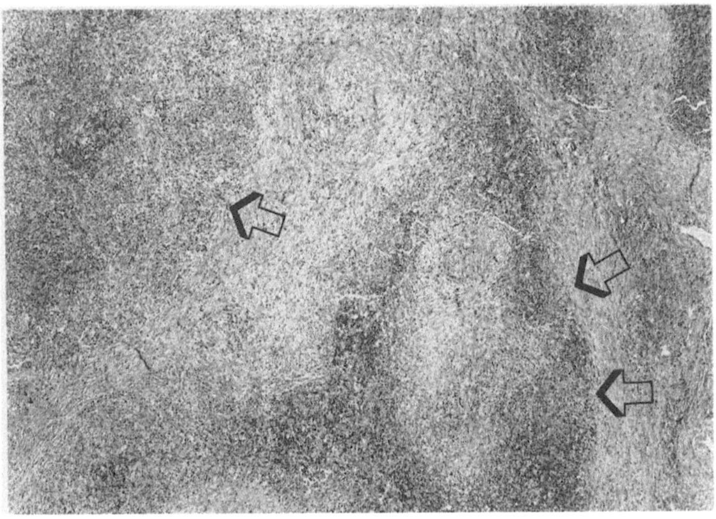

Fig. 50. Low power photomicrograph of nodular sclerosing Hodgkin's disease of the thymus. In contrast to thymoma, the cellular lobules have diffuse or rounded borders with intervening fibrous stroma *(arrows)*

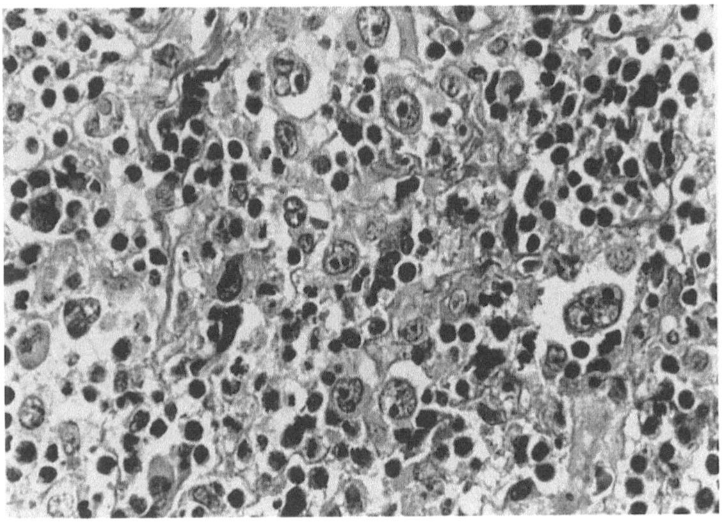

Fig. 51. Hodgkin's disease of the thymus. Classic Sternberg-Reed cells, with multilobulated, nucleolated nuclei, are admixed with reactive lymphocytes

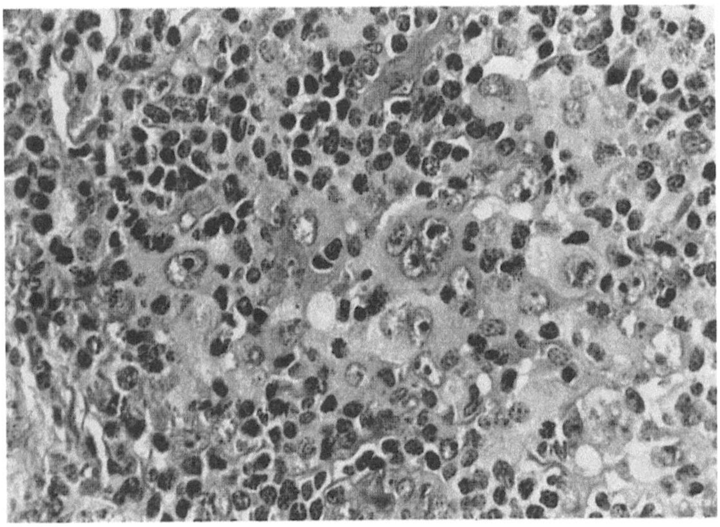

Fig. 52. Hodgkin's lymphoma of the mediastinum, showing focal syncytia of Sternberg-Reed cells. The latter differ cytologically from the tumor cells of thymoma

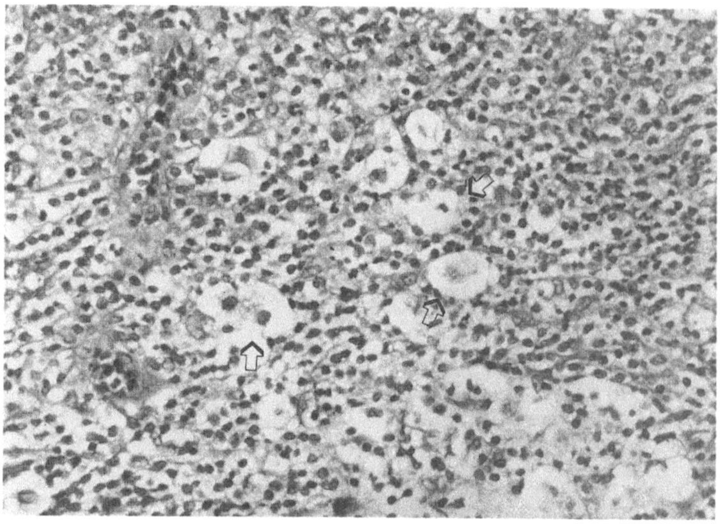

Fig. 53. "Lacunar" cells in nodular sclerosing Hodgkin's disease of the thymus *(arrows)*. These elements display artifactual but reproducible retraction of cellular cytoplasm from surrounding stroma, producing clear intracellular spaces

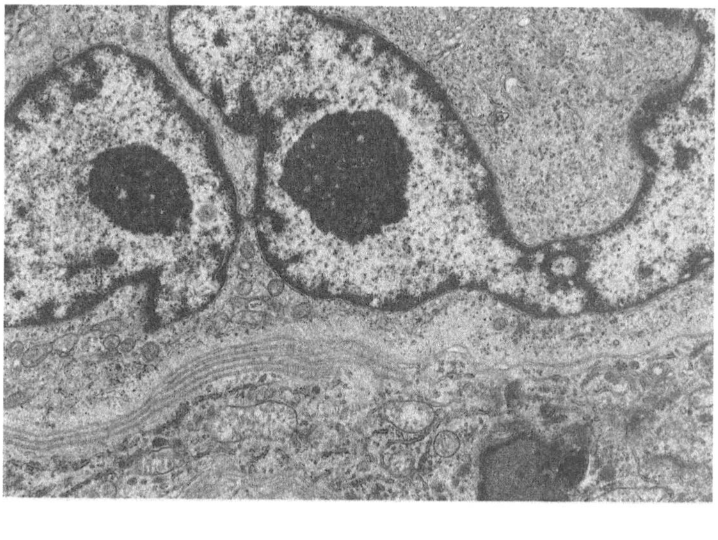

Fig. 54. Electron photomicrograph of Sternberg-Reed cell in thymic Hodgkin's disease. Cytoplasmic tonofilaments and intercellular junctions are lacking, and the nucleus is bilobed with prominent nucleoli

cludes classical Sternberg-Reed cells (which have at least two nuclear lobes, vesicular chromatin, and prominent eosinophilic nucleoli), atypical immunoblasts, plasma cells, small lymphocytes, eosinophils, and neutrophils (Figs. 51 and 52; Grogan 1985). Among these reactive elements, eosinophils have a special significance, for they are only rarely present in true thymomas (Rosai and Levine 1976). In addition, a peculiar cell type, possibly a fixation artifact, is present in NSHD, but not in thymomas. This is the "lacunar cell," in which the cytoplasm is retracted against the nuclear membrane, resulting in a clear intracellular space (Fig. 53; Grogan 1985).

Hassall's corpuscles and small cysts may be present as remnants of the normal thymus gland in NSHD. These should not be misinterpreted as being evidence for a thymic epithelial origin for such cases. Ultrastructurally, the Sternberg-Reed cells and atypical immunoblastic cells of NSHD contain irregularly shaped nuclei with prominent nucleoli, and abundant numbers of free polyribosomes (Fig. 54). Tonofilaments and desmosomes are uniformly absent, as are prolonged cytoplasmic extensions and basal lamina (Peiper and Kahn 1982).

Immunocytochemically, NSHD again differs conclusively from true thymoma. A monoclonal antibody directed at a monocyte-macrophage antigen, Leu-M1, binds uniformly to Sternberg-Reed cells and atypical immunoblasts (atypical Sternberg-Reed cells) (Hsu and Jaffe 1984), but does not recognize thymic epithelium (Fig. 55; Wick, unpublished work). NSHD displays binding of peanut agglutinin (Hsu and Jaffe 1984) whereas thymoma does not. Conversely, the EMA and cytokeratin positivity of thymoma is not

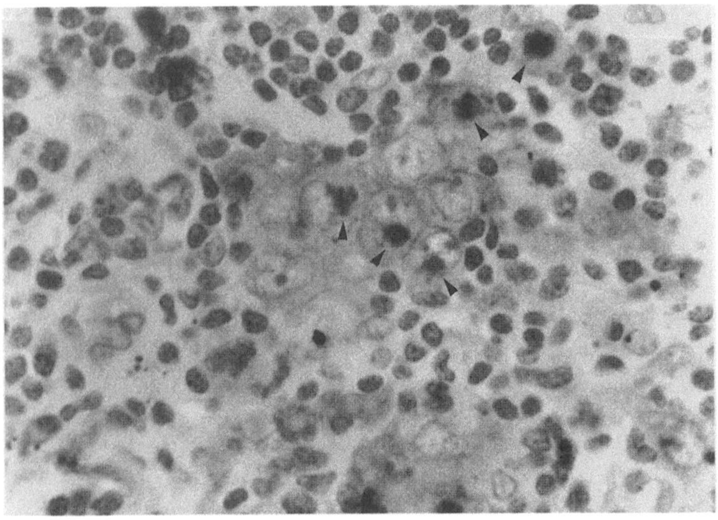

Fig. 55. Punctate perinuclear positivity for Leu-MI, in Sternberg-Reed cells of thymic Hodgkin's lymphoma. This antigen is not observed in thymoma

shared by HD of the thymus (Sloane and Ormerod 1981; Wick, unpublished work).

In confining our attention to the nodular sclerosing form of Hodgkin's lymphoma, we do not mean to imply that the other three variants of HD may not involve the thymus. However, these are much less common than NSHD, and confusion with thymoma is less likely. In any event, a discussion of the histopathologic spectrum of HD is beyond the scope of this chapter; the interested reader is referred to other sources for more information on this topic (Strum 1973; Colby et al. 1982; Grogan 1985).

Prognosis and Therapy

NSHD of the thymus frequently exists as stage I disease (no other locations) (Colby et al. 1982). However, as in any case of this disorder, clinical staging via laparotomy and splenectomy, computerized tomography and/or lymphangiography, and bone marrow biopsy is indicated. Patients with stage I or II disease are currently treated with radiotherapy (Hutchison et al. 1984) while stage III or IV involvement necessitates chemotherapy (Ferme et al. 1984).

Mauch and Hellman (1984) have recently reviewed the response of limited thymic NSHD to radiotherapy. They found that patients whose mediastinal masses measured less than one-third of the transverse thoracic diameter had an excellent outcome after irradiation, while those with larger tumors had a high risk of local relapse and progression, and required more aggressive treatment. Overall, the 5-year survival of stage I thymic NSHD currently approaches 90% (Colby et al. 1982).

Differential Diagnosis

The differential diagnosis considerations in cases of NSHD are rather limited. In addition to *thymoma,* which has already been dicussed, the other major alternative is a *granulomatous fibroinflammatory mass.* Hodgkin's disease may display epithelioid granulomas, which may be so prominent as to obscure the underlying lymphomatous process (Kadin et al. 1970). Consequently, if special stains and cultures for fungi and bacteria yield negative results, the pathologist should carefully reexamine any granulomatous mediastinal mass, with a diagnosis of Hodgkin's disease (or *seminoma*) in mind.

Non-Hodgkin's Lymphoma of the Thymus

Several subtypes of NHL may involve the thymus, and may present diverse problems in differential diagnosis with other lesions. Consequently, the discussion will be centered on this point.

Lymphoblastic, Small Lymphocytic, Small Noncleaved, and Small Cleaved Follicular Center Cell Diffuse Lymphomas

All of these subtypes are characterized by a monomorphic infiltrate of small lymphoid cells. They differ in terms of their nuclear morphology: lymphoblastic lymphoma (LBL) shows "convoluted" or round nuclei with a high mitotic rate (Fig. 56; Nathwani et al. 1976; Cossman 1985); small cell lymphocyte-like lymphoma (SCLLL) resembles an infiltrate of mature, reactive lymphocytes (Fig. 57; Pangalis et al. 1977); and small cleaved follicular center cell lymphoma (SCFCCL) shows discernible nuclear indentations in small lymphoid cells (Fig. 58; Mann et al. 1979). Occasional neoplasms show a uniform cell type with oval nuclei, peripherally clumped chromatin, and multiple nucleoli, and the regular distribution of tingible body macro-

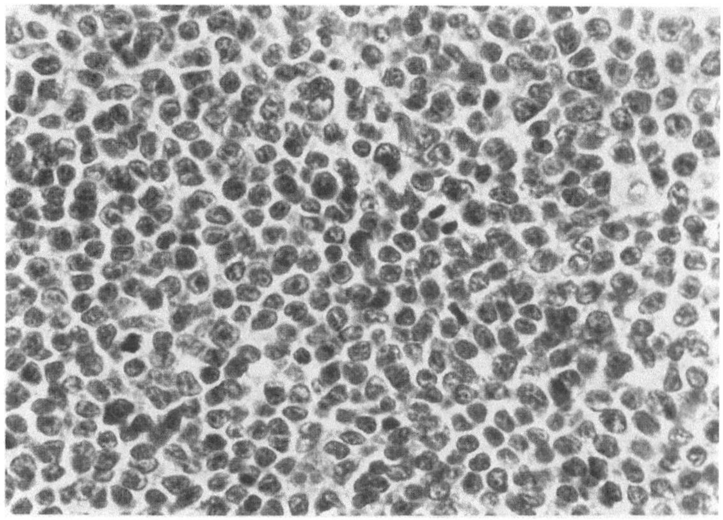

Fig. 56. Sheets of small lymphoid cells with "convoluted" nuclear membranes, in thymic lymphoblastic lymphoma. Mitoses are numerous

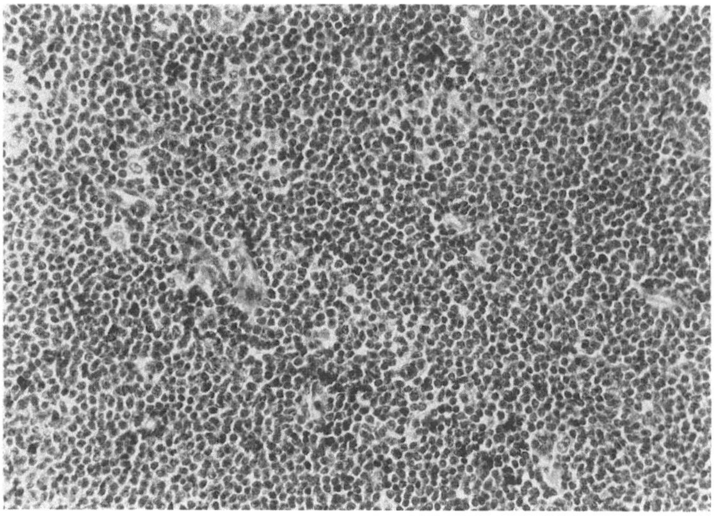

Fig. 57. Thymic infiltrate of small hympho-cyte-like lymphoma cells. In such cases, histologic separation from predominantly lymphocytic thymoma is difficult by conventional microscopy

Fig. 58. This thymic infiltrate of a small cleaved follicular center cell lymphoma shows cells with folded nuclear membranes ▼

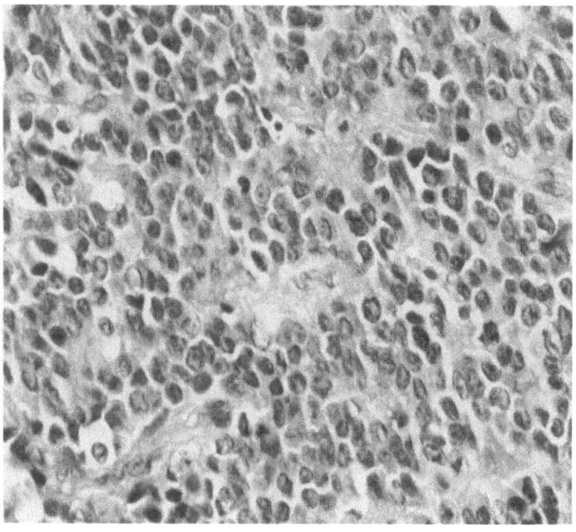

phages throughout (Fig. 59). These belong to the "Burkitt's-like" small noncleaved cell lymphoma category (Grogan et al. 1982).

The major importance of these forms of NHL lies in their potential confusion with *predominantly lymphocytic thymomas*. However, several points of pathologic distinction separate the two classes of tumors. NHL does not show the encapsulation or internal fibrous septation of thymoma, either grossly or microscopically, and it lacks perivascular serum lakes, microcysts, and foci of medullary differentiation (Rosai and Levine 1976). Ultrastructurally, there are no epithelial cells in NHL, which are recognized by desmosomal attachments, pericellular basal lamina, and cytoplasmic tonofilaments (Peiper and Kahn 1982). Finally, immunohistochemical stains do not reveal the same pat-

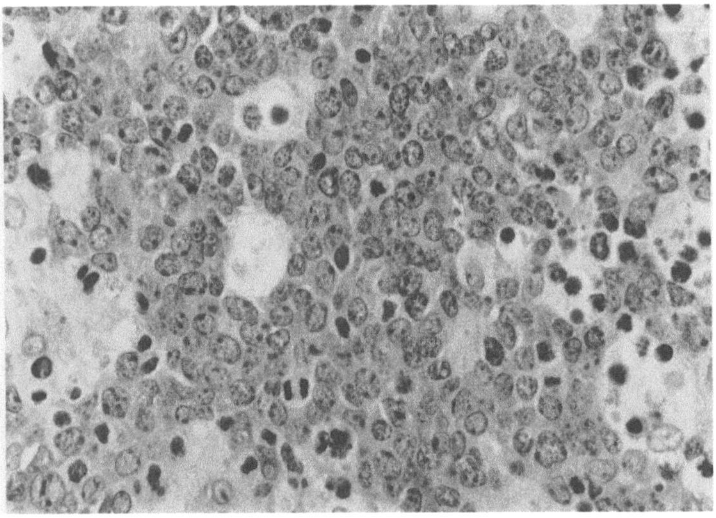

Fig. 59. A rare case of Burkitt's (small noncleaved follicular center cell) lymphoma of the thymus. The tumor cells have coarse, clumped nuclear chromatin, and prominent nucleoli. Mitotic figures are numerous. Admixed, reactive "tingible body" histiocytes give the neoplasm a "starry sky" appearance

tern of EMA- or cytokeratin-reactive tumor cells in NHL as they do in thymoma (Kurtin and Pinkus 1985). In NHL, residual thymic epithelial cells may indeed be entrapped by the lymphomatous infiltrate, but they do not show the regular dispersion which typifies predominantly lymphocytic thymoma (Wick, unpublished work).

Analysis of the lymphoid component by immunohistology may also provide useful differential diagnostic information (Knowles 1985). Most cases of SCLLL, Burkitt's lymphoma, and SCFCCL are B-cell neoplasms, and would be expected to display monotypic surface immunoglobulin and such marker antigens as BL-1 and BL-2. In contrast, the reactive cells of predominantly lymphocytic thymoma are T cells, and exhibit OKT3 reactivity (Chan et al. 1984). Unfortunately, this OKT3 reactivity may lead to confusion with LBL, which is a T-cell neoplasm in many cases. However, stains for the presence of terminal deoxynucleotidyl transferase (TdT), OKT6 antigen, and common acute lymphoblastic leukemia antigen (CALLA) often yield positive results in cases of LBL (Bollum 1979; Newman et al. 1980), but not in lymphocytic thymoma (Chan et al. 1984).

Involvement of the thymus by SCLLL, SCFCCL, and Burkitt's lymphoma is rare in the absence of extrathoracic nodal disease (Rosai and Levine 1976), and thus is less likely to cause diagnostic confusion. However, LBL commonly presents with disease confined within the mediastinum, and is centered in the thymus (Sternberg's sarcoma) (Smith et al. 1973).

The clinical features of these lymphoma variants are heterogeneous, and differ from those of thymoma. SCLLL and SCFCCL tend to occur in middle-aged or elderly individuals, and are more likely to produce nonspecific systemic complaints than symptoms and signs of a mediastinal mass at presentation (Patchefsky et al. 1974; Rausing 1976; Weisenburger et al. 1981). Thymic involvement is commonly detected on routine chest radiography in such cases. LBL is commoner in children and adolescents, and often presents with respiratory embarrassment due to a quickly growing thymic mass (Nathwani et al. 1976). Burkitt's lymphoma also occurs primarily in the pediatric age group and is rarely confined to the mediastinum at diagnosis, but more often involves this anatomic site only in the context of disseminated disease (Grogan et al. 1982). Even with appropriate chemotherapy, SCLLL and SCFCCL progress to involve multiple lymph node groups and the liver, spleen, and bone marrow in most cases, leading to death within 5-10 years after diagnosis (Patchefsky et al. 1974). LBL is a rapidly evolving, lethal neoplasm, which disseminates widely to lymph nodes, viscera, and bone marrow, commonly with the appearance of acute leukemia. Aggressive, multiagent chemotherapy must be instituted promptly after diagnosis to offer any chance of cure. However, the 5-year survival rate in cases of LBL is still well below 50% (Jaffe 1985). Likewise, Burkitt's lymphoma requires heroic therapeutic intervention, and has a poor prognosis (Grogan et al. 1982).

Mixed Small and Large Cell Lymphoma

Mixed small and large cell lymphomas (MSLCL) of the thymus are almost invariably B-cell neoplasms, and tend to occur in adult patients (Rosai and Levine 1976; Cossman 1985). Symptoms and signs of a mediastinal mass are inconstant, but such tumors may manifest themselves by the superior vena cava syndrome, or by chest and back pain, dyspnea, or cough.

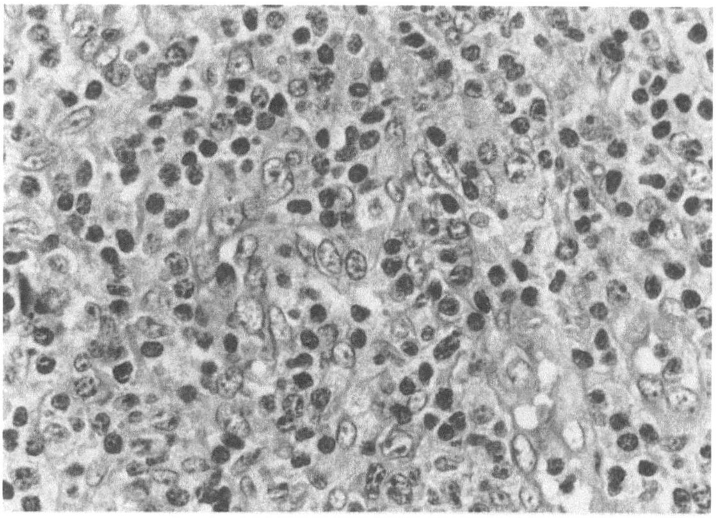

Fig. 60. Mixed small and large cell thymic lymphoma. Large lymphoid cels have irregular nuclear contours, coarse chormatin, and prominent nucleoli, unlike the epithelial cells of thymomas

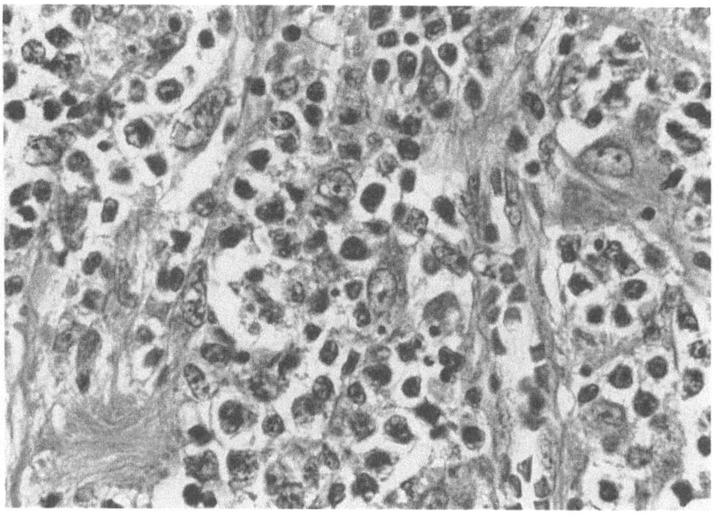

Fig. 61. This example of mixed small and large cell thymic lymphoma contains a lesser number of large epithelioid lymphoid cells. Confusion with thymoma may be avoided by attention to small lymphoid cells. Confusion with thymoma may be avoided by attention to small lymphoid cells, which are also atypical

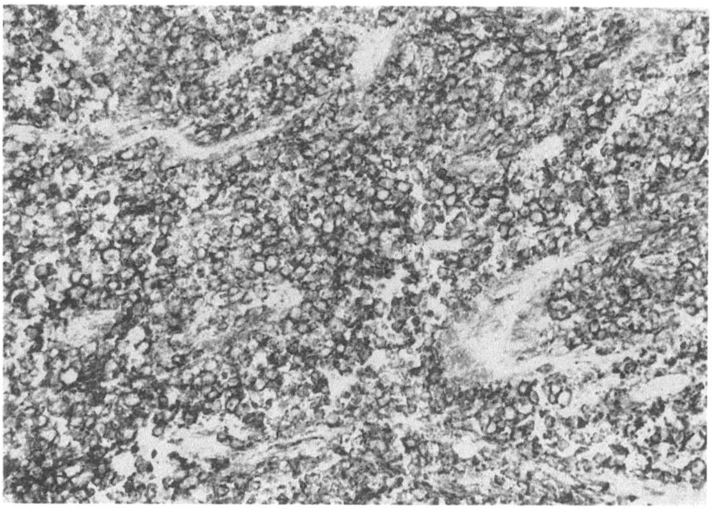

Fig. 62. Diffuse membrane-based immunoreactivity for common leukocyte antigen in small cell thymic lymphoma

The primary histologic differential diagnostic consideration in these cases is that of mixed lymphoepithelial thymoma. However, the same differences as those described for the gross appearance of SCLLL or SCFCCL and thymoma pertain to MSLCL and thymoma as well. Histologically, the "large" cells of MSLCL are cytologically atypical with vesicular nuclei, high nucleocytoplasmic ratios, and frequently prominent nucleoli (Figs. 60 and 61), unlike the epithelial cells of true thymoma.

Immunocytochemically, *all* cells in MSLCL of the thymus, both large and small, show lymphoid characteristics; i. e., they are common leukocyte antigen-positive (Fig. 62), and cytokeratin- and EMA-negative (Kurtin and Pinkus 1985; Wick, unpublished work). Monoclonal antibodies for B-cell antigens also label both cell populations (Knowles 1985).

Chemotherapy is the recommended treatment for these lesions. The response to treatment and the prognosis are variable, and depend on the relative proportions of small and large lymphoid cells (Fischer et al. 1981). Like SCLLL and SCFCCL, MSLCL commonly involves extrathoracic lymph node groups and viscera at diagnosis, in patients with mediastinal masses.

Large Cell Lymphoma

Clinical Features: Large cell lymphoma (LCL) is the type of NHL which, except for LBL, is most likely to present clinically with thymic and mediastinal disease (Lichtenstein et al. 1980; Levitt et al. 1982). Females are affected 1.2-2.5 times more frequently than males; the mean age at diagnosis is 27 years, although this tumor may occur in children and elderly individuals (Lichtenstein et al. 1980; Levitt et al. 1982). Unlike other types of NHL (aside from LBL), mediastinal LCL commonly produces symptoms and signs which are directly related to tumor growth, including superior vena cava obstruction, chest pain, dyspnea, and cough. These are generally of brief duration (1-8 weeks) before the patient comes to medical attention (Levitt at al. 1982). Evidence of extrathoracic disease is present at diagnosis in approximately 25% of cases (Perrone et al. 1986).

Pathologic Features

Grossly, mediastinal LCLs are typically large, somewhat lobulated, firm, gray-white masses which may show internal necrosis (Fig. 63). They are usually unencapsulated, and invade contiguous lung, great vessels, or pericardium. The internal fibrous bands of thymoma or NSHD are absent. Histologically, this variant of NHL is virtually always diffuse in its pattern of growth (Addis and Isaasson 1986), rather than nodular, as seen in some cases of SCFCCL and MSLCL. The tumor cells have indistinct borders, scanty amphophilic or slightly basophilic cytoplasm, and irregular nuclear outlines (Figs. 64 and 65). Nuclear chromatin may be vesicular or coarsely clumped with occasionally prominent nucleoli, and easily found mitoses. Multilobulated nuclear forms are also common. If nucleoli are uniformly evident, large, and eosinophilic, the diagnosis of the immunoblastic subtype of LCL should be considered (Cossman 1985).

Secondary features characteristic of thymic LCL are the persistence of focal thymic epithelium, with or without cyst formation, expanded thymic lobules and compartmentalizing fibrous stroma, which give the neoplasm a pseudoepithelial, clustered appearance (Fig. 66; Miller et al. 1981). Based on these findings, the unwary may render a diagnosis of *primary thymic carcinoma;* however, attention to other observations such as nuclear detail, and prominent invasion of

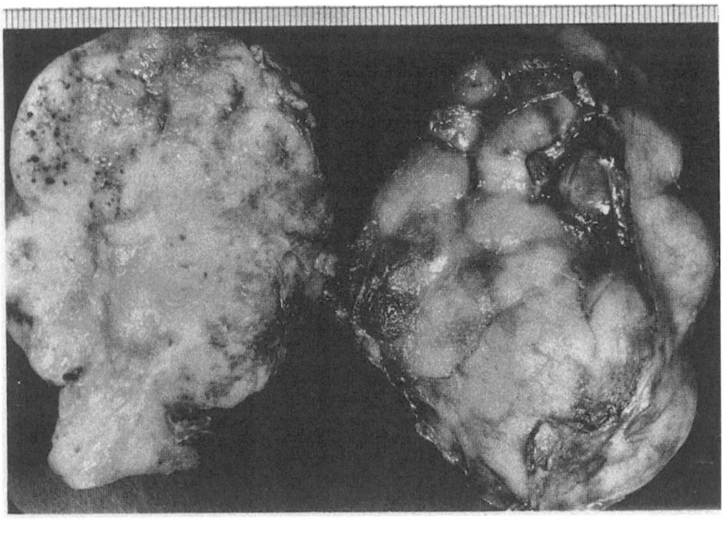

Fig. 63. Gross specimen of large cell thymic lymphoma. The tumor is lobulated, "fleshy," and focally hemorrhagic and necrotic. This appearance is similar to that of thymic carcinoma

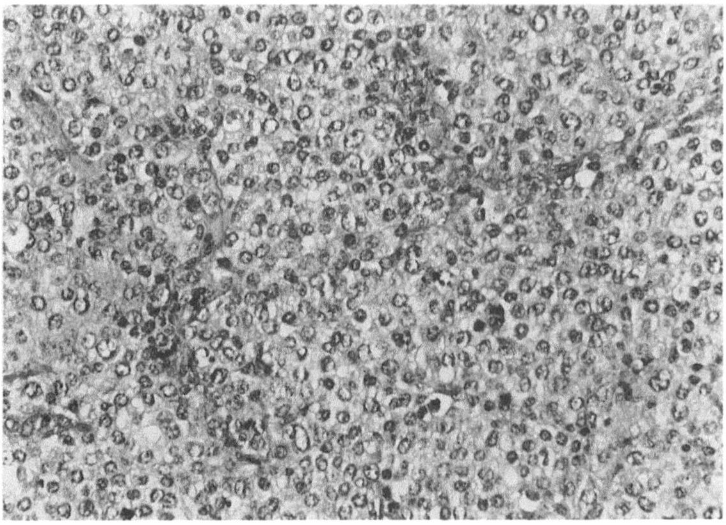

Fig. 64. Vague clustering of tumor cells in large cell thymic lymphoma. This attribute, in addition to cytologic features on low power microscopy, often leads to misinterpretation as lymphoepithelioma-like thymic carcinoma

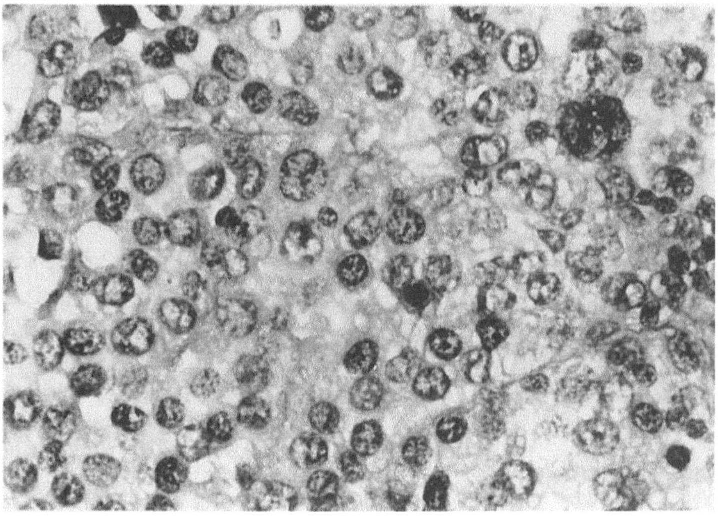

Fig. 65. Higher power view of tumor shown in Fig. 64. Close inspection shows greater nuclear pleomorphism than that seen in cells of thymic carcinoma, with slightly irregular nuclear contours

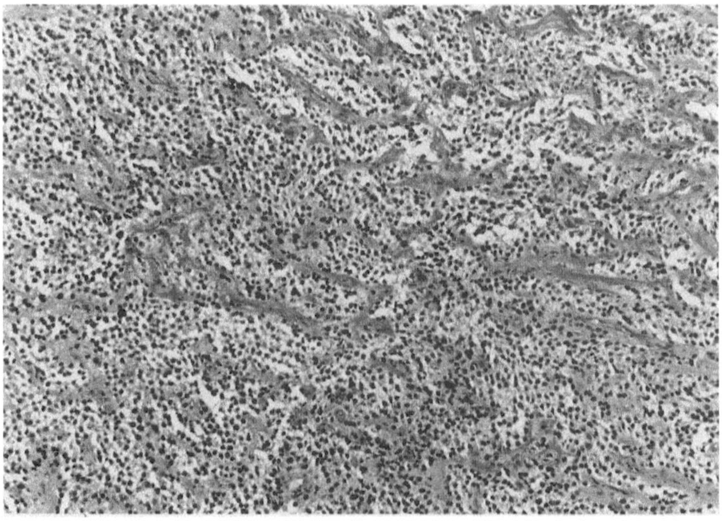

Fig. 66. Sclerotic, "compartmentalizing" stroma in large cell thymic lymphoma, which may lead to a misdiagnosis of thymic carcinoma

blood vessels walls or permeation of mediastinal fat, neither of which is common in thymic carcinoma, usually enables the pathologist to avoid error. Nonetheless, the occasional cases in which the distinction between LCL and thymic carcinoma is problematic with conventional microscopy can often be correctly diagnosed by electron microscopy and immunohistochemistry (Gatter et al. 1984; Perrone et al. 1986; Wick, unpublished work).

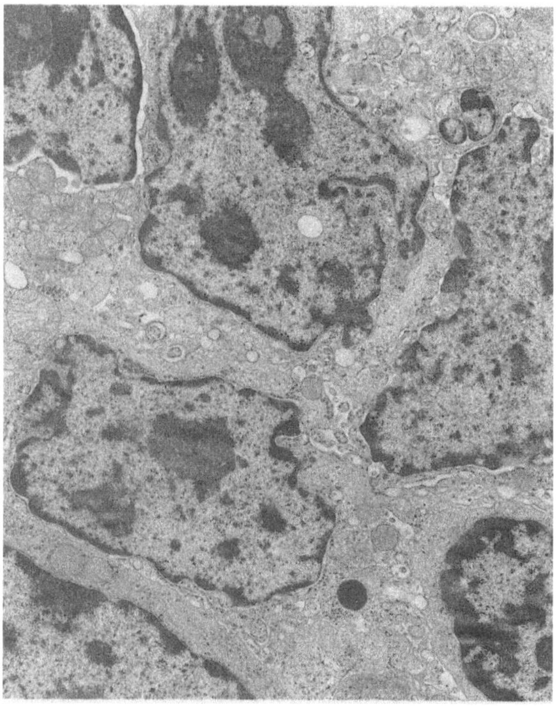

Fig. 67. Electron photomicrograph of large cell mediastinal lymphoma. Tumor cells have irregular nuclear outlines, and contain numerous polyribosomes. Tonofilaments and desmosomal intercellular attachments are absent

Ultrastructurally, thymic LCL does not show intercellular junctions in the vast majority of cases (Fig. 67). Rarely, appositional plaques may be observed between cells (Perrone et al. 1986); however, the well-formed cytoplasmic tonofilaments of thymic carcinoma are uniformly absent, as is the pericellular basal lamina. Furthermore, LCL exhibits a paucity of specialized intracellular organelles except fo free polyribosomes, and a limited amount of rough endoplasmic reticulum (Peiper and Kahn 1982).

Immunocytochemistry is perhaps the most useful tool in the differential diagnosis of carcinoma and LCL. Carcinoma displays reactivity for cytokeratin (Snover et al. 1982; Wick et al. 1982b; Kodama et al. 1986), while lymphoma expresses common leukocyte antigen (Fig. 68; Perrone et al. 1986). As stated previously in this chapter, these results are mutually exclusive. *Thymic seminoma,* which can enter the differential diagnosis in some cases, shows immunoreactivity for PLAP (Beckstead 1983; Manivel et al. 1987) which is lacking in lymphomas and thymic carcinomas (Wick, unpublished work). LCL of the mediastinum, as in other sites, is usually shown to be a B-cell neoplasm by cell marker studies (Addis and Isaacson 1986). However, a relatively greater proportion of thymic large cell lymphomas show a T-cell (Waldron et al. 1984) or true histiocytic phenotype than those in extrathoracic locations.

Behavior and Prognosis

Mediastinal LCL must be treated with aggressive multiagent chemotherapy protocols (Trump and Mann 1982); adjuvant radiotherapy has also been recommended (Perrone et al. 1986). Even with appropriate therapy, 20%-50% of patients will have subsequent mediastinal tumor recurrence, or will fail to show any

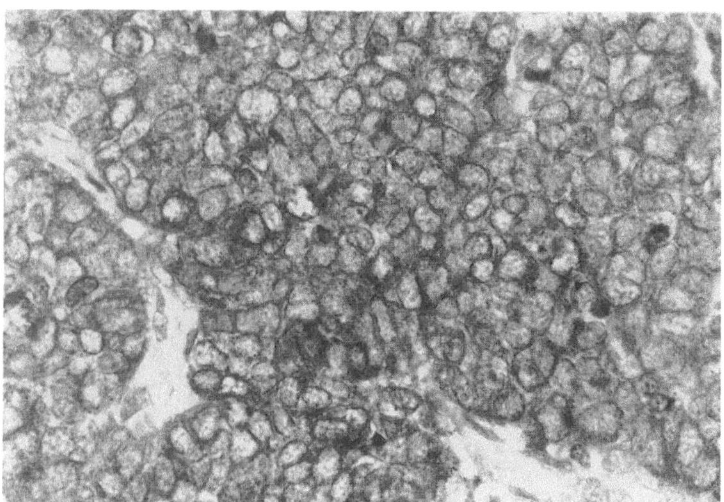

Fig. 68. Diffuse immunopositivity for common leukocyte antigen in large cell lymphoma of thymus. Such reactivity excludes a diagnosis of epithelial neoplasm

response at all (Lichtenstein et al. 1980; Levitt et al. 1982; Trump and Mann 1982; Perrone et al. 1986). In this instance, extrathoracic disease may appear in lymph nodes, kidney, liver, pancreas, gastrointestinal tract, and gonads (Perrone et al. 1986).

A recent study by Perrone et al. (1986) showed that the presence of extrathoracic disesase at diagnosis, incomplete response to initial therapy, and immunoblastic histologic features were poor prognostic indicators in thymic LCL, while the degree of intratumoral sclerosis correlated directly with a favorable response to treatment. The overall disease-free survival in 60 cases of thymic LCL in this series was 50%, at a median of 34.5 months after diagnosis and institution of chemotherapy and/or radiotherapy. Intrathoracic recurrence was omnious, in that 80% of such cases subsequently died of disease. We have already mentioned the greater tendency for LCL of the mediastinum to express a T-cell or histiocytic phenotype compared with this tumor type in extrathoracic sites. Since the prognosis of B-cell, T-cell, and true histiocytic LCL appears to vary, and different therapeutic protocols may be indicated for each of these (Cossmann et al. 1984; Weiss et al. 1986; Neimann 1986), cell marker studies are strongly recommended in all cases of mediastinal LCL (Van der Valk et al. 1983).

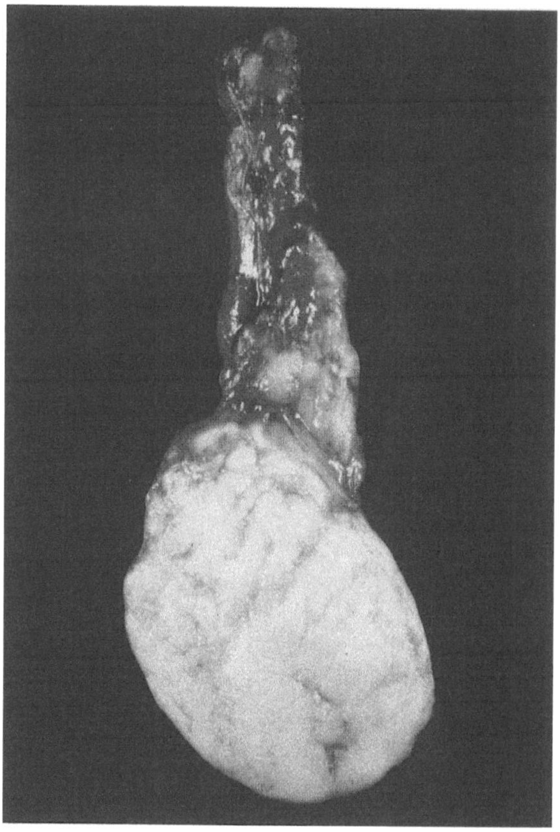

Fig. 69. Gross photograph of a thymolipoma. One lobe of the thymus is expanded by an internally lobulated, encapsulated mass which in, in the fresh state, was soft and yellow. A remnant of normal thymus is present at the top of the figure

Thymolipoma and Thymoliposarcoma

Thymolipoma

Thymolipoma, a tumor distinct from simple lipoma of the mediastinum, was first described by Lange in 1916. It is composed of both histologically normal thymic tissue and mature fat and is contained within the thymic capsule (Hall 1948; Faler and Fero 1956; Lattes 1962; Korhonen and Laustela 1968; Rosai and Levine 1976). However, the contention that the lesion is simply lipomatous is contradicted by the fact that the absolute mass of thymic tissue is increased in cases of thymolipoma (Rosai and Levine 1976). In addition, cases of aplastic anemia (Barnes and O'Gorman 1962), pure red cell aplasia (Otto et al. 1982), hypogammaglobulinemia (Otto et al. 1982), and myasthenia gravis (Reintgen et al. 1978; Otto et al. 1982) have been reported in association with thymolipoma, but not with lipomas of the mediastinum. Nevertheless, thymolipoma is not a form of thymoma, since its nonlipomatous, epithelial element has the configuration of non-neoplastic, nonhyperplastic thymic tissue. Hence, its histogenetic nature is still the subject of some controversy.

Thymolipoma may occur at any age, but the mean age for its appearance is 22 years (Trites 1966; Korhonen and Laustela 1968; Teplick et al. 1973). There is no sex predilection. In the majority of cases, the lesion is found incidentally on routine chest roentgenograms, but approximately 10% are associated with paraneoplastic syndromes or present with dyspnea and cough (Rosai and Livine 1976; Otto et al. 1982). Thoracic computerized tomography is capable of demonstrating the fatty density which characterizes thymolipoma.

Grossly, thymolipomas are lobated, yellowish, soft, and encapsulated (Fig. 69). They may be adherent to contiguous mediastinal structures, but are not invasive (Rosai and Levine 1976). Roughly 70% of thymolipomas weigh over 500 g, and 23% are in excess of 2000 g (Otto et al. 1982). Microscopically, 75%-90% of a given thymolipoma is made up of mature adipose tissue, while the remainder consists of unremarkable thymic tissue containing Hassall's corpuscles (Figs. 70 and 71). Germinal centers are never evident.

Because of this distinctive histologic appearance, differential diagnostic considerations are virtually nonexistent. As will be discussed shortly, a similar le-

spread) 9 months after surgery. The authors suggested that standard chemotherapy for the treatment of osteosarcoma should be employed in similar cases in the future.

References

Abell MR, Fayos JV, Lampe I (1965) Retroperitoneal germinomas (seminomas) without evidence of testicular involvement. Cancer 18: 273-290

Addis BJ, Isaacson PG (1986) Large cell lymphoma of the mediastinum: a B-cell tumor of probable thymic origin. Histopathology 10: 379-390

Adebonojo SA, Nicola ML (1976) Teratoid tumors of the mediastinum. Am Surg 42: 361-365

Altmannsberger M, Osborn M, Schauer A, Weber K (1981) Antibodies to different intermediate filament proteins: cell type-specific markers on paraffin-embedded human tissues. Lab Invest 45: 427-434

Aygun C, Slawson RG, Bajaj K, Salazar OM (1984) Primary mediastinal seminoma. Urology 23: 109-117

Azzopardi JG, Williams ED (1968) Pathology of "nonendocrine" tumors associated with Cushing's syndrome. Cancer 22: 274-286

Baker J, Holdaway IM, Jagusch M, Kerr AR, Donald RA, Pullan PT (1982) Ectopic secretion of ACTH and met-enkephalin from a thymic carcinoid. J Endocrinol Invest 5: 33-37

Barnes RDS, O'Gorman P (1962) Two cases of aplastic anemia associated with tumours of the thymus. J Clin Pathol 15: 264-268

Battifora H, Sheibani K, Tubbs RR, Kopinski MI, Sun TT (1984) Antikeratin antibodies in tumor diagnosis: distinction between seminoma and embryonal carcinoma. Cancer 54: 843-848

Beckstead JH (1983) Alkaline phosphatase histochemistry in human germ cell neoplasms. Am J Surg Pathol 7: 341-349

Bergh NP, Gatzinsky P, Larsson S, Lundin P, Ridell B (1978a) Tumors of the thymus and thymic region: II. Clinicopathological studies on Hodgkin's disease of the thymus. Ann Thorac Surg 25: 99-106

Bergh NP, Gatzinsky P, Larsson S, Lundin P, Ridbell B (1978b) Tumors of the thymus and thymic region: III. Clinicopathological studies on teratomas and tumors of germ cell type. Ann Thorac Surg 25: 107-111

Berry CL, Keeling J, Hilton C (1969) Teratoma in infancy and childhood: a review of 91 cases. J Pathol 98: 241-252

Bjornsson J, Scheithauer BW, Okazaki H, Leech RW (1985) Intracranial germ cell tumors: pathobiological and immunohistochemical aspects of 70 cases. J Neuropathol Exp Neurol 44: 32-46

Bollum FJ (1979) Terminal deoxynucleotidyl transferase as a hematopoietic cell marker. Blood 54: 1203-1215

Brown LR, Aughenbaugh GL, Wick MR, Baker BA, Salassa RM (1982) Roentgenologic diagnosis of primary corticotropin-producing carcinoid tumors of the mediastinum. Radiology 142: 143-148

Burt ME, Javadpour N (1981) Germ-cell tumors in patients with apparently normal testes. Cancer 47: 1911-1915

Burns BF, McCaughy E (1986) Unusual thymic seminomas. Arch Pathol Lab Med 110: 539-541

Buskirk SJ, Evans RG, Farrow GM, Earle JD (1982) Primary retroperitoneal seminoma. Cancer 49: 1934-1936

Canty TG, Siemens R (1978) Malignant mediastinal teratoma in a 15-year old girl. Cancer 41: 1623-1626

Carney JA, Thompson DP, Johnson CL, Lynn HB (1972) Teratomas in children: clinical and pathologic aspects. J Pediatr Surg 7: 271-282

Carter D, Bibro MC, Touloukian RJ (1982) Benign clinical behaviour of immature mediastinal teratoma in infancy and childhood: report of two cases and review of the literature. Cancer 49: 398-402

Chan WC, Zaatari GS, Tabei S, Bibb M, Brynes RK (1984) Thymoma: an immunohistochemical study. Am J Clin Pathol 82: 160-166

Chong GC, Beahrs OH, Sizemore GW, Woolner LH (1975) Medullary carcinoma of the thyroid gland. Cancer 35: 695-704

Cicciarelli FE, Soule EH, McGoon DC (1964) Lipoma and liposarcoma of the mediastinum: a report of 14 tumors including one lipoma of the thymus. J Thorac Cardiovasc Surg 47: 411-429

Cohen RB, Toll GD, Castelman B (1960) Bronchial adenomas in Cushing's syndrome: their relation to thymomas and oat cell carcinomas associated with hyperadrenocorticism. Cancer 13: 812-817

Colby TV, Hoppe RT, Warnke RA (1982) Hodgkin's disease: a clinicopathologic study of 659 cases. Cancer 49: 1848-1858

Cossman J (1985) Diffuse, aggressive non-Hodgkin's lymphomas. In: Jaffe ES (ed) Surgical pathology of the lymph nodes and related organs. Saunders, Philadelphia, pp 203-217

Cossman J, Jaffe ES, Fisher RI (1984) Immunologic phenotypes of diffuse, aggressive, non-Hodgkin's lymphomas: correlation with clinical features. Cancer 54: 1310-1317

Cox JD (1975) Primary malignant germinal tumors of the mediastinum: a study of 24 cases. Cancer 36: 1162-1168

Daniel RA Jr, Diveley WL, Edwards WH, Chamberlain N (1960) Mediastinal tumors. Ann Surg 151: 783-795

Dehner LP (1975) Tumor and tumorlike lesions. In: Dehner LP (ed) Pediatric surgical pathology. Mosby, St. Louis, pp 562-564

DeLellis RA, Wolfe HJ (1976) Calcitonin in spindle-cell thymic carcinoid tumors. Arch Pathol Lab Med 100: 340

DeLellis RA, Blount M, Tischler AS, Wolfe HJ, Lee AK (1983) Leu-enkephalin-like immunoreactivity in proliferative lesions of the human adrenal medulla and extra-adrenal paraganglia. Am J Surg Pathol 7: 29-37

DeSmet AA, Silver TM, Hart WR (1977) Endodermal sinus tumor of the anterior mediastinum. South Med J 70: 757-758

Donaldson MH, Duckett JW, Mulholland SG (1973) Malignant genitourinary tumors. In: Suton WW, Vieti JJ, Fernbach DJ (eds) Clinical pediatric oncology. Mosby, St. Louis, p 504

Dry J, Pradalier A, Herman D, Leynadier F (1976) La polyadénomatose endocrinienne avec tumeur carcinoïde. Sem Hôp Paris 52: 1691-1695

Duguid JB, Kennedy AM (1930) Oat-cell tumours of mediastinal glands. J Pathol Bacteriol 33: 93-99

Einhorn LH (1986) Cancer of the testis: a new paradigm. Hosp Pract [OFF] 21: 165-178

Engel RM, Elkins RC, Fletcher BD (1968) Retroperitoneal teratoma: review of the literature and presentation of an unusual case. Cancer 22: 1068-1073

Falor WH, Ferro FE (1956) Lipothymoma. Surgery 39: 291-296

Fechner RE (1969) Hodgkin's disease of the thymus. Cancer 23: 16-23
Ferme C, Teillet F, d'Agay MF, Gisselbrecht C, Marty M, Boiron M (1984) Combined modality in Hodgkin's disease: comparison of six versus three courses of MOPP with clinical and surgical restaging. Cancer 54: 2324-2329
Fetissof F, Boivin F, Jobard P, Arbeille-Brassart B; Romet JL, Maillet M (1982) Microfilamentous carcinoid of the thymus: correlation of ultrastructural study with Grimelius stain. Ultrastruct Pathol 3: 9-15
Fisher RI, Jones RB, DeVita VT, Simon RM, Garvin AJ, Berard CW, Young RC (1981) Natural history of malignant lymphomas with divergent histologies at staging evaluation. Cancer 47: 2022-2025
Fox MA, Vix VA (1980) Endodermal sinus (yolk sac) tumors of the anterior mediastinum. AJR 135: 291-294
Friedman NB (1951) The comparative morphogenesis of extragenital and gonadal teratoid tumors. Cancer 4: 265-276
Gatter KC, Alcock C, Heryet A, Pulford KA, Heyderman E, Taylor-Papadimitriou J, Stein H, Mason DY (1984) The differential diagnosis of routinely processed anaplastic tumors using monoclonal antibodies. Am J Clin Pathol 82: 33-43
Gillman J (1948) The development of the gonads in man, with a consideration of the role of fetal endovcrines and histogensis of ovarian tumors. Contrib Embryol 32 (no 210): 81-131
Glenner GS, Grimley PM (1974) Tumors of the extra-adrenal paraganglion system: supra-aortic and aortico-pulmonary paragangliomas. In: Atlas of tumor pathology, ser 2, fasc 9. Armed Forces Institute of Pathology, Washington, DC, pp 68-69
Golding PG, Elston CW, Levison VB, Bagshawe KD (1968) The diagnosis of trophoblastic tumours of testis. Br J Surg 55: 508-512
Gonzalez-Crussi F, Winkle RF and Mirkin DL (1978) Sacrococcygeal teratomas in infants and children: relationship of histology and prognosis in 40 cases. Arch Pathol Lab Med 102: 420-425
Gooneratne S, Keh P, Sreekanth S, Recant W, Talerman A (1985) Anterior medistinal endodermal sinus (yolk sac) tumor in a female infant. Cancer 56: 1430-1433
Greenwood SM, Goodman JR, Schneider G, Forman BH, Kress SC, Gelb AF (1971) Choriocarcinoma in a man. The relationship of gynecomastia to chorionic somatomammotropin and estrogens. Am J Med 51: 416-422
Grogan TM (1985) Hodgkin's disease. In: Jaffe ES (ed) Surgical pathology of the lymph nodes and related organs. Saunders, Philadelphia, pp 86-134
Grogan TM, Warnke RA, Kaplan HS (1982) A comparative study of Burkitt's and non-Burkitt's "undifferentiated" malignant lymphoma: immunologic, cytochemical, ultrastructural, cytologic, histopathologic, clinical and cell culture features. Cancer 49: 1817-1828
Hall GFM (1948) A case of thymolipoma with observations on a possible relationship to intrathoracic lipomata. Br J Surg 36: 321-324
Havlicek F, Rosai J (1984) A sarcoma of thymic stroma with features of liposarcoma. Am J Clin Pathol 82: 217-224
Ho FCS, Ho JCI (1977) Pigmented carcinoid tumour of the thymus. Histopathology 1: 363-369
Hodge J, Aponte G, McLaughlin E (1959) Primary mediastinal tumors. J Thorac Cardiovasc Surg 37: 730-744
Hsu SM, Jaffe ES (1984) Leu-Ml and peanut agglutinin stain the neoplastic cells of Hodgkin's disease. Am J Clin Pathol 82: 29-32
Hullin DA, Brown K, Kynoch PAM, Smith C, Thompson RJ (1980) Purification, radioimmunoassay, and distribution of human brain 14-3-2 protein (nervous-system specific enolase) in human tissues. Biochim Biophys Acta 628: 98-108
Huntington RW Jr, Bullock WK (1970) Yolk sac tumors of extragonadal origin. Cancer 25: 1368-1376
Hutchison GB (1984) Radiotherapy of stage I and II Hodgkin's disease: a collaborative study. Cancer 54: 1928-1942
Jacobsen GK, Jacobsen M, Praetorius-Clausen P (1981) Distribution of tumor-associated antigens in the various histologic components of germ cell tumors of the testis. Am J Surg Pathol 5: 257-266
Jaffe ES (1985) An overview of the classification of non-Hodgkin's lymphomas. In: Jaffe ES (ed) Surgical pathology of the lymph nodes and related organs. Saunders Co, Philadelphia, pp 135-145
Javadpour N (1979) Serum and cellular biologic tumor markers in patients with urologic cancer. Hum Pathol 10: 557-568
Kadin ME, Donaldson SS, Dorfman RF (1970) Isolated granulomas in Hodgkin's disease. N Engl J Med 283: 859-861
Katz A, Lattes R (1969) Granulomatous thymoma or Hodgkin's disease of thymus? A clinical and histologic study and a re-evaluation. Cancer 23: 1-15
Kay S, Willson MA (1970) Ultrastructural studies of an ACTH-secreting thymic tumor. Cancer 26: 445-452
Keller AR, Castelman B (1974) Hodgkin's disease of the thymus gland. Cancer 33: 1615-1623
Knapp RH, Fritz SR, Reiman HM (1982) Primary embryonal carcinoma and choriocarcinoma of the mediastinum: a case report. Arch Pathol Lab Med 106: 507-509
Knapp RH, Hurt RD, Payne S, Farrow GM, Lewis BD, Hahn RG, Muhm JR, Earle JD (1985) Malignant germ cell tumors of the mediastinum. J Thorac Cardiovasc Surg 89: 82-89
Knowles DM II (1985) Lymphoid cell markers. Their distribution and usefulness in the immunophenotypic analysis of lymphoid neoplasms. Am J Surg Pathol 9 [Suppl]: 85-108
Kodama T, Watanabe S, Sato Y, Shimosato Y, Miyazawa N (1986) An immunohistochemical study of thymic epithelial tumors. I. Epithelial component. Am J Surg Pathol 10: 26-33
Korhonen LK, Laustela E (1968) Thymolipoma: report of a case. Scand J Thorac Cardiovasc Surg 2: 147-150
Kurman RJ, Scardino PT, McIntire KR, Waldmann TA, Javadpour N (1977) Cellular localization of alpha-fetoprotein and human chorionic gonadotropin in germ cell tumors of the testis using an indirecte immunoperoxidase technique: a new approach to classification utilizing tumor markers. Cancer 40: 2136-2151
Kurtin PJ, Pinkus GS (1985) Leukocyte common antigen - a diagnostic discriminant between hematopoietic and nonhematopoietic neoplasms in paraffin sections using monoclonal antibodies: correlation with immunologic studies and ultrastructural localization. Hum Pathol 16: 353-365
Kuzur ME, Cobleigh MA, Greco A, Einhorn LH, Oldham RK (1982) Endodermal sinus tumor of the mediastinum. Cancer 50: 766-774
Lachman MF, Kim K, Koo BC (1986) Mediastinal teratoma associated with Klinefelter's syndrome. Arch Pathol Lab Med 110: 1067-1071
Lange I (1916) Über ein Lipom des Thymus. Zentralbl Allg Pathol 27: 97-101

Lattes R (1962) Thymoma and other tumors of the thymus: an analysis of 107 cases. Cancer 15: 1224-1260
Levine GD (1973) Primary thymic seminoma - a neoplasm ultrastructurally similar to testicular seminoma and distinct from epithelial thymoma. Cancer 31: 729-741
Levine GD, Rosai J (1976) A spindle cell variant of thymic carcinoid tumor: a clinical, histologic, and fine structural study with emphasis on its distinction from spindle cell thymoma. Arch Pathol Lab Med 100: 293-300
Levitt LJ, Aisenberg AC, Harris NL, Linggood RM, Poppema S (1982) Primary non-Hodgkin's lymphoma of the mediastinum. Cancer 50: 2486-2492
Lewis BD, Hurt RD, Payne WS, Farrow GM, Knapp RH, Muhm JR (1983) Benign teratomas of the mediastinum. J Thorac Cardiovasc Surg 86: 727-731
Leyton O, Turnbull HM, Bratton AB (1931) Primary cancer of the thymus with pluriglandular disturbance. J Pathol Bacteriol 34: 635-660
Lichtenstein AK, Levine A, Taylor CR, Boswell W, Rossman S, Feinstein DI, Lukes RJ (1980) Primary mediastinal lymphoma in adults. Am J Med 68: 509-514
Lokich JJ, Li F (1978) Carcinoid tumor of the thymus with hereditary hyperparathyroidism. Ann Intern Med 89: 364-365
Lowenhaupt E, Brown R (1951) Carcinoma of the thymus of granulomatous type: a clinical and pathological study. Cancer 4: 1193-1209
Lowenthal RM, Gumpel JM, Kreel L, McLaughlin JE, Skeggs DBL (1974) Carcinoid tumor of the thymus with systemic manifestations: a radiological and pathological study. Thorax 29: 553-558
Manes JL, Taylor HB (1973) Thymic carcinoid in familial multiple endocrine adenomatosis. Arch Pathol 95: 252-255
Manivel C, Wick MR, Abenoza P, Rosai J (1986) The occurence of sarcomatous components in primary mediastinal germ cell tumors. Am J Surg Pathol 10: 711-717
Manivel C, Jessurun J, Wick MR, Dehner LP (1987) Placental alkaline phosphatase immunoreactivity in testicular germ-cell neoplasms. Am J Surg Pathol 11: 21-29
Mann RB, Jaffe ES, Berard CW (1979) Maligant lymphomas: a conceptual understanding of morphologic diversity. Am J Pathol 94: 105-175
Marshall AHE, Wood C (1957) The involvement of the thymus in Hodgkin's disease. J Pathol Bacteriol 73: 163-166
Martini N, Golbey RB, Hajdu SI, Whitmore WF, Beattie EJ Jr (1974) Primary mediastinal germ cell tumors. Cancer 33: 763-769
Mauch P, Hellman S (1984) Mediastinal Hodgkin's disease. Significance of mediastinal involvement in early stage Hodgkin's disease. Hematol Oncol 2: 69-72
Mc Neil MM, Leong ASY, Sage RE (1981) Primary mediastinal embryonal carcinoma in association with Klinefelter's syndrome. Cancer 47: 343-345
Miettinen M, Partanen S, Lehto VP, Virtanen I (1983) Mediastinal tumors ultrastructural and immunohistochemical evaluation of intermediate filaments as diagnostic aids. Ultrastructrual Pathol 4: 337-347
Miller JB, Variakojis D, Bitran JD, Sweet DL, Kinzie JJ, Golomb HM, Ultmann JE (1981) Diffuse histiocytic lymphoma with sclerosis: a clinicopathologic entity frequently causing superior vena caval obstruction. Cancer 47: 748-756
Mostofi FK, Price EB (1973) Tumors of the male genital system. Embryonal carcinoma. In: Atlas of tumor pathology, ser 2, fasc 8. Armed Forces Institute of Pathology, Washington, DC, pp 40-52
Mukai K, Adams WR (1979) Yolk sac tumor of the anterior mediastinum: case report with light- and electron-microscopic examination and immunohistochemical study of alpha-fetoprotein. Am J Surg Pathol 3: 77-83
Nagasawa T, Abe T, Nakagawa T (1981) Pure red cell aplasia and hypogamma-globulinemia associated with $T\gamma$-cell chronic lymphocytic leukemia. Blood 57: 1025-1031
Nagle RB, McDaniel KM, Clark VA, Payne CM (1983) The use of antikeratin antibodies in the diagnosis of human neoplasms. Am J Clin Pathol 79: 458-466
Nathwani BN, Kim H, Rappaport H (1976) Malignant lymphoma, lymphoblastic. Cancer 38: 964-983
Neimann RC (1986) The peripheral T-cell lymphomas come of age. Mayo Clin Proc 61: 504-506
Newmann RA, Sutherland R, Greaves MF (1981) The biochemical characterization of a cell surface antigen associated with acute lymphoblastic leukemia and lymphocyte precursors. J Immunol 126: 2024-2030
Nogales-Fernandez F, Silverberg SG, Bloustein PA, Martinez-Hernandez A, Pierce GB (1977) Yolk sac carcinoma (endodermal sinus tumor): ultrastructure and histogenesis of gonadal and extragonadal tumors in comparison with normal human yolk sac. Cancer 39: 1462-1474
Norris HJ, Zirkin HJ, Benson WL (1976) Immature malignant teratoma of the ovary: a clinical and pathologic study of 58 cases. Cancer 37: 2359-2372
Null JA, LiVolsi VA, Glenn WWL (1977) Hodgkin's disease of the thymus (granulomatous thymoma) and myasthenia gravis: a unique association. Am J Clin Pathol 67: 521-525
Oberman HA, Libcke JH (1964) Malignant germinal neoplasms of the mediastinum. Cancer 17: 498-507
Okumori M, Mabuchi M, Nakagawa M (1983) Malignant thymoma associated with liposarcoma of the mediastinum: a case report. Jpn J Surg 13: 512-518
Olson JL, Salyer WR (1978) Mediastinal paragangliomas (aortic body tumor): a report of four cases and a review of the literature. Cancer 41: 2405-2412
Otto HF, Loning Th, Lachenmayer L, Janzen RWC, Gürtler KF, Fischer K (1982) Thymolipoma in association with myastenia gravis. Cancer 50: 1623-1628
Pachter MR, Lattes R (1963) Mesenchymal tumors of the mediastinum. I. Tumors of fibrious tissue, adipose tissue, smooth muscle, and striated muscle. Cancer 16: 74-94
Pachter MR, Lattes R (1964) "Germinal" tumors of the mediastinum: a clinicopathologic study of adult teratomas, teratocarcinomas, choriocarcinomas and seminomas. Am J Dis Chest 45: 301-310
Pangalis GA, Nathwani BN, Rappaport H (1977) Malignant lymphoma, well-differentiated lymphocytic: its relationship with chronic lymphocytic leukemia and macroglobulinemia of Waldenström. Cancer 39: 999-1010
Parker D, Holford CP, Begent RHJ, Newlands ES, Rustin GJS, Makey AR, Bagshawe KD (1983) Effective treatment for malignant mediastinal teratoma. Thorax 38: 897-902
Patchefsky AS, Brodovsky HS, Menduke H, Southard M, Brooks J, Nicklas D, Hoch WS (1974) Non-Hodgkin's lymphomas: a clinicopathologic study of 293 cases. Cancer 34: 1173-1186
Peck B (1977) Hypertrophic osteoartropathy with Hodgkin's disease in the mediastinum. JAMA 238: 1400-1401
Peiper SC, Kahn LB (1982) Ultrastructural comparison of Hodgkin's and non-Hodgkin's lymphomas. Histopathology 6: 93-109
Perrone T, Frizzera G, Rosai J (1986) Mediastinal diffuse large-cell lymphoma with sclerosis: a clinicopathologic study of 60 cases. Am J Surg Pathol 10: 176-191

Pugsley WS, Carleton RL (1953) Germinal nature of teratoid tumors of the thymus. Arch Pathol 56: 341-347

Rausing A (1976) Lymphocytic leukemia and lymphoma in the adult. Acta Med Scand [Suppl] 595: 1-270

Razzuk MA, Urschel HC Jr, Race GJ, Kingsley WB, Paulson DL (1971) Liposarcoma of the mediastinum: case report and review of the literature. J Thorac Cardiovasc Surg 61: 819-826

Recondo J, Libshitz HI (1978) Mediastinal extragonadal germ cell tumors. Urology 11: 369-375

Reintgen D, Fetter BF, Roses A, McCarty KS Jr (1978) Thymolipoma in association with myasthenia gravis. Arch Pathol Lab Med 102: 463-466

Remigio PA (1971) Granulomatous thymoma associated with erythroid hypoplasia. Am J Clin Pathol 55: 68-72

Reynolds TF, Yagoda A, Vurgin D, Golbey R (1979) Chemotherapy of mediastinal germ cell tumors. Semin Oncol 6: 113-115

Ringertz N, Lidholm SO (1956) Mediastinal tumors and cysts. J Thorac Cardiovasc Surg 31: 458-487

Rosai J (1981) Ackerman's surgical pathology, 6th edn, vol 1. Mosby, St. Louis, pp 871-902

Rosai J, Higa E (1972) Mediastinal endocrine neoplasm, of probable thymic origin, related to carcinoid tumor: clinicopathologic study of 8 cases. Cancer 29: 1061-1074

Rosai J, Levine GD (1976) Tumors of the thymus. In: Atlas of tumor pathology, ser 2, fasc 13. Armed Forces Institute of Pathology, Washington DC

Rosai J, Higa E, Davie J (1972) Mediastinal endocrine neoplasm in patients with multiple endocrine adenomatosis: a previously unrecognized association. Cancer 29: 1075-1083

Rosai J, Levine GD, Weber WR, Higa E (1976) Carcionoid tumors and oat cell carcinomas of the thymus. Pathol Annu 11: 201-226

Roslyn JJ, Gordon HE, Mulder DG (1983) Mediastinal parathyroid adenomas: a cause of persistent hyperparathyroidism. Am Surg 49: 523-527

Roth LM, Panganiban WG (1976) Gonadal and extragonadal yolk sac carcinomas: a clinicopathologic study of 14 cases. Cancer 37: 812-820

Russell CF, Edis AJ, Scholz DA, Sheedy PF, van Heerden JA (1981) Mediastinal parathyroid tumors. Experience with 38 tumors requiring mediastinotomy for removal. Ann Surg 193: 805-809

Sandhaus L, Strom RL, Mukai K (1981) Primary embryonal-choriocarcinoma of the mediastinum in a woman: a case report with immunohistochemical study. Am J Clin Pathol 75: 573-578

Sass M, Jao W, Horn T, Keh PC (1983) Mediastinal yolk sac tumor: ultrastructural and immunofluorescent studies. Ultrastruc Pathol 4: 67-73

Schantz A, Sewall W, Castleman B (1972) Mediastinal germinoma: a study of 21 cases with an excellent prognosis. Cancer 30: 1189-1194

Scholz DA, Bahn RC (1959) Thymic tumors associated with Cushing's syndrome: review of three cases. Mayo Clin Proc 34: 433-441

Sickels EA, Belliveau RE, Wiernik PH (1974) Primary mediastinal choriocarcinoma in the male. Cancer 33: 1196-1203

Sloane JP, Ormerod MG (1981) Distribution of epithelial membrane antigen in normal and neoplastic tissues and its value in diagnostic tumor pathology. Cancer 47: 1786-1795

Smith JL, Barker CR, Clein GP, Collins RD (1973) Characterisation of malignant mediastinal lymphoid neoplasm (Sternberg sarcoma) as thymic in origin. Lancet 1: 74-77

Snover DC, Levine GD, Rosai J (1982) Thymic carcinoma: five distinctive histological variants. Am J Surg Pathol 6: 451-470

Strum SB (1973) The natural history, histopathology, staging, and mode of spread of Hodgkin's disease. Ser Haematol 6: 20-115

Talerman A, Haije WG, Baggerman L (1977) Alpha-1 antitrypsin (AAT) and alphafoetoprotein (AFP) in sera of patients with germ-cell neoplasms: value as tumour markers in patients with endodermal sinus tumour (yolk sac tumour). Int J Cancer 19: 741-746

Tapia FJ, Polak JM, Barbosa AJA, Bloom SR, Marangos PJ, Dermody C, Pearse AGE (1981) Neuron-specific enolase is produced by neuroendocrine tumours. Lancet 1: 808-811

Teilmann I, Kassis H, Pietra G (1967) Primary germ cell tumor of the anterior mediastinum with features of endodermal sinus tumor (mesoblastoma vitellinum). Acta Pathol Microbiol Scand 70: 267-278

Teilum G (1959) Endodermal sinus tumors of the ovary and testis: comparative morphogenesis of the so-called mesonephroma ovarii (Schiller) and extraembryonic (yolk sac-allantoic) structures of the rat's placenta. Cancer 12: 1092-1105

Teplick JG, Nedwich A, Haskin ME (1973) Roentgenographic features of thymolipoma. AJR 117: 873-877

Trites AEW (1966) Thyrolipoma, thymolipoma and pharyngeal lipoma: a syndrome. Can Med Assoc J 95: 1254-1259

Trump DL, Mann RB (1982) Diffuse large cell and undifferentiated lymphomas with prominent mediastinal involvement: a poor prognostic subset of patients with non-Hodgkin's lymphoma. Cancer 50: 277-282

Ulbright TM, Loehrer PJ, Roth LM, Einhorn LH, Williams SD, Clark SA (1984) The development of non-germ cell malignancies within germ cell tumors: a clinicopathologic study of 11 cases. Cancer 54: 1824-1833

Uner R, Balim AI, Oktem K (1963) Mediastinal liposarcoma: report of a case. Am J Dis Chest 43: 103-105

Valderrama E, Kahn LB, Wind E (1983) Extraskeletal osteosarcoma arising in an ectopic hamartomatous thymus: report of a case and review of the literature. Cancer 51: 1132-1137

Van der Valk P, van den Besselaar-Dingjan G, Daha MR, Meijer CJLM (1983) Analysis of large-cell lymphomas using monoclonal and heterologous antibodies. J Clin Pathol 36: 44-50

Vogelzang NJ, Raghavan D, Anderson RW, Rosai J, Levitt SH, Kennedy BJ (1982) Mediastinal non-seminomatous germ cell tumors: the role of combined modality therapy. Ann Thorac Surg 33: 333-339

Vuletin JC, Rosen Y, Brigati DJ, Gourin A (1977) Endodermal sinus tumor of the mediastinum: ultrastructural study. Chest 72: 112-114

Waldron JA, Farber LL, Cadman E (1984) Primary large cell lymphomas of the mediastinum: an analysis of 18 cases. Lab Invest 50: 64A

Weisenburger DD, Nathwani BN, Diamond LW, Winberg CD, Rappaport H (1981) Malignant lymphoma, intermediate lymphocytic type: a clinicopathologic study of 42 cases. Cancer 48: 1415-1425

Weiss JW, Winter MW, Phyliky RL, Banks PM (1986) Peripheral T-cell lymphomas: histologic, immunohistologic and clinical characteriztion. Mayo Clin Proc 61: 411-426

Wenger ME, Dines DE, Ahmann DL, Good CA (1968) Primary mediastinal choriocarcinoma. Mayo Clin Proc 43: 570-575

Wick MR, Rosai J (in press) Endocrine pathology of the thymus: an update. In: Lechago J, Kameya T (eds) Endocrine pathology update. Field and Wood. Philadelphia
Wick MR, Scheithauer BW (1982b) Oat-cell carcinoma of the thymus. Cancer 49: 1652-1657
Wick MR, Scheithauer BW (1984) Thymic carcinoid: a histologic, immunohistochemical, and ultrastructural study of 12 cases. Cancer 53: 475-484
Wick MR, Siegal GP (1980) Primary mediastinal embryonal carcinoma. Minn Med 63: 723-726
Wick MR, Scott RE, Li CY, Carney JA (1980) Carcinoid tumor of the thymus: a clinicopathologic report of seven cases with a review of the literature. Mayo Clin Proc 55: 246-254
Wick MR, Bernatz PE, Carney JA, Brown LR (1982a) Primary mediastinal carcinoid tumors. Am J Surg Pathol 6: 195-205
Wick MR, Weiland LH, Scheithauer BW, Bernatz PE (1982b) Primary thymic carcinomas. Am J Surg Pathol 6: 613-630
Wick MR, Bahn RC, Scholz DA (1983a) Retrospective ultrastructural study of three thymic neoplasms associated with Cushing's syndrome: evidence of their neuroendocrine nature. Minn Med 66: 114-117
Wick MR, Scheithauer BW, Kovacs K (1983b) Neuron-specific enolase in neuroendocrine tumors of the thymus, bronchus and skin. Am J Clin Pathol 79: 703-707
Williams ED, Sandler M (1963) The classification of carcinoid tumors. Lancet 1: 238-239
Wilson BS, Lloyd RV (1984) Detection of chromogranin in neuroendocrine cells with an monoclonal antibody. Am J Pathol 115: 458-468
Woolner LB, Keating FR Jr, Black BM (1952) Tumors and hyperplasia of the parathyroid glands: a review of the pathological findings in 140 cases of primary hyperparathyroidism. Cancer 5: 1069-1088

11 Mediastinal Tumor-like Conditions and Tumors that can Simulate Thymic Neoplasms

Alberto M. Marchevsky

Introduction

Many of the neoplasms and tumor-like conditions that occur in the anterosuperior mediastinum may simulate thymic lesions on chest roentgenograms or even on computerized tomograms (CT) (Marchevsky and Kaneko 1984). They include inflammatory soft tissue lesions, malignant lymphomas and other lymphadenopathies, cysts, endocrine neoplasms, and tumors of mesenchymal or neurogenic origin. Patients with any of these conditions may undergo surgical intervention on a clinical diagnosis of thymoma, the correct diagnosis being established only after histologic examination of tissue obtained by biopsy or resection. Detailed descriptions of the pathologic features of all these diseases is beyond the scope of this chapter. Only the most important aspects of the most frequent or most interesting mediastinal lesions that are liable to simulate, clinically and roentgenologically, thymic tumors will be discussed (Table 1).

Table 1. Mediastinal lesions that may simulate thymic neoplasms and cysts on chest roentgenograms

Inflammatory tumor-like conditions
- Granulomatous mediastinitis with fibrosis
- Inflammatory pseudotumor of the thymus

Lymphadenopathies
- Malignant lymphomas
  - Hodgkin's disease
  - Non-Hodgkin's lymphoma
- Metastatic neoplasms
- Granulomatous lymphadenitis and lymphadenopathies
- Angiofollicular lymph node hyperplasia (Castleman's disease)

Cysts
- Congenital mediastinal cysts
  - Bronchogenic cysts
  - Gastroenteric cysts
  - Mesothelial cysts, other
- Acquired mediastinal cysts
  - Thoracic duct cysts, other

Endocrine lesions
- Thyroid lesions
  - Adenomatous multinodular goiters
  - Diffuse goiters
  - Follicular thyroid adenomas
  - Malignant thyroid neoplasms, other
- Parathyroid lesions
  - Adenomas
  - Lipoadenomas, other
- Paraganglial lesions
  - Paragangliomas (chemodectomas)
  - Pheochromocytomas

Mesenchymal tumors and tumor-like conditions
- Vascular mediastinal tumors
  - Lymphangiomas
  - Hemangiomas
  - Hemangiopericytomas
  - Hemangioendotheliomas, other
- Nonvascular mediastinal tumors
  - Tumors of adipose tissue origin
  - Fibrous histiocytomas
  - Eosinophilic granulomas, other

Neurogenic tumors
- Tumors of nerve origin
  - Schwannomas (neurilemomas)
  - Neurofibromas
  - Malignant tumors of nerve sheath origin, other
- Tumors of autonomic ganglia
  - Ganglioneuromas
  - Neuroblastomas
  - Ganglioneuroblastomas, other
- Tumor of paraganglia
- Tumors of probable Schwann cell origin

Rare thymic conditions
- Choristoma
- Spontaneous thymic hemorrhage

Inflammatory Tumor-like Conditions

Granulomatous Mediastinitis with Fibrosis

This syndrome is characterized by the development in the mediastinum of extensive and progressive fibrosis that may present roentgenologically and clinically as a neoplasm (Baum et al. 1960; Schowengerdt et al. 1969; Wieder and Rabinowitz 1977; Dines et al. 1979). It has been reported under various names: fibrous mediastinitis, granulomatous mediastinitis, idiopathic fibrosis of the mediastinum, mediastinal fibrosis complicating histoplasmosis and tuberculosis, mediastinal granuloma, and sclerosing mediastinitis (Strimlan et al. 1975; Light 1978). Its commonest cause in the United States of America is histoplasmosis (Strimlan et al. 1975). Tuberculosis, fungal infections such as aspergillosis, cryptococcosis, and mucormycosis, bacterial infections such as actinomycosis and nocardiosis, sarcoidosis, trauma, and drugs such as methysergide have also been incriminated. In some cases the cause is unknown. A delayed hypersensitivity reaction to an unidentified antigen has been postulated (Baum et al. 1960; Light 1978).

Pathologically, granulomatous mediastinitis with fibrosis appears as ill-defined infiltrating mediastinal tumor-like masses that slowly surround and compress mediastinal blood vessels and nerves as well as the trachea, esophagus, and heart (Marchevsky and Kaneko 1984). Biopsies show dense fibrosis, chronic inflammation, and epithelioid granulomas with or without central caseous necrosis. These granulomas may be present only focally in some lesions and their detection may then require the study of multiple histologic sections, special staining of which may show the presence of fungi or mycobacteria.

Clinically, the condition may present as a malignant neoplasm. It may cause superior vena cava obstruction, compression of pulmonary veins mimicking mitral valve stenosis, compression of pulmonary arteries with thrombosis and pulmonary hypertension, and other complications (Strimlan et al. 1975). Pulmonary interstitial fibrosis may develop in association (Light 1978). In most cases, however, granulomatous mediastinitis with fibrosis follows a slow, self-limiting clinical course and responds satisfactorily to surgical intervention (Strimlan et al. 1975).

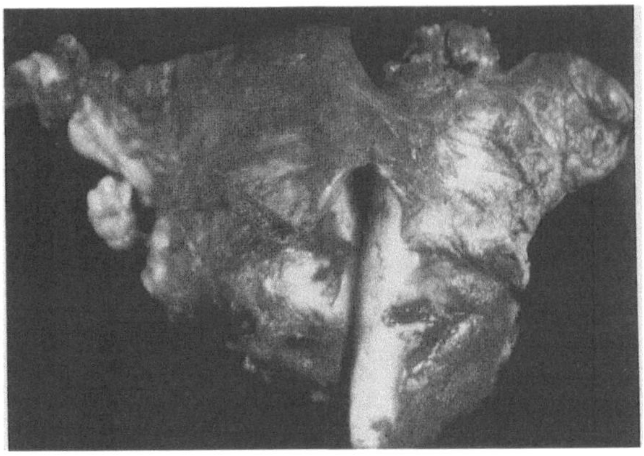

Fig. 1. Inflammatory pseudotumor of the thymus. The thymus is greatly enlarged, firm, and well encapsulated

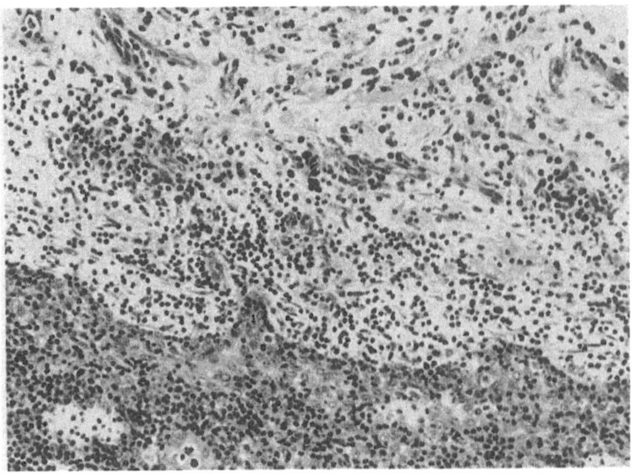

Fig. 2. Inflammatory pseudotumor of the thymus. The gland shows severe chronic inflammation. Focal hyperplasia of the thymic epithelium is seen in the lower third of the photomicrograph. Hematoxylin and eosin, ×100

Inflammatory Pseudotumor of the Thymus

We have recently had the opportunity to study a patient with a large inflammatory pseudotumor of the thymus simulating, clinically and on CT scans, a malignant thymoma (Fig. 1). The lesion consisted of a markedly enlarged thymus with extensive chronic inflammation and fibrosis (Fig. 2) and was eliminated by resection.

Lymphadenopathies

Lymphadenopathies are among the commonest causes of mediastinal tumors and tumor-like masses. Generally they affect the anterosuperior and middle mediastinal lymph nodes (Marchevsky and Kaneko 1984). Most mediastinal lymphadenopathies fall within one of three groups of diseases: malignant lymphomas, metastatic neoplasms, or granulomatous lymphadenitis and lymphadenopathies (Blank and Castellino 1977; Bragg 1978; Luosto et al. 1978). A rare lymphadenopathy that may occur in the mediastinum is angiofollicular lymph node hyperplasia (Castleman's disease) (Castleman et al. 1956).

Malignant Lymphomas

Malignant lymphomas are the most frequent malignant tumors of the mediastinum (Marchevsky and Kaneko 1984). They may arise primarily within the mediastinum, or be intrathoracic manifestations of a disseminated disease. Patients with primary mediastinal lymphomas (which constitute less than 10% of malignant thoracic lymphomas) present clinically with symptoms due to an enlarging mediastinal mass without evidence of tumor elsewhere (Lichtenstein et al. 1980).

Hodgkin's disease is the most frequent malignant lymphoma occurring in the mediastinum, chiefly in its nodular sclerosis form and usually affecting the prevascular, tracheobronchial, or paratracheal lymph nodes (Marchevsky and Kaneko 1984). Apart from the nodular sclerosis form, which is significantly commoner in young women, it affects the sexes equally (Ioachim 1982).

Pathologically, the principal feature of Hodgkin's disease is enlargement of lymph nodes and their partial or complete replacement by a mixed cell infiltrate composed of neoplastic mononuclear cells and neoplastic multinucleated cells mingled with inflammatory cells (lymphocytes, plasma cells, histiocytes, neutrophils, and eosinophils) (Ioachim 1982). The mononuclear cells (Hodgkin's or Dorothy Reed cells) have large clear nuclei with prominent basophilic nucleoli. The multinucleated cells (Sternberg-Reed cells) (Fig. 3) have similar nuclear features, but an amphophilic cytoplasm.

Hodgkin's disease is classified into four histopathological types: lymphocyte predominance; nodular sclerosis; mixed cellularity; and lymphocyte depletion. Four stages are recognized, depending on the extent of the disease (i.e., number of lymph nodes and organs affected) and patients are classified accordingly as being in stages I-IV (Ioachim 1982). Most cases of the nodular sclerosis form affect the mediastinum, which may also be affected in the mixed cellularity and lymphocyte depletion forms (Mauch et al. 1978; Lee et al. 1980; North et al. 1982).

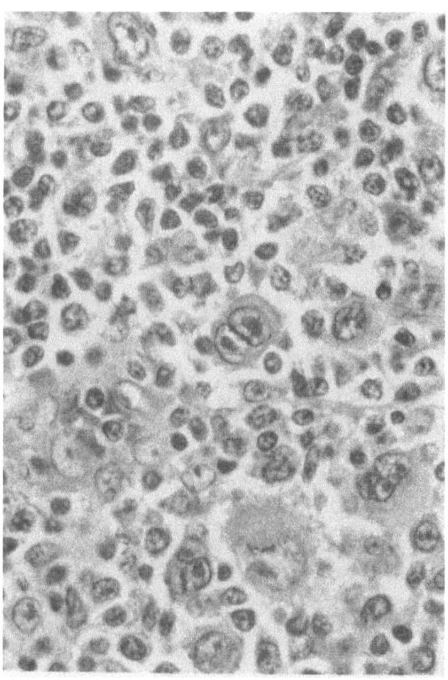

Fig. 3. Hodgkin's disease of the mediastinum. A lymph node is replaced by a pleomorphic lymphoid infiltrate containing large binucleated cells with prominent nucleoli (Sternberg-Reed cells). Hematoxylin and eosin, ×200

The prognosis in mediastinal Hodgkin's disease is influenced by the size of the mediastinal mass. A tumor is rated "large" if the ratio of its greatest transverse diameter to the transverse diameter of the thorax at T5-6 level exceeds 0.35. Patients with large tumors have higher relapse rates (74%) and shorter survival rates than patients with smaller tumors (Mauch et al. 1978; Lee et al. 1980; North et al. 1982).

The *non-Hodgkin's lymphomas* are a diverse group of neoplasms that have been classified in various ways - according to their clinicopathologic manifestations, or their morphological features, or the immunologic and physiologic characteristics of their tumor cells (Ioachim 1982). Table 2 shows the two classifications

Table 2. Working Formulation of Non-Hodgkin's Lymphomas for Clinical Usage: comparison with the Rappaport classification (Marchevsky and Kaneko 1984)

Working Formulation[a]	Rappaport classification[b]
Low grade	
A. *Malignant lymphoma* Small lymphocytic consistent with CLL-plasmacytoid	Lymphocytic, well differentiated
B. *Malignant lymphoma, follicular* Predominantly small cleaved cell; diffuse areas, sclerosis	Nodular, poorly differentiated lymphycytic
C. *Malignant lymphoma, follicular* Mixed, small cleaved and large cell; diffuse areas, sclerosis	Nodular, mixed, lymphohistiocytic
Intermediate grade	
D. *Malignant lymphoma, follicular* Predominantly large cell Diffuse areas Sclerosis	Nodular histiocytic
E. *Malignant lymphoma, diffuse* Small cleaved cell Sclerosis	Diffuse, poorly differentiated lymphocytic
F. *Malignant lymphoma, diffuse* Mixed, small and large cell Sclerosis Epithelioid cell component	Diffuse, mixed, lymphohistiocytic
G. *Malignant lymphoma, diffuse* Large cell Cleaved cell Noncleaved cell Sclerosis	Diffuse, histiocytic
High grade	
H. *Malignant lymphoma* Large cell, immunoblastic Plasmacytoid Clear cell Polymorphous Epithelioid cell component	Diffuse histiocytic

Working Formulation[a]	Rappaport classification[b]
I. Malignant lymphoma	Lymphoblastic
Lymphoblastic	
Convoluted cell	
Nonconvoluted cell	
J. Malignant lymphoma	Undifferentiated Burkitt's and undifferentiated non-Burkitt's
Small noncleaved cell	
Burkitt's	
Follicular areas	
Miscellaneous	
Composite	
Mycosis fungoides	
Histiocytic	
Extramedullary plasmacytoma	
Unclassifiable	
Other	

[a] National Cancer Institute
[b] Rappaport 1966

currently used in our institution, namely, the Working Formulation of Non-Hodgkin's Lymphomas for Clinical Usage proposed by a panel of experts sponsored by the National Cancer Institute (National Cancer Institute 1982) and the Rappaport classification (Rappaport 1966). Although the Working Formulation was not proposed as a new classification, but as "a means of translation among the various systems and to facilitate clinical comparisons of case reports and therapeutic trials," it provides a simple and reproducible presentation of this complex of neoplasms in categories with clear clinicopathologic correlations.

Median survivals of the 1175 patients included in the international study sponsored by the National Cancer Institute were: low grade, 5.1-7.2 years; intermediate grade, 1.5-3.4 years; high grade, 0.7-2.0 years (National Cancer Institute 1982). The clinicopathologic features of non-Hodgkin's lymphomas vary in different age groups (Ioachim 1982).

Child sufferers are usually over 2 years of age and symptomatic at the time of diagnosis (Elder and Touloukian 1979). They present with large anterior mediastinal masses most often located in the thymic area and compressing adjacent structures. Pathologically, the neoplasms are nearly always diffuse and of the lymphoblastic type, with convoluted and nonconvoluted nuclear features (Hausner et al. 1977: Weinstein et al. 1979; Mathew et al. 1980). Extrathoracic tumor growth in the central nervous system and the gonads generally occurs early in the disease. Acute lymphocytic leukemia often develops. The prognosis is poor, although encouraging results have been reported with chemotherapy protocols similar to those used in acute lymphocytic leukemia (Marchevsky and Kaneko 1984). Other non-Hodgkin's lymphomas such as the diffuse large cell type, the small cell noncleaved type, and undifferentiated lymphomas are less frequent in children than are those of the lymphoblastic type (Hausner et al. 1977; Weinstein et al. 1979; Mathew et al. 1980).

Mediastinal non-Hodgkin's lymphomas in adult patients generally have a diffuse histologic pattern. The commonest cell types are the diffuse large cell and the lymphoblastic (Fig. 4), the small cleaved cell and the small noncleaved cell types being less frequent (Nathwani et al. 1976; Lichtenstein et al. 1980; Miller et al. 1981; Nathwani et al. 1981). The patients present with large mediastinal masses and the clinical manifestations of compression of mediastinal structures, i.e., dyspnea, dysphagia, chest or shoulder pain, congestive heart failure, or the superior vena cava syndrome. Extensive mediastinal fibrosis with resultant compartmentalization of tumor cells by sclerosis is often a feature of the diffuse large cell lymphoma, the cell type most likely to produce the superior vena cava syndrome (Miller et al. 1981). The incidence of acute lymphocytic leukemia is lower in adults with mediastinal lymphoblastic lymphomas than in children with these tumors.

Rare mediastinal lesions that have to be distinguished from malignant lymphomas are extramedullary plasmacytomas (Arbona et al. 1980) and myeloblastomas (granulocytic sarcomas) occurring in patients with acute myelogenous leukemia (Banerjee and Silva 1981).

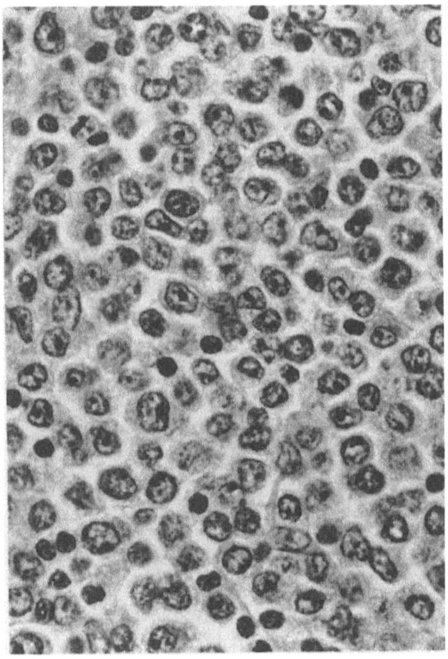

Fig. 4. Large cell immunoblastic lymphoma of the mediastinum. The lesion is composed of large lymphoid cells with basophilic cytoplasm and round vesicular nuclei with prominent nucleoli. Hematoxylin and eosin, × 200

Metastatic Neoplasms

Numerous intrathoracic and extrathoracic neoplasms metastasize to mediastinal lymph nodes, chiefly through lymphangitic spread. Most often they originate from primary malignancies in the lungs or esophagus, but secondary deposits from other sites, including the breast, the genitourinary tract, the neck, and the oral cavity, and from malignant melanoma, have been reported. Rarely, metastatic neoplasms simulate primary mediastinal neoplasms clinically (McLoud and Meyer 1982).

Granulomatous Lymphadenitis and Lymphadenopathies

Lymph node enlargement from granulomatous lymphadenitis and lymphadenopathies is a common cause of mediastinal masses (Marchevsky and Kaneko 1984). Granulomas are localized, dense collections of macrophages which may develop into epithelioid cells and giant cells. They are specialized immune reactions induced by insoluble or particulate substances (which ultimately undergo phagocytosis and mobilization by mononuclear cells) and resulting from a variety of infectious and noninfectious states (Ioachim 1983). Among the most frequent causes of mediastinal granulomatous lymphadenitis and lymphadenopathies roentgenologically simulating mediastinal new growths are fungal infections such as coccidioidomycosis, cryptococcosis, and histoplasmosis, sarcoidosis (Fig. 5), and tuberculosis (Bein et al. 1978; Ioachim 1983). Rarer causes include silicosis, Wegener's granulomatosis, and granulomas secondary to neoplasms.

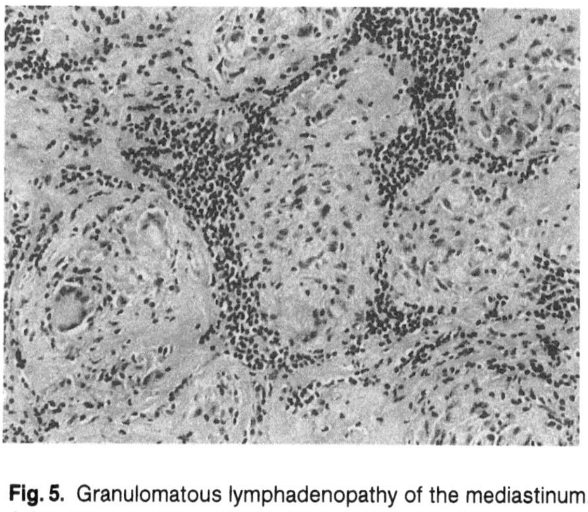

Fig. 5. Granulomatous lymphadenopathy of the mediastinum. A lymph node of a patient with sarcoidosis exhibits multiple noncaseating epithelioid cell granulomas. Hematoxylin and eosin, ×100

Angiofollicular Lymph Node Hyperplasia

Angiofollicular lymph node hyperplasia (Castleman's disease) is an unusual form of lymph node hyperplasia simulating thymoma, described by Castleman and associates in 1956. It has also been called angiomatous lymphoid hamartoma, giant lymph node hyperplasia, and lymphnodal hamartoma (Keller et al. 1972). Its cause and pathogenesis are unknown.

This condition has been reported in many locations in addition to the mediastinum, including cervical, mesenteric, and retroperitoneal lymph nodes, the spleen, and the soft tissues of the chest wall and extremities (Marchevsky and Kaneko 1984). The single or multiple lymph nodes affected are usually greatly enlarged, and may have diameters of up to 7 cm. Two histologic variants of the disease are recognized: the hyaline-vascular type, characterized by the replacement of the normal lymph node architecture by numerous small lymphoid follicles containing prominent capillaries surrounded by hyaline sheaths (lollipop follicle); and the plasma cell type, characterized by the presence of large sheets of mature and immature plasma cells in the interfollicular areas (Fig. 6; Keller et al. 1972; Gaba et al. 1978; Nordstrom et al. 1978).

Angiofollicular lymph node hyperplasia occurs in persons of both sexes and at all ages. The subjects are usually asymptomatic, a mediastinal mass being detected at routine chest roentgenography. Some pa-

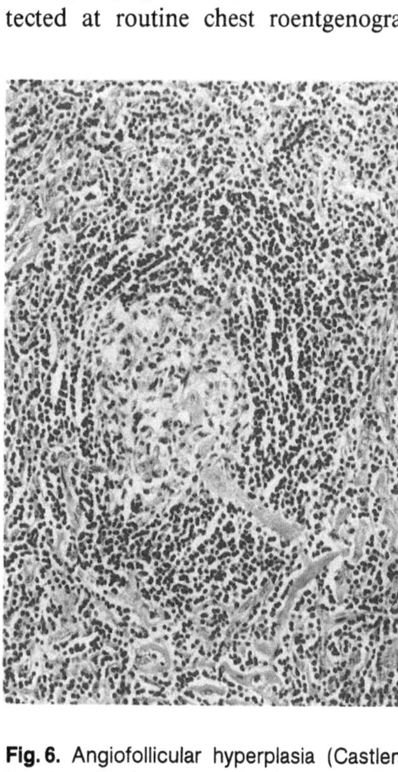

Fig. 6. Angiofollicular hyperplasia (Castleman's disease). A lymph node shows prominent neovascularity with vascularity of lymphoid follicle (lollipop follicle). Hematoxylin and eosin, ×100

ent sizes. Fetal, macrofollicular, microfollicular, and trabecular forms can be distinguished.

Malignant neoplasms of the thyroid are rarely primary in the mediastinum (Fish and Moore 1963). Although papillary and follicular thyroid carcinomas primary in the area have been described (Fig. 9; Waggoner 1958; Marchevsky and Kaneko 1984), thyroid carcinomas in the mediastinum should be considered metastatic until proved otherwise (Fig. 10; Marchevsky and Kaneko 1984).

Parathyroid Lesions

Ectopic parathyroid glands have been described in different parts of the mediastinum, but most frequently in the anterior mediastinum adjacent to or within the thymus. In fact, the inferior parathyroids have a common embryologic origin with the thymus. They derive from the third branchial pouches in close contact with the developing thymic anlage, and it is not uncommon to find small ectopic parathyroids in the thymic region (Nathaniels et al. 1970). Ectopic parathyroids have also been reported in other compartments such as the posterior mediastinum (Massac et al. 1982).

Mediastinal parathyroid adenomas, hyperplasia, lipoadenomas, and carcinomas have been described (Marchevsky and Kaneko 1984). The *adenomas,* which are the most frequent, are usually single, and approximately 20% are situated intrathymically (Fig. 11; Nathaniels et al. 1970). They present as well-encapsulated nodules composed of trabeculae, solid nests, and microacini lined with chief cells, oncocytic cells, or clear cells.

It is not easy to distinguish parathyroid adenomas from parathyroid hyperplasia on the basis of histologic findings alone. The diagnosis of adenoma requires that the lesion be single and the other three parathyroids normal, facts that can be confirmed by surgical exploration of all the parathyroids and biopsy of at least one parathyroid that is known to be normal.

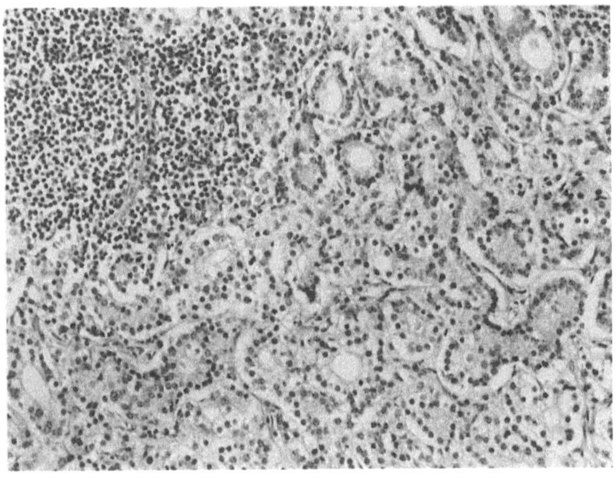

Fig. 11. Intrathymic parathyroid adenoma composed of trabeculae of clear and chief cells. Hematoxylin and eosin, ×100

Lipoadenomas are well-encapsulated lesions composed of parathyroid tissue and adipose tissue (Wolff and Goodman 1980), and are thought to represent benign tumors or parathyroid gland hamartomas. They are usually functional and associated with hyperparathyroidism. As they are generally small they are readily mistaken for normal parathyroids. However, the low power microscopic appearance of an encapsulated nodule distinct from the normal parathyroid tissue is characteristic. Parathyroid carcinomas rarely occur in the mediastinum.

Paraganglial Lesions

The paraganglia are structures of the diffuse neuroendocrine system. They occur scattered throughout the body and are composed of neuroepithelial cells with intracytoplasmic dense-core membrane-bound granules containing amines. In the mediastinum, parasympathetic paraganglia lie in close contact with the great vessels (aorticopulmonary, aortic body, paraganglia), and sympathetic paraganglia are located along the para-aortic ganglia (Marchevsky and Kaneko 1984).

Paragangliomas (chemodectomas) are infrequent tumors derived from paraganglia. They are encapsulated, highly vascular, and composed of nests of cuboidal cells with clear cytoplasm surrounded by vascularized fibrous septa (cell balls or *Zellballen*) (Pachter 1963; Enquist et al. 1974; Victor et al. 1975; Olson and Salyer 1978; Kawai et al. 1979). They may show areas of hemorrhage, mitosis, nuclear pleomorphism, and focal vascular invasion, features that do not necessarily indicate malignancy. They are usually benign, but about 10% are malignant and metastasize as malignant tumors (Enquist et al. 1974; Victor et al. 1975; Olson and Salyer 1978). Some 10% of paragangliomas are multiple (Marchevsky and Kaneko 1984), and may be associated with other endocrine abnormalities to constitute the multiple endocrine neoplasia syndrome. They have also been described as one of the elements in the so-called Carney's triad, the other two elements being pulmonary chondroma and gastric leiomyoblastoma (Dajee et al. 1982).

Pheochromocytomas are tumors with morphological features identical to those of paragangliomas (Marchevsky and Kaneko 1984), and characterized by the presence of intracytoplasmic epinephrine or norepinephrine. They usually arise from the adrenal glands, but have been described in extra-adrenal sites, including the anterior mediastinum where they may be confused roentgenologically with thymic tumors.

Mesenchymal Tumors and Tumor-like Conditions

Mesenchymal tumors account for less than 10% of mediastinal masses (Pachter and Lattes 1963a, b, c).

Vascular Mediastinal Tumors

Lymphangiomas are the most frequent mesenchymal tumors. Most often they are an intrathoracic extension of a cervical lymphangioma, sometimes they occur in the anterosuperior mediastinum simulating thymic lesions roentgenologically (Sumner et al. 1981), rarely they are multiple in patients with lymphangiomatosis (Marchevsky and Kaneko 1984). They are poorly circumscribed soft lesions, gray and sponge-like in appearance, containing chyle-filled spaces, and ranging in size from small to "giant" (Marchevsky and Kaneko 1984). They are called cystic hygromas when their cystic spaces are large, and cavernous lymphangiomas when the vessels are smaller and form a spongy mass. Histologically, lymphangiomas consist of irregular interconnecting vessels lined with endothelial cells, and surrounded by a stroma which often contains lymphoid infiltrates or lymphoid follicles. Other less frequent mediastinal vascular tumors are hemangiomas, hemangioendotheliomas, and hemangiopericytomas (Fig. 12; Marchevsky and Kaneko 1984).

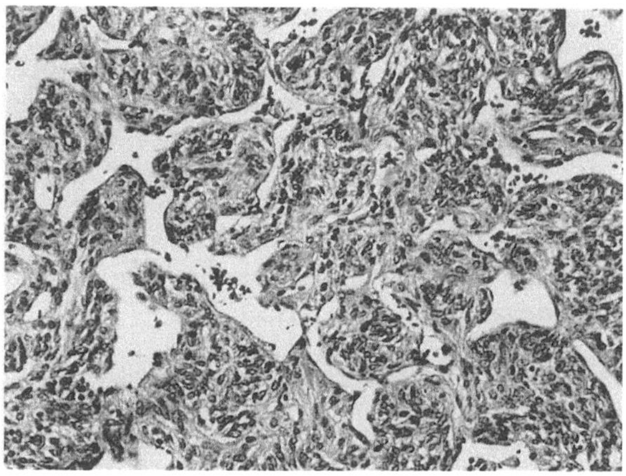

Fig. 12. Hemangiopericytoma of the anterior mediastinum. The lesion has abundant anastomosing vascular spaces lined by endothelial cells. The adjacent stroma has prominent spindle cells proliferating in an extravascular location. Hematoxylin and eosin, ×100

Nonvascular Mediastinal Tumors

Among nonvascular mediastinal mesenchymal tumors, mention should be made of tumors of adipose tissue origin such as lipomas, lipoblastomas, and liposarcomas, the last two of which are rare (Marchevsky and Kaneko 1984). Lipomas occur in the anterosuperior mediastinum, but their characteristic roentgenologic appearance and coefficient of density on computerized scans of the thorax minimize confusion with thymic lesions (Politis et al. 1979).

The mediastinum may also be the site of origin of chondrosarcomas, malignant fibrous histiocytomas, leiomyomas, leiomyosarcomas, mesenchymomas, osteogenic sarcomas, rhabdomyomas, and rhabdomyosarcomas, and of tumor-like conditions such as eosinophilic granuloma, extramedullary hematopoiesis, fibromatosis, and primary amyloidosis (Marchevsky and Kaneko 1984). Pleural fibromas may also present clinically as mediastinal tumors (Fig. 13).

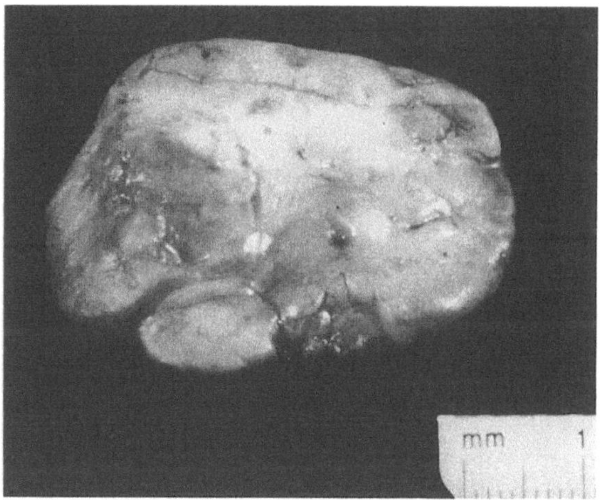

Fig. 13. Pleural fibroma that simulated roentgenologically an anterior mediastinal lesion. The lesion is firm, gray, and well encapsulated

Neurogenic Tumors

Up to 39% of mediastinal neoplasms are intrathoracic neurogenic tumors. They are most frequent in the posterior compartment, where they are unlikely to be mistaken roentgenologically for thymic tumors (Gale et al. 1974; Davidson et al. 1978; Chavez Espinosa et al. 1980; Stradling et al. 1981). They may, however, occur in other parts of the mediastinum, including the anterosuperior compartment. Mediastinal neurogenic tumors may be classified as tumors of peripheral nerves, of autonomic ganglia, of paraganglia, and of probable

Schwann cell origin (Table 3; Marchevsky and Kaneko 1984).

Table 3. Neurogenic tumors of the mediastinum (Marchevsky and Kaneko 1984)

Tumors of peripheral nerves		
	Benign	
		Schwannoma
		Melanotic schwannoma
		Neurofibroma
		Neurofibromatosis
		Pigmented neuroectodermal tumor
	Malignant	
		Tumor of nerve sheath origin
		Malignant melanocytic schwannoma
Tumors of autonomic ganglia		
	Benign	
		Ganglioneuroma
	Malignant	
		Neuroblastoma
		Ganglioneuroblastoma
Tumors of paraganglia		
		Paraganglioma
		Pheochromocytoma
Tumors of probable Schwann cell origin		
		Granular cell tumor

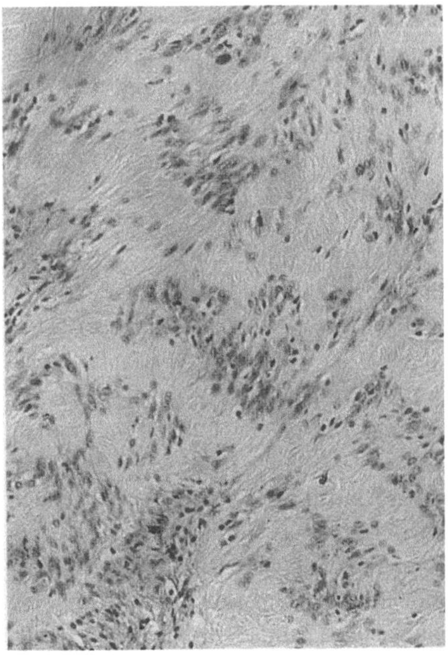

Fig. 14. Schwannoma composed of spindle cells with focal palisading and Verocay body formation. Hematoxylin and eosin, ×100

Tumors of Nerve Origin

Schwannomas (neurilemomas) are most frequent among neurogenic mediastinal tumors (Gale et al. 1974; Davidson et al. 1978). They arise from Schwann cells in nerve sheaths, and develop as well-encapsulated soft white or yellow tumors composed histologically of spindle cells with elongated, twisted nuclei arranged in bundles, short fascicles, or in a loose myxoid background (Fig. 14). Typical of schwannomas are Verocay bodies (oval structures composed of two compact rows of well-aligned spindle cells) and nuclear palisading. Schwannomas may be multiple in the mediastinum in patients with neurofibromatosis. They seldom undergo malignant transformation.

Neurofibromas are the second most frequent neurogenic tumors of the mediastinum, where they can occur as isolated tumors or as multiple thoracic manifestations of neurofibromatosis (von Recklinghausen's disease) (Stradling et al. 1981). They are soft, well-circumscribed, but not encapsulated white-gray neoplasms, usually fusiform, and composed of spindle cells with elongated, wavy nuclei dispersed in a loose connective tissue stroma containing "wire-like" collagen strands. Unlike schwannomas, they seldom exhibit nuclear palisading and they have no Verocay bodies. Ultrastructurally they are composed of Schwann cells, fibroblasts, and, again unlike schwannomas, neurites and mesoaxons. Neurofibromas are benign tumors that do not recur after resection and seldom become malignant, except in patients with neurofibromatosis, in whom the incidence of malignant transformation can be as high as 13% (Marchevsky and Kaneko 1984).

Malignant tumors of nerve sheath origin, tumors of autonomic ganglia, and tumors of probable Schwann cell origin are rare in the anterior mediastinum (Marchevsky and Kaneko 1984). Tumors of paraganglia were discussed in the section of this chapter dealing with endocrine tumors.

Rare Thymic Conditions: Choristoma of the Mediastinum

An extraskeletal osteosarcoma arising in ectopic hamartomatous thymic tissue located in the left pleural cavity and containing benign bone has been reported by Valderrama et al. (1983) (Fig. 15).

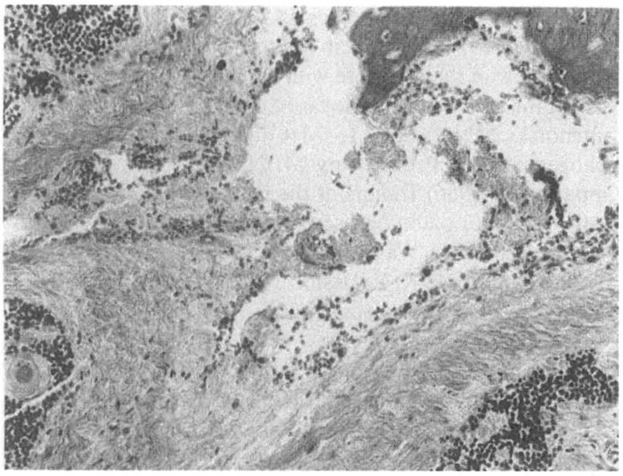

Fig. 15. Choristoma of the thymus. The lesion was located extrathymically and was composed of thymic tissue, fibrous tissue, and bone. Hematoxylin and eosin, × 100

References

Abell MR (1956) Mediastinal cysts. Arch Pathol 61: 360-379

Agha FP, Master K, Kaplan S, Cottrell TS (1975) Multiple bronchogenic cysts in the mediastinum. Br J Radiol 48: 54-57

Arbona GL, Lloyd TV, Lucas J (1980) Mediastinal extramedullary plasmacytoma. South Med J 73: 670-671

Banerjee D, Silva E (1981) Mediastinal mass with acute leukemia: myeloblastoma masquerading as lymphoblastic lymphoma. Arch Pathol Lab Med 105: 126-129

Baum GL, Green RA, Schwarz J (1960) Enlarging pulmonary histoplasmoma. Am Rev Respir Dis 82: 721-726

Bein ME, Putman CE, McLoud TC, Mink JH (1978) A reevaluation of intrathoracic lymphadenopathy in sarcoidosis. AJR 131: 409-415

Bernheim J, Griffel B, Versano S, Bruderman I (1980) Mediastinal leiomyosarcoma in the wall of a bronchial cyst. Arch Pathol Lab Med 104: 221

Blank N, Castellino RA (1977) Mediastinal lymphadenopathy. Semin Roentgenol 12: 215-223

Bragg DG (1978) The clinical, pathologic and radiographic spectrum of the intrathoracic lymphoma. Invest Radiol 13: 2-11

Castleman B, Iverson L, Pardo Menendez V (1956) Localized mediastinal lymph node hyperplasia resembling thymoma. Cancer 9: 822-830

Chavez Espinosa JI, Chavez Fernandez JA, Hoyer OHMP, Fernandez LG (1980) Endothoracic neurogenic neoplasm: (analysis of 30 cases). Rev Interam Radiol 5: 49-54

Chitale AR (1969) Gastric cyst of the mediastinum: a distinct clinicopathological entity. J Pediatr 75: 104-110

Dajee A, Dajee H, Hinrichs S, Lillington G (1982) Pulmonary chondroma, extra-adrenal paraganglioma, and gastric leiomyosarcoma: Carney's triad. J Thorac Cardiovasc Surg 84: 377-381

Davidson KG, Walbaum PR, McCormack RJM (1978) Intrathoracic neural tumours. Thorax 33: 359-367

Dines DE, Payne WS, Bernatz PE, Pairolero PC (1979) Mediastinal granuloma and fibrosing mediastinitis. Chest 75: 320-324

Elder JS, Touloukian RJ (1979) Surgical diagnosis of mediastinal lymphoma of childhood. Arch Surg 114: 54-58

Enquist RW, Tormey DC, Jenis EH, Warkel RL (1974) Malignant chemodectoma of the superior mediastinum with elevated urinary homovanillic acid. Chest 66: 209-211

Fish J, Moore RM (1963) Ectopic thyroid tissue and ectopic thyroid carcinoma: a review of the literature and report of a case. Ann Surg 157: 212-222

Gaba AR, Stein RS, Sweet DL, Variakojis D (1978) Multicentric giant lymph node hyperplasia. Am J Clin Pathol 69: 86-90

Gale AW, Jelinovsky T, Grant AF, Leckie BD, Nicks R (1974) Neurogenic tumors of the mediastinum. Ann Thorac Surg 17: 434-443

Glazer GM, Axel L, Moss AA (1982) CT diagnosis of mediastinal thyroid. AJR 138: 495-498

Gowar FJS (1978) Mediastinal thoracic duct cyst. Thorax 33: 800-802

Hausner RJ, Rosas-Uribe A, Wickstrum DA, Smith PC (1977) Non-Hodgkin's lymphoma in the first two decades of life: a pathological study of 30 cases. Cancer 40: 1533-1547

Ioachim HL (1982) Lymph node biopsy. JB Lippincott, Philadelphia, pp 183-215

Ioachim HL (1983) Granulomatous lesions of lymph nodes. In: Ioachim HL (ed) Pathology of granulomas. Raven, New York, pp 151-187

Kawai K, Kimura S, Miyamoto J, Sekiguchi T, Kano S, Ogawa Y, Fujii K, Yamada R, Kitagawa R, Ogata E (1979) A case of multiple extra-adrenal pheochromocytomas. Endocrinol Jpn 26: 693-696

Keller AR, Hochholzer L, Castleman B (1972) Hyaline-vascular and plasma-cell types of giant lymph node hyperplasia of the mediastinum and other locations. Cancer 29: 670-683

Lee CKK, Bloomfield CD, Goldman AI, Levitt SH (1980) Prognostic significance of mediastinal involvement in Hodgkin's disease treated with curative radiotherapy. Cancer 46: 2403-2409

Lichtenstein AK, Levine A, Taylor CR, Boswell W, Rossman S, Feinstein DI, Lukes RJ (1980) Primary mediastinal lymphoma in adults. Am J Med 68: 509-514

Light AM (1978) Idiopathic fibrosis of mediastinum: a discussion of three cases and review of the literature. J Clin Pathol 31: 78-88

Lillie WI, McDonald JR, Clagett OT (1950) Pericardial celomic cysts and pericardial diverticula: a concept of etiology and report of cases. J Thorac Surg 20: 494-504

Lindskog BI, Malm A (1965) Diagnostic and surgical considerations on mediastinal (intrathoracic) goiter. Am J Dis Chest 47: 201-207

Luosto R, Koikkalainen K, Jyrälä A, Franssila K (1978) Mediastinal tumours: a follow-up study of 208 patients. Scand J Thorac Cardiovasc Surg 12: 253-259

Marchevsky AM, Kaneko M (1984) Surgical pathology of the mediastinum. Raven, New York

Massac E Jr, Righini M, Seremetis M (1982) Mediastinal hyperfunctioning parathyroid adenoma. J Natl Med Assoc 74: 385-387

Mathew PM, Prangnell DR, Cole AJL, Hill FGH, Shah KJ, Jones PHM, Martin J, Palmer MK, Thompson EN, Eden OB, Mott MG, Mann JR (1980) Clinical, haematological, and radiological features of children presenting with lymphoblastic mediastinal masses. Med Pediatr Oncol 8: 193-204

Mauch P, Goodman R, Hellman S (1978) The significance of mediastinal involvement in early stage Hodgkin's disease. Cancer 42: 1039-1045

McLoud TC, Meyer JE (1982) Mediastinal metastases. Radiol Clin North Am 20: 453-468

Miller JB, Variakojis D, Bitran JD, Sweet DL, Kinzie JJ, Golomb HM, Ultmann JE (1981) Diffuse histiocytic lymphoma with sclerosis: a clinicopathologic entity frequently causing superior venacaval obstruction. Cancer 47: 748-756

Morris UL, Colletti PM, Ralls PW, Boswell WD, Lapin SA, Quinn M, Halls JM (1982) CT demonstration of intrathoracic thyroid tissue. J Comput Assist Tomogr 6: 821-824

Nathaniels EK, Nathaniels AM, Wang C (1970) Mediastinal parathyroid tumors: a clinical and pathological study of 84 cases. Ann Surg 171: 165-170

Nathwani BN, Kim H, Rappaport H (1976) Malignant lymphoma, lymphoblastic. Cancer 38: 964-983

Nathwani BN, Diamond LW, Winberg CD, Kim H, Bearman RM, Glick JH, Jones SE, Gams RA, Nissen NI, Rappaport H (1981) Lymphoblastic lymphoma: a clinicopathological study of 95 patients. Cancer 48: 2347-2357

National Cancer Institute (1982) National Cancer Institute sponsored study of classifications of non-Hodgkin's lymphomas: summary and description of a working formulation for clinical usage: the non-Hodgkin's lymphoma pathologic classification project. Cancer 49: 2112-2135

Nordstrom DG, Tewfik HH, Latourette HB (1978) Plasma cell giant lymph node hyperplasia responding to radiation therapy. Am J Roentgenol 130: 169-171

North LB, Fuller LM, Hagemeister FB, Rodgers RW, Butler JJ, Shullenberger CC (1982) Importance of initial mediastinal adenopathy in Hodgkin disease. AJR 138: 229-235

Olson JL, Salyer WR (1978) Mediastinal paragangliomas (aortic body tumor): a report of four cases and a review of the literature. Cancer 41: 2405-2412

Ovrum E, Birkeland S (1979) Mediastinal tumours and cysts: a review of 91 cases. Scand J Thorac Cardiovasc Surg 13: 161-168

Pachter MR (1963) Mediastinal nonchromaffin paraganglioma: a clinicopathologic study based on eight cases. J Thorac Cardiovasc Surg 45: 152-160

Pachter MR, Lattes R (1963a) Mesenchymal tumors of the mediastinum. I. Tumors of fibrous tissue, adipose tissue, smooth muscle, and striated muscle. Cancer 16: 74-94

Pachter MR, Lattes R (1963b) Mesenchymal tumors of the mediastinum. II. Tumors of blood vascular origin. Cancer 16: 95-107

Pachter MR, Lattes R (1963c) Mesenchymal tumors of the mediastinum. III. Tumors of lymph vascular origin. Cancer 16: 108-117

Politis J, Funahashi A, Gehlsen JA, DeCock D, Stengel BF, Choi H (1979) Intrathoracic lipomas: report of three cases and review of the literature with emphasis on endobronchial lipoma. J Thorac Cardiovasc Surg 77: 550-556

Ramenofsky ML, Leape LL, McCauley RGK (1979) Bronchogenic cyst. J Pediatr Surg 14: 219-224

Rappaport H (1966) Tumors of the hematopoietic system. In: Atlas of tumor pathology, sec 3, fasc 8. Armed Forces Institute of Pathology, Washington, pp 91-206

Salyer DC, Salyer WR, Eggleston JC (1977) Benign developmental cysts of the mediastinum. Arch Pathol Lab Med 101: 136-139

Schowengerdt CG, Suyemoto R, Main FB (1969) Granulomatous and fibrous mediastinitis: a review and analysis of 180 cases. J Thorac Cardiovasc Surg 57: 365-379

Stradling JR, Huddart S, Arnold AG (1981) Sleep apnoea syndrome caused by neurofibromatosis and superior vena caval obstruction. Thorax 36: 634-635

Strimlan CV, Dines DE, Payne WS (1975) Mediastinal granuloma. Mayo Clin Proc 50: 702-705

Sumner TE, Volberg FM, Kiser PE, Schaffner L de S (1981) Mediastinal cystic hygroma in children. Pediatr Radiol 11: 160-162

Tsuchiya R, Sugiura Y, Ogata T, Suemasu K (1980) Thoracic duct cyst of the mediastinum. J Thorac Cardiovasc Surg 79: 856-859

Valderrama E, Kahn LB, Wind E (1983) Extraskeletal osteosarcoma arising in an ectopic hamartomatous thymus. Report of a case and review of the literature. Cancer 51: 1132-1137

Victor S, Anand KV, Andappan P, Bharathy S, Rao S, Reddy KC (1975) Malignant mediastinal chemodectoma. Chest 68: 583-584

Waggoner LG (1958) Intralaryngeal intratracheal thyroid. Ann Otol Rhinol Laryngol 67: 61-71

Weinstein HJ, Vance ZB, Jaffe N, Buell D, Cassady JR, Nathan DG (1979) Improved prognosis for patients with mediastinal lymphoblastic lymphoma. Blood 53: 687-694

Weisenburger DD, DeGowin RL, Gibson DP, Armitage JO (1979) Remission of giant lymph node hyperplasia with anemia after radiotherapy. Cancer 44: 457-462

Wieder S, Rabinowitz JG (1977) Fibrous mediastinitis: a late manifestation of mediastinal histoplasmosis. Radiology 125: 305-312

Wolff M, Goodman EN (1980) Functioning lipoadenoma of a supernumerary parathyroid gland in the mediastinum. Head Neck Surg 2: 302-307

Part III

Related Diseases

12 Myasthenia Gravis

Robert P. Lisak

Introduction

Myasthenia gravis (MG) encompasses several disorders of the neuromuscular junction, characterized by impaired transmission with resulting weakness. The commonest form is an acquired disorder in which there is a decrease in available receptor for acetylcholine at the postjunctional muscle membrane, owing to autoantibodies to portions of that receptor.

MG is a relatively uncommon disease of the nervous system, occurring at an estimated prevalence rate of 0.5-5/100000 and an incidence rate of approximately 0.4/100000 (Hokkanen 1969; Kurtzke 1978). It has been suggested that there may be 2-3 times as many patients who have not been diagnosed. The disease occurs in several forms (see later in this chapter) and the age of onset ranges from birth for the congenital and the transient neonatal form to the seventh and even the eighth decade. The disease is commonest in women (3:1-4:1) in the first four decades of life; the incidence thereafter is essentially equal (Simpson 1981). There is no evidence for a geographically related effect on the incidence of MG, as there is for other diseases such as multiple sclerosis.

Pathogenesis

The arrival of an electrical impulse at the end of a motor nerve results in a concerted release of a large number of synaptic vesicles containing acetylcholine which then interact with the specific receptor in the postsynaptic (muscle) membrane. These receptors are concentrated on the terminal expansions of the postsynaptic folds of the neuromuscular junction. This interaction results in local depolarization, called the endplate potential (EPP). When sufficient in magnitude, the EPP will depolarize the surrounding muscle membrane beyond its excitation threshold. This results in an action potential which propagates along the muscle membrane, into the T-tubular system which then triggers contraction of that muscle cell. The current produced by the EPP above that required to cause depolarization ensures that a regenerative spike will be produced with each synaptic potential, even if there are minor fluctuations in transmitter release efficiency. This reserve current is the safety factor of neuromuscular transmission.

It is clear that presynaptic and postsynaptic events are complex and influenced by many factors, including divalent cations, temperature, rate of firing, etc. If a junction has a reduced margin of safety, as in MG, because of reduction of available receptors for acetylcholine, it will be susceptible to block due to the usually unimportant normal fluctuations seen at a healthy neuromuscular junction. Changes in other factors important for transmission or addition of agents that adversely affect net acetylcholine release, acetylcholine interaction with its receptor, or propagation of the depolarizing current that are normally tolerated can have a disastrous effect in junctions with a reduced safety factor.

Animal Models

A major breakthrough in our understanding of the immunopathogenesis of MG resulted in large part from the observation by Patrick and Lindstrom (1973) that rabbits sensitized with acetylcholine receptor from electric fish developed antibodies to the receptor, with weakness and fatigue of neuromuscular transmission that was reversed by anticholinesterases. This work was rapidly confirmed by other groups using several other species (Lennon et al. 1975; Tarrab-Hazdai et al. 1975a). Animals sensitized to nonmammalian receptor developed antibodies that also bound to receptor of the sensitized animal (Lennon et al. 1975; Grantano et al. 1976; Lindstrom et al. 1978).

Although disease can be transferred with unfractionated lymphocytes to naive animals (Tarrab-Hazdai et al. 1975b; Lennon et al. 1976), it has become clear that the disease, experimental autoimmune myasthenia gravis (EAMG), is due to the action of antibodies to acetylcholine receptor (AChR) rather than due to cytotoxic or delayed hypersensitivity mediated by AChR-specific T cells active at the neuromuscular junction (Engel et al. 1976; Lindstrom and Lambert

1978; Lennon 1976). However, since AChR is a protein antigen, it is not surprising that helper T cells and antigen-presenting and -processing cells are important in the development of this autoimmune disease (Christadoss et al. 1979).

Serum immunoglobulins from animals with EAMG readily transfer disease to recipient animals (Lindstrom et al. 1976a; Lennon 1976), and can also be shown to have in vitro effects similar to those observed with serum from patients with MG (Lennon 1976). The serum of animals with EAMG produces a decrease in available AChR via several mechanisms, including: (a) induction of complement-mediated membrane destruction; (b) induction of cell-associated destructive changes in muscle membrane which may represent interactions with antibody and activated complement and/or an antibody-determined cell-mediated cytotoxic reaction (ADCC); and (c) downregulation of AChR in the muscle membrane (Engel et al. 1976; Lindstrom et al. 1976a; Lennon 1976; Lindstrom and Lambert 1978; Lindstrom and Einarson 1979). There seems to be little evidence for a major pathogenic role for steric or allosteric blockade of the α-bungarotoxin-AChR binding (ligand binding) site on the AChR molecule in EAMG.

We have also gained insight into the action of antibodies to AChR as well as the nature of biologically important antigenic sites on the different peptide chains through the use of monoclonal antibodies to AChR. Many of the reported monoclonal antibodies seem to be directed at a sequence on the α-chains of AChR. Since MG patient sera and EAMG sera frequently have antibody to the same region, this has been called the main immunogenic region (Tzartos and Lindstrom 1980; Tzartos et al. 1982; Lindstrom 1985). It has been found that antibodies to non-ligand-binding portions of the molecule are capable of passively transferring EAMG, whereas monoclonal antibodies to the ACh binding site do not cause neuromuscular blockade when transferred to mammalian recipients (Lennon and Lambert 1980; Tzartos and Lindstrom 1980; Gomez et al. 1981; Lennon and Lambert 1981). However, it has been reported that monoclonal antibodies to the ACh binding site transfer a rapidly evolving block when administered to avian recipients (Gomez and Richman 1983). Thus, under certain circumstances, antibodies to the ligand binding site have the potential to mediate reduction of available AChR in vivo.

Immunopathogenic Mechanisms in MG

Studies in humans affected by MG have taught us a great deal about mechanisms by which anti-AChR decreases available AChR at the muscle endplate (Engel 1984; Ashizawa and Appel 1985). Serum Ig from patients with MG seems to be able to initiate several immunopathologic mechanisms. Among these are: (a) complement-mediated destruction of the muscle endplate (Engel et al. 1981); (b) steric and/or allosteric blocking of the ligand binding site (previously thought to have little if any importance in human MG); and (c) antigen-specific downregulation of membrane AChR initiated by cross-linking of identical epitopes on adjacent molecules of AChR, thus increasing the normal degradation rate of this molecule (Appel et al. 1977; Kao and Drachman 1977; Drachman et al. 1978; Bursztajn et al. 1983). The presence of anti-AChR that binds to the ligand binding site occurs in a minority of patients and in those patients such antibodies represent a small percentage of the total anti-AChR. The importance of antibodies to the ACh binding site is controversial in MG in humans (Ashizawa and Appel 1985; Levinson et al. 1987a). In vitro studies of anti-AChR have also shown that cross-linking of epitopes within the same molecule does not result in downregulation (Conti-Tronconi et al. 1982). Moreover, as with monoclonal antibodies raised against AChR, some antibodies may bind to sites on AChR that do not result in any biologically important effects. Patients have more than one antibody to AChR and frequently anti-AChR activity can be found in several subclasses of IgG. Serum Ig from patients with MG, but not controls, transfers neuromuscular block to immunosuppressed mice, but there is no correlation between anti-AChR titer and capacity to transfer disease (Toyka et al. 1975, 1977). When one remembers that local and systemic factors can also affect neuromuscular transmission in junctions with reduced safety factors for such transmission, it is not surprising that there is not a direct correlation between total anti-AChR titers and clinical severity of disease.

Increased cell-mediated reactivity to AChR has been reported by several groups studying the in vitro reactivity of peripheral blood mononuclear cells (PBM) from patients with MG (Abramsky et al. 1975; Richman et al. 1976; McQuillen et al. 1983; Sisley et al. 1987). Such increased reactivity is modest and likely represents, as in the EAMG model, reactivity of helper/inducer T cells that are important in anti-AChR production. However, there is no evidence of a direct cytotoxic effect or other AChR T cells being involved in the reduction of available AChR at the neuromuscular junction (Zweiman and Lisak 1986). There is also no evidence of an ADCC reaction at the endplate in humans. It should be noted, however, that there are no extensive studies of the endplate in patients with severe MG immediately following the onset of disease. Therefore, it is conceivable that an ADCC reaction could be important in recent onset disease.

Autoimmunity

Patients with MG have evidence of broad-based autoimmunity, suggesting defects in immunoregulation not limited to the autoimmune response to AChR (Lisak et al. 1982, 1985a; Levinson et al. 1985, 1987a). The serum of many patients contains elevated titers of antinuclear antibodies, anti-striated muscle (striatal) antibodies, anti-thyroglobulin, rheumatoid factor, etc. Moreover, there is an increase in associated putative autoimmune/immunopathologic disorders, including thyroid diseases, rheumatoid arthritis, systemic lupus erythematosus, etc. There is an increased frequency of *HLA* haplotypes *B8* and *DR3* among patients with MG without thymoma (Compston et al. 1980; Behan and Shields 1982). These same haplotypes are also associated with other immunopathologic diseases. Familial acquired myasthenia gravis is exceptional, but there seems to be an increased incidence in family members with other immunopathologic disorders. For those reasons, investigators have looked for broad-based qualitative and quantitative defects in immunoregulation in patients with MG.

Several investigators have studied PBM of patients with MG to determine if abnormalities of T-cell suppressor function are present. There is unfortunately no uniformity of opinions as to T-cell suppressor function, owing to use of different assays as well as to clinical differences in patients, including differences in therapy (Birnbaum and Tsairis 1976; Mischak et al. 1979; Shore et al. 1979). We have reported that there is an increase in the levels of PBM spontaneous immunoglobulin-secreting cells (IgSC) in some patients with MG (Levinson et al. 1981a, b). Spontaneous IgSC are felt to be a reflection of in vivo B-cell activation. It is not known whether the increase in spontaneous IgSC results from excess T-cell help, decreased suppression by T cells, monocytes, or other cells, inherent increase in B-cell activity and maturation toward terminally differentiated cells, or some combination of these possibilities. As noted later in this chapter, there is no evidence for an increase in B cells in the PBM of patients with MG by the usual criteria (surface Ig or IgM). We were unable to find a correlation between increased spontaneous IgSC and anti-AChR serum titers. There was a trend toward higher levels in patients with more severe disease.

There have been many studies of subpopulations of lymphocytes in the blood of patients with MG. There is no evidence for abnormalities of percentages of B cells or monocytes in PBM. It is possible that there are differences in subpopulations of B cells as assessed by newly described monoclonal antibodies. The future will likely see such studies of PBM (and thymus, see later in this chapter).

There have been several studies of T-cell subsets employing monoclonal antibodies which identify subsets with defined functional capacities. Some report a mild decrease in levels of $T8^+$ cells (suppressor/cytotoxic) (Bahir et al. 1981; Skolnik et al. 1982). There is no direct evidence that such modest decreases correlate with functional abnormalities. Some have reported decreased levels of $T3^+$ (Skolnik et al. 1982); others in helper T cells in older onset patients (Haynes et al. 1983). The serum of many patients with MG contains antibodies to lymphocytes (Lisak et al. 1979), but it is not known whether these antibodies are associated with or responsible for the lower levels of $T8^+$ cells or decreased total mature T cells ($T3^+$) or functional T-cell abnormalities reported by various investigators.

As detailed elsewhere in this volume, histologic abnormalities of the thymus are common in patients with acquired MG. We have reported increased levels of spontaneous IgSC in suspensions of thymic cells of patients with MG when compared with patients undergoing cardiac surgery (Levinson et al. 1984). These levels frequently exceed levels of IgSC of autologous PBM. Increased thymic spontaneous IgSC in comparison with autologous PBM was never detected in studies of cardiac surgery patients. These increased levels of spontaneous IgSC in thymic cell suspensions of MG patients are even more remarkable given the lack of differences in surface positive μ (B) cells between MG and normal thymuses and the relative paucity of B cells, by these criteria, in the thymus when compared with PBM. Differences in maturational state of thymic B cells in MG could be responsible for these findings, as could defects in T-cell regulatory functions or other changes in the intrathymic milieu in MG.

Incubation of thymic cells with the T-cell and monocyte-dependent polyclonal B-cell activator pokeweed mitogen (PWM) results in striking B-cell in vitro maturation and activation, both in patients with MG and in controls (Levinson et al. 1984). Thus, one could postulate that the potential for increased polyclonal B-cell activity exists in normal thymus as well as that of patients with MG. The increased polyclonal in vivo activity in MG may indicate that non-B-cell factors in the myasthenic thymus, absent in the control thymus, are responsible for the observed differences from normal subjects. Whether these differences reside in T-cell, epithelial cell, or accessory cell populations is not known. The role, if any, of AChR present in the thymus in an immunogenetically susceptible host in either in vivo or in vitro polyclonal or antigen-specific activation (see later in this chapter) is likewise not known. Recently, we have reported marked isotype restriction (IgG > IgM) of secreted immunoglobulins in PWM-stimulated thymic cell cultures from patients with MG in comparison with blood cells of MG patients and normal subjects (IgG = IgM) (Levinson et al. 1987b).

As noted, we have not found significantly increased levels of B cells in thymic cell suspensions obtained from patients with MG (Lisak et al. 1983a). However, in situ immunohistologic studies clearly demonstrate an increase in B cells, in a pattern similar to reactive lymph nodes, in the medullary germinal follicles in patients with MG (Kornstein et al. 1984). The dilution of these B cells by the overwhelming excess of T cells in the likely reason that an increase in B cells is not detected in thymic cell suspensions. We have also been unable to demonstrate differences in the levels of monocyte/macrophages (latex-ingesting and/or nonspecific esterase-containing cells) in thymic cell suspensions of patients with MG when compared with controls.

We and most others have been unable to detect differences in T-cell subpopulations between patients with MG and controls, either by thymic cell suspensions or by in situ studies (Lisak et al. 1983a; Stauver et al. 1985). Indeed, the in vitro response to PWM is somewhat surprising given the relative paucity of mature T cells ($T3^+$) when compared with PBM of autologous patients and controls. There may be functional differences in T cells of patients with MG and controls and/or qualitative differences in other T-cell subsets. It has become increasingly clear that $T4^+$ and $T8^+$ populations are themselves heterogeneous.

We first reported increased levels of major histocompatibility complex class II cells in thymic cell suspensions of some patients with MG when compared with age-matched controls (Lisak et al. 1983a). These cells could represent: (a) epithelial cells that passed through the steel mesh screen employed in preparing cell suspensions which had subsequently rounded up and thus no longer appeared as large flat cells; (b) monocyte/macrophages (unlikely given the paucity of such cells detected by the usual criteria); (c) dendritic cells similar to those seen in reactive lymph nodes; (d) B cells that do not bear the usual surface Ig or IgM because of maturational changes; and/or (e) T cells activated in vitro. We have recently noted that thymic cell suspensions have a significant number of $B1^+$ (a non-IgB-cell surface marker) IgM^- cells, whereas blood B cells are almost invariably $B1^+IgM^+$ (Zweiman et al., unpublished work). The role of such abnormal B cells is not known.

MG differs from most other immunopathologic/autoimmune diseases in that the clinically important autoantibodies have been clearly identified. This allows the study of potential abnormalities of immunoregulation that are specific to those autoantibodies as well as comparison with other more broad-based defects. We have recently reported that the PBM of many patients with MG synthesize anti-AChR in vitro, even in the absence of stimulation with PWM. Moreover, the addition of PWM to cultures of PBM from myasthenic patients results in increased levels of synthesized AChR. PBM of normal subjects rarely synthesize detectable levels of this autoantibody, even in the presence of PWM. The levels of in vitro anti-AChR secretion correlate with serum anti-AChR titers in individual patients, but not with the levels of in vitro secreted IgG in the same culture supernatants. Thus, we feel that the in vitro secretion of anti-AChR does not simply represent a nonspecific abnormal polyclonal response of PBM of patients with MG, and suggests that this assay can serve as a useful model for the investigation of immunoregulation of anti-AChR (Lisak et al. 1983b, 1984).

Depletion of $T8^+$ suppressor cells from cultures of PBM or normal individuals does not result in detectable increases in anti-AChR secretion in vitro, although such cells show an increase in polyclonal activation (increased levels of secreted IgG and increased frequency of PWM-activated IgSC) (Lisak et al. 1984). Therefore, the failure of PBM of normal subjects to secrete anti-AChR in vitro cannot be ascribed to the action of cells within that $T8^+$ population. We have also performed similar studies with the PBM of patients with MG. Depletion of $T8^+$ cells results in an increase in both secreted anti-AChR and polyclonal B-cell responses. These experiments demonstrate for the first time that anti-AChR-secreting B cells are under some immunologic suppressor control (Lisak et al. 1986a).

There has been interest in the capacity of thymic lymphocytes of patients with MG to synthesize anti-AChR in vitro as well as the capacity of these cells to induce (increase) the amount of antiAChR synthesized by PBM. Several groups have now demonstrated that thymic lymphocytes of patients with MG, but not controls, synthesize anti-AChR in vitro (Vincent et al. 1978; McLachlan et al. 1981; Newsom-Davis et al. 1981a, b; Lisak et al. 1983c, 1985a, 1986b). Newsom-Davis and colleagues have found that cells from patients with thymic hyperplasia synthesize anti-AChR, whereas cells from patients with thymoma do not do so. Others have reported that cell suspensions from thymomas synthesize anti-AChR, but less than non-thymoma cell suspensions (Fujii et al. 1984). The investigators at the Royal Free Hospital in London have also reported that incubation of thymic cell suspensions with PWM results in inhibition of in vitro anti-AChR synthesis. In contrast, we have found a heterogeneous response to PWM. Thymic cell suspensions of some patients are inhibited by incubation with PWM, others are stimulated to produce increased anti-AChR, while others are neither stimulated nor inhibited (Lisak et al. 1985b, 1986b, 1987).

There is also disagreement as to whether suspensions of thymic cells or PBM synthesize greater amounts of anti-AChR per cell. In our studies to date we have found that unstimulated cultures of thymic cells generally synthesize more anti-AChR than unstimulated autologous PBM. PWM-stimulated PBM synthesize greater amounts than PWM-incubated thymic cells, even in those instances in which thymic cells are stimulated by PWM to increase anti-AChR synthesis. The peak in vitro synthesis of anti-AChR is almost always greater in PBM cultures.

In our experience, there is more anti-AChR synthesized per nanogram IgG by thymus cell suspensions than autologous PBM. However, it has been demonstrated that other antibodies are synthesized by thymic cells in vitro. Newsom-Davis et al. (1981b) have reported synthesis of antibodies to influenza virus, and we have been able to demonstrate synthesis of anti-tetanus toxoid antibodies by thymic cell suspensions of patients who received a booster immunization with tetanus toxoid 2-4 weeks prior to thymectomy (Lisak et al. 1986b, 1987).

When thymic cells of patients are cocultured with PBM of autologous MG patients, there is an increase in synthesis of anti-AChR by PBM, but not anti-influenza antibodies (Newsom-Davis et al. 1981a, b). The nature of this interaction (T-cell help, presentation of antigen, AChR, by accessory cells, etc.) is not known (Wilcox et al. 1984). As yet, there are no published studies by other groups that address this phenomenon.

Clinical Signs, Symptoms, and Classification

MG is a disorder of neuromuscular transmission and, therefore, the symptoms are those related to muscle weakness. While other symptoms are occasionally reported, these are rare and generally not supported by objective criteria. Patients with MG have generally, although not invariably, fluctuating weakness. There is a high incidence of involvement of the muscles innervated by the cranial nerves, most commonly the extraocular muscles and the facial muscles, although any muscle groups can be involved. Uncontrolled weakness of bulbar and/or respiratory muscles may lead to aspiration or respiratory failure.

Involvement of the motor system classically affects proximal muscles, resulting in gait disability, difficulty in rising from chairs, climbing stairs, and problems with tasks involving keeping the arms elevated. In others, especially the more severely affected patients, distal weakness is present and can be very severe (Osserman 1958; Oosterhuis 1964; Lisak and Barchi 1982). There are many different ways of classifying patients with MG; one is presented in Table 1.

Table 1. Clinical classification of myasthenia gravis

Generalized
Neonatal myasthenia gravis
Congenital myasthenia gravis
Benign with ophthalmoparesis/ophthalmoplegia
Familial infantile
Juvenile myasthenia gravis
Adult generalized
Mild
Moderate
Severe
Late severe
Early atrophy
Ocular
Juvenile
Adult

Neonatal MG

Neonatal MG occurs in approximately 10%-20% of infants born to women with MG. It may be apparent from birth, but more frequently becomes manifest 24 h after delivery, and may occur up to 5 days postpartum. The severity varies and, in infants with marked involvement of bulbar and/or respiratory muscles, death may occur if correct diagnosis and treatment are delayed. Among the manifestations are feeding difficulties, weakness, hypotonia, and respiratory distress. Ophthalmoplegia and ptosis, which are among the commonest manifestations of other forms of myasthenia, are uncommon in neonatal MG. The clinical status of the mother, including severity, current and previous therapy, and the experience of prior pregnancies do not predict the occurrence and severity in an infant (Namba et al. 1970; Donaldson 1978). It now seems clear that the disease is caused by the transplacental transfer of IgG antibodies to AChR (Keesey et al. 1977; Donaldson et al. 1981). Diagnosis is easily made with edrophonium or neostigmine administration (see later). Treatment consists of therapy with anticholinesterase medications (see later), and the disease generally remits spontaneously within 21 days. Exchange transfusion or plasmapheresis are seldom necessary. Infants with neonatal MG are not at increased risk for subsequent development of acquired (juvenile or adult onset) MG.

Congenital MG

It is now quite clear that there are several types of congenital MG as well as other congenital disorders of neuromuscular transmission which have some clinical features in common with MG in its more classical acquired and congenital forms (Lisak and Barchi 1982). The various types of congenital MG are the rarest types of myasthenia. The most frequently encountered congenital myasthenic syndrome is characterized by symmetric and severe involvement of the extraocular muscles, frequently with complete external ophthalmoplegia. Other muscles may be involved to a varying degree, but bulbar involvement is less common and seldom severe. This variety of MG is rarely if ever life-threatening. While a reduced amount of acetylcholine at the endplate is involved in the pathogenesis, there are no circulating antibodies to AChR (Vincent and Newsom-Davis 1979) or antibodies bound to muscle endplate. Thus, it is not surprising that immunologic therapy (see later) is ineffective in the treatment of congenital MG.

The other congenital syndromes include: (a) a rare form which simulates neonatal MG, but occurs in infants of women who do not themselves have myasthenia (Greer and Schotland 1960; Conomy et al. 1975); (b) a disorder due to decreased acetylcholinesterase at the endplate; (c) a syndrome thought to be caused by a presynaptic defect of acetylcholine resynthesis or mobilization; and (d) a syndrome characterized by a decremental repetitive response (see later in this chapter), but which worsens with the administration of anticholinesterase medications. This latter entity is believed to result from congenital changes in the endplate structure, leading to a prolongation of the open time of the acetylcholine-induced ion channels, and defective transmission (Engel et al. 1977, 1979; Engel 1984).

Juvenile MG

Juvenile MG begins after 2 years of age and, unlike congenital forms, is not present, even retrospectively, from birth. It is an acquired disease and can either be restricted to a purely ocular form or be generalized. The defect in neuromuscular transmission is due to a defect in available AChR at the muscle endplate caused by antibodies to acetylcholine receptor. The age of onset can be any time from 2 years of age, and it is obvious that it is difficult to set an upper limit on the age of onset since it merges with adult onset myasthenia. Other than certain therapeutic considerations related to the use of certain treatment modalities in young patients, there is no reason to consider juvenile MG as being different from the commonly occurring acquired adult form (Teng and Osserman 1955; Fenichel 1978; Snead et al. 1980; Lisak and Barchi 1982).

Adult Generalized MG

The commonest form of generalized MG is the adult type. The degree of involvement varies from patient to patient, as does the severity. As noted earlier, symptoms and signs relate to the muscles involved in individual patients. In addition to ocular muscles (see later) patients complain of difficulty chewing, swallowing (dysphagia), speaking (dysarthria), drooling (facial weakness), and weakness of neck muscles, as a result of involvement of muscles innervated by cranial nerves V, VII, IX, X, XI, and XII. Weakness in muscles of the extremities and trunk leads to problems with walking, getting up from chairs, or using arms and hands. Dyspnea and respiratory failure can result from diaphragmatic and intercostal muscle weakness.

Spontaneous remissions occur in 15%-20% of patients with autoimmune (acquired non-neonatal) MG, but permanent spontaneous remissions are rare. The standard classification of Osserman (Table 2), or variations of it, is widely employed (Osserman 1958; Oosterhuis 1964). The major differentiation in that system is based on the presence or absence of bulbar and respiratory muscles (IIA versus IIB), although other differentiating points are late development of severe disease (IV), rapidity of disease development (III), and early atrophy (V). It is not clear that there are any im-

Table 2. Clinical classification of myasthenia gravis (Osserman 1958)

Pediatric
Neonatal
Juvenile
Adult
Group I (ocular, localized)
Group II (generalized with gradual onset)
A (no bulbar and/or respiratory involvement)
B (bulbar and/or respiratory involvement)
Group III (generalized; acute fulminating)
Group IV (late deterioration, ⩾2 years after onset, in group II patient)
Group V (significant muscle atrophy early in course)

munopathologic correlates to this classification. Moreover, aggressive therapy of early and mild disease has altered the natural history of MG. Indeed there are no good data on the "natural history" of MG or subtypes of MG in the modern era of therapy. Others have suggested a simpler classification (Lisak and Barchi 1982) or one based on disability (Szobar 1976).

Adult Ocular MG

Presentation of generalized MG frequently involves ptosis and/or varying degrees of ophthalmoplegia, sometimes as the only symptoms at onset. Patients with involvement of ocular muscles in ocular or generalized MG describe drooping of the lids (unilateral or bilateral) and diplopia. In 10%-20% of patients, the disease is clinically limited to the extraocular muscles and never progresses to the clinically generalized form. It is controversial as to what period of time must pass without generalized symptoms befor a patient can be assured that the disease will be restricted to the extraocular muscles. It is unusual after 5 years and rare after 7 years for ocular disease to become generalized (Osserman 1958; Lisak and Barchi 1982). There does not seem to be any predictive value in the level of antibodies to AChR, electrophysiologic, or pharmacologic studies (Bever et al. 1983). Abnormal motor point biopsies (see later in this chapter) have been reported in nonextraocular muscles in patients with clinical ocular myasthenia (Tsujihata et al. 1980).

Diagnostic Tests

There are three principal approaches to the diagnosis of MG in a patient suspected of having the disorder. These are pharmacologic, electrophysiologic, and immunologic. Certain tests combine two or more of these approaches (Lisak and Barchi 1982). For many, the diagnosis is still best established by demonstrating a temporary objective improvement in one or more signs after administration of intravenous edrophonium. In some patients with repeatedly normal tests with short-acting agent, intramuscular injection of neostigmine may be used. In patients with weakness predominantly of the extremities, this may allow for a more detailed and complete examination of the muscles. Simultaneous intramuscular administration of atropine is advisable in the neostigmine test to abrogate the muscarinic side effects, but is rarely necessary with edrophonium in patients without cardiac disease. In the rare patient who needs atropine under those circumstances, it should be administered 30 min before the edrophonium. Patients with MG are extremely sensitive to curare and curare-like agents. This is the basis of the systemic curare test which is now only occasionally performed. Some also employ a regional curare test in patients with uncertain diagnosis.

The classic neurophysiologic test for MG is repetitive stimulation of a nerve at a slow rate (generally 2-5 Hz), and recording over the surface of an appropriate muscle for that nerve. Patients with MG classically show a significant decrement (>10%-15%, depending on the laboratory) by the third or fourth response. The yield can be increased by testing several muscles if necessary and, when possible, testing a muscle that is clinically weak. Other procedures that have been employed in electrophysiologic testing are determining if there is prolonged post-tetanic stimulation exhaustion (or post-exercise), or augmentation of that phenomenon in an ischemic limb.

A newer technique is termed single-fiber electromyography. This requires special equipment and depends on a decrease in the number of paired muscle responses (increased blocking or "jitter") to stimuli. The test takes some time to perform and is not pathognomonic of MG since neurogenic diseases can result in increased jitter. However, the test can be useful in the proper clinical context, especially in patients with mild disease with predominantly ocular or cranial nerve findings who fail to give an unequivocally positive result with other testing modalities (Stålberg et al. 1971; Sanders et al. 1979).

In centers with special neuro-ophthalmologic expertise, pupillography, opticokinetic nystagmus testing, and testing for latent ocular divergence can be carried out. Abnormalities of these tests are reversed by administration of edrophonium in patients with MG and, therefore, these can be considered as extensions of pharmacologic tests. It should also be noted that repetitive stimulation can be combined with the regional curare test and edrophonium administration. Abnormal barium swallow reversed by anticholinesterase also can occasionally be useful.

A major advance in the diagnosis of MG is the testing of serum for antibodies to AChR (Appel et al. 1975). When human or fetal calf muscle is used as the source of the receptor-rich material, 75%-90% of patients with generalized MG have positive tests (Lindstrom et al. 1976b; Lefvert et al. 1978). In patients with ocular MG, the percentages are lower, 30%-50% being a more likely range. The most commonly employed assay is a radioimmunoassay in which receptor is labeled with iodinated α-bungarotoxin, reacted with the test sera, and then the immune complex precipitated with anti-immunoglobulin or staphylococcal protein A. Others have employed tests to detect blocking antibodies (antibodies to the α-bungarotoxin and/or ACh binding site) and ELISA assays as well. These are discussed elsewhere in this volume. There are several explanations for: (a) the failure of all patients with acquired MG to have detectable antibodies to acetylcholine receptor in their serum; and (b) the lack of direct correlation of titer and severity in patient groups, and even in individual patients. None of these explanations is fully satisfactory (see prior discussion and Chap. 19).

Testing for antibodies to skeletal muscle (the original autoantibodies of MG) has very limited use. Some 30% of patients with MG have such antibodies and if a myasthenic patient has a thymoma, the percentage increases to 90%-95%. However, 30% of patients with thymoma, but no MG also have such antibodies detectable in their serum. The usefulness is, therefore, currently limited to helping decide if a patient with MG has a thymoma since a negative test in a patient with MG is strong evidence against the presence of that tumor (Lisak and Barchi 1982). Aarli and his colleagues have reported that patients with MG and thymoma have a serum antibody to a citric acid extract of muscle which does not cross-react with the antistriatal antibodies. Anti-citric acid extract is rarely, if ever, seen in MG without thymoma, or thymoma in the absence of MG. Thus, a positive result with this test would indicate the presence of a thymoma in a patient with MG (Aarli et al. 1981). We will need to wait and see if this is supported when the test becomes more widely employed.

Routine muscle biopsy offers little help in the diagnosis of MG. In particularly difficult cases, biopsy of the motor point to determine if there is reduced binding of labeled α-bungarotoxin (decreased receptors for acetylcholine) has been employed (Pestronk et al. 1985). Electron microscopy can also be used to study the presynaptic and postsynaptic morphology and to determine if IgG and complement components are present at the postsynaptic junction (Engel et al. 1976; Engel 1984). This latter technique is limited to a very few centers.

Radiologic evaluation of patients with MG is considered elsewhere in this volume (Chaps. 16 and 17). However, I will briefly outline our approach. In our experience, 50% of patients with thymoma and MG will have positive findings on routine chest X-rays. If necessary (for preoperative evaluation), this can be readily confirmed by computerized tomographic (CT) scans of the chest. In our hands there have been no false-negative CT scans; we have not found an unsuspected thymoma in a patient undergoing therapeutic thymectomy for other indications (see later in this chapter). However, in the absence of calcifications or evidence of intrathoracic spread, the CT scan has false-positives. We have seen many patients with increased mediastinal density in the region of the thymus where only hyperplasia was found at surgery (Janssen et al. 1983). We feel that these are important considerations in a patient with MG who would not otherwise be a candidate for thymectomy (see later in this chapter).

Treatment

Anticholinesterase

The administration of anticholinesterase drugs frequently provides effective symptomatic therapy in the vast majority of patients with MG. In some instances, such drugs are capable of completely reversing symptoms of weakness. Unfortunately, in other patients additional therapy is required and/or side effects occur which cannot be adequately controlled by administration of atropine or atropine-like drugs. Because drugs such as pyridostigmine (Mestinon) or neostigmine (Prostigmin) do not treat the fundamental cause of acquired MG (autoantibodies directed against AChR binding to receptor at the endplate), some have suggested that anticholinesterase medication not be employed if possible. Unfortunately, in some patients therapy directed at the immune system, such as corticosteroids, or cytotoxic immunosuppressive drugs, produce greater side effects (both immediate and potential future effects) than the theoretical deleterious cholinergic effects on human muscle. In others, anticholinesterases are required in addition to corticosteroids, cytotoxic agents, and/or thymectomy.

The dose of anticholinesterases and the frequency of administration vary from patient to patient and may also vary in the same patient at different times. These medications are not well absorbed, and in those instances when oral medications cannot be employed, parenteral forms of neostigmine and pyridostigmine can be used at about $\frac{1}{30}$th of the oral dose.

Side effects include both muscarinic and nicotinic cholinergic excess. Muscarinic side effects include abdominal cramps, diarrhea, palpitations, lightheadedness, nausea, sweating, increased nasal and bronchial secretions, salivation, lacrimation, bradycardia, and increased urination. These can usually be controlled or lessened by the use of atropine, propantheline, etc. Patients receiving very large doses of anticholinesterases may also have trouble with nicotinic side effects.

Adjunct Therapy

During the era prior to the use of corticosteroids and widespread employment of thymectomy, patients who failed to achieve a satisfactory response to anticholinesterase medications were sometimes treated with other agents. These drugs included sympathetic amines such as ephedrine, which increases acetylcholine release, xanthines, potassium supplements, and spironolactone. Although these agents sometimes had some salutary effects, they were seldom striking and these drugs, including newer agents such as the aminopyridines, have not been a major advance in therapy of myastenic patients.

Corticosteroids

The use of corticosteroids has had a major impact on the therapy of patients with MG, although there are no large controlled randomized studies that prove the effectiveness of these agents in myasthenic patients. Nonetheless, patients frequently show dramatic improvement over a short period of time after having been doing poorly at a stable level for a prolonged period of time. In addition, other patients who, based on the experience of physicians with considerable expertise in treating patients with MG, would not have been expected to do well without these agents will frequently return to levels of normal function (Johns 1977; Drachman 1978; Lisak and Barchi 1982). It has been estimated that about 75% of patients will respond to corticosteroids (Johns 1987).

There are several suggested treatment protocols. Commencing therapy with daily corticosteroids (1 mg/kg/day prednisone or equivalent) seems to bring about the most rapid improvement and is strongly suggested for patients with significant generalized MG in whom a rapid improvement is desirable (Johns 1977). Beginning therapy at 2 mg/kg every other day (prednisone) will likely be slower, but after several months the patient should achieve the same level of improvement (Sghirlanzoni et al. 1984). It has been suggested that starting at 25 mg prednisone (or its equivalent) every other day and gradually increasing the dose until maximal improvement (Seybold and Drachman 1974) or 100 mg every other day reached results with a lower incidence of temporary worsening (Jenkins 1972; Warmolts et al. 1972). There are, however, no controlled studies to support this view. It should also be noted that lower doses of corticosteroids can be used from the beginning of therapy in some patients with predominantly or exclusively ocular involvement. In such patients, lower levels of corticosteroids are both effective and more reasonable to employ given the lack of risk of ocular MG and the often high incidence of side effects of large doses of corticosteroids.

The mechanisms responsible for the improvement induced by corticosteroids in patients with MG are not clear (reviewed in Lisak and Barchi 1982). It seems quite clear that long-term reduction in titers of AChR antibodies occurs and is likely the explanation for sustained improvement. It is probable that the drugs work in part by suppressing the T-helper cell population and thus affect the antibody titers as well as immunoglobulin production in general. However, many patients show rapid improvement at a time when no significant changes are seen in antibody titers. Thus, corticosteroid-induced improvement may well be due to other actions of these drugs. Corticosteroids have been shown to increase nerve conduction in experimental animals. It is also possible that these agents have a beneficial effect on phenomena taking place at the endplate as a result of the antigen-antibody reaction. Certain androgens have been shown to increase AChR channel function (Erulkar et al. 1984). It is not known if corticosteroids have such activity.

The explanation for temporary worsening induced in patients with MG is not clear. It has been shown that corticosteroids can have a local anesthetic-like effect on endplate function (Wilson et al. 1974) and patients with MG are quite sensitive to anything that further reduces the safety of neuromuscular transmission.

The long-term and short-term side effects of corticosteroids are well known and will not be listed here. They must be kept in mind when using these drugs. Because of these side effects, it is desirable to lower the dose gradually to the lowest amount that allows the patient to achieve a satisfactory level of function for that particular patient. In some patients, that dose may have virtually no significant side effects; in others this is not possible. As in all clinical medicine, one must try to achieve a reasonable balance for the individual patient. In my experience, patients who improve on corticosteroids will always need some dose of these medicines unless thymectomy has been performed or a corticosteroid-sparing agent is used. Unfortunately, not all patients who undergo thymectomy respond well enough to avoid corticosteroids or cytotoxic immunosuppressive drugs.

Immunosuppressants

There has been a recent increase in the use of cytotoxic immunosuppressive agents in the treatment of patients with MG, although the earliest reports date to the late 1960s (Mertens et al. 1969). There are still no published randomized prospective studies of such agents in MG. Nonetheless, several series have been published in which the effects of thymectomy, corticosteroids, and plasma exchange have been reasonably accounted for and in which immunosuppressants, generally azathioprine, seem to have been very useful (Matell et al. 1976; Mertens et al. 1981; Witte et al. 1984; Hohlfeld et al. 1985).

The indications for the use of azathioprine vary from one series to another. I use azathioprine: (a) to reduce the dose of corticosteroids in responsive patients who have unacceptable corticosteroid side effects; (b) in patients who have failed to improve with anticholinesterases, thymectomy, and/or corticosteroids; (c) with or without corticosteroids in patients with moderately severe or severe MG to decrease the frequency of plasma exchange; and (d) as a substitute for corticosteroids in nonurgent situations in which age or preexisting medical conditions make the use of corticosteroids risky. I do not use azathioprine in clinical ocular MG or in patients with mild generalized disease with control of bulbar or respiratory symptoms by other means.

The use of azathioprine is not without risk. Idiosyncratic reactions, including fever and hepatoxicity, occur and require the drug to be discontinued. Idiosyncratic elevations of hepatocellular enzymes may occur up to a few weeks after the beginning of therapy, especially when the drug is begun at a low dose and gradually increased. Other patients may have elevations of hepatocellular or obstructive hepatic enzymes, sometimes but not always in association with increases in dose of azathioprine. Anorexia, nausea, and rarely diarrhea are reported in patients treated with azathioprine. Discontinuing the drug for a week or so and then reinstituting therapy at a lower dose will frequently allow the continued use of azathioprine. Other side effects include decrease in white blood cells, hemoglobin, hematocrit, and red blood cells. This can often be handled by stopping the drug for a week and reinstituting azathioprine at a lower dose, after allowing the values to return to safe levels. We generally give a test dose of 50 mg for a few days and if there is no change in liver function tests, complete blood cell count (CBC), or platelets, we increase the dose over the next 2-3 weeks, monitoring the liver function tests, CBC, and platelets.

We have found that it may take 4-6 months to obtain a therapeutic effect which correlates well with the reported delay in decrease in serum titers of anti-AChR antibodies when azathioprine is used as a solitary immunosuppressive drug. The duration of therapy varies with the indications for therapy. In the absence of therapy with corticosteroids or thymectomy, we have found, as have others, that discontinuation of therapy is associated with exacerbation of the myasthenic symptoms. We have recently found that the development of macrocytosis is a useful indicator of therapeutic effect (Witte et al. 1986).

Because of the higher incidence of significant bone marrow suppression as well as alopecia and hemorrhagic cystitis, cyclophosphamide is used less frequently than azathioprine. We generally employ this drug in patients who require an immunosuppressive agent and cannot tolerate azathioprine, or who have failed to improve with azathioprine therapy. It should be pointed out that cyclophosphamide likely has some oncogenic potential. One should also be careful in the use of either drug, but especially cyclophosphamide, in women of childbearing age. In addition, cyclophosphamide may induce sterility. It has been suggested that intermittent pulsing with cyclophosphamide may have less long-term side effects than lower dose chronic therapy in autoimmune diseases. To our knowledge, this strategy has not been employed in patients with MG.

Cyclosporin A, a more selective immunosuppressive agent, has been shown to be effective in MG, and may be as effective as azathioprine (Tindall et al. 1987a, b; Goulon et al. 1987; Schalke et al. 1987). However, cyclosporin A is highly toxic and should not be considered a drug for early use (Drachman 1987). What is needed is a study that compares cyclosporin A with cyclophosphamide in patients who fail to improve after thymectomy, corticosteroids, and azathioprine (or cannot tolerate effective doses of these agents.

Apheresis

The use of plasma exchange has become an important part of the management of some patients with MG (reviewed in Lisak and Barchi 1982; Lisak 1984). We have found it useful under certain circumstances, including: (a) crisis or rapid deterioration, especially in the absence of an identifiable infection, but also in some patients in whom crisis is triggered by infection; (b) as an adjunct to low dose corticosteroids in a patient who would otherwise require high doses of these toxic agents; (c) if patients worsen during periods of corticosteroid tapering; (d) to improve patients' status for thymectomy; and (e) for post-thymectomy management. We do not find it to be of use in stable MG, especially at mild degrees of deficit (Lisak 1984).

There is some controversy over the need for obligatory use of corticosteroids and/or cytotoxic immunosuppressive agents in all patients who undergo plasmapheresis. Many patients are already being treated with corticosteroids when they are first referred for plasmapheresis. The question is, do patients not already receiving such agents who are to begin apheresis need to be placed on these agents? In patients with gradual decline or repeated periods of unexplained worsening, and in patients who clearly have demonstrated the need for frequent plasma exchange, there is little question of the need for these agents. Patients who have had thymectomy for thymoma generally have MG which is more difficult to manage. If undergoing plasma exchange and not already on corticosteroids or immunosuppressive agents, they will usually require these agents. On the other hand, we have seen many patients who are brought through a crisis or period of worsening and then are able to be treated with low levels of anticholinesterase, or go on to benefit from previous or subsequent thymectomy.

It had also been suggested that the use of corticosteroids and immunosuppressive agents at the time of plasma exchange would result in suppression of the autoimmune response at a particularly susceptible period. While suppression of the production of antibodies to AChR are thus achieved to some degree, many feel that the clinical improvement and antibody production inhibition benefit is independent of the interaction with plasma exchange. Although plasma exchange without concomitant immunosuppression may well lead to a return of titers to high levels, the return is not always associated with clinical deterioration, which is the important issue. In our experience, it is clear that the risk for patients receiving plasma exchange is almost exclusively related to the immunosuppressive anti-inflammatory drugs they receive. If such drugs are clearly necessary (as discussed earlier in this chapter), then that is a separate issue.

Other Therapy

It had been suggested that administration of gamma-globulin might have a beneficial effect in MG (Genkins et al. 1979), presumably by inhibiting anti-AChR antibody synthesis, along with "normal" immunoglobulins, by negative feedback. Despite a recent surge of interest in this form of therapy (Devathason et al. 1984; Fateh-Moghadam et al. 1984; Gajdos et al. 1984, 1987; Ippoliti et al. 1984; Besinger et al. 1987; Uchiyama et al. 1987), it is not clear that the improvement in some of the patients in these anectodal reports could be ascribed primarily to gamma-globulin therapy. In addition, the effect on immunologic parameters, such as anti-AChR antibody titers, was not consistent.

Splenic radiation and total lymphoid irradiation have also been proposed as therapeutic modalities in MG. Although such therapy might eventually be shown to play a role in a very select group of patients with MG, at the current time it should be considered a research modality and then only in patients who have life-threatening disease resistant to other forms of therapy.

Thymectomy

The role of thymectomy is covered elsewhere in this volume in detail. However, a brief outline of our use of thymectomy would seem to be an integral part of this chapter. I recommend thymectomy for patients with generalized MG, early in the course, at a time when we have found no major risk for such surgery. We employ plasma exchange and/or corticosteroids in those patients who otherwise might have difficulty with respiratory or bulbar function. We do not routinely employ these in all patients. I do not recommend thymectomy for patients with clinical ocular MG, even if they have pharmacologic or electrophysiologic abnormalities suggesting subclinical generalized disease (Papatestas et al. 1976) since it is not clear that these predict which patients will go on to clinical generalized MG (Bever et al. 1983). It has been recently reported that thymectomy may be of benefit for the ocular motor symptoms of ocular MG (Schumm et al. 1985). I also recommend thymectomy for all patients who have thymomas, on the basis of our previously published criteria (Janssen et al. 1983). There is a question of age in choosing patients for thymectomy. There is a hesitancy to perform thymectomy on patients prior to puberty, although there is no immunologic or clinical evidence to demonstrate that this would result in an immunosuppressed individual. Indeed, thymectomy likely has less side effects for a developing child or adolescent than high doses of corticosteroids. It is also not clear if there is an upper age limit. It had been suggested that 40 years of age was a reasonable cutoff, but we have done many thymectomies on patients in the fifth to the seventh decades of life without any difficulties and with evidence of therapeutic success. It is also clear that there are no prospective, randomized studies that prove that thymectomy is effective in MG. It would, therefore, seem reasonable, as with all therapy in MG, that one should not be dogmatic.

Conclusion

We have learned much about the pathogenesis of MG in the past 10-15 years and there have also been significant improvements in the result of treatment of patients with this disease. There are, as described in this chapter, many questions as yet unanswered, perhaps the most important being the origin of the autoimmune response to AChR. Moreover, we still have no cure for the disease and many of the effective forms of therapy are not universally effective, safe, or specific. However, because of the progress in our understanding of MG, further advances in this disorder should continue by employing the newly emerging techniques in cell biology, immunology, molecular biology, and genetics.

References

Aarli JA, Lefvert A-K, Tönder O (1981) Thymoma-specific antibodies in sera from patients with myasthenia gravis demonstrated by indirect haemagglutination. J Neuroimmunol 1: 421-427

Abramsky O, Aharonov A, Webb C, Fuchs S (1975) Cellular immune response to acetylcholine receptor-rich fraction, in patients with myasthenia gravis. Clin Exp Immunol 19: 11-16

Appel SH, Almon RR, Levy N (1975) Acetylcholine receptor antibodies in myasthenia gravis. N Engl J Med 293: 760-761

Appel SH, Anwyl R, McAdams MW, Elias S (1977) Accelerated degradation of acetylcholine receptor from cultured rat myotubes with myasthenia gravis sera and globulins. Proc Natl Acad Sci USA 74: 2130-2134

Ashizawa T, Appel SH (1985) Immunopathologic events at the endplate in myasthenia gravis. In: Steck AJ, Lisak RP (guest eds) Immunoneurology. Springer Semin Immunopathol 8: 177-196

Behan PO, Shields J (1982) Genetics. In: Lisak RP, Barchi RL (eds) Myasthenia gravis. Saunders, Philadelphia, pp 37-50

Berrih S, Gaud C, Bach M-A, Le Brigand H, Binet JP, Bach JF (1981) Evaluation of T cell subsets in myasthenia gravis using anti-T cell monoclonal antibodies. Clin Exp Immunol 45: 1-8

Besinger UA, Fateh-Moghadam A, Knorr-Held, Wick M, Kissel H, Albiez M (1987) Immunomodulation in myasthenia gravis by high-dose intravenous 7-5 immunglobulin. Ann NY Acad Sci 505: 828-831

Bever CT Jr, Aquino AV, Penn AS, Lovelace RE, Rowland LP (1983) Prognosis of ocular myasthenia. Ann Neurol 14: 516-519

Birnbaum G, Tsairis P (1976) Suppressor lymphocytes in mayasthenia gravis and effect of adult thymectomy. Ann NY Acad Sci 274: 527-535

Bursztajn S, McManaman JL, Elias SB, Appel SH (1983) Myasthenic globulin enhances the los of acetylcholine receptor clusters. Science 219: 195-196

Christadoss P, Lennon VA, David C (1979) Genetic control of experimental autoimmune myasthenia gravis in mice. I. Lymphocyte proliferative response to acetylcholine receptor is under *H*-2-linked Ir gene control. J Immunol 123: 2540-2543

Compston DAS, Vincent A, Newsom-Davis J, Batchelor JR (1980) Clinical, pathological, HLA antigen and immunological evidence for disease heterogeneity in myasthenia gravis. Brain 103: 579-601

Conomy JP, Levinsohn M, Fanaroff A (1975) Familial infantile myasthenia gravis: a cause of sudden death in young children. J Pediatr 87: 428-430

Conti-Tronconi BM, Gotti CM, Hunkapiller MW, Raftery MA (1982) Mammalian muscle acetylcholine receptor: a supramolecular structure formed by four related proteins. Science 218: 1227-1229

Devathasan G, Kueh YK, Chong PN (1984) High-dose intravenous gammaglobulin for myasthenia gravis. Lancet 2: 809-810

Donaldson JO (1978) Neurology of pregnancy. Saunders, Philadelphia, pp 62-65

Donaldson JO, Penn AS, Lisak RP, Abramsky O, Brenner T, Schotland DL (1981) Antiacetylcholine receptor antibody in neonatal myasthenia gravis. Am J Dis Child 135: 222-226

Drachman DB (1978) Myastenia gravis. N Engl J Med 298: 136-142; 186-193

Drachman DB (1987) Present and future treatment of myasthenia gravis. N Engl J Med 316: 743-745

Drachman DB, Angus CW, Adams RN, Michelson JD, Hoffman GJ (1978) Myasthenic antibodies cross-link acetylcholine receptors to accelerate degradation. N Engl J Med 298: 1116-1122

Engel AG (1984) Myasthenia gravis and myasthenic syndromes. Ann Neurol 16: 519-534

Engel AG, Tsujihata M, Lindstrom JM, Lennon VA (1976) The motor end-plate in myasthenia gravis and in experimental autoimmune myasthenia gravis: a quantitative ultrastructural study. Ann NY Acad Sci 274: 60-79

Engel AG, Lambert EH, Gomez MR (1977) A new myasthenic syndrome with end-plate acetylcholinesterase deficiency, small nerve terminals, and reduced acetylcholine release. Ann Neurol 1: 315-330

Engel AG, Lambert EH, Mulder DM, Torres CF, Sahashi K, Bertorini TE, Whitaker JN (1979) Investigations of cases of a newly recognized familial, congenital myasthenic syndrome. Ann Neurol 6: 146-147

Engel AG, Sahashi K, Fumagalli G (1981) The immunopathology of acquired myasthenia gravis. Ann NY Acad Sci 377: 158-174

Erulkar SD, Wetzel DM, Kilgren L, Rendt J, Parsons T, Yang S (1984) 5 α-Dihydrotestosterone modulates acetylcholine-activated single channels in myotubes cultured from adult male *Xenopus laevis* larynx. Neurosci Abst 10: 12

Fateh-Moghadam A, Wick M, Besinger U, Geursen RG (1984) High-dose intravenous gammaglobulin for myasthenia gravis. Lancet 1: 848-849

Fenichel GM (1978) Clinical syndromes of myasthenia in infancy and childhood: a review. Arch Neurol 35: 97-103

Fujii Y, Monden Y, Nakahara K, Hashimoto J, Kawashima Y (1984) Antibody to acetylcholine receptor in myasthenia gravis: production by lymphocytes from thymus or thymoma. Neurology 34: 1182-1186

Gajdos PH, Outin H, Elkharrat D, Brunel D, Rohan-Chabot P de, Raphael JC, Goulon-Goeau C, Morel E (1984) High-dose intravenous gammaglobulin for myasthenia gravis. Lancet 1: 406-407

Gajdos PH, Outin HD, Morel E, Raphael JC, Goulon M (1987) High-dose intravenous gamma globulin for myasthenia gravis: an alternative to plasma exchange? Ann NY Acad Sci 505: 842-844

Genkins G, Papatestas AE, Kornfeld P, Horowith SH (1979) Studies in myasthenia gravis: staging and gammaglobulin.

In: Dau PC (ed) Plasmapheresis and immunobiology of myasthenia gravis. Houghton Mifflin, Boston, pp 144-150
Gomez CM, Richman DP (1983) Anti-acetylcholine receptor antibodies directed against the α-bungarotoxin binding site induce a unique form of experimental myasthenia. Proc Natl Acad Sci USA 80: 4089-4093
Gomez CM, Richman DP, Burres SA, Arnason BGW, Berman PW, Fitch FW (1981) Monoclonal hybridoma anti-acetylcholine receptor antibodies: antibody specificity and effect of passive transfer. Ann NY Acad Sci 377: 97-109
Goulon M, Elkharrat D, Gajdos PH, Lokiec F, Morel E (1987) Preliminary results in myasthenia gravis treated with cyclosporin. Ann NY Acad Sci 505: 857-860
Granato DA, Fulpius BW, Moody JF (1976) Experimental myasthenia in Balb/c mice immunized with rat acetylcholine receptor from rat denervated muscle. Proc Natl Acad Sci USA 73: 2872-2876
Greer M, Schotland M (1960) Myasthenia gravis in the newborn. Pediatrics 26: 101-108
Haynes BF, Harden EA, Olanow CW, Eisenbarth GS, Weschler AS, Hensley LL, Roses AD (1983) Effect of thymectomy on peripheral lymphocyte subsets in mayasthenia gravis: selective effect on T-cells in patients with thymic atrophy. J Immunol 131: 773-777
Hohlfeld R, Toyka KV, Besinger UA, Gerhold B, Heininger K (1985) Myasthenia gravis: reactivation of clinical disease and of autoimmune factors after discontinuation of long-term azathioprine. Ann Neurol 17: 238-242
Hokkanen E (1969) Epidemiology of myasthenia gravis in Finland. J Neurol Sci 9: 463-478
Ippoliti G, Cosi V, Piccolo G, Lombardi M, Mantegaz R (1984) High-dose intravenous gammaglobulin for myasthenia gravis. Lancet 2: 809
Janssen RS, Kaye AD, Lisak RP, Schatz NJ, Arger PA, Savino PJ (1983) Radiologic evaluation of the mediastinum in maysthenia gravis. Neurology 33: 534-539
Jenkins RB (1972) Treatment of myasthenia gravis with prednisone. Lancet 1: 765-767
Johns TR (1977) Treatment of myasthenia gravis: long-term administration of corticosteroids with remarks on thymectomy. In: Griggs RC, Moxley RT III (eds) Advances in Neurology, vol 17. Raven, New York, pp 99-122
Johns TR (1987) Long-term corticosteroid treatment of myasthenia gravis. Ann NY Acad Sci 505: 568-583
Kao I, Drachman DB (1977) Myasthenic immunoglobulin accelerates acetylcholine receptor degradation. Science 196: 527-529
Keesey J, Lindstrom J, Cokely H, Herrmann C Jr (1977) Anti-acetylcholine receptor antibody in neonatal myasthenia gravis. N Engl J Med 296: 55
Kornstein MJ, Brooks JJ, Anderson AO, Levinson AI, Lisak RP, Zweiman B (1984) The immunohistology of the thymus in myasthenia gravis. Am J Pathol 117: 184-194
Kurtze JF (1978) Epidemiology of myasthenia gravis. In: Schoenberg BS (ed) Neurological epidemiology: principles and clinical applications. Advances in Neurology, vol 19. Raven, New York, pp 545-564
Lefvert AK, Bergström K, Matell G, Osterman PO, Pirskanen R (1978) Determination of acetylcholine receptor antibody in myasthenia gravis: clinical usefulness and pathogenetic implications. J Neurol Neurosurg Psychiat 41: 394-403
Lennon VA (1976) Immunology of the acetylcholine receptor. Immunol Commun 5: 323-344
Lennon VA, Lambert EH (1980) Myasthenia gravis induced by monoclonal antibodies to acetylcholine receptors. Nature 285: 238-240
Lennon VA, Lambert EH (1981) Monoclonal autoantibodies to acetylcholine receptors: evidence for a dominant idiotype and requirement of complement for pathogenicity. Ann NY Acad Sci 377: 77-95
Lennon VA, Lindstrom JM, Seybold ME (1975) Experimental autoimmune myasthenia: a model of myasthenia gravis in rats and guinea pigs. J Exp Med 141: 1365-1375
Lennon VA, Lindstrom JM, Seybold ME (1976) Experimental autoimmune myasthenia gravis: cellular and humoral immune responses. Ann NY Acad Sci 274: 283-299
Levinson AI, Dziarski A, Lisak RP, Zweiman B, Moskovitz AR, Brenner T, Abramsky O (1981a) Polyclonal B-cell activity in myasthenia gravis. Neurology 31: 1198-1201
Levinson AI, Dziarski A, Lisak RP, Zweiman B, Moskovitz AR, Brenner T, Abramsky O (1981b) Comparative immunoglobulin synthesis by blood lymphocytes of myasthenics and normals. Ann NY Acad Sci 377: 385-392
Levinson AI, Zweiman B, Lisak RP, Dziarski A, Moskovitz AR (1984) Thymic B-cell activation in myasthenia gravis. Neurology 34: 462-468
Levinson AI, Lisak RP, Zweiman B, Kornstein M (1985) Phenotypic and functional analysis of lymphocytes in myasthenia gravis. In: Steck AJ, Lisak RP (guest eds) Immunoneurology. Springer Semin Immunopathol 8: 209-233
Levinson AI, Zweiman B, Lisak RP (1987a) Immunopathogenesis and treatment of myasthenia gravis. J Clin Immunol 7: 187-197
Levinson AI, Zweiman B, Lisak RP (1987b) Isotype restriction of thymic B-cell immunoglobulin synthesis in myasthenia gravis. Ann NY Acad Sci 505: 701-703
Lindstrom J (1985) Immunobiology of myasthenia gravis, experimental autoimmune myasthenia gravis, and Lambert-Eaton syndrome. Annu Rev Immunol 3: 109-131
Lindstrom J, Einarson B (1979) Antigenic modulation and receptor loss in experimental autoimmune myasthenia gravis. Muscle Nerve 2: 173-179
Lindstrom JM, Lambert EH (1978) Content of acetylcholine receptor and antibodies bound to receptor in myasthenia gravis, experimental autoimmune myasthenia gravis, and Eaton-Lambert syndrome. Neurology 28: 130-138
Lindstrom JM, Engel AG, Seybold ME, Lennon VA, Lambert EH (1976a) Pathological mechanisms in experimental autoimmune myasthenia gravis. II. Passive transfer of experimental autoimmune myasthenia gravis in rats with anti-acetylcholine receptor antibodies. J Exp Med 144: 739-753
Lindstrom JM, Seybold ME, Lennon VA, Whittingham S, Duane DD (1976b) Antibody to acetylcholine receptor in myasthenia gravis: prevalence, clinical correlates, and diagnostic value. Neurology 26: 1054-1059
Lindstrom J, Einarson B, Merlie J (1978) Immunization of rats with polypeptide chains from torpedo acetylcholine receptor causes an autoimmune response to receptors in rat muscle. Proc Natl Acad Sci USA 75: 769-773
Lisak RP (1984) Plasma exchange in neurologic disease. Arch Neurol 41: 654-657
Lisak RP, Barchi RL (1982) Myasthenia gravis. Saunders, Philadelphia
Lisak RP, Mercado F, Zweiman B (1979) Cold reactive antilymphocyte antibodies in neurological disease. J Neurol Neurosurg Psychiatry 42: 1054-1057
Lisak RP, Levinson AI, Zweiman B (1982) Abnormalities of immunologic control mechanisms and autoimmunity in myasthenia gravis. In: Schotland DL (ed) Disorders of the motor unit. Wiley, New York, pp 257-265

Lisak RP, Zweiman B, Skolnik P, Levinson AI, Moskovitz AR, Guerrero F (1983a) Thymic lymphocyte subpopulations in myasthenia gravis. Neurology 33: 868-872
Lisak RP, Laramore C, Zweiman B, Moskovitz A (1983b) In vitro synthesis of antibodies to acetylcholine receptor by peripheral blood mononuclear cells of patients with myasthenia gravis. Neurology 33: 604-608
Lisak RP, Laramore C, Levinson AI, Zweiman B, Zembryki D, Moskovitz AR (1983c) In vitro synthesis of antibodies to acetylcholine receptor by thymic lymphocytes from patients with myasthenia gravis. Ann Neurol 14: 121
Lisak RP, Laramore C, Levinson AI, Zweiman B, Moskovitz AR, Witte A (1984) In vitro synthesis of antibodies to acetylcholine receptor by peripheral blood cells: role of suppressor T cells in normal subjects. Neurology 34: 802-805
Lisak RP, Levinson AI, Zweiman B, Kornstein M (1985a) In vitro synthesis of antibodies to acetylcholine receptor (anti-AChR) by thymic lymphocytes (TL) of patients with myasthenia gravis (MG). Neurology 35 [Suppl 1]: 101
Lisak RP, Levinson AI, Zweiman B (1985b) Autoimmune aspects of myasthenia gravis. In: Cruse JM, Lewis RE Jr (eds) Concepts in immunopathol, vol 2, Karger, Basel, pp 65-101
Lisak RP, Laramore C, Levinson AL, Zweiman B, Moskovitz AR (1986a) Suppressor T cells in myasthenia gravis and antibodies to acetylcholine receptor. Ann Neurol 19: 87-89
Lisak RP, Levinson AI, Zweiman B, Kornstein MJ (1986b) Antibodies to acetylcholine receptor and tetanus toxoid: in vitro synthesis by thymic lymphocytes. J Immunol 137: 1221-1225
Lisak RP, Levinson AI, Zweiman B, Kornstein MJ (1987) In vitro synthesis of IgG and antibodies to AChR by peripheral and thymic lymphocytes. Ann NY Acad Sci 505: 39-48
Matell G, Bergström K, Franksson C, Hammarström L, Lefvert AK, Möller E, von Reis G, Smith E (1976) Effects of some immunosuppressive procedures on myasthenia gravis. Ann NY Acad Sci 274: 659-676
McLachlan SM, Nicholson LVB, Venables G, Mastaglia FL, Bates D, Smith BR, Hall R (1981) Acetylcholine receptor antibody synthesis in lymphocyte cultures. J Clin Lab Immunol 5: 137-142
McQuillen DP, Koethe SM, McQuillen MP (1983) Cellular response to human acetylcholine receptor in patients with myasthenia gravis. J Neuroimmunol 5: 59-65
Mertens HG, Balzereit F, Leipert M (1969) The treatment of severe myasthenia gravis with immunosuppressive agents. Eur Neurol 2: 321-339
Mertens HG, Hertel G, Reuther P, Ricker K (1981) Effect of immunosuppressive drugs (azathioprine). Ann NY Acad Sci 377: 691-699
Mischak RP, Dau PC, Gonzalez RL, Spitler LE (1979) In vitro testing of suppressor cell activity in myasthenia gravis. In: Dau PC (ed) Plasmapheresis and the immunobiology of myasthenia gravis. Houghton Mifflin, Boston, pp 72-78
Namba T, Brown SB, Grob D (1970) Neonatal myasthenia gravis: report of two cases and review of the literature. Pediatrics 45: 488-504
Newsom-Davis J, Willcox N, Scadding G, Galder L, Vincent A (1981a) Anti-acetylcholine receptor antibody synthesis by cultured lymphocytes in myasthenia gravis: thymic and peripheral blood cell interactions. Ann NY Acad Sci 377: 393-402
Newsom-Davis J, Willcox N, Calder L (1981b) Thymus cells in myasthenia gravis selectively enhance production of anti-acetylcholine-receptor antibody by autologous blood lymphocytes. N Engl J Med 305: 1313-1318
Oosterhuis HJGH (1964) Studies in myasthenia gravis. Part 1. A clinical study of 180 patients. J Neurol Sci 1: 512-546
Osserman KE (1958) Myasthenia gravis. Grune and Stratton, New York, pp 79-86
Papatestas AE, Genkins G, Horowitz SH, Kornfeld P (1976) Thymectomy in myasthenia gravis: pathologic, clinical, and electrophysiologic correlations. Ann NY Acad Sci 274: 555-573
Patrick J, Lindstrom J (1973) Autoimmune response to acetylcholine receptor. Science 180: 871-872
Pestronk A, Drachman DB, Self SG (1985) Measurement of junctional acetylcholine receptors in myasthenia gravis: clinical correlates. Muscle Nerve 8: 245-251
Richman DP, Patrick J, Arnason BGW (1976) Cellular immunity in myasthenia gravis: response to purified acetylcholine receptor and autologous thymocytes. N Engl J Med 294: 694-698
Sanders DB, Howard JF Jr, Johns TR (1979) Single-fiber electromyography in myasthenia gravis. Neurology 29: 68-76
Schalke B, Kappos L, Dommasch D, Rohrbach E, Mertens HG (1987) Cyclosporin A treatment of myasthenia gravis: initial results of a double-blind trial of cyclosporin A versus azathioprine. Ann NY Acad Sci 505: 872-875
Schumm F, Wiethölter H, Fateh-Moghadam A, Dichgans J (1985) Thymectomy in myasthenia with pure ocular symptoms. J Neurol Neurosurg Psychiatry 48: 332-337
Seybold ME, Drachman DB (1974) Gradually increasing doses of prednisone in myasthenia gravis: reducing the hazards of treatment. N Engl J Med 290: 81-84
Sghirlanzone A, Peluchetti D, Mantegazza R, Fiacchino F, Cornelio F (1984) Myasthenia gravis: prolonged treatment with steroids. Neurology 34: 170:174
Shore A, Limatibul S, Dosch H-M, Gelfand EW (1979) Identification of two serum components regulating the expression of T-lymphocyte function in childhood myasthenia gravis. N Engl J Med 301: 625-629
Simpson JA (1981) Myasthenia gravis and myasthenic syndromes. In: Walton JN (ed) Disorders of voluntary muscle, 4th edn. Livingstone, Edingburgh, pp 585-624
Sisley A, Lisak RP, Brenner T (1987) Proliferative response of blood cells of patients with myastenia gravis to purified mammalian acetylcholine receptor. Ann Neurol 22: 139-140
Skolnik PR, Lisak RP, Zweiman B (1982) Monoclonal antibody analysis of blood T-cell subsets in myastenia gravis. Ann Neurol 11: 170-176
Snead OC III, Benton JW, Dwyer D, Morley BJ, Kemp GE, Bradley RJ, Oh SJ (1980) Juvenile myasthenia gravis. Neurology 30: 732-739
Stålberg E, Ekstedt J, Broman A (1971) The electromyographic jitter in normal human muscles. Electroencephalogr Clin Neurophysiol 31: 429-438
Stauver M, Hudson J, Tindall RSA (1985) Altered thymic cell populations in myasthenia gravis: characterization, localization, and relationship to AChR-bearing cells. Neurology 35 [Suppl 1]: 102
Szobor A (1976) Myasthenia gravis: a quantitative evaluation system: disability status scale (DSS) applied for myasthenia gravis. Eur Neurol 14: 439-446
Tarrab-Hazdai R, Aharonov A, Silman I, Fuchs S, Abramsky O (1975a) Experimental autoimmune myasthenia induced in monkeys by purified acetylcholine receptor. Nature 256: 128-130
Tarrab-Hazdai R, Aharonov A, Abramsky O, Yaar I, Fuchs S (1975b) Passive transfer of experimental autoimmune my-

asthenia gravis by lymph node cells in inbred guinea pigs. J Exp Med 142: 785-789

Teg P, Osserman KE (1955) Studies in myasthenia gravis: neonatal and juvenile types. J Mt Sinai Hosp 22: 711-727

Tindall RSA, Rollins JA, Phillips JT, Greenlee RG, Belendiuk G (1987a) A double-blind randomized placebo-controlled trial to assess the safety and efficacy of cyclosporin A in the treatment of myasthenia gravis. Ann NY Acad Sci 505: 854-856

Tindall RSA, Rollins JA, Phillips JT, Greenlee RG, Wells L, Belendiuk G (1987b) Preliminary results of a double-blind, randomized, placebo-controlled trial of cyclosporine in myasthenia gravis. N Engl J Med 316: 719-727

Toyka KV, Drachman DB, Pestronk A, Kao I (1975) Myasthenia gravis: passive transfer from man to mouse. Science 190: 397-399

Toyka KV, Drachman DB, Griffin DE, Pestronk A, Winkelstein JA, Fischbeck KH Jr, Kao I (1977) Myasthenia gravis: study of humoral immune mechanisms by passive transfer to mice. N Engl J Med 296: 125-131

Tsujihata M, Hazama R, Ishii N, Ide Y, Takamori M (1980) Ultrastructural localization of acetylcholine receptor at the motor endplate: myasthenia gravis and other neuromuscular diseases. Neurology 30: 1203-1211

Tzartos SJ, Lindstrom JM (1980) Monoclonal antibodies used to probe acetylcholine receptor structure: localization of the main immunogenic region and detection of similarities between subunits. Proc Natl Acad Sci USA 77: 755-759

Tzartos SJ, Seybold ME, Lindstrom JM (1982) Specificties of antibodies to acetylcholine receptors in sera from myasthenia gravis patients measured by monoclonal antibodies. Proc Natl Acac Sci USA 79: 188-192

Uchiyama M, Ichikawa Y, Takaya M, Moriuchi J, Shimizu H, Arimari S (1987) High-dose gammaglobulin therapy of generalized myasthenia gravis. Ann NY Acad Sci 505: 868-871

Vincent A, Newsom-Davis J (1979) Absence of anti-acetylcholine receptor antibodies in congenital myasthenia gravis. Lancet 1: 441-442

Vincent A, Scadding GK, Thomas HC, Newsom-Davis J (1978) In-vitro synthesis of anti-acetylcholine-receptor antibody by thymic lymphocytes in myasthenia gravis. Lancet 1: 305-307

Warmolts JR, Engel WK (1972) Benefit from alternate-day prednisone in myasthenia gravis. N Engl J Med 286: 17-20

Willcox HNA, Newsom-Davis J, Calder LR (1984) Cell types required for anti-acetylcholine receptor antibody synthesis by cultured thymocytes and blood lymphocytes in myasthenia gravis. Clin Exp Immunol 58: 97-106

Wilson RW, Ward WD, Johns TR (1974) Corticosteroids: a direct effect at the neuromuscular junction. Neurology 24: 1091-1095

Witte A, Cornblath DR, Parry GJ, Lisak RP, Schatz NJ (1984) Azathioprine in the treatment of myasthenia gravis. Ann Neurol 15: 602-605

Witte A, Cornblath DR, Lisak RP, Schatz NJ (1986) Monitoring azathioprine therapy in myasthenia gravis. Neurology

Zweiman B, Lisak RP (1986) Cell-mediated immunologic in neurologic diseases. In: Cohen S (ed) Cell-mediated immunity in human disease: Hum Pathol 17: 234-245

13 Pure Red Cell Aplasia

Sanford B. Krantz

Introduction

A severe anemia called pure red cell aplasia (PRCA) develops in 2%-6% of patients with thymomas (Jacobs et al. 1959; Schmid et al. 1965; Salyer and Eggelston 1976), and in certain patients after resection of thymomas (Hirst and Robertson 1967; Safder et al. 1970). Physicians who care for patients with thymomas must therefore be able to recognize PRCA, and must understand its pathogenesis and treatment.

In PRCA patients cease making new red cells, but continue to make white cells and platelets in normal quantity (Jacobs et al. 1959). In children the condition has been called transient erythroblastopenia of childhood (TEC) (Dessypris et al. 1982). Whereas in adults it often presents in a chronic form, requiring repeated cell transfusions, in children it is most often transitory with complete recovery in 2-3 months. Recent laboratory investigation has shown that in many cases PRCA and TEC are autoimmune diseases, with the erythroid cells of the bone marrow serving as the primary target cells for immune injury (Krantz et al. 1973; Dessypris et al. 1982).

Diagnosis

The blood reticulocyte count in PRCA is less than 1% in the presence of severe anemia, and the bone marrow has less than 0.5% of mature erythroblasts. In a few cases, 3%-4% of early erythroblasts, such as proerythroblasts and basophilic erythroblasts, may be present, producing a picture of "maturation arrest." Although an occasional bone marrow sample may have an increased number of small lymphocytes, it is the almost complete, selective absence of late erythroblasts, in which many microscopic fields have to be searched to find one mature erythroblast, that distinguishes PRCA from other blood disorders (Hirst and Robertson 1967; Marmont et al. 1975). A few patients may have mild leukopenia or thrombocytopenia, or mild leukocytosis or thrombocytosis, but most often the white cell and platelet counts are normal. The condition is therefore easily distinguished from aplastic anemia, in which very low white cell and platelet counts are evident. The bone marrow of a patient with PRCA is shown in Fig. 1. The marrow is very cellular because normal white cell, megakaryocyte, and lymphocyte production are maintained, and only erythropoiesis is absent. This is a far different picture from that seen in aplastic anemia, where the bone marrow is totally hypocellular because of reduced production of all hematopoietic cells.

Athough bone marrow biopsy and particle smear are important in the diagnosis of PRCA, other laboratory abnormalities may also occur. Paraproteinemia, hypogammaglobulinemia, decreased complement levels, anergy, and antinuclear antibodies have all been described in patients with PRCA, although in any single patient it is unusual to find more than one or two of these phenomena (Krantz and Zaentz 1977; Clark et al. 1984). In addition, patients with PRCA may have other autoimmune conditions, and may show laboratory evidence of pernicious anemia, autoimmune hypothyroidism, myasthenia gravis, multiple endocrine gland insufficiency, and autoimmune hemolytic anemia (Krantz and Dessypris 1985). Erythropoietin levels most often are increased in serum and urine, although two patients have been reported with antibody to the hormone and very low levels (Jepson and Lowenstein 1968; Peschle et al. 1975). Repeated red cell transfusions lead to increased iron deposition in the reticuloendothelial cells and to the laboratory manifestations of cirrhosis, diabetes mellitus, and cardiomyopathy with arrythmias.

PRCA occurs as a primary condition without known cause, or secondary to drugs, infections, or hemolytic anemias (Table 1). Drugs and chemicals associated with its onset are listed in Table 2. These cases are usually acute and self-limited. When the drug is removed or the infection or hemolysis clears, the PRCA disappears. A chronic form of PRCA may be associated with lupus erythematosus, rheumatoid arthritis, severe renal failure, or nutritional deficiencies such as marasmus and kwashiorkor, and with a wide variety of lymphoproliferative and nonhematologic malignancies (Table 1; Krantz and Zaentz 1977; Hilali

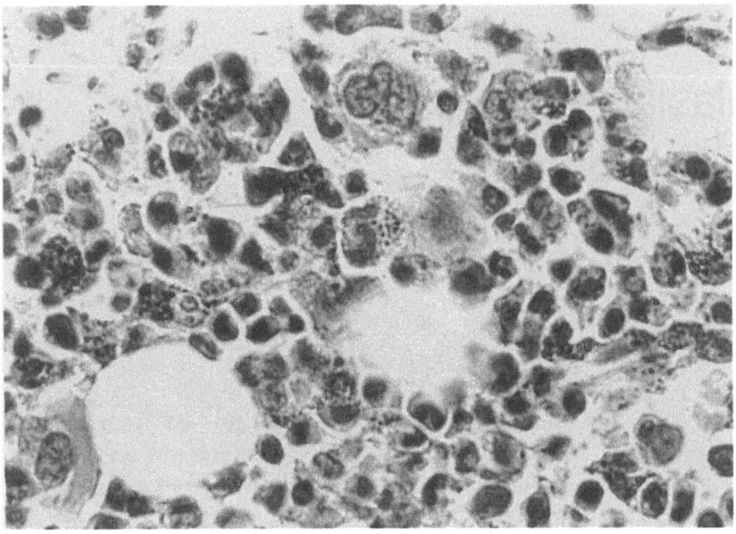

Fig. 1. Bone marrow particle section from patient with pure red cell aplasia. Normal cellularity with presence of multinucleated megakaryocytes, small lymphocytes, and granuloid cells, but no erythroblasts × 400

Table 1. Classification of pure red cell aplasia

Primary (includes transient erythroblastopenia of childhood)
Secondary
Drugs and chemicals
Infections
Parvovirus, mycoplasma, viral hepatitis, mumps, infectious mononucleosis, staphylococcemia, meningococcemia, human immunodeficiency virus
Neoplasms
Thymoma
Hematologic
Chronic lymphocytic and granulocytic leukemia, idiopathic myelofibroisis, lymphoma, multiple myeloma, angioimmunoblastic lymphadenopathy
Nonhematologic
Squamous and small cell carcinoma of the lung, carcinoma of the breast, stomach, or unknown primary site, Kaposi's sarcoma
Collagen vascular diseases
Systemic lupus erythematosus, rheumatoid arthritis
Hemolytic anemia (aplastic crisis)
Severe renal failure
Severe malnutrition

and Joyner 1983); primary treatment of the associated chronic condition is then usually necessary to produce a remission of the PRCA.

Of particular interest is the association of PRCA with thymomas. Thymoma has been reported in 50% of all cases of PRCA in the literature (Jacobs et al. 1959; Hirst and Robertson 1967), but this is probably an overstatement due to enhanced interest in the combined conditions. In our series of 37 consecutive patients with PRCA, one had a coexistent thymoma, and in one a thymoma was resected before PRCA developed (Clark et al. 1984). PRCA associated with thymoma, like primary PRCA, represents a chronic state of

Table 2. Drugs and chemicals associated with onset of pure red cell aplasia

Agent	Reference
Aminopyrine	Gasser 1957
Asphenamine	Sharff and Neumann 1944
Azathioprine	McGrath et al. 1975
Bromosulfonphtalein	Broccia and Dessalvi 1983
Calomel	Gasser 1957
Cephalothin	MacCulloch et al. 1974
Chenopodium	Gasser 1949
Chloramphenicol	Hirst and Robertson 1967; Vilan et al. 1973
Chlorpropamide	Recker and Hynes 1969
Co-trimoxazole	Stephens 1974
Dapsone	Nicholls and Concannon 1982
Diphenylhydantoin	Brittingham et al. 1964; Dessypris et al. 1985
Fenoprofen	Weinberger 1979; Reitz and Bottomly 1984
Gold	Reid and Patterson 1977
Halothane	Jurgensen et al. 1970
Isoniazid	Mielke 1958; Goodman and Block 1964
Methazolamide	Krivoy et al. 1981
Penicillin	Gasser 1949
Phenobarbital	Gasser 1949
Phenylbutazone	Swineford et al. 1958; Ibrahim et al. 1966
Salicylazosulfapyridine	Peschle et al. 1978
Santonin	Gasser 1957
Sodium valproate	MacDougall 1982
Sulfasalazine	Dunn and Kerr 1981
Sulfathiazole	Strauss 1943; Tsai and Levin 1957
Thiamphenicol	Cornet et al. 1974
Tolbutamide	Schmid et al. 1963

markedly reduced erythropoiesis. However, in 29% of these cases removal of the thymoma is followed by remission of the anemia (Jacobs et al. 1959) and often other therapies for PRCA are unsuccessful unless the thymoma is first resected (Roland 1964; Hirst and Robertson 1967). Thus, all patients with PRCA should have investigation to exclude thymoma.

Anterior mediastinal masses detected at chest roentgenography or lateral tomography in patients with PRCA should be resected. Patients with PRCA and no masses detectable by these means should nevertheless have computed tomography (CT) scans of the mediastinum. CT mediastinal scans can reveal thymomas with great sensitivity in patients over 40 years of age, but in those under 40, although they may exclude thymoma, they cannot diagnose it with a high degree of confidence because of the variable size of the normal thymus gland (Fon et al. 1982). Selective uptake of [^{75}Se] selenomethionine has also been used to detect this tumor (Min et al. 1978). Thymomas in PRCA have been predominantly of the epithelial spindle cell type, although some lymphocytic thymomas have been described (Roland 1964; Schmid et al. 1965). This is in contrast to the higher incidence of the lymphocytic type in patients with myasthenia gravis (LeGolvan and Abell 1977).

Pathogenesis

A remarkable feature of PRCA is the growth of erythroblasts after the marrow cells are incubated with erythropoietin in vitro. A large increase in hemoglobin synthesis and in the development of mature erythroblasts has been observed in liquid culture, and growth of erythroid colonies has been identified in plasma clot culture (Krantz and Kao 1967; Zaentz et al. 1975; Dessypris et al. 1982). Thus, erythroid progenitor cells are present in PRCA marrows, even when erythroblasts are absent. Development of mature erythroblasts in vitro by the patient's marrow cells is, however, inhibited by addition of the patient's plasma immunoglobulin (Ig)G, a fact which has been demonstrated by measuring hemoglobin synthesis with ^{59}Fe and by enumerating the development of erythroid colony-forming units (CFU-E) and erythroid burst-forming units (BFU-E) in the presence of PRCA IgG and normal IgG. After remission of the disease the IgG inhibitor is no longer present (Krantz et al. 1973; Cavalcant et al. 1978; Dessypris et al. 1982).

Theoretically, such an autoimmune inhibitor of erythropoiesis might act on the erythroid progenitor cells to prevent their maturation; it might be cytotoxic for the erythroblasts; or it might neutralize erythropoietin. Some patients with PRCA have IgG that is cytotoxic for their own erythroblasts in vitro while not affecting lymphocytes or red cells (Krantz et al. 1973). Where a small number of PRCA erythroblasts were still present IgG was demonstrated on their cytoplasmic membranes, but not on the erytroblasts when the patients were in remission (Bjorkholm et al. 1976; Romano et al. 1980). Other PRCA patients have IgG that inhibits the development of their own CFU-E or BFU-E, or both (Cavalcant et al. 1978; Messner et al. 1981; Dessypris et al. 1982).

This phenomenon was studied in a consecutive group of 12 children with TEC by all these methods. (Dessypris et al. 1982). Of the 12 children, 8 had an IgG inhibitor that prevented development of CFU-E or BFU-E. In two cases it inhibited BFU-E growth, but not CFU-E growth, and in two others it inhibited CFU-E, but not BFU-E. Three of the IgG inhibitors of the CFU-E were complement dependent, whereas one inhibited without the presence of complement. None of the IgG fractions neutralized erythropoietin and none were cytotoxic for erythroblasts, or prevented granulocyte-macrophage development. Thus, most of these TEC IgG fractions acted on the CFU-E or BFU-E either by direct cytotoxicity or by preventing further differentiation.

Most of these studies concerned patients with primary idiopathic PRCA, but one patient with systemic lupus erythematosus had an IgG inhibitor to BFU-E (Cavalcant et al. 1978), and Dessypris et al. (1984) found a similar inhibitor to BFU-E and CFU-E in one of three patients with rheumatoid arthritis. This specific inhibitor persisted in lower concentration even after an azathioprine-induced remission, suggesting a possible role in the chronicity of PRCA. The marrow of a patient with diphenylhydantoin-induced PRCA recovered after withdrawal of the drug (Dessypris et al. 1985). The patient's IgG, prepared at the time of diagnosis, suppressed the development of his blood BFU-E in vitro, but only in the presence of very small amounts of the drug which were not inhibitory without the IgG. The IgG and diphenylhydantoin together had no effect on granulocyte-macrophage development in vitro, nor did normal IgG, nor the patient's remission IgG, inhibit BFU-E development in the presence of the drug. The drug effect appeared to be immunologically mediated and to require the presence of the patient's IgG. The necessity for both may explain the rapid disappearance of PRCA when the drug was discontinued.

The possibility of other pathogenetic mechanisms for PRCA is also being explored, as IgG inhibitors are not found in all cases. Initial reports suggested that the blood lymphocytes of some PRCA patients inhibited erythropoiesis by normal marrow cells in vitro (Litman and Zanjani 1977), but subsequent studies have indicated that multiple blood transfusions lead to sensitization of blood lymphocytes, a fact which may explain the inhibition of allogeneic normal marrow cells (Torok-Storb et al. 1980). In a study of patients with PRCA and Tγ-cell chronic lymphocytic leukemia using autologous marrow cells, Nagasawa et al. (1981) and Lipton et al. (1983) froze the T cells and treated the patients to produce a remission of the PRCA. When the pretreatment T cells were incubated with the patient's own remission marrow cells, inhibition of erythropoiesis, but not of granulopoiesis, occurred. In one case, this inhibition was genetically restricted to cells from the patient and from partially human leukocyte antigen (HLA) identical subjects (Lipton et al. 1983). In similar studies in patients with primary PRCA and TEC, a decrease in T-cell inhibitory activity correlated with clinical improvement as the patients were either treated with immunosuppressive drugs (PRCA) or recovered spontaneously (TEC) (Hanada et al. 1984; 1985).

The pathogenetic relation of thymoma to PRCA is unknown. A serum IgG inhibitor of erythropoiesis was demonstrated in one patient, but was never tested on the patient's own marrow cells and might represent an allogeneic immune inhibitor unrelated to the disease. The fact that resection of a thymoma may not have an immediate effect, or any effect, on the PRCA suggests that these thymomas are not producing a direct inhibitor. Some thymomas might contribute to hypersensitivity of the immune system, or arise from a hypersensitive, hyperplastic system, instead of directly producing an inhibitor of erythropoiesis. More investigation is needed to clarify this relationship.

PRCA may have other causes. Of 28 patients with acute, self-limited PRCA associated with sickle cell hemolytic anemia, 24 were infected with the B19 parvovirus (Serjeant et al. 1981), whereas only 4 of 94 control subjects were so infected. Addition of serum containing this virus to normal marrow cells in vitro produced a marked reduction of CFU-E development. This was prevented by serum containing antibody to the virus (Young, Mortimer et al. 1984) and the virus was demonstrated in the marrow erythroblasts (Young, Harrison et al. 1984). Thus, although PRCA is morphologically "pure," its pathogenesis may vary.

Treatment

Since many cases of PRCA are secondary to drugs and infections and are acute and self-limited, initial therapy consists in maintenance of the hematocrit with red cell transfusions, withdrawal of all drugs or substitution of a different formulation, and observation for 1-2 months to determine if the PRCA will remit. In our series of 37 consecutive patients, vitamin B_{12} and folic acid were of no benefit, and androgens benefited only 1 of 22 patients (Clark et al. 1984). Rare cases of folate and vitamin B_{12} deficiency in association with PRCA have nevertheless been reported and serum blood levels should be measured when a deficiency is suspected (Pezzimenti and Lindenbaum 1972).

In view of the higher incidence of thymoma in PRCA a roentgenographic search should be made for this tumor. Resection of thymomas in PRCA has resulted in a 29% incidence of remission (Jacobs et al. 1959) and has improved the response to corticosteroids (Roland 1964; Hirst and Robertson 1967). Corticosteroids invoked a response in only 1 of 9 patients without prior removal of an apparent thymoma (Hirst and Robertson 1967), but induced remission in 10 of 22 patients without thymoma (Clark et al. 1984). In patients who cannot undergo thymectomy, the thymoma should be irradiated. This has not had a high yield of remissions (Roland 1964), but there have been some (Field et al. 1968). In the absence of remission, corticosteroids or cytotoxic immunosuppressive drugs, or both, should be administered (Roland 1964; Hamilton and Conley 1969; Marmont et al. 1975; Clark et al. 1984). Three elective resections of normal thymus glands in PRCA been done (Soutter and Emerson 1960; Zeok et al. 1979; Krantz and Zaentz, unpublished work), but no resultant remission of PRCA has been reported.

Because chronic primary PRCA appears to have an autoimmune pathogenesis, treatment in may cases has consisted mainly of corticosteroids, alone (Roland 1964; Schmid et al. 1965) or associated with cytotoxic immunosuppressive drugs (Krantz and Zaentz 1977; Clark et al. 1984). Since the latter are leukemogenic (Greene et al. 1982) and provoke infertility (Uldall et al. 1972; Fairley et al. 1972), it is best to begin with corticosteroids alone, especially in young subjects. Oral administration of 60 mg prednisone daily for 4 weeks brought about remission (defined as cessation of the need for red cell transfusion) in 10 of 22 patients (45%) with primary PRCA and in none of five patients with secondary PRCA (Clark et al. 1984). All remissions occurred within 4 weeks.

Patients who do not respond to corticosteroids, or who relapse after their discontinuation, should be treated with combined immunosuppressive chemotherapy. This generally consists in a constant oral dose of 30 mg prednisone daily, plus 50 mg oral cyclophosphamide or azathioprine daily, increasing gradually to 150 mg daily over 3 weeks (Clark et al. 1984; Krantz and Dessypris 1985). Blood counts are obtained each week to be sure that no leukocyte or platelet toxicity has occurred. If there is no undue toxicity, and no remission has occurred, these drugs are continued for an additional 8-10 weeks with blood counts, including reticulocyte counts, every 1-2 weeks. When erythropoiesis becomes normal, or the leukocyte count is below 2000 cells per microliter, the cytotoxic drug is stopped. If neither of these events occurs the cyclophosphamide or azathioprine is again increased by 50 mg increments every 2-3 weeks until either end point is reached.

Combined therapy with cytotoxic immunosuppressive drugs and prednisone, as described, led to remission in 13 of 23 patients (56%) with primary PRCA and in 5 of 9 patients (56%) with secondary PRCA (Clark et al. 1984). As six of these patients had relapsed after remission induced by corticosteroids, and six had failed to respond to corticosteroids, the use of combined therapy was clearly beneficial. A few patients had an early increase in reticulocytes after 2-4 weeks of treatment (Krantz and Kao 1967). In others, a gradual increase of reticulocytes did not begin until after 1-2 months of therapy, with no concomitant leukocyte or platelet toxicity (Hartmann and Krantz 1974). In some cases, however, cyclophosphamide or azathioprine have had to be increased over several months with the production of a leukocyte count of 2000 cells per microliter before reticulocytes appeared (Fig. 2). In the small number of patients in whom there was no erythropoietic response after the administration of a maximum amount of cyclophosphamide or azathioprine to the point of marrow toxicity and a leukocyte count of 2000 cells per microliter, the cytotoxic drug was stopped, and when marrow regeneration took place in 3-5 weeks it was sometimes accompanied by normal erythropoiesis (Krantz and Kao 1969).

In most cases these drugs were stopped after remission was induced, but 13 of 23 patients subsequently relapsed (Clark et al. 1984). As a result of retreatment, and in some cases initiation of maintenance immunosuppression with cyclophosphamide in patients with a tendency to relapse, 54% of the patients with induced remissions remained transfusion-free during most of a 2- to 252- (mean 90)-month follow-up period (Clark et al. 1984). Patients with repeated relapses were maintained on cyclophosphamide for 2-3 years and often remained in remission for years after its eventual discontinuation (Zaentz et al. 1976; Clark et al. 1984).

If the treatment methods described are not successful, there are still other therapeutic possibilities. Beneficial results in isolated cases have been reported with anti-human thymocyte globulin (Marmont et al. 1975), plasmapheresis (Messner et al. 1981), high dose intra-

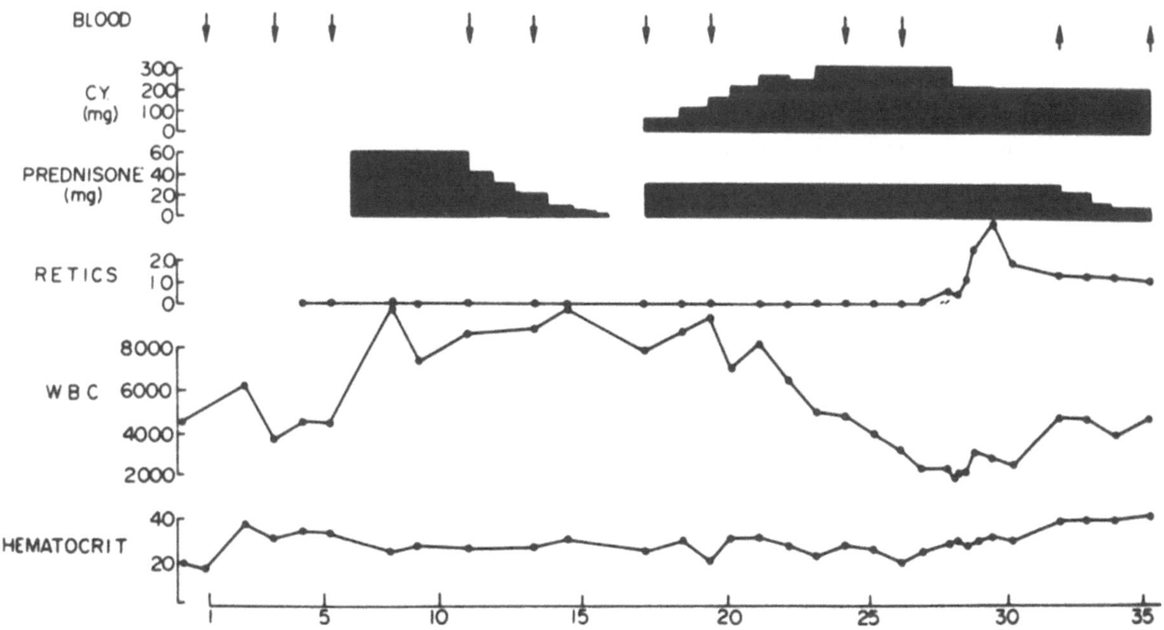

Fig. 2. Response of patient with pure red cell aplasia to prednisone and cyclophosphamide. This 38-year-old male had no remission with prednisone. He was then treated with prednisone and gradually increasing doses of cyclophosphamide for 10 weeks until the leukocyte count was 2000 cells per microliter and reticulocytes appeared in the blood. Cyclophosphamide was then reduced and prednisone discontinued. The patient was maintained on cyclophosphamide for 2 years and after its discontinuation he was still in remission when last seen 4 years later (Krantz 1978)

venous gammaglobulin (Clauvel et al. 1983), splenectomy (Zaentz et al. 1975), or cyclosporin (Tötterman et al. 1984; Debusscher et al. 1985). Certain patients who had no remission after splenectomy later responded to immunosuppressive drugs to which they had previously been resistant (Safdar et al. 1970; Clark et al. 1984). Thus, treatment for primary PRCA is similar to that for other hematopoietic autoimmune diseases such as autoimmune hemolytic anemia and autoimmune thrombocytopenic purpura.

Summary

PRCA is a condition with a selective absence of erythropoiesis. Many cases are acute and self-limited. They may be secondary to drug use or to infections, and rapidly disappear when the drug concerned is discontinued or the infection cured. Other cases of PRCA are chronic, and associated with malignancies or collagen vascular diseases. In many cases PRCA appears to have an autoimmune pathogenesis with an IgG inhibitor of erythropoiesis and a response to immunosuppressive therapy.

PRCA develops in 2%-6% of patients with thymomas and in some patients after resection of thymomas. It has been reported that 50% of patients with PRCA have thymomas and that resection of the thymoma has resulted in remission of the PRCA in 29% of these patients. Removal of normal thymus, in contrast, has not led to remission.

The pathogenetic relation between thymomas and PRCA is not known. Some thymomas have been associated with an inhibitor of erythropoiesis, but an autologous inhibitor has not been identified. The finding that thymomas have been resected with no immediate effect on PRCA suggests that other factors may be concerned. Whether some thymomas have an indirect effect on erythropoiesis, possibly through a modulation of the immune system, or arise from a hyperactive system, is not known. More work on the interaction between the immune system and erythropoiesis is needed before the precise biologic relation of thymomas to PRCA can be understood.

References

Bjorkholm M, Holm G, Mellsledt H, Carlberger G, Nisill J (1976) Membrane bound IgG on erythroblasts in pure red cell aplasia following thymectomy. A case report. Scand J Haematol 17: 341-346

Brittingham TE, Lutcher CL, Murphy DL (1964) Reversible erythroid aplasia induced by diphenylhydantoin. Arch Intern Med 113: 764-768

Broccia G, Dessalvi P (1983) Acute pure red cell aplasia following bromosulphonphtalein injection in a patient with non Hodgkin lymphoma. Haematologica [Pavia] 68: 680-683

Cavalcant J, Shadduck RK, Winkelstein A, Zeigler Z, Mendelow H (1978) Red-cell hypoplasia and increased bone marrow reticulin in systemic lupus erythematosus: reversal with corticosteroid therapy. Am J Hematol 5: 253-263

Clark DA, Dessypris EN, Krantz SB (1984) Studies on pure red cell aplasia. XI. Results of immunosuppressive treatment of 37 patients. Blood 63: 277-286

Clauvel JP, Vainchenker W, Herrera A, Dellagi K, Vinci G, Tabilio A, Lacombe C (1983) Treatment of pure red cell aplasia by high dose intravenous immunoglobulins. Br J Haematol 55: 380-382

Cornet A, Cornu P, Barbier JP, Favriel JM, Massouline G (1974) Un cas d'érythroblastopénie réversible due au thiamphénicol. Sem Hôp (Paris) 50: 1567-1570

Debusscher L, Paridaens R, Stryckmans P, Delwiche F (1985) Cyclosporine for pure red cell aplasia. Blood 65: 249

Dessypris EN, Krantz SB, Roloff JS, Lukens JN (1982) Mode of action of the IgG inhibitor of erythropoiesis in transient erythroblastopenia of childhood. Blood 59: 114-123

Dessypris EN, Baer MR, Sergent JS, Krantz SB (1984) Rheumatoid arthritis and pure red cell aplasia. Ann Intern Med 100: 202-206

Dessypris EN, Redline S, Harris JW, Krantz SB (1985) Diphenylhydantoin-induced pure red cell aplasia. Blood 65: 789-794

Dunn AM, Kerr GD (1981) Pure red cell aplasia associated with sulphasalazine. Lancet 2: 1288

Fairley KF, Barrie JU, Johnson W (1972) Sterility and testicular atrophy related to cyclophosphamide therapy. Lancet 1: 568-569

Field EO, Caughi MN, Blackett NM, Smithers DW (1968) Marrow-suppressing factors in the blood in pure red-cell aplasia, thymoma and Hodgkin's disease. Br J Haematol 15: 101-110

Fon GT, Bein ME, Mancuso AA, Kessey JC, Lupetin AR, Wong WS (1982) Computed tomography of the anterior mediastinum in myastenia gravis. Radiology 142: 135-141

Gasser C (1949) Akute Erythroblastopenie: 10 Fälle aplastischer Erythroblastenkrisen mit Riesenproerythroblasten bei allergisch-toxischen Zustandsbildern. Helv Paediatr Acta 2: 107-143

Gasser C (1957) Aplasia of erythropoiesis: acute and chronic erythroblastopenias or pure (red cell) aplastic anemias in childhood. Pediatr Clin North Am 4: 445-468

Goodman SB, Block MH (1964) A case of red cell aplasia occuring as a result of antituberculous therapy. Blood 24: 616-623

Greene MH, Boice JD Jr, Greer BE, Blessing JA, Dembo AJ (1982) Acute nonlymphocytic leukemia after therapy with alkylating agents for ovarian cancer: a study of five randomized clinical trials. N Engl J Med 307: 1416-1421

Hamilton CR Jr, Conley CL (1969) Pure red cell aplasia and thymoma. Johns Hopkins Med J 125: 262-269

Hanada T, Abe T, Nakamura H, Aoki Y (1984) Pure red cell aplasia: relationship between inhibitory activity of T cells to CFU-E and erythropoiesis. Br J Haematol 58: 107-113

Hanada T, Abe T, Takita H (1985) T-cell mediated inhibition of erythropoiesis in transient erythroblastopenia of childhood. Br J Haematol 59: 391-392

Hartmann RC, Krantz SB (1974) Paroxysmal nocturnal hemoglobinuria and pure red cell aplasia. Two rare anemias

with immunologic implications. Postgrad Med J 55: 141-147
Hilali MA, Joyner MV (1983) Pure red-cell aplasia secondary to angioimmunoblastic lymphadenopathy. J R Soc Med 76: 894-895
Hirst E, Robertson TI (1967) The syndrome of thymoma and erythroblastopenic anemia: a review of 56 cases including 3 case reports. Medicine (Baltimore) 46: 225-264
Ibrahim JM, Rawstron J, Booth J (1966) A case of red cell aplasia in a Negro child. Arch Dis Child 41: 213-215
Jacobs EM, Hutter RVP, Pool JL, Ley AB (1959) Benign thymoma and selective erythroid aplasia of the bone marrow. Cancer 12: 47-57
Jepson JH, Lowenstein L (1968) Panhypoplasia of the bone marrow. I. Demonstration of a plasma factor with anti-erythropoietin-like activity. Can Med Assoc J 99: 99-101
Jurgensen JC, Abraham JP, Hardy WW (1970) Erythroid aplasia after halothane hepatitis: report of a case. Am J Dig Dis 15: 577-581
Krantz SB (1978) Implications of studies on pure red cell aplasia (PRCA) for the study of aplastic anemia. In: Japan Medical Research Foundation (ed) Aplastic anemia. University of Tokyo Press, Tokyo, pp 305-319
Krantz SB, Dessypris EN (1985) Pure red cell aplasia. In: Golde DW, Takaku F (eds) Hematopoietic stem cells. Dekker, New York, pp 229-251
Krantz SB, Kao V (1967) Studies on red cell aplasia. I. Demonstration of a plasma inhibitor to heme synthesis and an antibody to erythroblast nuclei. Proc Nat Acad Sci USA 58: 493-500
Krantz SB, Kao V (1969) Studies on red cell aplasia. II. Report of a second patient with an antibody to erythroblast nuclei and a remission after immunosuppressive therapy. Blood 34: 1-13
Krantz SB, Zaentz SD (1977) Pure red cell aplasia. In: Gordon AS, Silber R, LoBue J (eds) The year in hematology - 1977. Plenum, New York, pp 153-190
Krantz SB, Moore WH, Zaentz SD (1973) Studies on red cell aplasia. V. Presence of erythroblast cytotoxicity in γG-globulin fraction of plasma. J Clin Invest 52: 324-336
Krivoy N, Ben-Arieh Y, Carter A, Alroy G (1981) Methazolamide-induced hepatitis and pure RBC aplasia. Arch Intern Med 141: 1229-1230
LeGolvan DP, Abell MR (1977) Thymomas. Cancer 39: 2142-2157
Lipton JM, Nadler LM, Canellos GP, Kudisch M, Reiss CS, Nathan DG (1983) Evidence for genetic restriction in the suppression of erythropoiesis by a unique subset of T lymphocytes in man. J Clin Invest 72: 694-706
Litman SD, Zanjani ED (1977) Lymphocytes suppressing both immunoglobulin production and erythroid differentiation in hypogammaglobulinemia. Nature 266: 57-58
MacCulloch D, Jackson JM, Venerys J (1974) Drug-induced red cell aplasia. Br Med J 4: 163-164
MacDougall LG (1982) Pure red cell aplasia associated with sodium valproate therapy. JAMA 247: 53-54
Marmont A, Peschle C, Sanguineti M, Condorelli M (1975) Pure red cell aplasia (PRCA): response of three patients to cyclophosphamide and/or antilymphocyte globullin (ALG) and demonstration of two types of serum IgG inhibitors to erythropoiesis. Blood 45: 247-261
McGrath BP, Ibels LS, Raik E, Hargrave M, Mahony JF, Stewart JH (1975) Erythroid toxicity of azathioprine: macrocytosis and selective marrow hypoplasia. Q J Med 44: 57-63
Messner HA, Fauser AA, Curtis JE, Dotten D (1981) Control of antibody-mediated pure red-cell aplasia by plasmapheresis. N Engl J Med 304: 1334-1338
Mielke HG (1958) Aplastische Anämie (Erythroblastophthise) nach INH-Behandlung. Folia Haematol: 2-10
Min KW, Waddell CC, Pircher FJ, Granville GE, Gyorkey F (1978) Selective uptake of ^{75}Se-selenomethionine by thymoma with pure red cell aplasia. Cancer 41: 1323-1328
Nagasawa T, Abe T, Nakagawa T (1981) Pure red cell aplasia and hypogammaglobulinemia associated with Tr-cell chronic lymphocytic leukemia. Blood 57: 1025-1031
Nicholls MD, Concannon AJ (1982) Maloprim-induced agranulocytosis and red-cell aplasia. Med J Aust 2: 564-566
Peschle C, Marmont AM, Marone G, Genovese A, Sasso GF, Condorelli M (1975) Pure red cell aplasia: studies on an IgG serum inhibitor neutralizing erythropoietin. Br J Haematol 30: 411-417
Peschle C, Marmont A, Perugini S, Bernasconi C, Brunetti P, Fontana G, Ghio R, Resegotti L, Rizzo SC, Condorelli M (1978) Physiopathology and therapy of adult pure red cell aplasia (PRCA): a cooperative study. In: Japan Medical Research Foundation (ed) Aplastic anemia. University of Tokyo Press, Tokyo, pp 285-303
Pezzimenti JF, Lindenbaum J (1972) Megaloblastic anemia associated with erythroid hypoplasia. Am J Med 53: 748-754
Recker RR, Hynes HE (1969) Pure red blood cell aplasia associated with chlorpropamide therapy. Arch Intern Med 123: 445-447
Reid G, Patterson AC (1977) Pure red-cell aplasia after gold treatment. Br Med J 2: 1457
Reitz CL, Bottomley SS (1984) Pure red cell aplasia associated with fenoprofen. Am J Med Sci 287: 62-63
Roland AS (1964) The syndrome of benign thymoma and primary aregenerative anemia: an analysis of forty-three cases. Am J Med Sci 247: 719-731
Romano E, Layrisse M, Romano M, Soyano A, Layrisse Z (1980) Electron microscopic demonstration of IgG antibodies directed to erythroblast in primary acquired pure red cell aplasia. Clin Immunol, Immunopathol 17: 330-334
Safdar SH, Krantz SB, Brown EB (1970) Successful immunosuppressive treatment of erythroid aplasia appearing after thymectomy. Br J Haematol 19: 435-443
Salyer WR, Eggleston JC (1976) Thymoma: a clinical and pathological study of 65 cases. Cancer 37: 229-249
Schmid JR, Kiely JM, Pease GL, Hargraves MM (1963) Acquired pure red cell agenesis: report of 16 cases and review of the literature. Acta Haematol (Basel) 30: 255-270
Schmid JR, Kiely JM, Harrison EG Jr, Bayrd ED, Pease GL (1965) Thymoma associated with pure red-cell agenesis: review of literature and report of 4 cases. Cancer 18: 216-230
Serjeant GR, Topley JM, Mason K, Serjeant BE, Pattison JR, Jones SE, Mohamed R (1981) Outbreak of aplastic crises in sickle cell anaemia associated with parvovirus-like agent. Lancet 2: 595-597
Sharff O, Neumann H (1944) Über eine seltene Form von Knochenmarkschädigung durch Salvarsan. Med Klin 40: 500
Soutter L, Emerson CP (1960) Elective thymectomy in the treatment of aregenerative anemia associated with monocytic leukemia. Am J Med 28: 609-614
Stephens MEM (1974) Transient erythroid hypoplasia in a patient on long-term co-trimoxazole therapy. Postgrad Med J 50: 235-237

computerized tomography, but was demonstrable at necropsy (Twomey et al. 1975; Socinski et al. 1983).

The spectrum of immune deficiencies accompanying thymoma may gradually appear over months or years. The commonest is an antibody deficiency syndrome with overt hypogammaglobulinemia or agammaglobulinemia, sometimes complicated, occasionally dominated, by deficiency of cell-mediated immunity (MacLean et al. 1956; Martin et al. 1956; Gafni et al. 1960; Robins-Browne et al. 1977; Kauffman et al. 1979). Myasthenia gravis is rare in subjects with antibody deficiency (Te Velde et al. 1966), although it has been reported in subjects with prominent cellular defects (Rowland et al. 1965). For simplicity, antibody deficiency and deficiency of cell-mediated immunity will be described separately. In reality they frequently overlap. In a substantial though undetermined proportion of cases, however, the lymphoid immune deficiency is complicated by loss of inflammatory cells (neutrophils, eosinophils, and basophils, Waldmann et al, 1967; Mitchell et al. 1983) and this may increase susceptibility to infection.

Antibody Deficiency Syndrome

Patients with thymoma and immunodeficiency most often present with recurrent mucosal infections, including paranasal sinusitis, bronchitis, otitis media, or conjunctivitis which tend to persist and become chronic despite the use of antimicrobials. Cultures usually show encapsulated pyogenic bacteria *(Streptococcus pneumoniae, Hemophilus influenzae,* and occasionally *Pseudomonas aeruginosa.)* These agents, that are also involved in the development of recurrent pneumonia and, rarely, of bacteremia, meningitis, of splenic abscess, predominate because the patients lack the functional opsonizing antibodies needed to direct the inflammatory response. Less commonly, viral infections - especially with enteroviruses such as the virus of poliomyelitis or the ECHO virus, or with adenoviruses - occur and lead to pneumonia or central nervous system disorders. Susceptibility to these viruses is thought to result from lack of virus-neutralizing antibodies. Also encountered in antibody-deficient patients are intestinal infestations with *Cryptosporidium* species and *Giardia lamblia.*

Clinical manifestations, usually attributed to infections for which the responsible organisms may not always be identifiable, include arthritis, cough, diarrhea (which may lead to a diagnosis, often erroneous, of nonspecific inflammatory bowel disease), dyspnea, fever of unexplained cause, or weight loss.

These infections usually persist unless adequate therapy directed at the underlying hypogammaglobulinemia is started. All too frequently the immune deficiency is unrecognized for some time, during which the patient sustains significant irreversible organ damage such as chronic paranasal sinusitis, bronchitis, bronchiectasis, or chronic pneumonia.

Deficiency of Cell-Mediated Immunity

Patients with the syndrome of thymoma with immune deficiency in whom cellular host defenses are lost often present with oral candidiasis and weight loss, which may be accompanied by dermatophytosis and onychomycosis. When thrush develops in the context of antibiotic use its significance may not be immediately appreciated by the clinician. It is usually easily controlled at first by standard antifungal agents, but recurrence after discontinuance of suppressive medications indicates severely compromised cell-mediated immunity. Later manifestations include local or disseminated infections with mycobacteria, cytomegalovirus, herpes simplex or varicella zoster virus, or human papilloma viruses (especially type-3-associated flat warts), other fungal infections (cryptococci or histoplasma), and *Pneumocystis carinii* pneumonia. Other microorganisms to be expected include *Legionella* species, *Listeria monocytogenes, Cryptosporidia,* and *Toxoplasma gondii.* Kaposi's sarcoma has been reported in this form of immunodeficiency (Mullins 1971; Hirst and Robertson 1967), as in certain other deficiencies of cell-mediated immunity such as acquired immune deficiency syndrome (AIDS) or after organ transplantation.

The prognosis is generally worse in patients with clinically important cellular immune defects than in those whose immunodeficiency is limited to hypogammaglobulinemia. This is partly because the obligate or facultative intracellular pathogens that are opportunistic in such patients are more difficult to manage than those commonly affecting antibody-deficient subjects. Immune globulin replacement, moreover, has no counterpart or utility in the reconstitution of cellular defects.

Differential Diagnosis

In subjects over the age of 40 years the processes leading to primary immune deficiency are few and relatively easily defined. The presence of an anterior mediastinal mass, absence or paucity of B cells and their precursors, or the development of candidiasis, generally suffice to establish the clinical diagnosis, which is sometimes supported by the presence of other associated disorders such as pure red cell aplasia.

The most frequent form of primary antibody deficiency, common variable immunodeficiency (CVI) as defined by a World Health Organization Expert Committee (World Health Organization 1978), generally begins in the second or third decade of life. It is a heterogeneous group of disorders characterized by measurable antibody deficiency, despite the presence of B cells. In most cases the B cells that are detected do not differentiate into plasma cells because of intrinsic defects (Siegal et al. 1978). Precursors of B cells can be demonstrated by sensitive laboratory techniques.

Patients with CVI do not develop thymomas, but they may have mediastinal adenopathy due to infection or lymphoma, and this may give rise to diagnostic difficulty and justify biopsy. Both Hodgkin's disease and non-Hodgkin's lymphoma are more frequent in sufferers from CVI than in normals. Autoimmune phenomena occurring in CVI may mimic, at least superficially, the hematopoietic lineage defects of the thymoma syndrome. I have seen two cases in which CVI, Coombs-positive hemolytic anemia, and steroid-responsive erythroid aplasia were associated. Other autoimmune disorders that may occur in patients with CVI (or their close relations) include type-1 (insulin-dependent) diabetes mellitus, Hashimoto's thyroiditis, Graves' disease, vitiligo, and rheumatoid arthritis. Infections associated with cellular immunodeficiency do not, as a rule, develop in these patients although, like patients with thymoma, they may be anergic and have T-cell subset disturbances and abnormalities of mitogen responsiveness.

Older adults with AIDS (Gottlieb et al. 1981; Siegal et al. 1981) may present with a clinical history indistinguishable from that of the thymoma syndrome in which cellular immunity is chiefly disturbed. I have observed male and female AIDS patients in their 50s and 60s with oral and esophageal candidiasis, Kaposi's sarcoma, and other opportunistic diseases. Non-Hodgkin's lymphoma, idiopathic thrombocytopenic purpura, and severe, progressive anemia are also associated with this disorder, which is now known to be caused by a specific group of retroviruses that infect and inactivate lymphocytes. Such patients seldom show a mediastinal mass on computerized tomography, but they do have antibodies to the human immunodeficiency virus (HIV). They have ample numbers of B cells and increased numbers of tissue plasma cells with a corresponding hypergammaglobulinemia (especially IgA). T-cell subset deviations, with depletion of CD4-positive (helper) T cells from the blood, are the rule by the time clinical manifestations of immune deficiency appear. The proportion of suppressor/cytotoxic (CD8-positive) T cells in blood and lymphoid tissues is increased and contributes to a low T-cell subset ratio. This may not be so at the time when symptoms occur in the thymoma syndromes, though mild T-cell subset changes do occur. Elderly patients with AIDS may appear to have no clear-cut risk factors for retroviral transmission, in which case a history of blood transfusion, homosexuality, intravenous drug abuse, or receipt of pooled clotting factors (Factor VIII or IX concentrates) should be sought.

Patients with lymphoproliferative diseases sometimes express secondary immune deficiency, initially suggesting a primary disorder. Thus, sufferers from chronic lymphocytic leukemia or non-Hodgkin's lymphoma may have hypogammaglobulinemia with typically associated infections. Multiple myeloma produces antibody deficiency despite the presence of a monoclonal spike protein, and myeloma has also been described in association with the thymoma syndrome. Patients with nonsecretory myeloma occasionally present with panhypogammaglobulinemia, and herpes zoster may develop in patients with Hodgkin's disease, but such infections are rarely severe before the underlying disease is itself manifest.

Pathology

The thymomas associated with immunodeficiency are usually described as containing "epithelial" or spindle cells, most often variably admixed with lymphocytes (whence "lymphoepithelioma") which have the cell surface marker characteristics of thymic T-lymphocytes (thymocytes). Thymic carcinoids and germ cell tumors have not been associated with these syndromes. The biology of thymomas cannot usually be predicted from their histologic appearance, but their morbidity can usually be gauged from the ease of removal, degree of encapsulation, and involvement of intrathoracic structures at the time of surgical exploration. Probably more than 90% are clinically benign: they can be removed in their entirety, do not recur, and are not found at necropsy. Even among thymomas thought to be malignant, few of those associated with immunodeficiency metastasize outside the chest cavity, though they may recur locally, with pleural implants of uncertain clinical significance. Truly malignant, distantly metastatic thymic carcinomas are rarely associated with immune deficiencies or related conditions.

The associated pathologic features relate to the absence of the B-cell lineage and to infectious processes resulting from the immunologic disorder. B-cell areas of lymphoid tissue (germinal centers of lymph nodes and spleen, and diffuse lymphoid tissues of bronchial tree and gastrointestinal tract) are depleted of cells and may be absent, except in cases in which cellular deficiency is marked. The bone marrow lacks pre-B cells, B cells, and plasma cells. Cases of thymoma with immune deficiency have been described in which the lamina propria of the intestine was a site of residual B-cell differentiation, and the only site of a small number of plasma cells (Broom et al. 1975; Platts-Mills et al. 1981), a finding that may depend more on the stage of evolution of the disease than on any special feature of the thymoma-immunodeficiency relation. Any deficiencies in other lineages - eosinophils, neutrophils, erythroid elements, megakaryocytes (Sundström et al. 1972) - depend on associated hematopoietic abnormalities. Bronchiectasis, chronic pneumonitis, and other manifestations of acute and chronic infection with viral, bacterial, protozoal, and fungal agents are usually present.

Clinical Immunology and Diagnostic Evaluation

Thymoma-associated immune deficiencies range from apparently pure deficiencies of B cells to pure defects of cellular immunity. Deficiency of other hematopoietic cell lineages, especially of the erythroid series, is commonly present or emerges during the disease.

The hallmark of immunodeficiency with thymoma is the antibody deficiency that is present in at least two-thirds of cases. The syndrome may be recognized clinically when the immune system is in decline, but not yet totally lost, recurrent severe infections even preceding measurable hypogammaglobulinemia. At this stage, tests for functional antibody deficiency (Table 1, Siegal et al. 1980) may give abnormal results, even in the absence of hypogammaglobulinemia, which only becomes evident in the course of months or years of follow-up. Absence of isohemagglutinins (titers below 1:4) suggests a failure of IgM antibody production. A positive Schick test indicates absence of IgG (tissue-diffusing) antibody to diphtheria toxin, normally present in immunized adults. Antibody deficiency is also suggested by failure to elicit antibody formation with pneumococcal, typhoid, brucella, or other vaccines, and inability to demonstrate the presence of virus-neutralizing antibodies to poliovirus or the presence of antibodies to other ubiquitous environmental microbes.

Serum protein electrophoresis on paper or cellulose acetate strips cannot always be depended on to define hypogammaglobulinemia; in general, the more sensitive quantitation of the major immunoglobulin classes (isotypes) by either radial immunodiffusion or nephelometry is needed to define the levels of IgG, IgA, and IgM. Immunoelectrophoresis provides a qualitative but not quantitative definition of the presence or absence of the gamma-globulins, and defines the presence of monoclonal proteins.

Hypogammaglobulinemia in the syndrome of thymoma with immunodeficiency is usually associated with absence of circulating and tissue B-lymphocytes as defined by cell surface marker analysis (Siegal et al. 1975; Siegal and Good 1977; Kauffmann et al. 1979; Litwin 1979; Siegal et al. 1980). These markers include

Table 1. Clinical characterization of humoral immunocompetence

Type of test	Method(s)	Comments
Immunoelectrophoresis	Analysis of precipitin arcs in agarose	Qualitative, defines monoclonal components
Immunoglobulin quantitation	Radial immunodiffusion, nephelometry	Defines levels of IgG, IgA, IgM, IgG1-3
	Enzyme-linked or radioimmunoassays (ELISA, RIA)	Defines levels of IgD, IgE, IgG4
Determination of preexisting antibodies	ELISA, hemagglutination, precipitation, RIA	Assesses prior immunization status
Response to immunization to new antigens	ELISA, hemagglutination, precipitation, RIA	Capacity to respond to a primary immunogen[a]
Enumeration of B cells and plasma cells in blood, gut, lymphoid tissues	Cell marker analysis for Ig, μ, δ, or with B-cell monoclonal antibodies; immunofluorescence, immunoperoxidase	Specificity of the reagents must be defined or results can be misleading
Assessment of pre-B cells in marrow	Immunofluorescence for cytoplasmic μ-chains or terminal deoxynucleotidyl transferase (TdT)	May be difficult if plasma cells are still present; TdT should resolve this

[a] For example, pneumococcal or brucella vaccines, keyhole limpet hemocyanin (KLH), bacteriophage φ-X 174

surface IgM and IgD, as well as certain monoclonal antibodies definitive for B cells. Plasma cells in bone marrow and most other sites are reduced in number or absent. However, the B cells and plasma cells of the intestinal lamina propria have been reported to be relatively spared. Typically, germinal centers of lymphoid tissues, the normal sites of B cell migration, are sparsely populated or absent. The few patients who have been studied also appear to have a paucity of B-cell precursors, the pre-B cells (Pearl et al. 1978). These cells, currently defined cytologically by the simultaneous presence of the nuclear enzyme terminal deoxynucleotidyl transferase (TdT) and of cytoplasmic μ-chains, normally account for up to 10% of marrow mononuclear cells. Thus, the entire immunoglobulin-producing cell lineage is usually lost, and with it the ability to make antibodies. Brenner et al. (1984) and I myself (unpublished work) have observed patients

Table 2. Clinical characterization of cell-mediated immunocompetence

Type of test	Method(s)	Comments
Delayed-type hypersensitivity to recall antigens	Intradermal testing with ubiquitous immunogens leading to induration at 48-72 h	Assesses prior state of immunization, residual T-cell competence; may still be present despite significant defects in evolving immunodeficiency
Skin sensitization with haptens	Immunization and subsequent challenge with dinitrochlorobenzene (DNCB)	Assesses ability to make primary cellular immune responses; sensitive to evolving immunodeficiency
Rejection of skin homograft	Transplant of allogeneic skin graft and observation of time to rejection	Determines capacity to recognize foreign cellular antigens and mobilize a rejection reaction; rarely done today (hepatitis transmission, etc.)
Enumeration of T, NK, and large granular lymphocytes and their subsets in blood, lymphoid tissues	Cell surface marker techniques with rosettes, monoclonal antibodies; immunofluorescence, immunoperoxidase	Determines presence of cell populations and their distribution
Lymphocyte proliferative response to mitogens	In vitro stimulation of cells with plant proteins (lectins) nonspecifically activating blast transformation and division with incorporation of radioactive thymidine indicating new DNA synthesis	Defines ability of lymphocytes to perform proliferative responses essential to the development of immunity: clonal enlargement and cellular differentiation
Lymphocyte proliferative response to antigens	In vitro stimulation, as above, with specific antigens[a]	Indicates ability of these cells to respond to antigenic specificities by division; comparison with skin tests may suggest functional abnormalities, e.g., serum inhibitors
Mixed lymphocyte culture	Mixture of cells from two genetically distinct subjects leads to cell division that is measured as are mitogen responses	Measures capacity of lymphoid cells to recognize alloantigens and undergo proliferative responses; correlate of homograft recognition
Cellular release of lymphokines in response to mitogens or antigens	In vitro bioassay or ELISA, RIA for the presence of soluble mediators of inflammation made by lmyphoid cells[b]	Tests capacity of lymphoid cells to communicate with other hematopoietic cells to recruit, activate, or suppress their activity appropriately
Cytotoxicity assays	Lymphocytes mixed with target cells (e.g., various cell lines, chicken red blood cells (RBC) prelabeled with radioactive chromate; target cells, when killed, release radioactivity that is measured	Measures capacity of various lymphoid cells to kill certain other cell types such as tumor lines

[a] For example, keyhole limpet hemocyanin, tetanus toxoid, *Candida albicans*

[b] For example alpha, gamma interferons; macrophage-activating factors (MAF) (largely interferons); macrophage migration inhibition factor (MIF); interleukin 2 (IL-2). Many other lymphokines described, each with its own bioassay for a particular type of cell-cell interaction

with symptomatic hypogammaglobulinemia who still had normal numbers of circulating B cells when the syndrome was initially recognized. Possibly these subjects were observed early in the decline of the lineage, before total depletion of the B cells.

Evidence of cellular immune deficiency in this syndrome is sometimes only indirect, as in vitro tests for it may give normal results. Loss of the T-cell lineage or of a T-cell subset analogous to the usual absence of B cells has not been reported. Cell-mediated immune defects are in fact suspected on clinical grounds because of the presence of candidiasis, cryptococcosis, cytomegalovirus, or herpes virus infections that immunologically intact persons resist through cellular, rather than humoral, host defences. Skin anergy (Table 2) is often present in these subjects, but not necessarily at the time of initial diagnosis. The numbers of T cells and T-cells subsets may be normal, or the proportion of helper cells may be depressed (Hayward et al. 1982). Lymphocyte responses to nonspecific mitogenic stimulation may be normal or reduced. Abnormal in vitro antigen-induced proliferation is more often described, and has been reported in association with serum inhibitors of proliferation (Geary et al. 1975; Twomey et al. 1975; Robins-Browne et al. 1977) that some investigators have thought to be immune complexes.

Two patients recently studied by us (Lopez C and Siegal FP, unpublished work) appear to have abnormalities of interferon-alpha (IFN-α) production (Lopez et al. 1983), a component of cellular immunity attributable to neither T nor B cells but to a large, granular lymphocyte (LGL) population. These cells, which normally produce IFN-α and probably other lymphokine activators of inflammatory responses,may represent yet another hematopoietic cell lineage that is defective or lost in patients with thymoma-related immune deficiencies.

Mechanisms of Disease

The process by which these immune dysfunctions develop is not known. The role of the thymic tumor is speculative. As thymomas do not occur secondarily in other hypogammaglobulinemic states, the thymic tumor is unlikely to be a compensatory response to the antibody deficiency. As in pure red cell aplasia (Chapt. 13), many phenomena may contribute to the pathogenesis of this heterogeneous syndrome.

Both cellular and humoral mechanisms for the destruction of stem cells or their progeny have been described. T cells from some thymoma patients suppress the in vitro terminal differentiation of B cells into plasma cells (Siegal et al. 1976; Waldmann et al. 1975; Litwin and Zanjani 1977; Siegal et al. 1978; Litwin 1979; Brenner et al. 1984). Some subjects with hypogammaglobulinemia and thymoma have no demonstrable suppressive T cells, although certain of them possess (whereas others completely lack) blood B-lymphocytes (Brenner et al. 1984; Siegal FP, unpublished work). In patients with erythroid aplasia and hypogammaglobulinemia suppressor T cells have been observed that were thought to inhibit both erythropoiesis and B-cell differentiation (Litwin and Zanjani 1977).

Since these patients generally lack circulating B cells, suppressor cell assays with normal mature B cells as their target are of questionable significance. Experiments by Hayward et al. (1982), however, in which normal marrow pre-B cells were cultured with T cells from hypogammaglobulinemic patients with thymoma, suggest that these less mature cells, as well as mature B-lymphocytes, may express structures that T cells can attack. If this syndrome were to be regarded as an autoimmune disorder, the varying manifestations from patient to patient would simply be a reflection of the specificity of the inhibiting mechanism (Waldmann et al. 1967; Mitchell et al. 1983).

The suggestion that the suppressor or cytotoxic T cell may play an important part in B lineage destruction receives some support from a case of thymoma syndrome that I have had occasion to study. The patient, a man whose monozygotic twin was normal, had radiosensitive suppressor T cells that inhibited terminal differentiation of his brother's normal B cells (Siegal et al. 1976, 1978). An attempt to reconstitute the patient's B-cell population through transplantation of his brother's bone marrow (without prior conditioning regimens such as irradiation) was unsuccessful. Nor did extracorporeal irradiation of the patient's blood before a second attempt at transplantation have any beneficial effect (Siegal FP, Rai KR, O'Reilly RJ, unpublished work). The suppressing T cells may have been the factor that led to resistance to engraftment.

In pure red cell aplasia, antibody-mediated mechanisms have also been implicated in the destruction of the lineage. Paradoxically, even in patients with severe hypogammaglobulinemia, autoantibodies against some component of the B-cell lineage may play a pathogenetic role. Degos et al. (1982) have described a woman who had combined cellular and humoral immune deficiency and severe neutropenia. Her serum contained IgG that inhibited both B-cell differentiation and granulocyte colony formation in vitro. The neutropenia responded to plasmapheresis, and a few B cells appeared in the blood, but the hypogammaglobulinemia did not improve. This suggests that antibodies directed against some stage of B-cell differentiation have a causative role in the development of the syndrome. On the other hand, in a female patient we studied (Siegal et al. 1975; Zanjani ED and Siegal FP, unpublished work) with agammaglobulinemia, erythroid aplasia, and eventually pancytopenia, we could not demonstrate serum factors suppressing in vitro erythropoiesis. Since the patient's remaining blood cells were virtually all T cells, it is possible that a purely cellular mechanism was responsible. One of the difficulties in elucidating the precise mechanism of immunosuppression in the syndrome of thymoma and immune deficiency is the relative rarity of the cases and the special in vitro systems that are needed to define them. It has not been possible to demonstrate a consistent pattern, partly because the techniques and target cells needed are not all immediately available when the opportunity for study arises. The interpretation of apparently autoimmune phenomena that may in fact be only secondary abnormalities is another problem. In chickens deprived of their B-cell lineage by bursectomy "suppressor cell" populations develop as a consequence of the loss of B cells (Blaese et al. 1974, 1975). Transfer of the suppressor cells to normal chickens leads to hypogammaglobulinemia. These apparently "autoimmune" cells are not, however, causally concerned in the pathogenesis of the agammaglobulinemia in the original bursectomized chicks, but are a consequence of the bursectomy itself. By analogy, in persons who lose a lineage as a result of viral infection or some other primary insult, "autoimmune" phenomena might develop secondarily, simply because the antigenic components characteristic of that lineage are no longer "self." This leads to a break in tolerance, with immunization by cross-reactive environmental antigens as a possible consequence. For example, some boys with congenital agammaglobulinemia (a hereditary, X-linked disease in which B cells are lacking but pre-B cells populate the marrow in normal numbers) have suppressor T cells similar to those seen in thymoma patients; others with the same disorder have no suppressor cells. The suppressor phenomenon noted in this setting may be consequent on the primary B-cell defect, as in the bursectomized chicks (Siegal et al. 1978).

Therapy

Conventional management of the syndrome of thymoma with immunodeficiency generally includes recognition and removal, if possible, of the thymic tumor. The view that early thymomectomy may at least stabilize the disease and prevent progression is attractive, but to compare it to early thymectomy for myasthenia gravis would not be appropriate. Several considerations militate against routine excision: 1. Immune deficiency (and also the other complications of thymoma) may arise, or may progress, months or years after apparently complete and successful removal of a thymic tumor. In other words, thymomectomy does not guarantee that associated syndromes will not develop. 2. No case in which immune defects have reversed as a result of thymomectomy has been reported. In this respect, the syndrome differs from pure red cell aplasia, which sometimes does seem to respond, at least transiently, to extirpation of the thymoma. 3. Even with the more aggressive thymic lesions, it is usually susceptibility to infection rather than the neoplasm itself that determines the course of the disease and the quality of life. In fact, the thymoma is more often detected as an incidental finding at roentgenography performed on account of infection than as a result of symptoms directly attributable to spread of the tumor or its involvement of adjacent structures. Thymomas tend to grow slowly or to remain static, as is evidenced by their retrospective visualization on chest films made many years before their clinical recognition. In some cases computerized axial tomography shows an encapsulated primary lesion and tumor-free thoracic cavities and mediastinal structures. 4. Patients with the thymoma-immunodeficiency syndrome may be severely ill with chronic or acute infections, and these, or age and general condition, may make operation inadvisable.

These arguments suggest that evaluation of each patient individually, with estimation of the risk: benefit ratio, is the most reasonable course to follow. In general, it is advisable to remove a tumor because it is there, and might become aggressive or malignant, but with the full realization that little immediate or even long-term benefit may accrue. For elderly subjects, or patients in poor general condition, a surgical approach is not mandatory.

Surgical intervention in patients with hypogammaglobulinemia should be carried out under cover of adequate levels of passively administered immune globulin. If there is severe bronchopulmonary disease or other infection it should be controlled as well as possible before the elective operation. Coexisting thrombocytopenia and anemia should also be corrected. Roentgentherapy has been shown to shrink thymomas, but, as with surgical treatment, there is no evidence that it benefits the immune system.

Medical management is determined by the type of immunologic defect present. It is easiest in patients with abnormalities confined to B cells leading to hypogammaglobulinemia. In such cases the method of choice, minimizing the tendency to progressive lung and paranasal sinus disease otherwise associated with antibody deficiency, is full-scale replacement of IgG by intravenous administration of immune (gamma-) globulin in sufficient amount to raise serum IgG levels into the normal range (Cunningham-Rundles et al. 1984). This can usually be achieved with a dosage of about 100 mg intravenous immune globulin per kilogram body weight per week, infused every 2–4 weeks according to local availability, serum levels being measured just before the next infusion. Satisfactory levels should be reached by the third or fourth infusion, unless there is an associated protein-losing state. This method is, unfortunately, expensive.

Immune globulin given by the intramuscular route is less satisfactory than when it is given intravenously, but clearly better than no treatment, as it prevents most episodes of conjunctivitis, pneumonia, bacteremia, viremia, and their complications. Its utility is less evident in bronchial and paranasal sinus disease. If only intramuscular immune globulin is available, it should be given in as large a dose, and at as short time intervals, as the patient can tolerate. Conventionally accepted intramuscular dosage regimens such as 0,6 ml per kilogram per month after a loading dose are suboptimal.

Gamma-globulin therapy is most effective if begun early in the disease; once irreversible bronchial damage (bronchiectasis, chronic bronchitis) has developed, chronic bronchorrhea is common. Physicians and surgeons should not be discouraged by continued sputum production, which may continue indefinitely. The full benefits of immune globulin treatment may not be manifest for 6–12 months. Even then, certain symptoms, such as diarrhea due to *Giardia lamblia* may not respond to this therapy, which is directed only at the volume of distribution of IgG.

In the meantime, the judicious, frequently empirical use of safe oral antibiotics, generally on a rotating schedule, to suppress acute bronchial and paranasal sinus infections and minimize sputum production is indicated. Personally, I rely on ampicillin/amoxycillin, tetracyclines, and trimethoprim-sulfamethoxazole at standard oral doses. Each is given for up to a maximum of 14 days, but not beyond the 3rd or 4th day if by then there is no visible reduction in sputum volume, color, and tenacity. Postural drainage regimens, nebulized saline, and bronchodilators are sometimes useful as adjunctive measures. Ideally, antimicrobials for the treatment of pneumonitis should be selected on the basis of sputum Gram's stain, clinical presentation and, if necessary, bronchoscopy and transbronchial biopsy. In this case empiricism is sometimes justified; the spectrum of microorganisms likely to infect the patient depends on whether cellular or antibody deficiency predominates, as well as on the presence of neutropenia, which predisposes to dissemination of *Candida albicans, Staphylococcus aureus,* and *Pseudomonas aeruginosa,* and to infections with *Mucor* spp. Diarrheal states require etiologic definition and here again an empirical approach to treatment of intestinal bacterial overgowth, gluten-sensitive enteropathy, parasitic infestations, and other intestinal disorders may be appropriate. Any associated diseases such as pernicious anemia with achlorhydria, erythroid aplasia, and thrombocytopenia should, of course, also be treated.

In the presence of clinically significant cellular immune defects management is more difficult. Generally, these defects are not responsive to immune globulin, although immune globulin is often essential when a combined humoral and cellular immune disorder is present. The intracellular pathogens complicating cellular immunodeficiency must be treated, if possible, with available antivirals, antimycobacterials, and antifungals. Oral thrush can generally be suppressed by the chronic use of clotrimazole troches or, if complicated by onychomycosis, with ketoconazole. Recurrent herpes simplex that ulcerates, or severe herpes zoster are treated with oral acyclovir, and mycobacterial infections with combinations including isoniazid, rifampicin, or its derivatives such as ansamycin. Currently, experimental antivirals such as ganciclovir [9-(1,3-dihydroxy-2-propoxymethyl) guanine, DHPG] may be able to contain cytomegaloviral diseases. No satisfactory regimen for the long-term control of cellular immunodeficiency with thymoma has yet been devised. Transfer factor or related substances, thymic humoral factors, thymic transplantation, and immunoaugmenting agents such as isoprinosine have a place in clinical trials, but have not reached the practical stage.

The fact that these disorders may have an autoimmune basis may justify the seemingly paradoxical approach of immunosuppressive therapy with corticosteroids, plasmapheresis, leukapheresis, or even cytostatic drugs. Although so far there has been no notable repair of the defective lymphoid components of the syndrome, other clinically important benefits may result, such as alleviation of anemia or of life-threatening neutropenia (Degos et al. 1982). These experimental efforts seem abundantly justified in patients who have more than just antibody deficiency.

The prognosis in thymoma with immune deficiency depends chiefly on the severity of the immune defects. For patients with an isolated antibody deficiency, IgG replacement therapy and, if possible, removal of the thymoma, may be sufficient to provide an essentially normal life. For those with cell-mediated immune deficiency, the prognosis is generally worse, regardless of the progress of the tumor itself. Such patients tend eventually to succumb either to an intractable infection or to some other associated opportunistic disorder such as Kaposi's sarcoma.

Conclusions

The syndrome of thymoma and immunodeficiency is part of a larger pattern of apparently autoimmune diseases associated with tumors of the thymus. It presents many clinical and scientific challenges to the physician, and causes much morbidity and mortality in its victims. The most perplexing among the problems it poses is the nature of the relation between the thymic tumor and the associated disorder of the immune system, a puzzle still awaiting solution.

References

Blaese RM, Weiden PL, Koski I, Dooley N (1974) Infectious agammaglobulinemia: transmission of immunodeficiency with grafts of agammaglobulinemic cells. J Exp Med 140: 1097-1101

Blaese RM, Peng JW, Muchmore A, Dooley N, Koski I (1975) T-suppressor cells as mediators of infectious agammaglobulinemia. Fed Proc 34: 1031

Brenner MK, Reittie JGE, Chadda HR, Pollock A, Asherson GL (1984) Thymoma and hypogammaglobulinemia with and without T suppressor cells. Clin Exp Immunol 58: 619-624

Broom BC, de la Concha EG, Webster ADB, Loewi G, Asherson GL (1975) Dichotomy between immunoglobulin synthesis by cells in gut and blood of patients with hypogammaglobulinaemia. Lancet 2: 253-256

Cunningham-Rundles C, Siegal FP, Smithwick EM, Lion-Boulé A, Cunningham-Rundles S, O'Malley J, Barandun S, Good RA (1984) Efficacy of intravenous immunoglobulin in primary humoral immunodeficiency disease. Ann Intern Med 101: 435-439

Degos L, Faille A, Housset M, Boumsell L, Rabian C, Parames T (1982) Syndrome of neutrophil agranulocytosis, hypogammaglobulinemia, and thymoma. Blood 60: 968-972

Gafni J, Michaeli D, Heller H (1960) Idiopathic acquired agammaglobulinemia associated with thymoma: report of two cases and review of the literature. New Engl J Med 263: 536-541

Geary CG, Byron PR, Taylor G, MacIver JE, Zervas J (1975) Thymoma associated with pure red cell aplasia, immunoglobulin deficiency and an inhibitor of antigen-induced lymphocyte transformation. Brit J Haematol 29: 479-485

Good RA (1954) Agammaglobulinemia: a provocative experiment of nature. Bull Univ Minn Hosp Min Med Found 26: 1-19

Gottlieb MS, Schroff R, Schanker HM, Weisman JD, Fan PT, Wolf RA, Saxon A (1981) *Pneumocystis carinii* pneumonia and mucosal candidiasis in previously healthy homosexual men. N Engl J Med 305: 1425-1431

Hayward AR, Paolucci P, Webster ADB, Kohler P (1982) Pre-B cell suppression by thymoma patient lymphocytes. Clin Exp Immunol 48: 437-442

Hirst E, Robertson TI (1967) The syndrome of thymoma and erythroblastopenic anemia: a review of 56 cases including 3 case reports. Medicine (Baltimore) 46: 225-264

Kauffman CA, Linnemann CC Jr, Alvira MM (1979) Cytomegalovirus encephalitis associated with thymoma and immunoglobulin deficiency. Am J Med 67: 724-728

Litwin SD (1979) Immunodeficiency with thymoma: failure to induce IgG production in immunodeficient lymphocytes cocultured with normal T cells. J Immunol 122: 728-732

Litwin SD, Zanjani ED (1977) Lymphocytes suppressing both immunoglobulin production and erythroid differentiation in hypogammaglobulinaemia. Nature 266: 57-58

Lopez C, Fitzgerald PA, Siegal FP (1983) Severe acquired immune deficiency syndrome in male homosexuals: diminished capacity to make interferon-alpha in vitro associated with severe opportunistic infections. J Infect Dis 148: 962-966

MacLean LD, Zak SJ, Varco RL, Good RA (1956) Thymic tumor and acquired agammaglobulinemia: a clinical and experimental study of the immune response. Surgery 40: 1010-1017

Martin CM, Gordon RS, McCullough NB (1956) Acquired hypogammaglobulinemia in an adult: report of a case, with clinical and experimental studies. N Engl J Med 254: 449-456

Mitchell EB, Platts-Mills TAE, Pereira RS, Malkovska V, Webster AD (1983) Acquired basophil and eosinophil deficiency in a patient with hypogammaglobulinaemia associated with thymoma. Clin Lab Haematol 5: 253-257

Mullins JF (1971) Discussion of paper by Schoch EP Jr. Arch Dermatol 103: 318-319

Pearl ER, Vogler LB, Okos AJ, Crist WM, Lawton AR III, Cooper MD (1978) B lymphocyte precursors in human bone marrow: an analysis of normal individuals and patients with antibody-deficiency states. J Immunol 120: 1169-1175

Platts-Mills TAE, de Gast GC, Webster ADB, Asherson GL, Wilkins SR (1981) Two immunologically distinct forms of late onset hypogammaglobulinaemia. Clin Exp Immunol 44: 383-388

Robins-Browne RM, Green R, Katz J, Becker D (1977) Thymoma, pure red cell aplasia, pernicious anaemia and candidiasis: a defect in immunohomeostasis. Br J Haematol 36: 5-13

Rowland LP, Griffiths CO, Kabat EA (1965) Myasthenia gravis, thymoma and cryptococcal meningitis. N Engl J Med 273: 620-627

Siegal FP, Good RA (1977) Human lymphocyte differentiation markers and their application to immune deficiency and lymphoproliferative diseases. Clin Haematol 6: 355-422

Siegal FP, Wernet P, Dickler HB et al. (1975) B lymphocytes lacking surface Ig in patients with immunodeficiency: initiation of Ig synthesis in culture in cells from a patient with thymoma. Birth Defects 2: 40-44

Siegal FP, Siegal M, Good RA (1976) Suppression of B-cell differentiation by leukocytes from hypogammaglobulinemic patients. J Clin Invest 58: 109-122

Siegal FP, Siegal M, Good RA (1978) Role of helper, suppressor and B-cell defects in the pathogenesis of the hypogammaglobulinemias. N Engl J Med 299: 172-178

Siegal FP, Pahwa S, Pahwa R (1980) Congenital and acquired primary disorders of B and T lymphocyte function. In: Grieco MH (ed) Infections in the abnormal host. Yorke Medical Books, New York, pp 129-162

Siegal FP, Lopez C, Hammer GS, Brown AE, Kornfeld SJ, Gold J, Hassett J, Hirschmann SZ, Cunningham-Rundles C, Adelsberg BR, Parham DM, Siegal M, Cunningham-Rundles S, Armstrong D (1981) Severe acquired immunodeficiency in male homosexuals, manifested by chronic perianal ulcerative herpes simplex lesions. N Engl J Med 305: 1439-1444

Socinski MA, Ershler WB, Frankel J-P, Albertini RJ, Ciongoli AK, Krawitt EL, Burns SL, Mangan KF (1983) Pure RBC aplasia and myasthenia gravis: coexistence of two diseases associated with thymoma. Arch Intern Med 143: 543-546

Souadjian JV, Enriquez P, Silverstein MN, Pépin J-M (1974) The spectrum of diseases associated with thymoma: coincidence or syndrome? Arch Intern Med 134: 374-379

Sundström C, Lundberg D, Werner I (1972) A case of thymoma in association with megakaryocytopenia. Acta Pathol Microbiol Immunol Scand A 80: 487-490

Te Velde K, Huber J, van der Slikke LB (1966) Primary acquired hypogammaglobulinemia, myasthenia, and thymoma. Ann Intern Med 65: 554-559

Twomey JJ, Waddell CC, Krantz S, O'Reilly R, L'Esperance P, Good RA (1975) Chronic mucocutaneous candidiasis with macrophage dysfunction, a plasma inhibitor, and co-existent aplastic anemia. J Lab Clin Med 85: 968-977

Waldmann TA, Strober W, Blaese RM, Strauss AJL (1967) Thymoma, hypogammaglobulinemia, and absence of eosinophils. J Clin Invest 46: 1127-1128

Waldmann TA, Broder S, Durm M, Blackman M, Krakauer R, Meade B (1975) Suppressor T cells in the pathogenesis of hypogammaglobulinemia associated with a thymoma. Trans Assoc Am Physicians 88: 120-134

Wick MR, Scheithauer BW, Dines DE (1982) Thymic neoplasia in two male siblings. Mayo Clin Proc 57: 653-656

World Health Organization (1978) Immunodeficiency: report of a WHO scientific group. WHO Tech Rep Ser 630

Additional Reading

Buckley RH (1988) Humoral immunodeficiency. Clin Immunol Immunopathol 40: 13-24

Buff DD, Greenberg SD, Loong P, Palumbo FS (1988) Thymoma, *Pneumocystis carinii* pneumonia, and AIDS. NY State J Med 88: 276-277

Davila DG, Ryan DH (1986) Thymoma, hypogammaglobulinemia, and pernicious anemia. South Med J 79: 904-906

Ectivill X, Gonzalez D, Solar J, Mones J, Pujol-Moix N (1984) Thymoma associated with erythroblastopenia and hypogammaglobulinemia with an increase in the T8+ lymphocyte subpopulation (letter) (in Spanish). Med Clin (Barc) 92: 334

Fujimura S, Kondo T, Yamauchi A, Handa M, Nakada T (1985) Experience with surgery for thymoma associated with pure red blood cell aplasia. Report of three cases. Chest 88: 221-225

Gupta S, Savorymutta SH, Gibbs JS, Evans DJ, Hodgson HJ (1985) Watery diarrhea in a patient with myasthenia gravis, thymoma, and immunodeficiency. Am J Gastroenterol 90 (11): 877-881

Hoxio JA, Flaherty LE, Haggarty BS, Rackowski JL (1986) Infection of T4 lymphocytes by HTLV-III does not require expression of the OKT4 epitope. J Immunol 136 (2): 361-363

Kirkpatrick CH (1984) Host factors in defense against fungal infections. Am J Med 77 (40): 1-12

Kornstein MJ, Hoxio JA, Levinson AI, Brooks JJ (1985) Immunohistology of human thymomas. Arch Pathol Lab Med 109 (5): 480-483

Lohtonon A, Soppi E, Panalius M (1984) Myasthenia gravis, thymoma and immunodeficiency (in Finnish). Duodecim 100 (22): 1544-1550

Lovinson AI, Hoxio JA, Kornstein MJ, Zombryki D, Matthews DM, Schreiber AD (1985) Absence of the OKT4 epitope on blood T cells and thymus cells in a patient with thymoma, hypogammaglobulinemia, and red blood cell aplasia. J Allergy Clin Immunol 75 (3): 433-439

Mangan KF, Volkin R, Winkelstein A (1986) Autoreactive erythroid progenitor-T suppressor cells in the pure red cell aplasia associated with thymoma and panhypogammaglobulinemia. Am J Hematol 23 (2): 167-173

Manzanoll C, Moroll A, Koller H (1985) Immune defect following thymoma. Case description and review (in German). Schweiz Med Wochenschr 115 (40): 1393-1401

Murakami M, Catheart MK (1986) Suppression of polyclonal immunoglobulin production by a soluble factor produced by a human thymus hybridoma. Immunopharmacology 11 (3): 141-154

Namura M, Nunoda S, Taga K, Gonda A, Takeda R, Okada Y (1985) A case of malignant thymoma associated with massive pericardial effusion, hypogammaglobulinemia and disseminated cytomegalovirus infection (in Japanese). Nippon Naika Gakkai Zasshi 74 (6): 799-807

Rosenow EC 3d, Hurley BT (1984) Disorders of the thymus. A review. Arch Intern Med 144 (4): 763-770

Soler J, Ectivill X, Ayato R, Brunct S, Pujol-Moix N (1985) Chronic T-cell lymphocytosis associated with pure red cell aplasia, thymoma and hypogammaglobulinemia [letter]. Br J Haematol 81 (3): 582-584

Soppi E, Eskola J, Roytta M, Varomaa T, Pancluis M, Lohtonon A (1985) Thymoma with immunodeficiency (Good's syndrome) associated with myasthenia gravis and benign IgG gammopathy. Arch Intern Med 145 (8): 1704-1707

15 Other Conditions Associated with Thymic Disorders

Charles Ruchti and Max W. Hess

Introduction

The physiologic role of the thymus and its better known connections with certain disease entities have been discussed in preceding chapters. What remain, under the heading of "other conditions associated with thymic disorders," may at first sight appear to be a haphazard grouping of diseases whose only common denominator is the sometimes chance finding of thymic changes, notably neoplasms, during their course. Study of these conditions is, however, not unrewarding. It provides additional evidence in favor of the concepts that: (a) the thymus's two components, cortex and medulla, are distinct entities, each with its own histology, function, and reactivity; and (b) certain apparently "thymic" changes may not be truly intrathymic, but may in fact be the reflection of changes in the adjacent parathymic lymph nodes.

In this introduction we shall present evidence that intrathymic changes, and reactions of the "thymic complex" (i. e., the thymus and the neighboring parathymic lymph nodes) are consequences, not causes, of a range of chronic diseases with an immunologic component. These changes and reactions rarely affect the thymic cortex, which should be regarded as the real seat of the thymus's physiologic activity, but are generally confined to the adjacent lymph nodes or to the thymic medulla, a part of the gland that behaves much like a peripheral lymphoid organ. They often lead to enlargement of the "thymic complex" - enlargement variously termed "thymic hyperplasia," "thymitis," or "lymphofollicular hyperplasia of the thymus" (Chap. 7) - and are therefore of interest to surgeons.

The thymus is often referred to as being "primary" or "central" because of the absence of evident antigenic influence on proliferation and differentiation of T-lymphocyte precursors within the thymus. However, blood-borne materials can penetrate the thymic medulla, but not the thymic cortex, with relative ease (Raviola and Karnovsky 1972). This may explain, at least in part, why the medulla can become the site of intensive plasma cell proliferation during chronic infection (Heiniger et al. 1965), and why its response to local antigen injection is very similar to that of lymph nodes (Jankovic et al. 1971).

Thus, to be precise, the attribute "central" should be reserved for the thymic cortex, which appears to be effectively protected from stimulants both by a blood-thymus barrier excluding antigens (Marshall and White 1961), and by the immunologic immaturity of cortical thymocytes (Raff 1973). However, even the protection of the cortex is only relative, under certain conditions. Intra-abdominally injected particulate material is rapidly cleared from the peritoneal cavity and reaches the draining parathymic lymph nodes in large amount. Thence, smaller amounts translocate via lymphatics through the thymic capsule to enter the cortical parenchyma within less than 2 h, preferentially in the vicinity of the lymph nodes (Eggli et al. 1987). Later the injected material may also be found in association with medullary blood vessels in a distribution pattern indistinguishable from that observed after intravenous injection (Raviola and Karnovsky 1972). When stimulants were given via the intra-abdominal route, cortical thymocytopoiesis was enhanced in the segment adjacent to parathymic lymph nodes (Müller et al. 1987).

It thus appears that protection of the thymus against peripheral stimulants is effective, although not absolute. The protective mechanisms function differently in medulla and cortex. Whereas the blood-thymus barrier gives relatively good protection to the cortex, it is "leaky" with regard to the medulla. The existence of a "leaky" capsule-thymus barrier has also to be taken into account in assessing the possibility that cortical function may be influenced by exogenous stimulation, particularly as parathymic lymph nodes are an important drainage area for the peritoneal cavity. The relatively effective protection of the thymic parenchyma against extrathymic stimulants explains why intrathymic immune reactions are rare, in contrast to parathymic lymph nodes in which immunologic changes may reach such proportions that they appear on histologic evaluation to be located in the thymic medulla, if one does not carefully distinguish the thymus from these lymph nodes.

A knowledge of physiologic, age-dependent, thymic involution, of the cortex in particular, is necessary if the thymic changes that occur during certain diseases

and germinal centers in the thymic medulla in up to one-third of cases (Habu et al. 1971; Mizuno et al. 1976; Nicholson 1978; Bergmann et al. 1982). Enlargement without evidence of a "medullary" immune reaction is, however, also observed. There seems to be a general consensus that the thymic changes are the consequence rather than the cause of the underlying disease. Thus, no improvement is to be expected following thymectomy.

Among other thymus-associated endocrinopathies, a case of idiopathic Addison's disease in a patient with myasthenia gravis and a predominantly lymphocytic thymoma was reported by Salyer and Eggleston in 1976. *Thymic carcinoid tumors* responsible for Cushing's syndrome due to ectopic ACTH production have been observed (Lowry et al. 1976; Wick et al. 1980). Carcinoid tumors of foregut origin are nonargentaffin; it is therefore conceivable that they are not associated with a carcinoid syndrome. Rarely, they have been observed in cases of multiple endocrine neoplasia (MEN) syndrome type I (Wermer's syndrome; Rosai et al. 1972) and type II (Sipple's syndrome; Marchevsky and Dikman 1979).

Cutaneous Disorders

Pemphigus (in various forms) (Beutner et al. 1968; Peck et al. 1968) and *lichen planus* (Aronson et al. 1978) have been described in patients with thymomas. In many instances, myasthenia gravis was also present, and the dermatologic symptoms appeared after thymectomy. The rare combination of *juvenile pemphigoid* and autoimmune hemolytic anemia observed in an 8-month-old infant with thymic hypoplasia by Bloomfield et al. (1982) probably resulted from an inborn T-cell deficiency.

Miscellaneous Parathymic Disorders

Other diseases that have been found to be associated with thymoma with more than chance frequency include: *giant cell myocarditis* (usually present concurrently with autoimmune diseases such as myasthenia gravis, systemic lupus erythematosus, or dermatomyositis; Legg and Brady 1965; Rogers et al. 1968; Burke et al. 1969), *nephrotic syndrome* (Karcher et al. 1982); and *megaesophagus* (Demos et al. 1966). The association of thymoma and follicular thymic hyperplasia with *intestinal and hepatic diseases* has also been reported.

The intestinal disorders (Tsuchiya 1984) include: *ulcerative colitis* (Schmid 1970; Habu et al. 1971; Mizuno et al. 1976); *nontropical sprue, Whipple's disease,* and the *malabsorption syndrome* (Legg and Brady 1965; Gilbert et al. 1968). That these diseases may be both the cause and the consequence of humoral immunodeficiency must be taken into account when their causal relation with thymic changes is assessed.

Thymic changes in chronic liver diseases (Kamegaya et al. 1971) have rarely been sought or described. They have been reported in *hepatic cirrhosis* (Corridan 1963) and in *lupoid hepatitis* (Linke 1965). The incidence of *extrathymic neoplasms* in patients with thymomas or other thymic changes is controversial. Current estimates run from "a few" to 20% (Otto 1984; Rosenow and Hurley 1984).

Conclusions

The list of parathymic disorders in this chapter is incomplete by necessity. This, like their heterogeneous nature, is due to the fact that, in general, thymic changes are neither expected by clinicians nor routinely looked for by pathologists.

The information available leads to the conclusion that two categories of change in the thymic complex tend to be associated with extrathymic disease, namely: (a) thymomatous lesions which usually, but not always, benefit from thymectomy or thymomectomy, and (b) nonthymomatous lesions, which occur mainly in the form of "lymphofollicular hyperplasia" of the medulla or of parathymic lymph nodes, which may be regarded as the consequence rather than the cause of the associated diseases, and in which thymectomy is ineffective, with the exception of myasthenia gravis where the autoimmune reaction may be directed against antigens present in the thymic medulla itself.

References

Aronson IK, Soltani K, Paik KI, Rubenstein D, Lorincz AL (1978) Triad of lichen planus, myasthenia gravis, and thymoma. Arch Dermatol 114: 255-258

Bergman TA, Mariash CN, Oppenheimer JH (1982) Anterior mediastinal mass in a patient with Graves' disease. J Clin Endocrinol Metab 55: 587-588

Beutner EH, Chorzelski TP, Hale WL, Hausmanowa-Petrusewicz I (1968) Autoimmunity in concurrent myasthenia gravis and pemphigus erythematosus. JAMA 203: 845-849

Biggart JD, Nevin NC (1967) Hyperplasia of the thymus in progressive systemic sclerosis. J Pathol Bacteriol 93: 334-337

Bloomfield S, Stockdill G, Barnetson RSC (1982) Thymic hypoplasia, autoimmune haemolytic anaemia and juvenile pemphigoid in an infant. Br J Dermatol 106: 353-355

Burke JS, Medline NM, Katz A (1969) Giant cell myocarditis and myositis: associated with thymoma and myasthenia gravis. Arch Pathol Lab Med 88: 359-366

Corridan M (1963) The thymus in hepatic cirrhosis. J Clin Pathol 16: 445-447
Dawkins RL (1975) Experimental autoallergic myositis, polymyositis and myasthenia gravis: autoimmune muscle disease associated with immunodeficiency and neoplasia. Clin Exp Immunol 21: 185-201
Demos NJ, Yadusky RJ, Timmes JJ, Poulos PP (1966) Thymoma associated with megaesophagus: a case report. J Thorac Cardiovasc Surg 51: 708-713
Eggli P, Schaffner Th, Gerber HA, Hess MW, Cottier H (1987) Accessibility of thymic cortical lymphocytes to particles translocated from the peritoneal cavity to parathymic lymph nodes. Thymus 8: 129-139
Friedman NB (1967) Tumors of the thymus. J Thorac Cardiovasc Surg 53: 163-182
Gilbert EF, Harley JB, Anido V, Mengoli HF, Hughes JT (1968) Thymoma, plasma cell myeloma, red cell aplasia and malabsorption syndrome. Am J Med 44: 820-829
Goldstein G, Mackay IR (1969) The human thymus. Heinemann, London, pp 207-220
Habu S, Kameya T, Tamaoki N (1971) Thymic lymphoid follicles in autoimmune disease. I. Quantitative studies with special reference to myasthenia gravis. Keio J Med 20: 45-56
Heiniger HJ, Cottier H, Hess M, Stoner RD (1965) Zellkinetik der Plasmazellen mit Russelschen Körperchen: autoradiographische Untersuchungen mit Hilfe von Thymidin-^{3}H an älteren Mäusen mit experimenteller chronischer Trichinosis. Schweiz Med Wochenschr 95: 1424-1426
Henry K (1981) The human thymus in disease with particular emphasis on thymitis and thymoma. In: Kendall MD (ed) The thymus gland. Academic, London, pp 85-111
Jankovic BD, Isakovic K, Petrovic S (1971) Cellular and immunological events following injection of antigen into the chicken thymus. In: Lindahl-Kiessling K, Alm G, Hanna MG Jr (eds) Morphological and functional aspects of immunity. Plenum, London, pp 197-201
Janzen RWCh, Lachenmayer L (1976) Parathymische Syndrome. Dtsch Med Wochenschr 101: 1292-1294
Kamegaya K, Tsuchiya M, Sambe K (1971) Thymic abnormalities and the chronicity of liver disease: report of 10 cases and follow-up study. Keio J Med 20: 77-90
Karcher DS, Pearson CE, Butler WM, Hurwitz MA, Cassell PF (1982) Giant lymph node hyperplasia involving the thymus with associated nephrotic syndrome and myelofibrosis. Am J Clin Pathol 77: 100-104
Ketz E, Fopp M, Weissert M, Bekier A (1979) Polymyositis, myasthenic syndrome and thymoma in a patient with defective cell-mediated immunity. Acta Neurol Belg 79: 469-474
Kirkpatrick CH, Windhorst DB (1979) Mucocutaneous candidiasis and thymoma. Am J Med 66: 939-945
Krantz SB, Moore WH, Zaentz SD (1973) Studies on red cell aplasia. V. Presence of erythroblast cytotoxicity in G-globulin fraction of plasma. J Clin Invest 52: 324-336
Lattes R (1962) Thymoma and other tumors of the thymus: an analysis of 107 cases. Cancer 15: 1224-1260
Legg MA, Brady WJ (1965) Pathology and clinical behavior of thymomas: a survey of 51 cases. Cancer 18: 1131-1144
Linke A (1965) Thymustumor mit lupoider Hepatitis. Schweiz Med Wochenschr 95: 1492-1494
Lowry PJ, Rees LH, Tomlin S, Gillies G, Landon J (1976) Chemical characterization of ectopic ACTH purified from a malignant thymic carcinoid tumor. J Clin Endocrinol Metab 43: 831-835
Marchevsky AM, Dikman SH (1979) Mediastinal carcinoid with an incomplete Sipple's syndrome. Cancer 43: 2497-2501
Marshall AHE, White RG (1961) The immunological reactivity of the thymus. Br J Exp Pathol 42: 379-385
Mizuno Y, Shimabukuro K, Kurita K, Tsuchiya M (1976) Thymus abnormalities in ulcerative colitis - comparative study with other auto-immune diseases. Gastroenterol Jap 11: 208-214
Müller Ch, Tschumper A, Tschumper J-C, Hess MW, Cottier H (1987) Parathymic lymph node-oriented proliferative response of the murine thymic cortex to intraperitoneal stimulation. Thymus 9: 3-12
Nicholson RL (1978) Thymic hyperplasia in thyrotoxicosis. J Can Assoc Radiol 29: 264-265
Otto HF (1984) Pathologie des Thymus. In: Doerr W, Seifert G, Uelinger E (eds) Spezielle Pathologische Anatomie, vol 17. Springer, Berlin Heidelberg New York
Peck SM, Osserman KE, Weiner LB, Lefkovits A, Osserman RS (1968) Studies in bullous diseases: immunofluorescent serologic tests. N Engl J Med 279: 951-958
Raff MC (1973) T and B lymphocytes and immune responses. Nature 242: 19-23
Raviola E, Karnovsky MJ (1972) Evidence for a blood-thymus barrier using electron-opaque tracers. J Exp Med 136: 466-498
Rogers BHG, Manaligod JR, Blazek WV (1968) Thymoma associated with pancytopenia and hypogammaglobulinemia: report of a case and review of the literature. Am J Med 44: 154-164
Rosai J, Higa E, Davie J (1972) Mediastinal endocrine neoplasm in patients with multiple endocrine adenomatosis. Cancer 29: 1075-1083
Rosenow EC III, Hurley BT (1984) Disorders of the thymus: a review. Arch Intern Med 144: 763-770
Salyer WR, Eggleston JC (1976) Thymoma: a clinical and pathological study of 65 cases. Cancer 37: 229-249
Schmid KO (1970) Thymus und Colitis ulcerosa. Verh Dtsch Ges Pathol 54: 313-319
Simeone JF, McCloud T, Putnam CE, Marsh J (1975) Thymoma and systemic lupus erythematosus. Thorax 30: 697-700
Souadjian JV, Enriquez P, Silverstein MN, Pépin JM (1974) The spectrum of diseases associated with thymoma: coincidence or syndrome? Arch Intern Med 134: 374-379
Theofilopoulos AN, Dixon FJ (1985) Murine models of systemic lupus erythematosus. Adv Immunol 37: 269-390
Tosi P, Kraft R, Luzi P, Cintorino M, Fankhauser G, Hess MW, Cottier H (1982) Involution patterns of the human thymus. I. Size of the cortical area as a function of age. Clin Exp Immunol 47: 497-504
Tsuchiya M (1984) Immunological abnormalities involving the thymus in ulcerative colitis and therapeutic effects of thymectomy. Gastroenterol Jp 19: 232-346
Wegelin C (1918) Über Lymphfollikel mit Keimzentren im Thymusmark. Zentralbl Allg Pathol 29: 441-447
Wick MR, Scott RE, Chin-Yang LI, Carney JA (1980) Carcinoid tumor of the thymus. A clinicopathologic report of seven cases with a review of the literature. Mayo Clin Proc 55: 246-254
Wilkins EW Jr, Castleman B (1979) Thymoma: a continuing survey at the Massachusetts General Hospital. Ann Thorac Surg 28: 252-256

Part IV

Clinical Investigations

16 Conventional Radiology

Louis Kreel

Introduction

In many ways there is no normal radiology of the adult thymus. It is not usually visible on an adult chest film, in either frontal or lateral projections, nor on fluoroscopy or conventional tomography as its flattened margins are buried within the contours of the mediastinum. The thymus does not impinge on the normal cardiovascular silhouette, its soft tissue density is indistinguishable from the surrounding structures and there is no contrast agent that produces a thymic blush (Kreel 1969).

In young children however the thymus forms a major component of the mediastinum. Its morphology is by far the most inconstant of the body organs varying not merely with age, but with stress, drugs and nutrition; it is a barometer of well-being in infancy (Caffey 1978). No wonder that sudden death in this age group was attributed to "status thymicolymphaticus" the most notorious of non-disease entities - the large normal thymus was far too prominent not to be considered pathological. For a period this non-disease, status thymicolymphaticus, was treated with radiotherapy, causing thyroid cancer some 15-20 years later (Hammar 1923).

In normal young adults, particularly in women, a minor problem exists when the left lobe of the thymus mimics an enlarged pulmonary artery and, if not recognised as a normal variant, can lead to unnecessary investigations (Kreel 1970). Radiologically the major concern in adults is to identify tumours in the thymus such as thymoma, carcinoid and lymphoma. Most are visible on chest radiographs and their characteristic features are readily recognised (Kreel 1970). Computed tomography has replaced venography, arteriography and pneumomediastinography to investigate the thymus (Kreel 1978). Some basic observations nevertheless remain pertinent to modern practice, even though more relevant to the parathyroids or mediastinal pathology.

Anatomy

The thymus, thyroid and parathyroids are closely related in their development.

Not surprisingly, they have aspects of their arterial supply and venous drainage in common (Williams and Warwick 1980). The two-lobed thymus is ensheathed in loose areolar tissue of the anterior mediastinum, lying between the sternum and great vessels; in front of and between the pleura and lungs, it reaches from above the innominate artery to the pericardium below. From above downwards it is related posteriorly to the trachea, inferior thyroid veins, the innominate and left carotid arteries, the aorta and pericardium.

The size and shape of the thymus changes remarkably with age. Comparing infants, adolscents and adults, the thymus is approximately 0.8% of total body weight at birth, falling to 0.08% at puberty and 0.01% in the mature adult (Goldstein and MacKay 1969). The change in comparative size is matched by a change in shape in infancy through to the young adult. In the sagittal plane the adult gland is no more than a thick ribbon or band (see Fig. 14). Prolongations of the gland or the thymothyroid ligament, when it is replaced by fibrous tissue lying immediately in front of the left recurrent laryngeal nerve, attach the left lobe to the inferior pole of the thyroid or inferior parathyroid (parathyroid III).

Up to the age of 20 years each lobe of the two-lobed thymus is enclosed in a thick fibrous capsule giving off delicate septa dividing the gland into lobules. The septa disappear in the middle-aged and elderly as the thymus diminishes in size and weight being gradually replaced by fatty tissue (Williams and Warwick 1980). The thymus is slightly larger in males than females and the left lobe usually reaches somewhat more caudally than the right. One more anatomical observation is extremely relevant to radiology. The gland is soft and pliant, impressed and indented by adjacent organs, changing shape during respiration, but not displacing or deforming abutting structures (Caffey 1978; Day and Gedgandas 1984). Furthermore, however large the normal thymus, it is not a cause of respiratory distress.

Radiological Appearances

In infancy, usually up to 2 years, but on occasions to an even older age, the thymus can form a prominent part of the mediastinal shadow on the chest radiograph. It is extremely variable in size and shape and there is, in fact, no prominent thymus in about half the cases, bilateral prominence in about a fifth (Fig. 1) and right-sided prominence in a quarter (Fig. 2). Left-sided prominence occurs in about 8% (Fig. 3, Day and Gedgandas 1984). Although a completely absent thymic shadow occurs in the rare aplasia syndromes, it is much more commonly absent owing to stress from infection, malnutrition or drug therapy (Caffey 1978). Removal of these factors allows regrowth of the thymus and the reappearance on chest radiographs often with rebound to a size greater than originally present (Chap. 7; Cohen et al. 1980). It is important to bear this fact in mind, to avoid unnecessary thoracotomies (Handmaker und O'Mara 1977). Furthermore, this regrowth can also take up ^{67}Ga citrate, causing possible confusion with mediastinal lymphomas.

The silhouette of the thymus merges with that of the heart, frequently and particularly on the right there is an intervening notch or angle at the junction (Caffey 1978; Kreel 1969, 1970). Occasionally the thymicocardiac shadow on the frontal view suggests the presence of marked cardiomegaly. The correct interpretation can be made on the lateral view as the thymus produces an anterior retrosternal density whereas cardiac enlargement, in a true lateral view, will overlap the spine (Caffey 1978; Day and Gedgandas 1984).

While this is so in the vast majority of cases, very rarely in infants or young children there is a prolongation of the thymus into the posterior mediastinum. On the lateral view this can mimic cardiomegaly (Cohen et al. 1983; Saade et al. 1976). A steroid test was often performed before the advent of modern imaging to shrink the thymus so as to distinguish cardiomegaly from a posteriorly situated thymus.

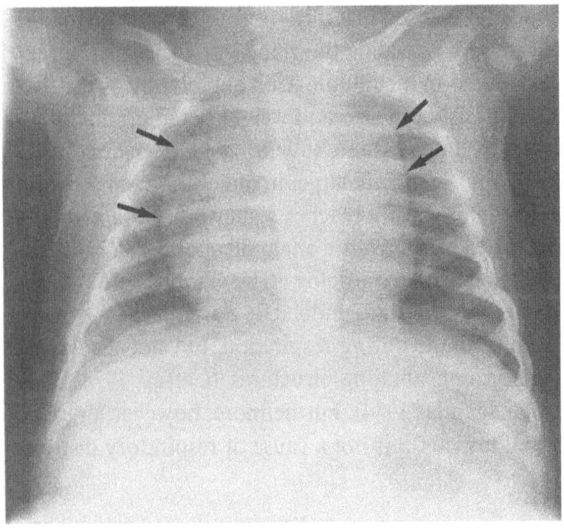

Fig. 1. Normal thymus of infancy - bilateral prominence *(arrows)* occurring in about 20%

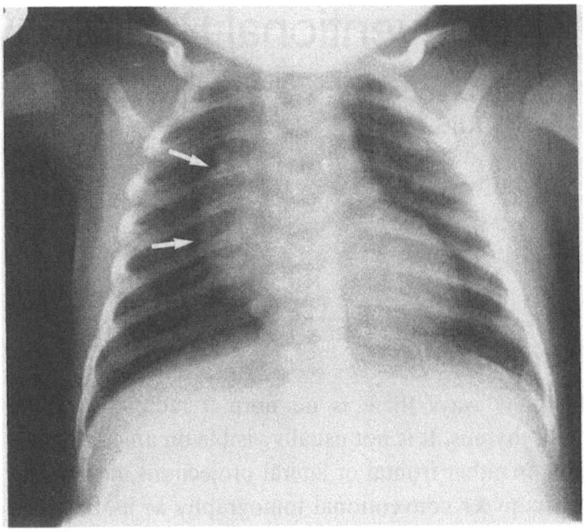

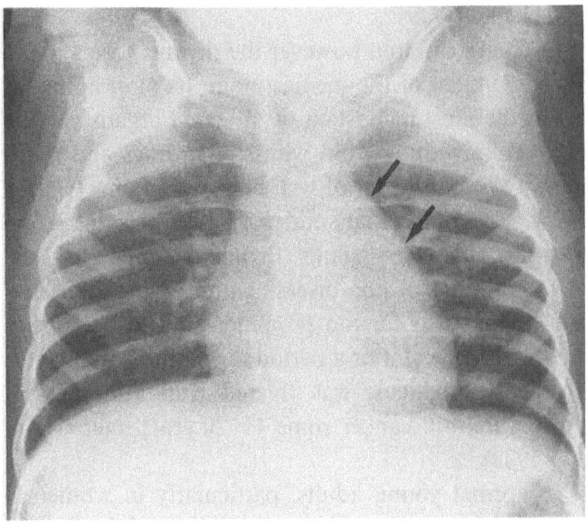

Fig. 3. Left-sided prominence of normal infant thymus *(arrows)* occurring in about 8%

There are other signs besides the notch between thymus and heart, which may be bilateral or single and obvious or slight, to identify the thymus. In about 5% a "sail-shaped" configuration is produced, more commonly on the right (Fig. 4). The lateral prolongation from the mediastinum may extend into and along the lesser fissure simulating a pleural effusion or the sha-

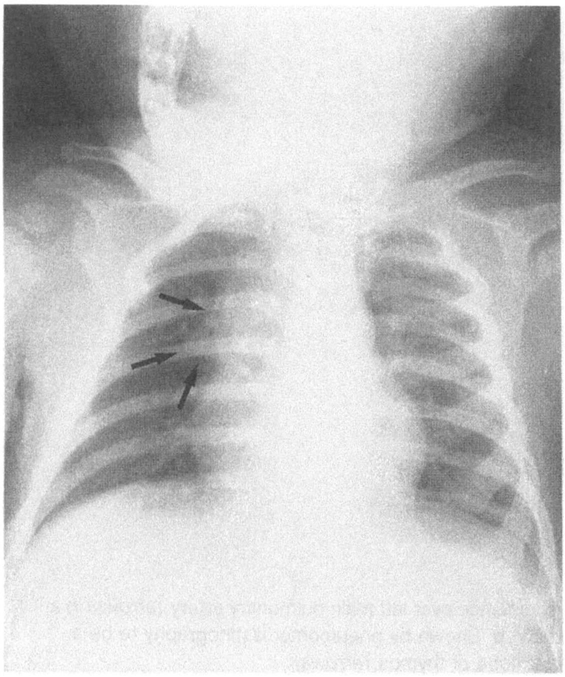

Fig. 4. "Sailshaped" right lobe of thymus *(arrows)* present in about 5% of normal infants

dow may be mistaken for right upper lobe consolidation. When large the thymus abuts upon the ribs; the impressions formed on it by the ribs produce a ripple or scalloped margin seen best on an oblique view and usually on the left. Another sign that may be of help is the variation in shape of the thymus with respiration (Caffey 1978; Day and Gedgandas 1984).

With mediastinal emphysema, gas outlines the whole thymus as it becomes displaced laterally to produce the appearance of "angle's wings" or "floating" thymus and the characteristic thymic shape is then particularly well seen on the lateral view as it is separated from the sternum anteriorly and the ascending aorta posteriorly.

The variability of the size of the thymus has been stressed repeatedly, however measurements of the cardiothymic/thoracic ratio (CT/T) can be of diagnostic importance. This ratio is taken as the mediastinal diameter at the carina divided by the internal diameter of the thorax at the level of the diaphragm, in inspiration on a nonrotated view. On supine anteroposterior film in normal neonates on day 1 the CT/T is 0.35 (S. D. 0.08). However in respiratory distress syndrome (RDS) this ratio can be 0.46, but if the mother receives prenatal steroids which have a protective action on RDS the CT/T is invariably normal. The CT/T can furthermore be of some predictive value for the development of RDS. If the CT/T is greater than 0.46 then RDS becomes three times more likely and if less than 0.30 is two-and-a-half times less likely for the same degree of prematurity (Gewolb 1979).

In childhood the thymus can become prominent owing to a number of conditions such as Addison's disease, gigantism (hyperpituitarism with excess growth hormone), hyperthyroidism or successful treatment of hypothyroidism with thyroxine, recovery from malnutrition, thermal burns and chronic illness (Yulish and Owens 1980). The mediastinum becomes widened hiding the border of the ascending aorta on the right and occupying the aortopulmonary bay on the left (Caffey 1978). A thymic cyst produces a much more localised bulge, its rounded margin projecting from the mediastinum, and can be demonstrated by sonography as an anechoic mass lying anterior to the heart.

The assessment of abnormality in infancy is extremely difficult because of the wide normal variation from invisibility to extreme prominence. Conversely in the adult a visible thymus on the chest radiograph spells abnormality, apart from one particular circumstance. In young adults, particularly in women, a prominence in the region of the main pulmonary artery can be due to a normal left lobe of thymus, and is not too infrequently seen on routine chest films (Fig. 5; Kreel 1968). Poststenotic dilatation of the pulmonary artery and pulmonary hypertension are readily excluded excluded by absence of clinical and radiographic signs as are conditions producing pulmonary plethora such as left-to-right shunt.

A false impression of pulmonary artery enlargement may also be given when it is more cranially placed than usual, an anatomical variant noted on computerised tomography examinations (Mencini and Proto 1982).

Abnormalities of the thymus shown on chest radiographs in the adult are almost exclusively due either to tumours or cysts. The commonest tumour is thymoma associated with myasthenia gravis, but carcinoid, lymphoma, metastases, dermoid and primary teratoma have been well documented (Rosai et al. 1972). The benign thymolipoma is rare, but can be extremely large (Winario et al. 1982). Thymic cysts also occur as well as haemorrhage into the thymus itself and postoperatively into the thymic bed (Kreel 1969; Kreel 1970; Moskowitz et al. 1980; Young et al. 1973). While thymic lymphofollicular hyperplasia is a common finding on histology, especially in myasthenia gravis, enlargement due to true hyperplasia is often confined to patients with thyrotoxicosis (Golstein and MacKay 1969).

The majority of tumours of the thymus can be demonstrated on chest radiographs, producing a characteristic appearance because the basic shape of the thymus

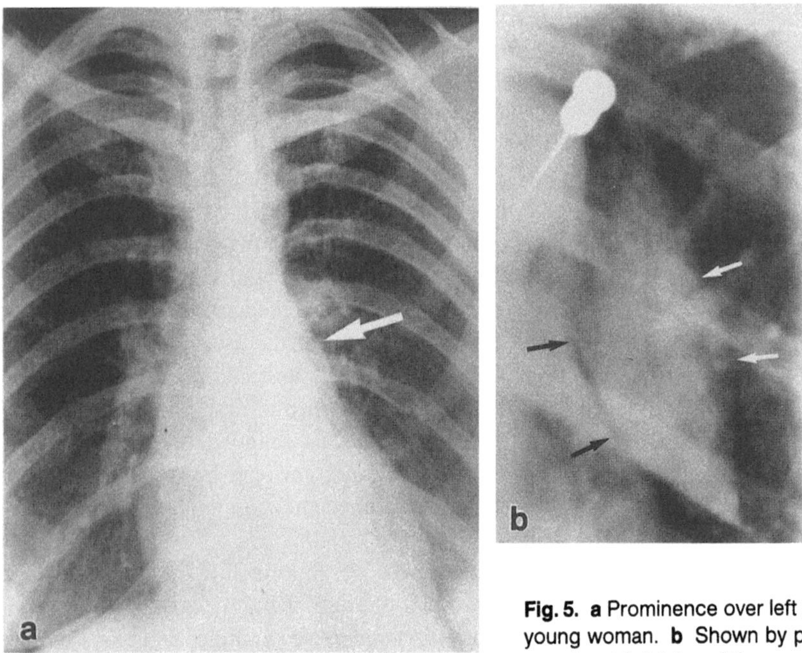

Fig. 5. a Prominence over left main pulmonary artery *(arrows)* in a young woman. **b** Shown by pneumomediastinography to be a prominent left lobe of thymus *(arrows)*

is retained (Brown et al. 1980). In hyperplasia or lymphoma the enlargement tends to be bilateral whereas thymoma, carcinoid, metastases or teratoma produce unilateral enlargement.

On the right the expanding lobe of the thymus obscures the margin of the ascending aorta and right atrium (Fig. 6) and on the left obscures the main pulmonary artery and upper border of the left ventricle (Fig. 7) forming a notch where it joins the heart shadow. Because the thymus lies anteriorly the thymic mass as well as the thymicocardiac notch is accentuated on oblique chest views. About 40% of thymomas have a lobulated contour.

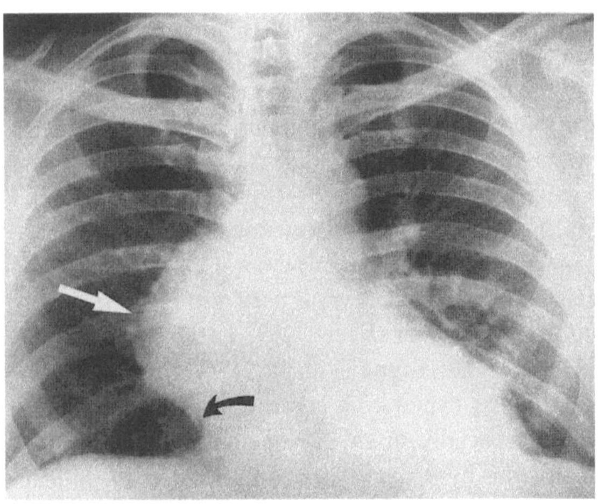

Fig. 6. Right-sided thymoma *(white arrow)* obscuring ascending aortic and right atrial contours with a pronounced notch of its junction with a right heart border *(black arrows)*

These are the common appearances of thymic tumours, but other features have also been encountered. A thymoma may appear as a small rounded mediastinal mass mimicking a paravertrebral tumour, but on the lateral view is seen to lie retrosternally (Brown et al. 1980). Almost all thymic tumours are in the upper or mid-retrosternal region, however about 5% overlie the heart and may even reach the diaphragm, suggesting right atrial or left ventricular enlargement on the

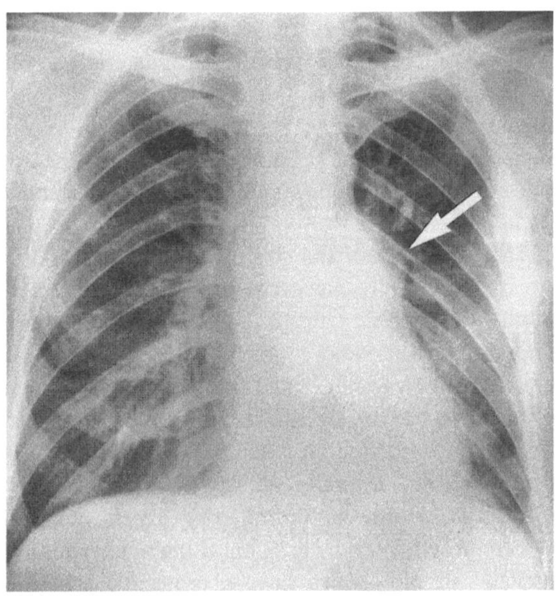

Fig. 7. Small left thymoma causing a bulge over the pulmonary artery *(arrows)*

frontal view, but on a well-penetrated film a vertical tissue plane may be seen between the thymic tumour and the cardiac contour.

Similarly the normal pulmonary artery will be visible through the mass in almost half the cases, particularly on the left where the thymoma overlies the main pulmonary artery and left main trunk when appearances may be mistaken for a dilated "pulmonary conus". As shown previously, a similar appearance can be found as a normal variant in young healthy women.

Slighter degrees of thymic enlargement are visible more frequently on the left than on the right because the pulmonary bay below the aortic knuckle becomes filled in, whereas on the right the enlarging thymus merges with the shadow of the ascending aorta, nestling in the angle between the pulmonary and aortic roots anteriorly. Thymic tumours are seen lying in front of the aortic shadow on the lateral view and then to have a relatively straight margin inferiorly at their base which has a sharp angle anteriorly and a rounded margin posteriorly.

A post-thymectomy effusion into the thymic bed, expanding the anterior medaistinal shadow, produces the characteristic thymic shape (Fig. 8) that is accentuated in the oblique position. The notch at the junction with the pericardium can be particularly well demonstrated on fluoroscopy. Transmitted pulsation is quite frequent with right-sided tumours, raising the possibility of an aneurysm of the ascending aorta (Fig. 9; Kreel 1969, 1970). The notch and the appearance on the lateral view should decide the issue, but computed tomography, digital substraction arteriography or ultrasonography may be required for the diagnosis.

Approximately 15% of thymomas show calcification, usually amorphous patches with irregular strands suggesting a local nodule (Fig. 10) possibly due to previous necrosis or haemorrhage, not to be mistaken for calcified lymph nodes (Brown et al. 1980; Harper and Guyer 1965). Curvilinear calcification on the margin of a thymic cyst also occurs and occasionally a dense

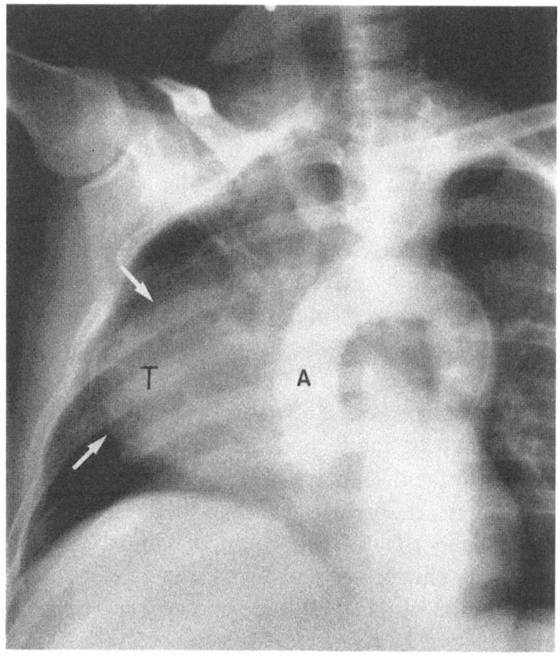

Fig. 9. Right thymoma *(T, arrows)* that showed marked transmitted pulsation. Aortogram clearly shows mass separable from aorta *(A)* on retrograde aortography. More recently less invasive methods such as computed tomography, digital subtraction arteriography or cardiac sonography would be used

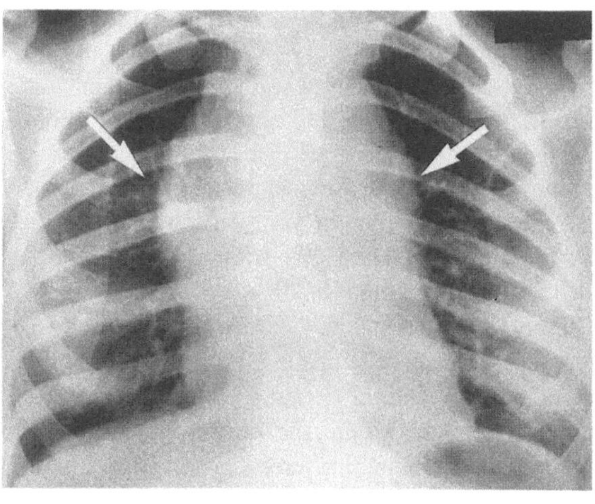

Fig. 8. Typical thymic shape *(arrows)* produced by haemorrhage into the thymic bed that occurred post-thymectomy

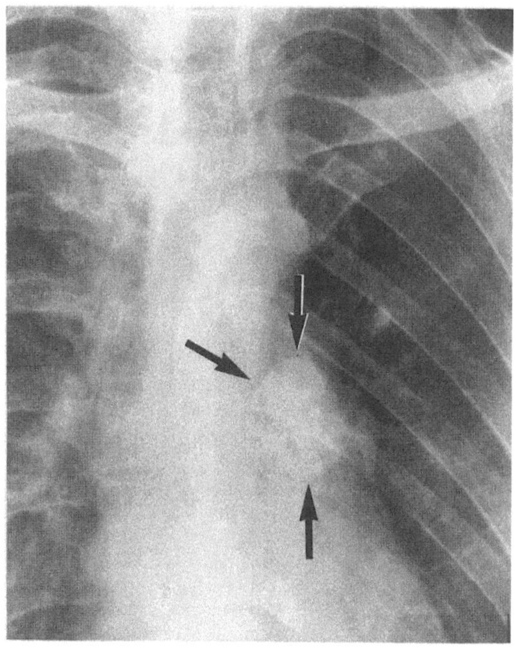

Fig. 10. Irregular strands of calcification in a thymoma *(arrows)* suggesting a localised nodule of tumour

mass of calcification in a tumour. Smaller areas of calcification will only be shown on the lateral or on a well-penetrated frontal view. Calcification whether large or small, regular or irregular, does not help to distinguish between benign and malignant thymoma. In fact there are no reliable features of the mass itself in predicting the biological outcome of these tumours.

Thymic carcinoid tumours are thought to be derived from neural crest anlage and behave quite differently from the epithelially derived thymoma. The former can be decidedly malignant while the latter are relatively benign. Carcinoid shows marked local invasion, produces pleural effusions, pulmonary nodules and bone metastases whereas thymomas are locally invasive and produce pleural seeding shown as typical pleural-based lesions, but distant metastases are rare (Chaps. 9, 10; Levine and Rosai 1978).

While carcinoid and thymoma have quite distinct biological behaviours, the appearance of the primary tumour in the thymus is similar. As mediastinal invasion progresses, the enlarging mass produces a number of secondary effects. The mediastinum and trachea are displaced, phrenic nerve paralysis with an elevated diaphragm occurs (Fig. 11) and superior vena cava obstruction may be produced.

While the invasive nature of a thymoma cannot be predicted by its radiological appearances, statistics show that clearly defined tumours less than 5 cm diameter, are likely to be benign or noninvasive, but if greater than 8 cm, flat, irregular or poorly defined, over 50% will be invasive (Brown et al. 1980). Moreover the flat, plaque-like tumours are the most difficult to visualise on chest radiographs.

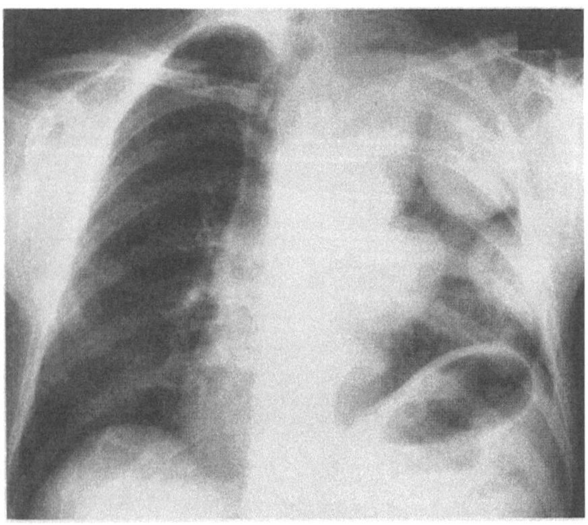

Fig. 11. Invasive thymoma in a late stage showing characteristic features of mediastinal mass displacing trachea, with an elevated left hemidiaphragm and typical pleural-based nodules due to pleural seeding

Thymic tumours, particularly lymphoma, not uncommonly contain small cysts, but the shape of the tumour within the thymus is unaltered (Keller and Castelman 1974). Large cysts in the thymus produce a circular contour when the diagnosis can be suggested on the chest radiograph, particularly if curvilinear calcification at the margin is also present. The rare benign thymolipoma is usually very large, enclosing the heart and giving the false impression of gross cardiomegaly. The fatty nature of the tumour can be suspected from the relatively low density of the tumour and confirmed by sonography when it produces highly reflective echoes, or by the low attenuation on computed tomography (Winario et al. 1982).

Very rarely myasthenia gravis is caused by ectopic thymus located within the lung. Intrapulmonary thymoma may be perihilar or more laterally placed and seen as single or multiple lung nodules (Kung et al. 1985). More commonly a myasthenia-like syndrome is produced by a bronchial carcinoma. The radiological signs on the chest radiograph may be quite minimal such as slightly increased density of the hilum, or minimal linear collapse, or the signs may be obvious such as collapse or consolidation.

In some 90% of cases of myasthenia gravis a thymoma, if present, is visible on the chest radiograph or on fluoroscopy (Caffey 1978; Harper and Guyer 1965). Conventional tomography is seldom of help in detecting an occult tumour. In the past mediastinal pneumography, venography and arteriography were undertaken to demonstrate tumours not visible on fluoroscopy or on frontal and lateral chest radiographs. These tumours are usually less than 4 cm diameter and are now demonstrable by computed tomography.

Lymphoma can affect the thymus, be it Hodgkin's or non-Hodgkin's disease, can be confined to the thymus, be associated with lymphadenopathy or produce only adjacent lymph node enlargement. Lymphoma usually produces diffuse thymic enlargement of both lobes, but a well-recognised variety of Hodgkin's disease, the nodular sclerosing type producing "granulomatous thymoma" is often confined to one lobe and produces a bumpy or bosselated appearance. Small cysts are not uncommon in lymphoma, but it occasionally presents as a large cyst within which are only small foci of lymphoma (Smith et al. 1983).

Primary teratocarcinoma of the thymus produces, thymic enlargement indistinguishable from other thymic tumours, but the dermoid of the anterior mediastinum can lie within the thymus producing a rounded mass containing areas of calcification not infrequently with a "popcorn" appearance. Sarcoid can also enlarge the thymus and thyrotoxicosis is a well-recognised cause of moderate diffuse enlargement due to hyperplasia of the thymus.

Thymic Venography (Kreel 1967; 1969)

The central thymic vein (the great vein of Keynes) can be selectively catheterised from the left subclavian via the median basilic vein (Fig. 12) or from the superior vena cava via the right femoral vein and inferior vena cava, traversing the right atrium. Injection of contrast medium performed very gently during a Valsalva manoeuvre outlines the main vein and its two major branches with draining veins encircling the outer margin of each lobe of the thymus, their lateral components forming the lateral thymic vein which empties on the left into the brachiocephalic vein and on the right into the superior vena cava. Either lateral vein may communicate with or empty into an inferior thyroidal vein. In localising a parathyroid adenoma positive venous sampling may thus reflect either an intrathymic or intrathyroidal gland.

A thymoma is diagnosed by curvilinear displacement of major thymic veins, occasionally by a plexus of coarse veins (Fig. 13) and infiltrating carcinoid has been shown with filling of a periaortic venous plexus of the ascending aorta. However, since the advent of computed tomography, venography is no longer used to diagnose thymic tumours.

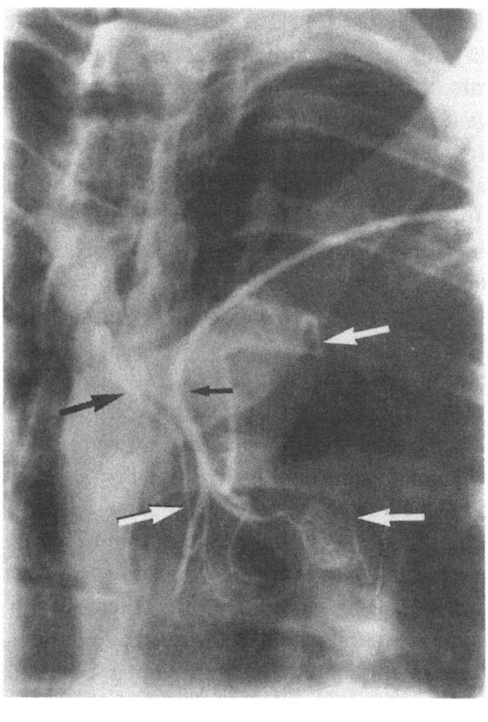

Fig. 12. Normal thymic venogram via left subclavian vein showing a central great vein of Keynes *(small black arrow)*, dividing into two major tributaries and the lateral thymic veins; the right *(black arrows)* draining into the superior vena cava and the left *(white arrows)* into the left brachiocephalic vein

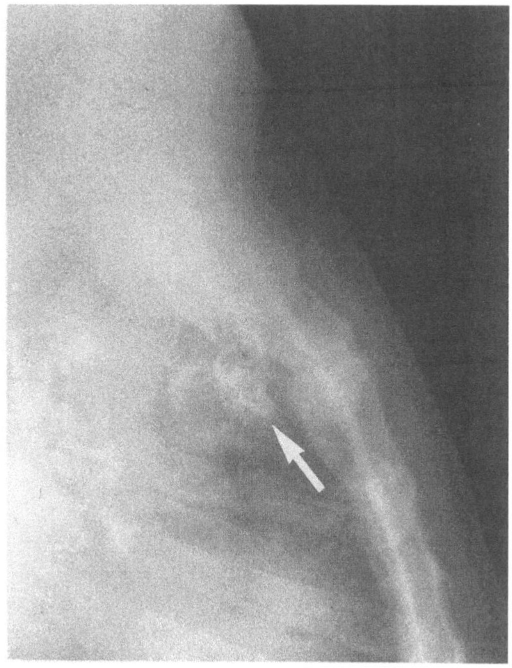

Fig. 13. Lateral view of thymic venogram demonstrating small thymoma *(arrow)* shown as a coarse network of veins within the tumour

Pneumomediastinography (Kreel 1965, 1968)

The injection of gas into the mediastinum and around the thymus can be by either the suprasternal or transsternal route; fluoroscopy with spot films and lateral and prone frontal tomography is then undertaken (Fig. 14). Like venography and arteriography, this ex-

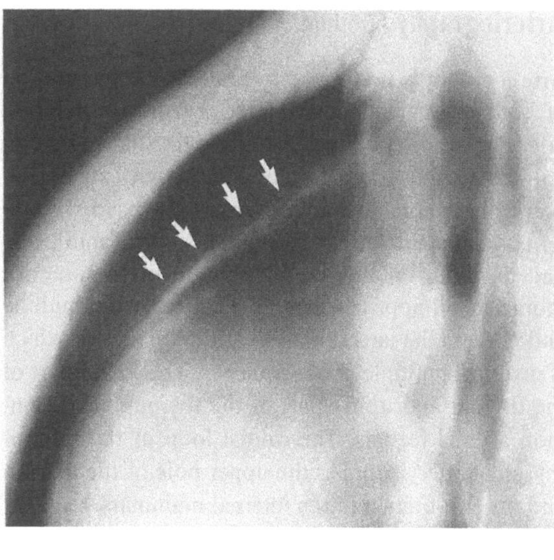

Fig. 14. Normal mature thymus *(arrows)* in myasthenia gravis shown by pneumomediastinum with lateral tomography

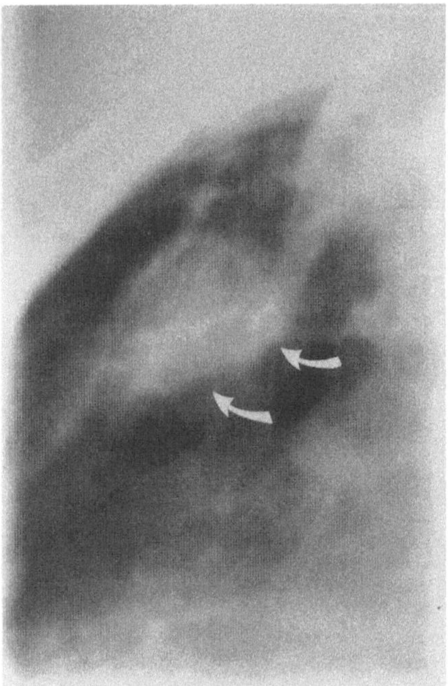

Fig. 15. Moderate-sized thymoma *(arrows)* shown on a pneumomediastinogram with lateral fluoroscopic spot film

amination has been superseded by computed tomography.

Tumours are shown as a localised bulge on the thymus (Fig. 15) and pneumomediastinography was used only when a tumour was not shown on chest radiographs of fluoroscopy. Superiorly the left brachiocephalic vein could mimic a superiorly located thymoma, and was distinguished by contrast injection into the left basilic vein.

Arteriography (Göthlin et al. 1977)

Arteriography is performed by selective catheterisation of both internal mammary arteries from the femoral artery or by injection into the subclavian artery by digital subtraction arteriography. Subclavian catheterisation from the brachial artery can also be used. The internal mammary artery is normally 1-1.5 mm wide and descends on the internal margin of the anterior thoracic wall approximately 2-4 cm from the midline and close to the lateral margin of the thymus to which is gives off multiple small branches. The lower part of the thyroid and upper part of the thymus have common arterial feeders. The caudal loop of the inferior thyroidal artery supplies the upper pole of the thymus and the first branch of the internal mammary gives off a superior branch to the inferior pole of the thyroid.

Tumours are shown by displaced vessels being streched around the margin and by neovascularity. A tumour stain may also occur. Carcinoid tumours tend to have greater neovascularity and tumour blush. Thymic granulomatous disease (nodular sclerosing Hodgkin's disease) produces similar appearances.

Nuclear Medicine (Handmaker and O'Mara 1977)

Gallium-67 citrate (^{67}Ga) is taken up by lymphoma and may thus show thymic infiltration, bearing in mind that in children the normal thymus also takes up this isotope, particularly in the presence of sepsis.

Bone scans are often positive; thymomas only very rarely produce distant metastases, but carcinoid of thymus, although a much less common tumour, frequently metastasises to lung and bone. The bone metastases are usually sclerotic, frequently affecting the axial skeleton like most hormonal tumours.

Conclusions

Modern scanning methods, particularly computed tomography, have made invasive investigations of the thymus obsolete. Nevertheless, conventional or normal radiology still has an important role in the evaluation of the thymus almost exclusively by chest radiography and fluoroscopy. The variable size of the normal thymus is particularly relevant in children; under 2 years of age thethymus is prominent and however large it may appear, it is almost certainly normal, with only a few exceptions such as haemorrhage into the thymus or formation of a cyst. However, the infant thymus fluctuates in size, being diminished by stress, malnutrition infection and steroids, but subsequently regrowing as normality is restored and even showing rebound to form a larger component of the thymicocardiac shadow than previously.

The cardiothymic/thoracic (CT/T) ratio can be of assistance in assessing the respiratory distress syndrome. Clear visualisation of the whole thymus indicates a pneumomediastinum. The large thymus must be differentiated from cardiomegaly, almost always possible on the lateral view, bearing in mind the rare posterior prolongation of a large thymus in infancy which may need the steroid test for differentiation. The prominence in the region of the main and left pulmonary artery in adolescents and young adults is usually a normal variant whether due to a prominent left lobe of the thymus or a "high" position.

Thymic tumours and cysts can usually be recognised on conventional radiography by their characteristic shape and 90% of thymomas associated with myasthenia gravis can be detected on chest films or fluoroscopy and seeding to the pleura by invasive thymomas can also be shown, but at a later stage than on computed tomography.

Calcification in thymomas occurs in 15%, but does not differentiate between benign and invasive tumours although marginal curvilinear calcification is characteristic of a cyst and "popcorn" calcification of a dermoid. Pleural effusions, bone and liver metastases indicate that a thymic tumour is likely to be a carcinoid and two-lobed tumours suggest lymphoma. A major problem nevertheless remains unresolved. How can an invasive tumour be distinguished from a benign tumour? If greater than 8 cm with irregular flat contours (and certainly when there are metastases, a pleural effusion or phrenic nerve palsy) it should be considered invasive and if a clearly defined mass less than 5 cm and no signs of distant spread it is statistically benign, but even these criteria of benignancy may be in doubt, not to speak of the grey area between 5- and 8-cm tumours. Histology is also unhelpful and at present surgery is always indicated.

References

Brown LR, Muhm JR, Gray JE (1980) Radiographic detection of thymoma. AJR 134: 1181-1188

Caffey J (1978) Thymus in pediatric X-ray diagnosis: a textbook for students and practioners of pediatrics, surgery and radiology, 7th edn, vol 1. Year Bood Medical, Chicago, pp 510-526

Cohen M, Hill CA, Cangir A, Sullivan MP (1980) Thymic rebound after treatment of childhood tumours. AJR 135: 151-156

Cohen MD, Weber TR, Sequeira FW, Vane DW, King H (1983) The diagnostic dilemma of the posterior mediastinal thymus: CT-manifestations. Radiology 146: 691-693

Day DL, Gedgaudas E (1984) The thymus. Radiol Clin North Am 22: 519-538

Gewolb IH, Lobowitz RL, Taeusch HW (1979) Thymus size and its relationship to the respiratory distress syndrome. J Pediatr 95: 108-111

Goldstein G, Mackay IR (1969) The human thymus. Heinemann, London

Göthlin J, Jonsson K, Lunderquist A, Rausing A, Alburquerque LM (1977) The angiographic appearance of thymic tumours. Radiology 124: 47-52

Hammer JA (1921) The new views as to the morphology of the thymus gland and their bearing on the problem of the function of the thymus. Endocrinology 5: 543-573, 731-760

Handmaker H, O'Mara RE (1977) Gallium imaging in pediatrics. J Nucl Med 18: 1057-1063

Harper RAK, Guyer PB (1965) The radiological features of thymic tumours: a review of sixtyfive cases. Clin Radiol 16: 97-105

Keller AR, Castleman B (1974) Hodgkin's disease of the thymus gland. Cancer 33: 1615-1623

Kreel L (1965) Pneumomediastinography in myasthenia gravis. Proceedings of the 11th International Congress of Radiology. Excerpta Medica International Congress Series No 105: 55-56

Kreel L (1967) Selective thymic venography: new method for visualisation of the thymus. Br Med J 1: 406-407

Kreel L (1968) Radiology in myasthenia gravis. Proc R Soc Med 61: 754-757

Kreel L (1969) Radiology in diagnosis. In: Green R (ed) Myasthenia gravis, chap 5. Heinemann, London, pp 43-69

Kreel L (1969) Radiology in diagnosis. Chapter 5 in myasthenia gravis. Ed. Green R. William Heinemann Medical Books Ltd, London pp 43-69

Kreel L (1970) Radiology of the thymus. Trans Med Soc Lond 86: 96-103

Kreel L (1978) Computed tomography of the thorax. Radiol Clin North Am 16 575-584

Kung I, Loke SL, So SY, Lam WK, Mok CK, Aung Khin M (1985) Intrapulmonary thymoma: report of two cases. Thorax 40: 471-474

Levine GD, Rosai J (1978) Thymic hyperplasia and neoplasia: a review of current concepts. Hum Pathol 9: 495-515

Mencini RA, Proto AV (1982) The high left and right pulmonary arteries: a CT pitfall. J Comput Assist Tomogr 6: 452-459

Moskowitz PS, Noon MA, McAlister WH, Mark JBD (1980) Thymic cyst hemorrhage: a case of acute symptomatic mediastinal widening in children with aplastic anemia. AJR 134: 832-836

Rosai J, Higa E, Davie J (1972) Mediastinal endocrine neoplasm in patients with multiple endocrine adenomatosis. A previously unrecognised association. Cancer 29: 1075-1083

Saade H, Whitten DM, Necheles TF, Leape L, Darling D (1976) Posterior mediastinal accessory thymus. J Pediatr 88: 71-72

Smith PLC, Jobling C, Rees A (1983) Hodgkin's disease in a large thymic cyst in a child. Thorax 38: 392-393

Williams PL, Warwick K (1980) The thymus in grays anatomy, 36th edn. Churchil-Livingstone, Edinburgh, pp 780-784

Winarso P, Isherwood I, Photiou S, Donnelly RJ (1982) Thymolipoma simulating cardiomegaly: use of computed tomography in diagnosis. Thorax 37: 941-942

Young R, Pochaczevsky R, Pollak L, Bryk D (1973) Cervicomediastinal thymic cysts. AJR 117: 855-860

Yulish BS, Owens RP (1980) Thymic enlargement in a child during therapy for primary hypothyroidism. AJR 135: 157-158

17 Computed Tomography and Magnetic Resonance Imaging

Pierre Schnyder and Gordon Gamsu

Introduction

The thymus is the major structure within the anterior mediastinum which is bounded by the sternum anteriorly, the heart, aorta, and great vessels posteriorly, and the lungs laterally. Imaging of the thymus was very difficult prior to the advent of computed tomography (CT) and magnetic resonance (MR) imaging. Buried in the mediastinal fat, the normal and minimally abnormal thymus is rarely seen on conventional chest radiographs or conventional tomograms after the first decade of life. Imaging of the thymus by pneumomediastinograms is possible, but has not gained widespread acceptance (Sone et al. 1980). The unique transaxial display and contrast resolution of CT and MR are ideally suited for imaging the thymus. Improvements in spatial resolution of CT scanners and MR imagers in the early 1980's have also enabled improved detection and evaluation of thymic abnormalities (Schnyder and Candardjis 1987).

CT and MR Anatomy

The CT and MR appearance and relative size of the normal thymus is closely related to the age of the patient being examined. At birth, the thymus weighs 10-15 g, increasing to its maximum weight of 25-35 g around puberty (Baron et al. 1982a; Heiberg et al. 1982; Francis et al. 1985; Moore et al. 1983). However, there is some variability in the size of a child's thymus, and a gland of up to 40 g can be found in about 5% of children or adolescents (Kendall et al. 1980; Siegelmann et al. 1984; Young and Turnbull 1931). The thymus does not appear to increase in size after the age of 3 years on CT or MR studies, explained by the more rapid enlargement of the thorax than of the thymus gland. The normal thymus can be demonstrated by CT and MR in 100% of subjects under the age of 20 years (Heiberg et al. 1982).

Originating from the left and right third pharyngeal pouches, the thymus has two distinct lobes. However, in the infant and young child this feature cannot be recognized on CT or MR images. The neonatal and childhood thymus appears to fill the mediastinum between the great vessels and aorta posteriorly and the sternum anteriorly (Fig. 1), making the detection of abnormality at this age difficult. The anterior aspect of each thymic lobe is molded to the inner anterior chest wall and the sternum. The lateral margins of the thymus are convex and can be seen on CT to impinge on the medial portions of the lungs. The CT density (attenuation) of the thymus in the very young is 20-40 Hounsfield units (HU) and therefore distinctly greater than fat, and almost equal to the density of muscle. In one study including children and adolescents, the CT density of the gland varied between 20 and 119 HU before intravenous infusion of contrast material and was slightly greater afterward (Heiberg et al. 1982). On MR images, the normal young thymus is homogeneous and appears less intense than subcutaneous fat or mediastinal fat. It is clearly seen in all children and infants. Its dimension and contour are similar in both MR and CT examinations.

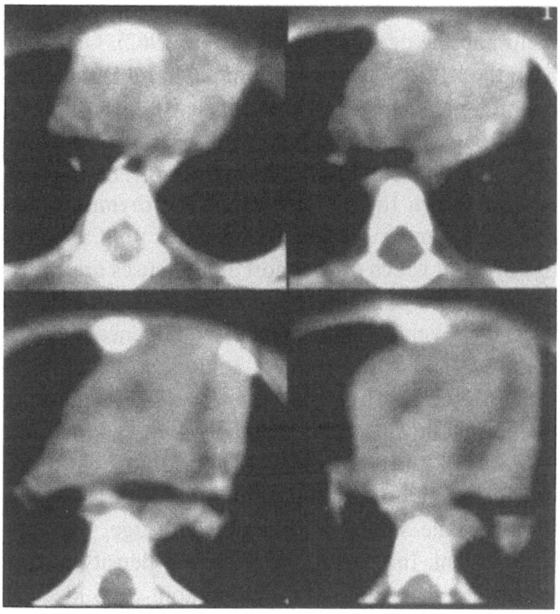

Fig. 1. Normal thymus. Serial CT scans in a 3-year-old show a normal thymus filling the anterior mediastinum and bulging to both sides

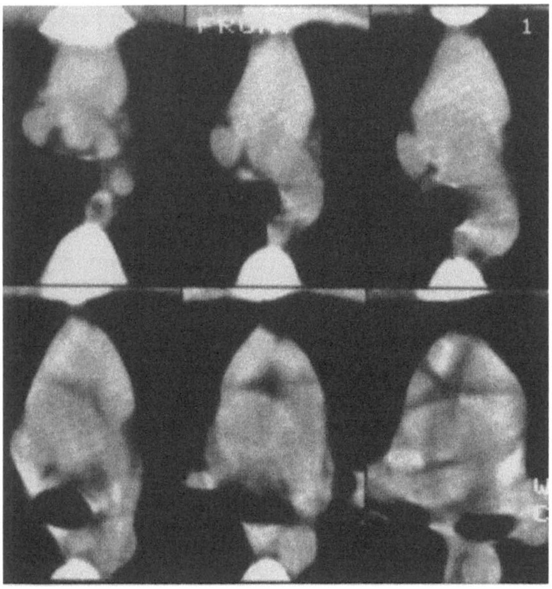

Fig. 2. Normal thymus. Serial CT scans show the normal thymus in a 9-year-old. The gland is more adult in shape and is beginning to assume a two-lobed appearance

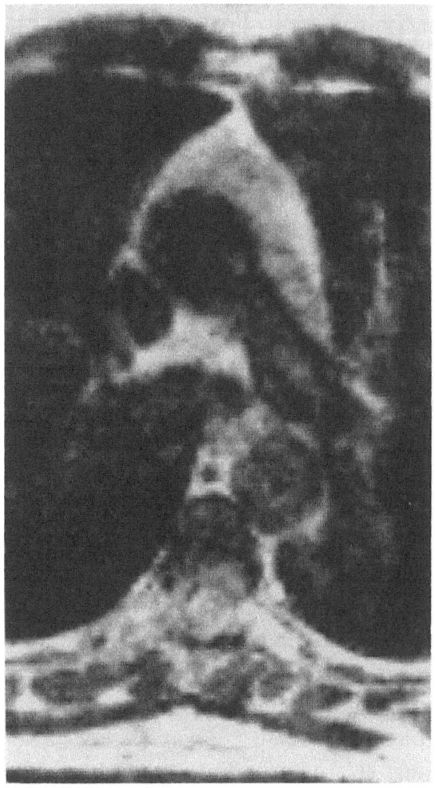

Fig. 3. Normal thymus. MR image (S. E. 500/28) in a young adult shows the thymus sharply contrasted with mediastinal fat. The dominant left lobe is more apparent than the right

With increasing age through adolescence, the thymus reaches a more predictable adult shape (Fig. 2). In the adult, the shape is either of two separate lobes or appears like an arrowhead. When two-lobed, each lobe may be oval, elliptical, triangular, or semilunar (Baron et al. 1982a). In general, the lateral margins are straight or concave. The two lobes usually remain in close proximity to the ascending aorta and main pulmonary artery. The thymus is surrounded by a fibrous capsule with attachments to the sternopericardial ligament and the pericardium (Rouvière 1962). On CT or MR, the left lobe is usually dominant and is more frequently seen than the right lobe (Fig. 3).

Both on CT and MR the thymus begins to show fatty involution from around the age of 20. The frequency with which the CT density of the thymus is less than water and more like fat increases until after the age of 50, at which time almost all thymuses are entirely fatty in composition (Dixon et al. 1981). On MR images, the thymus usually appears homogeneous and is readily visible in the younger adult against the background of mediastinal fat. The T_1 relaxation time of the normal thymus varies markedly with age (de Geer et al. 1985). It is usually over 1000 ms in the child and decreases to around 250 ms in middle age. The T_2 relaxation time similarly decreases with age, but to a lesser extent. In general, the hydrogen density of thymus is less than that of fat and on spin-echo MR images the thymus has a less intense signal than fat, irrespective of the recovery times used for the imaging sequences (Fig. 4).

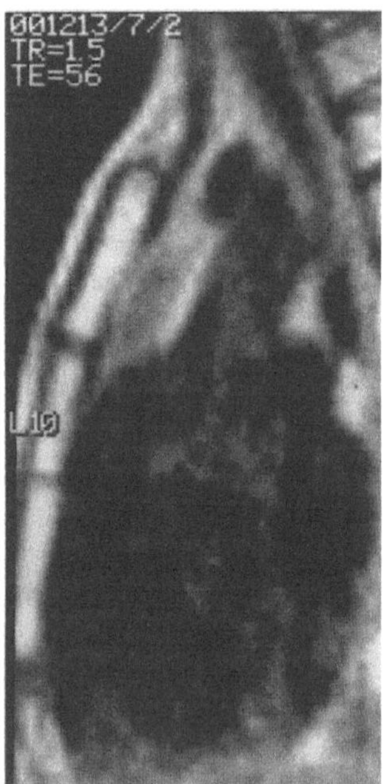

Fig. 4. Normal thymus. Sagittal MR image (S. E. 1500/56) shows the normal thymus clearly seen against mediastinal fat and the vessels that contain flowing blood, and thus no signal

Both on CT and MR the frequency with which the thymus is confidently indentified, decreases with age as the gland involutes. Even with modern high resolution CT scans and thin slices, the thymus is not seen in every elderly individual. While it is demonstrated on CT in all individuals under 30 years of age, it can only be seen in about three-quarters of subjects between 30 and 50 years old, and in less than half of normal subjects over 50 (Baron et al. 1982 a). On MR images, spatial resolution is poorer than on CT, but contrast resolution is better. Thus, in the adult the larger left lobe of the thymus is more readily seen than the smaller right lobe.

The measured size of the normal thymus, as displayed on CT or MR images, also depends on the age of the subject and decreases with time. On CT scans (when demonstrated), the anteroposterior length of the right thymic lobe measures about 2 cm (the left is about 1 cm longer) before adulthood and decreases to about 1.5 cm bilaterally by the age of 50. The transverse thickness of the normal thymus is about 1 cm in adolescents, and this dimension decreases to about 0.5 cm by 50 years of age (Fig. 5). On MR images, the thymus has slightly larger dimensions, probably because of motion artifacts. The left lobe, paralleling the aortic arch, is seen more frequently on MR than is the right lobe. The major difference between the MR and the CT appearance of the normal thymus is that MR can discriminate involuted thymus from mediastinal fat more readily than can CT.

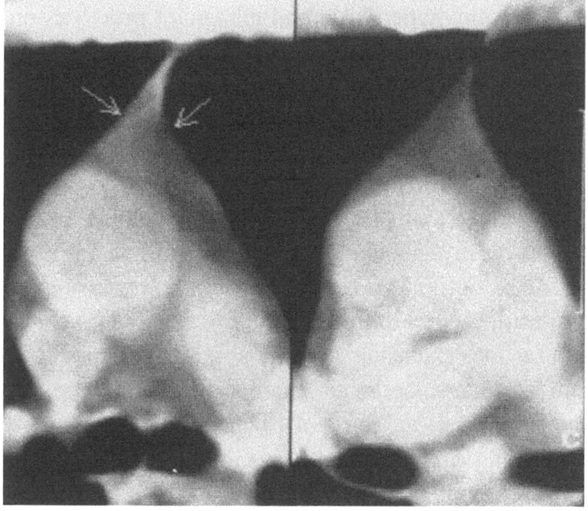

Fig. 5. Normal thymus. Thin-section CT scans in a 65-year-old show the normal involuted left and right lobes of the thymus

Technique

Computed Tomography

CT examination of the thymus is usually undertaken as an examination of the entire thorax. It should include scans extending from the lung apices to the depths of posterior pleural sulci. In general the patient is supine and the arms are extended above the head. The highest possible resolution should be used and rapid scan times are advised to decrease motion artifacts. Usually 1-cm contiguous scans are obtained. When necessary, the immediate site of the thymus (thoracic inlet to aortic root) can be rescanned with scans that are 5 mm thick or less. Radiographic contrast material is usually injected intravenously to opacify the mediastinal vessels and more easily localize the thymus. Abnormal thymic lesion may enhance their CT density after infusion of intravenous contrast material. However, this is not a specific indication of malignancy or of a specific disease. Enhancement with intravenous contrast material will more readily outline cystic and necrotic areas within thymic masses. In young children sedation or even general anesthesia may be necessary. However, thymic tumors are rare in the very young and CT or MR are not commonly undertaken in the young child for thymic abnormalities.

Magnetic Resonance

The best MR techniques for thymic imaging have yet to be determined. Most MR imaging of the thorax uses the spin-echo technique with variable recovery times (T_R) and echo times (T_E) (Gamsu et al. 1983; Schulthess et al. 1986). In general, a short recovery time ($\leqslant$0.5 s) will improve contrast between mediastinal fat and thymus, while a long T_R ($\geqslant$1.5 s) will improve signal-to-noise ratios and thus the clarity of the images. Although MR has the advantage of enabling imaging in sagittal or coronal planes, transaxial imaging remains the favored plane for thymic abnormalities. In most circumstances, cardiac gating has not been used for MR imaging of the thymus. Nevertheless, lesions low in the anterior mediastinal compartment will be more clearly displayed with cardiac gatings, and this modification is advised. The measurement of proton relaxation times is possible with MR scanning, but there are not yet sufficient data to demonstrate whether these measurement can characterize desease.

Indications for CT or MR in Thymic Disease

The role of transaxial imaging modalities is dependent on the patient's clinical status and the results of other imaging studies. In the case of thymoma or suspected thymoma, CT or MR can be used to detect an occult tumor. It can also suggest invasion of the mediastinum or adjacent structures by an invasive tumor. Detection of regional and distant metastases is most precisely defined by CT or MR. In other tumors or lymphoma, CT or MR are again the most precise methods of defining the extent of tumor. As with most mediastinal masses detected because of symptoms or as an incidental finding on a chest radiograph, CT can be useful to characterize the tumor.

At this time, CT has slightly better spatial resolution than MR and defines the wall and edges of lesions to a better extent. The MR characteristics of tumors give better contrast resolution than their CT density. However, at present, MR shows no clear advantages over CT. In the future, improvements in MR and the introduction of MR spectroscopy may open new fields of tissue characterization and response to treatment.

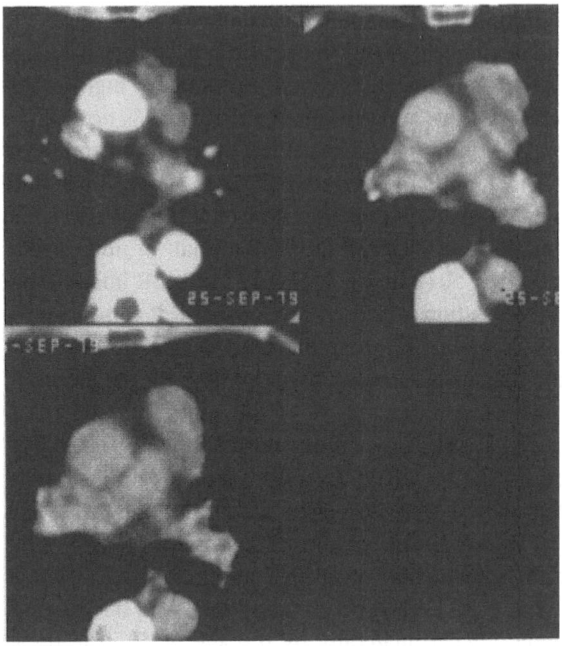

Fig. 6. Thymic hyperplasia. Selected CT scans in a 62-year-old woman with myasthenia gravis show hyperplasia of the thymus, confirmed by surgery and histology

Thymic Abnormalities

Thymic Hyperplasia

Thymic hyperplasia, also known as lymphofollicular hyperplasia, is characterized by an enlargement of the thymus with preservation of the gland's general architecture. The lymphoid follicles are hyperplastic and the thymic medulla is diffusely infiltrated with lymphocytes and plasma cells. The association of lymphofollicular hyperplasia with myasthenia gravis on the one hand and true thymic hyperplasia with thyrotoxicosis on the other hand is well known (Franken 1968; Gunn et al. 1964; Van Herle and Chopra 1971; Janssen et al. 1983).

In about half of patients with thymic hyperplasia, the gland will be sufficiently enlarged to produce an anterior mediastinal mass on chest radiographs. In virtually all patients the hyperplasia will be detected with CT. The long and short axes of each lobe are substantially increased when compared with age-matched normal individuals (Baron et al. 1982b; Walter 1983). The greater than normal thickness (short axis) of at least one lobe is more striking. In an occasional patient thymic hyperplasia will appear as a rounded mass on transverse axial CT images (Fig. 6). The CT density of thymic hyperplasia is similar to that of chest wall muscle and thus is similar to the normal young thymus. In some patients small calcifications are evident on high resolution CT images, and in others cystic degeneration of the germinal centers may produce an inhomogeneous appearance in the hyperplastic thymus.

The MR proton spin-echo appearance of thymic hyperplasia has not been described, but the resolution capabilities of units in the 0.3-1.5 T range should be sufficient to image thymic hyperplasia. From our knowledge of the intensity of the normal thymus, it should be relatively easy to image thymic hyperplasia with MR. Whether MR will be able to discriminate between thymic hyperplasia and malignant processes on the basis of relaxation times is still not known.

Thymoma

The role of CT or MR in thymomas is twofold. In patients with myasthenia gravis the demonstration of an otherwise occult mass may indicate the necessity for thymectomy. In addition, CT and MR may be able to demonstrate extension of a thymoma to the mediastinum or pleura, and thus change the therapeutic approach. About one-third of thymomas are malignant (Castleman and Norris 1949; Goldman et al. 1975; Baron et al. 1982b; Fon et al. 1982). The differentiation between benign thymoma and invasive thymoma may be difficult histologically. Thus, the prognosis and therapeutic approach are frequently determined by the extent of invasion of the thymoma, and the concept of extension through its fibrous capsule is of major importance. CT and MR have become the preferred modalities for the presurgical determination of this extension.

Noninvasive Thymoma

The majority of noninvasive thymomas appear on transaxial images as a round or oval, well-circumscribed mass arising within a lobe of the thymus (Fig. 7). Thymomas less than 2 cm diameter may appear as no more than a focal bulge on the contour of the normal thymus. The CT density (attenuation) of a thymoma is similar to that of a normal young thymus. It is usually unaffected or only slightly affected by the administration of intravenous contrast material. Intratumoral calcifications are found in about one-quarter of noninvasive thymomas (Baron et al. 1982b; Harper and Guyer 1965; Walter 1983). Their presence however, is not indicative of benignancy. Areas of cystic degeneration are also found within noninvasive thymoma and appear on CT as areas of lower density. Their appearance on CT is similar to the degenerative changes seen with thymic hyperplasia.

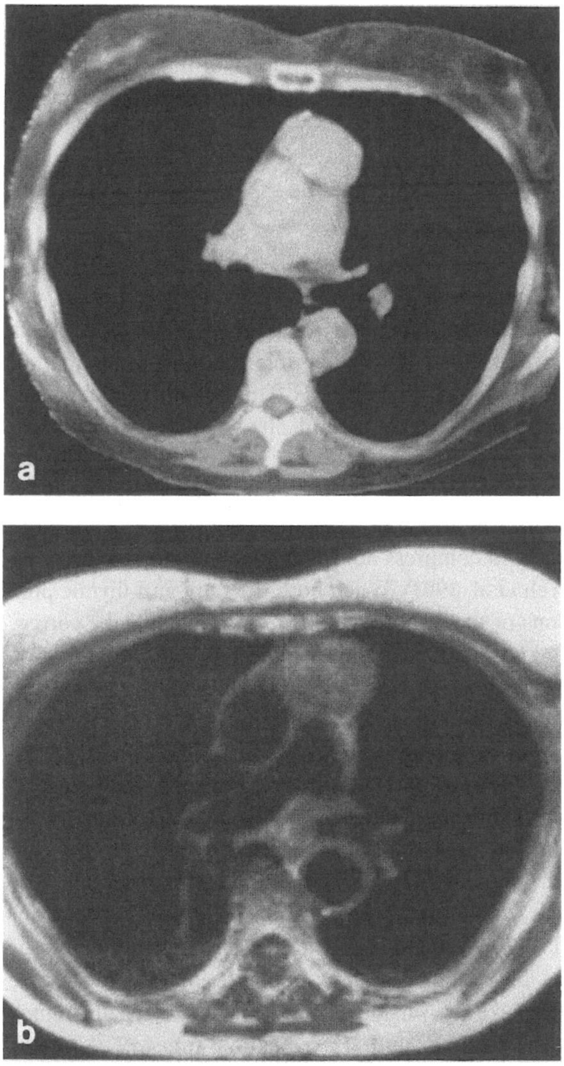

Fig. 7 a, b. Noninvasive thymoma in an asymptomatic 56-year-old woman. CT scans (**a**) demonstrates a well-circumscribed mass in front of the aorta and pulmonary artery. The mass appears well delineated from adjacent mediastinal fat. MR images (**b**) (S. E. 1500/28) shows the mass as inhomogeneous in intensity and not as well delineated from the adjacent soft tissues

Thymomas may occur anywhere along the thymolymphatic duct and are not exclusively limited to a preaortic site. They are commonest in an inverted U around the base of the heart, but can arise from the thoracic inlet to low in front of the pericardium (Walter 1983). They may even arise in the middle mediastinum. Thus, transaxial imaging for detection of thymoma must encompass the entire mediastinum.

Administration of intravenous contrast material only slightly enhances the CT density of the tumor but when combined with thin sections (less than 5 mm thick) CT can help to delineate the capsule of a tumor from pericardium, pleura, and mediastinal contents. The ability of CT to demonstrate the noninvasive nature of a thymoma is most important, as less than 2% of encapsulated thymomas will recur after surgery (Fechner 1969).

The published information on the MR demonstration of thymoma is limited. In the published cases the lesions were well demarcated within the anterior mediastinum (Gamsu et al. 1984; Ross et al. 1984). Thymomas had a short T_1 relaxation time, but still showed contrast from mediastinal fat at $T_R = 500$ ms. In another case that we have seen, similar imaging characteristics were found. Whether MR will be as good or better than CT in defining capsular invasion by thymomas, is not presently known.

Invasive Thymoma

CT is the most precise method available for the detection of local and regional spread of invasive thymoma. Invasive thymoma appears on CT as an irregular, ill-defined mass, usually within the anterior (prevascular) mediastinum. The hallmark of mediastinal invasion by this tumor is obliteration of the tissue planes defined by mediastinal fat (Baron et al. 1982b; Otto and Hüsselmann 1978). However, this may be difficult to detect and false-negative results on CT are not uncommon. Close attention must be paid to the mediastinal recesses that surround the aorta, pulmonary arteries, and superior vena cava.

The mediastinal organs most readily invaded by a thymoma are the trachea, great arteries and veins, the

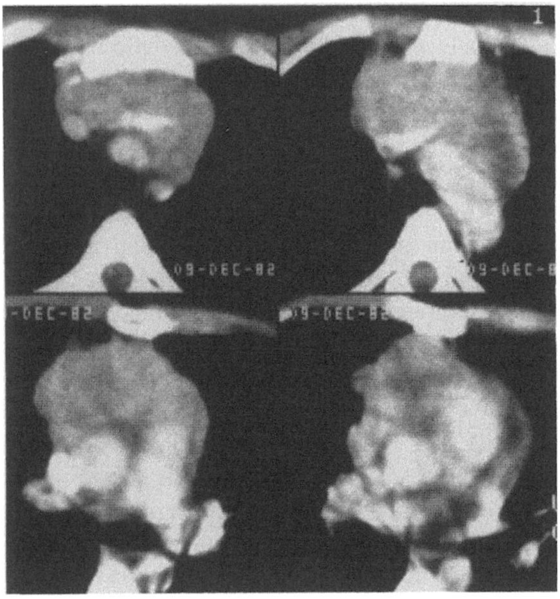

Fig. 8. Invasive thymoma. Serial CT scans show a large anterior mediastinal mass displaying and surrounding the great arteries and veins. The tumor also extends to the pericardium

mediastinal pleura, and pericardium (Fig. 8). Once the tumor reaches the pleural surface it can extend anteriorly around the chest wall, posteriorly along the mediastinal pleura (Zerhouni et al. 1982), or inferiorly, through the diaphragm (Scatarige et al. 1985). An alternative mode of pleural extension is across the pleura by droplet spread, without continuity with the primary tumor (McCrea and Maslar 1982).

CT is the best nonsurgical method of detecting extension to the pleura and transpleural spread (Zerhouni et al. 1982). CT or MR examination of the thorax in patients with suspected invasive thymoma should thus always encompass the entire thorax to the most inferior extent of the posterior diaphragmatic sulci (a favored site for transpleural seeding of tumor).

Invasive thymoma can extend directly across the pleura to the pulmonary parenchyma, although this is less common than mediastinal or pleural spread. Extrathoracic extension of invasive thymoma is rare. Nevertheless, invasion through the diaphragm to the abdomen or through the aortic or esophageal hiatuses have been reported (Siegelmann et al. 1984). Again, CT is the most sensitive noninvasive method of detecting transdiaphragmatic spread of tumor. When diaphragmatic deposits of tumor are found with CT or MR, the examination should be extended to include the abdomen.

The CT density of invasive thymoma is in the 35-60 HU range and not specific for this tumor. The CT appearance is usually more heterogeneous than noninvasive thymoma, although this finding is not by itself indicative of an invasive neoplasm. Areas of tumor necrosis are usually more clearly demonstrated after intravenous bolus injection or infusion of contrast material. The tumor usually becomes denser as it enhances, while the necrotic areas do not change in density. The contrast between the tumor, mediastinal fat, and vessels is also increased.

On CT, intratumoral calcifications and areas of cystic degeneration are equally common in invasive and noninvasive thymoma. The only definitive diagnostic indications of invasive disease are detection of regional or distant metastases (Baron et al. 1982b; Gamsu 1983; Moore et al. 1982). The MR appearance of invasive thymoma have not been published. In two cases we have observed that the tumor was readily delineated from mediastinal fat. Neither of our cases had the short T_1 relaxation time reported once in the literature (Ross et al. 1984).

Thymolipoma

Thymolipoma (lipothymoma) is a usually benign, anterior mediastinal mass arising from the thymus. It has a well-formed fibrous capsule that surrounds mature fat containing thymic rests. This lesion produces relatively few symptoms, and 50% of thymolipomas are first detected from chest radiographs as an asymptomatic mediastinal mass (Peake and Zeigler, 1977; Teplick et al. 1973). They may, however, reach a large size and compress adjacent vessels, and even the heart (Yeh et al. 1983). When both the fatty and thymic portions of the tumor are shown on CT scans, the correct diagnosis can be strongly suspected. The CT density of the fatty areas will be -100 to -60 HU while the thymic components are between $+30$ and $+160$ HU. In our experience, the thymic components may not be very evident, and the tumor cannot be distinguished on its imaging characteristics from a mediastinal lipoma. The prevascular site of origin is a clue to the correct diagnosis. As with thymomas, tumoral calcification can be found (Peake and Zeigler, 1977; Teplick et al. 1973; Walter 1983). The MR findings of thymolipoma have not been described. Presumably, the tumor will have the imaging characteristics of a fatty tumor with short T_1 and T_2 relaxation times. The tumor should appear intense of T_1-weighted images.

Myasthenia Gravis

The role of CT or MR in the evaluation of patients with myasthenia gravis will depend on the approach to this clinical problem in any given institution. A thymoma or thymic hyperplasia is found in about 10%-20% of patients with myasthenia gravis and one-third to one-half of these thymomas will be invasive (Batata et al. 1974; Goldman et al. 1975; Moore et al. 1982; Rosai and Levine 1976; Wechsler and Olanow 1980). When chest radiographs demonstrate an anterior mass, CT or MR should be obtained to determine the extent of the abnormality and detect possible occult metastases. If no mass is evident and thymectomy will be performed routinely, CT or MR are probably not indicated. Otherwise, we would advocate CT or MR to detect small thymomas that could be invasive and are not evident on standard chest radiographs. In the clinical context of myasthenia gravis, CT is virtually 100% sensitive and relatively specific in detecting small thymomas (Moore et al. 1982). Contiguous thin sections should be obtained to show thymic hyperplasia or thymoma. In most circumstances the demonstration of thymoma will indicate the need for surgery, even though the prognosis for patients with myasthenia gravis is less good with a thymoma than without one (Gamsu 1983). Removal of the tumor does not necessarily improve the prognosis.

Hodgkin's Disease and Lymphoma

Primary Hodgkin's disease of the thymus is rare. The CT appearance has only been briefly reported (Baron et al. 1982b; Federle and Callen 1979; Walter 1983; Lindfors et al. 1985); and the MR findings are not yet documented. The commoner CT finding is of a well-defined mass in the anterior mediastinum that enhances slightly after intravenous injection of contrast material. Regional lymphadenopathy may be evident on CT. In one case, the tumor had undergone cystic degeneration providing a large multicystic mediastinum mass, with no other specific findings (Federle and Callen 1979). In the usual clinical circumstances, CT cannot specifically diagnose a mass as Hodgkin's disease and CT is obtained to display the extent and stage of the abnormality. CT is by far the most precise method of defining lymphadenopathy at other sites within the mediastinum and thorax.

Although the MR imaging characteristics of thymic lymphoma have not been described, we have studied several cases of mediastinal lymphoma. These neoplasms have a T_1 relaxation time that is shorter than carcinoma of the lung, but longer than inflammatory processes. They have an MR intensity that is similar to muscle and readily contrasts with mediastinal fat. It is unlikely that with conventional proton spin-echo MR imaging, we will be able to discriminate between lymphoma and other causes of a mediastinal mass.

Other Neoplasms

Several other tumors can arise within or around the thymus. The commonest of these are germ cell and carcinoid tumors. The germ cell tumors arise from primitive germ cells, and when these are neoplastic, they produce benign or malignant teratomas, dermoid cysts, embryonal carcinomas, seminomas, endodermal sinus tumors, and choriocarcinomas. Some 80% of the germ cell tumors are benign and consist of dermoids and teratomas. The cystic and fatty components of these tumors are readily identified on CT scans and presumably MR images, but these are not specific for benignancy. Thin-walled cystic teratomas are, however, usually benign and although they do not invade adjacent structures, CT can demonstrate compression of adjacent structures and organs by large benign teratomas.

The more malignant of these germinal cell tumors have all the CT and presumably MR characteristics of invasive thymomas. They may have low density (intensity) necrotic areas, areas of cystic degeneration, and even intratumoral calcifications. They can invade the mediastinum, pleura, and pericardium and produce a CT or MR appearance indistinguishable from invasive thymoma. The only clearly differentiating feature is that they do not have the propensity for transpleural droplet spread. Seminomas are similar in imaging characteristics to the other germinal cell tumors (Levitt et al. 1984; Livesay et al. 1979; Walter 1983). They may be inhomogeneous, contain cystic areas, and calcifications within the tumor are frequent (Fig. 9). En-

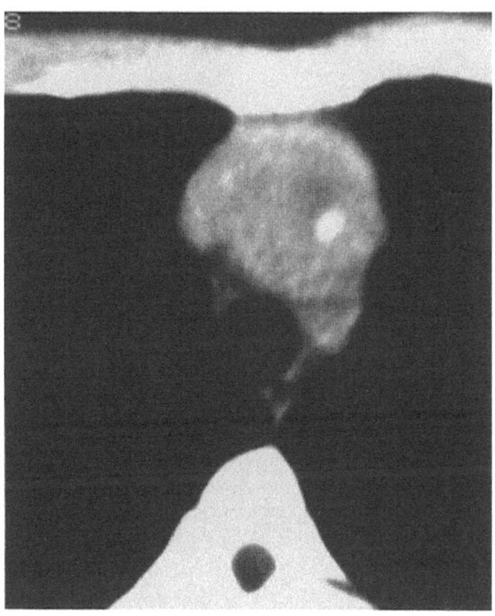

Fig. 9. Thymic seminoma. CT scan demonstrate an anterior mediastinal mass with low density areas representing necrosis and calcification. Surgery revealed a thymic seminoma

hancement of the solid portions of the tumor after infusion of contrast material occurs, but is not diagnostically specific. Invasion by this malignant tumor is diagnosed with CT and MR images by obliteration of tissue planes and replacement of mediastinal fat by tumor. Vascular invasion may be seen on CT after infusion of contrast material, and more readily with MR images.

Carcinoid tumors arising in the thymus are rare and often associated with multiple endocrine neoplasia (MEN) syndromes types I and II (Birnberg et al. 1982). About 40% of these patients have Cushing's syndrome, but none have been reported with a carcinoid syndrome. Thymic carcinoids are both locally aggressive and readily metastasize to distant sites. Their CT findings are similar to invasive thymoma, and superior vena cava obstruction is a surprisingly common finding. The conventional chest radiograph may be normal and the thymus should be evaluated with CT or MR, as a site for a tumor causing an unexplained Cushing's syndrome.

Thymic Cysts

True or congenital thymic cysts are exceedingly rare (Rosai and Levine 1976); most cysts within the thymus are degenerative. They are found within tumors such as thymomas, or can occur after radiation therapy for Hodgkin's disease (Baron et al. 1981). Congenital thymic cysts are commonest in the usual site of the thymus, but can occur anywhere along the thymolymphatic duct. Most thymic cysts are asymptomatic and seen on a chest radiograph or CT scans as an unexpected finding. Their CT density is usually in the range of water (0-15 HU), but may be higher or lower (Fig. 10; Siegelmann et al. 1984; Walter 1983). Increased density of up to 50 HU represents hemorrhage or cellular debris within the cysts. Low values of up to −30 HU indicate cholesterol within the cyst. Although the MR characteristics of congenital thymic cysts have not been described, the known feature of these types of cysts would be apparent. Thymic cysts should appear intense on both T_1- and T_2-weighted images. These findings were seen in the one case we have observed.

On CT, the wall of a thymic cyst is thin (1-2 mm) and sharply defined. It may be enhanced by a bolus of intravenous contrast material. Most cysts are unilocular, but multilocular cysts have also been described (Wychulis et al. 1971). These cysts are not uncommonly surrounded by a small amount of normal thymic tissue.

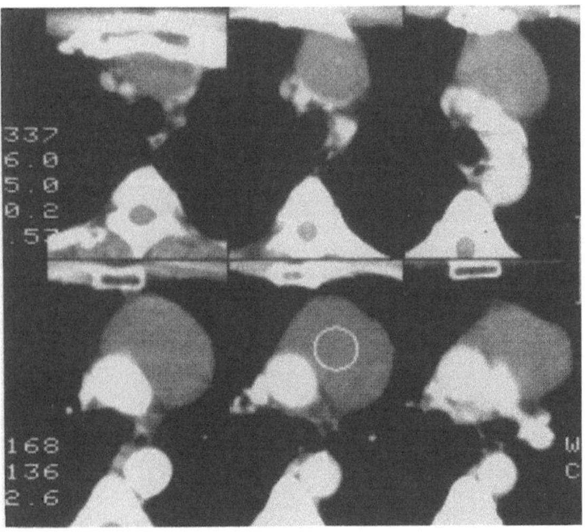

Fig. 10. Thymic cyst. A series of CT scans show a large, low density (6 HU), thin-walled structure within the anterior mediastinum. Although this lesion has all the characteristics of a thymic cyst, cystic degeneration of a thymoma could look identical

References

Baron RL, Sagel SS, Baglan RJ (1981) Thymic cysts following radiation therapy for Hodgkin's disease. Radiology 141: 593-597

Baron RL, Lee JKT, Sagel SS, Peterson RR (1982a) Computed tomography of the normal thymus. Radiology 142: 121-125

Baron RL, Lee JKT, Sagel SS, Levitt RG (1982b) Computed tomography of the abnormal thymus. Radiology 142: 127-134

Batata MA, Martini N, Huvos AG, Aguilar RI, Beattie EJ (1974) Thymomas: clinicopathologic features, therapy and prognosis. Cancer 34: 389-396

Birnberg FA, Webb WR, Selch MT, Gamsu G, Goodman PC (1982) Thymic carcinoid tumors with hyperparathyroidism. AJR 139: 1001-1004

Castleman B, Norris EH (1949) Pathology of the thymus in myasthenia gravis: a study of 35 cases. Medicine (Baltimore) 28: 27-58

De Geer G, Webb WR, Gamsu G (1986) Normal thymus: assessment with MR and CT Radiology 158: 313-317

Dixon AK, Hilton CJ, Williams GT (1981) Computed tomography and histological correlation of thy thymic remnant. Clin Radiol 32: 255-257

Fechner RE (1969) Recurrence of noninvasive thymomas. Report of four cases and review of the literature. Cancer 23: 1423-1427

Federle MP, Callen PW (1979) Cystic Hogdkin's lymphoma of the thymus: computed tomography appearance. J Comput Assist Tomogr 3: 542-544

Fon GT, Bein ME, Mancuso AA, Keesey JC, Lupetin AR, Wong WS (1982) Computed tomography of the anterior mediastinum in myasthenia gravis. Radiology 142: 135-141

Francis IR, Glazer GM, Bookstein FL, Gross BH (1985) The thymus: reexamination of age-related changes in size and shape. AJR 145: 249-254

Franken EA Jr (1968) Radiologic evidence of thymic enlargement in Graves's disease. Radiology 91: 20-22
Gamsu G (1983). Thymoma. In: Moss AA, Gamsu G, Genant HK (eds) Computed tomography of the body. Saunders, Philadelphia, pp 247-249
Gamsu G, Webb WR, Sheldon P, Kaufman L, Crooks LE, Birnberg FA, Goodman P, Hinchcliffe WA, Hedgecock M (1983) Nuclear magnetic resonance imaging of the thorax. Radiology 147: 473-480
Gamsu G, Stark DD, Webb WR, Moore EH, Sheldon PE (1984) Magnetic resonance imaging of benign mediastinal masses. Radiology 151: 709-713
Goldman AJ, Herrmann C Jr, Keesey JC Jr, Mulder DG, Brown WJ (1975) Myasthenia gravis and invasive thymoma: a 20 years experience. Neurology 25: 1021-1025
Gunn A, Michie W, Irvine WJ (1964) The thymus in thyroid disease. Lancet 2: 776-778
Harper RAK, Guyer PB (1965) The radiological features of thymic tumours. A review of sixty-five cases. Clin Radiol 16: 97-105
Heiberg E, Wolverson MK, Sundaram M, Nouri S (1982) Normal thymus: CT characteristics in subjects under age 20. AJR 138: 491-494
Janssen RS, Kaye AD, Lisak RP, Schatz NJ, Arger PA, Savino PJ (1983) Radiologic evaluation of the mediastinum in myasthenia gravis. Neurology 33: 534-539
Kendall MD, Johnson HRM, Singh J (1980) The weight of the human thymus gland at necropsy. J Anat 131: 483-497
Levitt RG, Husband JE, Glazer HS (1984) CT of primary germ-cell tumors of the mediastinum. AJR 142: 73-78
Lindfors KK, Meyer JE, Dedrick CG, Hassell LA, Harris NL (1985) Thymic cysts in mediastinal Hogdkin's disease. Radiology 156: 37-41
Livesay JJ, Mink JH, Fee HJ, Bein ME, Sample WF, Mulder DG (1979) The use of computed tomography to evaluate suspected mediastinal tumors. Ann Thorac Surg 27: 305-311
McCrea ES, Maslar JA (1982) Thymoma with distant intrathoracic implants, with CT confirmation. Cancer 50: 1612-1614
Moore AV, Korobkin M, Powers B, Olanow W, Ravin CE, Putman CE, Breiman RS, Ram PC (1982) Thymoma detection by mediastinal CT: patients with myasthenia gravis. AJR 138: 217-222
Moore AV, Korobkin M, Olanow W, Heaston DK, Ram PC, Dunnick NR, Silverman PM (1983) Age-related changes in the thymus gland: CT-pathologic correlation. AJR 141: 241-246
Otto HF, Hüsselmann H (1978) Klinisch-pathologische Studie zur Klassifikation und Prognose von Thymustumoren. I. Histologische und ultrastrukturpathologische Untersuchungen. Z Krebsforsch 91: 81-102
Peake JB, Zeigler MG (1977) Thymolipoma: report of three cases. Am Surg 43; 477-479
Rosai J, Levine GD (1976) Tumors of the thymus. In: Altas of tumor pathology. Armed Forces Institute of Pathology, Washington DC, p 31
Ross JS, O'Donovan PB, Novoa R, Mehta A, Buonocore E, MacIntyre WJ, Golish JA, Ahmad M (1984) Magnetic resonance fo the chest: initial experience with imaging and in vivo T1 and T2 calculations. Radiology 152: 95-101
Rouvière H (1962) Anatomie humaine descriptive et topographique. Masson, Paris, p 465
Scatarige JC, Fishman EK, Zerhouni EA, Siegelman SS (1985) Transdiaphragmatic extension of invasive thymoma. AJR 144: 31-35
Schnyder P, Candardjis G (1987) Computed tomography of thymic abnormalities. Eur J Radiol 7: 107-113
von Schulthess GK, McMurdo K, Tscholakoff D, De Geer G, Gamsu G, Higgins CB (1986) Mediastinal masses: MR imaging. Radiology 158: 289-296
Siegelmann SS, Scott WW Jr, Baker RR, Fishman EK (1984) CT of the thymus. In: Siegelmann SS (ed) Computed tomography of the chest. Churchill Livingstone, Edinburgh, pp 233-271
Sone S, Higashihara T, Morimoto S, Yokota K, Ikezoe J, Masaoka A, Monden Y, Kagotani T (1980) Normal anatomy of thymus and anterior mediastinum by pneumomediastinography. AJR 134: 81-89
Teplick JG, Nedwich A, Haskin ME (1973) Roentgenographic features of thymolipoma. AJR 117: 873-877
Van Herle AJ, Chopra JJ (1971) Thymic hyperplasia in Graves' disease. J Clin Endocrinol Metab 32: 140-146
Walter E (1983) Computertomographische Diagnostik des Thymus. In: Jahrbuch der Schweizerischen Gesellschaft für Radiologie und Nuklearmedizin. Huber, Bern, pp 25-34
Wechsler AS, Olanow CW (1980) Myasthenia gravis. Surg Clin North Am 60: 931-945
Wychulis AR, Payne WS, Clagett OT, Woolner LB (1971) Surgical treatment of mediastinal tumors. J Thorac Cardiovasc Surg 62: 379-392
Yeh HC, Gordon A, Kirschner PA, Cohen BA (1983) Computed tomography and sonography of thymolipoma. AJR 140: 1131-1133
Young M, Turnbull HM (1931) An analysis of the data collected by the Status Lymphaticus Investigation Committee. J Pathol Bacteriol 34: 213-258
Zerhouni EA, Scott WW Jr, Baker RR, Wharam MD, Siegelmann SS (1982) Invasive thymomas: diagnosis and evaluation by computed tomography. J Comput Assist Tomogr 6: 92-100

18 Methods for Neurophysiological Investigation

Joseph A. M. Bergmans

Abbreviations

ACh, acetylcholine; antiChE, anticholinesterases; EMG, electromyography; ELS, Eaton-Lambert syndrome; MAP, muscle action potential; MG, myasthenia gravis; NERA, nerve evoked repetitive activity; NM, neuromuscular; PTE, post-tetanic exhaustion; PTF, post-tetanic facilitation.

Clinical neurophysiology occupies a key position in the diagnosis and the management of MG. Jolly first described the abnormal fatigability of the contractile muscle response during repetitive stimulation (the so-called myasthenic reaction), with recovery after a short period of rest, in 1895. Harvey and Masland (1941a, b) elaborated the techniques to assess NM function in MG with evoked EMG, and Harvey et al. (1942) were the first to describe the changes occurring after thymectomy.

In this book centred around surgery of the thymus, this chapter will illustrate from a practical standpoint the role of clinical neurophysiology in the management of a patient with MG. We will limit ourselves to the classical autoimmune form of MG, which is the only form where the indication for thymectomy is presently recognized. The newly described congenital myasthenic syndromes (Engel et al. 1981; Engel 1984) and ELS (Lambert et al. 1961; Lambert and Rooke 1965; Engel 1984) will be mentioned only briefly when problems of differential diagnosis are involved.

Diagnosis of Mysthenia Gravis

In the daily clinical setting, evoked EMG techniques represent the most practical way to confirm the diagnosis and to follow a myasthenic pathology. More specialized techniques (single muscle fibre EMG), or techniques studying specific muscle groups not accressible with evoked EMG testing will also be described.

Nerve Stimulation Techniques (Evoked EMG)

The diagnosis of MG rests on the neurophysiological demonstration of a partial NM block in given muscle groups. This demonstration requires the activation, with an electrical stimulus, of a set of motor nerve fibres, while recording the activity of the corresponding muscles: this is currently feasible for proximal and distal limb muscles, the orbicularis oculi muscle (Botelho et a. 1952), the platysma muscle (Krarup 1977) and the trapezius muscle (Schumm and Stohr 1984. Some muscle groups frequently involved in MG (external eye muscles and pharyngeal muscles) are not accessible to evoked EMG testing.

Response to Single Activation

The existence of a partial NM block at rest in a given proportion of muscle fibres is demonstrated by the lower amplitude of the MAP in response to supramaximal nerve stimulation, and by the fact that this MAP is enhanced by the administration of antiChE (Harvey et al. 1941a). In distal hand muscles, a lower amplitude of the MAP is only demonstrated statistically (Lambert et al. 1961; Borenstein and Desmedt 1973); in proximal muscles, though, there is a clear separation between the normal population and a population of patients with MG (Borenstein and Desmedt 1973; Desmedt 1981, 1983). Due to this partial block existing at rest, myasthenic muscles frequently display EMG patterns analogous to those seen in myopathies, namely motor unit potentials of low amplitude, of short duration, and with an increased incidence of polyphasic forms (Oosterhuis et al. 1972). This can occasionally lead to an erroneous diagnosis. The functional nature of these alterations is demonstrated by the fact than they can be reversed by antiChE (Pinelli 1978) or by cooling the muscle (Desmedt 1981, 1983), a procedure which decreases the NM block (Borenstein and Desmedt 1975).

Response to Repetitive Stimulation

During repetitive stimulation, myasthenic muscles show typical decrementing responses, similar to those seen in curarized muscles (Harvey and Masland

1941b; Harvey et al. 1941a), which can be explained by the relative emptying of presynaptic stores of transmitter by the stimulation. A two-store model can account for the observed data: the nerve impulse liberates a given amount of transmitter from a small store of immediately releasable ACh, and this store is refilled from a large main presynaptic store by a process called mobilization; the large store is then refilled by synthesis of new transmitter (Bergmans et al. 1972, 1973a, b).

Programs of short-lasting repetitive stimulation allow the study of the kinetics of release of transmitter from the store of immediately releasable ACh, while programs of long-lasting repetitive stimulation study the kinetics of release from the main presynaptic store. Both kinds of stimulation programs can be used for diagnostic purposes.

Short Trains of Volleys

The typical pattern seen in MG during short trains (up to 40 nerve volleys) of repetitive stimulation is a gradual decrease of the amplitude of the responses, followed by a plateau from the fourth or fifth response onwards (Harvey and Masland 1941b). Evoked EMG techniques were standardized by Desmedt (1961, 1966, 1973a), who recommended a frequency of 2-5/s to detect a NM block, since this frequency corresponds to the interval of maximal depression on double-shock stimulation (Harvey and Masland 1941b; Desmedt 1966, 1973a). The decrease of the responses is formulated either by the percentage ratio of the amplitude (or area, see below) of the fifth to the first MAP, or by subtracting this percentage from 100%, which yields the so-called decrement.

In normal subjects, a facilitation of the amplitude of the MAP can be observed during short trains of volleys, specially at higher frequencies of stimulation: the increase in amplitude is accompanied by a decrease in duration (the area remaining practically constant), indicating that it is due to a better synchronization of the action potential in the muscle fibres (Harvey et al. 1941a; Desmedt 1958); hence the name of pseudofacilitation. This phenomenon may lead to an incorrect assessment of the state of NM transmission in patients with MG, as shown in Fig. 1, where an important facilitation of amplitude is present at higher frequencies; however, at all frequencies, the area of the MAP shows the typical decremental pattern of MG.

Ideally, therefore, the area of the MAP should be used for decrement measurements. During stimulation at 3/s, normal subjects may present decrements of up to 20% (10% when using amplitude measurements: Desmedt and Borenstein 1976), particularly at the level of the hand muscles. A decrement below this limit

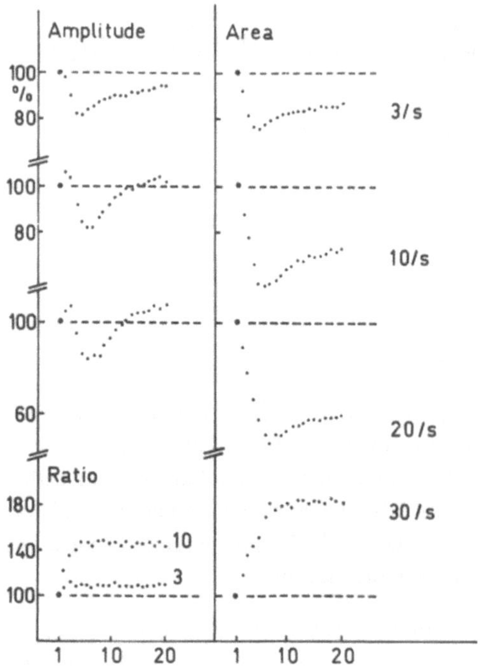

Fig. 1. Pseudofacilitation in MG: responses to short trains of 20 volleys at 3, 10, 20 and 30/s in an untreated patient. Supramaximal stimulation of the median nerve at the wrist, recording in thenar muscles. *Upper part:* amplitude and area of individual responses (trains at 3, 10 and 20/s). *Lower part:* ratio of the amplitude to the area in trains at 3, 10 and 30/s

should thus always be confirmed with sensitization tests (see below). Amplitude measurements should be included in the evaluation, however: in some muscles of patients with MG a decrement in amplitude may be seen with no decrement in area, because components of the MAP (in particular the peak) are shifted from the early to the later part of the MAP. In extreme cases, neither a change in amplitude nor a change in area of the MAP is observed, but simply an increase in latency (see Fig. 2) which corresponds to a triggering of the MAP on later points of the end-plate potential (see Fig. 9.1 in Sanders 1983). This phenomenon may be of diagnostic value when it is observed at low frequencies in the absence of other signs. It is never seen at 3/s in normal subjects.

Corresponding to the most prevalent clinical picture of MG, in which involvement of limb muscles is most pronounced proximally, decrements in short volleys at 3/s are usually more pronounced in these muscles (Özdemir and Young 1976; Desmedt and Borenstein 1976; Borenstein and Desmedt 1973; Desmedt 1981, 1983). However, this is not a general rule, and occasionally patients with MG may be seen with no decrement in proximal muscles and clear decrements in hand muscles (Fig. 3), corresponding to a clinical pic-

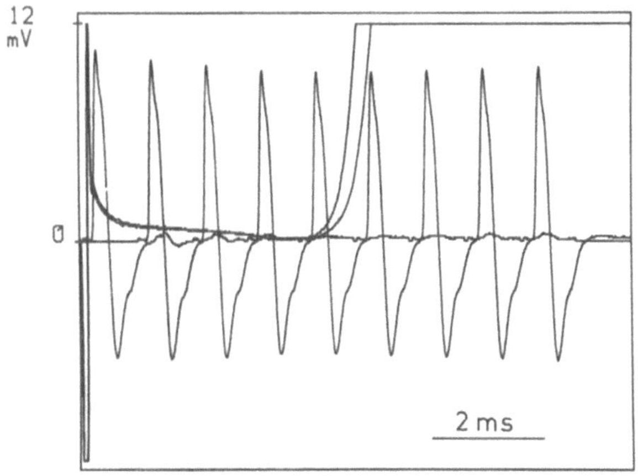

Fig. 2. Change in latency of the MAP in short train of volleys at 3/s in an untreated patient with MG. Stimulation of right median nerve, recording in thenar muscle. Superimposed records: (a) on a slow time base, the nine responses in the train (amplitude calibration on left), (b) on a fast time base (time calibration below) and at higher amplification, the response to the first and the fifth volley in the train: only the ascending limb of these responses in visible

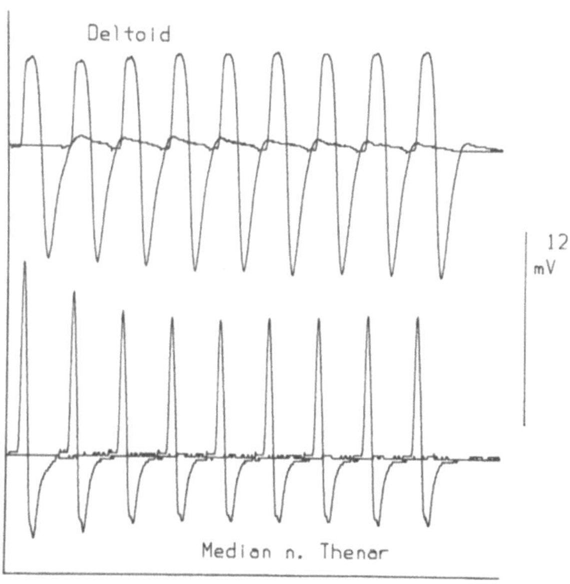

Fig. 3. Responses to a short train of volleys at 3/s in the deltoid muscle and median nerve-innervated thenar muscles in the same untreated MG patient

ture of predominantly, distal involvement (see also Denys et al. 1979). We have seen a patient with MG whose only complaint was a unilateral foot drop: in this subject decrements were present only in the corresponding anterior tibial muscle. The neurophysiological examination should thus be guided by the clinical data, especially in a disease with such a polymorphic presentation: for every patient an individualized diagnostic approach is needed.

Changes in muscle temperature markedly influence the NM block (Borenstein and Desmedt 1973, 1975; Stålberg 1980; Stålberg and Sanders 1983), which is reduced with the low muscle temperatures frequently present in unheated muscles during routine clinical examinations. Adequate control of muscle temperature is thus mandatory.

If stimulation at 3/s is adequate to disclose a NM block, higher frequencies of stimulation have to be included in the diagnostic programs to identify particular types of NM block. In this situation, measurements of the area of the MAP become mandatory, since pseudofacilitation phenomena are more marked (Fig. 1). Prominent facilitation is disclosed with high frequencies of stimulation in ELS, the two other, diagnostic features being the low amplitude of the MAP to single activation and the presence of a decrement at 3/s (Lambert et al. 1961; Lambert and Rooke 1965). Patients with MG may present at some stage of their disease a decrease in amplitude of the MAP to single activation, together with the appearance of facilitation phenomena at high frequencies of stimulation (Takamori and Gutmann 1971; Boiardi et al. 1979). On the other hand, cases of MG have been described with low amplitude of the MAP (as seen in ELS), and no facilitation at high frequencies of stimulation: instead, the MAP decreases during repetitive stimulation at all frequencies, and the minimal level is attained only around the 20th response. A coexisting other defect

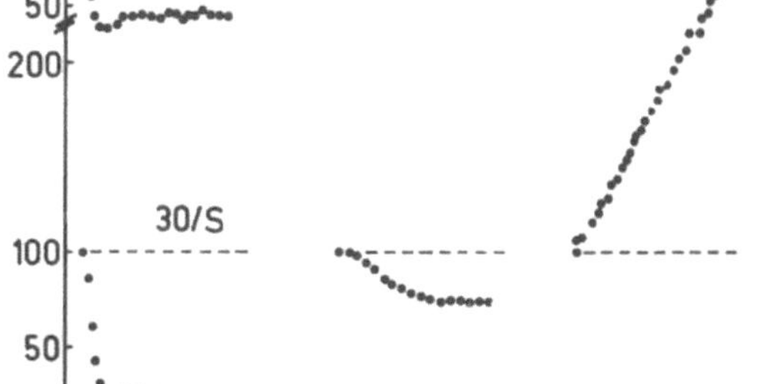

Fig. 4 a–c. Responses to trains of 40 volleys at 3, 10 and 30/s in median nerve - innervated thenar muscles. **a** In a patient with classical MG: **b** in a patient with myasthenia with assumed deficient mobilization of transmitter, **c** in a patient with ELS. Amplitude of initial response: **a** 10.5 mV, **b** 2 mV, **c** 1.5 mV. All patients untreated

has been assumed in these cases, possibly deficient mobilization of transmitter from the main presynaptic store to the store of immediately releasable transmitter (Bergmans et al. 1975a). Figure 4 illustrates tests at 3, 10 and 30/s in one case each of typical MG, ELS, and this latter form of atypical MG.

Long-Lasting Repetitive Stimulation

In patients with MG (Bergmans et al. 1972, 1973a) and in normal curarized subjects (Bergmans et al. 1976), long-lasting repetitive stimulation produces an important depletion of the transmitter stores, with slow recovery, which can be exploited to devise sensitization procedures to detect NM block in muscles not disclosing a decrement at rest (Desmedt 1966, 1973a, 1981, 1983; Desmedt and Borenstein 1976; Borenstein and Desmedt 1973).

Figure 5 illustrates the gradual decline of responses observed when a myasthenic muscle is stimulated at 2,4 and 8/s for several minutes (Bergmans et al. 1972; see also Johns et al. 1956). At long intervals, a plateau is reached which corresponds to equilibrium between the quantities of transmitter mobilized from the main presynaptic store towards the store of immediately releasable ACh and the quantities of transmitter which enter the main store by synthesis of new transmitter. This terminal plateau level is not observed in the congenital myasthenic syndrome with deficient synthesis of transmitter (Hart et al. 1979; Engel et al. 1981). When a repetitive series is interrupted, as at point 2 in Fig. 5e, the decrement present at rest remains temporarily increased for a prolonged period, indicating slow recovery of the normal quantities of transmitter in the main presynaptic store. A sensitization test relies on the demonstration of this higher value of decrement after conditioning with repetitive stimulation.

Depletion of transmitter in the main presynaptic store can also be evoked by short periods of high-frequency stimulation, or by its physiological equivalent, namely a period of maximal voluntary innervation

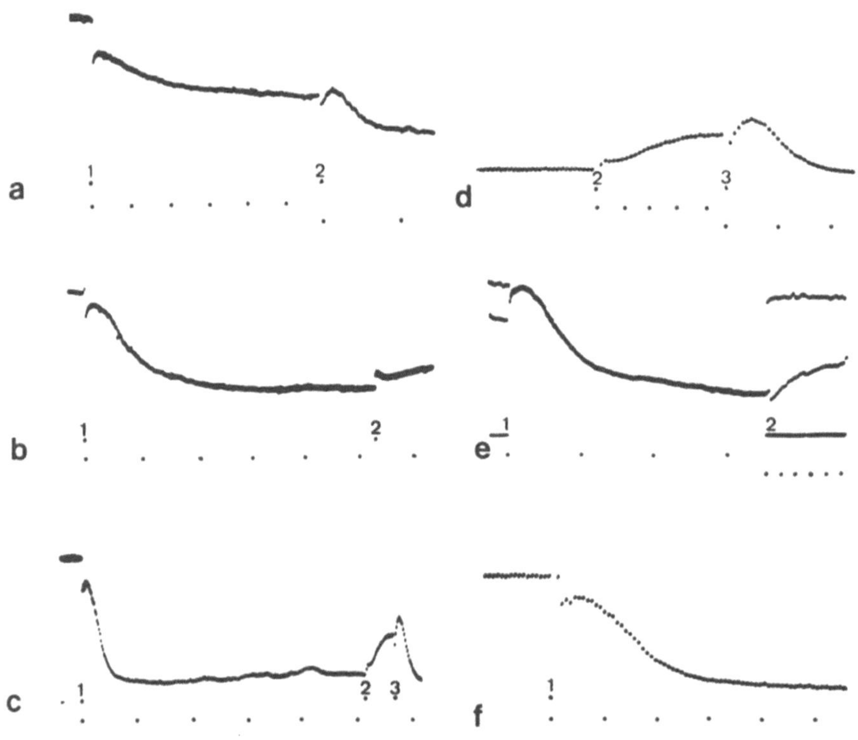

Fig. 5 a–f. Long-lasting repetitive stimulation in an untreated patient with MG. All records are the consecutively measured values of area of the MAP in thenar muscles, *(ordinate)* against time *abscissa)*. Continuous stimulation of the median nerve, between points 1 and 2: **a** 2/s, **b, e** 4/s, **c** 8/s. The numbered dots represent the zero level for the area measurements, and the other dots are time calibration marks (5-min intervals). Control values of the area of the MAP in response to testing volleys given every 10 s are illustrated to the left of point 1 in **a, b, c and f.** In **e**, to the left of point 1 and to the right of point 2 are illustrated the area of the first response *(upper line)* and of the fifth response *(lower line)* in a train of five volleys at 3/s repeated every minute (time calibration after point 2 at 5-min intervals). **f** An expanded trace of the beginning of **e** (time calibration at 1-min intervals). At point 2 in traces **a**, **b** and **c**, the stimulation frequency is switched to 4/s **(a, c)** or 2/s **(b)**. At point 3 in **c** it is switched to 8/s. **d** An expanded trace of the switching phase of trace **c** (time calibration at 1-min intervals between points 2 and 3, at 2-min intervals after point 3). (From Bergmans et al. 1972 with permission)

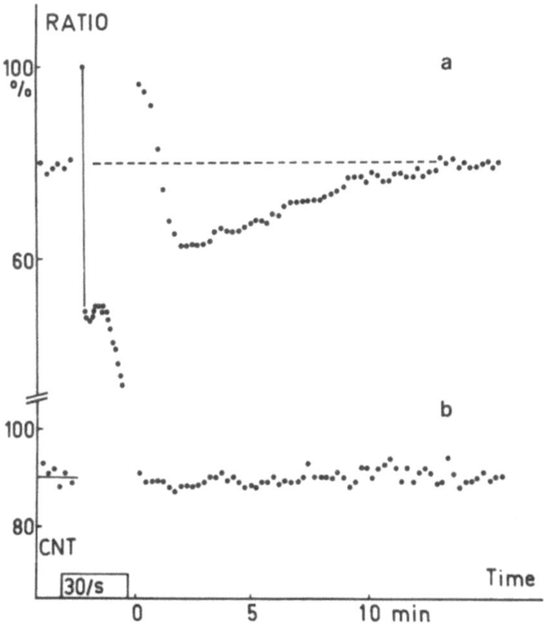

Fig. 6 a, b. Changes in NM block induced by a short period of high-frequency stimulation in a normal subject submitted to computer-controlled curarization (pancuronium bromide), which ensures a constant level of NM block. **a** Level of NM block in the left median nerve before and after a period of repetitive stimulation at 30/s for 17 s. The changes in area of the responses during the stimulation at 30/s are also illustrated. **b** The ratio of the area of the fifth to that of the first response in median nerve-innervated muscles of the right arm, to monitor the NM block. *CNT*, control values before repetitive stimulation. (From Bergmans et al. 1976 with permission)

(Desmedt 1966). In this situation, the prominent period of depression (identical to that seen after low-frequency stimulation) is preceded by a period of facilitation, during which the amplitude of the MAP is increased and the decrement during trains at 3/s is decreased. This is illustrated in Fig. 6 for a normal human curarized subject.These two phases have been named respectively post tetanic and postactivation facilitation (Johns et al. 1955) and exhaustion (Desmedt 1957, 1966).

In our laboratory, current sensitization procedures use conditioning with either stimulation at 3/s for 10 min, with measurement of the decrement 4 min (PTE) after the end of this stimulation, or stimulation at 50/s for 15 s, with measurement of amplitude and decrement 15 s (PTF) and 10 min (PTE) after the end of the stimulation. In normal subjects, the post-tetanic fifth to first response ratio does not differ from the control by more than 5%. In cases of suspected ELS, the measurement of PTF is an important element of diagnosis: a facilitation of amplitude of the response of more than 220% is seen in this syndrome (Lambert and Rooke 1965).

More efficient sensitization procedures can be devised when repetitive stimulation is combined with ischaemia (Borenstein and Desmedt 1966, 1973; Desmedt and Borenstein 1977), which blocks the replenishment of the main presynaptic store depleted by the stimulation (see Fig. 1 in Bergmans et al. 1973a). Different sensitization techniques have been developed: the technique devised by Borenstein and Desmedt (1973) combines a first period of stimulation at 3/s for 4 min, which may disclose a NM block in a fraction of subjects with MG, followed by a second identical period under ischaemia ("two-step test"): this approach does not give false-positive results in normal subjects (Desmedt and Borenstein 1976, 1977). In the protocol devised by Bergmans et al. (1973a), stimulation at 4/s for 8 min is given under ischaemia, with short trains at 3/s testing for a NM block at the 8th, 9th and 10th min of ischaemia. With this approach a NM block was demonstrated in a small proportion (5 of 150) of normal subjects (false positives), where decrement values between 10% and 19% were seen in trains at 3/s given at the 10th min of ischaemia (Bergmans et al. 1975b). Comparison of the two protocols in the same subject with mainly localized forms of MG indicates that some patients remain negative in the two-step test, and are positive in the protocol with longer repetitive stimulation under ischaemia (false negatives in the two-step test). There is thus an overlap between a normal population and a population of patients with MG, also observed when the sensitivity to systemic administration of curare is tested: 3%-4% of normal subjects present a curare sensitivity of the order of that seen in MG patients (Pelikan et al. 1953; see also Hertel et al. 1977). It is thus impossible to devise a test detecting all subjects with MG which remains negative in all normal subjects.

The NM block is increased only slightly or not at all by repetitive stimulation under ischaemia in ELS (Bergmans et al. 1975b), which was originally considered a useful differential diagnostic feature. The same observation has, however, been made in subjects with MG with low amplitude of the MAP (Bergmans, unpublished observations), which would be an extreme example of the known inverse relation between the amount of PTE and the level of initial response (Desmedt 1973a, 1983).

The results of evoked EMG studies must be interpreted in relation to clinical data: a NM block indistinguishable from that seen in MG can be observed occasionally in motor neuron disease (Hodes 1948; Mulder et al. 1959; Desmedt 1973b, 1981; Denys and Norris 1979; Özdemir and Young 1976), in polyneuropathy (Simpson 1966; Niakan et al. 1981) and in multiple sclerosis (Patten et al. 1972; Chaco 1974; Aita et al. 1974; Achari et al. 1976).

Single Fibre EMG

Single fibre EMG relies on the recording, using a special needle with a laterally positioned recording surface of 25 μm in diameter, of the activity of individual muscle fibres. This needle can be positioned so as to record simultaneously from two muscle fibres belonging to the same motor unit. During voluntary activation of the motor unit, a fluctuation of the interval between the discharge of these two fibres is observed, which has been called jitter (Stålberg and Trontelj 1979). Jitter is increased in curarization (Ekstedt and Stålberg 1969; Stålberg et al. 1975; Stålberg 1978) and in MG (Ekstedt and Stålberg 1967; Stålberg et al. 1974; Stålberg and Trontelj 1979; Sanders et al. 1979; Stålberg 1980; Sanders 1983), and occasional blockings of the second response are observed. Single fibre EMG is a very sensitive technique for the detection of pathology occurring at the NM junction, which has, among other things, allowed the detection of subclinical involvement in patients with clinical remission (Sanders et al. 1979; Stålberg 1980) and in relatives of patients with MG (Stålberg et al. 1976; Pirkanen et al. 1981). As for evoked EMG studies, single fibre EMG is only one element of the global neurophysiological evaluation. Abnormal jitter may be observed in myopathies, neuropathies and anterior horn disease (Stålberg and Trontelj 1979; Stålberg 1980; Sanders 1983); these possibilities must thus first be excluded by thorough clinical and neurophysiological examination.

Measurements of jitter are more demanding than evoked EMG testing; furthermore, they require excellent patient cooperation. For serial measurements, they do not compare favourably with evoked EMG testing, which achieves a global assessment of the muscle, while jitter measurements are the result of a statistical sampling.

Other Diagnostic Techniques

Curare Sensitivity

Patients with MG present higher sensitivity to competitive NM blocking substances, and this property can be used as a diagnostic test (Bennett and Cash 1943; Pelikan et al. 1953; Rowland et al. 1961; Hertel and Ricker 1977). This testing can be done more safely by injecting curare intravenously in an ischaemic limb, and measuring either muscular force (Foldes et al. 1968) or the NM block with evoked EMG testing (Horowitz et al. 1975; Boiardi et al. 1977); ocular forms of MG, however, often go undetected with this technique (Horowitz et al 1975; Horowitz and Sivak 1978).

Extraocular Muscles

Different parameters of extraocular muscle function are altered in MG and respond favourably to antiChE. Positive response to antiChE has thus been considered as a diagnostic test for MG with the following parameters: fatigue of the amplitude and the velocity of ocular saccades (Baloh and Keesey 1976); ocular deviation, as measured by Lancaster red-green test (Retzlaff et al. 1969; Kelly et al. 1982). AntiChE also evoke in MG patients an increase in amplitude of optokinetic nystagmus (Spector et al. 1975; Spector and Daroff 1976) and an increase in intraocular pressure (Campbell et al. 1970). These tests have potential value for the evaluation of localized ocular MG.

Stapedius Reflex Fatigability

This technique measures the changes in acoustic impedance of the middle ear, resulting from the contraction of the stapedius muscle in response to an acoustic stimulus. The stimulus can be presented either as a prolonged (30-60 s) continuous tone (Blom and Zakrisson 1974; Warren et al. 1977) or as pulsed tones given during a period of 300 s (Kramer et al. 1981; Sanders 1983). With both techniques, a decrement of the stapedius reflex is evidenced in MG, and this decrement is reversed, at least partially, by the injection of Tensilon (edrophonium chloride). This technique appears useful in predominantly ocular and oropharyngeal forms of MG.

Follow-Up of Patients with MG

Periodic neurophysiological monitoring of patients with MG permits both ascertainment of the quality of therapeutic control and detection of overdosage to antiChE.

AntiChE Evoked Repetitive Discharges

AntiChE administered intra-arterially evoke, in normal subjects, nerve-evoked repetitive activity (NERA) (Harvey et al. 1941b). NERA ist not observed in MG in these conditions (Harvey et al. 1941a), and appears during the period of amelioration which follows thymectomy (Harvey et al. 1942). The appearance of NERA during treatment with antiChE, together with a reduction of the MAP amplitude, is a good indicator of incipient overdosage (Roberts and Wilson 1969).

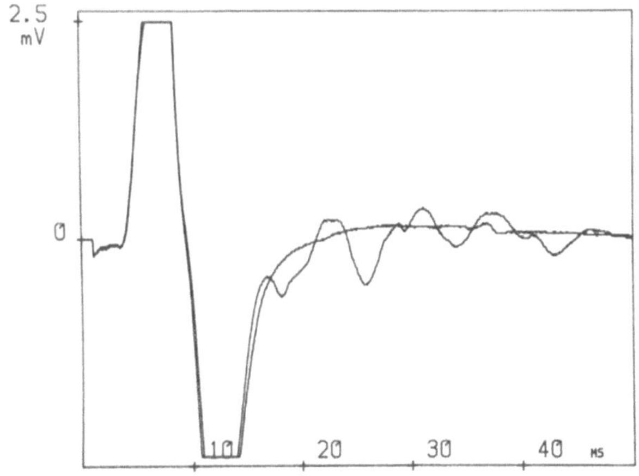

Fig. 7. Neurophysiological signs of overdosage with antiChE in a patient with MG treated with 120 mg pyridostigmine bromide every 3 h and examined 1 h after a last dose. The responses of thenar muscles to two supramaximal stimuli at 3/s applied to the median nerve are illustrated. The first response gives way to a repetitive discharge

NERA due to antiChE is illustrated in Fig. 7, where several repetitive discharges can be seen following the main MAP. On double shock stimulation, NERA to the second volley is obliterated for 10 s, corresponding to the period of depression of transmitter release after a single volley. In the wake of a period of voluntary activation or of short-duration, high-frequency stimulation, a potentiation of this repetitive discharge is observed during PTF and a depression during PTE. The depression on double stimulation is useful to detect this response when it is present at a low level. Analogous NERA is present without treatment in the congenital myasthenic synstome with acetylcholinesterase deficiency (Engel et al. 1977, 1981) and in the slow-channel syndrome (Engel et al. 1981, 1982).

The Monitoring of AntiChE Treatment

In addition to careful clinical evaluation (Oosterhuis 1984), the follow-up of a patient with MG treated with antiChE includes on one hand the measurement of responses to short trains of volleys in muscles presenting a decrement, and on the other hand the search for NERA in less involved muscles. In patients with poor therapeutic response to antiChE, it may be worthwhile to measure neurophysiologically the time course of the response to oral administration of a test dose of antiChE. This allows the evaluation, in the individual patient, of the exact time course of the effect, and adaptation of the rhythm of administration. The effect on NM block is directly related to the antiChE concentration in the serum (Chan and Calvey 1977; Calvey et al. 1979): clinical neurophysiology allows the direct monitoring of the effect on the target organs of drugs whose absorption and elimination are known to be variable (Kornfeld et al. 1970; Calvey and Chan 1977; Cohan et al. 1977; Aquilonius et al. 1979).

The Follow-Up of a Patient with MG in Relation to Thymectomy

In every surgical operation on a patient with MG, one has to take into consideration the depression of NM transmission induced by practically all anaesthetics. The techniques to cope with this problem are now well established (see reviews in Matthews and Derrick 1957; Foldes and McNall 1962). Thus peroperative monitoring of the level of NM block (Bergmans 1980) is not mandatory. However, some operations on patients with MG require the use of curarizing drugs (abdominal surgery). In this situation one can consider the use of small doses of classical competitive curarizing drugs (Foldes et al. 1962; Blitt et al. 1975) or of the new generation of competitive curarizing drugs which are rapidly degraded by Hofmann elimination (Bell et a. 1984), but only if continuous peroperative monitoring of the NM blocks is carried out.

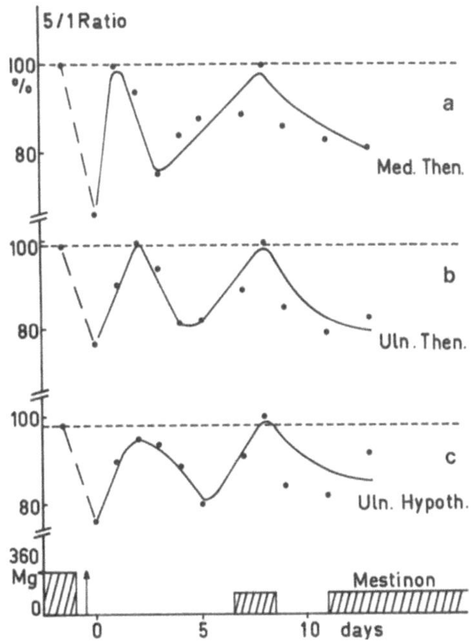

Fig. 8 a–c. Postoperative monitoring of the level of NM block, in the median nerve-innervated thenar muscles and the ulnar nerve-innervated thenar and hypothenar muscles (area of fifth response as percentage of area of first response in a train of five volleys at 3/s). Treatment was 60 mg pyridostigmine (Mestinon) every 3 h in the preoperative period and 30 mg every 3 h in the postoperative period, at the indicated intervals. (From Bergmans 1980 with permission)

The immediate postoperative period creates special problems, since it is known that a temporary remission of the disease sometimes occurs at this time (Genkins et al. 1960; Head 1964). The time course of this remission can be followed accurately with evoked EMG testing: it usually starts on the 1st postoperative day, and lasts either a very short time or up to 2-3 weeks (Bergmans 1980). In view of this variability, neurophysiological monitoring is mandatory, and allows precise adaptation of the antiChE medication. In the patient whose case is illustrated in Fig. 8, the fifth to first response ratio fell to low values on the operative day, due to withdrawal of antiChE treatment (Bergmans 1980). A spontaneous improvement ensued, peaking on the 2nd postoperative day. Treatment at low dosage was resumed on the 6th postoperative day and led to a decrease of the NM block peaking on the 8th postoperative day, together with the appearance of NERA, which led to the decision to temporarily discontinue the antiChE treatment.

The Monitoring of Plasmapheresis, of Corticosteroid or Immunosuppressive Treatment and of the Long-term Effects of Thymectomy

Clinical amelioration seen with plasmapheresis is reflected in a decrease of the decrement (Denys et al. 1979; Arrigo et al. 1979; Nielsen et al. 1982), and a neurophysiological improvement is similarly observed during the remission following thymectomy (Genkins et al. 1975; Pinelli et al. 1975; Papatestas et al. 1976; Horowitz et al. 1976).

Neurophysiological monitoring is helpful at two critical stages of therapy with corticosteroids. During the early phase of exacerbation which is observed when an initial high-dosage schedule is applied (Brunner et al. 1976), repeated measurements of the level of NM block can aid in adapting the dosage of antiChE. During the later phase of gradual improvement (Brunner et al. 1976) we have found the NM responses during sensitization procedures to be the best guide for the gradual tapering of the dosage of corticosteroids; insufficient dosage is followed by a deterioration of the neurophysiological parameters after only 15-30 days, preceding in most cases the clinical aggravation. With regular neurophysiological monitoring, the appropriate therapeutic decisions can thus be taken in good time.

References

Achari AN, Trontelj JV, Campos RJ (1976) Multiple sclerosis and myasthenia gravis. A case report with single fiber electromyography. Neurology 26: 544-546

Aita JF, Snyder DH, Reichl W (1974) Myasthenia gravis and multiple sclerosis: an unusual combination of diseases. Neurology 24: 72-75

Aquilonius SM, Eckernas AS, Hartvig P, Hultman J, Lindström B, Osterman PO (1979) A pharmacokinetic study of neostigmine in man using gas chromatography-mass spectrometry. Eur J Clin Pharmacol 15: 367-371

Arrigo A, Ascari E, Ippoliti G, Piccolo G, Pinelli P, Ruberto MG (1979) The effect of plasmapheresis on myasthenic blocking of neuromuscular transmission: a follow-up electromyographical examination. In: Dau PC (ed) Plasmapheresis and the immunobiology of myasthenia gravis. Houghton Mifflin Medical, Boston, pp 216-228

Baloh RW, Keesey JC (1976) Saccade fatigue and response to edrophonium in the diagnosis of myasthenia gravis. Ann NY Adac Sci 274: 631-641

Bell CF, Florence AM, Hunter JM, Jones RS, Utting JE (1984) Atracurium in the myasthenic patient. Anaesthesia 39: 961-968

Bennett AE, Cash PT (1943) Myasthenia gravis. Curare sensitivity: a new diagnostic test and approach to causation. Arch Neurol Psychiat 49: 537-547

Bergmans J (1980) Apport des techniques neuro-physiologiques à la surveillance de patients myasthéniques, en particulier à l'occasion de la thymectomie. Ann Chir Thorac Cardiovasc 34: 182-187

Bergmans J, Rosselle N, Verheyen G, Schellens L (1972) The kinetics of transmitter release in myastehnia gravis. I. An electrophysiological analysis of the storage of transmitter. Electromyogr Clin Neurophysiol 12: 443-488

Bergmans J, Rosselle N, Verheyen G, Schellens L (1973a) The kinetics of transmitter release in myasthenia gravis. II. An electrophysiological analysis of the replenishment of transmitter stores. Electromyogr Clin Neurophysiol 13: 3-58

Bergmans J, Rosselle N, Verheyen G, Schellens L (1973b) The kinetics of transmitter release in myasthenia gravis. III: An electrophysiological analysis of the release of transmitter. Electromyogr Clin Neurophysiol 13: 145-173

Bergmans J, Cleppe D, Diniz P, Rosselle N (1975a) Atypical myasthenia gravis. A neurophysiological and pharmacological study. Electromyogr Clin Neurophysiol 15: 271-277

Bergmans J, Diniz P, Fannes-Breselow C, Rosselle N (1975b) The effect of ischaemia on neuro-muscular transmission in the Lambert-Eaton syndrome. Electromyogr Clin Neurophysiol 15: 279-283

Bergmans J, Fannes-Breselow C, Gribomont B (1976) A reassessment of the neurophysiological evidence for a presynaptic defect in myastenia gravis. Electromyogr Clin Neurophysiol 16: 337-351

Blitt CD, Wright WA, Peat J (1975) Pancuronium and the patient with myasthenia gravis. Anesthesiology 42: 624-626

Blom S, Zakrisson JE (1974) The stapedius reflex in the diagnosis of myasthenia gravis. J Neurol Sci 21: 71-76

Boiardi A, Bussone G, Negri S (1977) Critical assessment of the local curare test in myasthenia gravis. Eur Neurol 15: 275-280

Boiardi A, Bussone G, Negri S (1979) Alternating myasthenia and myastheniform syndrome in the same subject. J Neurol 220: 57-64

Borenstein S, Desmedt JE (1966) Sensibilisation par l'ischémie de la réaction de l'épuisement de post-activation dans la myasthénie humaine. C R Acad Sci [D] 262: 1472-1475
Borenstein S, Desmedt JE (1973) New diagnostic procedures in myasthenia gravis. In: Desmedt JE (ed) New developments in electromyography and clinical neurophysiology. Karger, Basel, pp 350-374
Borenstein S, Desmedt JE (1975) Local cooling in myasthenia. Arch Neurol 32: 152-157
Botelho SY, Deaterly CF, Austin S, Comroe JH (1952) Evaluation of the electromyogram of patients with myasthenia gravis. AMA Arch Neurol Psychiat 67: 441-450
Brunner NG, Berger CL, Namba T, Grob D (1976) Corticotropin and corticosteroids in generalized myasthenia gravis: comparative studies and role in management. Ann NY Acad Sci 274: 577-595
Calvey TN, Chan K (1977) Plasma pyridostigmine levels in patients with myasthenia gravis. Clin Pharmacol Ther 21: 187-193
Calvey TN, Wareing M, Williams NE, Chan K (1979) Pharmacokinetics and pharmacological effects of neostigmine in man. Br J Clin Pharmacol 7: 149-155
Campbell JJ, Simpson E, Crombie AL, Walton JN (1970) Ocular myasthenia: evaluation of Tensilon tonography an electromystagmography as diagnostic tests. J Neurol Neurosurg Psychiatry 33: 639-646
Chaco J (1974) Multiple sclerosis with impaired neuromuscular transmission. Confin Neurol 36: 182-185
Chan K, Calvey TN (1977) Plasma concentration of pyridostigmine and effects in myasthenia gravis. Clin Pharmacol Ther 22: 596-601
Cohan SL, Dretchen KL, Neal A (1977) Malabsorption of pyridostigmine in patients with myasthenia gravis. Neurology 27: 299-301
Denys EH, Norris FH (1979) Amyotrophic lateral sclerosis: impairment of neuromuscular transmission. Arch Neurol 36: 202-205
Denys EH, Dau PC, Lindstrom JM (1979) Neuromuscular transmission before and after plasmapheresis in myasthenia gravis and myasthenic syndrome. In: Dau PC (ed) Plasmapheresis and the immunobiology of myasthenia gravis. Houghton Mifflin Medical, Boston, pp 248-257
Desmedt JE (1957) Nature of the defect of neuromuscular transmission in myasthenic patients: Post-tetanic exhaustion. Nature 179: 156-157
Desmedt JE (1958) Méthodes d'étude de la fonction neuromusculaire chez l'homme. Myogramme isométrique, électromyogramme d'excitation et topographie de l'innervation terminale. Acta Neurol Psychiatr Belg 58: 977-1017
Desmedt JE (1961) Neuromuscular defect in myasthenia gravis: Electrophysiological and histopathological evidence. In: Viets HR (ed) Myasthenia gravis. Thomas, Springfield, pp 150-178
Desmedt JE (1966) Presynaptic mechanisms in myasthenia gravis. Ann NY Acad Sci 135: 209-246
Desmedt JE (1973a) The neuromuscular disorder in myasthenia gravis. I. Electrical and mechanical response to nerve stimulation in hand muscles. In: Desmedt JE (ed) New developments in electromyography an clinical neurophysiology. Karger. Basel, pp 241-304
Desmedt JE (1973b) The neuromuscular disorder in myasthenia gravis. II. Presynaptic cholinergic metabolism, myasthenic-like syndromes and a hypothesis. In: Desmedt JE (ed) New developments in electromyography and clinical neurophysiology. Karger. Basel, pp 305-342
Desmedt JE (1981) How to validate myasthenia gravis in the patient with a diagnostic problem. Ann NY Acad Sci 377: 583-605
Desmedt JE (1983) The electrophysiological validation of myasthenia gravis. In: Albuquerque EX, Eldefrawi AT (eds) Myasthenia gravis. Chapman and Hall, London, pp 249-273
Desmedt JE, Borenstein S (1976) Diagnosis of myasthenia gravis by nerve stimulation. Ann NY Acad Sci 274: 174-188
Desmedt JE, Borenstein S (1977) Double-step nerve stimulation test for myasthenic block: sensitization of postactivation exhaustion by ischaemia. Ann Neurol 1: 55-64
Ekstedt J, Stålberg E (1967) Myasthenia gravis. Diagnostic aspects by a new electrophysiological method. Opuscula Med 12: 73-76
Ekstedt J, Stålberg E (1969) The effect of non-paralytic doses of *d*-tubocurarine on individual motor end-plates in man, studied with a new electrophysiological method. Electroencephalogr Clin Neurophysiol 27: 557-562
Engel AG (1984) Myasthenia gravis and myasthenic syndromes. Ann Neurol 16: 519-534
Engel AG, Lambert EH, Gomez MR (1977) A new myasthenic syndrome with end-plate acetylcholinesterase deficiency, small nerve terminals, and reduced acetylcholine release. Ann Neurol 1: 315-330
Engel AG, Lambert EH, Mulder DM, Gomez MR, Whitaker JN, Hart Z, Sahashi K (1981) Recently recognized congenital myasthenic syndromes: (a) end-plate acetylcholine (ACh) esterase deficiency, (b) putative abnormality of the ACh induced ion channel, (c) putative defect of ACh resynthesis or mobilization. Clinical features, ultrastructure and cytochemistry. Ann NY Acad Sci 377: 614-639
Engel AG, Lambert EH, Mulder DM, Torres CF, Sahashi K, Bertorini TE, Whitaker JN (1982) A newly recognized congenital myasthenic syndrome attributed to a prolonged open time of the acetylcholine-induced ion channel. Ann Neurol 11: 553-569
Foldes FF, McNall PG (1962) Myasthenia gravis: a guide for Anesthesiologists. Anesthesiology 23: 837-872
Foldes FF, Klonymus DH, Maisel W, Osserman KE (1968) A new curare test for the diagnosis of myasthenia gravis. JAMA 203: 649-653
Genkins G, Kreel I, Jacobson E, Osserman KE, Baronofsky ID (1960) Studies in myasthenia gravis: technical care of the thymectomy patient. Bull NY Acad Med 36: 826-834
Genkins G, Papatestas AE, Horowitz SH, Kornfeld P (1975) Studies in myasthenia gravis: early thymectomy. Am J Med 58: 517-524
Hart Z, Sahashi K, Lambert EH, Engel AG, Lindstrom J (1979) A congenital, familial myasthenic syndrome caused by a presynaptic defect of transmitter resynthesis or mobilization. Neurology 29: 556-557
Harvey AM, Masland RL (1941a) A method for the study of neuromuscular transmission in human subjects. Bull Johns Hopkins Hosp 68: 81-93
Harvey AM, Masland RL (1941b) The electromyogram in myasthenia gravis. Bull Johns Hopkins Hosp 69: 1-13
Harvey AM, Lilienthal JL Jr, Talbot SA (1941a) Observations on the nature of myasthenia gravis: The phenomena of facilitation and depression of neuromuscular transmission. Bull Johns Hopkins Hosp 69: 547-565
Harvey AM, Lilienthal JL Jr, Talbot SA (1941b) On the effects of the intra-arterial injection of acetylcholine and prostigmine in normal man. Bull Johns Hopkins Hosp 69: 529-546

Harvey AM, Lilienthal JL Jr, Talbot SA (1942) Observations on the nature of myasthenia gravis. The effect of thymectomy on neuromuscular transmission. J Clin Invest 21: 579-588
Head JM (1964) Respiratory failure after thymectomy for myasthenia gravis. Ann Surg 160: 123-130
Hertel G, Ricker K (1977) Der Curare-Test in der Diagnostik der Myasthenia gravis. Dtsch Med Wochenschr 102: 90-92
Hertel G, Ricker K, Hirsch A (1977) The regional curare test in myasthenia gravis. J Neurol 214: 257-265
Hodes R (1948) Electromyographic study of defects of neuromuscular transmission in human poliomyelitis. Arch Neurol Psychiatr 60: 457-473
Horowitz SH, Sivak M (1978) The regional curare test and electrophysiologic diagnosis of myasthenia gravis: further studies. Muscle Nerve 1: 432-434
Horowitz SH, Genkins G, Kornfeld P, Papatestas AE (1975) Regional curare test in evaluation of ocular myasthenia. Arch Neurol 32: 84-88
Horowitz SH, Genkins G, Papatestas AE, Kornfeld P (1976) Electrophysiologic evaluations of thymectomy in myasthenia gravis. Preliminary findings. Neurology 26: 615-619
Johns RJ, Grob D, Harvey MA (1955) Symposium on myasthemia gravis: electromyographic changes in myasthenia gravis. Am J Med 19: 679-683
Johns RJ, Grob D, Harvey MA (1956) Studies in neuromuscular function. II: Effects of nerve stimulation in normal subjects and in patients with myasthenia gravis. Bull Johns Hopkins Hosp 99: 125-135
Jolly F (1895) Ueber Myasthenia gravis pseudoparalytica. Berl Klin Wochenschr 32: 1-7
Kelly JJ, Daube JR, Lennon VA, Howard FM, Younge BR (1982) The laboratory diagnosis of mild myasthenia gravis. Ann Neurol 12: 238-242
Kornfeld P, Samuels AJ, Wolf RL, Osserman KE (1970) Metabolism of 14C-labeled pyridostigmine in myasthenia gravis. Evidence for multiple metabolites. Neurology 20: 634-641
Kramer LD, Ruth RA, Johns ME, Sanders DB (1981) A comparison of stapedial reflex fatique with repetitive stimulation and single-fiber electromyography in myasthenia gravis. Ann Neurol 9: 531-536
Krarup C (1977) Electrical and mechanical responses in the platysma and in the adductor pollicis muscle in patients with myasthenia gravis. J Neurol Neurosurg Psychiatry 40: 241-249
Lambert EH, Rooke ED, (1965) Myasthenic state and lung cancer. In: Lord Brain, Norris FH Jr (eds) The remote effects of cancer on the nervous system. Grune and Stratton, New York, pp 67-80
Lambert EH, Rooke ED, Eaton LM, Hodgson CH (1961) Myasthenic syndrome occasionally associated with bronchial neoplasm: neurophysiologic studies. In: Viets HR (ed) Myasthenia gravis. Thomas, Springfield, pp 362-410
Mathews WA, Derrick WS (1957) Anesthesia in the patient with myasthenia gravis. Anesthesiology 18: 443-453
Mulder DW, Lambert EH, Eaton LM (1959) Myasthenic syndrome in patients with amyotrophic lateral sclerosis. Neurology 9: 627-631
Niakan E, Bertorini TE, Acchiardo SR, Werner MF (1981) Procainamide-induced myasthenia-like weakness in a patient with peripheral neuropathy. Arch Neurol 38: 378-379
Nielsen VK, Paulson OB, Rosenkvist J, Holsoe E, Lefvert AK (1982) Rapid improvement of myasthenia gravis after plasma exchange. Ann Neurol 11: 160-169
Oosterhuis HJ (1984) Myasthenia gravis. Churchill Livingstone, Edinburgh (Clinical neurology and neurosurgery monographs)
Oosterhuis HJ, Hootsmans WJ, Veenhuyzen HB, Zadelhoff I (1972) The mean duration of motor unit action potentials in patients with myasthenia gravis. Electroencephalogr Clin Neurophysiol 32: 697-700
Özdemir C, Young RR (1976) The results to be expected from electrical testing in the diagnosis of myasthenia gravis. Ann NY Acad Sci 274: 203-222
Papatestas AG, Genkins G, Horowitz SH, Kornfeld P (1976) Thymectomy in myasthenia gravis: pathologic, clinical, and electrophysiological correlations. Ann NY Acad Sci 274: 555-573
Patten BM, Hart A, Lovelace R (1972) Multiple sclerosis associated with defects in neuromuscular transmission. J Neurol Neurosurg Psychiatry 35: 385-394
Pelikan EW, Tether JE, Unna KR (1953) Sensitivity of myasthenia gravis patients to tubocurarine and decamethonium. Neurology 3: 284-296
Pinelli P (1978) The effect of anticholinesterases on motor unit potentials in myasthenia gravis. Muscle Nerve 1: 438-441
Pinelli P, Arrigo A, Moglia A (1975) Myasthenia decrement and myasthenic myopathy. A study on the effects of thymectomy. J Neurol Neurosurg Psychiatry 38: 525-532
Pirkanen R, Bergström K, Hammarström L, Knutsson E, Lefvert AK, Matell G, Nilsson BY, Smith CI (1981) Neuromuscular safety margin: genetical, immunological, and electrophysiological determinants in relatives of myasthenic patients. A preliminary report. Ann NY Acad Sci 377: 606-613
Retzlaff JA, Kearns TP, Howard FM, Cronin ML (1969) Lancaster red-green test in evaluation of edrophonium effect in myasthenia gravis. Am J Ophthalmol 67: 13-21
Roberts DV, Wilson A (1969) Electromyography in diagnosis and treatment. In: Greene R (ed) Myasthenia gravis. Lippincott, Philadelphia, pp 29-42
Rowland LP, Aranow H, Hoefer PFA (1961) Observations on the curare test in differential diagnosis of myasthenia gravis. In: Viets HR (ed) Myasthenia gravis. Thomas, Springfield, pp 411-434
Sanders DB (1983) Electrodiagnosis of myasthenia gravis: Recent techniques. In: Albuquerque EX, Eldefrawi AT (eds) Myasthenia gravis. Chapman and Hall, London, pp 275-295
Sanders DB, Howard JF, Johns TR (1979) Single-fiber electromyography in myasthenia gravis. Neurology 29: 68-76
Schumm F, Stohr M (1984) Accessory nerve stimulation in the assessment of myasthenia gravis. Muscle Nerve 7: 147-151
Simpson JA (1966) Disorders of neuromuscular transmission. Proc R Soc Med 59: 993-998
Spector RH, Daroff RB (1976) Edrophonium infrared optokinetic nystagmography in the diagnosis of myasthenia gravis. Ann NY Acad Sci 274: 642-651
Spector RH, Daroff RB, Birkett JE (1975) Edrophonium infrared optokinetic nystagmography in the diagnosis of myasthenia gravis. Neurology 25: 317-321
Stålberg E (1978) Neuromuscular transmission studied with single-Fiber electromyography. Acta Anaesth Scand [Suppl] 70: 112-117
Stålberg E (1980) Clinical electrophysiology in myasthenia gravis. J Neurol Neurosurg Psychiatry 43: 622-633
Stålberg E, Sanders DB (1983) Electrophysiological tests of neuromuscular transmission. In: Stålberg E, Young RR (eds) Clinical neurophysiology. Butterworths, London, pp 88-116 (Butterworths international medical reviews)

Stålberg E, Trontelj JV (1979) Single fiber electromyography. Old Woking, Eng: Mirvalle; Pleasentiville, New-York, 1-244

Stålberg E, Ekstedt J, Broman A (1974) Neuromuscular transmission in myasthenia gravis studied with single fibre electromyography. J Neurol Neurosurg Psychiatry 37: 540-547

Stålberg E, Schiller HH, Schwarz MS (1975) Safety factor in single human motor end-plates studied in vivo with single fibre electromyography. J Neurol Neurosurg Psychiatry 38: 799-804

Stålberg E, Trontelj J, Schwartz MS (1976) Single-muscle-fiber recording of the jitter phenomenon in patients with myasthenia gravis and members of their families. Ann NY Acad Sci 274: 189-202

Takamori M, Gutmann L (1971) Intermittent defect of acetylcholine release in myasthenia gravis. Neurology 21: 47-54

Warren WR, Gutmann L, Cody RC, Flowers P, Segal AT (1977) Stapedius reflex decay in myasthenia Gravis. Arch Neurol 34: 496-497

19 Dosage of Serum Acetylcholine Receptor Antibodies

Bernard W. Fulpius

Introduction

Anti-acetylcholine receptor antibodies are usually polyclonal antibodies which are directed against the nicotinic acetylcholine receptor (nAChR) glycoprotein. This definition does not mean that these antibodies necessarily interact with functional parts of the receptor molecule. Anti-nAChR antibodies belong to the G or M class of immunoglobulins, and to any one of their subclasses. Thus, these antibodies represent a rather heterogeneous population of molecules with possibly very different properties if one considers their molecular size, ability to cross the foetoplacental barrier, half-life, resistance to proteolysis, tendency to aggregate and form complexes, capacity to bind complement factors and affinity for the receptor molecule.

Experimental Studies

Anti-nAChR antibodies can be raised experimentally, for example by the active immunization of rabbits with injections of nAChR purified from specific sources, usually the electric organs of *Torpedo* fishes or the skeletal muscles of mammals (Vincent 1980). This immunization procedure leads to a pathological condition called experimental autoimmune myasthenia gravis. Rabbits suffering from it will develop a flaccid paralysis and usually die. The clinical signs are preceded by the appearance of serum anti-nAChR antibodies. This experimental condition resembles, but is not identical to myasthenia gravis, a human muscle disease which has a prevalence of about 5-7 per 100000 and which is characterized by weakness and abnormal fatiguability of voluntary muscles with recovery of motor power on resting as well as positive response to treatment with anticholinesterase drugs.

Myasthenia Gravis

Anti-nAChR antibodies are also present in the serum of patients with myasthenia gravis. They are detected in more than 90% of these patients. The measured titres may differ widely from one case to another and vary during the course of the disease of any individual. At the present time, anti-nAChR antibody determination is considered to be an almost specific and highly sensitive method of confirming or suspecting the diagnosis of myasthenia gravis as these antibodies are virtually absent in normal controls or in patients with other neurological or immunological diseases, although they have been detected in a few very rare conditions such as patients with thymoma, but without myasthenia gravis (Cuénoud et al. 1980), aged individuals and patients with Down's syndrome (Tanaka and Miyatake 1983), patients on long-term neuroleptics and suffering from tardive dyskinesia (Lieberman et al. 1984) and bone-marrow-grafted patients without myasthenia gravis (Smith et al. 1985).

Anti-nAChR antibodies found in the serum of myasthenic patients are autoantibodies. They can interact with the patient's own receptors (Drachman 1981). As a matter of fact anti-nAChR antibodies which leave the vascular compartment may diffuse into the extracellular space and enter the narrow synaptic cleft where they can reach the receptor molecules located at the top of the postsynaptic folds and, alone or in conjunction with complement factors, cause synaptic dysfunction. This finding is of considerable interest. It demonstrates that muscle weakness, the cardinal feature of the disease, arises from a reduced number of functional nAChRs at the neuromuscular junctions brought about by an antibody-mediated autoimmune reaction.

The discovery of the existence in myasthenia gravis of autoantibodies that might be pathogenic raised a great deal of interest among clinicians in consideration of the following question: would the level of measured anti-nAChR antibodies be related to the patient's clinical status? This question is of fundamental importance. As a matter of fact, a positive correlation would permit one to control the evolution of the disease, to predict the occurrence of relapses, and to test whether the therapy has been appropriately selected. Unfortunately, most of the data published in this context have been disappointing and one has to admit, for the most part, that the level of serum anti-nAChR antibodies does not correlate with the clinical severity of the disease, with the exceptions of cases of ocular myasthenia which show rather low titres and cases of generalized myasthenia with an early onset which show rather high titres. This lack of correlation can be explained by several factors: (a) the assays currently used do not detect specifically the subset (or subsets) of anti-nAChR antibodies which are pathogenic; (b) the level of circulating antibodies does not necessarily reflect the level existing in the vicinity of the receptor, (as a matter of fact an uptake of antibodies at affected end-plates might significantly deplete the circulation of appreciable amounts of anti-nAChR antibodies) and (c) anti-nAChR antibodies circulating as immune complexes escape detection.

Thymus

In myasthenic patients the thymus can show two types of histologic abnormalities: (a) lymphofollicular hyperplasia associated with the development of germinal centres which resemble active secondary follicles in peripheral lymphoid organs. This alteration is found in the majority of myasthenic patients, predominantly females, with an early onset of symptoms; (b) thymoma which may belong to various cellular types. This is found in about 10% of myasthenic patients. The thymus can also simply involute, as is the case in patients, predominantly males, with a late onset of symptoms.

The clinical condition of myasthenic patients often improves after thymectomy. Such a beneficial effect can be observed when the operation is performed on patients with early or late onset as well as on patients bearing a thymoma. Although there is no clear correlation between the serum level of anti-nAChR antibodies and the pathology of the thymus, with the exception of very high concentrations of these autoantibodies that are generally related to the presence of a thymoma (Limburg et al. 1983), measurements of anti-nAChR antibodies routinely before and after thymectomy may yield valuable prognostic data. As a matter of fact, Vincent et al. (1983) reported a significant correlation between clinical state and serum anti-nAChR titres in patients, mostly with an early onset, studied for 1-3½ years after thymectomy although the correlation was weak in some individuals. On the other hand and according to Olanow et al. (1982), the titres did not change after thymectomy although the clinical condition improved when patients with a late onset underwent the operation. A similar observation was made for patients after thymectomy for a thymoma (Limburg et al. 1983). There are two main lines of evidence that the thymus itself participates in the production of anti-nAChR antibodies:

1. The nicotinic cholinergic receptor seems to be present within the thymus. This finding is supported by several experiments performed by different investigators which describe binding of α-bungarotoxin to a thymic extract, to thymic epithelial cells and to cultured thymic myoid cells. This neurotoxin, a specific nicotinic cholinergic antagonist, is one of the main protein constituents that can be easily purified from the venom of the snake ***Bungarus multicinctus.*** It is regularly used as an iodinated derivative to identify specifically nAChR in mixtures of proteins or in given tissues because of its high specificity, its high affinity and its very slow dissociation rate. The presence of nAChR within the thymus is also supported by experiments in which anti-nAChR antibodies or sera from patients with myasthenia gravis were shown to react with a large proportion of thymocytes, some epithelial cells and Hassalls' corpuscles (Pizzighella et al. 1983). In this context, the beneficial effect of thymectomy could, at least in part, be due to the removal, with the thymus, of a source of continuing antigenic stimulation. Whether nAChR found within the thymus is a nonfunctioning membrane structure or a functioning receptor remains to be clarified.
2. Anti-nAChR antibodies seem to be produced within the thymus. This second finding is supported by the direct demonstration of these autoantibodies in a thymic extract and by experiments illustrating the spontaneous production of anti-nAChR antibodies by cultured thymic lymphocytes from myasthenic patients, in one case even by thymoma cells (Fujii et el. 1984). In this context, the beneficial effect of thymectomy could be due to the removal of an important source of cells secreting the anti-nAChR antibodies. This possibility was formulated by Tindall (1980) who suggested that the thymus could have been a major site of anti-nAChR antibody synthesis in patients who experienced a rapid reduction of their titre after thymectomy.

Pathogenic Role

The emergence of anti-nAChR antibodies does not seem to represent the primary event in myasthenia gravis. According to Lefvert et al. (1978), the synthesis of these antibodies is triggered by antigenic stimuli such as the release of nAChR from damaged end-plates or myoid cells within the thymus although, as yet, there has been no demonstration of the existence of specific factors, such as viruses, that could have led to synaptic or cellular damage. Such a pathogenic mechanism is probably not unique and more complex sequences of events should also be envisaged, as it is admitted that forms of the disease, different from generalized myasthenia gravis, such as congenital myasthenia or myasthenia associated with a thymoma might have different aetiologies. As a possible mechanism one should consider the neoplastic development of an anti-nAChR antibody-producing clone which could initiate complement activation locally on the postsynaptic membrane and cause the liberation of nAChR-containing fragments into the surrounding tissue and circulation. This would then present the receptor together with other antigens from the skeletal muscle tissue to the immune system and generate additional antibody responses. In the case of antibodies directed against antigen different from nAChR, they will certainly not contribute to the pathogenesis of the myasthenic symptoms, even if they are present and may be detected, often in large amounts, in the vascular compartment (Gilhus et al. 1983).

Circulating anti-nAChR antibodies can be pathogenic by interacting in situ with the receptor, hence impairing its specific role in synaptic transmission. The resulting synaptic dysfunction can be caused by one, two or three of the following mechanisms, each of them leading to a diminution of available and functional nAChRs on the postsynaptic membrane: (a) an alteration of the turnover of nAChR which can be due to a decrease in the rate of receptor synthesis, an increase in the rate of receptor degradation or both simultaneously; (b) a complement-mediated muscle membrane destruction followed by a remodelling in the region of the synaptic junction with a broadening of the synaptic cleft; (c) a blockade of the acetylcholine binding site on the receptor.

Circulating anti-nAChR antibodies can be pathogenic in another manner, namely, as immune complexes. As such, they would cause less specific damage than free anti-nAChR antibodies, since receptors for these complexes are known to occur in several anatomical areas. This would lead, in those places, to immune complex deposition and tissue injury. Practically, very little is known of these specific complexes in myasthenia gravis as the methods used so far to quantify them are nonspecific and all kinds of complexes, whatever the antigen involved, will be detected.

There must exist several clones of antibodies directed agains nAChR, each of them being specific for an antigenic determinant on the receptor molecule, but not all of them being pathogenic. This heterogeneity of anti-nAChR antibodies is very marked since, in addition, not all of them belong to the same class or subclass of immunoglobulins (Lefvert et al. 1981) and every subpopulation of anti-nAChR antibodies has a given affinity against the antigen (Bray and Drachman 1982). It follows that the design of general and reliable assays to measure circulating anti-nAChR antibodies is complicated. At present, these antibodies can be identified by several methods. All of them, however, depend on the use of α-bungarotoxin for labelling the antigen specifically.

Identification

Immunoprecipitation assays are the most widely used (Lindstrom 1977; Monnier and Fulpius 1977). They require first labelling the receptor glycoproteins with ^{125}I-labelled α-bungarotoxin. Anti-nAChR antibodies that combine with the toxin-receptor complexes obtained in such a way are then precipitated by adding the appropriate anti-human IgG (or IgM) serum. They are found in 90%–95% of patients with myasthenia gravis when the selected receptor glycoproein is that which is solubilized with non-ionic detergents from human skeletal muscles. Lower percentages are found when the receptor is extracted from monkey, calf or rat skeletal muscles or when it is obtained from the electric organ of *Torpedo* fishes. This type of assay, however, underestimates the actual amount of anti-nAChR antibodies that circulate free in the serum because ^{125}I-labelled α-bungarotoxin bound to nAChR may alter or sterically occlude antigenic determinants recognized by particular subpopulations of anti-nAChR antibodies. This is particularly true of the antibodies that specifically block the binding of acetylcholine, the natural ligand, to the receptor. This subpopulation of antibodies deserves special attention because it could act by causing an immunopharmacological blockade. In order to detect the antibodies that block acetylcholine binding, one has to use inhibition assays (Fulpius et al. 1980). They consist of a quantitative evaluation of the competition between antibodies and α-bungarotoxin for binding to nAChR from different sources. It is difficult to evaluate quantitatively the inhibition by antibodies of toxin binding to nAChR because anti-nAChR antibodies can also inhibit toxin fixation by steric mechanisms (when they are directed against sites adjacent to the toxin binding site) or by allosteric mechanisms (when they are directed against remote portions of the receptor molecule, a situation more likely to occur when the receptor is solubilized by detergent and hence loses its native conformation to "some" degree). It follows that appropriate inhibition assays are difficult to perform since they must meet at least two requirements: (a) the receptor must be in its native environment as is the case in intact cells or membrane fragments: (b) cross-reactivity with human anti-nAChR antibodies should be restricted to the ligand binding site as seems to be the case with *Torpedo* electric organs and cultured chick muscle cells. Further difficulties are encountered while performing inhibition assays, namely to obtain and to purify large amounts of antigen, to reach an adequate sensitivity and to purify large amounts of high titre IgG from myasthenic patients. Finally, as the acetylcholine binding site is not strictly equal to the α-bungarotoxin binding site, it is necessary to test, in an additional step, small cholinergic ligands. It follows that the development of suitable specific immunodiagnostic methods for routine detection of antibodies directed against the cholinergic binding site is still needed. In this respect, one should consider of great potential value the development of monoclonal antibodies directed against the cholinergic binding site of the receptor (Tzartos et al. 1982).

Conclusion

Anti-nAChR antibody determination, as it is performed at the present time, is without any doubt extremely useful to confirm the diagnosis of myasthenia gravis. However, it is not much help in ascertaining the gravity of the disease or following its evolution because of an obvious lack of correlation between observed levels of anti-nAChR antibodies and the clinical status. The use, in assays performed at different times or in different laboratories of antigens from different sources, implies that some form of standardization should always be performed with, for example, sera of well-established activity, to make valid comparisons between titres measured in different individuals or on different occasions, in a given patient. Assays using well-defined monoclonal antibodies directed against the human antigen will probably solve many of the problems encontered at the present time. They are, however, not available yet.

References

Bray JJ, Drachman DB (1982) Binding affinities of anti-acetylcholine receptor autoantibodies in myasthenia gravis. J Immunol 128: 105-110

Cuénoud S, Feltkamp TEW, Fulpius BW, Oosterhuis HJGH (1980) Antibodies to acetylcholine receptor in patients with thymoma but without myasthenia gravis. Neurology 30: 201-203

Drachman DB (1981) The biology of myasthenia gravis. Annu Rev Neurosci 4: 195-225

Fujii Y, Monden Y, Nakahara K, Hashimoto J, Kawashima Y (1984) Antibody to acetylcholine receptor in myasthenia gravis: production by lymphocytes from thymus or thymoma. Neurology 34: 1182-1186

Fulpius BW, Miskin R, Reich E (1980) Antibodies from myasthenic patients that compete with cholinergic agents for binding to nicotinic receptors. Proc Natl Acad Sci USA 77: 4326-4330

Gilhus NE, Aarli JA, Matre R (1983) Myasthenia gravis. Antibodies to skeletal muscle cell surface antigens. J Neuroimmunol 5: 239-249

Lefvert AK, Bergström K, Matell G, Osterman PO, Pirskanen R (1978) Determination of acetylcholine receptor antibody in myasthenia gravis: clinical usefulness and pathogenetic implications. J Neurol Neurosurg Psychiatry 41: 394-403

Lefvert AK, Cuénoud S, Fulpius BW (1981) Binding properties and subclass distribution of anti-acetylcholine receptor antibodies in myasthenia gravis. J Neuroimmunol 1: 125-135

Lieberman JA, Bradley RJ, Rubinstein M, Kane JM (1984) Antibodies to acetylcholine receptors in tardive dyskinesia. Lancet I: 1066

Limburg PC, The TH, Hummel-Tappel E, Oosterhuis HJGH (1983) Anti-acetylcholine receptor antibodies in myasthenia gravis. Part 1. Relation to clinical parameters in 250 patients. J Neurol Sci 58: 357-370

Lindstrom J (1977) An assay for antibodies to human acetylcholine receptor in serum from patients with myasthenia gravis. Clin Immunol Immunopathol 7: 36-43

Monnier VM, Fulpius BW (1977) A radioimmunoassay for the quantitative evaluation of anti-human acetylcholine receptor antibodies in myasthenia gravis. Clin Exp Immunol 29: 16-22

Olanow CW, Lane RJM, Roses AD (1982) Thymectomy in late-onset myasthenia gravis. Arch Neurol 39: 82-83

Pizzighella S, Riviera AP, Tridente G (1983) Thymic involvement in myasthenia gravis. Study by immunofluorescent and immunoperoxidase staining. J Neuroimmunol 4: 117-127

Smith CIE, Hammarström L, Lefvert AK (1985) Bone-marrow grafting induces acetylcholine receptor antibody formation. Lancet I: 978

Tanaka M, Miyatake T (1983) Anti-acetylcholine receptor antibody in aged individuals and in patients with Down's syndrome. J Neuroimmunol 4: 17-24

Tindall RSA (1980) Humoral immunity in myasthenia gravis: effect of steroids and thymectomy. Neurology 30: 554-557

Tzartos SJ, Seybold ME, Lindstrom JM (1982) Specificities of antibodies to acetylcholine receptors in sera from myasthenia gravis patients measured by monoclonal antibodies. Proc Natl Acad Sci USA 79: 188-192

Vincent A (1980) Immunology of acetylcholine receptors in relation to myasthenia gravis. Physiol Rev 60: 756-824

Vincent A, Newsom-Davis J, Newton P, Beck N (1983) Acetylcholine receptor antibody and clinical response to thymectomy in myasthenia gravis. Neurology 33: 1276-1282

Part V

Surgical Procedures

20 Indications for Thymectomy

Jean-Claude Givel

The usual procedure in thymic surgery is complete resection of the gland. Its aim is most often either treatment of myasthenia gravis or resection of a thymic tumour. Thymectomy is only exceptionally performed for other reasons.

The indication for thymectomy in myasthenia gravis (MG) stems from Sauerbruch's observation in 1911 (Schumacher and Roth 1912): he performed a thymectomy on a young girl who suffered from hyperparathyroidism and MG and noted, to his astonishment, an improvement in her MG. In 1936 Blalock removed a cystic thymic tumour from a 19-year-old myasthenic patient and noted an improvement in her neuromuscular function (Blalock et al. 1939). Since then, many others have contributed to the acknowledgement of the value of thymectomy in the treatment of MG.

The outcome of the neurological deficit following thymectomy varies from one subject to another. It is therefore important to rely on precise criteria to decide on surgical indications in myasthenic patients. Age, sex, duration and severity of disease, and the presence or absence of a thymoma are the factors which all determine the postoperative outcome of MG patients who undergo thymectomy. They must be taken into account when deciding the indication for surgery.

The natural history of untreated MG is death in approximately 40% at 10 years (Simpson et al. 1966). Spontaneous remission can occur in around 25% of all cases, but is most often seen in the purely occulomotor form of the disease (Osserman's class I) and tends to be frequently short-lived. In a randomized study, Buckingham et al. (1976) demonstrated the better remission and survival rates of patients who underwent thymectomy compared to those under medical therapy. These results have since been confirmed by many studies (Masaoka and Monden 1981; Mulder et al. 1983; Papatestas et al. 1987 a).

Over the past 10 years the indications for thymectomy have changed significantly, and they are still somewhat variable among different departments. Papatestas et al. have since 1976 recommended early thymectomy for all patients with generalized MG. While there is still disagreement whether thymectomy should be performed for the purely occulomotor forms of MG, this is not the case for slight or moderate forms of generalized MG, for it can cause complete remission or prevent the progression of disease in most cases (Olanow et al. 1982; Huang et al. 1988). Several studies seem to demonstrate that the results of surgery are better when preoperative symptoms were of short duration (Genkins et al. 1975; Olanow et al. 1982). Thus, thymectomy is performed in conjunction with appropriate medical therapy in MG patients between the ages of 14 and 65 years (Huang et al. 1988). Jaretzki et al. (1988) think that age in itself is not a contraindication to surgery, which is preferable to severe symptoms of MG or to high doses of corticosteroids at both extremes of life. Elderly patients all have residual thymic epithelial tissue and, even if at higher risk, tolerate thymectomy well, and results are usually as good as in younger patients. Furthermore, Jaretzki et al. recommend wide resection of the thymus in these patients.

The operative trauma of thymectomy is no longer a major concern. Both preoperative preparation and the improvement in the intra- and postoperative management of these patients have considerably reduced the morbidity and mortality associated with thymectomy in MG. Preoperative plasmapheresis can considerably alleviate symptoms and simplify the perioperative management of MG patients, and is certainly a great step forward in reducing morbidity (Cooper et al. 1988; Huang et al. 1988).

The choice between the cervical or the transsternal approach also plays a part in the decision making and is the subject of controversy. This is more a problem of technique than of surgical indications, and is discussed in Chaps. 21 and 22. However, some of the arguments of the proponants of both techniques are relevant to surgical indications (Jaretzki, in Cooper et al. 1988):

1. After incomplete resection, it is often necessary to reoperate for recurring or persistent symptoms; at surgery, residual thymic tissue is the rule.
2. As little as 3 g residual thymic tissue can cause considerable symptoms, which resolve following resection.
3. After incomplete resection, transient remission or worsening of symptoms can occur.

4. The less thymic tissue resected, the worse the results of surgery.

The proponents of cervicotomy think that this operation, with its less traumatic incision, causes less morbidity and shorter hospital stays, while offering similar results to transsternal thymectomy. It is thus more acceptable to both patients (especially young women) and their physicians, and encourages early surgery (Cooper et al. 1988). Others think that only "maximal" thymectomy can give the best results and avoid recurrences due to residual thymic tissue, and think that this is the only rational form of treatment (Jaretzki et al. 1988).

Thymomas are commonly associated with MG, especially in medically treated patients. These tend to be slow-growing neoplasms which should be resected. Papatestas et al. (1987 b) have shown that the neurological course in patients with small tumours is more favourable, and that up to 26% of tumours less than 5 cm in diameter can escape preoperative detection. This is a further reason to recommend early thymectomy in MG patients.

In patients with purely occulomotor MG (Osserman's class I), the initial treatment should be medical. If there is no improvement after 1 year, if symptoms become generalized or recur, then thymectomy should be performed (Cooper et al. 1988).

Whenever the presence of residual thymic tissue is suspected, because a patient fails to respond to thymectomy or has an early relapse or deterioration of symptoms, transsternal re-exploration of the mediastinum should be performed and all residual tissue resected. This decision depends on the patient's clinical condition and on the type of initial resection.

Thymomas should always be completely resected whenever possible, whether or not there are associated symptoms. It is equally important that all thymic tissue be resected, for variable degrees of thymic epithelial hyperplasia can be seen in association with thymomas; MG can occur in approximately 6%-10% of subtotal thymectomies for thymoma (Jaretzki et al. 1988).

All tumours of the thymus should always be as completely resected as possible, regardless of associated symptoms. Surgery is the only way to reach a precise diagnosis and determination of the extent of disease. Furthermore, whether the tumour be an invasive thymoma or another more rare histological type, surgery is still one of the mainstays of treatment, and survival tends to be better with aggressive surgical treatment followed by radio- and/or chemotherapy.

While the indications for thymectomy in patients with MG are clear, this is not the case with many of the other rare syndromes associated with thymic pathologies. In pure red cell aplasia thymectomy is indicated only if there is an associated thymoma; otherwise thymectomy does not seem to confer any benefit, apart from the above-mentioned proviso that some thymomas escape detection. Neither the hypoglammaglobulinaemias nor the other syndromes discussed in Chap. 15 seem to benefit from thymectomy.

References

Blalock A, Mason MF, Morgan HJ, Riven SS (1939) Myasthenia gravis and tumors of the thymic region: report of a case in which the tumor was removed. Ann Surg 110: 544-561

Buckingham JM, Howard FM, Bernatz PE, Payne WS, Harrison EG, O'Brien PC, Weiland LH (1976) The value of thymectomy in myasthenia gravis: a computer-assisted matched study. Ann Surg 184: 453-457

Cooper JD, Al-Jilaihawa AN, Pearson FG, Humphrey JG, Humphrey HE (1988) An improved technique to facilitate transcervical thymectomy for myasthenia gravis. Ann Thorac Surg 45: 242-247

Genkins G, Papatestas A, Horowitz S (1975) Studies in myasthenia gravis. Am J Med 58: 517-524

Huang MH, King KL, Hsu WH, Huang BS, Hsu HK, Wang LS, Chien KY (1988) The outcome of thymectomy in nonthymomatous myasthenia gravis. Surg Gynecol Obstet 166: 436-440

Jaretzki A III, Penn AS, Younger DS, Wolff M, Olarte MR, Lovelace RE, Rowland LP (1988) "Maximal" thymectomy for myasthenia gravis. J Thorac Cardiovasc Surg 95: 747-757

Masaoka A, Monden Y (1981) Comparison of the results of transsternal simple, transcervical simple and extended thymectomy. Ann NY Acac Sci 377: 755-765

Mulder DG, Hermann C Jr, Keesey J, Edwards H (1983) Thymectomy for myasthenia gravis. Am J Surg 146: 61-66

Olanow CW, Wechsler AS, Roses AD (1982) A prospective study of thymectomy and serum acetylcholine receptor antibodies in myasthenia gravis. Ann Surg 196: 113-121

Papatestas AE, Genkins G, Horowitz SH, Kornfeld P (1976) Thymectomy in myasthenia gravis. Ann NY Acad Sci 274: 555-576

Papatestas AE, Genkins G, Kornfeld P, Eisenkraft JB, Fagerstrom RP, Pozner J, Anfoes Jr AH (1987 a) Effects of thymectomy in myasthenia gravis. Ann Surg 206: 79-88

Papatestas AE, Pozner J, Genkins G, Kornfeld P, Matta RL (1987 b) Prognosis in occult thymomas in myasthenia gravis following transcervical thymectomy. Arch Surg 122: 1356

Schumacher ED, Roth J (1912) Thymektomie bei einem Fall von Morbus Basedowi mit Myasthenie. Mitteil Grenzgeb Med Chir (Jena) 25: 746-765

Simpson JA, Westenberg MR, Magee HR (1966) Myasthenia gravis: an analysis of 195 cases. Acta Neurol Scand 42: 7-27

21 Surgical Approaches

Marco Merlini and David B. Clarke

General Considerations

The best surgical approach to the thymus can be a difficult choice. Apart from biopsy, possibly done by mediastinoscopy or anterior mediastinotomy, the only procedure performed on the gland is thymectomy. However, this term can cover different procedures ranging from simple thymectomy (excision of the thymus with its macroscopic capsule) to extended thymectomy (resection of the thymus with exenteration of the anterior mediastinal fat from the lower poles of the thyroid to diaphragm and from hilum to hilum).

The surgical decision is influenced by different criteria, the extent of the planned resection (simple or extended thymectomy) or the suspicion of a thymoma are the most important ones. Other factors such as the general and respiratory condition of the patient or the cosmetic appearance of the incision must also be considered. We are therefore dealing with a subject of some controversy (Rowland 1980). In this chapter, an effort has been made to collect different opinions and to summarize the reasons which govern this surgical choice.

Thymectomy is mainly carried out by two approaches: transsternal or transcervical. The technical details of these procedures are described in Chap. 22. However, combined transsternal and transcervical thymectomy is convincingly defended by some authors (Jaretzki 1977) and will be discussed. Finally, other approaches such as horizontal and lateral thoracotomies sometimes have good indications.

The thymus is situated astride two anatomical regions, the neck and the mediastinum, each having a different surgical approach. This particular position constitutes one cause of the controversy. The best approach to the median part of the neck is a transverse incision. However, after a low cervicotomy, retraction of the strap muscles and division of the deep cervical fascia, only the cranial poles of the thymus appear. The rest of the gland which is hidden by the sternum must be drawn up to be delivered. The approach to the anterior mediastinum is generally a vertical skin incision and sternotomy. However, the caudal poles of the thymus extend in most cases no further than the fourth intercostal space (Baron 1982) and a total sternotomy may seem to be an excessively large incision for access to the thymus alone.

Before the era of thoracic surgery, thymectomy was performed through a cervical incision. Later, when a thoracotomy became technically possible, the usual access to the thymus was by median sternotomy. In the late 1960's however, Kirschner and Kark (1969, 1971) returned to transcervical thymectomy mainly because the postoperative course of myasthenic patients was smoother after this more limited approach.

The precise indications for thymectomy have also varied over the last few decades. The procedure has had an empirical basis for many years and consequently simple thymectomy was generally accepted (Papatestas et al. 1978; Papatestas et al. 1981). More recently, anatomical variations of the gland were described with the probability of finding extracapsular thymic tissue (Masaoka et al. 1975; Jaretzki et al. 1977; Hankins et al. 1985) and the risk of leaving thymic remnants if only a simple thymectomy is performed (Masaoka et al. 1982; Austin et al. 1983; Rubin 1985, personal communication). Thus, the tendency to extend the resection to anterior mediastinal fat gained popularity. However, this extended procedure is difficult to perform without a median sternotomy. Moreover, the current development of noninvasive radiological imaging is sometimes of help in the choice of the surgical procedure. Every myasthenic patient planned for operation undergoes a mediastinal scan. Thus, a thymic enlargement, a suspected or overt thymoma can be demonstrated beforehand. With the suspicion of a thymoma, the transsternal approach is indicated.

Pulmonary function is a deciding factor in the choice of surgical approach. Preoperative respiratory insufficiency limits the indications for a thoracotomy. The myasthenic patient is particularly at risk of postoperative respiratory failure (Ip et al. 1985). Thus, the operative risk has to be assessed thoroughly (Mittman 1961; Diener 1973): the general category of high risk for thoracic surgery is defined when the maximum voluntary ventilation is less than 50% of the predicted value, the forced expiratory volume in 1 s is less than

2 l, the arterial PCO_2 is higher than 45 mm Hg and PO_2 lower than 50 mm Hg (Tisi 1979). Therefore, it has first to be determined if the myasthenic is in this high risk category (Eisenkraft et al. 1986). Furthermore, the mechanical impairment of ventilation induced by muscular section or thoracic destabilization must be carefully considered. It is low or nonexistent for a cervicotomy: thus, a cervical incision is tolerated by the myasthenic patient with impaired respiratory function. Median sternotomy temporarily destabilizes the thoracic cage; however, no muscular section is carried out. This procedure is thus acceptable for the myasthenic patient with a compensated respiratory function. A lateral thoracotomy involving muscular sections and operative unilateral lung collapse is most prone to cause respiratory complications and can be planned only with good respiratory and muscular function (Leuenberger 1985, personal communication).

A thymectomy for a noncompensated myasthenic patient must be carefully considered. If it is admitted that early thymectomy is mandatory (Genkins et al. 1975; Gamondès 1985, personal communication), the myasthenia must be stabilized before the operation. The medical treatment is well standardized nowadays with anticholinesterase drugs and corticoids (Johns 1977; Bolooki and Schwarzmann 1978; Heiser et al. 1982). Myasthenics may be prepared a few days in advance with plasmapheresis (Dau et al. 1977; Gracey 1984a; Spence et al. 1984; d'Empaire et al. 1985; Thorlacius et al. 1985). The details of optimal preoperative management are explained elsewhere in this book. Thus, the myasthenic patient is better prepared than in the past. During the procedure, recent neuromuscular blocking agents can be administered selectively (Bergmans 1980; Baraka and Dajani 1984; Ward and Wright 1984; Buzello et al. 1986; Murphy and Magner 1986; Eisenkraft 1987). Muscular relaxation can be monitored precisely (Ali 1985). After the operation most patients can be mechanically ventilated for a few hours and then be safely extubated (Leventhal et al. 1980; Gracey et al. 1984b; Younger et al. 1984). When artificial ventilation is necessary for a longer period, endotracheal tubes with low pressure cuffs avoid the need for tracheostomy.

The choice of the approach may become more complex when the additional criterion of cosmesis is introduced. The final decision is now more difficult because vital criteria can compete in the surgical balance with aesthetic ones. Many myasthenic patients are young women and form, by their age and sex, a quite different category from those usually amenable to a median sternotomy for an aortocoronary bypass or cardiac valve replacement. The incision of a cervicotomy, paralleling the lines of minimal extensibility of the skin, leaves a more acceptable scar than a vertical presternal incision (Egloff 1985, personal communication). This latter is visible with any open collar and is likely to cause psychological problems. Therefore, for young women, an appropriate approach must be seriously considered (Crucitti 1985, personal communication).

Transsternal Thymectomy

For the majority of surgeons, median sternotomy is the standard incision (Neville 1984). This approach allows total access to the anterior mediastinum and also gives adequate exposure of the lower part of the neck which according to many experienced authors is the only way the entire thymus can be removed (Austin 1985; Gamondès 1985; Neville 1985, personal communications). The left lobe, larger than the right, extends laterally close to the phrenic nerve (Mulder et al. 1983). Furthermore, the thymus is somewhat difficult to differentiate from perithymic fat; thus, the dissection is easier by median sternotomy. Opening the left pleura permits recognition of the nerve; thymus and fat are lifted up *en bloc* (Mulder 1985, personal communication). The same is possible for the caudal poles, which are also difficult to separate from the perithymic fat, especially in the elderly (Doglietto et al. 1983). All these manoeuvres are feasible only by this approach. Moreover, the gland can be safely separated from the innominate vein with good vascular control.

When an undiagnosed small thymoma is discovered, the resection can be complete. For a suspected thymoma, median sternotomy is mandatory (Cohn et al. 1974; Mulder 1985; Neville 1985, personal communications): tumour extension and pleural, pericardial or vascular invasion is defined and resectability assessed. With the current preoperative management of myasthenia gravis, the risk of respiratory failure and other morbidity is low (Neville 1984; Mulder and Rubin 1985, personal communication). Most patients leave the hospital after 4–7 days.

Special mention should be made regarding the magnitude of resection possible by median sternotomy. This approach gives the possibility of simple or extended thymectomy. The long-term results obtained by one method or the other can also influence the general choice of approach and technique. Results of simple thymectomy in a few series can be seen in Table 1. Those of extended thymectomy are found in Table 2.

Table 1. Results of transsternal simple thymectomy in non-thymomatous and thymomatous myasthenia gravis

	No. of patients	No. of thymomas	Follow-up (years)	Mean (years)	No. of patients improved[a]	No. of patients in remission[b]
Gamondès et al. 1981	54	0	0.5-26	7	53 (98%)	34 (63%)
	7	7	0.5-26	7	2 (28%)	1 (14%)
Masaoka and Monden 1981	23	0	0.25-10	–	16/19 (84%)[c,d]	12/19 (63%)
Papatestas et al. 1981	105	0	1-5	–	–	18/75 (24%)[d,e]

[a] Including patients with remission
[b] No symptoms, no anticholinesterase therapy
[c] Follow-up at 5 years on 19 of 23 patients
[d] Results at 5 years
[e] Follow-up at 5 years on 75 of 105 patients

Table 2. Results of extended thymectomy in non-thymomatous and thymomatous myasthenia gravis

	No. of patients	No. of thymomas	Follow-up	Mean (years)	No. of patients improved	No. of patients in remission
Clark et al. 1980	20	1	5-88 months	2.7	18 (90%)	11 (55%)
Fisher et al. 1987	27	3	–	–	24 (90%)	14 (52%)
Masaoka and Monden 1981	95	0	3 months-5 years	–	16/18 (89%)[a,b]	10/18 (56%)
Monden et al. 1984	46	46	3 months-5 years	–	(84%)[a]	(26%)
Mulder et al. 1983	198	0	–	7.5	181 (91%)	107 (54%)
	51	51	–	7.5	35 (68%)	19 (37%)
Olanow et al. 1982	47	9	6-51 months	2.1	46 (98%)	29 (61%)
Rubin et al. 1981	22	1	6 months-15 years	5.5	20 (91%)	10 (45%)

[a] Results at 5 years
[b] Follow-up at 5 years on 18 of 95 patients

Transcervical Thymectomy

This approach is used for routine thymectomy in myasthenia gravis in several centers, including one with an experience of over 1000 cases (Papatestas 1987a). Among these large series, even thymomas were removed transcervically. Most of these were discovered at the time of surgery. In specialized institutions where all myasthenic patients now undergo early thymectomy, the percentage of thymomas is probably lower than elsewhere and thus the cervical approach appears more tempting (Papatestas 1987b). This approach is difficult and requires a perfect understanding of mediastinal surgery (Crile 1966; Paletto and Maggi 1974; Levasseur and Le Brigand 1975; Papatestas et al. 1975; Le Brigand 1982). Understandably, it is defended by authors from specialized centres who have mastered the technique and the blunt dissection it involves around vascular structures. The procedure is easier in children and young adults with an elastic thoracic cage (Maggi 1985, personal communication). In older adults, access to the distal part of the thymus is more challenging, particularly if perithymic tissue resection is required. Surgeons using this technique often split the manubrium sterni and some have a special retractor to widen the operative field (Maggi et al. 1982; Paletto and Maggi 1982; Donnelly 1985, personal communication).

In experienced hands, this method is safe. It also has the undisputed advantages of a painless postoperative course and an aesthetic scar (Donnelly et al. 1984). It bears the danger of haemorrhage, pneumothorax and the risk of leaving thymic remnants. When the postoperative clinical resolution of myasthenia gravis is unsatisfactory, the suspicion of remnants or regrowth arises and with it the difficult decision concerning the indication and timing of a second surgical exploration (Henze et al. 1984). Some authors prefer to start with a transcervical approach while being prepared to proceed to an immediate transsternal exploration if unsatisfied by the cervical access. Rosenberg et al. (1983) thus start by a cervicotomy; in case of acci-

Table 3. Results of transcervical thymectomy in non-thymomatous myasthenia gravis

	No. of patients	Follow-up (years)	Mean (years)	No. of patients improved	No. of patients in remission
Doglietto et al. 1983	28	–	4	27 (96.4%)	6 (21.4%)
Donnelly et al. 1984	22	–	0.5	17 (77%)	3 (13%)
Maggi et al. 1982	242	1-8	–	196 (80.9%)	60 (24.7%)
Papatestas et al. 1981	358	1-5	–	–	14/58 (24%)[a,b]

[a] Follow-up at 5 years on 58 of 358 patients
[b] Results at 5 years

dental capsular tear, even if minute, sternotomy is carried out. By using this method, sternotomy is avoided in about 50% of his cases (Rosenberg 1985, personal communication).

Several authors think that the transcervical approach is inadequate for routine thymectomy in myasthenia gravis and contraindiated if a thymoma is present (Austin 1985; Clark 1985; Miller 1985; Neville 1985, personal communications). The results of the transcervical approach are reported in Table 3.

Extended Thymectomy

Extended thymectomy associates extracapsular resection with anterior mediastinal fat exenteration from neck to diaphragm and hilum to hilum. The mediastinal exenteration is only possible by total median sternotomy. This technique probably contributes to the excellent remission rate, about 60%, in non-thymomatous myasthenia gravis and currently better results in thymomatous myasthenia gravis are obtained than with other methods (Masaoka 1985, personal communication).

Recurrence cannot be totally excluded as thymic tissue can exist outside the mediastinum (Gilmour 1941). However, a radical resection is most satisfactory in that it eliminates most of the mediastinal fat. There is no theoretical argument against it (Austin 1985; Jaretzki 1985; Neville 1985, personal communications) and fewer recurrences are presently reported with this method.

Combined Thymectomy

When neck exposure is considered insufficient through a presternal incision, it is possible to combine it with a transverse cervicotomy. Jaretzki defends this approach arguing that the gland has many cervical and mediastinal variations. His patients have a remission rate of over 60% with 2-4 years of follow-up (personal communication). In a published series of 47 cases (6 with thymoma) operated on with a relatively short follow-up of 1½ years, (Penn et al. 1981) noted an improvement in 41 patients (87.2%) including 20 (42.5%) remissions or "asymptomatic" patients.[1]

Special Approaches

Median Sternotomy T-Incision

This approach has been described by Miller (1981) (Fig. 1). The skin incision is T-shaped, the horizontal limb overlying the second costal cartilage. A skin flap is elevated from the horizontal limb, to the suprasternal notch and the sternum is partially sectioned. A small retractor is then inserted. Miller has performed 55 procedures without mortality or complications. This T-incision has the advantages of median sternotomy with good exposure of the mediastinum, safe resection of the thymus and a gratifying cosmetic aspect (Miller 1985, personal communication).

Transverse Submammary Thoracotomy

This approach was first used for cardiac surgery in children and young women. However, it can be performed for anterior mediastinum exploration. A horizontal incision is made at the upper border of the sixth rib (Fig. 2), Brutel de la Rivière et al. 1981; Mulder 1986; Bédard et al. 1986). The incision is upwardly curved at its extremities. The upper flap is elevated and held by traction. Sternotomy is performed vertically. Laks and Hammond (1980) propose a transverse incision in the submammary skin fold, which rises in

[1] Asymptomatic: "slight residual facial muscle weakness; uses of anticholinesterase only occasionally; no corticoids"

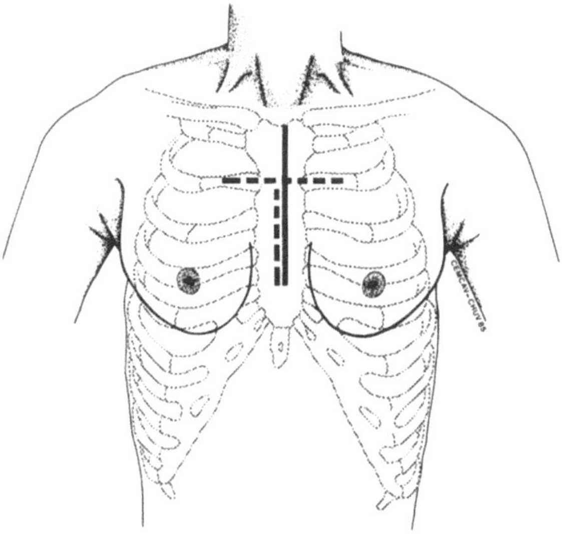

Fig. 1. Surgical approach according to Miller et al. (1981). *Broken line* skin incision; *full line* sternum section

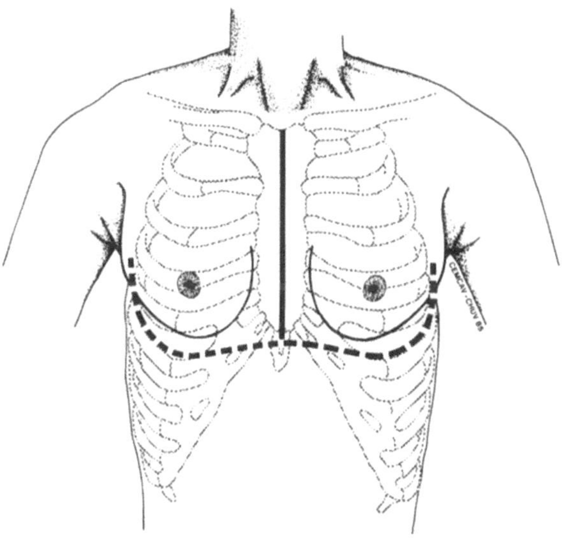

Fig. 2. Surgical approach according to Brutel de la Rivière et al. (1981). *Broken line* skin incision; *full line* sternum section

the midline to the level of the nipples (Fig. 3). The skin flaps are mobilized, superiorly to the suprasternal notch and inferiorly to the tip of the xiphoid process. The sternum is also split vertically.

These incisions do not show with a low-necked dress and are indicated in young women. Brom et al. point out the gratitude of their patients (1985, personal communications). The technique must be scrupulous as risk of postoperative haematoma, infection and skin flap necrosis exists (Laczkovics et al. 1983). It also leaves a small area of insensibility between the breasts in nearly 50% of patients.

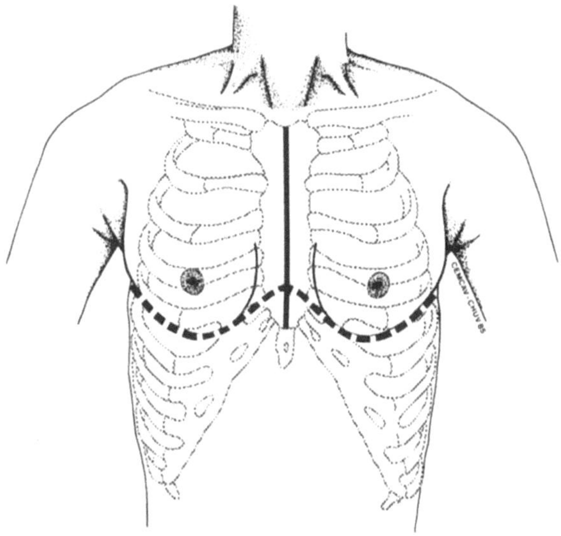

Fig. 3. Surgical approach according to Laks and Hammond (1980). *Broken line* skin incision; *full line* sternum section

Horizontal Thoracotomy and Sternotomy

A horizontal approach was described by Waddell and reported by Heiser and Rutherford (1982) with a transverse skin incision (15-20 cm long) at the sternomanubrial junction (Fig. 4). The sternum is transected in the shape of an inverted V. The chest is opened transversally and thymectomy performed leaving an aesthetic scar. The V section of the sternum allows perfect reduction and postoperative stability of the chest. By this approach a "thorough exploration" of the mediastinum is possible.

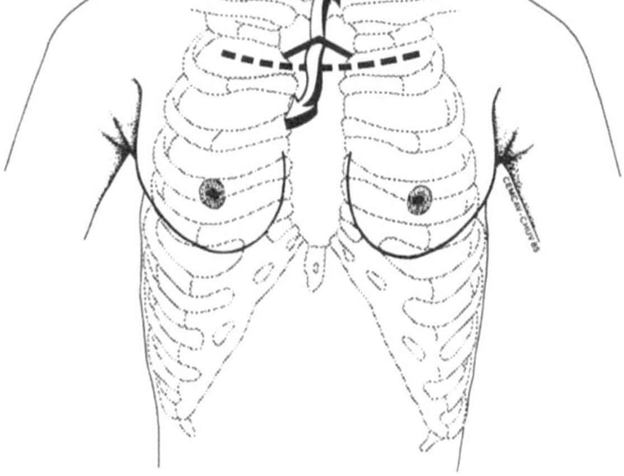

Fig. 4. Surgical approach according to Waddell (Heiser et al. 1982). *Broken line* skin incision; *full line* sternum section

Anterolateral Thoracotomy

A high anterolateral thoracotomy for a nonenlarged gland is used by only a few authors (Le Brigand et al. 1980). The incision is hidden in the submammary fold. It gives an excellent view of the mediastinum. However, the exploration of the cranial poles of the thymus seems to be difficult by this approach.

Thymomas

When a malignancy of the thymus is suspected, mediastinoscopy can confirm the diagnosis. For a confirmed thymoma a median sternotomy is the incision of choice, providing good access for tumour resection. Radical exenteration of the anterior mediastinum is strongly recommended for thymic tumours without myasthenia gravis (Jaretzki 1985, personal communication). Lateral thoracotomies are appropriate for anterior large lateralized thymomas. The *posterolateral approach* was reported many years ago by Clagett and Root (1944). It can be indicated for tumours suspected of encroaching upon the pulmonary pedicle or invading the lung parenchyma. Good preoperative imaging of the tumour extension (computerized tomography or magnetic resonance imaging) is necessary before deciding upon this approach because of the respiratory impairment a posterolateral thoracotomy is likely to cause.

References

Ali HH (1985) Monitoring of neuromuscular function. Clin Anesthesiol 3: 451-454

Austin EH, Olanow CW, Wechsler AS (1983) Thymoma following transcervical thymectomy for myasthenia gravis. Ann Thorac Surg 35: 548-550

Baraka A, Dajani A (1984) Atracurium in myasthenics undergoing thymectomy. Anesth Analg 63: 1127-1130

Baron RL, Lee JKT, Sagel SS, Peterson RR (1982) Computed tomography of the normal thymus. Radiology 142: 121-125

Bédard P, Keon WJ, Brais MP, Goldstein W (1986) Submammary skin incision as a cosmetic approach to median sternotomy. Ann Thorac Surg 41: 339-341

Bergmans J (1980) Apport des techniques neuro-physiologiques à la surveillance des patients myasthéniques, en particulier à l'occasion de la thymectomie. Ann Chir 34: 182-187

Bolooki H, Schwarzmann RJ (1978) High dose steroids patients with myasthenia gravis undergoing thymectomy. J Thorac Cardiovasc Surg 75: 754-757

Brutel de la Riviere A, Brom GHM, Brom AG (1981) Horizontal submammary skin incision for median sternotomy. Ann Thorac Surg 32: 101-104

Buzello W, Noeldge G, Krieg N, Brobmann GF (1986) Vecuronium for muscle relaxation in patients with myasthenia gravis. Anesthesiology 64: 507-509

Clagett OT, Root GT (1944) Surgical approach for tumors of the thymus. Surg Gynecol Obstet 78: 397-401

Clark RE, Marbarger JP, West PN, Spratt JA, Florence JM, Roper CL, Ferguson TB, Weldon CS (1980) Thymectomy for mysthenia gravis in the young adult. Long-term results. J Thorac Cardiovasc Surg 80: 696-701

Cohn HE, Solit RW, Schatz NJ, Schlezinger N (1974) Surgical treatment in myasthenia gravis. A 27 year experience. J Thorac Cardiovasc Surg 68: 876-885

Crile G (1966) Thymectomy through the neck. Surgery 59: 213-215

Dau PC, Lindstom JM, Cassel CK, Denys EH, Shev EE, Spitler LE (1977) Plasmapheresis and immunosuppressive drug therapy in myasthenia gravis. N Engl J Med 297: 1134-1140

D'Empaire G, Hodgkin DC, Perlo VP, Pontoppidan H (1985) Effects of prethymectomy plasma exchange on postoperative respiratory function in myasthenia gravis. J Thorac Cardiovasc Surg 89: 592-596

Diener CF (1973) Evaluation of disability and assessment of operative risk. Med Clin North Am 53: 763-770

Doglietto GB, Bellantone R, Tonali P, Sofo L, Crucitti F (1983) La via cervicale e quella sternotomica per l'accesso al timo non neoplastico nella miastenia. Minerva Chir 38: 1-3

Donnelly RJ, Laquaglia MP, Fabri B, Hayward M, Florence AM (1984) Cervical thymectomy in the treatment of myasthenia gravis. Ann R Coll Surg Engl 66: 307-308

Eisenkraft JB (1987) Myasthenia gravis and thymic surgery anesthetic considerations. In: Gothard JWW (ed) Baillière's clinical anesthesiology, vol 1. Thoracic anesthesia. Tindall, London

Eisenkraft JB, Papatestas AE, Kahn CH, Mora CT, Fagerstrom R, Genkins G (1986) Predicting the need for postoperative mechanical ventilation in myasthenia gravis. Anesthesiology 65: 79-82

Fischer JE, Grinvalski HT, Nussbaum MS, Sayers HJ, Cole RE, Sanaka FJ (1987) Aggressive surgical approach for drug-free remission from myasthenia gravis. Ann Surg 205: 496-503

Gamondès JP, Maret H, Maret G (1981) Soixante-et-une thymectomies pour myasthénie. Tactique opératoire et résultats. Chirurgie 107: 215-218

Genkins G, Papatestas AE, Horowitz SH, Kornfeld P (1975) Studies in myasthenia gravis: early thymectomy. Electrophysiologic and pathologic correlations. Am J Med 58: 517-524

Gilmour JR (1941) Some developmental abnormalities of the thymus and parathyroids. J Pathol Bacteriol 52: 213-218

Gracey DR, Howard FM Jr, Divertie MB (1984a) Plasmapheresis in the treatment of ventilator-dependent myasthenia gravis patients. Reports of four cases. Chest 85: 739-743

Gracey DR, Divertie MB, Howard FM, Payne WS (1984b) Postoperative respiratory care after transsternal thymectomy in myasthenia gravis. A 3-year experience in 53 patients. Chest 86: 67-71

Hankins JR, Mayer RF, Satterfield JR, Turney SZ, Attar S, Sequeira AJ, Thompson BW, McLaughlin JS (1985) Thymectomy for myasthenia gravis: 14-year experience. Ann Surg 201: 618-625

Heiser JC, Rutherford RB, Ringel SP (1982) Thymectomy for myasthenia gravis. A changing perspective. Arch Surg 117: 533-537

Henze A, Biberfeld P, Christensson B, Matell G, Pirskanen R (1984) Failing transcervical thymectomy in myasthenia gravis. Scand J Thorac Cardiovasc Surg 18: 235-238
Ip MSM, So SY, Lam WK (1985) Respiratory problems in myasthenia gravis. Ann Acad Med Singapore 14: 442-445
Jaretzki A, Bethea M, Wolff M, Olarte MR, Lovelace RE, Penn AS, Rowland L (1977) A rational approach to total thymectomy in the treatment of myasthenia gravis. Ann Thorac Surg 24: 120-130
Johns TR (1977) Treatment of myasthenia gravis: long-term administration of corticoids with remarks on thymectomy. In: Griggs RC, Moxley TR (eds) Advances in Neurology, vol 17. Raven, New York, pp 99-122
Kark AE, Kirschner PA (1971) Total thymectomy by the transcervical approach. Br J Surg 58: 321-326
Kirschner PA, Osserman KE, Kark AE (1969) Studies in myasthenia gravis. Transcervical total thymectomy. JAMA 209: 906-910
Laczkovics A, Krisch I, Miholic J, Klepetko W, Domanig E (1983) Ein kosmetisch vorteilhafter Zugang zur medianen Sternotomie. Wien Klin Wochenschr 95: 678-679
Laks H, Hammond GL (1980) A cosmetically acceptable incision for the median sternotomy. J Thorac Cardiovasc Surg 79: 146-149
Le Brigand H (1982) Evolution of the indications and results of treatment of myasthenia by thymectomy. Int Surg 67: 9-11
Le Brigand H, Levasseur P, Miranda AR, Gaud C, Wojakowski I (1980) Résultats du traitement chirurgical de la myasthénie. Semin Hôp Paris 56: 1502-1505
Levasseur P, Le Brigand H (1975) La thymectomie par voie cervicale. Nouv Presse Méd 4: 2591-2593
Leventhal SR, Orkin FK, Hirsch RA (1980) Prediction of the need for postoperative mechanical ventilation in myasthenia gravis. Anesthesiology 53: 26-30
Maggi G (1982) L'exeresi del timo per via cervicale. Archivio ed atti della società italiana di chirurgia. Ottantaquattresimo Congresso, Rom 19-23 Oct 1982. Masson, Milan, pp 889-896
Maggi G, Paletto AE, Casadio C, Pischedda F, Trifiletti G (1982) Résultats de 368 thymectomies pour myasthénie. Lyon Chir 78: 101-104
Masaoka A, Monden Y (1981) Comparison of the results of transsternal simple, transcervical simple, and extended thymectomy. Ann NY Acad Sci 377: 755-765
Masaoka A, Nagaoka Y, Kotake Y (1975) Distribution of thymic tissue at the anterior mediastinum. Current procedures in thymectomy. J Thorac Cardiovasc Surg 70: 747-754
Masaoka A, Monden Y, Seike Y, Tanioka T, Kagotani K (1982) Reoperation after transcervical thymectomy for myasthenia gravis. Neurology 32: 83-85
Miller JI, Mansour KA, Hatcher CR (1981) Median T sternotomy incision for thymectomy in myasthenia gravis. Ann Thorac Surg 34: 473-474
Mittman C (1961) Assessment of operative risk in thoracic surgery. Am Rev Respir Dis 84: 197-207
Monden Y, Nakahara K, Kagotani K, Fujii Y, Masaoka A, Kawashima Y (1984) Myasthenia gravis with thymoma: analysis of and postoperative prognosis for 65 patients with thymomatous myasthenia gravis. Ann Thorac Surg 38: 46-52
Mulder DG, Herrmann C, Keesey J, Edwards H (1983) Thymectomy for myasthenia gravis. Am J Surg 146: 61-66
Mulder DG, White K, Herrmann C (1986) Thymectomy. Surgical procedures for myasthenia gravis. AORN J 43: 640-646
Murphy DF, Magner JB (1986) Neuromuscular blockade with atracurium besylate in a patient with myasthenia gravis. Ir J Med Sci 155: 202-203
Neville WE (1984) Topography of the mediastinum, thymectomy and excision of primary mediastinal masses. In: Nyhus LM, Baker RJ (eds) Mastery of surgery. Little, Brown, Boston, pp 289-298
Olanow CW, Wechsler A, Roses AD (1982) A prospective study of thymectomy and serum acetylcholine receptor antibodies in myasthenia gravis. Ann Surg 196: 113-121
Paletto AE, Maggi G (1974) La tecnica della timectomia per via cervicale con o senza split del manubrio sternale. Minerva Med 65: 4309-4314
Paletto AE, Maggi G (1982) Thymectomy in the treatment of myasthenia gravis: results in 320 patients. Int Surg 67: 13-16
Papatestas AE, Genkins G, Kornfeld P, Horowitz S, Kark AE (1975) Transcervical thymectomy in myasthenia gravis. Surg Gynecol Obstet 140: 535-540
Papatestas AE, Genkins G, Jaretzki A (1978) Cervical thymectomy. Pro and Con. In: Duvoisin RC (ed) Transactions of the American Neurological Association. Springer, New York, 103: 286-291
Papatestas AE, Genkins G, Kornfeld P (1981) Comparison of the results of the transcervical and transsternal thymectomy in myasthenia gravis. Ann NY Acad Sci 377: 766-778
Papatestas AE, Genkins G, Kornfeld P, Eisenkraft J, Fagerstrom RP, Pozner J, Aufses AH (1987a) Effects of thymectomy in myasthenia gravis. Ann Surg 206: 79-88
Papatestas AE, Pozner J, Genkins G, Kornfeld P, Matta RJ (1987b) Prognosis in occult thymomas in myasthenia gravis following transcervical thymectomy. Arch Surg 122: 1352-1356
Penn AS, Jaretzki A, Wolff M, Chang HW, Tennyson V (1981). Thymic abnormalities: antigen or antibody? Response to thymectomy in myasthenia gravis. Ann NY Acad Sci 377: 786-804
Rosenberg M, Jauregui WO, de Vega ME, Herrera MR, Roncoroni AJ (1983) Recurrence of thymic hyperplasia after thymectomy in myasthenia gravis. Its importance as a cause of failure of surgical treatment. Am J Med 74: 78-82
Rowland L (1980) Controversies about the treatment of myasthenia gravis. J Neurol Neurosurg Psychiatry 43: 644-659
Rubin JW, Ellison RG, Moore HV, Pai G (1981) Factors affecting response to thymectomy for myasthenia gravis. J Thorac Cardiovasc Surg 82: 720-728
Spence PA, Morin JE, Katz M (1984) Role of plasmapheresis in preparing myasthenic patients for thymectomy: initial results. Can J Surg 27: 303-305
Thorlacius S, Aarli UJA, Jacobson H, Halversen K (1985) Plasma exchange in myasthenia gravis: clinical effect. Acta Neurol Scand 72: 464-468
Tisi GM (1979) Preoperative evaluation of pulmonary function. Am Rev Respir Dis 119: 293-310
Ward S, Wright DJ (1984) Neuromuscular blockade in myasthenia gravis with atracurium besylate. Anesthesia 39: 51-53
Younger DS, Braun NMT, Jaretzki A, Penn AS, Lovelace RE (1984) Myasthenia gravis: determinants for independent ventilation after transsternal thymectomy. Neurology 34: 336-340

22 Technical Aspects of Thymectomy

David B. Clarke

Introduction

Surgical excision of the virtually normal thymus encountered in the patient with myasthenia gravis presents few challenges. Even the presence of a benign tumour adds little to the difficulties of this straightforward operation. It is only when surgeons elect to remove invasive tumours that their technical resources will be stressed. Much of the safety of thymectomy is derived from improvements in the preoperative and postoperative management. During the early days of surgery for myasthenia, it was not unusual for weakness of the respiratory muscles to make postoperative ventilator support essential. Red rubber endotracheal tubes were poorly tolerated for more than a day or two so that tracheostomy was performed frequently with all its attendant complications. Modern practice has virtually eliminated the need for long-term ventilation and it is many years since the author performed a tracheostomy following thymectomy.

Preoperative and Postoperative Management

Thymic tumours are occasionally associated with pancytopenia, red cell hypoplasia, Cushing's syndrome, Addison's disease and hypogammaglobulinaemia. Preoperative assessment should alert the surgeon to these conditions and as far as possible, they should be corrected prior to surgery. The use of muscle relaxant drugs can be part of routine anaesthetic practice. However, these drugs potentiate the disorder of neuromuscular transmission in the myasthenic patient and will have prolonged effects which will certainly extend into the postoperative period and compel the anaesthetist to institute positive pressure ventilation. The demands for drugs used in the treatment of myasthenia fluctuate after surgery. Initially, motor power may return to nearly normal levels for the first few postoperative days, only to be followed by a return of weakness and eventually to slow inprovement. It may be weeks before the benefits of the operation are apparent. The reintroduction of neostigmine or pyridostigmine after surgery is a matter of clinical judgment, based upon physical examination of the patient and titrated against the patient's needs. Excessive medication with neostigmine may itself lead to interference with neuromuscular conduction and prolong the need for ventilation. It follows, therefore, that management of the patient's drug regime through surgery is of vital importance and should be based upon close cooperation between the neurologist and the surgeon. Since the introduction of the new generation of relaxant drugs such as atracurium we have maintained the preoperative regime of pyridostigmine into the postoperative period and reduced or withdrawn this therapy during the following weeks or months, dictated by the clinical evaluation of the patient. Anaesthesia for patient undergoing thymectomy is considered in Chapt. 23.

Surgical Anatomy

Surgery of the thymus demands familiarity with the anatomy of the neck, the thoracic inlet and the anterior mediastinum. When planning access to these regions account should be taken of the direction of Langer's lines so that an optimal cosmetic result will be obtained. The standard transverse skin incision is ideal for the cervical approach. Vertical incisions over the sternum will usually leave a fine scar in their upper portion, but when extended to the xiphisternum and epigastrium the scars frequently become hypertrophic or keloid. Transverse incisions over the upper chest anteriorly tend to become stretched and unsightly in the midline and, particularly when a bilateral submammary incision is used which has an upward convexity over the sternum, interference with lymphatic drainage may produce swelling of the inferior skin flap.

Deep to the platysma lie the sternothyroid and sternohyoid muscles with sternomastoid muscles lateral to them. All are invested by fascia with large veins running over the surface. By keeping strictly to the midline when separating the strap muscles these veins are avoided and a relatively bloodless plane can be followed until the pretracheal fascia, which invests the thyroid and trachea, is encountered. In the suprasternal notch lie a transverse vein and the interclavicular ligaments. These structures must be divided when performing a median sternotomy.

The manubrium sterni articulates with the medial ends of the clavicles and the costal cartilages of the first and second ribs, the latter being at the level of the manubriosternal joint (the angle of Louis). The blood supply of the manubrium and the body of the sternum (the gladiolus) is derived from branches of the internal mammary artery which runs a finger breadth lateral to the bone. These branches lie at the level of the intercostal spaces, deep to the intercostal muscles.

The thymus gland is the most anterior structure in the superior mediastinum, but it is unusual for it to be in contact with the deep surface of the sternum. It is usually separated from it by fat, or if the anaesthetist inflates the lungs, these may meet in the midline and can be injured when the sternum is divided.

The thymus itself is a greyish pink structure. Its lower poles are broad and flattened. They lie on the pericardium, but seldom extend lower than the third costal cartilage (Fig. 1). The right and left lobes can be separated, but are usually fused at the level of the brachiocephalic vein. The upper poles extend as thin ribbons up into the neck as far as the lower poles of the thyroid gland. Laterally the gland blends with fat and the plane of separation is not clearly defined. The surgeon must be aware that the phrenic nerves are important posterolateral relations of the thymus and if the dissection proceeds too far laterally they may be injured. The left brachiocephalic (innominate) vein lies deep to the midportion of the gland and in immediate relationship to it. Sometimes a tongue of thymic tissue passes deep to the vein. Its junction with the right brachiocephalic vein to form the superior vena cava lies to the right and posteriorly so that it is not usually at risk during routine thymectomy. The anatomy of the venous drainage of the thymus is variable. It may be represented by two short veins which drain from the right and left lobes directly into the brachiocephalic vein or by a single common vein which lies between the lobes and accepts branches from each of them. In addition, smaller veins may drain into the brachiocephalic vein more laterally and unless these are indentified and ligated formally they will tear when traction is applied to the gland. The arterial supply is derived from numerous small branches coming from the internal mammary and inferior thyroid arteries and pericardial branches of the phrenic artery. These are seldom large enough to require formal ligation and division. While the aorta and the great vessels arising from the arch are important posterior relations, they are only of surgical consequence during the extended dissection required when removing large or invasive tumours. The ascending aorta lies within the pericardial sac, the pericardial reflection being at the level of the arotic arch. Similarly, the trachea which passes into the mediastinum in a posteroinferior direction and lies deep to the brachiocephalic vein is only a close relation of the upper pole of the thymus in the neck.

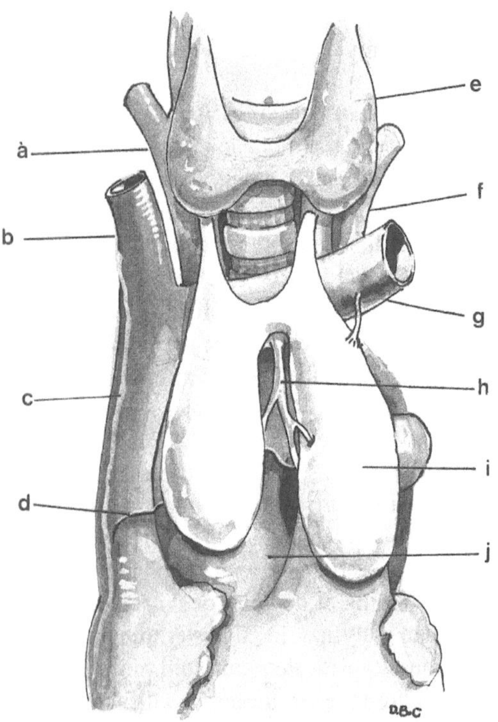

Fig. 1. Surgical anatomy of the thymus. *a* brachiocephalic artery; *b* right brachiocephalic vein; *c* phrenic nerve lying on superior vena cava; *d* Pericardial reflection; *e* thyroid gland; *f* left subclavian artery; *g* left brachiocephalic vein; *h* thymic vein; *i* thymus; *j* ascending aorta

Operative Surgery: The Choice of Approach

(see Chap. 21)

Blalock first demonstrated the benefit of thymectomy for myasthenia in 1939 (Blalock et al. 1939). For many years excision of the thymus was performed through a median sternotomy. Although the approach is simple and provides excellent access, there is no doubt that the stability of the thoracic skeleton is impaired and there may be some interference with breathing and coughing after surgery. In order to reduce this disadvantage, it has been our practice to divide only the upper half of the sternum and we have had no reason to feel dissatisfied with the technique. An alternative was suggested in 1968 (Carlens 1968; Papatestas et al. 1975). The gland is removed through a transverse cervical incision. Although the inferior poles must be freed by blind dissection, and the method is usually thought to be unsuitable for the removal of tumours of any size, there is no impairment of the patient's respiratory function. Against this must be set the possibility that the thymus may not be removed in its entirety and the need for a formal exploration of the anterior mediastinum must be accepted if the patient fails to improve after surgery (Henze et al. 1984). Each techniques has its persuasive advocates and both methods will be described (Masaoka and Monden 1981; Matell et al. 1981). Younger et al. (1987) recommend "maximum thymectomy" which involves resecting not only the gland, but also the surrounding mediastinal fat which may constain small foci of thymic tissue. This involves a combined cervical and transsternal approach. It is claimed that 96% of patients benefit from this procedure (Jaretzki et al. 1988).

Occasionally, the nature of a mediastinal mass cannot be determined by investigations. A tissue diagnosis of anterior mediastinal tumours is most easily obtained through a short anterior thoractomy (anterior mediastinotomy). Mediastinoscopy is not appropriate for the investigation of these tumours as the plane of exploration follows the line of the trachea and there is poor access to the anterior mediastinum. If there is also superior vena caval obstruction, mediastinoscopy can be dangerous. However, sometimes abnormal tissue can be felt in the suprasternal notch and the method can be useful.

There are occasions when a standard posterolateral thoractomy is the incision of choice. Large tumours of the lower pole of the thymus rarely present as masses projecting from the cardiac silhouette on the plain chest radiograph and it may not be possible to differentiate these from other mediastinal or pulmonary tumours. A thoractomy provides the most versatile approach when the nature of the pathology is uncertain and thymectomy can be performed without difficulty through this incision.

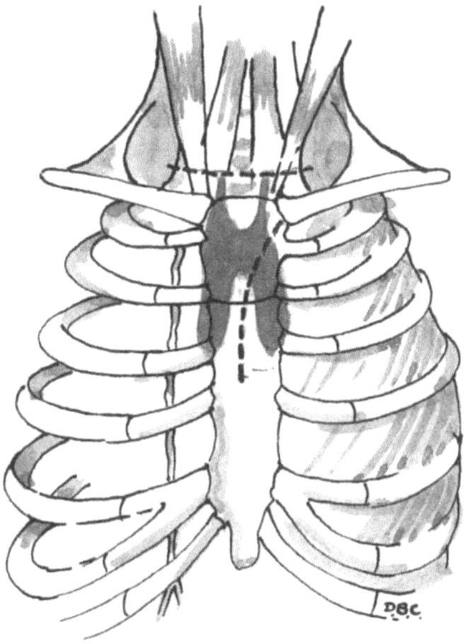

Fig. 2. The skin incision for transsternal and transcervical thymectomy

Transsternal Thymectomy

The skin incision commences at the sternoclavicular joint and swings to the midline. Its lower end is level with the fourth costal cartilage (Fig. 2). This gives a better cosmetic result than the standard midline incision. As contraction of the wound occurs with healing it will be almost invisible when the patient wears an open-neck garment. Diathermy is used to divide the periosteum between the attachment of the pectoral muscles to the sternum and the upper end of the sternum is displayed with blunt dissection. Some venous bleeding is not unusual, but is readily controlled with diathermy. The third intercostal space is defined by palpation and a transverse incision through the pectoral muscles exposes the lateral borders of the sternum at this level. Curved forceps are passed round the edges of the sternum on each side, keeping close to the bone to avoid injuring the internal mammary vessels. Some bleeding from sternal branches of these vessels is not unusual, but is readily controlled. The sternum is now divided transversely and then longitudinally to meet the transverse incision. There is no doubt that a power saw makes this part of the operation very easy, but a Gigli saw can serve nearly as well (Fig. 3). A cholecystectomy forceps is passed round the sternum, keeping its tip closely applied to the posterior surface of the bone to avoid injuring underlying structure. It is used to draw the Gigli saw round the sternum. After transverse division of the bone, the manubrium is levered forward and forceps are passed behind the sternum from below until the tips appear in the suprasternal space. The Gigli saw is drawn down behind the manubrium, which is now divided longitudinally. A Lebsch chisel serves equally well. Bleeding from the posterior periosteum is arrested with diathermy and bone wax is used to control oozing from the bone marrow. A self-retaining retractor is now inserted and the superior mediastinal contents are displayed. If it is anticipated that wider exposure will be needed, the sternum is divided throughout its length. The layer of fascia which covers the thymus is identified and divided in the midline. Blunt dissection is used to identify the plane of separation between the two lobes of the thymus. Dissection proceeds inferiorly, freeing the inferi-

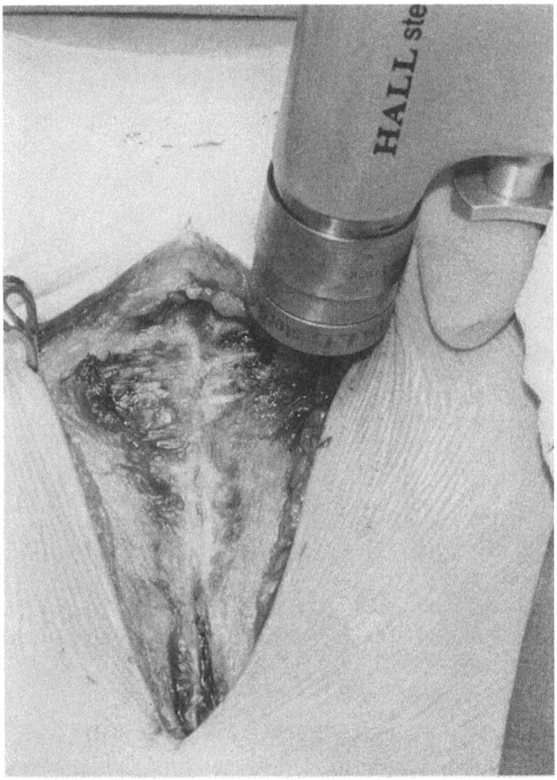

Fig. 3. Transverse division of the sternum with a power saw

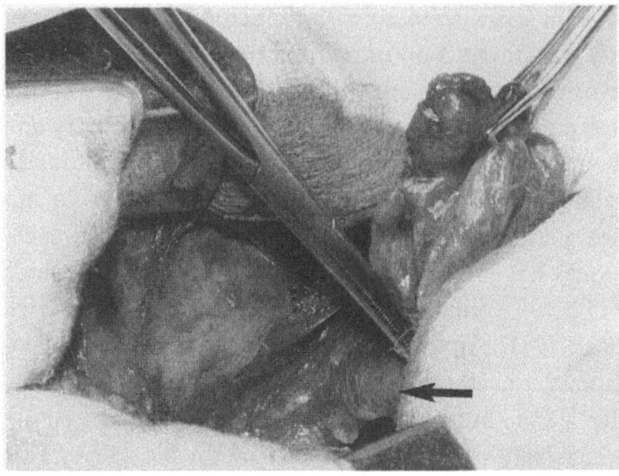

Fig. 4. The lower poles of the thymus are elevated and the left brachiocephalic vein is demonstrated *(arrow)*

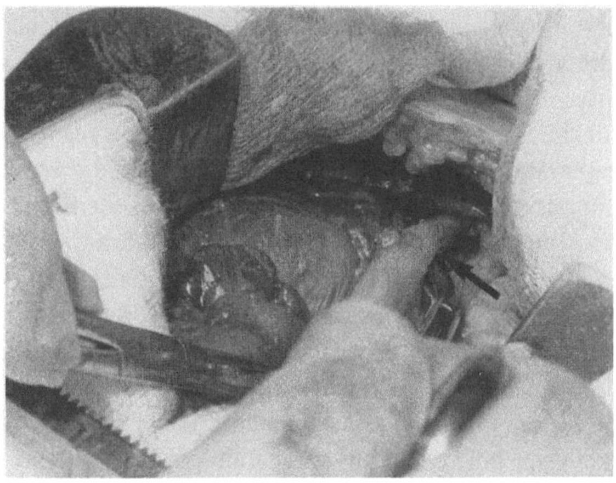

Fig. 5. The upper poles of the thymus are freed as they run up into the neck *(arrow)*

or poles of the gland from the pericardium and then following the lateral borders round on each side in turn. The plane of separation between the thymus and mediastinal fat is not always easy to define, but the difference in texture is readily discerned by palpation and the lateral margin of the gland is mobilized by a combination of dissection and rubbing between finger and thumb. Care should be taken not to wander out into the fat as damage to the phrenic nerve may result. When both lower poles are mobilized, they are elevated with tissue forceps and dissection proceeds behind the gland until the left brachiocephalic (innominate) vein is exposed (Fig. 4). This is a key manoeuvre in the operation - inadvertant injury to this large vein may provoke torrential bleeding. Localization of the vein can sometimes be more easily achieved by continuing to separate the two lobes in the midline and following the thymic vein which runs between them until it enters the brachiocephalic vein. The venous drainage of the gland is commonly by two veins which are identified, ligated and divided. Mobilization can then proceed up towards the neck. The upper poles narrow into two ribbons of tissue which run up towards the thyroid. These are freed by blunt dissection as far as possible, and finally released by gentle traction (Fig. 5). Occasionally, a minute portion of the gland is left behind, but is not usually clinically significant. The arterial supply of the gland is represented by small branches of the internal mammary and inferior thyroid arteries and these are secured with electrocoagulation. After complete haemostastis has been obtained, the wound is checked to confirm whether the pleura has been opened. Small holes can be sutured and the wound closed with a narrow bore suction drain (e. g. Redivac) to the anterior mediastinum. Wide breaches into the pleura are better managed by the insertion of a standard intercostal drain into the appropriate pleural cavity. This is particularly important if the surface of the lung has been injured. The develepment of a postoperative pneumothorax can be of serious consequence to the patient with impaired ventilatory function.

The divided sternum is approximated with interrupted wire sutures, two to the transverse component

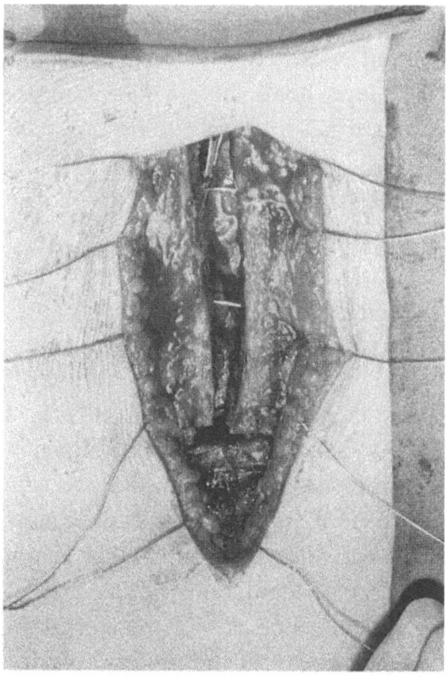

Fig. 6. Approximation of the divided sternum with wire sutures

of the sternotomy and three to the manubrium (Fig. 6). These may either be passed through the bone with the aid of an awl or heavy duty needles swaged to the wire can be used. Passing sutures round the bone can lead to brisk haemorrhage from the internal mammary artery. The pectoral muscles are sutured together in the midline and the subcutaneous tissues and skin are closed.

Some authors are firm believers in "maximum thymectomy" which is in fact a mediastinal exenteration (Jaretzki et al. 1988). This operation requires total sternotomy which is easy to perform with a power saw. After spreading the edges of the sternum, the mediastinum is completely exposed. The resection of the thymus proceeds as described already. However, the localization and dissection of the phrenic nerves is a particularly important step. Then, all the mediastinal fatty tissue from the lower poles of the thyroid gland to the diaphragm is removed. Laterally, the dissection is carried out as fas as possible from hilum to hilum, from within the pleural cavities.

Transcervical Thymectomy

The procedure is carried out under general anaesthesia, utilizing new short-acting muscle relaxant agents. The patient is in a supine position with the neck hyperextended. Neck and chest are prepared and draped as for a mediastinoscopy. The surgeon faces the head and the assistant is on the surgeon's left. The anaesthesist is placed on the left or the right, towards the feet of the patient. A transverse collar incision, 6-7 cm long is made at the supraclavicular notch. The subcutaneous fat and platysma are sectioned and haemostasis is achieved. A superior 4-cm flap is elevated. The cervical fascia is opened longitudinally in the midline and strap muscles (sternohyoid and sternothyroid) are retracted or detached from their sternal origin. The loose prethymic fascia is then opened with fine scissors and the upper poles of the thymus can be identified because they are firmer and more pinkish then the surrounding fat. The upper poles of the gland are separated from thyroid lobes and elevated. A parathyroid gland is sometimes visualized and must be preserved. The posterior border of the thymus is freed from the posterior aspect of the sternum by finger dissection so as to insert an angulated retractor. Strong retraction is very useful with an elastic chest, as in young people or children. However, it may not widen the approach at all if used on a rigid thoracic cage. One thymic lobe is dissected after the other: the left one is generally larger. It is a process of sharp and blunt dissection. The lobes are first prepared posteriorly and laterally and the small lateral arterioles from the internal mammary artery to the gland are coagulated. The thymic lobes are then dissected on their medial and anterior aspect and progressively retracted and delivered by positioning serial clamps. The innominate vein is reached and, must be recognized. In the vast majority of cases (98% according to Papatestas et al. 1975), it lies behind the thymus. However, in a few, one or both lobes can be behind the vein and this particular situation has to be recognized. The vein of Keynes, which drains the gland, ends in the innominate vein. At this level, the lobes tend to fuse (transverse limb of the H). Both upper lobes are dissected before dividing the vein of Keynes. By slight traction the vein is now exposed and ligated or clipped. The final dissection is delicate as distinction between the lower poles and the mediastinal fat is difficult. Care must be taken not to tear the thymic capsule.

In the event of difficult exposition, the manubrium sterni can be sectioned. Certain authors do it frequently (Maggi et al. 1980); the inferior skin flap is also elevated and periosteum electrocoagulated. The manubrium is freed posteriorly and sawn. A deep strong retractor is applied. After thymectomy, the superior mediastinum is inspected. The mediastinoscope can be used because of its angulated light (Klingen et. al. 1977). Occasional pleural tears can be sutured; otherwise, a thoracic drain is passed through the chest into the pleural space. The collar incision is closed in two planes with a small suction drain for 24 h.

Mediastinoscopy

Formal mediastinoscopy, in which the plane of dissection follows the trachea, gives poor access to the anterior mediastinum. Sometimes a thymic tumour extends into the neck where it may be palpable in the suprasternal notch. In such cases, material may be obtained for histological examination trough a transverse incision one finger breadth above the notch. The strap muscles are separated in the midline until the isthmus of the thyroid is seen. This is displaced upwards and the sleeve of pretracheal fascia is divided thereby baring the anterior surface of the trachea. Abnormal tissue may be encountered at any stage of the dissection and a biopsy taken, but if the lesion has not been seen, the index finger is advanced along the anterior surface of the trachea to develop a plane into the superior mediastinum. Palpation provides the most reliable guide to the presence of a mediastinal mass and if such a mass is felt, gentle blunt dissection with the finger is used to clear its surface of surrounding tissues. The examining finger is then removed and a mediastinoscope is inserted. Every thoracic surgeon will have heard stories of inadvertent biopsy of the arch of the aorta even if he or she has not had personal experience of this catastrophe. Every care should be taken, both by palpation and inspection, to differentiate the suspect lesion from the aorta, and if doubt still exists, a trial aspiration with a long needle should be carried out.

Anterior Mediastinotomy

This method provides safe access to the anterior mediastinum and can be performed easily and quickly. The approach is through the bed of a resected costal cartilage. The appropriate cartilage is selected after study of the chest radiograph or computerized tomographic (CT) scan; the second or third rib is most commonly chosen. With the patient under general anaesthesia, a transverse incision is made over the cartilage and the pectoralis major is split in the line of its fibres. A self-retaining retractor is inserted. The perichondrium is incised with diathermy and peeled from the cartilage with a periosteal elevator. The freed cartilage is divided at the costochondral junction and its sternal attachment and removed. The underlying internal mammary vessels are divided between ligatures. The pleural cavity may have been entered, but if the pleura is intact, it can be brushed laterally to expose the anterior mediastinum. Although the access afforded is rather limited, it is adequate to obtain biopsy material and to permit a digital estimate of the extent and fixation of the lesion and even to evaluate invasion of structures in the hilum of the lung or the anterior wall of the chest. The wound is closed with continuous sutures. The intercostal layer holds sutures poorly; repair of the pectoralis major is all that is required. A tube drain is inserted into the chest if the surface of the lung has been injured or if bleeding from the biopsy site has been troublesome.

Anterior Thoractomy

The indications for this approach to the thymus must be very limited. Access is poor and the incision is neither easy to make nor to close. The claim that it is cosmetically superior is dubious, but it is undoubtedly useful if the patient has a tracheostomy which might infect the preferred median sternotomy approach.

The skin incision commences at the manubriosternal junction and runs parallel to the sternum. At the fourth intercostal space it swings laterally and continues in the line of the ribs to the anterior axillary line. The pectoralis major is divided 1 cm from its attachment to the sternum, and freed along its inferior border. Brisk bleeding from perforating branches of the internal mammary artery is controlled.

The flap of skin and pectoral muscle is swung upwards to reveal the anterior chest wall. The fourth intercostal space is defined, retracting the anterior margin of the latissimus dorsi to expose its lateral extent. The intercostal muscle is incised throughout its length, with a finger inside the chest to protect the lung and to ensure that division of the intercostals proceeds exactly between the ribs. Failure to do this will denude the rib of muscle and lead to difficulties in closing the wound. The internal mammary vessels are ligated and divided. The second, third and fourth costal cartilages are divided obliquely close to their attachments to the sternum. These oblique cuts run from medial to lateral, thereby leaving wedges of cartilage attached to the sternum against which the mobilized anterior chest wall will abut when the wound is closed. If the cartilages are simply divided transversely, the anterior chest wall tends to become displaced inwards, thereby leading to an unsightly depression. A stout suture is passed through the first intercostal space and tied round the ribs, bundling them together like the slats of a Venetian blind.

The surgeon now has a wide, triangular exposure of the anterior chest, but unfortunately structures behind the sternum are inaccessible. A standard posterolateral thoractomy, in the author's vew, has all the claimed advantages of the anterior thoracotomy and none of its disadvantages. In closing the anterior thoracotomy, two or three pericostal sutures are needed to supplement the flimsy and friable intercostal muscle layer. Much of the strength of the closure depends upon the accurate reattachment of the pectoralis major muscle.

Surgery for Malignant Tumours of the Thymus

Some controversy exists regarding the role of surgery for thymic malignancy. The differentiation between invasive and encapsulated tumours rests more upon the macroscopic assessment of invasion of the tumor at the time of operation than upon histological appearances. While this information may be obtained at a limited exploration through an anterior mediastinotomy, the true nature of the tumour may only be appreciated when a formal exposure of the gland has been carried out. Widely invasive tumours are probably best treated with radiotherapy with or without cytotoxic drugs, but if complete surgical extirpation is technically feasible the long-term results are superior. In a series of 30 patients treated at the Walter Reed Army Medical Center and the National Naval Center, Bethesda (Cohen et al. 1984) it was concluded that complete surgical excision offered the best chance of long-term survival when compared with partial excision and postoperative irradiation (see chap. 31).

Local invasion of the capsule of the gland or the adjacent pericardium presents few technical difficulties. Wider involvement of the structures in the mediastinum or the lung can present the surgeon with a major challenge. It would be impossible to detail every aspect of such surgery, but some problems which may be encountered are worthy of consideration.

Involvement of the pericardium is frequently associated with a pericardial effusion, but seldom with direct invasion of the heart. The pericardium is opened at a point distant from the tumour and with a finger inside the sac as a guide, the mass is mobilized with the anterior pericardium *en bloc* (Fig. 7). The phrenic nerves should be identified and preserved, if at all possible, to prevent postoperative respiratory difficulties. There is no compelling reason to repair the defect so created, but sheets of bovine pericardium are available which can be sutured to the edges of the incision. Limited invasion of the lungs may be found along the medial aspects of the upper lobes.

A wedge excision of pulmonary tissue by means of a curved vascular clamp adds little to the procedure. The cut surface of the lung is repaired with a running mattress suture followed by a simple over-and-over stich or indeed, by any other technique (e.g. staples) with which the surgeon is familiar. More extensive involvement may dicatate that the whole lobe is re-

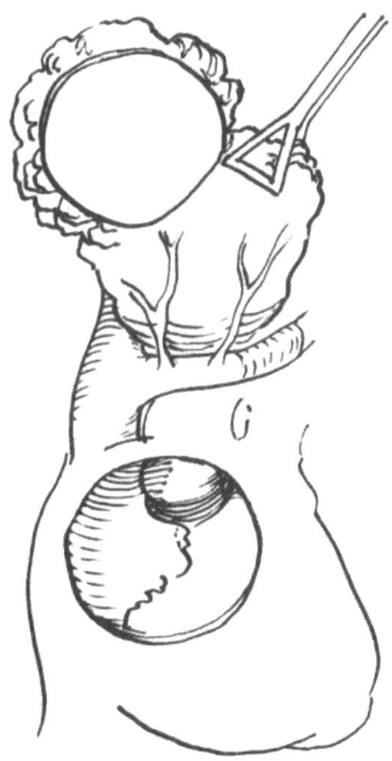

Fig. 7. Diagram showing mobilization of a thymic tumour with a disc of involved pericardium

moved. An upper lobectomy can be performed through a median sternotomy, but access to structures in the major fissure and at the lung hilum is not easy. The ability to collapse the lung by a double-lumen endotracheal tube improves the view considerably. Tumours which involve the left lung often extend posteriorly along the aortic arch. The recurrent laryngeal nerve may be involved, but if possible, it should be identified and spared as difficulty with effective coughing can be of grave consequence to the myasthenic patient.

Superior vena caval obstruction is easily recognized on clinical examination and many surgeons would regard this as a contraindication to surgery for a thymic tumour. However, the decision may not be so clear cut in practice. Investigations including CT scanning may indicate a mass in the anterior mediastinum, but fail to demonstrate its nature. The mass may be benign and eminently resectable. Anterior mediastinotomy through the bed of the resected second or third costal cartilage can provide additional and sometimes conclusive information, but there will certainly be occasions when the surgeon will consider that a formal exploration of the anterior mediastinum in the presence of superior vena caval obstruction is in the best interests of his patient.

Fierce bleeding from venous collaterals must be controlled during the skin incision and division of the sternum. Prelimininary dissection establishes the position of the right and left brachiocephalic veins as they enter the tumour and these vessels are encircled with tapes. The superior vena cava below the tumour is exposed within the pericardium. A tape can be passed round it at its junction with the right atrium without difficulty, but there is an advantage in identifying the azygos vein as it enters the posterior aspect of the cava and passing the tape cephalad to this vessel. This ensures that when vascular clamps are applied, an important collateral venous pathway from the head remains open. In the presence of established caval obstruction, clamps can be applied without the need for establishing a shunt to conduct the venous return from the upper half of the body (Fig. 8).

Mobilization of the tumour can now proceed with the assurance that major haemorrhage from the great veins can speedily be controlled. The surgeon may be pleasantly surprised to find that the tumour is compressing these vessels without invading them. On one occasion, the author encountered local invasion of the left brachiocephalic vein by a long tongue of tumour which passed into the vena cava. It was possible to extract this tumour and reconstruct the vein. When it is apparent that only resection of part of the vena cava or its two tributaries will alow the tumour to be excised, the surgeon will be faced with the task of replacing these vessels. Unfortunately, the vascular prostheses used in arterial reconstructions are unsuccessful when used as vein substitutes. I have had some success

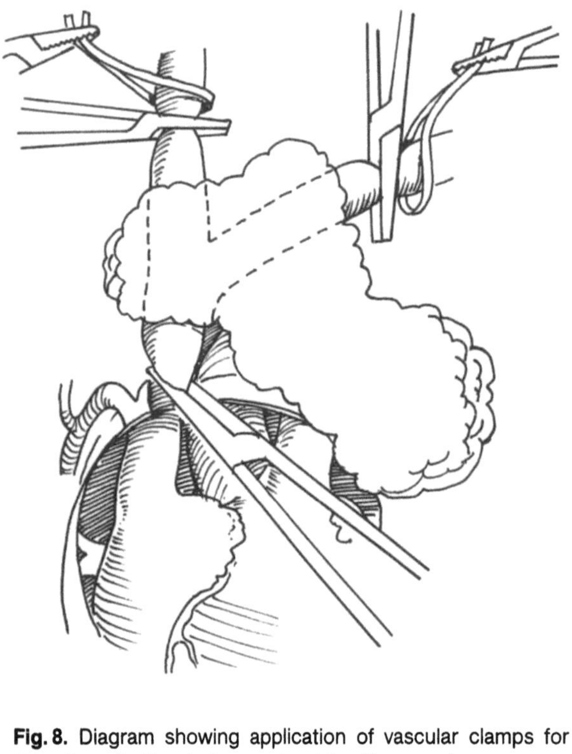

Fig. 8. Diagram showing application of vascular clamps for resection of a thymic tumour involving the superior vena cava

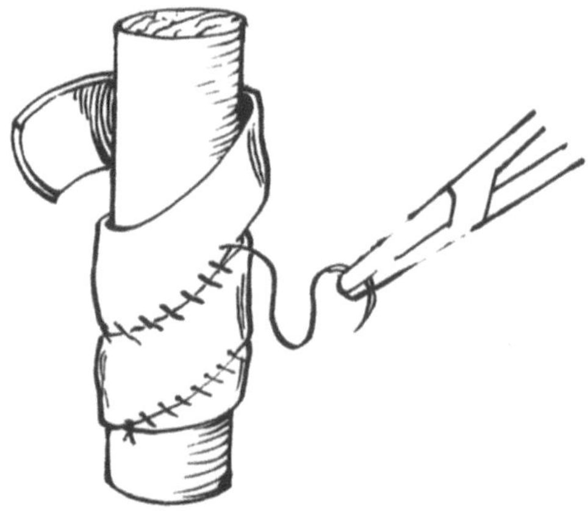

Fig. 9. Construction of a vena caval replacement with a ribbon of saphenous vein sutured round a stent

using a woven silastic rubber prosthesis. There have been encouraging reports of replacement of the superior vena cava by prostheses constructed from bovine pericardium; or with the patient's own common femoral vein harvested distal to its saphenous and profunda branches. Alternatively, autologous saphenous vein is split longitudinally and the ribbon thus formed is sutured as a spiral round a stent of appropriate size. (Fig. 9). If these extended and technically demanding operations are successful in achieving complete removal ot the thymus, a 5-year survival rate of 60% may be anticipated. Incomplete removal justifies the use of postoperative radiotherapy.

References

Blalock A, Mason MF, Morgan HJ, Riven SS (1939) Myasthenia gravis and tumors of thymic region; report of case in which tumor was removed. Ann Surg 110: 544-61

Carlens E (1968) Thymectomy for myasthenia gravis with the aid of mediastinoscopy. Opuscula. Med 13: 175

Cohen DJ, Ronnigen LD, Graeber GM, Deshong JL, Jaffin J, Burge JR, Zajtchuk R (1984) Management of patients with malignant thymoma. J Thorac Cardiovasc Surg 87: 301-307

Henze A, Biberfeld P, Christensson B, Matell G, Pirskanen R (1984) Failing transcervical thymectomy in myasthenia gravis. An evaluation of transsternal re-exploration. Scand J Thorac Cardiovasc Surg 18: 235-238

Jaretzki A, Penn AS, Younger DS, Wolff M, Olarte MR, Lovelace RE, Rowland LP (1988) "Maximal" thymectomy for myasthenia gravis: results. J Thorac Cardiovasc Surg 95: 747-757

Klingen G, Johansson L, Westerholm CJ, Sunderström C (1977) Transcervical thymectomy with the aid of mediastinoscopy for maysthenia gravis: eight years experience. Ann Thorac Surg 23: 342-347

Masaoka A, Monden Y (1981) Comparison of the results of transsternal simple, transcervical simple and extended thymectomy. Ann NY Acad Sci 377: 755-765

Maggi G, Casadio C, Pischedda F, Casalegno PA, Saini U (1980) Indication et technique chirurgical de la thymectomie chez les myasthéniques. Ann Chir 34: 164-168

Matell G, Lebram G, Osterman PO, Pirskanen R (1981) Follow-up comparison of suprasternal vs transsternal method for thymectomy in myasthenia gravis. Ann NY Acad Sci 377: 844-845

Papatestas AE, Genkins G, Kornfeld P, Horowitz S, Kark AE (1975) Transcervical thymectomy in myasthenia gravis. Surg Gynecol Obstet 140: 535-540

Younger DS, Jaretzki A, Penn AS (1987) Maximum thymectomy for myasthenia gravis. Ann NY Acad Sci 505: 832-835

23 Anaesthesia for Thymectomy

T. Hilary Howells and Gabriel S. Shuster

Introduction

There are many problems which the anaesthetist has to face when considering anaesthesia for thymectomy. Some of these are very special to thymectomy and others are more general. The commonest reason for thymectomy is as a part of treatment of myasthenia gravis, a condition which provides a challenge to the anaesthetist (Papatestas et al. 1987). Most of this chapter will be concerned with problems related to myasthenia. Other medical conditions may also be encountered, some of which are associated with myasthenia gravis and others which may be purely coincidental.

The anaesthetist needs to provide the best possible operating conditions. This will depend on the surgical approach to be taken and will involve factors such as the control of systemic blood pressure and respiration. Additionally the anaesthetist has to deal with the purely anaesthetic problems such as the choice of premedicant and anaesthetic drugs.

The anaesthetist's responsibility can be conveniently considered in three parts corresponding to the preoperative, the perioperative and the postoperative periods. In the management of myasthenic patients there is considerable overlap in the expertise of physicians, surgeons and anaesthetists and the patient will benefit from a shared approach to the overall problems.

Preoperative Period

The preoperative period provides an opportunity for planning between nurses, physiotherapists, surgeons, physicians and anaesthetists and is a chance to prepare the patient physically and psychologically for surgery. Personal contact between the patient and members of staff who will later become involved is very important. The anaesthetist's preoperative visit can do much to reduce the anxiety level of the patient. Sensible discussion of methods of analgesia and postoperative pain expectations can actually reduce the amount of analgesia required later. If it is anticipated that the patient will be nursed on an intensive care ward and possibly require ventilatory support, then this is best explained by the staff who will later nurse the patient. A meeting with the physiotherapist may be beneficial and some concepts such as deep breathing and incentive spirometry can be introduced. Visits of this nature encourage continuity of care and greatly enhance staff satisfaction. Whilst this outline of management benefits all patients in general, it is vital to the myasthenic patient in whom anxiety can precipitate a myasthenic crisis.

Assessment

The anaesthetist will make a personal assessment of the patient, but it is also necessary to seek the opinions of the medical and surgical teams. Intercurrent medical conditions should be identified, as should any particular anaesthetic hazards. A drug history is important. Steroid therapy can cause adrenal suppression and it is widely held that patients who have recently received courses of steroids may not be able to produce an adequate surge of endogenous glucocorticoids to meet the stress imposed by surgery. It is usual therefore to administer parenteral hydrocortisone to such patients in the perioperative period. Work by Lloyd (1981) suggests that this practice is probably rarely necessary. However, a common practice is to administer 25 mg hydrocortisone at induction of anaesthesia, as well as 100 mg hydrocortisone over the next 24 h (in addition to the usual dosage) if the patient has received corticosteroids for over 1 month during the preceding 6-12 months (White and Kumagai 1979; Symreng et al. 1981).

Large thymic masses may cause tracheobronchial compression, superior vena caval obstruction or even cardiac tamponade. Tracheobronchial compression may be asymptomatic, but there is frequently a tell tale wheeze. Penetrated lateral chest radiographs plus thoracic inlet views are helpful, but tomography and computerised axial tomography can more clearly delineate tracheobronchial compression. Anaesthesia may precipitate or exacerbate airway obstruction in these patients and the obstruction is not always relieved by tracheal intubation. An inhalational induction is recommended for such patients. Alternatively awake intubation under topical anaesthesia, with fibre optic bronchoscopy, is a very safe technique. Ketamine induction followed by blind nasal intubation under topical anaesthesia has also been advocated. It is said that long thin tubes with side ports can be manipulated so as to allow ventilation distal to the sites of tracheobronchial compression. In extreme cases extracorporeal circulation has been established prior to anaesthesia.

Superior vena caval obstruction causes oedema of the head, neck and arms. Respiratory embarrassment is common and severe hypotension can occur under anaesthesia. Drugs and fluids should not be given via the veins of the upper limbs and central venous catheterisation is dangerous. Bleeding is likely to be considerable during surgery. Preoperative radiotherapy or chemotherapy will markedly reduce the anaesthetic risks. Mackie and Watson (1984) have written an excellent review of these problems.

Rheumatoid arthritis, Hashimoto's thyroiditis and thyrotoxicosis can all be associated with myasthenia gravis and these conditions pose their own problems to the anaesthetist. The myasthenic patient is more at risk from the complications of intercurrent respiratory disease or from respiratory embarrassment due to obesity or depressant drugs. It is important to assess the likelihood of the myasthenic patient requiring postoperative ventilatory support. Many attempts have been made to identify the predisposing factors, but none have been totally satisfactory. Unfortunately this type of work depends upon the retrospective analysis of data collected from relatively small numbers of cases over a number of years. There have been five such studies. Loach et al. (1975) suggested that the high rist factors were: age greater than 50 years; vital capacity less than 2 l; bulbar weakness; the use of a sternum-splitting surgical approach; and the presence of a thymoma. Leventhal et al. (1980) applied multivariate discriminant analysis to the data from 24 patients. They were unable to demonstrate an increased risk associated with the Loach factors apart from a low vital capacity. They identified four risk factors which they weighted with a points system such that a total score of greater than 10 should indicate a need for postoperative ventilatory support. The factors were as follows: myasthenia diagnosed more than 5 years previously (12 points); chronic respiratory disease (10 points); maintenance dose of pyridostigmine greater than 750 mg/day (8 points); and vital capacity less than 2.9 l (4 points). This scoring system was evaluated by Grant and Jenkins (1982) who found a reasonable correlation, but with a few false negatives and a few false positives. Two more recent studies (Gracey et al. 1984; Younger et al. 1984) have failed to substantiate the Leventhal factors. Younger et al. (1984) suggest that clinical criteria are nearly useless as predictors of postoperative ventilatory performance. They suggest that the most powerful predictor is the static maximum expiratory force which should be greater than 40 cm H_2O. This measurement relates well to coughing ability which reflects the ability to clear secretions - probably the key to postoperative independence from ventilatory support.

The condition of the patient should be optimal prior to surgery, particularly with regard to the control of myasthenia and freedom from respiratory tract infections. Routine biochemical and haematological investigations should yield normal results. Hypokalaemia is to be particularly avoided as this will exacerbate myoneural weakness. The nutritional status of the patient should be good. Lung function tests do not contribute very usefully to the assessment as they do not measure respiratory muscle fatiguability. Physiotherapy, bronchodilators and antibiotics have traditionally been used to improve preoperative respiratory function. Plasma exchange is now being used for this purpose with promising results (Gracey et al. 1984, Younger et al. 1984).

Tailoring the pharmacological treatment of myasthenia during the perioperative period is still controversial. The following problems are encountered: a postoperative change in the anticholinesterase requirement; an extreme sensitivity to neuromuscular blocking agents; a real danger of precipitating a cholinergic crisis postoperatively; and an increase in bronchial secretions whenever cholinergic drugs are used. These problems have been faced in various ways. Earlier authors recommended cessation of all therapy preoperatively followed by elective mechanical ventilation, often via tracheostomy. This method is said to rest the neuromuscular junction and to provide muscle relaxation during surgery. The great bonus of this technique is the minimisation of bronchial secretions. Work in children (Davies and Steward 1973) suggests that withdrawal of treatment 24 h before surgery can reduce postoperative pulmonary complications. The major disadvantage is that the resultant muscle weakness may precipitate respiratory failure. At the Royal Free Hospital we continue anticholinesterase therapy right up until the time of operation.

Steroid therapy is a useful part of the treatment of some myasthenic patients. Very high doses of steroids have been given to patients in the perioperative period. There is evidence that these patients have fewer postoperative pulmonary complications and that it may be possible to withdraw their anticholinesterase drugs prior to surgery without causing problems (Bolooki and Schwartzman 1978).

Plasma exchange is likely to become a more important part of the preoperative preparation in severe myasthenia. Fresh frozen plasma or purified human albumin are given in exchange for the patient's own plasma. There are theoretical risks from removing the patients's own plasma proteins, namely decreased resistance to infection and reduced coagulability. There are also risks of transmitting blood-borne infections such as serum hepatitis or AIDS via the replacement plasma. A small retrospective study to evaluate the role of plasma exchange (Spence et al. 1984), indicates that it may be a useful and safe adjuvant to preoperative treatment of severe myasthenia.

Premedication

The purpose of a premedication is to produce a calm and cooperative patient who may have some amnesia of the preoperative period and who will benefit from a smooth induction of anaesthesia. Anticholinergic drugs are often included in premedication because they carry additional advantages. These are: a reduction in the volume of salivary and bronchial secretions (but at the cost of an increase in viscosity); some protection against vagal reflexes; and a limited antiemetic effect. The analgesic properties of opiate premedicant drugs may reduce the requirement for anaesthetic agents during surgery and may carry through into the early postoperative period. Unfortunately opiates depress respiratory drive which is an important consideration in myasthenia gravis. Likewise benzodiazepines, which are useful sedatives, are unsuitable for myasthenic patients. There are some authorities who recommend atropine only as a premedicant for myasthenic patients (Davies and Steward 1973; Girnar and Weinreich 1976). In our experience the majority of adults presenting for thymectomy can safely be given a premedication containing papaveretum (10-20 mg) and hyoscine (0.2-0.4 mg).

Perioperative Period

General Management

An intravenous infusion should be set up before the induction of anaesthesia. Invasive cardiovascular monitoring is not usually required unless a difficult surgical dissection is anticipated. If necessary this is performed after the induction of anaesthesia. An electrocardiograph and noninvasive recording of blood pressure will normally provide adequate monitoring of the cardiovascular system. Bradycardias are common and may occur during induction (Florence 1984), but are seldom severe. A small dose of atropine intravenously at induction will protect against bradycardias. Information regarding ventilatory adequacy can be obtained via routine capnography or transcutaneous blood gas measurement.

Neuromuscular blocking drugs are best avoided altogether when dealing with myasthenic patients because adequate muscle relaxation can be achieved without them and their effects are wholly unpredictable. There may be resistance to suxamethonium, but there is a risk of developing a prolonged "phase two block" (Feldman 1984; Miller and Lee 1981). Myasthenic patients have a greatly increased sensitivity to nondepolarising neuromuscular blocking agents. This is the basis of one of the more hazardous tests for myasthenia gravis. The short-acting, nondepolarising agent, atracurium, has been reportedly used without complications in myasthenic patients for non-thymic surgery (Ward and Wright 1984).

All volatile anaesthetic agents have a direct depressant effect on the neuromuscular junction which can be monitored by transcutaneous neurostimulation (Relaxograph) (Eisenkraft 1987). Isoflurane and enflurane have a greater effect than halothane. The use of volatile agents with myasthenic patients greatly reduces muscle tone and facilitates smooth anaesthesia. Deep anaesthesia can be achieved most rapidly with halothane because it can be given in concentrations of greater relative potency than either enflurane or isoflurane and it is less likely to cause respiratory irregularities during induction. Repeated exposure to halothane must be avoided as the risk of hepatitis is real (Neuberger and Williams 1984). Recovery from isoflurane and from enflurane anaesthesia is faster than from halothane. A good technique for smooth, deep anaesthesia is thus a combination of inhaled O_2-N_2O-isoflurane and injected alfentanil (a very short-acting opiate), with the addition of small doses of atracurium if necessary. The global depression of the neuromuscular junction is constantly monitored by transcutaneous neurostimulation.

Anaesthesia for thymectomy can be conducted without volatile agents. Total intravenous anaesthesia techniques without neuromuscular block and neuroleptanaesthesia have been described. A combination of the short-acting opiate, fentanyl, and either etomidate or Althesin (a mixture of the steroids alphaxolone and alphadolone) by infusion was reported in a series of 22 patients undergoing transcervical thyroidectomy (Florence 1984). However, Althesin has been withdrawn from some markets owing to anaphylactic reactions to it, and etomidate is usually not used by infusion to avoid depression of the hypothalamo-pituitary-adrenal axis. Over 70% of these patients required an opiate antagonist at the end of surgery and this is probably because a large dose of fentanyl was given at induction. The group who received Althesin made a faster recovery than those receiving etomidate. None of the patients in this study required postoperative mechanical ventilation and neither were opiate analgesics required. It is probable that the low invasiveness of the surgical technique was a factor in the success of this study.

Special Management

There are three surgical approaches to the thymus gland. The most conservative is the transcervical in which access is gained through the sternal notch. The sternum is retracted anteriorly and surgery is performed through the retrosternal tunnel created. For this surgical technique the anaesthetist usually allows spontaneous ventilation. More common is the radical approach involving thoracotomy through a total sternal split which gives generous surgical access. Anaesthetic management is as for any formal thoracotomy and controlled ventilation by a mechanical ventilator is the rule. The third approach is through a partial sternotomy which provides a compromise access to the thymus. It is also the most challenging for the anaesthetist because allowing the patient to breathe spontaneously results in significant paradoxical ventilation while instituting mechanical controlled ventilation causes the medial lung edges to blow into the wound and obscure the field of operation.

Partial sternotomy was favoured at the Royal Free Hospital until 1986. For this approach we used intermittent manually controlled ventilation with a circle system and a carbon dioxide absorber. From the onset of anaesthesia we aimed to achieve hyperventilation such that the $PaCO_2$ was maintained at about 3.5 kPa. The FIO_2 was kept at O.35. This state allowed intermittent periods of apnoea to be provided during critical surgical manipulations. Ventilation then proceeded intermittently by hand, with breath-by-breath control, keeping the surgical progress in continuous view. Since 1987 we have used thoracotomy by total sternal split.

Our current anaesthetic technique involves propofol induction which facilitates initial hand ventilation by mask and early establishment of light inhalational anaesthesia. A second dose of propofol then gives excellent conditions for tracheal intubation. Neuromuscular blocking agents are never used either for intubation or the maintenance of controlled ventilation during anaesthesia.

Towards the end of surgery volatile anaesthetic agents are withdrawn and controlled ventilation is diminished until spontaneous respiration returns. Because we have maintained our patients on optimal anticholinesterase therapy up to the induction of anaesthesia, we expect them to demonstrate at least as good (if not better) muscle power immediately after thymectomy.

Surgical Complications

There are surgical complications which may arise at the time of operation and will involve the anaesthetist. Blood loss is usually low in adults and transfusion is seldom necessary. However, there are many potential sources of catastrophic bleeding close to the thymus gland. In contrast, children often require transfusion during thymectomy (Davies and Steward 1973).

Air embolism is extremely rare in thymic surgery. Air enters the venous circulation through a cut vein, but can only do so if the venous pressure is subatmospheric and the walls of the vein are prevented from collapsing. To prevent this, surgery can be performed with the patient in a slightly head-down position. If the volume of air is large enough it will cause an airlock in the right ventricular outflow tract. A large fall in cardiac output will occur accompanied by arrythmias and gaseous exchange will be greatly diminished. If a stethoscope is placed over the precordium or if an oesophageal stethoscope is in use, then a loud "millwheel murmur" will be heard. A sharp fall in end-tidal PCO_2 can be detected with a capnograph. A Doppler ultrasound probe can be placed over the right ventricle and will provide the most sensitive method of detection. Once air embolism has been detected wet packs should be pressed over the wound to prevent the entry of more air. The patient should be tilted head down and on the left side. If a central venous line is advanced into the right ventricle it may be possible to aspirate air.

Postoperative Period

Respiratory failure is particularly prone to occur within the first 24 h and it is this period with which the anaesthetist is most concerned. All of our patients are transferred to the intensive therapy unit for close supervision during this period. A small minority of patients are electively ventilated postoperatively. The majority of patients are extubated in theatre having first demonstrated that they are making adequate respiratory effort. If there is any doubt then we apply our criteria which are fulfilled when there is a vital capacity greater than 15 ml/kg, maximal inspiratory and expiratory pressures greater than 30 cm H_2O and a respiratory rate less than 30 per minute.

The particular problems of the early postoperative period are as follows: the effects of residual anaesthetic drugs, the control of pain, clearance of bronchial secretions and the altered anticholinesterase requirement. There is experimental evidence that most of the commonly used intravenous induction agents cause postsynaptic depression at the neuromuscular junction, but the clinical significance is doubtful (Torda and Gage 1977). Thiopentone has a particularly long elimination half-life of 18 h and can theoretically cause sedation, respiratory depression and antanalgesia during the recovery period.

Large amounts of halothane are dissolved in the tissues during anaesthesia and are gradually released into the circulation over hours or even days following an anaesthetic. Bergmans (1980) has monitored neuromuscular transmission in a group of myasthenic patients undergoing thymectomy with halothane anaesthesia. He was able to demonstrate that neuromuscular depression increased with the duration of anaesthesia and took several hours to recover.

The pain of thymectomy is greatest if the sternum is completely divided and least if the transcervical approach is used. Wound pain may inhibit deep breathing and coughing, thus predisposing to sputum retention, atelectasis and infection. Opiate analgesics are antitussive and depress respiration. Nevertheless, analgesia will permit better chest movement and coughing and is particularly useful during physiotherapy. High thoracic epidural anaesthesia, with 0.25% bupivacaine (D6-7) in the postoperative period has been reported to offer a good solution to this problem (Ferretti et al. 1987).

Alterations in the postoperative anticholinesterase requirement are anticipated. This often takes the form of a temporary reduction, but it cannot be relied upon to occur. Our policy is to replace the quantity of anticholinesterase that has been omitted during surgery with intramuscular neostigmine according to the formula: 0.5 mg neostigmine intramuscularly = 60 mg pyridostigmine orally. Regular edrophonium testing (2 mg followed by 8 mg) enables us to determine the frequency of further doses of anticholinesterase drugs which are given in as small doses as possible. Oral pyridostigmine should be recommenced within a few hours of surgery. One of the greatest dangers of this period is over-treatment of myasthenia which causes an increase in bronchial and salivary secretions and eventually a cholinergic crisis. Interpretation of the edrophonium test may be straightforward. The patient often has a correct subjective impression and there may be an obvious clinical change. Measurements made before and after the test may be helpful, but it must be realised that the respiratory musculature may have a different sensitivity to anticholinesterases than other muscle groups. The grip strength can be measured with a simple dynamometer. An anaesthetic face mask can be used in order to measure the vital capacity and the maximal inspiratory and expiratory forces. A Wright's respirometer and a pressure gauge will be required. Practice is needed to take these measurements and they can be taken much more easily from the intubated patient.

Even with faultless management of the anticholinesterase regime, a few patients will develop respiratory muscle fatigue and will require ventilatory support. This may occur up to 24 h after surgery. An increasing respiratory rate together with a fall in vital capacity and a fall in expiratory or inspiratory force is a reliable indication of fatigue and must be taken seriously.

Regular chest physiotherapy is likely to help in the clearance of secretions. Davies and Steward (1973) have suggested that the benefit of physiotherapy can be enhanced when it follows an edrophonium test combined with a small dose of intravenous pethidine. Atropine may be given in the postoperative period to reduce the volume of secretions (Girnar and Weinreich 1976). Glycopyrrolate has a stronger but similar effect. Aminoglycosides and tetracycline antibiotics have some curariform activity. They should be avoided where possible although the extent to which these drugs are dangerous is not clear.

After 24-48 h the patient can usually be transferred to a general ward and may well move out of the anaesthetist's sphere of influence. A few unfortunate patients will require prolonged ventilatory support on the intensive care ward. In our unit tracheostomy is reserved for those who make a slow recovery. Modern plastic endotracheal tubes which have high volume, low pressure cuffs, can be used for prolonged periods without causing permanent tracheal damage. In the long term, tracheostomy is better tolerated by the patient and permits oral feeding. In addition the spontaneously breathing tracheostomised patient can have bronchial secretions aspirated easily, and can be reconnected rapidly to a ventilator if required. Diligent observation and clinical acumen are required to steer the patient safely through the postoperative course. Once again combined management with the surgical and medical teams is required to ensure that a satisfactory outcome from thymectomy may be achieved.

References

Bolooki H, Schwartzman RJ (1978) High-dose steroids for perioperative management of patients with myasthenia gravis undergoing thymectomy. A preliminary report. J Thorac Cardiovasc Surg 75: 754-757

Bergmans J (1980) Apport des techniques neuro-physiologiques à la surveillance de patients myasthéniques, en particulier à l'occasion de la thymectomie. Ann Chir 34: 182-187

Davies DW, Steward DJ (1973) Myasthenia gravis in children and anaesthetic management for thymectomy. Can Anaesth Soc J 20: 253-258

Eisenkraft JB (1987) Myasthenia gravis and thymic surgery - anaesthetic considerations. Baillières Clin Anaesth 1: 133-162

Feldman SA (1984) Neurological conditions and anaesthesia. In: Churchill-Davidson HC (ed) A practice of anaesthesia, 5th edn. Saunders, Philadelphia, pp 739-340

Ferretti F, Crestani S, Rodriguez NJ, Tosi C, Martinoli S (1987) Peut-on employer l'analgésie épidurale thoracale haute dans les soins intensifs postopératoires du myasthénique après thymectomie transsternale? Schweiz Med Wochenschr 117: 438-441

Florence AM (1984) Anaesthesia for transcervical thymectomy in myasthenia gravis. Ann R Coll Engl 66: 309-312

Girnar DS, Weinreich AI (1976) Anesthesia for transcervical thymectomy in myasthenia gravis. Anesth Analg 55: 13-17

Gracey DR, Divertie MB, Howard FM Jr, Payne WS (1984) Postoperative respiratory care after transsternal thymectomy in myasthenia gravis. A 3-year experience in 53 patients. Chest 86: 67-71

Grant RP, Jenkins LC (1982) Prediction of the need for postoperative mechanical ventilation in myasthenia gravis: thymectomy compared to other surgical procedures. Can Anaesth Soc J 29: 112-116

Leventhal SR, Orkin FK, Hirsh RA (1980) Prediction of the need for postoperative mechanical ventilation in myasthenia gravis. Anesthesiology 53: 26-30

Lloyd EL (1981) A rational regimen for perioperative steroid supplements and a clinical assessment of the requirement. Ann R Coll Surg Engl 63: 54-57

Loach AB, Young AC, Spalding JMK, Smith AC (1975) Postoperative management after thymectomy. Br Med J 75: 309-312

Mackie AM, Watson CB (1984) Anaesthesia and mediastinal masses. A case report and review of the literature. Anaesthesia 39: 899-903

Miller J, Lee C (1981) Muscle diseases. In: Katz J, Benumof J, Kadis LB (eds) Anesthesia and uncommon diseases. Pathophysiologic and clinical correlations, 2nd edition. Saunders, Philadelphia, pp 550-554

Neuberger J, Williams R (1984) Halothane anaesthesia and liver damage. Br Med J 298: 1136-1139

Papatestas AE, Genkins G, Kornfeld P, Eisenkraft JB, Fagerstrom RP, Pozner J, Aufses AH (1987) Effects of thymectomy in myasthenia gravis. Ann Surg 206: 79-88

Spence PA, Morin JE, Katz M (1984) Role of plasmapheresis in preparing myasthenic patients for thymectomy: initial results. Can J Surg 27: 303-305

Symreng T, Karlberg BE, Kågedal B, Schildt B (1981) Physiological cortisol substitution of long-term steroid-treated patients undergoing major surgery. Br J Anaesth 53: 949-954

Torda TA, Gage PW (1977) Postsynaptic effect of i. v. anaesthetic agents at the neuromuscular junction. Br J Anaesth 49: 771-776

Ward S, Wright DJ (1984) Neuromuscular blockade in myasthenia gravis with atracurium besylate. Anaesthesia 39: 51-53

White VA, Kumagai LF (1979) Preoperative endocrine and metabolic considerations. Med Clin North Am 63: 1321-1334

Younger DS, Braun NMT, Jaretzki III A, Penn AS, Lovelace RE (1984) Myasthenia gravis: determinants for independent ventilation after transsternal thymectomy. Neurology 34: 336-340

24 Postoperative Care

Dominique Thorin

Introduction

The perioperative mortality of myasthenia gravis patients has declined tremendously since the introduction of effective ventilatory assistance, but there is still a good deal of morbidity associated with this disease. A sound knowledge of its pathophysiology and of the postoperative respiratory distress which is one of its common features should allow the medicosurgical team to anticipate postoperative complications and thus reduce this morbidity.

Several factors influence the short and midterm postoperative outcome of myasthenic patients. The clinical stage of the disease particularly as regards cranial nerve dysfunction - the duration of its evolution, its response to treatment, the type of operation planned and the experience of the medicosurgical team together all play an important role.

Osserman's classes III and IV myasthenia correspond to severe disease and often imply that ventilatory assistance will be required for the first few days after surgery. Class II disease has a more variable outcome. It is usually the degree to which the oropharyngeal muscles are affected and the risk of bronchoaspiration associated with dysphagia which determine the need for postoperative ventilation.

Postoperative Care

Preoperative Medical Therapy

Oral administration of anticholinesterase drugs such as pyridostigmine (60 mg q 3-4 h) is the mainstay of medical therapy for myasthenia gravis. The total dose of pyridostigmine should be reduced by 20%-40% before the operation, either by reducing each dose or by increasing the time interval between doses, despite the patient's probable psychological dependence on medication (Havard and Scadding 1983). The administration of neostigmine to overcome residual relaxation at the end of an operation can be dangerous and cause an overdose of anticholinesterases, inducing a cholinergic crisis with attendant increase in muscle weakness. It must be remembered that 2 mg pyridostigmine administered intravenously is equivalent to 60 mg per os (Stoelting et al. 1988). The muscarinic effects of acetylcholine can be dangerous when there is an overdose of anticholinesterase drugs. Diarrhea, colic, myosis, hypersalivation and lacrimation are the classic signs of overdose. Atropine can be used occasionally to overcome these symptoms but should not be administered routinely.

Although plasmapheresis is useful in alleviating the symptoms of myasthenia gravis, its use during the perioperative period is still limited to the high-risk patients in Osserman's classes III and IV (Cooper et al. 1988). In these patients it can shorten the postoperative need for mechanical ventilation (d'Empaire et al. 1985).

One study showed that administration of high doses of corticosteroids (1 g methylprednisone) reduced morbidity due to neurological and respiratory complications following transsternal thymectomy (Bolooki and Schwartzman 1978). However, these results need to be confirmed by further studies.

Certain drugs have an inherent depressant effect on the neuromuscular junction and must be used with considerable caution in myasthenic patients. These are notably the aminoglycoside antibiotics (gentamicin), diuretics which cause hypokalaemia, antiarrythmic agents (quinidine and procainamide), and calcium channel blockers.

Anaesthesiological Techniques

The anaesthesiological technique must be taken into account when planning the postoperative care of a myasthenic patient. Locoregional anaesthesia should be preferred whenever allowed by the patient's clinical condition and the type of operation, as the lack of intubation and the postoperative analgesia can be advantageous. However, it must be remembered that the toxicity of the ester group of local anaesthetics (2-chloroprocaine, for example) can be increased because their hydrolysis is diminished by the administration of anticholinesterases.

So as to have all substances which depress neuromuscular function completely eliminated by the end of the operation, the technique of general anaesthesia which is currently recommended uses a short-acting agent for induction, followed by a volatile agent to maintain anaesthesia (Eisenkraft 1987). However, some patients will require hypnosedatives and/or opiates, and their muscle strength may be depressed longer than is necessary.

More than all the preceding factors, careful *pre*operative clinical observation is fundamental to an appreciation of the myasthenic patient's need for postoperative mechanical ventilation. The severity of bulbar dysfunction with dysarthria and dysphagia (Osserman's classes III and IV) is one of the best predictive factors. The measurement of expiratory respiratory function and maximal static expiratory pressure, both of which are important to produce a productive cough with clearing of the airways, are useful paraclinical tests (Younger et al. 1984).

Extubation

It is usually possible to extubate myasthenic patients immediately, but occasionally this must be deferred for a few hours or, in exceptional cases, days. Medical therapy is reintroduced before extubation only if it is imperative for respiratory function. It is usually administered after extubation either orally (or through the nasogastric tube) or parenterally (1/30th of the oral dose).

The criteria for extubation depend mainly on clinical observation. In doubtful cases it can be helpful to measure the respiratory parameters usual for evaluation of the respiratory capacity of an intubated patient: a vital capacity of over 20 ml/kg, an inspiratory/expiratory force of under/over $-25/+25$ cm H_2O, an unassisted minute ventilation of less than 10 ml/min and voluntary ventilation over 20 l/min are all favourable (Gracey et al. 1984). Furthermore, a check of arterial blood gases and of the degree of respiratory fatigue during spontaneous ventilation will permit extubation to be carried out under good conditions.

Postoperative Analgesia

Postoperative analgesia is usually satisfactory with parenteral administration of opiates; doses should be reduced by approximately one-third in patients who are taking anticholinesterases (Foldes and Nagashima 1984). Extradural administration of opiates can also be quite useful in myasthenic patients, particularly after thoracotomies, although there are no controlled studies on this subject.

Postoperative Respiratory Complications

Symptoms

Sudden respiratory decompensation after surgery requires the distinction to be made between a myasthenic crisis and a cholinergic crisis. As the requirements for pyridostigmine vary considerably during the postoperative period, it can be necessary to evaluate this need with an intravenous edrophonium test (10 mg). This test is also useful to differentiate a myasthenic crisis, which will be rapidly alleviated by the administration of edrophonium, from a cholinergic crisis, in which symptoms remain unchanged or become transiently worse after injection of the drug.

It is possible that, despite all these precautions, the neuromuscular deficit worsens and hitherto unaffected muscle groups such as the respiratory muscles become involved. In addition, tracheobronchial secretions can become particularly abundant and troublesome.

The symptoms of respiratory decompensation are shared by both types of crisis. First of all, there is tachypnoea of unknown origin. It can be caused by afferent signals from the tired respiratory muscles or from intrapulmonary receptors stimulated by microatelectases, which are themselves favoured by the decrease in vital capacity (Gibson et al. 1977). It is to be noted that many patients have a greater decrease in vital capacity than predicted, due to a reduction in the compliance of both lungs and the chest wall. The cause of this diminished compliance of the lungs is not known, but is surely related to the diffuse microatelectases which can be seen at autopsy (De Troyer et al. 1980). The compliance of the chest wall is reduced by the ankylosis and fibrosis of the costovertebral and sternal articulations. Furthermore, postoperative diaphragmatic dysfunction can contribute to the respiratory distress, particularly after abdominal surgery, through the inhibition of phrenic nerve conduction by a reflex stimulation of visceral and somatic efferents (Ford et al. 1983).

Progressively, there is a dissociation between the thoracic and abdominal components of respiration, which first becomes alternate, then paradoxical. Paradoxical respiration is the clinical sign of weak or nonexistent diaphragmatic contraction. The period of weaning from the ventilator may be accompanied by asynchronous or paradoxical movements of the chest and abdomen, and it is well established that this clinical state is due to fatigue of the inspiratory muscles. A cyclical alteration, which alternates between the diaphragm and the other inspiratory muscles, precedes the fatigue of muscles caused by the inspiratory resistance. However it is to be noted that the appearance of this respiratory cycle is not predictive of the success or failure of ventilator weaning (Cohen et al. 1982).

Thus, the appearance of asyncronous or paradoxical repiratory movements between the diaphragm and the chest wall are the sign that the relative load of the inspiratory muscles is increased, but not necessarily to a degree which induces exhaustion. However it is important to note these abnormal repiratory movements and to know that they are the clinical sign of muscle fatigue.

Careful clinical observation and measurement of arterial blood gases allow respiratory decompensation to be recognized in time and mechanical ventilatory assistance to be started.

Protection of the airway is another reason why intubation may be desirable. Patients with dysarthria and dysphagia, either initially or during a myasthenic crisis, have pathological swallowing and cough mechanisms which expose them to repetitive bronchoaspiration.

Treatment

It is important to explain to the patient the reasons why it is necessary to revert to mechanical ventilation, and that this should not be considered as failure.

The treatment of respiratory decompensation is straightforward. It includes intermittent positive pressure breathing (IPPB), bronchial aspiration and appropriate antibiotics. It is not necessary to administer pyridostigmine during the period of mechanical ventilation. Treatment is usually resumed during or after weaning from the ventilator.

Neuromuscular diseases, particularly myasthenia gravis, imply certain features which distinguish them from other chronic lung diseases, especially chronic obstructive lung disease, during ventilatory weaning. Firstly, the pulmonary deficit in myasthenia gravis is restrictive and is characterized by progressive reduction of the vital capacity. However, this is not a good predictor of the deterioration of muscle strength, unless the vital capacity is very small (≤ 20 ml/kg) (Loach et al. 1975). Secondly, since expiration is a passive function and inspiration is an active one, it is the latter which is usually less perturbed by the pathological process. This is because the inspiratory muscles are better "trained" than the expiratory ones. As expiration is particularly important to generate an effective cough, the myasthenic patient cannot develop a sufficient maximal expiratory pressure ($P_E$max) because he is incapable of inspiring to total lung capacity. Thus, the dynamic compression of air during the cough is less efficient, and therefore the speed of the expired air is reduced (De Troyer and Pride 1985).

Like all other muscle groups, the respiratory muscles which have been fatigued by the underlying disease process and by the perioperative stress require a rest period for recuperation.

Two facts are well recognized at present. The first is that an occasional maximal effort is all that is required for a muscle to maintain its tonus. The other is that the best way for a muscle group to acquire endurance is to perform tiring exercise followed by a period of complete rest (Muller 1970).

These two observations make intermittent mandatory ventilation (IMV) an unsatisfactory modality during weaning for myasthenic patients. This mode of ventilation neither allows maximal muscular exercise nor complete rest, but requires on the contrary constant effort from potentially fatigued muscles. Brief periods of continuous positive airway pressure, alternating with periods of complete mechanical ventilation, are thus probably preferable to decreasing IMV for patients with neuromuscular diseases.

While these comments allow the weaning off the ventilator to be tailored to the neuromuscular patient's individual needs, obviously the usual criteria for extubation remain valid for these patients.

Surgery

When myasthenic patients undergo surgical procedures other than thymectomy, all the respiratory difficulties mentioned above and the reduced vital capacity are present and can require postoperative mechanical ventilatory support, especially following thoracic and abdominal surgery. When operations on the digestive tract are performed, it is probably better to avoid the administration of anticholinesterases as much as possible during the immediate postoperative period, for it seems that the use of these drugs can be associated with an increased incidence of anastomotic leaks (Bell and Lewis 1968).

Pregnancy

Pregnancy has an unpredictable influence on the course of myasthenia gravis. It provokes no more remissions than relapses. Furthermore, the way the myasthenia is influenced by a first pregnancy is in no way predictive of its behaviour during a subsequent one.

Lastly, it seems that deterioration is more frequent in the postpartum period, due to the normalization of the mother's hormonal status (Frenkel and Ehrlich 1964). Thus, whatever the surgery performed, these patients require the full attention of their attending physicians as described above.

If an operation is required during the first months of pregnancy, interruption of the pregnancy should be seriously considered.

Myasthenia and the Newborn

Myasthenia gravis in the newborn is a transient condition that affects approximately 12% of children born of myasthenic mothers. The transplacental transfer of maternal antibodies is responsible for the generalized muscle weakness, the hyporeflexia and the respiratory distress of the newborn baby. Although most cases are seen within 24 h of birth, neonatal myasthenia can appear up to 4 days post partum, the delay being due to the transplacental transfer of cholinesterases (Namba et al. 1970).

If the clinical condition warrants it, an edrophonium test (0.5-1 mg i. m.) should be carried out.

Even though this condition is transitory, 80% of these neonates will require anticholinesterase treatment for 2-4 weeks (Rudolph and Hoffman 1982).

References

Bell CMA, Lewis CB (1968) Effect of neostigmine on integrity of ileorectal anastomosis. Br Med J 3: 587-588

Bolooki H, Schwartzman RJ (1978) High-dose steroids for perioperative management of patients with myasthenia gravis kundergoing thymectomy. A preliminary report. J Thorac Cardiovasc Surg 75 (5): 754-757

Cohen CA, Zagelbaum G, Gross D, Roussos C, Macklem PT (1982) Clinical manifestations of inspiratory muscle fatigue. Am J Med 73 (3): 308-316

Cooper JD, Al-Jilaihawa AN, Pearson FG, Humphrey JG, Humphrey HE (1988) An improved technique to facilitate transcervical thymectomy for myasthenia gravis. Ann Thorac Surg 45 (3): 242-247

D'Empaire G, Hoaglin DC, Perlo VP, Pontoppidan H (1985) Effect of prethymectomy plasma exchange on postoperative respiratory function in myasthenia gravis. J Thorac Cardiovasc Surg 89 (4): 592-596

De Troyer A, Borenstein S, Cordier R (1980) Analysis of lung volume restriction in patients with respiratory muscle weakness. Thorax 35 (8): 603-610

De Troyer A, Pride NB (1985) The respiratory system in neuromuscular disorders. In: Roussos C, Macklem PT (eds) The thorax (Part B). Dekker, New York, pp 1089-1121

Eisenkraft JB (1987) Myasthenia gravis and thymic surgery - anaesthestic considerations. Ballieres Clin Anaesth 1 (1): 133-162

Foldes FF, Nagashima H (1984) Myasthenia gravis and anesthesia. In: Oyama T (ed) Endocrinology and the anaesthetist. Elsevier, New York (Monographs in anaesthesiology, vol 11, pp 171-203)

Ford GT, Riveout KS, Bozdeck LK et al. (1983) Inhibition of breathing arising from the gallbladder. Physiologist 26: A 38

Frenkel M, Ehrlich EN (1964) The influence of progesterone and mineralocorticoids upon myasthenia gravis. Ann Intern Med 60 (6): 971-981

Gibson GJ, Pride NB, Newsom Davis J, Loh LC (1977) Pulmonary mechanics in patients with respiratory muscle weakness. am Rev Respir Dis 115 (3): 389-395

Gracey DR, Divertie MB, Howard FM, Payne WS (1984) Postoperative respiratory care after transsternal thymectomy in myasthenia gravis. A 3 year experience in 53 patients. Chest 86 (1): 67-71

Havard CWH, Scadding GK (1983) Myasthenia graivs: pathogenesis and current concepts in management. Drugs 26: 174-184

Loach AB, Young AC, Spalding JMK, Crampton Smith A (1975) Postoperative management after thymectomy. Br Med J I: 309-312

Muller EA (1970) Influence of training and of inactivity on muscle strength. Arch Phys Med 51: 449-462

Namba T, Brown SB, Grob D (1970) Neonatal myasthenia gravis: report of two cases and review of the literature. Pediatrics 45: 488-504

Rudolph AM, Hoffman JIE (eds) (1982) Pediatrics, 17th edn. Appleton-Century Crofts, Norwalk, Conn., p 1688

Stoelting RK, Dierdorf SF, McCammon AL (1988) Skin and musculoskeletal diseases. In: Stoelting RK, Dierdorf SF (eds) Anesthesia and co-existing diseases. Churchill Livingston, New York, pp 545-587

Younger DS, Braun NMT, Jaretski A, Penn S, Lovelace RE (1984) Myasthenia gravis: determinants for independant ventilation after transsternal thymectomy. Neurology 34 (3): 336-340

25 Thymectomy in Childhood

Claude P. Le Coultre

Introduction

Surgery of the thymus in childhood is uncommon. Thymectomy may be indicated for true thymic hyperplasia, myasthenia gravis, thymic tumors (benign or malignant), thymic cysts, and other rare conditions. Thymic lesions may involve a normally located gland or ectopic thymic tissue. The principal difference between adult and childhood thymic surgery concerns the pathology and the surgical indications. Once thymectomy or thymic surgery has been considered, the surgical technique is similar to that in adults.

Enlarged Thymus and Thymic Hyperplasia

The median weight of a normal thymus varies from 22 to 55 g during the first 3 years of life (Boyd 1932). A normal thymus frequently extends up to the neck on either side (Ravitch 1986). An enlarged thymus in infancy and early childhood is the commonest cause of a mediastinal mass (Lamesch 1983).

The previous practice of irradiating an enlarged thymus and its disastrous consequences (high incidence of subsequent thyroid carcinoma) are now well documented and condemned (La Franchi and Fonkalsrud 1973). The supposed connection between enlarged thymus and sudden infant death syndrome has also been refuted. Welch et al. (1979) and Ravitch (1986) have emphasized that a normal thymus does not cause respiratory distress in infants and that an enlarged thymus mistaken for a surgical lesion is likely to be only an incidental finding in such patients.

Occasionally a large anterior mediastinal mass, that cannot be definitely identified as the thymus, presents a diagnostic problem and may require further noninvasive clinical investigations such as a computerized tomographic (CT) or nuclear magnetic resonance (NMR) scan. Injection of air into the mediastinum (pneumomediastinum) for diagnostic purposes has been reported by some authors (Cumming and Simpson 1975; Lamesch 1983), but is not in common practice anymore. In any case, one should never operate on an infant only on the basis of the eccentricity or predominance of one lobe (Figs. 1 and 2). Therapeutic trials with steroids (prednisone 1.5 mg/kg for 5 days) have been known to produce a rapid decrease in the size of the enlarged gland (Lamesch 1983; Cuendet and Braun 1982; Kuhn 1985).

True *thymic hyperplasia* or *massive thymic enlargement* however, does exist and can provoke symptoms which require surgery. Lack (1981) distinguishes the following two types of hyperplasia: the first, *true thymic hyperplasia*, is an increase in volume and weight of the gland, albeit with normal histology. The increase in size is due to the formation of new cellular elements. The second, *lymphofollicular hyperplasia*, is characterized by the presence of lymphoid follicles, with germinal centers. This type of hyperplasia may be associated with myasthenia gravis (as discussed later).

True hyperplasia is extremely rare. It may cause respiratory distress through displacement and compression of the bronchopulmonary system. Steroid therapy is usually ineffective. Lack (1981) reported two cases (11- and 14-year-old boys) with true hyperplasia and thymic glands which weighed respectively 324 and 490 g. Katz et al. (1977) recorded one case of massive thymic enlargement of 224 g. This child also had lym-

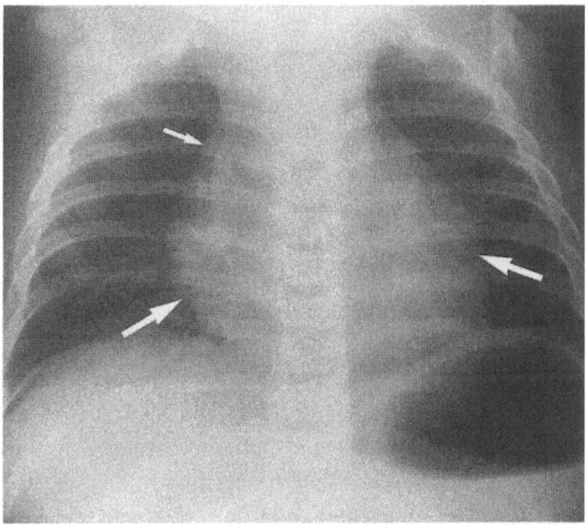

Fig. 1. Thymus considered of normal size in a 6-month-old boy. (Courtesy of Dr. D. Nusslé, Department of Pediatric Radiology)

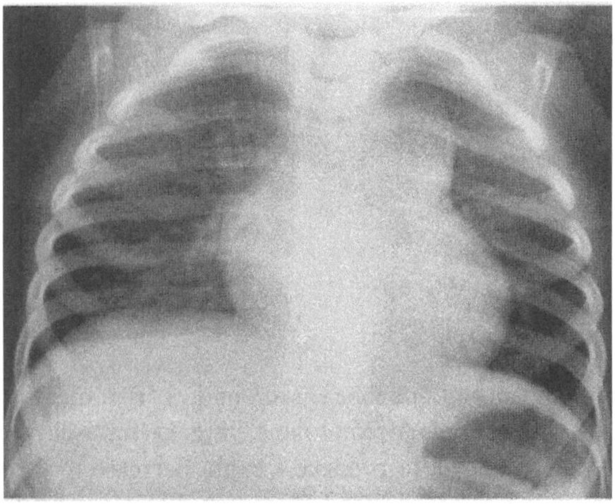

Fig. 2. Left anterior mediastinal mass in a 4-year-old girl. CT scan helped to confirm a simply enlarged thymic lobe; no surgery was necessary. (Courtesy of Dr. D. Nusslé, Department of Pediatric Radiology)

phocytosis, both in peripheral blood and bone marrow smears, which disappeared after thymectomy. Lee et al. (1979) described the case of a 22-month-old infant with a hyperplastic thymus of 550 g. These children were all symptomatic and required surgery. Blasimann et al. (1977) documented 14 cases of thymic hyperplasia; 2 cases presented with lobular atelectasis of a lung (without clinical signs of respiratory distress). The experience of these authors led them to draw up outlines for surgical indications:

1. Persistence of the mediastinal mass in spite of steroid therapy and persistence of stridor regardless of treatment;
2. The presence of calcifications within the mass, indicating the possibility of a nonthymomatous tumor;
3. Persistence of hyperplasia for over 2 years.

However, these indications are rare, for Haller et al. (1969), in a series of 80 children with a mediastinal mass, found 8 with thymic hyperplasia (4 newborns and 4 children up to 5 years) none of which required surgery.

Surgical Approach

Surgery for true thymic hyperplasia can be performed either by sternotomy or by lateral thoracotomy. The choice of procedure depends on the location of the mass and the surgeon's preference. In some cases the mass has been extirpated through a cervical incision (Blasimann et al. 1977).

Myasthenia Gravis

Myasthenia gravis is quite seldom recognized in early childhood. The first deliberate thymectomy for the treatment of myasthenia gravis was reported by Blalock et al. in 1941. The surgical decision is difficult because of the relatively small number of children presenting with the condition and thus the lack of controlled studies. Some authors treat their patients medically as long as they can, while others prefer thymectomy early in the course of the disease. Most large series deal with adult patients among whom there are a few childhood cases (Blalock et al. 1941; Cohn et al. 1974; Fenichel 1978; Fraser et al. 1978; Clark et al. 1980; Rubin et al. 1981; Olanow et al. 1982).

The review of the results from several large pediatric centers has led Fonkalsrud et al. (1970) and Youssef (1983) to recommend thymectomy in young patients presenting with a short duration of myasthenia gravis, with progressive symptoms and an unstable response to medication. It would appear from their data that most young patients with a short history of myasthenia gravis do benefit from early surgery. A remission or improvement rate of 70% can be expected, although Ravitch (1986) disagrees with these optimistic figures.

In a series of 14 children reported by Fonkalsrud et al. (1970), 3 were younger than 4 years and 2 had thymomas. Improvement or remission was observed in the majority of cases. Youssef (1983) reported a series of 8 children (6 girls, 2 boys) with a mean age of 11 years, all with negative antibodies; 4 had lymphofollicular hyperplasia, 3 a normal thymus, and 1 an atrophic gland. All improved dramatically after surgery. In all series, there were more girls than boys. In children, the association of thymoma with myasthenia gravis is rare and only a few cases have been recorded in the literature. Slater et al. (1978), in a review of 141 patients with thymoma and myasthenia gravis, found only 2 children.

Steroid Therapy

Some authors have recommended the use of steroid therapy, pre-, peri-, or postoperatively (Sarnat et al. 1977; Bolooki and Schwartzman 1978). Fenichel (1978) suggests its use in the postoperative period. Clark et al. (1980) have a protocol with thymectomy as the initial major therapeutic approach, followed by short-term anticholinesterase and long-term prednisone administration. A few days of systemic steroid treatment may cause involution of the thymus and thus facilitate complete surgical removal. In Bolooki's series of 32 patients treated with high doses of corticosteroids perioperatively, it was possible to extubate these patients within 2 h of surgery. On the other hand, Olanow et al. (1982) follow a protocol with repeated plasmapheresis before surgery, with good results.

Surgical Approach

Transcervical thymectomy has been advocated by Campbell et al. (1983), who reported in their series identical long-term results with a transcervical or transsternal approach. However, Masaoka et al. (1975) found thymic remnants in the extrathymic mediastinal fat in 13 of 18 patients. The cervical approach has been reported to accomplish only subtotal or partial resection (Jaretzki et al. 1977; Youssef 1983). Experimentally, autoimmune myasthenia gravis in the neonate cannot be induced after total thymectomy, though it can be if only partial thymectomy is performed (Jaretzki et al. 1977). There are reports of recurrence of myasthenia gravis in which residual thymic tissue has been found (Joseph and Johns 1973; Youssef 1983). Most authors stress the importance of the complete excision of the thymus. All thymic tissue, as well as all mediastinal fat, should be removed *en bloc* from hilum to hilum and from neck to diaphragm. Sternotomy is therefore preferred for full excision of the thymus and radical exenteration of anterior mediastinal soft tissue. Wide exposure of the mediastinum is necessary for this total dissection (Fonkalsrud et al. 1970; Bolooki and Schwartzman 1978; Clark et al. 1980; Youssef 1983).

Mortality has been estimated at less than 4% with modern anesthetic techniques. The critical postoperative period is identical for both children and adults. All authors agree on the necessity of careful intensive care, which is mandatory in this type of surgery (Millichap and Dodge 1960).

Thymic Tumors

In children, thymic tumors represent only 5%-10% of mediastinal masses (La Franchi and Fonkalsrud 1973). These tumors are described in the pathology section of this book.

Thymoma

They must be considered in the differential diagnosis of anterior mediastinal masses, which include malignant lymphomas, Hodgkin's disease, thymic hyperplasia, germ cell tumors, sarcomas, pleuropericardial cysts, and mediastinal lipomas (Levine and Rosai 1978; Welch et al. 1979). Thymomas are uncommon pediatric tumors and very few cases have been reported under the age of 18. They may be silent or inapparent and may be an incidental X-ray finding. They can also produce the following symptoms: cough, dyspnea, cyanosis, wheezing, or superior vena cava compression syndrome.

Thymoma can be of epithelial nature, lymphocytic, or lymphoepithelial. Some tumors may contain calcifications. The association with myasthenia gravis is rare and usually involves benign thymomas (Blasimann et al. 1977; Clark et al. 1980). Other occasional associations described with thymomas are erythrocyte aplasia, agammaglobulinemia, megaesophagus, lupus erythematosus, and various collagen disorders (Welch et al. 1979; Smith et al. 1983; Valderrama et al. 1983).

In children, the outlook for *infiltrating thymomas* is very poor. The course is faster and the prognosis poorer than in adults. Approximately 80% die within 6 months. We biopsied a thymoma in a 13-year-old North African boy in 1973. He had a nonresectable infiltrating thymoma with metastasis to the iliac bone, a superior vena cava syndrome and a most unusual hypertrophic osteoarthropathy (Marie-Bamberger syndrome) (Figs. 3 and 4). He received 4000 rads to the mediastinum and 3600 rads to the iliac crest, which was well tolerated. The thymic mass regressed dramatically as did the osteous apposition. Pathologic diagnosis was a lymphoepithelial thymoma. The child died 10 months later.

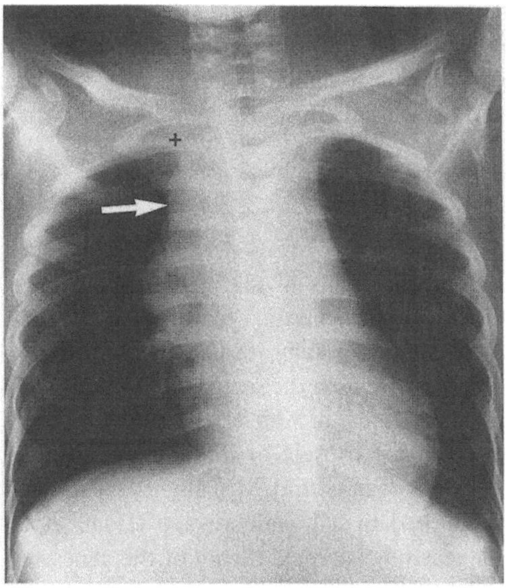

Fig. 3. Homogeneous mass *(arrow)* with displacement of mediastinal pleura *(cross)* in a 13-year-old boy. The mass was an invasive thymoma. (Courtesy of Dr. D. Nusslé, Department of Pediatric Radiology)

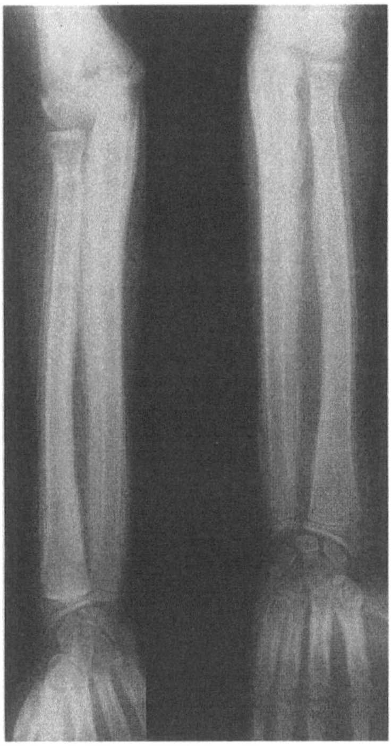

Fig. 4. Hypertrophic osteoarthropathy. (Courtesy of Dr. D. Nusslé, Department of Pediatric Radiology)

La Franchi and Fonkalsrud (1973) reported a series of 18 children with thymic masses, among whom they found 10 cases of true thymic hyperplasia, 4 benign and 3 infiltrating thymomas, and 1 case of Hodgkin's disease. The youngest infant reported to have an infiltrating thymoma was 8 months old (Deshpande et al. 1981). Bowie et al. (1979) recorded the case of a 9-year-old boy with a similar tumor, presenting with pleural and pericardial effusions.

Germ Cell Tumors

Primary germ cell tumors of the mediastinum represent less then 1% of mediastinal tumors (Knapp et al. 1985). These tumors, usually located in the testes or the ovaries, may occur in the mediastinum and occasionally in the thymus, in which case they are totally confined within the capsule or intimately associated with the thymus (Burns and McCaughey 1986) and not only attached to a thymic vestige (Dyan et al. 1976). The generally accepted theory of the genesis of extragonadal germ cell tumors is that they arise from primitive germ cells which descend in the mediastinum with the thymic anlage (Recondo and Libshitz 1978; Bergh et al. 1978b; Knapp et al. 1985). Primitive germ cells migrate along the urogenital ridge to the gonadal ridge. As the urogenital ridge extends from the sixth cervical to the third lumbar vertebra, an arrest in the migration of these cells could explain the occurrence of germ cell tumors in the mediastinum, peritoneal organs, and retroperitoneum. These tumors include teratomas (mature or immature), teratocarcinomas, seminomas, embryonal carcinomas, choriocarcinomas, and endodermal sinus or yolk sac tumors (Oberman and Libcke 1964; Kuhn 1985).

In spite of the fact that teratomas are usually pediatric tumors, very few pediatric patients have been reported to present germ cell tumors of the thymus. Most affected children are asymptomatic. When present, symptoms are nonspecific and depend on compression of surrounding structures (chest pain, cough, hemoptysis, loss of weight, lymphadenopathy, superior vena cava syndrome). Symptoms are more frequent in the presence of malignant lesions (Whittaker and Lynn 1973).

Teratoma. This is an embryonal neoplasm that contains tissue of ectodermal, endodermal, and mesodermal origin. Although the commonest location is sacrococcygeal, Grosfeld et al. (1976) report an incidence of 11.7% of teratomas located in the media^tinum. Rupture of the teratoma into the tracheobronchial tree causing expectoration of hair has been reported (Thompson and Moore 1969). The X-ray finding on a plain film of teeth or skeletal elements is diagnostic (Kuhn 1985).

Seminoma. Primary seminoma of the mediastinum in childhood has been reported by Polansky et al. in 1979. The tumor is radiologically indistinguishable from lymphoma and biopsy is required for diagnosis (Kuhn 1985). An occult testicular tumor must always be excluded (Cox 1975; Kuhn 1985; Burns and McCaughey 1986).

Yolk Sac Tumors. These tumors may arise from poorly differentiated embryonal carcinoma (Teilum 1965; Norgaard-Pedersen et al. 1975; Gooneratne et al. 1985). They are usually associated with an elevated serum level of α-fetoprotein. The prognosis is poor.

Treatment. Discovery of a germ cell tumor is an indication for its removal, because malignancy may be present or develop and continued tumor growth may lead to symptoms. Excision through thoracotomy is recommended, which is curative for benign lesions and even some immature teratomas. Although the outcome for children presenting malignant germ cell tumors has improved over the past years with new chemotherapy management, these tumors are aggressive and prognosis remains uncertain (Carter et al. 1982; King 1986; Ravitch 1986).

Thymolipoma

Thymolipomas represent only 2%-9% of thymic tumors. A little over 60 patients have been reported with this condition - mainly adults, few children (Ringe et al. 1979; Dyon et al. 1979). Such tumors are usually asymptomatic or may occasionally give rise to symptoms such as dyspnea, pain, or cough and less frequently fatigue, dysphagia, hemoptysis. Thymolipomas have never been reported in conjunction with myasthenia gravis and they are a definite indication for surgical excision in order to establish the correct histological diagnosis.

Surgical Approach

In principle, thymic tumors should be excised at the earliest opportunity for some prove to be malignant. Either median sternotomy or lateral thoracotomy can be used. Benign tumors are usually easy to remove and do not present a major problem. On the other hand, locally invasive tumors can be more difficult to excise. The outlook is generally poor and, when feasible, total excision should be carried out. This may require opening of the pericardium or excision of part of the pleura or lung. Additional radiotherapy and chemotherapy are often necessary in such cases (Haller et al. 1969; Fonkalsrud et al. 1970; La Franchi and Fonkalsrud 1973; Rose et al. 1978; Welch et al. 1979).

Cystic Lesions of the Thymus

Thymic embryology explains the possible extramediastinal location of thymic tissue, and remnants may appear anywhere along its path of migration (Lamesch et al. 1974; Reiner and Beck 1980; Jensen et al. 1983; Graeber et al. 1984). Cystic thymic masses can be distributed from the upper neck to the lower mediastinum. However, most of them are located in the upper anterior mediastinum. They may extend to the neck or be entirely cervical.

When they are located within the *mediastinum*, the differential diagnosis must be made with other anterior mediastinal tumors (Lamesch et al. 1974). Patients may be asymptomatic or present with a swelling at the base of the neck. A soft bulging mass can also be seen or palpated in the suprasternal fossa, particularly during episodes of crying.

Cervical Thymic Cysts

Cervical thymic cysts usually present as a mass deep in the anterior cervical triangle, in contact with the carotid sheath or under the sternocleidomastoid muscle. These cysts are mostly asymptomatic, but may undergo rapid expansion either by internal hemorrhage or in association with respiratory infection. The differential diagnosis most often considered includes cystic hygroma, branchial cyst, benign teratoma, parathyroid, thyroid or thyroglossal duct cyst. The diagnosis is rarely made preoperatively.

The histologic finding of thymic tissue with Hassall's corpuscles within the wall of the cyst confirms its nature. Cholesterol crystals may also be found within the wall. The majority of these cysts are multilocular and contain a yellowish-brown fluid. They are lined by epithelium which is often ciliated. Solid extension of the cyst wall may reach the mediastinum. Visible connections with the normal mediastinal thymus may also be seen. Embryonic remnants, degenerating Hassall's corpuscles, neoplastic processes, and tissue sequestration during involution of the gland have all been considered as a possible origin of cervical thymic cysts (Graeber et al. 1984).

Thymic Cysts

Thymic cysts are most often found in children, with an average age of diagnosis between 7 and 10 years (Reiner and Beck 1980; Jensen et al. 1983; Graeber et al. 1984). Graeber et al. (1984) reported a series of 46 patients with a cystic mass of the thymus. Of these, 30 were limited to the mediastinum, 9 were large enough to extend either into the neck or the mediastinum, and 7 were cervical. The majority of patients were asymptomatic and 21 were under 15 years of age. The symptoms most often recorded were dysphagia, hoarseness, and cervical pain. Welch et al. (1979) in a review of 17 thymic cysts found 12 benign and 5 malignant neoplasms; 14 were solid and 3 were cystic. The patients were between 2 months and 17 years old. A total of 7 patients presented with no symptoms, 6 had cervical swelling which increased during coughing, crying, or the Valsalva maneuver. Diagnostic modalities include X-ray of the neck and chest, ultrasound, thymic scan, and NMR. CT scan can be of considerable diagnostic aid.

Surgical Approach

Localized cervical thymic cysts can be excised by a cervical incision. Occasionally two parallel incisions for a lesion extending from the submandibular area to the thoracic inlet have been proposed (Welch et al. 1979). Mediastinal masses should be removed through a sternotomy or a lateral thoracotomy. However, Ane et al. (1984) have reported the removal of a mediastinal thymic cyst through a cervical incision. Very large mediastinal masses extending to the neck may also require sternotomy and an additional cervical incision for optimal removal.

Other Rare Diseases of the Thymus

Granulomatous lesions of the thymus have been reported. They are often cases of Hodgkin's disease, but can occasionally be seminomas (Burns and McCaughey 1986) and should be treated as appropriate. Smith et al. (1983) reported the rare case of a 14-year-old boy who presented with Hodgkin's disease within a large thymic cyst. Valderrama et al. (1983) reported a unique case of an osteosarcoma arising within a hamartoma of the thymic gland, located in the pleural cavity of an 11-year-old girl. Woolley et al. (1974) recorded two unique cases of spontaneous bleeding in the thymus in the neonatal period. In each case the left mediastinal pleura ruptured, resulting in a left hemothorax. Both infants required surgery and in both instances the origin of the bleeding was found to be a hemorrhagic thymus.

Conclusions

Thymectomy in childhood is more a problem of deciding when to operate than a problem of surgical technique. The borderline between a "normally" enlarged thymus and true thymic hyperplasia is not always obvious, but differentiation is important as the former should not be excised. An enlarged thymus has not been known to cause respiratory distress. Steroid therapy can be a useful diagnostic aid in this case.

Invasive thymomas have a poor prognosis and should be rapidly excised, whereas benign thymomas are slow growing, noninvasive and usually have an excellent prognosis. Again the differentiation between the two types of thymoma is difficult to establish preoperatively.

The results of thymectomy in myasthenia gravis are not always predictable and there is as yet no consensus as to its place in the treatment of the disease. However, the current tendency is to perform thymectomy early in the course of generalized myasthenia gravis; furthermore, the importance of perioperative and postoperative care cannot be overemphasized.

References

Ane P, de Firmas JL, Oksman A, Roisan J (1984) Une volumineuse tumeur médiastinale peut être enlevée par cervicotomie. J Fr Otorhinolaryngol 33: 49-51

Bergh NP, Gatzinsky P, Larsson S, Lundin P, Ridell B (1978 a) Tumors of the thymus and thymic region. I. Clinicopathological studies on thymomas. Ann Thorac Surg 25: 91-98

Bergh NP, Gatzinsky P, Larsson S, Lundin P, Ridell B (1978 b) Tumors of the thymus and thymic region. III. Clinicopathological studies on teratomas and tumors of germ cell type. Ann Thorac Surg 25: 107-111

Cohn HE, Solit RW, Schatz NJ, Schlezinger N (1979) Surgical treatment in myasthenia gravis. A 27 year experience. J Thorac Cardiovasc Surg 68: 876-885

Cox JD (1975) Primary malignant germinal tumors of the mediastinum. A study of 24 cases. Cancer 36: 1162-1168

Cuendet A, Braun P (1982) Tumoren der Thymusdrüse. In: Bettex M, Genton N, Stockmann M (eds). Kinderchirurgie. Thieme, Stuttgart, pp 540-549

Cumming WA, Simpson JS (1975) Diagnostic pneumomediastinum. J Pediatr Surg 10: 971-972

Deshpande GN, Fisher JE, Jewett TC, Freeman AI (1981) Malignant thymoma in an eight-month-old boy. J Surg Oncol 18: 61-66

Dyan A, de Saint Florent G, Martyn X, Brouet G (1976) Difficultés du diagnostic entre kystes simples du thymus et dysembryomes intrathymiques. Nouv Presse Med 5: 28-30

Dyon JF, Paramelle B, Perdrix A, Pasquier B, Sarrazin R (1979) Un cas de thymolipome chez l'enfant. J Chir (Paris) 116: 123-128

Fenichel GM (1978) Clinical syndromes of myasthenia in infancy and childhood. A review. Arch Neurol 35: 97-103

Fonkalsrud EW, Herrmann C, Mulder DG (1970) Thymectomy for myasthenia gravis in children. J Pediatr Surg 5: 157-165

Fraser K, Simpson JA, Crawford J (1978) The place of surgery in the treatment of myasthenia gravis. Br J Surg 65: 301-304

Gooneratne S, Keh P, Sreekanth S, Recant W, Talerman A (1985) Anterior mediastinal endodermal sinus (yolk sac) tumor in a female infant. Cancer 56: 1430-1433

Blalock A, Harvey AM, Ford FR, Lilienthal JL (1941) The treatment of myasthenia gravis by removal of the thymus gland: preliminary report. JAMA 117: 1529-1533

Blasimann B, Kuffer F, Bettex M (1977) Chirurgische Betrachtungen über die Thymushyperplasie. Z Kinderchir 21: 214-230

Bolooki H, Schwartzman RJ (1978) High-dose steroids for perioperative management of patients with myasthenia gravis undergoing thymectomy. J Thorac Cardiovasc Surg 75: 754-757

Bowie PR, Teixeira OHP, Carpenter B (1979) Malignant thymoma in a nine-year-old boy presenting with pleuropericardial effusion. J Thorac Cardiovasc Surg 77: 777-781

Boyd E (1932) The weight of the thymus gland in health and in disease. Am J Dis Child 43: 1162-1214

Burns BF, McCaughey WTE (1986) Unusual thymic seminomas. Arch Pathol Lab Med 110: 539-541

Campbell JR, Bisio JM, Harrison MW, Campbell TJ (1983) Surgical treatment of myasthenia gravis in childhood. J Pediatr Surg 18: 857-861

Carter D, Bibro MC, Touloukian RJ (1982) Benign clinical behavior of immature mediastinal teratoma in infancy and

childhood: report of two cases and review of the literature. Cancer 49: 398-402
Clark RE, Marbarger JP, West PN, Spratt JA, Florence JM, Roper CL, Ferguson TB, Weldon CS (1980) Thymectomy for myasthenia gravis in the young adult. Long-term results. J Thorac Cardiovasc Surg 80: 696-701
Graeber GM, Thompson LD, Cohen DJ, Ronnigen LD, Jaffin J, Zajtchuk R (1984) Cystic lesion of the thymus. An occasionally malignant cervical and/or anterior mediastinal mass. J Thorac Cardiovasc Surg 87: 295-300
Grosfeld JL, Ballantine TVN, Lowe D, Baehner RL (1976) Benign and malignant teratomas in children: analysis of 85 patients. Surgery 80: 297-305
Haller JA, Mazur DO, Morgan WW (1969) Diagnosis and management of mediastinal masses in children. J Thorac Cardiovasc Surg 58: 385-393
Jaretzki III A, Bethea M, Wolff M, Olarte MR, Lovelace RE, Penn AS, Rowland L (1977) A rational approach to total thymectomy in the treatment of myasthenia gravis. Ann Thorac Surg 24: 120-130
Jensen JH, Larsen JL, Asschenfeldt P (1983) Congenital thymic cysts in the neck. Int J Pediatr Othorhinolaryngol 6: 95-100
Joseph BS, Johns TR (1973) Recurrence of nonneoplastic thymus after thymectomy for myasthenia gravis. Report of two cases. Neurology 23: 109-116
Katz SM, Chatten J, Bishop HC, Rosenblum H (1977) Massive thymic enlargement. Am J Clin Pathol 68: 786-790
King DR (1986) Ovarian cysts and tumors. In: Welch KJ, Randolph JG, Ravitch MM, O'Neill JA, Rowe MI (eds) Pediatric surgery, 4th edn. Year Book Medical Publishers, Chicago, pp 1341-1352
Knapp RH, Hurt RD, Payne WS, Farrow GM, Lewis BD, Hahn RG, Muhm JR, Earle JD (1985) Malignant germ cell tumors of the mediastinum. J Thorac Cardiovasc Surg 89: 82-89
Kuhn JP (1985) The mediastinum. In: Silverman FN (ed) Caffey's pediatric X-ray diagnosis, 8th edn. Year Book Medical Publishers, Chicago, pp 1302-1350
Lack EE (1981) Thymic hyperplasia with massive enlargement. Report of 2 cases with review of diagnosis criteria. J Thorac Cardiovasc Surg 81: 741-746
La Franchi S, Fonkalsrud EW (1973) Surgical management of lymphatic tumors of the mediastinum in children. J Thorac Cardiovasc Surg 65: 8-14
Lamesch AJ (1983) Massive thymic hyperplasia in infants. Z Kinderchir 38: 16-18
Lamesch A, Capesius C, Theisen-Aspesberro MC (1974) Cervical thymic cysts in infants and children. Z Kinderchir 14: 213-219
Lee Y, Moallem S, Clauss RH (1979) Massive hyperplastic thymus in a 22-month-old infant. Ann Thorac Surg 27: 356-358
Levine GD, Rosai J (1978) Thymic hyperplasia and neoplasia: a review of current concepts. Hum Pathol 9: 495-515
Masaoka A, Nagaoka Y, Kotake Y (1975) Distribution of thymic tissue at the anterior mediastinum. J Thorac Cardiovasc Surg 70: 747-754
Millichap JG, Dodge PR (1960) Diagnosis and treatment of myasthenia gravis in infancy, childhood and adolescence. Neurology 10: 1007-1014
Norgaard-Pedersen B, Albrechtsen R, Teilum G (1975) Serum alpha-foetoprotein as a marker for endodermal sinus tumour (yolk sac tumour) or a vitelline component of "teratocarcinoma". Acta Pathol Microbiol Scand [A] 83: 573-589
Oberman HA, Libcke JH (1964) Malignant germinal neoplasms of the mediastinum. Cancer 17: 498-507
Olanow CW, Wechsler AS, Roses AD (1982) A prospective study of thymectomy and serum acetylcholine receptor antibodies in myasthenia gravis. Ann Surg 196: 113-121
Polansky SM, Barwick KW, Ravin CE (1979) Primary mediastinal seminoma. AJR 132: 17-21
Ravitch MM (1986) Mediastinal cysts and tumors. In: Welch KJ, Randolph JG, Ravitch MM, O'Neill JA, Rowe MI (eds) Pediatric surgery 4th edn. Year Book Medical Publishers, Chicago, pp 602-618
Recondo J, Libshitz HI (1978) Mediastinal extragonadal germ cell tumors. Urology 11: 369-375
Reiner M, Beck AR (1980) Cervical thymic cysts in children. Am J Surg 139: 704-707
Ringe B, Dragojevic D, Frank G, Borst HG (1979) Thymolipoma - a rare, benign tumor of the thymus gland. Two case reports and review of the literature. J Thorac Cardiovasc Surg 27: 369-374
Rose JS, McCarthy J, Mutchler RW, Velcek FT (1978) Thymoma in childhood. NY State J Med 78: 82-84
Rubin JW, Ellison RG, Moore HV, Pai GP (1981) Factors affecting response to thymectomy for myasthenia gravis. J Thorac Cardiovasc Surg 82: 720-728
Sarnat HB, McGarry JD, Lewis JE (1977) Effective treatment of infantile myasthenia gravis by combined prednisone and thymectomy. Neurology 27: 550-553
Slater G, Papatestas AE, Genkins G, Kornfeld P, Horowitz SH, Bender A (1978) Thymomas in patients with myasthenia gravis. Ann Surg 188: 171-174
Smith PLC, Jobling C, Rees A (1983) Hodgkin's disease in a large thymic cyst in a child. Thorax 38: 392-393
Teilum G (1965) Classification of endodermal sinus tumour (mesoblastoma vitellinum) and so-called "embryonal carcinoma" on the ovary. Acta Pathol Microbiol Scand [A] 64: 407-429
Thompson DP, Moore TC (1969) Acute thoracic distress in childhood due to spontaneous rupture of a large mediastinal teratoma. J Pediatr Surg 4: 416-423
Valderrama E, Kahn LB, Wind E (1983) Extraskeletal osteosarcoma arising in an ectopic hamartomatous thymus. Report of a case and review of the literature. Cancer 51: 1132-1137
Welch KJ, Tapper E, Vawter GP (1979) Surgical treatment of thymic cysts and neoplasms in children. J Pediatr Surg 14: 691-698
Whittaker LD, Lynn HB (1973) Mediastinal tumors and cysts in the prediatric patient. Surg Clin North Am 53: 893-904
Woolley MM, Isaacs H, Lindesmith G, Vollmer DM, Van Adelberg S (1974) Spontaneous thymic hemorrhage in the neonate: report of two cases. J Pediatr Surg 9: 231-233
Youssef S (1983) Thymectomy for myasthenia gravis in children. J Pediatr Surg 18: 537-541

26 Thymic Transplantation for Relief of Immunodeficiency

Richard Hong

Introduction

When MacLean et al. (1957) removed the thymus gland from adult rabbits without any effect on the immune system, they concluded that the organ did not play a significant role in the development of the immune response. Unfortunately, they did not appreciate what is well known today, i. e. that T-lymphocytes peripheralize and accomplish their function (at least in part) by long-lived cell populations. The maintenance of T-cell functions by long-lived mature populations has confounded many interpretations of mechanisms of reconstitution by various modalities, as we shall see later. It was some years before Miller (1961), Good et al. (1962), and Waksman et al. (1962) were able to pinpoint the role of the thymus. Extirpation experiments in newborn animals, or in thymectomized irradiated adults produced a defect of the T-cell system which was lethal and corrected by thymus transplantation. Results of studies in the newborn, when considered in light of those in adults, demonstrated that thymic dependence of the immune system could be shown if organ removal occurred prior to adequate development of a post-thymic population. Studies in thymectomized irradiated adults confirmed these notions by removing the site of mature T-cell genesis and the post-thymic population as well.

This discovery was applied in the clinical setting by Rosen et al. (1962) and Hitzig et al. (1965). At first fetal thymuses were used, in part because of availability, in part because of fear of graft-versus-host (GVH) disease, and perhaps in part because of hope for greater differentiation capability of fetal tissues. Unfortunately, the full delineation of T- and B-cell had not been accomplished at that time and therefore, thymus transplantation was not in all cases the appropriate reconstitution modality. For this and other reasons, early attempts with thymus transplantation met with failure. In 1976, I utilized fragments of postnatal thymus, maintained in tissue culture, in a child with severe combined immunodeficiency (SCID) (Hong et al. 1976). The events leading to that trial, the results of cultured thymic fragment therapy, and the future hopes for that form of immunologic reconstitution comprise the substance of this chapter.

Fetal Thymus

When the tissues of the original cases of combined immunodeficiency were described, profound dysplasia of the thymus was a constant feature (Cottier 1958). With the experimental evidence that was accumulating concerning the central role of the thymus in the development of the immune system (Miller 1961; Good et al. 1962; Waksman et al. 1962), it was only natural that thymus transplantation would be attempted. No benefit was seen for several reasons.

Originally, fetal thymus slices were inserted into the rectus abdominus muscle, perhaps, in part, because of the success observed when parathyroid glands are reimplanted in muscles should they inadvertently be removed in surgery. Whether this subliminally presaged the later appreciation of hormonal function of the thymus is unknown. The intramuscular site should have worked, for the route of transplantation of thymus seemed not to make a difference in mouse studies described by Metcalf (1966). However, the exhaustive testing used today was not available then and it seems possible that some differences might be discernible by modern evaluation of transplanted animals.

If one examines the histology of transplanted thymuses, one is impressed with the tremendous amount of necrosis which occurs prior to establishment of the graft as a viable organ (Dukor et al. 1964). Also, the possibility of a local GVH reaction, wherein T cells of the thymus would react against the host, either within or near the gland, seems very likely. I believe that this local reaction could have harmed the gland sufficiently to impair its function. In the older literature, it was concluded that allogeneic grafts could not reconstitute athymic nude mice. We know today that cultured grafts (devoid of mature T cells) are very effective in this regard (Hong et al. 1979). Therefore, it is possible that the large number of mature T cells persisting in the graft prior to transplantation are not biologically insignificant and could cause a local GVH reaction.

Also, in the mid 1960s, fetal tissue was available only in England and there was an appreciable interval between the time of tissue harvest and transplantation. With the striking success of bone marrow transplantation in 1968, further attempts at thymus transplantation ceased. Furthermore, the fact that bone marrow alone could achieve a long-lasting cure led to the conviction that combined immunodeficiency disease was a stem cell disorder and that the thymic abnormalities were secondary to lack of stem cell ingress. This concept was based upon the histological appearance of mouse thymus which was maintained in culture and kept devoid of stem cells (Owen and Ritter 1969). Thus, thymus transplantation became relegated to a secondary form of treatment.

However, a reasonably large donor pool was prevented by histocompatibility restrictions. On a theoretical basis, 25% of the siblings could donate, but other factors, such as small family size, kept the actual numbers of donors very small. The overwhelming majority of patients were without donors. Thus, some form of alternative therapy was still needed.

A resurgence of interest in thymic transplantation occurred when Ammann et al. (1973), believing that the route of administration was important, injected fetal thymus intraperitoneally to a patient with combined immunodeficiency disease. The lymphocytes of this patient after transplantation possessed the ability to respond in vitro to phytohemagglutinin (PHA) and allogeneic cells, but not to antigens. The patient did not acquire the ability to demonstrate cutaneous delayed hypersensitivity; however, a persistent fungal infection of the skin cleared 4 weeks after implantation. The child remained fairly well for 4 more years, but finally died of *Pseudomonas* pneumonia. T cells of donor origin were observed with the acquisition of positive in vitro tests and persisted for the remainder of his life. No effect on immunoglobulins was observed and gamma-globulin injections were required. Following this partial success, two additional cases of fetal thymus transplants in patients with combined immunodeficiency disease were reported (Rachelefsky et al. 1975; Shearer et al. 1978). In the first, chimerism was again demonstrated; no changes in immunoglobulin were observed and gamma-globulin injections were required. The child is still alive, but suffers from chronic encephalopathy. In the second patient only E-rosette cells (T cells) increased in number, but the child was absolutely well for a period of 4 years, at which time she died suddenly from an overwhelming cytomegalovirus infection.

Insight into the immunologic events of these transplants was provided by our in vitro cultured thymus work beginning a few years later. In thymic fragments being cultured, we see a tremendous outpouring of thymocytes from small fragments. Small thymic fragments in culture appear to be fountains, raining thymocytes into the surrounding medium. The Ammann transplant can be likened to delayed-release medication capsules, spraying millions of thymocytes into the peritoneal cavity. As an aside, I mention that fetal liver cell transplants likewise resulted in no benefit until an intraperitoneal route was employed. It may be that special routes of traffic are favored by an intraperitoneal route. In examining the results of the fetal thymus transplant the striking characteristic seen was that T cells of the donor were easily found and apparently demonstrated PHA responsiveness. Therefore, this form of reconstitution was essentially a small allogeneic T-cell infusion which did not produce fatal GVH disease (subsequent experience did indicate that thymuses from fetuses over 14 weeks of age could cause fatal GVH disease). The three published reports of fetal thymus transplants in SCID all showed the same characteristics: T-cell engraftment, some functional responses, and no B-cell reconstitution. Thus, intraperitoneal fetal thymus injections may be considered small transfusions of allogeneic T cells which persist to produce lymphoid chimeras. When present in sufficiently low numbers, they do not induce GVH disease.

The major change in assessment of these patients was the acquisition of some positive in vitro responses characteristic of normal T cells. However, reconstitution of sufficient quality to allow an infection-free life was not seen. A site for maturation is not engrafted, and whatever T-cell benefit is obtained results from the small numbers of T cells which have survived the transplantation procedure. It is assumed, but not proven, that replication of the infused cells occurs, since chimerism persists for many years. Persistent lymphopenia, however, suggests that long-lived T cells may account for the observed phenomena, rather than proliferation. What is clear, nevertheless, is that a gradual increase in T-cell capability does not seem to occur and the amount of T-cell reconstitution is fixed at the level attained shortly after transplantation and is consistent with a rather restricted population of T cells. The lack of B-cell benefit can be explained on the basis of genetic restriction which prevents full and vigorous T-B-macrophage cooperation necessary for complete antibody responses (Zinkernagel et al. 1978 b). The attractiveness of fetal thymus as a therapeutic modality was based on the hope that fetal T cells were less capable of causing GVH disease and that fetal tissue might be tolerized by the host. Unfortunately, as mentioned previously, cells from older fetuses are potentially lethal. Furthermore, the thymus of a less than 14-week-old fetus is simply not large enough to effect a vigorous reconstitution. In any event, in my judgment, unless it becomes engrafted as a solid intact organ, fetal thymic tissue cannot become an effective form of treatment for T-cell deficiency.

Cultured Thymus Fragments: Experimental Considerations

Jacobs and Huseby (1967) first showed that organ culture of ovarian fragments permitted their engraftment across histocompatibility barriers. Opelz and Terasaki (1974) then showed that a short period of tissue culture decreased the stimulatory capacity of human peripheral blood monocytes. Lafferty et al. (1975) and subsequently Talmage et al. (1976) extended the work to thyroid fragments and provided the first insights into the mechanism for enhanced graft acceptance following organ culture. It appears quite certain now that the macrophages and B-lymphocytes play the major role in the initiation of the allograft rejection by an immunocompetent host. The culture period results in the death of the lymphocytes and macrophages contained in the organ. The usual serologically defined histocompatibility antigens can still be demonstrated (Talmage and Dart 1978); thus, the allograft rejection requires augmentation antigens, not usually detected by ordinary anti-HLA antisera.

Although in severe combined immunodeficiency, organ rejection is not a problem, we still thought that cultured thymus might be an interesting form of reconstitution to investigate further. We chose for our experimental model the congenitally athymic nude mouse. These animals had been studied extensively and syngeneic thymus transplantation was known to be curative. In the human situation, one does not have the luxury of inbred strains and we therefore were interested in the quality of reconstitution which could be obtained by allogeneic tissue. Previous studies suggested that allogeneic thymus was inferior in nude mice reconstitution (Kindred and Loor 1974; Loor et al. 1976). We were gratified to find that immune function and clinical health of the animals were exactly the same whether the recipients were syngeneic or allogeneic to the thymus donor. All transplanted animals showed normal longevity in an unprotected environment (Hong et al. 1979).

During this period, the phenomenon of genetic restriction was delineated by the seminal work of Zinkernagel et al. (1978 b, c). The principle has finally evolved that T cells respond to certain antigens only in the context of major histocompatibility antigens. In earlier studies, Zinkernagel et al. (1978 b, c) found that the relevant histocompatibility antigens were not those genetically endowed, but were dictated by the histocompatibility of the thymus in which the stem cell matured. The phenomenon of genetic restriction was strikingly illustrated in killing of virally infected target cells. If an animal was sensitized to a virus, its T-killer cells would kill viral targets only if they bore the "correct" histocompatibility antigens, i.e., the ones to which the animal was absolutely restricted by virtue of its thymus. The clinical consequence of this phenomenon was that we could never achieve a clinically significant reconstitution unless there was at least haploidentity between donor and recipient (Zinkernagel 1978 a).

These findings completely perplexed us, for our reconstituted nude mice were in excellent health and by then, we had transplanted our first patient who had shown an excellent response both clinically and by in vitro testing. We infected transplanted nude mice with vaccinia virus and found that they survived the infection and could destroy virally infected targets. In our experiments, we found the restriction to be to that of the host and not to the thymic donor. Similar results were subsequently published by Zinkernagel et al. (1980).

Further dissection of the phenomenon has determined that the thymus does indeed determine restriction elements, but these are in addition to the genetic histocompatibility. Thus, an allogeneic thymus transplant actually increases the repertoire of potential target cells and does not compromise an animal's ability to interact appropriately with his genetically determined self. Whether the thymic donor's histocompatibility matches with the recipient's in any way is of no consequence for the length or degree of T-cell reconstitution.

Cultured Thymus Transplants: Human Experience

Severe Combined Immunodeficiency

We transplanted our first patient with SCID in 1976 (Hong et al. 1976). At that time, the prevailing concept of the cause of SCID was that a stem cell fault was the most likely cause. Therefore, we expected, at best, only a T-cell response. To our pleasant surprise, a remarkable T- and B-cell response occurred. This observation provided clinical confirmation, at a functional level, of notions set forth by the observations of Pyke et al. (1975) and Seeger et al. (1976), wherein a major T-cell defect was observed in SCID. Pyke et al. (1975) showed that incubation of bone marrow cells with the supernatant of a thymic monolayer or the monolayer itself resulted in a small increase in numbers of cells bearing a mature T-cell marker, that for E-rosettes. Seeger et al. (1976), using normal T-helper cells, were able to induce immunoglobulin production of B cells obtained from a child with SCID.

At first, we observed gratifying results with both T- and B-cell benefit in approximately 30% of patients who were in good health at the time of transplantation (Hong 1981 a). Detailed results of these patients are shown in Fig. 1-4. It can be seen that variable degrees of reconstitution are achieved. Certainly 100% normality is not the rule. Nevertheless, it is important to emphasize that the children were able to live at home in an unprotected environment and, except for lack of free open contact with all other children, had little restriction on their daily lives. They were essentially infection free. An important conclusion to draw from these data is that complete normality of lymphocyte function tests is not necessary for at least a reasonable quality of life.

Another interesting point is that functional IgA responses, as measured by *Escherichia coli* isotype responses, are virtually nil in these patients. This would be consistent with the extreme dependence of IgA on T-helper activity, and with previous suggestions that sometimes selective IgA deficiency could be a manifestation of a primary T-cell defect (Horowitz and Hong 1975). The high association of IgA deficiency in ataxia telangiectasia would be a case in point (Epstein et al. 1966).

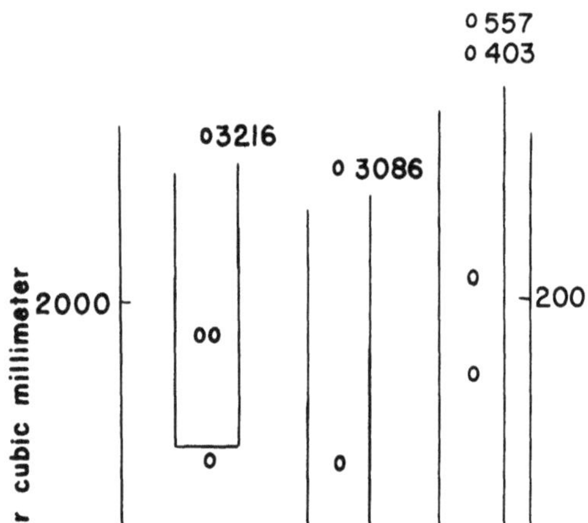

Fig. 1. Lymphocyte count, E-rosette number, and SIg^+ cells in eight surviving patients after CTF transplantation. The lower limits of normal values are shown by the bottom portion of the *open bar.* The same patient population is illustrated in Figs. 1-4. (Figs. 1-4 from *Proceedings of the 8th International Convocation on Immunology.* Basel, S. Karger, 1983, reproduced with permission)

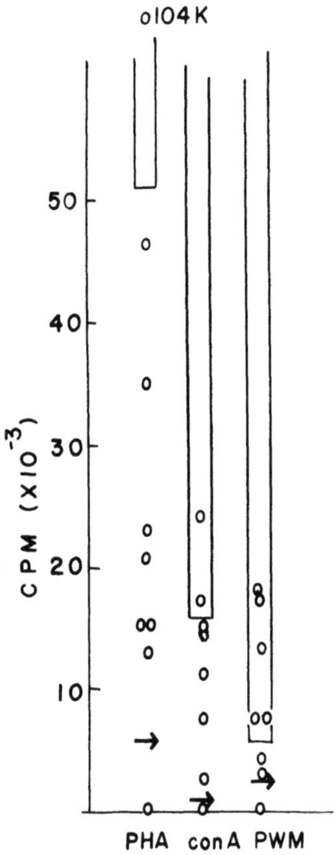

Fig. 2. Proliferation responses. The lower limits of normal responses are indicated by the bottom of the *open bar.* The *horizontal arrows* show the highest values ever attained by any SCID patients studied over the past 8 years ($N=43$). PHA phytohemagglotinin; con A concanavalin A; PWM pokeweed mitogen

However, as these children have been followed for longer periods of time, it seems that there is a decrease in thymic function. One patient, cared for in collaboration with Dr. E. R. Stiehm, was transplanted in 1978. He showed a marvelous response at first; he even recovered from hepatitis A infection and demonstrated an appropriate antibody response. Subsequently however, he experienced a chronic diarrheal state. Finally, intravenous hyperalimentation was necessary to achieve reasonable nutrition. Repeat thymic transplantations were ineffective and he ultimately died.

In 1984, only four of the eight transplanted patients were alive. One was malnourished, but without infection, one was in excellent health, one had recurrent diarrhea, and one had stage IV Hodgkin's disease. The development of Hodgkin's disease illustrated in a vivid way for us the precarious state of health of these patients, even though they appeared amazingly well. Prior to development of this complication, the patient seemed in perfect health and had been free of significant infection for over 3 years. This patient was started on a course of cyclic chemotherapy, but ultimately died.

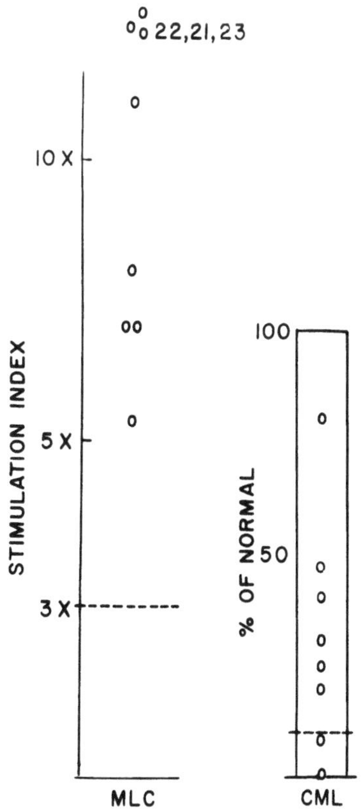

Fig. 3. Responses to allogeneic cells. Mixed leukocyte culture (MLC) responses shown as stimulation indices, defined as counts per minute of stimulated cultures/counts per minute of resting cultures. Values over 3 × are in normal range. Cell-mediated lympholysis (CML) is the percentage of specific release from chromium-labeled targets of the same individual used to stimulate a given responder (the transplanted patients). Normal values vary from day to day. The patients' values shown are expressed as a percentage of the normal individual's response to the same target on the day of the test. *Broken line* shows 10% of a normal response

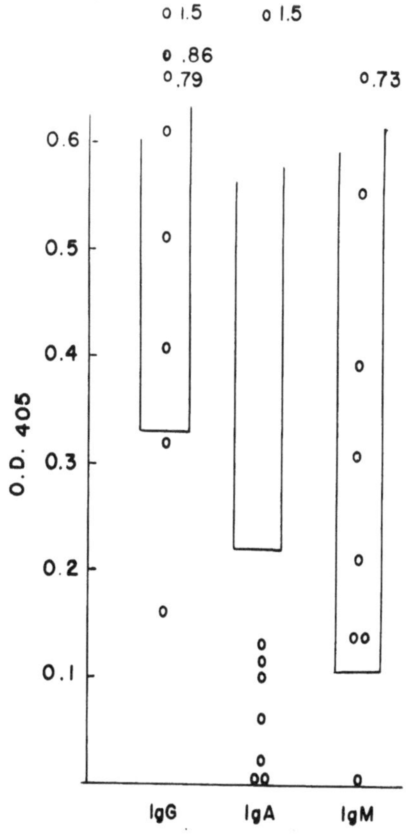

Fig. 4. Isotype responses to *E. coli* determined by ELISA assay. Values are expressed as optical density at 405 nm. The lower limits of the normal range are shown by the bottom portions of the *open bars*

Because of this unnerving complication, and in view of our recent gratifying results with haplo-identical bone marrow transplants, we elected to prepare another of the long-term survivors for bone marrow transplantation. It was necessary to ablate the child prior to transplantation because of immunity conferred by the previous thymic transplant. Thus, thymic transplantation created a paradox in that we produced a patient with too much immunity to allow transplantation without fear of rejection, but not enough immunity to permit complete freedom from complications of immunodeficiency. The price of the disease-free survival was ablative medication prior to transplantation. However, ultimately, this has not proven to be an unacceptable price. Two of the remaining patients have been successfully treated with monoclonal antibody-treated haplo-identical bone marrow transplants.

The accomplishment of successful bone marrow transplantation from a haplo-identical donor marks the end of the era of thymus transplantation for combined immunodeficiency. In light of the success of others using lectin-depleted marrow (Reisner et al. 1981) and ourselves using monoclonal antibody-treated inocula, I do not believe there is further indication for thymic transplantation in this disease.

Unresolved, in my mind at least, is the reason that thymus alone corrected both B- and T-cell deficiencies, yet no bone marrow transplant has required thymic transplantation to attain full T-cell function. In one patient, we biopsied the thymus after bone marrow transplantation and demonstrated normal histology (Moen et al. 1985), providing partial support for the concept that the morphology of the thymus is secondary rather than primary. In that case, the interpretation was flawed by the fact that a pretransplantation specimen was not obtained. A pretransplantion biopsy taken from his immunodeficient brother was typically dysplastic, however.

Other Diseases

The DiGeorge syndrome has repeatedly been presented as the prototype of pure T-cell deficiency. The fundamental defect is an embryologic maldevelopment of derivatives of the third and fourth pharyngeal pouches, which results in abnormalities of the parathyroid and thymus glands as well as facial and cardiac anomalies. The basic problem in assessing efficacy of therapy in the DiGeorge syndrome is the highly variable degree of the defect (Lischner 1972). In many cases (most, in my experience), the immunologic defects are trivial or spontaneously revert to normal. Of six patients with the DiGeorge syndrome whom I have examined or whose immunologic status I have evaluated, not one has required immunologic intervention. The presence of immunoglobulins or reasonable numbers of lymphocytes ($>1000\ mm^3$ usually indicates that a spontaneous regression will occur. The tendency for spontaneous reversal of the disease and the variable degree of the deficiency makes the DiGeorge syndrome a most undesirable disease for assessment of thymic capability of reconstitution.

The Nezelof syndrome is defined as a disorder in which there is incomplete B-cell development, but immunoglobulins are present, originally thought to be the typical phenotype of an isolated T-cell defect. We now know that there are many reasons for this type of inadequate immunoglobulin response, so that the fundamental fault is insufficiently delineated to allow informative assessment of therapy. For example, when the Nezelof syndrome was originally described, enzyme deficiency (e. g., adenosine deaminase or purine nucleoside phosphorylase) were unknown. Some cases classified under the category of the Nezelof syndrome were probably due to enzyme disease. Of four patients with the Nezelof syndrome transplanted with cultured thymus, not one showed any benefit whatever. Thus, paradoxically, in a situation where some B-cell function was observed and the disorder appeared to be ideal for thymic replacement therapy, we had uniformally dismal results. As will be seen later, a reasonable explanation for this failure could be rejection of the thymus.

We have also employed cultured thymus fragment (CTF) transplants in other less classic immunodeficiency states. Because of the findings that chronic lymphocytic leukemia (CLL) was associated with a measurable T-cell defect (Chiorazzi et al. 1979), we transplanted thymus in a male patient with CLL who had hypogammaglobulinemia and was requiring nearly monthly admissions to the hospital for serious pneumonia despite gamma-globulin replacement therapy. Return of T-cell proliferation tests to normal and clinical well-being was observed following the transplant. After 1 year, however, his immunity waned, he acquired overwhelming pneumonia, and died. No remnants of the transplant were seen at autopsy.

Chronic GVH disease is a major problem affecting the long-term outcome of bone marrow transplantation in adult leukemia patients. The incidence of chronic GVH disease is correlated with thymic deficiency (Fass et al. 1973). Atkinson et al. (1982) utilized cultured thymus fragment transplants to augment thymic function in bone marrow transplant patients. There was no evidence of any benefit and in the few instances where biopsy was performed, no transplanted tissue was found.

It finally occurred to us that the possibility of a graft rejection should be considered. In the transplants in children with severe combined immunodeficiency, no immunity was present and transplantation could be accomplished without any immunosuppression. However, in patients such as those with leukemia, and possibly Nezelof syndrome, such profound defects did not exist. Consequently, the grafts ultimately were lost.

A most gratifying experience was seen in a patient with chronic mucocutaneous candidiasis who had acquired the complication of oral cancer in the area of chronic infection (Hong and Dibbell 1981 b). His immunity to candida was restored and the candidiasis became very easy to control on minimal medication. About 1½ years later, his candida infections became more florid, and cancer was found in the buccal mucosa on the other side. A repeat transplant was performed. Because of our feeling that rejection was a real possibility, he was placed on low dose azathioprine therapy to inhibit rejection. His candida has again become controllable and he has remained free of malignant disease. Some 6 years after this transplant he remains well. As a result we believe that more attention must be paid to the possibility of rejection of CTF transplants than in the past.

An observation by Ready et al. (1984), showing that culture of thymus in deoxyguanosine allows transplantation across major histocompatibility barriers to immunologically normal recipients without immunosuppression provides a stimulus for further attempts to transplant thymuses in relatively immunocompetent recipients, following different culture techniques.

The Future

The future of thymus transplantation will be restricted to attempts to treat mild T-cell defects. As mentioned already, the use of post-transplantation immunosuppression is indicated. Another trial in bone marrow

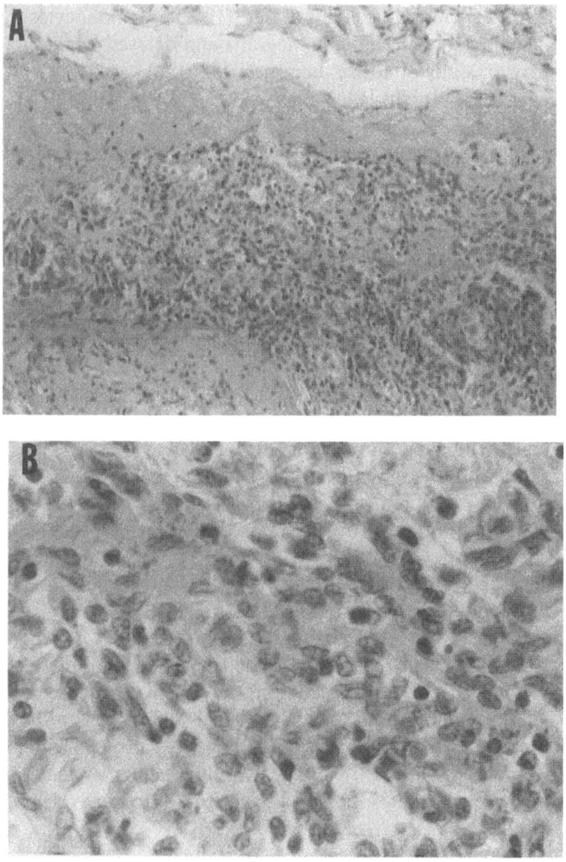

Fig. 5 A, B. Views of thymus biopsy from patient with AIDS transplanted with cultured thymus 3 months previously. The transplant is well engrafted, but alymphoid. **A** ×100, **B** ×400

transplantation is indicated, especially with the common usage of cyclosporin A to control GVH disease. Chronic mucocutaneous candidiasis which does not respond to ketoconazole therapy is another disorder which should benefit.

We recently transplanted thymuses in three patients with AIDS. All died. However, in the last patient we had the opportunity to review the site of transplantation (Fig. 5). Although the transplant has not become lymphoid, it is clearly present and engrafted. Perhaps in conjunction with an antiviral agent, lymphoid repopulation could occur. This is probably only a stopgap holding action and not a definitive cure. Nevertheless, such interim therapy has allowed a number of children with SCID, formerly uniformly fatal, to survive to a time when definitive cures could be given.

References

Ammann AJ, Wara DW, Salmon S, Perkins H (1973) Thymus transplantation: permanent reconstitution of cellular immunity in a patient with sex-linked combined immunodeficiency. N Engl J Med 289: 5-9

Atkinson K, Storb R, Ochs HD, Goehle S, Sullivan KM, Witherspoon RP, Lum LG, Tsoi MS, Sanders JE, Parr M, Stewart P, Thomas ED (1982) Thymus transplantation after allogeneic bone marrow graft to prevent chronic graft-versus-host disease in humans. Transplantation 33: 168-173

Chiorazzi N, Fu SM, Montazeri G, Kunkel HG, Rai K, Gee T (1979) T cell helper defect in patients with chronic lymphocytic leukemia. J Immunol 122: 1087-1090

Cottier H (1958) Zur Histopathologie des Antikörpermangelsyndroms. In: Trans Sixth Cong Europ Soc Haematol, Copenhagen 1957. Karger, Basel, pp 41-46

Dukor P, Miller JFAP, House W, Allman V (1965) Regeneration of thymus grafts. I. Histological and cytological aspects. Transplantation 3: 639-668

Epstein WL, Fudenberg HH, Reed WB, Boder E, Sedgwick RP (1966) Immunologic studies in ataxia-telangiectasia. I. Delayed hypersensitivity and serum immune globulin levels in probands and first-degree relatives. Int Arch Allergy Appl Immunol 30: 15-29

Fass L, Ochs HD, Thomas ED, Mickelson E, Storb R, Fefer A (1973) Studies of immunological reactivity following syngeneic or allogeneic marrow grafts in man. Transplantation 16: 630-640

Good RA, Dalmasso AP, Martinez C, Archer OK, Pierce JC, Papermaster BW (1962) The role of the thymus in development of immunologic capacity in rabbits and mice. J Exp Med 116: 773-796

Hitzig WH, Kay HEM, Cottier H (1965) Familial lymphopenia with agammaglobulinemia: An attempt at treatment by implantation of foetal thymus. Lancet 2: 151-154

Hong R (1981 a) Present and future status of thymus transplantation. Ann Clin Res 13: 350-357

Hong R, Dibbell DG (1981 b) Cultured thymus fragment transplant in chronic candidiasis complicated by oral carcinoma. Lancet 1: 773-774

Hong R, Santosham M, Schulte-Wissermann H, Horowitz S, Hsu SH, Winkelstein JA (1976) Reconstitution of B and T lymphocyte function in severe combined immunodeficiency disease after transplantation with thymic epithelium. Lancet 2: 1270-1272

Hong R, Schulte-Wissermann H, Jarrett-Toth E, Horowitz SD, Manning DD (1979) Transplantation of cultured thymic fragments II. Results in nude mice. J Exp Med 149: 398-415

Horowitz SD, Hong R (1975) Selective IgA deficiency - some perspectives. In: Bergsma D (ed) Immunodeficiency in man and animals. Sinauer, Sunderland Ma, pp 129-133

Jacobs BB, Huseby RA (1967) Growth of tumors in allogeneic hosts following organ culture explantation. Transplantation 5: 410-419

Kindred B, Loor F (1974) Activity of host-derived T cells which differentiate in nude mice grafted with co-isogenic or allogeneic thymuses. J Exp Med 139: 1215-1227

Lafferty KL, Cooley MA, Woolnough J, Walker KZ (1975) Thyroid allograft immunogenicity is reduced after a period in organ culture. Science 188: 259-261

Lischner HW (1972) DiGeorge syndrome(s). J Pediatr 81: 1042-1044

Loor F, Kindred B, Hägg LB (1976) Incomplete restoration of T-cell reactivity in nude mice after neonatal allogeneic thymus grafting. Cell Immunol 26: 29-46

Maclean LD, Zak SJ, Varco RL, Good RA (1957) The role of the thymus in antibody production; an experimental study of the immune response in thymectomized rabbits. Transplant Bull 4: 21-22

Metcalf D (1966) The nature and regulation of lymphopoiesis in the normal and neoplastic thymus. In: Wolstenholme GEW, Porter R (eds) Ciba foundation symposium on the thymus, experimental and clinical studies. Churchill, London, pp 242-263

Miller JFAP (1961) Immunological function of the thymus. Lancet 2: 748-749

Moen R, Hong R, Stiehm ER, Billing R, Shearer W, Winkelstein J, Johnson J (1985) Theoretical and biologic considerations in successful mismatched bone marrow transplantation. Pediatr Res 19: 278 a

Opelz G, Terasaki PI (1974) Lymphocyte antigenicity loss with retention of responsiveness. Science 184: 464-466

Owen JJT, Ritter MA (1969) Tissue interaction in the development of thymus lymphocytes. J Exp Med 129: 431-442

Pyke KW, Dosch HM, Ipp MM, Gelfand EW (1975) Demonstration of an intrathymic defect in a case of severe combined immunodeficiency disease. N Engl J Med 293: 424-428

Rachelefsky GS, Stiehm ER, Ammann AJ, Cederbaum SD, Opelz G, Terasaki PI (1975) T-cell reconstitution by thymus transplantation and transfer factor in severe combined immunodeficiency. Pediatrics 55: 114-118

Ready AR, Jenkinson EJ, Kingston R, Owen JJT (1984) Successful transplantation across major histocompatibility barrier of deoxyguanosine-treated embryonic thymus expressing class II antigens. Nature 310: 231-233

Reisner Y, Kapoor N, Kirkpatrick D, Pollack MS, Dupont B, Good RA, O'Reilly RJ (1981) Transplantation for acute leukaemia with HLA-A and B nonidentical parental marrow cells fractionated with soybean agglutinin and sheep red blood cells. Lancet 2: 327-331

Rosen FS, Gitlin D, Janeway CA (1962) Alymphocytosis, agammaglobulinaemia, homografts and delayed hypersensitivity; study of a case. Lancet 2: 380-381

Seeger RC, Robins RA, Stevens RH, Klein RB, Waldman DJ, Zeltzer PM, Kessler SW (1976) Severe combined immunodeficiency with B lymphocytes: in vitro correction of defective immunoglobulin production by addition of normal T lymphocytes. Clin Exp Immunol 26: 1-10

Shearer WT, Wedner HJ, Strominger DB, Kissane J, Hong R (1978) Successful transplantation of the thymus in Nezelof's syndrome. Pediatrics 61: 619-624

Talmage DW, Dart GA (1978) Effects of oxygen pressure during culture on survival of mouse thyroid allografts. Science 200: 1066-1067

Talmage DW, Dart GA, Radovich J, Lafferty KJ (1976) Activation of transplant immunity: effect of donor leukocytes on thyroid allograft rejection. Science 191: 385-388

Waksman BH, Arnason BG, Jankovic BD (1962) Role of the thymus in immune reactions in rats. III. Changes in the lymphoid organs of thymectomized rats. J Exp Med 116: 187-206

Zinkernagel RM (1978) Thymus function and reconstitution of immunodeficiency. N Engl J Med 298: 222 (letter)

Zinkernagel RM, Callahan GN, Althage A, Cooper S, Klein PA, Klein J (1978 b) On the thymus in the differentiation of "H-2 self-recognition" by T cells: evidence for dual recognition? J Exp Med 147: 882-896

Zinkernagel RM, Callahan GN, Althage A, Cooper S, Streilein JW, Klein J (1978 c) The lymphoreticular system in triggering virus plus self-specific cytotoxic T cells: evidence for T help. J Exp Med 147: 897-911

Zinkernagel RM, Althage A, Waterfield E, Kindred B, Welsh RM, Callahan G, Pincetl P (1980) Restriction specificities, alloreactivity, and allotolerance expressed by T cells from nude mice reconstituted with H-2-compatible or -incompatible thymus grafts. J Exp Med 151: 376-399

Part VI

Other Therapeutic Modalities

27 Chemotherapy for Invasive Thymomas

Sushil Bhardwaj and A. Philippe Chahinian

Introduction

Invasive thymomas are usually slowly growing tumors that tend to recur within the thoracic cavity (Le Golvan et al. 1977; Wilkins et al. 1966). The overall 5-year survival varies between 23% and 60% (Batata et al. 1974; Bernatz et al. 1961, 1973; Legg et al. 1965; Namba et al. 1978; Otto et al. 1978; Slater et al. 1978). Approximately one-third of patients with thymoma have myasthenia gravis, and one-tenth of patients with myasthenia gravis have a thymoma (Namba et al. 1978). The presence of myasthenia gravis in patients with thymoma adversely affected survival in some series (Wilkins et al. 1966), but not in others (Bernatz et al. 1973). Surgery and radiotherapy have been the major therapeutic modalities that have been used in the management of invasive thymoma. These modalities are discussed at length elsewhere in the text; however, some points deserve further mention. Repeat thoracotomy for recurrent intrathoracic thymoma is not unusual and adjuvant radiotherapy has been recommended by several authors (Wilkins et al. 1966; Bernatz et al. 1961, 1973; Goldman et al. 1975; Penn et al. 1972; Ariaratnam et al. 1979). Radiotherapy can be curative when the tumoral volume allows delivery of adequate doses. Its results remain poor, however, in cases of late recurrent disease after surgery (Penn et al. 1972).

Information regarding the efficacy of chemotherapy as a modality of treatment in the management of invasive thymoma was relatively scarce until very recently (Chahinian et al. 1981). The initial reports largely included case reports of individual patients. Since 1980 there have been several reports describing the effectiveness of chemotherapy of invasive thymoma in series consisting of larger numbers of patients. There is increasing evidence to support the role of chemotherapy as an important modality in the management of invasive thymoma, by itself in a patient with metastatic disease and as a component of a multi-modality approach including surgery and/or radiation therapy in a patient with advanced intrathoracic invasive thymoma.

Chemotherapeutic Agents

Single Agents

The activity of single agents for chemotherapy of thymoma is summarized in Table 1. In a review by Boston in 1976, 12 evaluable cases treated with chemotherapy were described. The longest remission (13 months) occurred in a patient treated with cisplatin (Talley et al. 1973). The activity of cisplatin has since been confirmed by others (Needles et al. 1981; Shetty and Arora 1981; Baum et al. 1981; Cocconi et al. 1982), including a report of a complete remission of greater than 10 months duration in a patient with thymoma metastatic to the kidney treated with cisplatin at a dose of 120 mg/m^2 at 3-week intervals (Needles et al. 1981). Levin et al. (1982) have reported a prolonged (24 months) remission in a patient with malignant thymoma metastatic to the pleura. The patient received combined modality therapy with cisplatin followed by radiation therapy, surgical excision, postoperative radiotherapy, and three additional cycles of treatment with cisplatin.

Other single agents with activity in invasive thymoma have been described. Boston (1976) reported a partial response of 1 months duration in a patient with metastatic thymoma who received doxorubicin 0.4 mg/kg every 8 h for six doses. Maytansine, an ansa macrolide, which produced atrophy of the thymus in rats (Mugera et al. 1977), has been reported to have resulted in objective remissions of 6–18 weeks duration in two of three patients with invasive thymoma (Chahinian et al. 1979, 1981; Jaffrey et al. 1980). L-Asparaginase resulted in a minor remission of 4 weeks duration in one of two patients with invasive thymoma (Chahinian et al. 1981).

The "thymolytic" effect of corticosteroids has been demonstrated (Claman 1972). Significant tumor reduction has been achieved in cases of thymoma with adrenocorticotropic hormone (Soffer et al. 1952) or corticosteroids alone (Green and Forman 1974; Almog et al. 1978; Posner et al. 1977; Shellito et al. 1978; Hu and Levine 1986). Whether this represents a direct oncolytic effect of corticosteroids or a decrease in the lymphocytic component of the tumor is unknown at the present time.

Table 1. Single-agent chemotherapy for invasive thymomas

Drug	Dose and schedule	No. of patients	Response (duration)	Reference
Cisplatin	4, 6, 10 mg m^{-2} day^{-1} × 5 days q 4 weeks; 10 treatment cycles	1	PR (13 months)	Talley et al. 1973
	120 mg/m^2 q 3 weeks; 4 treatment cycles	1	CR (10 months)	Needles et al. 1981
	100 mg/m^2 q 3 weeks; 2 treatment cycles	1	PR (?)	Shetty and Arora 1981
	3-4 mg/kg q 3 weeks; 1 treatment	1	PR (1 month)	Baum et al. 1981
	50-100 mg/m^2; 9 treatments	1	CR (>20 months)	Cocconi et al. 1982
	3 mg/kg, surgery, radiotherapy, and 4 more cycles of cisplatin	1	CR (24 months)	Levin et al. 1982
Doxorubicin	0.4 mg/kg q 8 h	1	PR (1 month)	Boston 1976
Maytansine	0.7-1.1 mg m^{-2} $week^{-1}$	3	2 PR (6 and 18 weeks)	Chahinian et al. 1981; Jaffrey et al. 1980

CR complete response; PR partial response

Combination Chemotherapy

Combination chemotherapy has been successful in effecting durable remissions in many neoplasms and in curing some of them (Holland 1983). Boston (1976) reported on the effectiveness of two different combinations. Doxorubicin, lomustine, vincristine, and bleomycin produced a partial remission for 7 weeks in one patient who also received concomitant radiotherapy. Nitrogen mustard, vincristine, vinblastine, and procarbazine was given to two patients with partial remission of 3 weeks and 3 months duration, respectively. A similar combination produced no response in another patient (Ariaratnam et al. 1979). The combination of cyclophosphamide, vincristine, and prednisone has been effective in one patient with invasive thymoma and pleural effusion, however the follow-up did not exceed 6 months (Griffin et al. 1978).

In 1980, Evans et al. reported objective tumor regression (partial remissions) in four of five patients with invasive thymoma treated with a combination of cyclophosphamide, vincristine (Oncovin), prednisone, and procarbazine (COPP). All five patients were previously untreated with chemotherapy and radiation therapy. In all four patients who responded, the COPP chemotherapy was followed by radiation therapy and surgery in two of the four patients. Three patients were free of disease at the time of the report at 3 months, 33 months, and 34 months.

In 1981, Chahinian et al. reported their experience with a combination of bleomycin, doxorubicin (Adriamycin), cisplatin, and prednisone (BAPP) which was begun in 1974 and produced a partial remission in two of five patients with invasive thymoma. The duration of response was 12 and 14 months, respectively. Four of the five patients who were treated with BAPP had received prior radiation therapy. Since this early report, we have now treated 16 patients with invasive thymoma with BAPP chemotherapy. In order to avoid potential pulmonary toxicity, bleomycin was omitted in two patients who had undergone prior pneumonectomy. Overall results revealed eight complete responses (50%) and five partial responses (31%) for an overall objective response rate of 81%. Consolidation radiotherapy to the mediastinum and/or restaging thoracotomy were carried out whenever technically feasible. Seven patients remained alive 6-130 months after chemotherapy (median 36 months). The other nine patients died 7-43 months after chemotherapy (median 26 months). Six patients had myasthenia gravis resistant to conventional medical treatment. Two of these patients who had a complete response to chemotherapy also had complete disappearance of symptoms of myasthenia following chemotherapy.

Campbell et al. (1981) reported a complete response following chemotherapy with a combination of cyclophosphamide, doxorubicin (Adriamycin), and cisplatin (Platinex) (CAP) in a patient with invasive thymoma metastatic to the lung. The remission duration was over 1 year with an overall survival from the onset of chemotherapy of over 23 months.

Shetty and Arora (1981) reported on a combination chemotherapy regimen of doxorubicin and cisplatin which resulted in a partial response (4 months duration), in a patient with metastatic thymoma which had recurred after having initially responded to cisplatin alone. In another case report (Thomas et al. 1983), the latter combination also resulted in a partial remission of 3 months duration. In a recent report describing a combination of doxorubicin and cisplatin at a higher dose (doxorubicin 80 mg/m^2 and cisplatin 120 mg/m^2), two patients with invasive thymoma achieved a complete response of over 4 and 12 months, respectively. One patient who had responded initially for 12 months, went on to a second complete response of over 8 months after retreatment with the same combination at the time of relapse (Klippstein et al. 1984).

The combination of doxorubicin and cyclophosphamide resulted in a complete remission of over 13 months in a patient with metastatic thymoma reported by Butler et al. (1982). In a review of 25 cases, Appleqvist et al. (1982) reported on the ineffectiveness of three different combinations: Bleo-CHOP (bleomycin, cyclophosphamide, doxorubicin, vincristine (Oncovin), and prednisone), COP (cyclophosphamide, vincristine, and prednisone) and cisplatin, vinblastine, and bleomycin in the management of metastatic thymoma. Hu and Levine (1986) reported a patient with malignant thymoma treated with a combination of cyclophosphamide, doxorubicin, vincristine (Oncovin), and prednisone (CHOP) who had an initial minor response followed by tumor progression after three cycles of chemotherapy. The details of the chemotherapy and patient characteristics were not described in either paper.

In 1983, Daugaard et al. reported a series of nine patients with invasive thymoma who were treated with a combination of vincristine, cyclophosphamide, lomustine, and prednisone in six of the nine patients. Four complete responses ranging from 31 to 62 months were described in addition to one partial response of 2 months duration.

In 1984, Fornasiero et al. reported 11 patients with invasive thymoma who were treated with a combination of cisplatin, doxorubicin, vincristine, and cyclophosphamide. A 91% objective response rate (four complete and six partial responses) was observed with a median duration of response of 18.5 months (range 5-29 months) for complete responders, and 10.5 months (range 5-22 months) for partial responders. Giaccone et al. (1985) have reported four patients with invasive thymoma who were treated with a combination of etoposide (VP 16) and cisplatin. One partial response of over 27 months was noted in addition to two minor responses. Hu and Levine (1986) described one patient with malignant thymoma unresponsive to chemotherapy with a combination of cisplatin and etoposide.

Uematsu and Kondo (1986) have reported a series of 11 patients with invasive thymoma, who were treated with radiotherapy. Intensive combination chemotherapy was administered to two patients with recurrent disease and they achieved complete remissions. One patient (a 27-year-old woman) who was found to have extensive intrathoracic metastases at thoracotomy achieved a partial remission with three cycles of VEP chemotherapy (1 mg vincristine intravenously on day 1, 100 mg cyclophosphamide, and 20 mg prednisone orally on days 1-7) administered postoperatively. This was followed by radiation therapy (1500 cGy) to the entire hemithorax initially with subsequent reduction of the radiation fields to cover the whole mediastinum (3000 cGy). The patient achieved complete remission following the radiation therapy and was administered an additional four cycles of VEP chemotherapy. She was disease free at 65 months at the time of the report.

A second patient (a 62-year-old man), with extensive invasive thymoma involving the anterior mediastinum with extension to left pleura, left lung, and pericardium, who underwent a macroscopic complete resection (positive microscopic surgical margin) followed by postoperative radiation therapy (4500 cGy in 25 fractions to the whole mediastinum and bilateral supraclavicular fossae) developed recurrent pleural thymoma 2 years later associated with myasthenia. CHOP chemotherapy (doxorubicin 50 mg/m^2 intravenously on day 1, cyclophosphamide 750 mg/m^2 intravenously on day 1, vincristine 1.4 mg/m^2 intravenously on day 1, and prednisone 50 mg/m^2 orally on days 1-5) was administered for five cycles with complete remission documented by chest X-rays and computerized tomographic (CT) scans. He received an additional two cycles of CHOP and remained in complete remission for 12 months when he developed recurrence of myasthenia associated with recurrence of pleural masses on CT scan. He was retreated with a combination of CHOP chemotherapy and entire hemithorax irradiation (1000 cGy), achieved a third remission, and was alive and well at the time of the report.

Uematsu and Kondo (1986) conclude that intensive combination chemotherapy before radiotherapy may be helpful in shrinking tumor masses in patients with multiple tumors. Lewis (1987) reported that either surgery and/or chemotherapy must follow debulking radiotherapy. Maggi et al. (1986) have reviewed the surgical treatment of 169 patients with thymoma, spanning a 28-year period. Postoperative chemotherapy with or without radiation therapy was administered to seven patients. Response was noted in: three patients who received radiation therapy and cisplatin; one patient who received radiation therapy plus combination chemotherapy with cisplatin and etoposide; and two patients who received postoperative cisplatin and etoposide alone without radiotherapy. One additional patient who received postoperative vincristine and radiation therapy was not benefited. Details of dose, schedule, and response were not provided.

Table 2. Combination chemotherapy for invasive thymomas: cisplatin-based regimens

Regimen	No. of patients	Response (duration)	Reference
BAPP	16	8 CR (median 18 months)	Chahinian 1988,
Bleomycin 12 mg/m^2 day 1		5 PR (median 5 months)	personal communication
Doxorubicin 50 mg/m^2 day 1			Chahinian et al. 1981, 1983
Cisplatin 50 mg/m^2 day 1			
Prednisone 40 mg/m^2 days 1-5			
CAP	1	1 CR (>12 months)	Campbell et al. 1981
Cyclophosphamide 600 mg/m^2 day 1			
Doxorubicin 50 mg/m^2 day 1			
Cisplatin 75 mg/m^2 day 1			
AP			
Doxorubicin[a]	1	1 PR (6 months)	Shetty and Arora 1981
Cisplatin[a]	1	1 PR (3 months)	Thomas et al. 1983
	2	2 CR (>4, >12 months)	Klippenstein et al. 1984
ADOC	11	4 CR (5->29 months)	Fornasiero et al. 1984
Doxorubicin 40 mg/m^2 day 1		6 PR (>5-22 months)	
Cisplatin 50 mg/m^2 day 1			
Vincristine 0.6 mg/m^2 day 3			
Cyclophosphamide 700 mg/m^2 day 4			
EP	4	1 PR (>27 months)	Giaccone et al. 1985
Etoposide 120 mg/m^2 days 4, 6, 8			
Cisplatin 60 mg/m^2 day 1			

CR complete response; PR partial response; [a] Different doses and schedules

Table 3. Combination chemotherapy for invasive thymomas: non-cisplatin regimens

Regimen	No. of patients	Response (duration)	Reference
MVPV	2	2 PR (3 months and 3 weeks)	Boston 1976
Nitrogen mustard			
Vincristine			
Procarbazine			
Vinblastine			
ACVB	1	1 PR (7 weeks)	Boston 1976
Doxorubicin 40 mg/m^2			
Lomustine 50 mg/m^2			
Vincristine 0.5 mg			
Bleomycin 5 mg			
COPP	5	4 PR	Evans et al. 1980
Cyclophosphamide		Given prior to radiotherapy NED at	
Vincristine		34 and 33 months	
Prednisone			
Procarbazine			
AC	1	1 CR (13 months)	Butler et al. 1982
Doxorubicin 50 mg/m^2			
Cyclophosphamide 750 mg/m^2			
VCC ± P	9	4 CR (31-62 months)	Daugaard et al. 1983
Vincristine 1.3 mg/m^2 day 1		1 PR (2 months)	
Cyclophosphamide 1 g/m^2 day 1			
Lomustine 70 mg/m^2 day 1			
Prednisone 40 mg/m^2 days 1-7 (6 patients)			
CHOP	1	1 CR (12 months)	Uematsu and Kondo 1986
Cyclophosphamide 750 mg/m^2 day 1			
Doxorubicin 50 mg/m^2 day 1			
Vincristine 1.4 mg/m^2 day 1			
Prednisone 50 mg/m^2 days 1-5			

CR complete response; PR partial response; NED no evidence of disease

The details of the various combination chemotherapy regimens are summarized in Tables 2 and 3. The overall cumulative objective response rate for the cisplatin-based regimens is 81% (15 complete responses and 14 partial responses in a total of 36 patients). The overall cumulative objective response rate for the noncisplatin regimens is 74% (6 complete responses and 8 partial responses in a total of 19 patients).

Based on our experience with the treatment of patients with metastatic thymoma, we recommend a combination chemotherapy program comprising bleomycin, doxorubicin, cisplatin, and prednisone (BAPP) (Table 2). BAPP is well tolerated. Nausea, vomiting, and alopecia occur in varying degree in practically all patients. Mild to moderate reversible hematologic toxicity is seen in most patients. Pulmonary, cardiac, or renal toxicity have not been observed. The total bleomycin dose used is less than 150 units and doxorubicin is discontinued prior to the cardiotoxic threshold dose of 450 mg/m^2.

Immunotherapy

MER (methanol extraction residue of bacillus Calmette Guérin) and *Corynebacterium parvum* were administered to two patients (one patient each) with metastatic thymoma with no evidence of response in the paper by Chahinian et al. (1981). Other interesting developments with possible implications for use in metastatic thymoma include the interferons which have been successful in the treatment of hairy cell leukemia, renal cell carcinoma, melanoma, and T-cell lymphoma. Interleukin 2 with lymphokine-activated killer cells is another innovative cancer treatment modality. However, this would have to be tested in experimental study prior to clinical use as the lymphocytes in thymomas are T-lymphocytes and could perhaps be activated by interleukin 2.

Summary

In conclusion our own experience as well as that of others reveals that invasive thymomas respond reasonably well to chemotherapy. This should be one of the essential components of the primary treatment for patients who present with large bulky unresectable mediastinal masses, or those with metastases. A combined modality program using consolidation radiotherapy and/or restaging surgery can further increase the complete response rates, and potentially cure some of these patients. Myasthenia gravis, which is often not well controlled with conventional medical management in these patients, can also improve and even disappear following chemotherapy.

References

Almog C, Pik A, Weisberg D, Herczeg E (1978) Regression of malignant thymoma with metastases after treatment with adrenocortical steroids. Isr J Med Sci 14: 476-480

Appelqvist P, Kostiainen S, Franssila K, Mattila S, Gröhn P (1982) Treatment and prognosis of thymoma: a review of 25 cases. J Surg Oncol 20: 265-268

Ariaratnam LS, Kalnicki S, Mincer F, Botstein C (1979) The management of malignant thymoma with radiation therapy. Int J Radiat Oncol Biol Phys 5: 77-80

Batata MA, Martini N, Huvos AG, Aguilar RI, Beattie EJ Jr (1974) Thymomas: clinicopathologic features, therapy and prognosis. Cancer 34: 389-396

Baum ES, Gaynon P, Greenberg L, Krivit W, Hammond D (1981) Phase II trial of cis-platin in refractory childhood cancer: children's cancer study group report. Cancer Treat Rep 65: 815-822

Bernatz PE, Harrison EG, Clagett OT (1961) Thymoma: a clinicopathologic study. J Thorac Cardiovasc Surg 42: 424-444

Bernatz PE, Khonsari S, Harrison EG, Taylor WF (1973) Thymoma: factors influencing prognosis. Surg Clin North Am 53: 885-892

Boston B (1976) Chemotherapy of invasive thymoma. Cancer 38: 49-52

Butler WM, Diehl LF, Taylor G, Weltz MD (1982) Metastatic thymoma with myasthenia gravis. Complete remission with combination chemotherapy. Cancer 50: 419-422

Campbell MG, Pollard R, Al-Sarraf M (1981) A complete response in metastatic malignant thymoma to cis-platinum, doxorubicin and cyclophosphamide. A case report. Cancer 48: 1315-1317

Chahinian AP, Bhardwaj S, Meyer RJ, Jaffrey IS, Kirschner PA, Holland JF (1981) Treatment of invasive or metastatic thymoma: report of eleven cases. Cancer 47: 1752-1761

Chahinian AP, Holland JF, Bhardwaj S (1983) Chemotherapy for malignant thymoma. Ann Intern Med 99: 736

Chahinian AP, Nogeire C, Ohnuma T, Greenberg ML, Sivak M, Jaffrey IS, Holland JF (1979) Phase I study of weekly maytansine given by iv bolus or 24-hour infusion. Cancer Treat Rep 63: 1953-1960

Claman HN (1972) Corticosteroids and lymphoid cells. N Engl J Med 287: 388-397

Cocconi G, Corrado B, Cuomo A (1982) Long-lasting response to cis-platinum in recurrent malignant thymoma. Case report. Cancer 49: 1985-1987

Daugaard G, Hansen HH, Rorth M (1983) Combination chemotherapy for malignant thymoma. Ann Intern Med 99: 189-190

Evans WK, Thompson DM, Simpson WJ, Feld R, Phillips MJ (1980) Combination chemotherapy in invasive thymoma, role of COPP. Cancer 46: 1523-1527

Fornasiero A, Daniele O, Sperandio P, Morandi P, Fosser VP, Cartei G, Fiorentino MV (1984) Chemotherapy of invasive or metastatic thymoma: report of 11 cases. Cancer Treat Rep 68: 1205-1210

Giaccone G, Musella R, Bertetto O, Donadio M, Calciati A (1985) Cis-platin containing chemotherapy in the treatment of invasive thymoma: report of five cases. Cancer Treat Rep 69: 695-697

Goldman AJ, Herrmann C Jr, Keesey JC, Mulder DG, Brown WJ (1975) Myasthenia gravis and invasive thymoma: a 20 year experience. Neurology 25: 1021-1025

Green JD, Forman WH (1974) Response of thymoma to steroids. Chest 65: 114-116

Griffin JD, Aisenberg AC, Long JC (1978) Lymphocytic thymoma associated with T-cell lymphocytosis. Am J Med 64: 1075-1079

Holland JF (1983) Breaking the cure barrier. J Clin Oncol 1: 75-90

Hu E, Levine J (1986) Chemotherapy of malignant thymoma. Case report and review of the literature. Cancer 57: 1101-1104

Jaffrey IS, Denefrio JM, Chahinian AP (1980) Response to maytansine in a patient with malignant thymoma. Cancer Treat Rep 64: 193-194

Klippstein TH, Mitrou PS, Kochendorfer KJ, Bergmann L (1984) High-dose Adriamycin (ADM) and and Cis-P (DDP) in advanced soft-tissue sarcomas and invasive thymomas. A pilot study. Cancer Chemother Pharmacol 13: 78-81

Legg MA, Brady WJ (1965) Pathology and clinical behavior of thymomas. A survey of 51 cases. Cancer 18: 1131-1144

LeGolvan DP, Abell MR (1977) Thymomas. Cancer 39: 2142-2157

Levin L, Sealy R, Barron J (1982) Syndrome of inappropriate antidiuretic hormone secretion following cis-dichlorodiammineplatinum II in a patient with malignant thymoma. Cancer 50: 2279-2282

Lewis JE, Wick MR, Scheithauer BW, Bernatz PG, Taylor WF (1987) Thymoma. A clinicopathologic review. Cancer 60: 2727-2743

Maggi G, Giaccone G, Donadio M, Ciuffreda L, Dalesio O, Leria G, Trifiletti G, Casadio C, Palestro G, Mancuso M, Calciati A (1986) Thymomas. A review of 169 cases, with particular reference to results of surgical treatment. Cancer 58: 765-776

Mugera GM, Ward JM (1977) Acute toxicity of maytansine in F344 rats. Cancer Treat Rep 61: 1333-1338

Namba T, Brunner NG, Grob D (1978) Myasthenia gravis in patients with thymoma, with particular reference to onset after thymectomy. Medicine 57: 411-433

Needles B, Kemeny N, Urmacher C (1981) Malignant thymoma: renal metastases responding to cis-platinum. Cancer 48: 223-226

Otto HF (1978) Klinisch-pathologische Studie zur Klassifikation und Prognose von 57 Thymus Tumoren. II. Prognostische Kriterien. Z Krebsforsch 91: 103-115

Penn CRH, Hope-Stone HF (1972) The role of radiotherapy in the management of malignant thymoma. Br J Surg 59: 533-539

Posner JB, Howieson J, Cvitkovic E (1977) "Disappearing" spinal cord compression: oncolytic effect of glucocorticoids (and other chemotherapeutic agents) on epidural metastases. Ann Neurol 2: 409-413

Shellito J, Khandekar JD, McKeever WP, Vick NA (1978) Invasive thymoma responsive to oral corticosteroids. Cancer Treat Rep 62: 1397-1400

Shetty MR, Arora RK (1981) Invasive thymoma treated with cis-platin. Cancer Treat Rep 65: 531

Slater G, Papatestas AE, Genkins G, Kornfeld P, Horowitz SH, Bender A (1978) Thymomas in patients with myasthenia gravis. Ann Surg 188: 171-174

Soffer LJ, Gabrilove JL, Wolf BS (1952) Effect of ACTH on thymic masses. J Clin Endocrinol Metab 12: 690-696

Talley RW, O'Bryan RM, Gutterman JU, Brownlee RW, McCredie KB (1973) Clinical evaluation of toxic effects cis-diamminedichloroplatinum (NSC-119875) - phase I clinical study. Cancer Chemother Rep 57: 465-471

Thomas J, De Wolf-Peeters C, Tricot G, Bekaert J, Broeckaert-Van Orshoven A (1983) T-cell chronic lymphocytic leukemia in a patient with invasive thymoma in remission with chemotherapy. Cancer 52: 313-317

Uematsu M, Kondo M (1986) A proposal for treatment of invasive thymoma. Cancer 58: 1979-1984

Wilkins EW Jr, Edmunds LH Jr, Castleman B (1966) Cases of thymoma at the Massachusetts General Hospital. J Thorac Cardiovasc Surg 52: 322-330

28 Radiotherapy of Thymic Tumors

W. John Simpson

Introduction

Benign or invasive malignant thymomas constitute the majority of tumours which arise in the thymus gland, but squamous and undifferentiated cancers, carcinoid and other tumours may also develop in thymic tissue. The principles of management and the indications for radiotherapy are the same for the latter tumour types as when they occur at other sites. Accordingly, this chapter will focus on the role of radiotherapy in managing differentiated thymomas. The discussion excludes undifferentiated or anaplastic tumours (thymic carcinomas) which exhibit a more aggressive behaviour and a poorer response to therapy than thymomas.

Indications for Radiotherapy

There is no need for adjuvant treatment of small (less than 5 cm diameter) thymomas which exhibit no extracapsular invasion and are totally excised. However, larger noninvasive tumours may have a greater likelihood of recurring locally (Lewis et al. 1987), which irradiation may reduce or prevent (Monden et al. 1985). In our experience, local recurrence frequently results in a fatal outcome, although this may not be apparent for many years. Monden et al. (1985) reported a similar outcome with 20 of 24 patients with recurrent or persistent thymoma dead of this tumour.

Extracapsular tumour invasion is a much stronger indication for adjuvant therapy. The addition of preoperative or postoperative radiotherapy reduces the frequency of local recurrence when the tumour has invaded the adjacent fat and connective tissue (Weissberg et al. 1973; Monden et al. 1985). When the thymoma invades pleura, pericardium, aorta, etc., the need for adjuvant treatment is clear (Batata et al. 1974; Monden et al. 1985), even when a grossly total excision has been achieved. In this situation, the presence of microscopic residual disease is shown by tumour at, or within several millimetres of a resection margin in many patients. Of 33 Princess Margaret Hospital (PMH) patients with extensively invasive (stage III) thymomas, 26 were found to have residual microscopic disease following grossly total resections. In the PMH patients with no residual disease histologically, the frequency of local recurrence was higher than in patients who undergo total excision of stage II thymomas (Table 1 indicates the staging used in our analyses). Bergh et al. (1978) reported pleural spread at surgery in eight of eleven stage III patients.

Table 1. Staging system for thymomas used in the analysis of PMH patients (After Masaoka et al. 1981)

Stage I	Encapsulated, noninvasive tumour
Stage II	Localized invasion (into mediastinal fat and connective tissue)
Stage III	Extensive invasion (into mediastinal pleura, pericardium, blood vessels, nerves or adjacent lung)
Stage IV	a) Distant pleural metastases. b) Extrathoracic metastases or discrete lung metastases (not invasion from pleura)

The optimum management of unresectable invasive thymomas is controversial. In the past, unresectability was determined at surgical exploration, or by the presence of superior vena caval obstruction, etc. Computerized tomography (CT) and magnetic resonance imaging (MRI) provide more reliable information than previous radiological studies, but still cannot differentiate with certainty the loss of tissue planes due to dense adherence of the fibrotic capsule to pleura, pericardium or great vessels from that due to tumour invasion of these structures (Stark 1987). Accordingly, patients with thymomas of borderline resectability may be advised to undergo surgical exploration in the hope of achieving a total resection, or at least debulking the tumour to facilitate subsequent treatment.

An alternative approach to the management of patients with unresectable or borderline tumours is to advise initial treatment with radiotherapy and/or chemotherapy. When chemotherapy is indicated, it is given first, with the intention of reducing tumour bulk prior to the administration of radiotherapy, thereby reducing significantly the volume of lung parenchyma irradiated. We recommend C-MOPP (cyclophosphamide, vincristine (Oncovin), procarbazine and prednisone) because this regimen is less toxic, particularly to the heart, than those containing doxorubicin or cisplatin. Three cycles are given before radiotherapy is initiated, provided that some shrinkage of the tumour occurs after the first cycle.

If complete disappearance of the thymoma occurs after three cycles of chemotherapy, we believe that surgical exploration is contraindicated, but radiotherapy should be given to consolidate the remission, with a dose appropriate for the management of microscopic disease. A partial response is more often observed, requiring the delivery of a higher radiation dose. A month after completing the radiotherapy, patients are reassessed with a view to surgical excision, if that is now feasible. Again, surgical exploration is unnecessary if CT scanning shows complete disappearance of the thymoma.

Prognostic Factors

Wilkins et al. (1966), Batata et al. (1974), Verley and Hollmann (1985), Lewis et al. (1987), and others have suggested that tumour size, histological subtype, etc., are of prognostic significance for thymoma patients. However, multivariate analysis of age at diagnosis, sex, tumour size, histological subtype and stage in 93 PMH patients with differentiated thymomas showed that only stage (Table 1) was an independent prognostic factor for cause-specific survival. Tumours with no extracapsular invasion or invasion limited to adjacent fat and connective tissue had a significantly greater 10-year cause-specific survival rate (over 90%) than those with tumours invading pericardium, pleura or great vessels, or with distant pleural deposits (approximately 75% 10-year cause-specific survival).

When postoperative status was added to this multivariate analysis, it became the only independent variable, with 10-year cause-specific survival rates of 100% for patients with no residual disease, 88% for those with microscopic residual disease, but only 40% for patients with gross residual disease or unresectable tumours (Fig. 1). Cohen et al. (1984) and others have arrived at the same conclusion based on overall survival rates. Nevertheless, prognostic factors by univariate analysis (diameter greater than 5 cm, extent of extracapsular invasion, predominantly epithelial histology) should be considered when the need for adjuvant treatment is under discussion.

Radiotherapy Techniques

The simplest technique is an anterior-posterior parallel pair of treatment portals encompassing the entire mediastinum (Figs. 2 and 3). Because of the propensity for transcoelomic spread of thymomas, it is important to include the entire pericardium in the target volume. This technique is suitable for patients with known or suspected microscopic postoperative disease, including those with stage III disease thought to have had a total excision. High energy radiation (18-25 MV) is preferred in order not to exceed spinal cord tolerance. If 4-6 MV X-rays or 60 Co radiation is used, a posterior spinal cord shield should be in place for several treatments if the anteroposterior separation exceeds 16 cm. We prescribe a tumour dose of 4000 cGy/20 fractions/4 weeks, although others suggest higher doses (Arriagada et al. 1984; Uematsu and Kondo

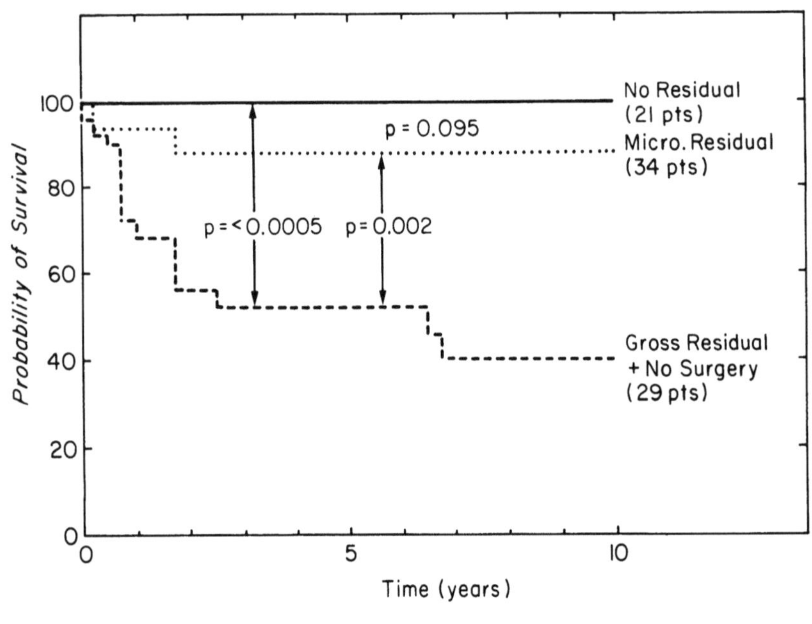

Fig. 1. Influence of postoperative status on cause-specific survival of patients with differentiated thymoma

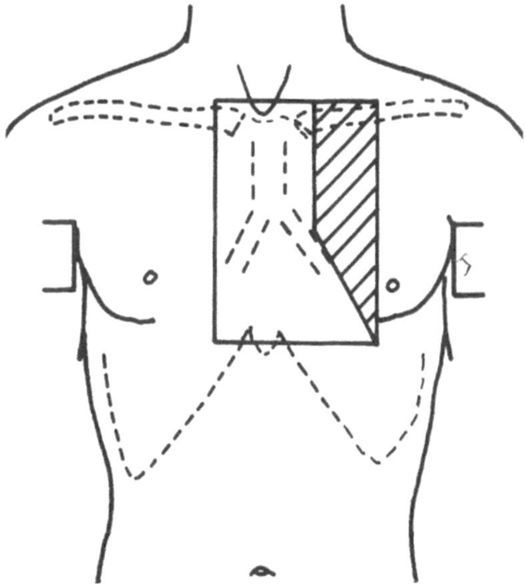

Fig. 2. Radiotherapy technique for anterior and posterior portals, which may be augmented by the addition of right and left lateral portals to provide a "boost" dose

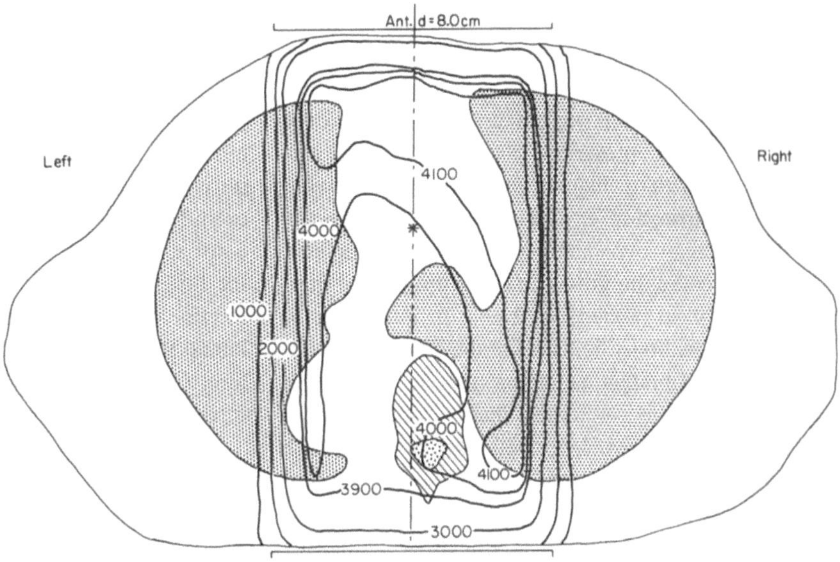

Fig. 3. Isodose curves for anterior and posterior portals; high energy radiation, suitable for treating patients with microscopic residual disease

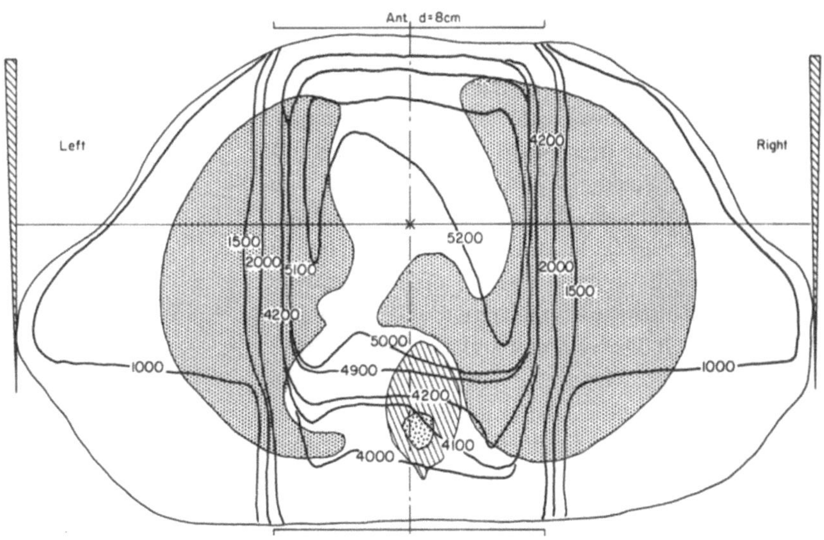

Fig. 4. Isodose curves for anterior and posterior portals (as in Fig. 3) supplemented by small lateral portals to encompass gross disease, with a small margin. Note that neither spinal cord nor lung tolerance is exceeded

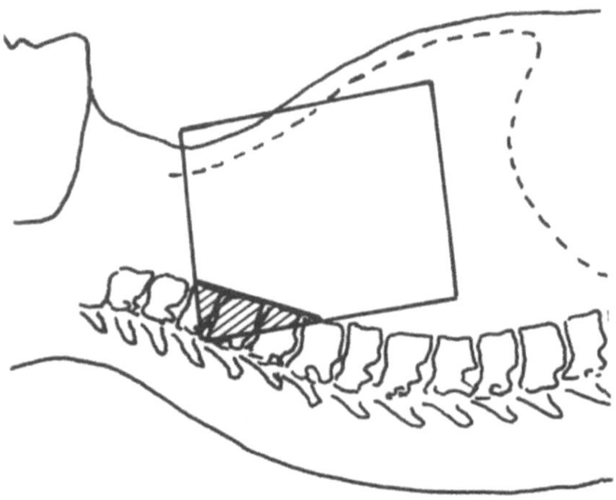

Fig. 5. Depending upon the spinal curvature in the lateral treatment portals, shielding may be necessary to prevent excessive radiation doses to the spinal cord

1986, etc). Our results, and those reported by many others, do not confirm better results with higher tumour doses.

When gross disease is present, a higher tumour dose is required. We prescribe 5000 cGy/20 fractions/4 weeks, although a higher total dose was recommended by Arriagada et al. (1984). This can be obtained by adding two lateral portals of smaller size, designed to cover the gross tumour with a small margin of uninvolved tissue (Figs. 2 and 4). The posterior borders of these boost fields are at the anterior surface of the vertebral bodies. Shielding may be required to achieve this (Fig. 5). The main tumour dose (4000 cGy/20 fractions/4 weeks) is delivered through the anterior and posterior portals; the boost (1000 cGy/10 fractions) is delivered *concurrently* through the lateral portals on alternate treatment days. Thus, neither lung nor spinal cord tolerance is exceeded.

The optimum tumour dose for the control of microscopic or gross tumour in thymoma patients remains unknown. Because invasive thymomas are uncommon, there have been no prospective studies, and no single institution has treated a large number of patients within one or two decades. However, there are many case reports in the medical literature in which complete tumour regression of gross disease, often permanent, was observed after the administration of doses ranging from 3500 to 7000 cGy (Penn and Hope-Stone 1972; Batata et al. 1974; Marks et al. 1978; Ariaratnam et al. 1979; Chahinian et al. 1981; McCrea and Maslor 1982; Stoll et al. 1984; Kersh et al. 1985), but the same reports include failures throughout the same dose ranges, including local mediastinal recurrences after tumour doses exceeding 5000 cGy and failure to achieve complete regression of gross tumour with tumour doses as high as 5800 cGy (Arriagada et al. 1984).

Unfortunately, almost all of these reports are impossible to relate to the management of differentiated thymomas because of the use of overall survival rates rather than cause-specific rates, or the inclusion of undifferentiated thymic cancers which have a much worse prognosis than the differentiated thymomas which require a totally different approach to treatment and prognosis. For these reasons, our recommendations for radiation doses of 4000 cGy in 20 fractions for patients with microscopic tumour, or 5000 cGy in 20 fractions for those with gross disease, are proposed in order to achieve maximum tumour response with minimum morbidity. A lower dose may be desirable if chemotherapy is given concurrently or sequentially.

More controversial is the practice of irradiating a hemithorax when pleural invasion has occurred, in the hope of preventing the pleural spread of the thymoma. Although we have used this technique frequently, and others have recommended it (Weissberg et al. 1973; Ariaratnam et al. 1979; Uematsu and Kondo 1986), its efficacy is not proven and it may result in serious complications. If this approach is implemented, the anterior and posterior portals are enlarged and a lung attenuator is used (Fig. 6) to decrease the radiation dose to the lungs to the appropriate level. Note the very low inferior margins required to include the medial and lateral insertions of the diaphragmatic pleura. A planning CT is desirable for the four-field technique descried earlier, and is essential for this technique.

The radiation dose is carried to the limits of tolerance - a lung dose corrected for tissue density of

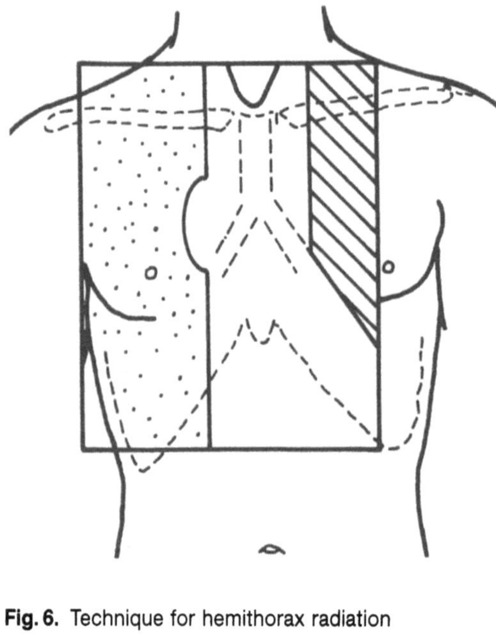

Fig. 6. Technique for hemithorax radiation

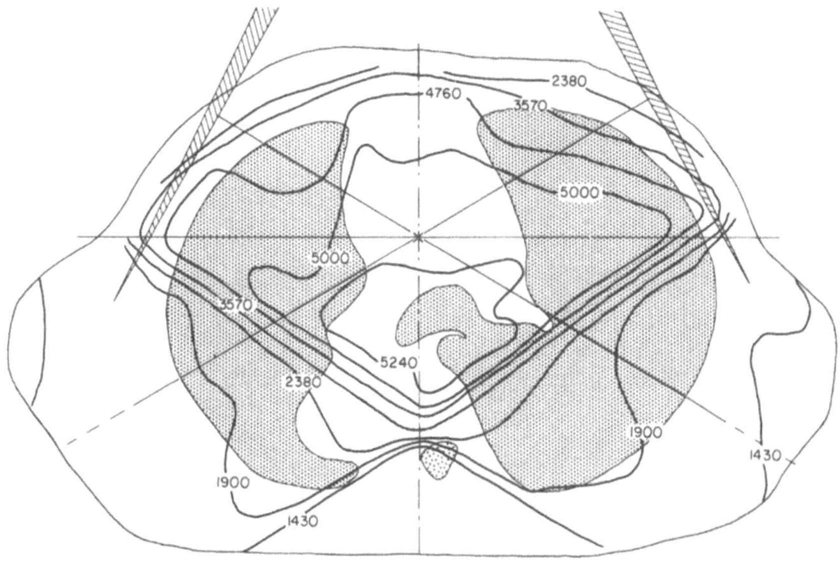

Fig. 7. Isodose curves for an anterior wedged pair of portals to treat the entire mediastinum illustrate the excessive radiation dose to almost all of the lung parenchyma

1800 cGy/20 fractions/4 weeks in patients with healthy lungs, but lower in those also treated by chemotherapy or who suffer from chronic obstructive lung disease, diabetes mellitus, etc. When one pleural deposit is detected on CT scanning, a boost dose of electrons should be given concurrently through a small portal, bringing the total dose to the deposit to 5000 cGy/20 fractions/4 weeks. If there are more than one gross pleural deposits, surgical excision should be recommended for the risk of fatal radiation pneumonitis is very high when several deposits are irradiated to a high dose. Batata et al. (1974) suggested the use of intrapleural radioactive phosphorus, but this would be appropriate only for patients without nodular pleural deposits or pleural adhesions.

Finally, we do not recommend the technique which uses an anterior wedged pair of oblique portals (Penn and Hope-Stone 1972; Mantell 1986). As shown in Fig. 7, this technique results in a much larger volume of lung tissue being irradiated to doses which exceed lung tolerance, leading to radiation pneumonitis and pulmonary fibrosis, which could prove to be fatal.

Complications

Acute

Acute complications include fatigue, oesophagitis and tracheitis. Fatigue usually develops in the last 1-2 weeks of treatment and clears rapidly after the completion of therapy. Infrequently, it is profound and persists for several months. Dysphagia due to radiation oesophagitis occurs during the last 2 weeks of treatment, subsiding promptly thereafter, and is usually accompanied by anorexia of moderate degree. Most patients tolerate a bland, soft diet with the aid of mild analgesics such as aspirin chewing gum. Rarely is the dysphagia so severe that hospitalization and intravenous fluids are required. Tracheitis follows a similar time sequence and patients may require a soothing cough syrup. Tracheitis predisposes patients to bacterial and fungal infections which must be treated promptly with antibiotic and antifungal agents. Nausea and vomiting are usually absent or mild, and readily managed by standard antiemetic drugs.

Delayed

Delayed complications may involve lung parenchyma, spinal cord or myocardium. Long-term oesophageal dysfunction has not been encountered following the radiation time-dose schedules described in this chapter.

Radiation pneumonitis develops within 3-6 months, involving retrocardiac lung parenchyma. It is usually asymptomatic and requires no treatment. When larger volumes of lung are irradiated to high doses, the pneumonitis and subsequent fibrosis may cause unproductive cough and dyspnoea, and may be fatal if large volumes of lung are affected. Forty-five PMH patients were treated with hemithorax or whole thorax radiotherapy, by the technique described earlier. Two of these patients (4.4%) died of radiation pneumonitis. Both were elderly (over 70 years); one was hypertensive and the other had been treated with six cycles of chemotherapy (cyclophosphamide, vincristine, pro-

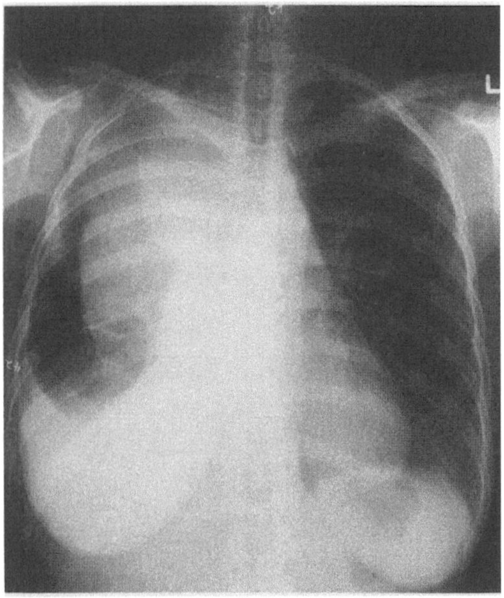

Fig. 8. Chest radiograph of a huge thymoma (predominantly lymphocytic) filling most of the right hemithorax

carbazine and prednisone). One of these was included in the three radiation-related deaths reported by Shamji et al. (1984), but the other two deaths included in that report were due to tumour and surgery-related complications (bronchopleural fistula and empyema). Treatment with steroids may be beneficial in the pneumonitis phase. Superinfections are common and require prompt treatment with antibiotics. This situation is encountered when a large unresectable thymoma, which fails to respond to chemotherapy, extends far into the pleural cavity, making it impossible to shield much of the lung (Fig. 8). There is little information on the lung toxicity of combined treatment with radiotherapy and chemotherapy, but it is probable that all chemotherapeutic agents except prednisone add to the radiation-induced damage (Phillips 1979). The tolerance of normal lung should be assumed to be lower, perhaps by 25%, when the two modalities are combined.

Radiation-induced spinal cord necrosis results in paraplegia and loss of bladder and bowel function. Its onset is usually within 9-18 months. Because of the devastating effects of spinal cord necrosis, it must be avoided by careful treatment planning. Here too, it must be assumed that chemotherapy adds to the toxicity, especially if a neurotoxic drug such as vincristine is part of the regimen (Byfield 1979; Goldberg et al. 1982; Cohen et al. 1983).

Cardiac damage is not usually encountered when the specified radiation schedules are employed. However, pericardial effusions have been observed in several patients with pericardial invasion by the thymoma. Myocardial radiation tolerance must be assumed to be lower when combined treatment is undertaken, particularly when the cardiotoxic drug doxorubicin is employed (Carter 1979; Phillips 1979).

Treatment Results

It is not possible to define clearly the role of external radiation in the management of thymomas for there have been no randomized prospective trials, and radiotherapy has been administered to patients believed to have poor prognostic factors or whose tumours were not resectable. Moreover, most authors have reported overall survival rates which would appear to be inappropriate because more than half the deaths of thymoma patients are due to causes unrelated to the thymomas or their treatment. Verley and Hollmann (1985) reported that only 25 of the 67 deaths in their series were due to uncontrolled tumour or treatment complications. Among the PMH patients, 27 of the 42 deaths were from unrelated causes, which included myasthenia gravis and red cell aplasia. Therefore, cause-specific survival should be used to determine the efficacy of treatment. Salyer and Eggleston (1976) stressed the need to use cause-specific survival rates. However, it is difficult, if not impossible, to obtain groups of patients with similar clinical features, but with different treatment regimens, to study the effects of those regimens.

A different approach to determine the efficacy of treatment is to examine the failure patterns of the various treatment groups. Of the 93 PMH patients with differentiated thymomas, followed for 4-24 years, 11 were treated initially by surgery alone; 8 were stage I (noninvasive) tumours. Four of them recurred locally in the mediastinum and a fifth patient relapsed simultaneously in the mediastinum and at a distant site. Fifty-nine patients were treated by total excision and preoperative or postoperative radiotherapy; 14 were stage I thymomas, but over half (33) had stage III disease. Of the 14 stage I patients, there were two recurrences, one in the mediastinum (a 19 cm mixed lymphocytic-epithelial thymoma with preoperative radiotherapy) and the other concurrently in the mediastinum and in bone in a patient with a 10 cm epithelial thymoma. In the 45 stage II and III patients, there were two mediastinal recurrences and two concurrent mediastinal and distant sites. Six patients were treated preoperatively with chemotherapy and radiotherapy; one patient was found to have no invasion beyond the capsule at the time of surgery. One of these patients suffered recurrence in the mediastinum subsequently.

These groups are not comparable. In particular, several of the "surgery only" patients were referred at the time of relapse and undoubtedly many other "surgery only" patients were never referred because they did not relapse, as reported by Maggi et al. (1986). Nevertheless, the results in the surgery plus radiotherapy patients suggest that radiotherapy was of some benefit, as claimed by Monden et al. (1985).

The response of gross tumour is easier to assess. Five PMH patients had residual gross disease following subtotal resection of extensive thymomas. Three of four patients treated with radiotherapy achieved complete responses. The fourth patient and the patient treated with both chemotherapy and radiotherapy showed partial responses. Of 23 PMH patients with unresectable thymomas, 15 achieved a complete response following radiotherapy. Chemotherapy was also used in five of these patients, and two others underwent post-radiation surgery with grossly total tumour resections. Only 2 of the 23 patients failed to show considerable tumour regression. Six patients were irradiated for recurrent thymoma. Five achieved complete remission of the tumour; chemotherapy was used in one of these and another underwent post-radiation surgery.

These results indicate that the majority of thymomas respond to external radiation and that gross tumour can be eradicated frequently, sometimes with the help of chemotherapy or post-radiation surgery. Similar results have been reported by Wilkins et al. (1966), Batata et al. (1974), Marks et al. (1978), Ariaratnam et al. (1979), Chahinian et al. (1981), Appelqvist et al. (1982), Arriagada et al. (1984), Stoll et al. (1984), Kersh et al. (1985), Uematsu and Kondo (1986) and others.

References

Appelqvist P, Kostiainen S, Franssila K, Matilla S, Gröhn P (1982) Treatment and prognosis of thymoma: a review of 25 cases. J Surg Oncol 20: 265-268

Ariaratnam LS, Kalnicki S, Mincer F, Botstein C (1979) The management of malignant thymoma with radiation therapy. Int J Radiat Oncol Biol Phys 5: 77-80

Arriagada R, Bretel JJ, Cailaud JM, Garetta L, Guerin RA, Laugier A, Le Chevalier T, Schlienger M (1984) Invasive carcinoma of the thymus. A multicenter retrospective review of 56 cases. Eur J Cancer Clin Oncol 20: 69-74

Batata MA, Martini N, Huvos AG, Aguilar RI, Beattie EJ (1974) Thymomas: clinicopathologic features, therapy, and prognosis. Cancer 34: 389-396

Bergh NP, Gatzinsky P, Larsson S, Lundin P, Ridell B (1978) Tumors of the thymus and thymic region. I. Clinicopathological studies on thymomas. Ann Thorac Surg 25: 91-98

Byfield JE (1979) Central nervous system toxicities from combined therapies. In: Vaeth JM (ed) Combined effects of chemotherapy and radiotherapy on normal tissue tolerance. Karger, Basel, pp 228-240

Carter SK (1979) Perspectives on combined modality treatment with emphasis on radiation therapy and chemotherapy. In: Vaeth JM (ed) Combined effects of chemotherapy and radiotherapy on normal tissue tolerance. Karger, Basel, pp 1-5

Chahinian AP, Bhardwaj S, Meyer RJ, Jaffrey IS, Kirschner PA, Holland JF (1981) Treatment of invasive or metastatic thymoma: report of eleven cases. Cancer 47: 1752-1761

Cohen DJ, Ronnigen LD, Graeber GM, Deshong SJL, Jaffin J, Burge JR, Zajtchuk R (1984) Management of patients with malignant thymoma. J Thorac Cardiovasc Surg 87: 301-307

Cohen ME, Duffner PK, Terplan KL (1983) Myelopathy with severe structural derangement associated with combined modality therapy. Cancer 52: 1590-1596

Goldberg ID, Bloomer WD, Dawson DM (1982) Nervous system toxic effects of cancer therapy. JAMA 247: 1437-1441

Kersh CR, Eisert DR, Hazra TA (1985) Malignant thymoma: role of radiation therapy in management. Radiology 156: 207-209.

Lewis JE, Wick MR, Scheithauer BW, Bernatz PE, Tylor WF (1987) Thymoma. A clinicopathologic review. Cancer 60: 2727-2743

Maggi G, Giaccone G, Donadio M, Ciuffreda L, Dalesio O, Leria G, Trifiletti G, Casadio C, Palestro G, Mancuso M, Calciati A (1986) Thymomas. A review of 169 cases, with particular reference to results of surgical treatment. Cancer 58: 765-776

Mantell BS (1986) Thymic tumours. In: Hope-Stone HF (ed) Radiotherapy in clinical practice. Butterworth, London, pp 170-173

Masaoka A, Monden Y, Nakahara K, Tanioka T (1981) Follow-up study of thymomas with special reference to their clinical stages. Cancer 48: 2485-2492

Marks RD, Wallace KM, Pettit HS (1978) Radiation therapy control of nine patients with malignant thymoma. Cancer 41: 117-119

McCrea ES, Maslar JA (1982) Thymoma with distant intrathoracic implants, with CT confirmation. Cancer 50: 1612-1614

Monden Y, Nakahara K, Iioka S, Nanjo S, Ohno K, Fujii Y, Hashimoto J, Kitagawa Y, Masaoka A, Kawashima Y (1985) Recurrence of thymoma: clinicopathological features, therapy and prognosis. Ann Thorac Surg 39: 165-169

Penn CRH, Hope-Stone HF (1972) The role of radiotherapy in the management of malignant thymoma. Br J Surg 59: 533-539

Phillips TL (1979) Small animal model systems for testing combined modality treatment effects on normal tissue. In: Vaeth JM (ed) Combined effects of chemotherapy and radiotherapy on normal tissue tolerance. Karger, Basel, pp 6-8

Salyer WR, Eggleston JC (1976) Thymoma. A clinical and pathological study of 65 cases. Cancer 37: 229-249

Shamji F, Pearson FG, Todd TRJ, Ginsberg RI, Ilves R, Cooper JD (1984) Results of surgical treatment of thymoma. J Thorac Cardiovasc Surg 87: 43-47

Stark P (1987) Imaging mediastinal tumors. CA 37: 211-224

Stoll DB, Lublin F, Brodovsky H, Laucius JF, Patchefsky A, Cooper H (1984) Association of subacute neuronopathy with thymoma. Cancer 54: 770-772

Uematsu M, Kondo M (1986) A proposal for treatment of invasive thymoma. Cancer 58: 1979-1984

Verley JM, Hollmann KH (1985) Thymoma. A comparative study of clinical stages, histologic features, and survival in 200 cases. Cancer 55: 1074-1086

Weissberg D, Goldberg M, Pearson FG (1973) Thymoma. Ann Thorac Surg 16: 141-147

Wilkins EW, Edmunds LH Jr, Castleman B (1966) Cases of thymoma at the Massachusetts General Hospital. J Thorac Cardiovasc Surg 52: 322-330

29 Treatment of Myasthenia Gravis After Thymectomy

Pierre-Antoine Uldry and Franco Regli

The principal drugs used for the treatment of myasthenia gravis (MG) are presented in Chap. 12. We consider here the practical treatment of patients in the weeks and months following thymectomy.

General Considerations

There are no universally accepted criteria for the timing and sequence of therapy in MG but three principles are now recognized (Drachman 1987; Rowland 1980):

1. Anticholinesterase drugs are useful in all clinical forms of the disease; particularly, they are the mainstay in ocular MG.
2. Immunosuppressants increase the frequency of remissions, but have some detrimental side effects.
3. Plasma exchange has only transient effects and does not confer greater long-term protection than do immunosuppressants alone.

Treatment After Thymectomy

Retrospective comparison of thymectomy and medical treatment has clearly demonstrated the benefits of surgery, even in MG with purely ocular symptoms. The pooled results of several large series suggest a remission rate of about 25% marked improvement in 45% and no effect in the remaining 30% (Papatestas et al. 1987; Scadding et al. 1985; Schumm et al. 1985). After surgery, signs of improvement can be noted as early as the first day or week, but it would seem that several months is the usual time it takes to appreciate the full benefit of thymectomy.

After thymectomy, remission of symptoms or substantial improvement allows a reduction in dosage with the aim of stopping the treatment or defining the effective minimal dose. However, general rules cannot be established because every patient has an individual course of myasthenia and therefore needs individually tailored therapy (Oosterhuis 1981; Newsom-Davis 1986):

- In patients with only anticholinesterase therapy before thymectomy, the drugs are given in the lowest possible dose, and the treatment can be tapered and withdrawn in the days following surgery in individuals who respond well. However, a certain proportion of patients require higher doses after surgery. This requirement can be transient, but is unfortunately permanent in some.
- In patients treated with corticosteroids, prednisone can be reduced quickly if azathioprine is given simultaneously. It is rarely necessary to give steroids for more than 4 to 6 weeks after thymectomy. Azathioprine is then gradually discontinued (by 2.5 mg every 3 months).
- If symptoms recur, treatment (anticholinesterase drugs and prednisone, then azathioprine) should be immediately reintroduced and the dose increased until control is reestablished. A further trial of drug reduction should be attempted after 1-3 months. Remission after thymectomy can occur up to 1-3 years after surgery, so repeated trials of drug reduction are warranted.
- If the patient does not improve after thymectomy and anticholinesterases are insufficient, prednisone is added first, and if there is still no improvement or there are important side effects, azathioprine is introduced.

Anticholinesterase drugs, corticosteroids, noncorticosteroid immunosuppressants and plasma exchange all remain acceptable forms of therapy for patients with MG after surgery.

Anticholinesterases

Cholinesterase inhibitors (pyridostigmine, neostigmine ambenonium) are the mainstay of symptomatic treatment for MG, and act by inhibiting the enzyme cholinesterase which normally hydrolyses acetylcholine at the neuromuscular junction. Pyridostigmine is preferred because of its longer action. There is still no way to determine the optimal dosage of anticholinesterases except by a trial that depends upon the patient's individual response (Davison et al. 1981; White et al. 1981; Aquilonius et al. 1983).

With pyridostigmine, a dosage of 60-120 mg per day is necessary at the beginning; the maintenance dose is 300-400 mg/day. The oral dose of neostigmine ranges from 7.5 to 45 mg, given every 2-6 h; the average maintenance dose is approximately 100 mg/day.

Corticosteroids

Notable clinical improvement induced by prednisone correlates with a decrease in antibody titer, which usually occurs over 3-6 months, and is observed in over 70% of patients. Because exacerbation of symptoms may occur during induction of treatment, patients with appreciable weakness will often require hospitalization. Increasing the dose in 10-mg steps from a low initial value, with alternate-day treatment, reduces side effects and the risk of initial deterioration (Johns 1987; Pascuzzi et al. 1984; Sghirlanzoni et al. 1984).

The indications for corticosteroid treatment are:

A. With thymectomy

- Before surgery: respiratory weakness.
- Soon after thymectomy: life-threatening complications
- Later after surgery (3 to 6 months): incapacitating or life-threatening complications

B. As an alternative to thymectomy when surgery is contraindicated

The efficacy of alternate-day prednisone therapy is now well recognized. A single dose of 100 mg prednisone every second day, like 50 mg daily, gives good results in most cases, even if some patients require a small dose (5-10 mg) on the "off" day. Conversely, a lower alternate-day or daily dose is often sufficient.

Nonsteroid Immunosuppressive Drugs

Because of the delayed response to azathioprine compared with prednisone, it has been suggested that initial treatment with both immunosuppressants and corticosteroids should be employed. The prednisone dose can then be reduced slowly and eventually discontinued once azathioprine has become effective. However, a few individuals require concomitant steroid therapy for longer than 6 months.

Azathioprine

Azathioprine appears to be a reasonable choice for long-term therapy in many patients who have failed to respond satisfactorily to prednisone and in those who have relapsed following prednisone and plasma exchange therapy (Howard 1982a; Witte et al. 1984; Hohlfeld et al. 1988; Michels et al. 1988).

A dosage of 1.5-2.5 mg/kg per day gives good results in most patients. Improvement is gradual, usually beginning after 2-6 months with maximal response within 1 year. Improvement seems to occur earlier in patients whose disease is of shorter duration. The development of macrocytosis is a good indicator of therapeutic effect. The improvement tends to persist for as long as the drug is continued. Relapses rarely occur in patients on a fixed dose who have previously achieved a state of improvement, but may occur 2-3 months after a reduction in the dose or discontinuation of azathioprine. In a few cases (less than 10%), it has been possible to discontinue the drug for periods of up to 3.5 years without relapse.

Cyclosporine

Cyclosporine has yielded good results in clinical trials involving heart, kidney and liver transplantation. Recent studies have shown that cyclosporine is probably a useful drug in some cases of MG, especially for the visual and bulbar symptoms (Nyberg-Hansen and Gjerstad 1988; Tindall et al. 1987). The efficacy of cyclosporine treatment has been demonstrated both by decrease muscle of weakness, and by improvement in the titer of circulating acetylcholine receptor antibodies. The effects can be seen as early as 4 weeks after the initiation of treatment.

The maintenance dosage should be kept as low as possible, 5 mg/kg per day or less, but clinical efficacy has often been sustained with trough levels below 200 ng/ml. Renal function must be carefully monitored. Although cyclosporine appears to be efficacious in some patients, the ultimate role of this drug in the treatment of MG remains to be established.

Plasma Exchange

A course of plasma exchange (55 ml/kg daily for 5 days) (Newsom-Davis et al. 1979; Howard 1982b; Nielsen et al. 1982; Rodnitzky and Bosch 1984) produces an improvement which is observed 24-48 h after the first plasmapheresis but is short-lived, lasting less than 1 month. Plasma exchange is currently used in the following circumstances in patients with MG after thymectomy:

- In myasthenic crisis
- In rapidly progressive MG, especially with uncontrolled bulbar or respiratory muscle compromise

- To avoid the use of corticosteroids in cases with relative contraindications for these drugs until the effect of thymectomy is seen
- To decrease the level of corticosteroids in those who do not tolerate the levels of corticosteroids required, or during the tapering off of corticosteroids if sudden and severe worsening occurs
- In patients with severe disease refractory to all other modalities
- In pregnancy when there is exacerbation of myasthenic symptoms (Levine and Keesey 1986)

The improvement in the clinical status is corroborated by a 70% reduction in the antiacetylcholine receptor levels after plasmapheresis. However, there is no correlation between the percentage of reduction in titer after plasma exchange and the maximal clinical response. In view of the risks of intensive daily immunosuppression, continuation of intermittent plasma exchange can be an interesting alternative provided the interval between exchanges is relatively long. Rodnitzky and Bosch (1984) reported two exchange-dependent patients in whom plasma exchange had been used for 5 years to control symptoms. In both patients, who also received azathioprine, the interval between exchanges gradually lengthened to 9 and 12 weeks over 2 and 3 years respectively, without the introduction of new immunosuppressants. However, the long-term response was no better than that produced by medication alone.

Episodes of acute myasthenic weakness have occurred during plasma exchange in some patients, presumably owing to the abrupt withdrawal of circulating cholinesterase inhibitors. However, acute cholinergic weakness of varying severity has also been reported in patients continuing to receive cholinesterase inhibitors during plasma exchange.

Other Treatments

Antilymphocyte and antithymocyte globulin infusions, gammaglobulin injections, mediastinal, splenic and total body irradiation and thoracic duct drainage have been reported to be of benefit in the management of myasthenic patients not responding to other therapy (Howard 1982a; Engel 1984; Drachman 1987). However, these treatment modalities are still regarded as experimental.

References

Aquilonius SM, Eckernäs SA, Hartvig P, Lindström B, Osterman PO, Stalberg E (1983) Clinical pharmacology of pyridostigmine and neostigmine in patients with myasthenia gravis. J Neurol Neurosurg Psychiatry 46: 929-935

Davison SC, Hyman NM, Dehghan A, Chan K (1981) The relationship of plasma levels of pyridostigmine to clinical effect in patients with myasthenia gravis. J Neurol Neurosurg Psychiatry 44: 1141-1145

Drachman DB (1987) Present and future treatment of myasthenia gravis. N Engl J Med 316: 743-745

Engel AG (1984) Myasthenia gravis and myasthenic syndromes. Ann Neurol 16: 519-534

Hohlfeld R, Michels M, Heininger K, Besinger U, Toyka KV (1988) Azathioprine toxicity during long-term immunosuppression of generalized myasthenia gravis. Neurology 38: 258-261

Howard JF Jr (1982a) Nonsteroidal immunosuppressive therapy for myasthenia gravis. Semin Neurol 2: 265-269

Howard JF Jr (1982b) Treatment of myasthenia gravis with plasma exchange. Semin Neurol 2: 273-279

Johns TR (1987) Long-term corticosteroid treatment of myasthenia gravis. Ann NY Acad Sci 505: 568-583

Levine SE, Keesey JC (1986) Successful plasmapheresis for fulminant myasthenia gravis during pregnancy. Arch Neurol 43: 197-198

Michels M, Hohlfeld R, Hartung HP, Heininger K, Besinger UA, Toyka KV (1988) Myasthenia gravis: discontinuation of long-term azathioprine. Ann Neurol 24: 798 (letter)

Newsom-Davis J (1986) Diseases of the neuromuscular junction. In: Asbury AK, McKhann GM, McDonald WI (eds) Diseases of the nervous system, vol 1. Heinemann Medical, London, pp 269-282

Newsom-Davis J, Wilson SG, Vincent A, Ward CD (1979) Long-term effects of repeated plasma exchange in myasthenia gravis. Lancet 1: 464-468

Nielsen VK, Paulson OB, Rosenkvist J, Holsoe E, Lefvert AK (1982) Rapid improvement of myasthenia gravis after plasma exchange. Ann Neurol 11: 160-169

Nyberg-Hansen R, Gjerstad L (1988) Myasthenia gravis treated with cyclosporin. Acta Neurol Scand 77: 307-313

Oosterhuis HJ (1981) Observations of the natural history of myasthenia gravis and the effect of thymectomy. Ann NY Acad Sci 377: 678-690

Papatestas AE, Genkins G, Kornfeld P, Eisenkraft JB, Fagerstrom RP, Pozner J, Aufses AH Jr (1987) Effects of thymectomy in myasthenia gravis. Ann Surg 206: 79-88

Pascuzzi RM, Coslett HB, Johns TR (1984) Long-term corticosteroid treatment of myasthenia gravis: report of 116 patients. Ann Neurol 15: 291-298

Rodnitzky RL, Bosch EP (1984) Chronic long-interval plasma exchange in myasthenia gravis. Arch Neurol 41: 715-717

Rowland LP (1980) Controversies about the treatment of myasthenia gravis. J Neurol Neurosurg Psychiatry 43: 644-659

Scadding GK, Havard CWH, Lange MJ, Domb I (1985) The long term experience of thymectomy for myasthenia gravis. J Neurol Neurosurg Psychiatry 48: 401-406

Schumm F, Wiethölter H, Fateh-Moghadam A, Dichgans J (1985) Thymectomy in myasthenia with pure ocular symptoms. J Neurol Neurosurg Psychiatry 48: 332-337

Sghirlanzoni A, Peluchetti D, Mantegazza R, Fiacchino F, Cornelio F (1984) Myasthenia gravis: prolonged treatment with steroids. Neurology 34: 170-174

Tindall RSA, Rollins JA, Phillips JT, Greenlee RG, Wells L, Belendiuk G (1987) Preliminary results of a double-blind, randomized, placebo-controlled trial of cyclosporine in myasthenia gravis. N Engl J Med 316: 719-724

White MC, De Silva P, Havard CWH (1981) Plasma pyridostigmine levels in myasthenia gravis. Neurology 31: 145-150

Witte AS, Cornblath DR, Parry GJ, Lisak RP, Schatz WNJ (1984) Azathioprine in the treatment of myasthenia gravis. Ann Neurol 15: 602-605

Part VII

Post-Thymectomy Evolution

30 Value of Thymectomy for Myasthenia Gravis

Philippe Levasseur and Henri Le Brigand*

Introduction

Although the beneficial effect of thymectomy on myasthenia gravis (MG) has been proven with good immunologic arguments, this fact has not always been sufficiently clear. Many years have now elapsed since the time when Blalock pioneered thymic resection for MG (Blalock et al. 1939, 1941; Blalock 1944), and subsequently many other authors contributed in establishing the role of thymectomy in the treatment of MG (Keynes 1946, 1949; Eaton and Clagett 1955; Simpson 1958, 1960; Viets and Schwab 1960). Since then, many series have shown the superiority of early surgical treatment in comparison with long-term medical therapy and, with the tremendous decrease in operative mortality, even the most hesitant neurologists have been convinced.

Indication, Timing, and Preparation for Thymectomy

The timing of the procedure is not yet standardized and still varies from one center to another. When the presence of a thymoma is certain or suspected, thymectomy should be performed as soon as possible. For generalized MG without suspicion of a thymic tumor, it is admitted that in most cases thymectomy ought to be carried out without delay on the condition that the patient is stabilized with anticholinesterase drugs for this seems to give the best long-term results (Maggi et al. 1982; Mulder et al. 1983; Otto and Strugalska 1987; Papatestas et al. 1987). In our center, surgery is recommended for patients with MG after 6 months of evolution, even if they are responding well to anticholinesterase treatment. We also perform thymectomy in patients with isolated ocular symptoms although Osserman's class I MG is known not to respond as well to surgical treatment; the good results obtained in our recent cases convinced us of the benefit of early thymectomy in these patients. Papatestas et al. (1987) have also recommended this aggressive approach to purely ocular disease. Maggi et al. (1982) have also reported that this is their preferred treatment for all patients with purely ocular disease except for children and adults over 60. Patients with severe MG are prepared with three or four plasmaphereses. Immunosuppressive drugs and corticosteroids are not used preoperatively whenever possible.

Prognosis After Surgical or Medical Treatment

The first and most important comparative study between thymectomy and medical treatment was published by Perlo et al. (1966). Their follow-up was less than 5 years in 25% of survivors, 5-15 years in 50%, and over 15 years in 25%. This study showed improvement in 89% (including the 32% in remission) for thymectomized patients, whereas only 32% of those treated medically were improved. Furthermore, better results were observed following surgery in all of the subgroups with similar severity of disease.

Later, Buckingham et al. (1976) reported a randomized series with a mean follow-up of 19.5 years for the surgical patients and 23 years for the medical ones, which confirmed the better remission, improvement, and survival rates obtained with thymectomy. Papatestas et al. (1987) compared the outcome of 1100 medically treated MG patients with that of 962 patients who underwent thymectomy between 1951 and 1985. There was an overall remission rate of 21% in the surgical series as opposed to only 13% in the other. Good results of thymectomy in children with MG have been reported by Rodriguez et al. (1983) in a study with a mean follow-up of 17 years.

Operative Mortality

This was high in the early days of thymectomy, particularly between 1940 and 1950. Blalock (1944) reported a 20% mortality rate, essentially due to postoperative respiratory complications. Since the early 1960s, operative mortality has decreased to 2%-5% (Perlo et al.

* Deceased

Table 1. Operative mortality for thymectomy in myasthenia gravis

Reference	Patients	Mortality (%)
Rzepecki et al. 1980	136	2.2
Sturridge 1980	129	0
Mulder et al. 1983	249	0.8
Levasseur 1985, unpublished work	550	0.5
Maggi 1985, personal communication	500	1.6
Papatestas et al. 1987	962[a+b]	3[a]
		0[b]

[a] 302 patients before 1973, [b] 660 after 1973

1966; Cohn et al. 1974). Later on this decreasing trend continued (Austin et al. 1983). Table 1 shows the mortality rates in several large series; it is currently 0%–2%. In two large series of 962 (Papatestas et al. 1987) and 550 (Levasseur 1985, unpublished work) it is respectively 1.1% and 0.5%, and all deaths occurred before 1973 (Papatestas et al. 1987) or 1975 (Levasseur 1985).

This low operative mortality is influenced mainly by two factors:

1. Surgical approach: the reported mortality for the transcervical approach (0.4%) is lower than that for the transthoracic approach (3%) (Slater et al. 1978). Maggi (1985, personal communication) also related a significant difference: 1.4% mortality following cervicotomy, 1.3% after cervicomanubriotomy, 2.5% for total sternotomy.
2. Presence of a thymoma: in a series of 500 cases of MG, 120 with and 380 without a thymoma, Maggi (1985, personal communication) noted 4 operative deaths in each group, a mortality of respectively 3.3% and 1.05%.

However, these factors are not independent; only a small proportion (25%) of patients with a thymoma can be operated on via cervicotomy whereas 83% of non-thymomatous thymuses can be resected by this approach. Furthermore, cervicotomy patients tend to have milder disease, and thymomas are commoner in patients with severe disease of long duration (Papatestas et al. 1987). In addition a significant proportion of thymomas are invasive lesions requiring more aggressive surgical resections, which obviously adversely affects operative mortality.

Late Mortality

Late mortality varies after thymectomy from 3% (Mulder et al. 1983; Levasseur 1985, unpublished work) to 14.1% (Maggi 1985, personal communication). This divergence is explained by the difference of severity of MG in the different series, the presence or absence of a thymoma, and the length of postoperative follow-up. Papatestas et al. (1987) noted an overall mortality rate of 6% for mild disease (Osserman's classes I A or II A) and 14% for severe disease in the absence of a thymoma. When MG occurred with a thymoma these figures were respectively 23% and 47%. Furthermore, in most series it is often difficult to separate overall mortality from death due to MG, and this has an obvious influence on the figures.

Postoperative Results

The postoperative evaluation determines the following categories:

Remission: no signs or symptoms of MG with no treatment whatsoever.

Improvement: no (or slight) symptoms or signs of MG with small doses of anticholinesterases. Marked improvement: normal or slightly reduced activity under decreased doses of anticholinesterases. Moderate improvement: clinical improvement with the same doses of anticholinesterases.

Failure: no improvement of symptoms with the same doses of anticholinesterases (no change); higher doses or additional immunosuppressive treatment required.

Table 2. Results of thymectomy for myasthenia gravis

Reference	Patients	Good results (%)
Keynes 1949	200[b]	92
Perlo et al. 1966	188[b]	89[c]
Papatestas et al. 1971	111[b]	87
Cohn et al. 1974	57	73
Buckingham et al. 1976	80[b]	66
Le Brigand et al. 1980	248	79.8
Sturridge 1980	129	70
Rzepecki et al. 1981	126[b]	76
Mulder et al. 1983	249	87
Monden et al. 1984b	80	94
Maggi 1985, personal communication	500	83
Levasseur 1985, unpublished work	170	87
Otto and Strugalska 1987	317	97
Jaretzki 1988	72[b]	96
	8[d]	87.5
	15[e]	86

[a] Remission or improvement
[b] MG without thymoma
[c] Women only
[d] MG without thymoma, repeat surgery for persistent symptoms
[e] MG with thymoma

Thymectomy is generally followed by good results. Table 2 shows the postoperative remission and improvement rates in several series. A few series dealt exclusively with non-thymomatous MG and the postoperative results were very good. However, in several series good results (remission or improvement) were reported in 83%-87% of patients, even though cases of thymomatous MG were included (Mulder et al. 1983; Maggi 1985, personal communication; Levasseur 1985, unpublished work).

Remission After Thymectomy

The postoperative improvement is not immediate. Remission rates in the first month are low (8.5% at 2 weeks; Otto and Strugalska 1987). The delay before clinical improvement or remission can be very long, sometimes taking several years. Maggi (1985, personal communication) reported remission in only one-third of his patients at 7 years. For Papatestas et al. (1971) remission rates increase as follows: 26% at 3 years, 41% at 5 years, 54% at 7 years. Monden et al. (1984b) had a remission rate of around 15% at 3 months, 40% at 3 years, and 50% at 5 years. Jaretzki et al. (1988) reported remission rates of approximately 10% at 10 months, 40% at 50 months, and 85% at 90 months in a series of 72 patients with non-thymomatous MG who underwent "maximal" thymectomy. A series of 34 patients in remission (out of 248) within a 10-year period of follow-up is presented in Fig. 1; a total of 16 patients (47%) reached their remission in the first postoperative year. The other 18 (53%) passed through stages of moderate to marked improvement before achieving remission in 4,5, or more years (Le Brigand et al. 1980). Thus, the ultimate results of thymectomy occur after an extremely variable length of time in each patient (months to many years). A reasonable length of time to wait before considering the results to be definite is probably 5 years.

Table 3 shows the remission rates in several published series. The large variation of reported results is due to the different definition of the term "remission" used by the various authors: some include patients who are asymptomatic, but still require anticholinesterases. Some of the series have short follow-ups, which lowers remission rates.

Table 3. Remission after thymectomy

Reference	Remission (%)
Buckberg et al. 1967	8.3
Cohn et al. 1974	31
Buckingham et al. 1976	33
Mulder et al. 1983	51
Monden et al. 1984b	50
Maggi 1985, personal communication	29
Levasseur 1985, unpublished work	9
Otto and Strugalska 1987	12
Papatestas et al. 1987	23[a]
	17[b]
Jaretzki et al. 1988	46[a]
	12.5[c]
	13[b]

[a] MB without thymoma
[b] MG with thymoma
[c] MG without thymoma, repeat surgery for persistent symptoms

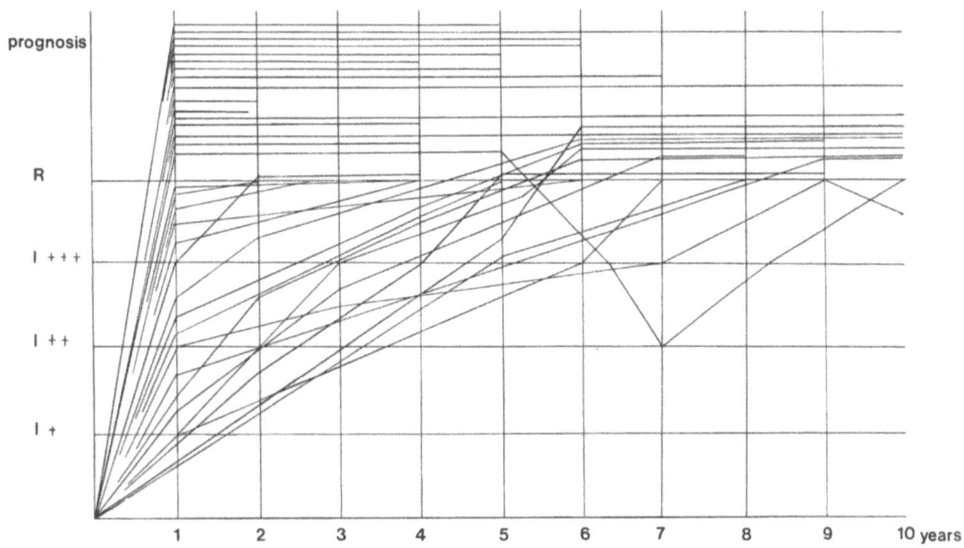

Fig. 1. Course after thymectomy in the 34/248 cases with complete remission. *R* remission; *I*+ + + very great improvement; *I*+ + great improvement; *I*+ moderate improvement

Factors Influencing the Prognosis of Thymectomy

Severity of MG

Buckberg et al. (1967) reported similar results following thymectomy for MG in patients with mild (Osserman's classes II A and II B) and severe disease (Osserman's classes III and IV): there were respectively 62% and 64% good results. Le Brigand et al. (1980) had 79% good results in mild disease and 83% good results in severe disease. Rodriguez et al. (1983) reported that by far the best results were seen in children with severe disease: 68% were in remission within 3 years, but only 28% of those without bulbar dysfunction achieved remission.

Papatestas et al. (1987) had less good results in patients with severe disease in their series of 962 patients who underwent thymectomy: 23% of patients with mild disease achieved remission, and only 17% with severe disease did so. This is attributed to two factors: patients with severe disease tended to have a longer preoperative course of MG, and thymomas were more frequent in this group - both factors adversely influence the prognosis.

Sex

It used to be reported that results were better in women (Keynes 1949; Eaton and Clagett 1955; Simpson 1958). In 1972 we reported 73% good results in women as opposed to only 55% in men (Levasseur et al. 1972). Mulder et al. (1983) also noted a better outcome in women (91% vs 75%) in their series with a mean follow-up of 7.5 years. Papatestas et al. (1987) and Jaretzki et al. (1988) did not find a significant relationship between sex and outcome in two large series with long follow-ups. This apparent discrepancy may be due to a sampling error for MG is far more frequent in women than in men.

Age

Maggi (1985, personal communication) reported a remission rate of 38.8% in patients under 40, but only 24.4% in older patients. Likewise, we have had similar results (Levasseur 1985, unpublished work). Papatestas et al. (1987) and Jaretzki et al. (1988) reported that age is not a significant prognostic factor. This does not mean that older patients do as well as younger ones, but rather that stepwise regression analysis has shown that thymomas are more frequent in older patients, and have an adverse effect on outcome. Taking this into account explains why age per se does not influence outcome.

Preoperative Evolution of MG

In several series, the remission rate after thymectomy is higher and mortality due to MG lower when the preoperative duration of symptoms is short (Osserman and Genkins 1971; Rodriguez et al. 1983; Mulder et al. 1983, Maggi 1985, personal communication). This observation is not constant (Schwab and Passouant 1952; Mulder et al. 1974; Buckingham et al. 1976). However, Otto and Strugalska (1987) have shown that there is a highly significant ($P = 0.001$) correlation between short duration of symptoms before thymectomy and good results. With symptoms for less than 12 months there were 96% good results (remission or great improvement). With MG for 12-24 months, 25-48 months, or more than 48 months the percentage of good results dropped to respectively 91%, 78%, and 48%.

Thymic Histology

Germinal Centers

The germinal centers and their prognostic significance have been extensively studied (Sloan 1943; Castleman and Norris 1949; Mackay et al. 1968; Papatestas et al. 1971; Buckingham et al. 1976; Slater et al. 1978; Monden et al. 1984a). The number of germinal centers increases with the preoperative duration of symptoms (Monden et al. 1984b). On the other hand, early remission in relation to the number of germinal centers is still controversial (Papatestas et al. 1971; Rubin et al. 1981; Otto and Strugalska 1987) as is the postoperative survival (Papatestas et al. 1971; Buckingham et al. 1976).

Lymphofollicular Hyperplasia

It still remains a matter of debate whether hyperplasia affects the prognosis. In 1971 Alpert et al. noted a different response to thymectomy, with better prognosis when hyperplasia was present. Later on Mulder et al. (1983) and Rodriguez et al. (1983) did not confirm this observation, reporting similar rates of remission with normal thymus or hyperplasia.

Thymoma

The presence of a thymoma clearly adversely affects the prognosis of MG. We observed 77% good results in the absence of thymoma, but only 53% with thymoma (Levasseur et al. 1972). Mulder et al. (1983) reported that in non-thymomatous MG the remission rate was 54% as opposed to 37% with thymoma. Papatestas et al. (1987) also reported important differences in the long-term outcome with and without thymomas: 10% remission in thymomatous MG as opposed to 23% without thymoma. In recent years, this difference has tended to decrease, probably in relation to better surgical technique in radically resecting thymomas and better treatment of their recurrences.

Acetylcholine Receptor Antibodies

Measurement of acetylcholine receptor antibodies (AChR-Ab) seems to yield prognostic data which as yet are not definitive, and this is also the subject of controversy. After thymectomy, there is a trend toward decreasing levels of AChR-Ab, though this change can take months. Rubin et al. (1981) did not find detectable AChR-Ab levels in patients in complete remission, whereas patients with residual symptoms still had measurable levels. Olanow et al. (1982) also noted a postoperative decrease in AChR-Ab levels which did not reach statistical significance. Furthermore, this decrease was not constant and, indeed, some patients had a increase in AChR-Ab levels along with evident clinical improvement. The current data therefore suggest that there is a correlation between falling AChR-Ab levels and the clinical course, but that it is inconstant. Furthermore, other considerations such as thymic factor may play an as yet undefined role (Olanow et al. 1982).

Other Autoimmune Diseases

Few publications deal with this issue other than anecdotally, making it difficult to draw meaningful conclusions. Rodriguez et al. (1983) studied the association of MG and other autoimmune diseases in children. There were 5 cases of rheumatoid arthritis, 3 of juvenile diabetes, 3 of asthma, and 3 of thyroid dysfunction. Of these 14 patients 12 underwent thymectomy with a 50% remission rate (better than for the patients without an associated autoimmune disease).

Monden et al. (1986) specifically studied this issue. In their series of 277 patients who underwent thymectomy for MG, there were 33 patients with 37 associated autoimmune disorders (3 patients had 2 or 3), not including diabetes mellitus (5 additional cases). Of these disorders, 9 occured after thymectomy. A second autoimmune disorder was significantly ($P = 0.007$) more frequent in patients without thymomas (15.1%) than in patients with thymomas (3.8%). Likewise, there were significantly ($P = 0.018$) more women affected (15.3% of females, 5.3% of males), and germinal centers were seen more frequently in the thymuses of the patients with a second autoimmune disorder ($P = 0.020$).

The rate of remission of MG after thymectomy was not significantly different for the patients with a second autoimmune disorder. The remission rate at 5 years was 40% for patients with (and 55% for those without) a second autoimmune disorder. The palliation rates at 5 years were respectively 90% and 97%. The course of the associated autoimmune disorders was unaffected by thymectomy in all patients.

Surgical Approach

The surgical approach does affect the prognosis and operative morbidity and mortality rates. The pros and cons of cervicotomy, cervicomanubriotomy, sternotomy, and the more or less radical resections of the mediastinum have been discussed in other chapters, and are the subject of great controversy. Maggi et al. (1982) and Papatestas et al. (1987) believe that cervicotomy gives just as good results with less morbidity than sternotomy. However, Masaoka and Monden (1981) as well as Mulder et al. (1983) and Jaretzki et al. (1988) have reported significantly better long-term results following *en bloc* mediastinal exenteration ("maximal" thymectomy).

References

Alpert LI, Papatestas AE, Kark A (1971) A histologic reappraisal of the thymus in myasthenia gravis. A correlative study of thymic pathology and response to thymectomy. Arch Pathol 91: 55-61

Austin EH, Olanow CW, Wechsler AS (1983) Thymoma following transcervical thymectomy for myasthenia gravis. Ann Thorac Surg 35: 548-550

Blalock A, Mason MF, Morgan HJ, Riven SS (1939) Myasthenia gravis and tumors of the thymic region: report of a case in which the tumor was removed. Ann Surg 110: 544-561

Blalock A, Harvey AM, Ford FR, Lilienthal JL jr (1941) The treatment of myasthenia gravis by removal of the thymus gland: preliminary report. JAMA 117: 1529-1533

Blalock A (1944) Thymectomy in the treatment of myasthenia gravis: report of 20 cases. J Thorac Surg 13: 316-339

Buckberg GD, Herrmann C jr, Dillon JB, Mulder DG (1967) A further evaluation of thymectomy for myasthenia gravis. J Thorac Cardiovasc Surg 53: 401-411

Buckingham JM, Howard FM jr, Bernatz PE, Payne WS, Harrison EG, O'Brien PC, Weiland LH (1976) The value of thymectomy in myasthenia gravis. A computer assisted matched study. Ann Surg 184: 453-458

Castleman B, Norris EH (1949) Pathology of the thymus in myasthenia gravis: study of 35 cases. Medicine (Baltimore) 28: 27-58

Cohn HE, Solit RW, Schatz NJ, Schlezinger N, Fineberg CH (1974) Surgical treatment in myasthenia gravis: a 27 year experience. J Thorac Cardiovasc Surg 68: 876-885

Eaton LM, Clagett OT (1955) Present status of thymectomy in the treatment of myasthenia gravis. Am J Med 19: 703-717

Jaretzki A, Penn AS, Younger DS, Wolff M, Olarte MR, Lovelace RE, Rowland LP (1988) "Maximal" thymectomy for myasthenia gravis. J Thorac Cardiovasc Surg 95: 747-757

Keynes G (1946) The surgery of the thymus gland. Br J Surg 32: 201-214

Keynes G (1949) The results of thymectomy in myasthenia gravis. Br Med J 2: 611-616

Le Brigand H, Levasseur P, Rojas-Miranda A, Gaud C, Wojanowski I (1980) Résultats du traitement chirurgical de la myasthénie (248 cas de thymectomies). Ann Chir 34: 169-172

Levasseur P, Noviant Y, Rojas-Miranda A, Merlier M, Le Brigand H (1972) Thymectomy for myasthenia gravis: long-term results in 74 cases. J Thorac Cardiovasc Surg 64: 1-5

Mackay IR, Whittingham S, Goldstein G, Curie TT, Hare WSV (1968) Myasthenia gravis: clinical, serological and histological studies in relation to thymectomy. Aust Ann Med 17: 1-11

Maggi G, Paletto AE, Casadio C, Pischedda F, Trifiletti G (1982) Résultats de 368 thymectomies pour myasthénie. Lyon Chir 78: 101-104

Masaoka A, Monden Y (1981) Comparison of the results of transsternal simple, transcervical simple and extended thymectomy. Ann NY Acad Sci 377: 755-765

Monden Y, Nakahara K, Kagotani K, Fujii Y, Masaoka A, Kawashima Y (1984a) Myasthenia gravis with thymoma: analysis of and postoperative prognosis for 65 patients with thymomatous myasthenia gravis. Ann Thorac Surg 38: 46-52

Monden Y, Nakahara K, Kagotani K, Fujii Y, Nanjo S, Masaoka A, Kawashima Y (1984b) Effects of preoperative duration of symptoms on patients with myasthenia gravis. Ann Thorac Surg 38: 287-291

Monden Y, Uyama T, Nakahara K, Fujii Y, Hashimoto J, Ohno K, Masaoka A, Kawashima Y (1986) Clinical characteristics and prognosis of myasthenia gravis with other autoimmune diseases. Ann Thorac Surg 41: 189-192

Mulder DG, Herrmann C, Buckberg GD (1974) Effect of thymectomy in patients with myasthenia gravis. A 16 year experience. Am J Surg 128: 202-206

Mulder DG, Herrmann C, Keesey J, Edwards H (1983) Thymectomy for myasthenia gravis. Am J Surg 146: 61-66

Olanow CW, Wechsler AS, Roses AD (1982) A prospective study of thymectomy and serum acetylcholine receptor antibodies in myasthenia gravis. Ann Surg 196: 113-121

Osserman KE, Genkins G (1971) Studies in myasthenia gravis: review of a 20 year experience in over 1200 patients. Mt Sinai J Med 38: 497-537

Otto TJ, Strugalska H (1987) Surgical treatment for myasthenia gravis. Thorax 42: 199-204

Papatestas AE, Alpert LI, Osserman KE, Osserman RS, Kark AE (1971) Studies in myasthenia gravis: effects of thymectomy. Results on 185 patients with non-thymomatous and thymomatous myasthenia gravis, 1941-1969. Am J Med 50: 465-474

Papatestas AE, Genkins G, Kornfeld P, Eisenkraft JB, Fagerstrom RP, Pozner J, Aufses AH (1987) Effects of thymectomy in myasthenia gravis. Ann Surg 206: 79-88

Perlo VP, Poskanzer DC, Schwab RS, Viets HR, Osserman KE, Genkins G (1966) Myasthenia gravis: evaluation of treatment in 1355 patients. Neurology 16: 431-439

Rodriguez M, Gomez MR, Howard FM jr, Taylor WF (1983) Myasthenia gravis in children: long-term follow-up. Ann Neurol 13: 504-510

Rubin JW, Ellison RG, Moore HV, Pai GP (1981) Factors affecting response to thymectomy for myasthenia gravis. J Thorac Cardiovasc Surg 82: 720-728

Rzepecki W, Lukasiewicz M, Emeryk B (1981) Appréciation du traitement de la myasthénie par la thymectomie. Ann Chir 35: 561-563

Schwab RS, Passouant P (1952) Les indications de la thymectomie au cours de la myasthénie. Presse Méd 60: 1501-1503

Simpson JA (1958) An evaluation of thymectomy in myasthenia gravis. Brain 81: 112-144

Simpson JA (1960) Myasthenia gravis: a new hypothesis. Scot Med J 5: 419-436

Slater G, Papatestas AE, Genkins G, Kornfeld P, Horowitz SH (1978) Thymectomy in patients more than 40 years of age with myasthenia gravis. Surg Gynecol Obstet 146: 54-56

Sloan HE jr (1943) The thymus in myasthenia gravis with observations on the normal anatomy and histology of the thymus. Surgery 13: 154-174

Sturridge MF (1980) La thymectomie dans le traitement de la myasthénie grave. Sem Hop Paris 56/37-38: 1506-1508

Viets HR, Schwab RS (1960) Thymectomy for myasthenia gravis. Thomas, Springfield

31 Postoperative Evolution and Prognosis of Thymic Tumors

Mohamed Boumghar and Michael Dusmet

Thymomas

Thymomas are relatively rare but, in adults, they are the commonest tumors of the anterosuperior mediastinum where they represent 29%-47% of all neoplasms (Rubush et al. 1973; Mullen and Richardson 1986). However, these tumors are far less frequently seen in children (Mullen and Richardson 1986), and most cases are actually misdiagnosed lymphoblastic lymphomas of the thymus (Rosai 1981). True thymomas in children tend to be aggressive lesions with a poor prognosis (ibid).

In adults thymomas tend to be slow-growing tumors (Allum and Watson 1983; Shamji et al. 1984; Verley and Hollmann 1985). Their behavior can be at times surprising with long, uneventful remissions after partial resection and radiotherapy of bulky, infiltrating lesions; on the other hand, small, well-encapsulated, easily resected tumors can recur rapidly (Le Brigand et al. 1979). Equally intriguing is the extremely aggressive course of the few thymomas which occurred during pregnancy (Argubright et al. 1984): all were associated with extensive local or distant disease and five of seven patients died within 6 months of delivery.

Two important aspects of the clinical assessment of thymomas are the degree of local invasion and the association with a paraneoplastic syndrome such as myasthenia gravis (MG) or pure red cell aplasia. The surgeon's evaluation of invasion of adjacent structures is more important than the histological assessment of the leading edge of these tumors (Verley and Hollmann 1985). Fibrous adhesions to adjacent structures can cause confusion with true invasion. Four stages were described by Masaoka et al. in 1981: I, complete encapsulation; II, macroscopic invasion of surrounding fat or pleura, microscopic invasion of capsule; III, macroscopic invasion of surrounding organs; and IV, pleural or pericardial dissemination, distant metastases. The thymoma is considered to be a stage II lesion if separation of the tumor from the pleura is difficult, or if the tumor capsule is not distinct. In one series (Verley and Hollmann 1985), fibrous adhesions to adjacent structures did not seem to alter the prognosis, and there was no significant difference in survival between patients in stages I and II in the series reported by Masaoka et al. (1981). However, there were only 2/37 recurrences in stage I disease as opposed to 3/13 in stage II disease. Furthermore, in the Mayo Clinic series (Lewis et al. 1987), there were more recurrences (9/45 vs 11/142) for adherent tumors as opposed to nonadherent lesions; moreover, death due to disease was respectively 2/42 and 2/142.

The importance of clearly distinguishing invasive and/or metastasizing thymomas from thymic carcinoma has been emphasized in Chap. 9. This has unfortunately not always been the case in the literature, both lesions being grouped together under the ambiguous term "malignant thymoma." This makes valid comparisons between different series difficult, and does not help the clinician in decision making. True thymic carcinomas, i.e., lesions with clear *cytologic* features of malignancy, have a dismal prognosis (Shimosato et al. 1977; Snover et al. 1982; Wick et al. 1982b; Verley and Hollmann 1985). On the other hand, invasive and/or metastatic thymomas, i.e., cytologically bland lesions with invasion of adjacent structures or distant dissemination, are lesions which are often responsive to radiotherapy and chemotherapy with significant long-term tumor-free survival in as many as two-thirds of patients (Masaoka et al. 1981; Verley and Hollmann 1985; Maggi et al. 1986; Uematsu and Kondo 1986). There are no reliable histologic criteria which predict recurrence or metastases. However, Lewis et al. (1987) postulate that there is a continuum between thymoma and thymic carcinoma with a no-man's-land between them, classified as thymomas, but with slight signs of atypia. In their experience these lesions merit special postoperative surveillance and have a clinical course similar to their histologic appearance, i.e., intermediate between frankly benign thymomas and clear-cut thymic carcinoma. This is in complete agreement with the findings of Gray and Gutowski (1979) and Verley and Hollmann (1985). This concept is borne out by a recent morphometric study of thymomas (Nomori et al. 1988): invasive thymomas had a significantly higher nucleocytoplasmic ratio than noninvasive ones. In the series reported by Fujimura et al. (1987) two-thirds of metastatic lesions showed varying degrees of atypia.

As discussed in this chapter and by several authors (Bernatz et al. 1973; Chahinian et al. 1981, Verley and Hollmann 1985; Fujimura et al. 1987; Lewis et al. 1987) the pedominantly epithelial thymomas tend to be more invasive and aggressive. Furthermore, as reported by Fujimura et al. (1987), it is the epithelial component of mixed lymphoepithelial lesions that demonstrates various degrees of atypia.

The influence of histologic subtype on prognosis is controversial. Verley and Hollmann (1985) reported better survival in patients with spindle cell and predominantly lymphocytic lesions (5- and 10-year survival of 80% and 75%, respectively) than for those with predominantly epithelial thymomas (5- and 10-year survival of 72% and 50%). Furthermore, these authors noted that invasive tumors tended to be predominantly epithelial. Lewis et al. (1987) reviewed the Mayo Clinic experience (283 cases), and found that the death rates were 44 per 1000 patient years for predominantly lymphocytic thymomas, 76 for mixed lymphoepithelial lesions, and 93 for predominantly epithelial ones. Spindle cell tumors tended to be well encapsulated and slow growing. Masaoka et al. (1981) also reported poorer survival for patients with predominantly epithelial tumors. On the other hand, in a review of 169 cases, Maggi et al. (1986) found that survival was worst for those with lymphoepithelial lesions (5- and 10-year survival of 76% and 55%), as opposed to 5- and 10-year survivals of 88% and 88% for predominantly lymphocytic thymomas, and respectively 88% and 79% for predominantly epithelial ones. On the basis of these figures it would not seem that the histologic subtype is as important a prognostic factor as invasiveness. Indeed, Lewis et al. (1987) state that "because predominantly epithelial tumors also tend to be more invasive at diagnosis, histologic subtype does not appear in our predictive model of tumor behavior as this factor is largely included in the factor of invasion." It is interesting to note that these same authors point out that 5 of the 8 cases in their series with extrathoracic spread were predominantly epithelial. Guillan et al. (1971) also reported that 8 of 12 cases of thymomas with extrathoracic metastasis were predominantly epithelial.

These findings have been confirmed by the analysis of a recent series of 141 patients with thymomas (Nakahara et al. 1988). There was no significant difference in survival between the three different histologic subtypes if the completely resected lesions were studied separately from the incompletely resected ones. However, whereas 33/36 (92%) of the predominantly lymphocytic lesions were completely resectable, only 61/77 (79%) of the mixed lymphoepithelial and 18/26 (69%) of the predominantly epithelial lesions were amenable to complete resection. Thus, the 10-year survival was respectively 88%, 86%, and 66% for the three different subtypes, which reflects the 10-year survival rates of 94% for completely resected lesions as opposed to 68% after subtotal resection.

Regression analysis of the Mayo Clinic series (Lewis et al. 1987) identified four independent prognostic variables: (a) the presence of invasion or metastasis; (b) the presence of symptoms (*not* paraneoplastic syndromes, but symptoms directly due to the tumor itself such as chest pain dyspnea, weight loss, night sweats); (c) age under 30; and (d) lack of total surgical excision. The relative weight of these four factors was 2.4 for the first and 1 for all three others. When these factors are summed the 10-year survival was over 95% for a total score of 1, 90% for a score of 2 or 2.4, 57% for 3.4, and 43% for 4.4 or 5.4. Size of the tumor, reported to be a major prognostic indicator by Papatestas et al. (1987b), was not an independent prognostic variable in the Mayo Clinic series, for large tumors tended to be invasive.

Another baffling feature of thymomas is the occurrence of MG following excision of the lesion (Appelquist et al. 1982; Allum and Watson 1983; Papatestas et al. 1987b). This has been reported to occur in 3%–9% of cases (Denayer et al. 1986; Maggi et al. 1986; Papatestas et al. 1987b), and is often not associated with recurrence of thymoma (Namba et al. 1978; Maggi et al. 1986). Both sexes are equally affected and the age of onset of MG ranges from 30 to 73 years. The interval between thymectomy and the first symptoms of MG varies from 2 months to 22 years, and in a majority of cases the initial lesion was a well-encapsulated thymoma (Namba et al. 1978). The response of MG to treatment does not seem to be affected by this curious clinical course. In our series, there were three cases of MG which occurred in the immediate postoperative course, 3 and 12 years following the removal of an infiltrating thymoma. Furthermore, a 72-year-old woman presented slight transient symptoms of MG following the excision of a predominantly lymphocytic thymoma (Table 1). These patients are described in Table 1. Obviously, the relapse of MG can also herald the recurrence of a thymoma (Le Brigand et al. 1980; Allum and Watson 1983; Maggi et al. 1986; Rosenberg et al. 1986).

Rosenow and Hurley (1984) reviewed the association of paraneoplastic syndromes and thymomas (see also Chaps. 12–15). We would like to reiterate that the spindle cell thymomas tend to be slow-growing, encapsulated lesions which are commonly associated with paraneoplastic syndromes, including MG (Masaoka et al. 1981; Verley and Hollmann 1985; Lewis et al. 1987). Furthermore, most of these symptoms are re-

Table 1. Description of patients with myasthenia gravis occurring after excision of a thymoma

Sex	Female	Female	Male	Female
Age (years)	43	62	67	72
Thymoma	Invasive, predominantly epithelial	Invasive, mixed lympho-epithelial	Invasive, mixed lympho-epithelial	Encapsulated, predominantly lymphocytic
Time from thymectomy to MG	9 years	3½ years	A few weeks after surgery	Immediately after surgery
Outcome	Died 16 years after thymectomy - heart failure. Recurrent tumor in chest at autopsy	Mastectomy for breast cancer 1 year after thymectomy; no evidence of disease when last seen	Died 3 months after thymectomy - right heart failure	Died in a road accident

lieved by thymectomy, except hypogammaglobulinemia. Rosenow could not find a single case of reversal of hypogammaglobulinemia following thymectomy. However, it has been demonstrated in several large series that the presence or absence of a paraneoplastic syndrome does not significantly influence the survival of patients with thymomas (Verley and Hollmann 1985; Maggi et al. 1986, Lewis et al. 1987).

One particular association that has obvious prognostic implications is the frequent occurence of a second primary malignancy in patients with thymomas. The reported incidence in the Mayo Clinic series (Lewis et al. 1987) was 17%. In a review of 2062 myasthenic patients, Papatestas et al. (1987a) noted 131 cases of extrathymic neoplasms. Of these, 89 occurred in patients who had not undergone thymectomy, whereas there were only 42 cases among the 962 patients who did so. Earlier appearance of tumors was also noted for those patients with thymomas. Papatestas et al. (1987a) concluded that early thymectomy might prevent the occurrence of extrathymic second primaries in these patients through unknown mechanisms. Table 2 shows our experience with extrathymic second primaries, illustrated by Fig. 1.

Table 2. Second primary tumors in patients with thymomas

	Second primary	Time between thymectomy and second primary
Invasive thymomas (24)	Carcinoid in Meckels's diverticulum	2 years
	Carcinoma of the prostate	7 years
	Fibrous hystiocytoma (thorax)	1 year
	Anorectal leiomyosarcoma	2 months
	Breast cancer	1 year
	Carcinoma of the bladder	Synchronous
Encapsulated thymomas (21)	Mediastinal lymphosarcoma	8 years
	Basocellular carcinoma (skin)	1 year
	Gastric adenocarcinoma	Synchronous

Noninvasive Thymomas

These tend to be slow growing tumors, which in 38%-52% of cases are not associated with paraneoplastic syndrome (Masaoka et al. 1981; Shamji et al. 1984; Verley and Hollmann 1985) and can be asymptomatic for long periods of time. Complete resection is usually curative (Salyer and Eggleston 1976; Shamji et al. 1984; Nakahara et al. 1988), however, in most large series 2%-12% recur locally, sometimes as late as 10 years postoperatively (Fechner 1969; Masaoka et al. 1981; Verley and Hollmann 1985; Maggi et al. 1986; Lewis et al. 1987). In the Mayo Clinic series (Lewis et al. 1987), the comparison of survival curves shows that excess death due to thymoma as compared with those for age- and sex-matched controls extends for approximately 15 years after diagnosis, and there was one case of recurrence 26 years after surgery. In our experience with 24 noninvasive thymomas (Table 3), 2 recurred in the mediastinum and in the thoracotomy scar respectively 1 and 14 years following surgery. Overall, 5- and 10-year survival was 63% and 37%. Because of this small but definite tendency for local recurrence of noninvasive lesions some authors recommend the removal of all mediastinal fat at the initial operation, for this can harbor thymic rests (Masaoka et al. 1981; Mulder et al. 1983); some authors even recommend routine adjuvant radiotherapy (Nakahara et al. 1988). However, this approach seems excessive of one bears in mind the local complications due to radiotherapy reported by Arriagada et al. (1981) and the 2 deaths caused by radiotherapy of these tumors

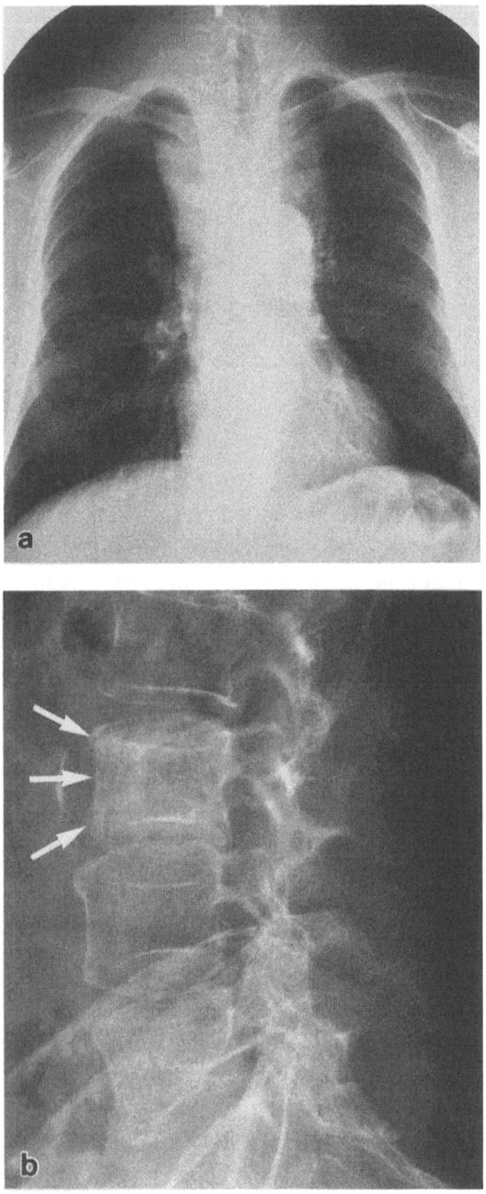

Fig. 1 a, b. This 55-year-old patient underwent subtotal excision of a mixed lymphoepithelial thymoma, followed by radiotherapy. He was operated on for carcinoma of Meckel's diverticulum 4 years later, and for carcinoma of the prostate 7 years after thymectomy. He died with extensive pleural, visceral, and spinal metastases 8 years after thymectomy. **a** preoperative chest X-ray, **b** metastasis to L-3 from the thymoma

Table 3. Patients with thymomas

	Patients	With MG	Without MG
Encapsulated thymomas	24	6	18
Invasive thymomas	21[a]	4	16
Total	45	10[a]	34

[a] An additional patient had hypogammaglobulinemia

reported by Shamji et al. (1984), especially since there were only 3 cases of recurrence following the complete removal of 191 occult thymomas in 996 patients who underwent thymectomy for MG without any postoperative radiotherapy or chemotherapy (Papatestas et al. 1987 b).

Special postoperative follow-up is warranted for patients with moderate histologic features of atypia, as discussed already in this chapter and by Lewis et al. (1987). The relative merits of complete *en bloc* exenteration of the mediastinum vs thymectomy via cervicotomy are discussed in Chaps. 20-22 and 30. Papatestas has stressed in two publications (Papatestas et al. 1987 a, b) the lack of benefit in long-term patient survival with the more invasive transsternal approach, which requires longer hospital stays and is therefore more costly. This, however, is in contradiction with the results published by Monden et al. (1984) who found that extended thymectomy gave much better long-term remission rates in both thymomatous and nonthymomatous MG.

It has been shown in several series that the overall survival of patients with paraneoplastic syndromes is the same as for those who do not present with such symptoms (Masaoka et al. 1981; Shamji et al. 1984; Verley and Hollmann 1985; Maggi et al. 1986; Lewis et al. 1987). However, the presence or absence of MG or another paraneoplastic syndrome is obviously an important prognostic factor (Masoaka et al. 1981). The prognosis of a patient presenting with a small, noninvasive, completely resected thymoma and MG or pure red cell aplasia is more reserved than for an asymptomatic patient with a similar lesion. Conversely, in patients with unresectable invasive or metastatic thymomas, tumor control is the major prognostic determinant (Bernatz et al. 1973; Gray and Gutowski 1979; Masoaka et al. 1981; Verley and Hollmann 1985; Maggi et al. 1986; Fujimura et al. 1987). This was clear in the 141 cases reported by Nakahara et al. (1988): 1 patient with stage I disease (out of 42) died of tumor progression, 7 of their paraneoplastic syndromes. Of 33 cases of stage II disease there were 4 tumor deaths and 4 paraneoplastic ones. There were 35 patients with stage III disease (5 tumor deaths and 1 paraneoplastic one) and 13 cases of stage IV disease with 4 tumor deaths (none due to paraneoplastic syndromes). Thus, the tumor per se was responsible for 6 deaths in patients who underwent complete resection (and paraneoplastic syndromes for 13 deaths), whereas these figures were respectively 7 and 0 for patients undergoing subtotal resection, and 10 and 0 for patients who had a biopsy without resection of their tumor. In our experience 3 patients had paraneoplastic syndromes and a noninvasive thymoma. One died of respiratory failure due to MG and one from immunologic complications of hypogammaglobulinemia.

Thus, the overall survival for patients with noninvasive thymomas is 85%-96% at 5 years, and 67%-80% at 10 years (Masaoka et al. 1981, Shamji et al. 1984; Verley and Hollmann 1985; Maggi et al. 1986), whether or not they presented with MG or another paraneoplastic syndrome. Nakahara et al. (1988) reported actuarial survival rates of 100% of 5 and 10 years and 86% at 15 years for stage I thymomas, and 91.5% at 5 years, 84.4% at 10 years, and 70.4% at 15 years for stage III disease. Furthermore, in all reported series many deaths in this group of patients are totally unrelated to thymectomy or MG.

Invasive and/or Metastatic Thymomas

The incidence of invasive thymomas varies from 7% to 67% with most series reporting 25%-60% (Bernatz et al. 1973; Rosai and Levine 1976; Wilkins and Castleman 1979; Verley and Hollmann 1985; Lewis et al. 1987). This demonstrates the difficulty in assessing invasiveness both grossly and microscopically. As mentioned already, the surgeon's careful evaluation of invasiveness is the most important prognostic criterion for the patient (Maggi et al. 1986). In our experience with 21 cases of invasive thymomas (Table 3) there was no histologic evidence of invasion of neighboring structures in five cases.

In several large series MG and other paraneoplastic syndromes are seen less frequently in patients with invasive thymomas than in those with encapsulated lesions (Masaoka et al. 1981; Shamji et al. 1984; Verley and Hollmann 1985; Nakahara et al. 1988). However, Maggi et al. (1986) reported that there was not a significant difference in the frequency of MG in invasive and noninvasive thymomas.

Metastases occur outside the chest in 1.5%-15.5% of invasive thymomas (José et al. 1980), usually in the liver, bones, brain, lymph nodes, and kidneys. They are often multiple, but occasionally present as a single pulmonary coin lesion (Cohen et al. 1984). The spine is the preferred location for bone metastasis which can be osteolytic or osteoblastic.

Totally encapsulated lesions which are completely resected can also metastasize, as in one case reported by Verley and Hollmann (1985). Lewis et al. (1987) also had three cases in their series of encapsulated, totally resected tumors which metastasized 2-8 years later (one tumor was adherent to adjacent structures without frank invasion). Of these three patients, one survived 21 years, one died of disease 3 years later, and one survived with disease to last follow-up at 11 years.

In our series of 21 invasive thymomas, 2 died with metastatic disease to the spine and brain 8 and 10 years after total resection and radiotherapy of their tumors. Furthermore, we have noted the presence of tumor floating in the innominate vein, and tumor obstruction of the main vein of tumor drainage without metastasis. The overall survival in our group of patients was 44% at 5 years, 27% at 10 years, and 0% at 20 years.

Radiotherapy has been used with inconsistent results, but is believed to be useful as adjuvant therapy for invasive thymomas (Chahinian et al. 1981; Monden et al. 1984; Fujimura et al. 1987; Nakahara et al. 1988). Uematsu and Kondo (1986) reported excellent response of incompleteley resected tumors to radiotherapy. The precise role and technique of radiotherapy are discussed in Chap. 28. However, one must bear in mind that radiotherapy is not without danger, as alluded to already as well as by Fujimura et al. (1987) who also had one patient who died of treatment complications. In our experience, two patients died of septic complications of actinic lung damage 3 and 8 years after surgery and radiotherapy. Furthermore, a third patient of ours died 9 years after irradiation of an intrathoracic lymphosarcoma that was probably radioinduced (unpublished work).

Chemotherapy is probably also a useful adjuvant treatment modality for invasive and metastatic thymomas. Hu and Levine (1986) pointed out in a recent review of the literature that cisplatin and prednisone seem to have unique potential in regard to most single or multiple drug regimens reported to date. In our experience, chemotherapy was totally ineffective in two cases. A third case was a 53-year-old man with a predominantly lymphocytic thymoma who presented 2 years after surgery with three successive pleural recurrences which were treated with vincristine, methotrexate, and cyclophosphamide in 4- to 5-week cycles. The patient was still alive and disease-free 6 years after treatment for his last recurrence.

The prognosis of invasive thymomas depends largely on the resectability of the lesion. In several large series, 7%-36% of invasive thymomas recurred after resection and/or radiotherapy (Masaoka et al. 1981; Shamji et al. 1984; Verley and Hollmann 1985; Lewis et al. 1987), but were still amenable to treatment (surgery, radiotherapy, and chemotherapy). In our series of 21 invasive lesions, 9 (32%) recurred 2 months to 10 years after surgery (unpublished work). Maggi et al. (1986) reported that the 5-year survival was 80% for completely resected lesions, 59% following subtotal resection and radiotherapy, and only 45% when the primary treatment was nonsurgical following biopsy of an unresectable mass. Masaoka et al. (1981) reported respective 5-year survivals of 89%, 7/13 (54%), and 2/8 (25%). However, Verley and Hollmann (1985) reported that survival did not depend on resectability, and attributed this apparent contradiction to the recent progress in radiotherapy and chemotherapy programs. But in spite of this progrees these authors reported a similar difference in survival between invasive and noninvasive thymomas. Nahakara et al. (1988) found that the actuarial survival rate of completely resected stage III disease (100% at 5 years, 95% at 10 and 15 years) was not significantly different from that of stage I and II lesions. However, patients with tumors that were not completely resected had survival rates of 80% at 5 and 10 years and 0% at 15 years. Stage IV disease led to 46.5% 5- and 10-year survival rates (0% and 15 years), and not a single patient who underwent biopsy without resection survived longer than 8 years.

Thymic Carcinoma

True thymic carcinomas, which are not to be confused with invasive and/or metastatic thymomas, are extremely rare tumors. The largest series is from the Mayo Clinic and it comprises 20 cases collected over 75 years (Wick et al. 1982b). Thus, it is difficult to make valid statements concerning the prognostic implications about the various subtypes described in Chap. 9.

Symptoms are usually due to the tumor mass itself: chest pain, cough, dyspnea, superior vena cava syndrome, pleural effusion, shoulder stiffness or pain, and general symptoms such as weight loss, night sweats, fever, fatigue. Paraneoplastic syndromes occur only occasionally: there were none in the cases reported by Shimosato et al. (1977), Snover et al. (1982) or Wick et al. (1982b). However, Verley and Hollmann (1985) reported 4 cases of MG in 14 cases of "type 4 thymoma," which would seem to meet the histopathologic criteria for thymic carcinoma. Thomas and Manivel (1987) reported a case of aplastic anemia in association with a thymic carcinoma.

Despite aggressive multimodality therapy (surgery, radiotherapy and chemotherapy), the prognosis is usually dismal: Wick et al. (1982b) reported an average survival of 18 months for the 18/20 patients who died, 1 patient survived 18 months to last follow-up with disease, and there was 1 long-term (43 month) disease-free survivor.

In Verley and Hollmann's series (1985) all patients died in less than 4 years. Snover et al. (1982) reported two patients surviving 2 and 2½ years without evidence of disease in a series of eight patients (one lost to follow-up). The only series which showed any significant hope for these patients were the eight described by Shimosato et al. (1977): these patients all had squamous cell lesions. Six patients were alive without disease 1-12 years (mean 4.3 years) after diagnosis, one died at 11 months and another at 21 months. However, it is possible that some of these cases should be classified as thymomas rather than as thymic carcinomas.

Thymolipoma and Thymoliposarcoma

Thymolipomas are rare tumors which are often large, asymptomatic, slow growing and can mimic either a normal thymus gland, or cardiomegaly. Pleural or pericardial adhesions are frequent, as is the displacement of adjacent mediastinal structures, but invasion of surrounding structures has never been described (Saegesser and Zoupanos 1970; Reintgen et al. 1978; Otto et al. 1982). These tumors have been associated with aplastic anemia (Barnes and O'Gorman 1962), pure red cell aplasia (Otto et al. 1982), hypogammaglobulinemia (Otto et al. 1982), MG (Reintgen et al. 1978; Otto et al. 1982), and Graves' disease (Benton and Gerard 1966). Excision is usually curative (Korhonen and Laustela 1968; Reintgen et al. 1978), and the paraneoplastic syndromes can remit following excision of these tumors (Reintgen et al. 1978; Otto et al. 1982).

We have seen two cases of thymolipoma without associated paraneoplastic syndromes. An 11-year-old girl underwent the excision of a large thymolipoma which was discovered during investigations for suspected cardiomegaly. Her postoperative course was uneventful. A 48-year-old man has undergone eight thoracotomies in 6 years for relatively rapid recurrences of a thymolipoma. These were also treated with radiotherapy, and there was a transformation to liposarcoma which was probably radioinduced.

Havlicek and Rosai (1984) have reported two cases of thymoliposarcoma. The first recurred after 25 years, was reexcised, then presented 6 years later with a probable spinal metastasis to T-5 treated by radiotherapy. The clinical course of the second patient was not described.

Neuroendocrine Tumors of the Thymus

As stated by Rosai et al. (1976) all carcinoid tumors are potentially malignant. The most undifferentiated are called grade III carcinoid or either oat cell or small cell carcinoma. Fortunately, this last entity is exceedingly rare in the thymus. Wick and Scheithauer reported a case in 1982 and found only six other cases in a review of the literature. The outlook for these patients does not seem as dismal as one might expect, for two cases responded well to single-agent chemotherapy. An interesting feature of Wick and Scheithauer's case was the association with a malignant pancreatic islet cell tumor and a family history suggestive of a familial multiple endocrine neoplasia (MEN) syndrome.

Carcinoid tumors which are not frankly anaplastic were extensively reviewed by Wick et al. in 1980. They reported that 20%-30% of these tumors metastasize, commonly to the skin and bones, as long as 10 years postoperatively. In their review of institutional cases and the literature they found that 38% of these tumors were associated with Cushing's syndrome or another endocrinopathy, and the behavior of the tumor was malignant in 64% of these cases, with a 65% mortality rate at 10 years. When these tumors are associated with Cushing's syndrome, complete excision causes remission of the endocrinopathy, but its reappearance can herald tumor recurrence (Engel and Kahana 1963). Some 45% were not associated with an endocrine abnormality, in which case only 48% behaved in a malignant fashion with a 10-year mortality rate of 29%. The remaining 17% occurred as part of a MEN syndrome and 67% of these lesions were malignant with a 10-year mortality of 50% (Wick et al. 1980).

Rosai and Higa (1972) studied the outcome of these tumors following total vs partial excision in 8 personal cases and a literature review of 8 cases. Overall there were 12 cases which were completely excised. Follow-up was available for 11, and 9 survived with no evidence of disease for 1-8 years (mean 4.6 years). Two totally excised tumors recurred either locally or in supraclavicular lymph nodes. However, one must bear in mind that the follow-up is too short to consider any of these cases as cured. There were four cases of tumors which were only partially excised, with adjuvant radiotherapy, and in two cases, chemotherapy. Two of these patients died of disease, one survived to last follow-up with disseminated disease, and one died of complications from radiotherapy 8 years postoperatively with no evidence of disease (no autopsy). These results seem encouraging. Unfortunately, they are not confirmed by the Mayo Clinic experience reported by Wick (Wick et al. 1982a). A total of 15 cases were seen in 50 years. Three tumors were discovered at autopsy in patients who died of Cushing's syndrome. Of the 12 remaining patients, 11 underwent complete or extensive resection of their tumors (the number of complete resections is not specified). Adjuvant radiotherapy and/or chemotherapy was administered to 9 of these 11 patients; nonetheless, 7 developed progressive metastasis. The patient who did not undergo surgery was treated with chemotherapy to no avail. Thus, metastasis developed in 73% of these cases, 7 died of local recurrence, metastasis, or metabolic complications of their tumors (6 cases) or myocardial infarction (1 case - lung metastasis at autopsy). Five survived with metastasis (which occurred as late as 8 years postoperatively, and only one of the three survivors with no evidence of disease has over 5 years of follow-up. Thus, only one in eight of the patients with a least 5 years of follow-up was "cured," and there was only one in seven who responded to adjuvant therapy. As if these figures were not gloomy enough, the only 15-year survivor presented with cervical lymph node metastasis 10 years postoperatively.

We have seen two cases of thymic carcinoids. One was a 44-year-old woman seen in 1957 with Cushing's syndrome. Following excision of the tumor and radiotherapy, she survived 13 years without evidence of disease. The initial diagnosis was pure epithelial thymoma without lymphocytic elements, but was in all likelihood an unrecognized carcinoid. The second case was a 19-year-old girl with a superior vena cava syndrome of recent onset and a mediastinal tumor which was partially resected via a right thoracotomy followed by radiotherapy and chemotherapy. The histologic diagnosis was neuroendocrine thymic carcinoma. She died of disease 11 months postoperatively.

Malignant Lymphomas

For many years the nodular sclerosing type of Hodgkin's disease (HD) of the thymus was considered to be a form of thymoma (Boumghar and Saegesser 1982). It is now recognized that this is not the case.

Hodgkin's Disease

HD of the anterior mediastinum is most often of the nodular sclerosing subtype and is often seen as stage I disease (Keller and Castleman 1974; Bergh et al. 1978; Colby et al. 1982). These lesions are usually single and encapsulated, can be partially cystic and quite large, with or without similar adjacent lymph nodes in roughly one-half of all cases (Keller and Castleman 1974; Bergh et al. 1978). Bergh et al. (1978) noted invasion of the superior vena cava in 1 case and direct invasion of the lung parenchyma in six (of 17 cases). Aggressive surgical therapy followed by radiotherapy (and chemotherapy in two cases) led to three early deaths and one late death. There were three recurrences, with long-term survival reported for two (one unspecified), which all occurred in patients with direct invasion of the lungs. The long-term outcome of patients with mediastinal HD is no different from that of patients with stage I disease in other locations (Colby et al. 1982; Hutchison 1984), and they should be treated in a similar manner (staging laparotomy, radiotherapy) following excision of their primary tumor. Chemotherapy is reserved for stage III and IV disease to avoid treatment-induced leukemias (Hutchison 1984). Currently, the 5-year survival for stage I HD is approximately 90%. The fact that the majority of these patients have the nodular sclerosis form of HD puts them in a better prognostic category (Colby et al. 1982). Mauch and Hellman (1984) found that the size of the initial lesion is a major prognostic indicator: lesions which measure less than one third of the transverse thoracic diameter are amenable to radiotherapy whereas larger lesions tend to recur unless treated more aggressively. North et al. (1987) reported that relapse was twice as likely to occur if there is residual mediastinal widening on chest X-rays after completion of therapy.

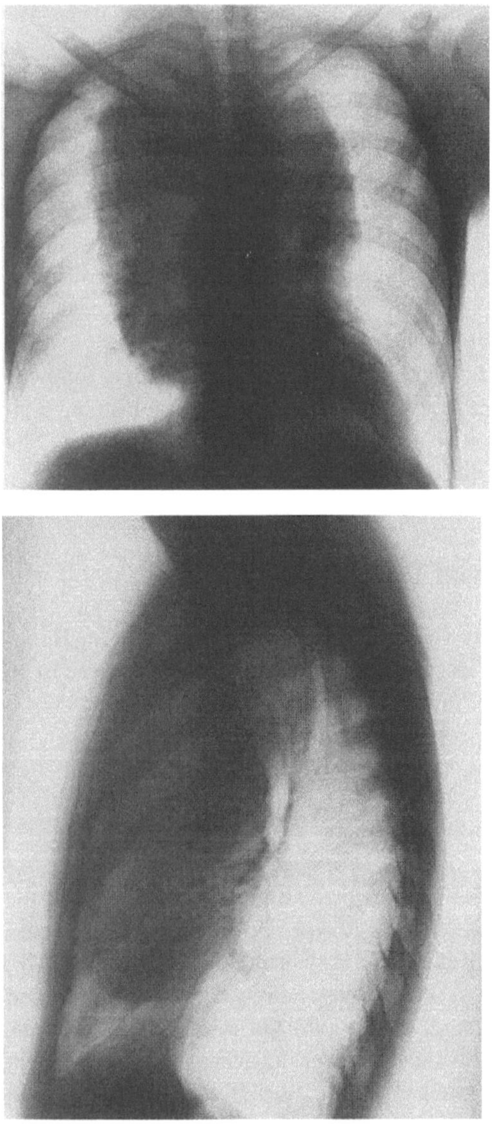

Fig. 2. Chest X-rays of a 35-year-old patient with Hodgkin's disease of the thymus which caused mediastinal compression, and was partially excised with postoperative radiotherapy and chemotherapy. The patient died after 5 months of progressive cachexia. At autopsy there was no extrathoracic disease

We have seen 12 cases of thymic HD. There was one perioperative death due to uncontrollable hemorrhage from a heavily infiltrated large vessel. A second patient died of progressive cachexia and cardiopulmonary failure 5 months after the subtotal excision, radiotherapy, and chemotherapy of a large mediastinal mass producing a mediastinal compression syndrome (Fig. 2). In both cases autopsy failed to reveal any evidence of extrathoracic disease. There were three cases of recurrence. In the first one, generalized disease (lungs and bones) led to death in 18 months despite surgery, radiotherapy, and chemotherapy. In the second one, a cervical lymph node recurrence which appeared a few months after an uneventful pregnancy was excised 8 years after initial surgery. Adjuvant chemotherapy was administered. Follow-up to date is 22 years without evidence of disease. In the third case, staging laparotomy 6 months after thoracotomy revealed extensive disease (liver, spleen, lymph nodes). Of 12 patients, 7 are alive 6-12 years after excision of the primary tumor, staging laparotomy, radiotherapy, and chemotherapy without evidence of disease. Riddel and Larsson (1980) have reported a case of HD coexisting in the same thymus with a small, encapsulated thymoma. Follow-up was not reported. This must not be taken to mean that thymic HD is a form of thymoma.

Non-Hodgkin's Lymphoma

Non-Hodgkin's lymphoma (NHL): the majority of these lesions, which account for less than 5% of all cases of NHL, are diffuse large cell lymphomas (often of B-cell origin) and they tend to behave aggressively in spite of therapy (Waldron et al. 1984; Addis and Isaacson 1986; Menestrina et al. 1986). According to Waldron et al. (1984), the T-cell lymphomas respond better to multi-agent chemotherapy. Menestrina et al. (1986) reported on eight cases with large (over 10 cm) masses and no extrathoracic disease at diagnosis. Despite aggressive treatment there was dissemination in seven patients. Partial remission was seen in four patients, three died of disease (mean survival 9 months) and five survived an average of 13 months (three disease-free survivals of respectively 4, 7, and 21 months). Addis and Isaacson (1986) reported on 15 patients. Follow-up was too short or unavailable for many cases, but overall the outcome was equally dismal. Trump and Mann (1982) reported similar results - 9/11 patients died within 26 months of diagnosis despite aggressive treatment.

Perrone et al. (1986) have published a report on mediastinal diffuse large cell lymphomas with sclerosis (60 cases). This seems, to be a less aggressive lesion which typically occurs in young women; 79% responded to initial therapy, 40% relapsed (80% mortality). However one-half of their patients were alive without disease with a mean follow-up of 34.5 months. All first relapses occurred within 19 months of diagnosis (median 9). Patients aged under 25, or with extrathoracic disease at diagnosis, or who responded incompletely to initial therapy tended to do poorly. These results are more encouraging than those reported by Miller et al. (1981). Of seven patients with diffuse hystiocytic lymphomas with sclerosis only two showed a significant response to treatment.

Germ Cell Tumors

Benign Teratomas

In two large reviews of surgical experience with mediastinal tumors, germ cell tumors represented 10% (Wychulis et al. 1971) and 14.4% of all mediastinal neoplasms (Mullen and Richardson 1986). Both reported that approximately 80% of these tumors are benign teratomas. Lewis et al. (1983) reported the Mayo Clinic experience with 86 cases of these rare tumors, which are slow growing, often asymptomatic, and frequently cystic. When symptoms are present they are due to tumor mass (substernal pain, dyspnea). A pathognomonic symptom is the expectoration of hair or sebaceous material (trichoptysis). These tumors occur most often in young adults, equally in males and females, are exceptional in the posterior mediastinum, and in 23% the operating surgeon "commented specifically on the close association between the tumor and the thymus. In several instances the tumor seemed to arise directly from the thymus" (Lewis et al. 1983). Complete resection is curative in all cases, but this is often technically difficult for almost all of these tumors are densely adherent to vital thoracic structures, requiring pulmonary lobectomy, pericardectomy, or sacrifice of a phrenic nerve in 15% of all cases, and only subtotal resection was feasible in seven cases. There were no cases of recurrence, and the only mortality is related to surgical complications (Lewis et al. 1983). These findings are confirmed by a collective review published in 1986 by Mullen and Richardson.

Malignant Primary Germ Cell Tumors

Malignant primary germ cell tumors of the mediastinum are rare. Aygun et al. (1984) found reports of a total of 319 cases, with 124 of pure *seminoma* (39%). Thus, the percentage of pure seminoma is the same as in the testes, and these are the commonest pure malignant germ cell tumors of the mediastinum. In their literatur review these authors noted that chest pain was the most frequent symptom, followed by cough and dyspnea. The superior vena cava syndrome is also frequent (Knapp et al. reported in 1985 that only 3/24 patients were asymptomatic). Only 28/127 (22%) of these tumors were resectable; 13 of these patients had adjuvant radiotherapy and 15 had none. Of these first 13 patients, 11 survived a mean of 9 years, 1 died at 11 months, and 1 survived 3 years without disease following therapy for metastasis developed after initial treatment. For the second 15 patients there was follow-up information on 13. Of these, 1 died postoperatively, and 12 survived for a mean of 9.3 years. The remaining patients underwent partial resection or biopsy only. Follow-up was available for 64, of whom 18 died of disease, 3 died of intercurrent illness, and 9 survived with metastasis. Thus, the overall "cure" rate was 65%, but a formal 5-year survival was not reported. Local recurrence was noted in 7 patients, and when there were metastases these were usually seen within 2 years; however, metastasis occurred 40 months, 4 years, and 10 years later in 3 patients. Knapp et al. (1985) reported that complete excision was possible in 9/24 patients (2 were not pure seminomas), and radiotherapy was administered to 21. They reported that 12 patients survived without disease for an average of 143 months, the tumor progressed in 3, and 9 died a mean of 50 months after diagnosis. Poor prognostic factors were age over 35, superior vena caval obstruction, lymphadenopathy, fever, and hilar disease on chest X-rays. Raghaven and Barrett (1980) reported similar results. Lee and Jackson (1985) saw six patients with pure primary mediastinal seminoma. All received radiotherapy and one also had chemotherapy. Five were alive without disease after 2.5-7 years and one had a spinal metastasis after 1 year.

We have seen two cases of mediastinal seminoma. The first (Fig. 3) was a 25-year-old man who underwent left pneumonectomy and pericardectomy with postoperative radiotherapy. After 3 years a mixed testicular tumor (seminoma plus embryonal carcinoma)

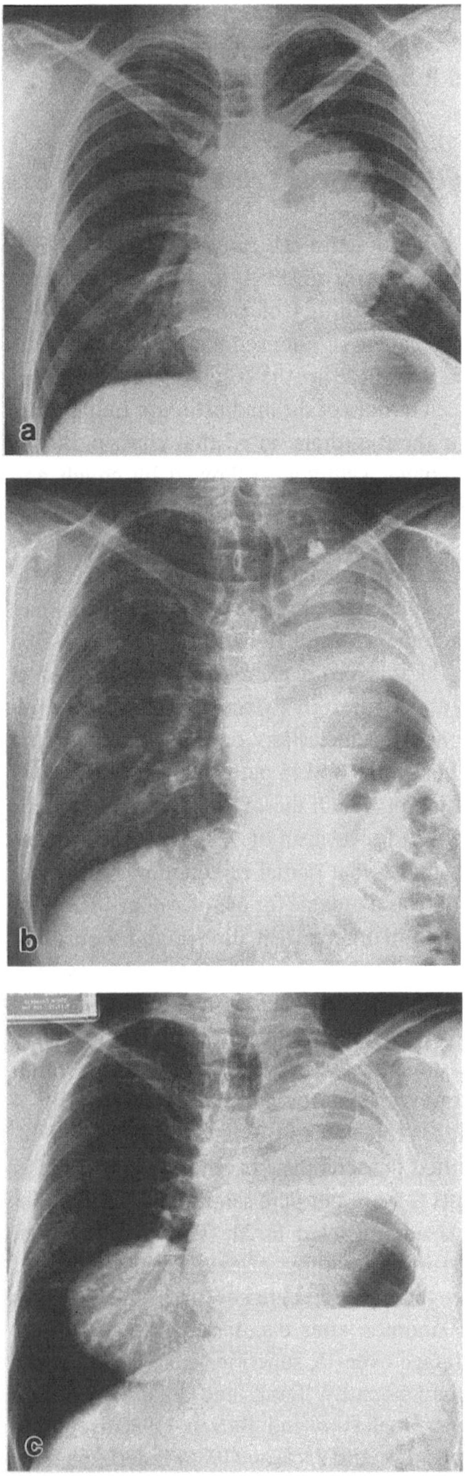

Fig. 3 a–c. Chest X-rays of a 25-year-old patient who underwent a left pneumonectomy and radiotherapy for a pure seminoma of the thymus in 1972 (**a** preoperative X-ray). In 1975 a testicular mixed germ cell tumor (seminoma and embryonal carcinoma) was resected. In 1976 (**b**), he presented with multiple pulmonary and retroperitoneal metastases which responded to chemotherapy. In 1977 (**c**) a single pulmonary "coin lesion" which did not respond to chemotherapy was seen. He died with disseminated disease in 1979

was resected, and inguinocrural lymphadenectomy performed; 1 year later he presented with pulmonary metastasis which disappeared for 1 year after chemotherapy was administered. He finally died 7 years after the initial diagnosis of disseminated disease (multiple metastases of the embryonal carcinoma were noted at autopsy). The second patient underwent subtotal resection of an asymptomatic mediastinal pure seminoma 10 years ago, followed by radiotherapy. Four relapses (distant metastasis to the lower spine and pelvis, then intrathoracic and lymph node metastasis) have been treated by radiotherapy and chemotherapy as well as by surgery, with complete remission and return of elevated β-human chorionic gonadotropin levels to normal each time. He is currently alive with disease and about to undergo chemotherapy for a fifth recurrence.

Embryonal carcinoma (EC) occurred in 17 cases among the 56 patients reported by Knapp et al. (1985). There were 9 cases of pure EC, the rest were mixed tumors. Vogelzang et al. (1982) reported 2 cases of mixed EC (with yolk sac tumors). Knapp et al. had follow-up data on 15 patients: 12 died, on average 10 months after diagnosis. One survived 36 months with "reasonable control of tumor." Two are disease-free 8 and 102 months after diagnosis. Complete resection of the tumor was possible in the second case. Neither case reported by Vogelzang et al. (1982) survived.

Yolk sac tumors (YST), also known as endodermal sinus tumors, often occur as mixed tumors. Knapp et al. (1985) reported three cases of pure YST, which were all rapidly fatal, as were the two cases reported by Vogelzang et al. (1982). Kuzur et al. (1982) reported ten cases of mediastinal YST. All were unresectabe, and eight were fatal within 23 months; one patient survived with disease for 21 months, and there was one 5-year survivor without disease. Gooneratne et al. (1985) reported a similarly reserved outlook for these patients, as did Truong et al. (1986).

Choriocarcinoma is another aggressive lesion, which is also exceedingly rare in a pure form. Knapp et al. (1985) reported three cases, which were invariably and rapidly fatal. We do not know of any significant long-term survivors.

Mixed Tumors

Not only can the various types of germ cell tumors be mixed together, but one occasionally sees other malignant elements within these tumors (sarcomas, carcinomas). These are extremely rare lesions, but they are not invariably fatal (Ulbright et al. 1984; Knapp et al. 1985; Manivel et al. 1986). We have seen four cases of malignant, nonseminomatous germ cell tumors of the mediastinum. Despite aggressive treatment (surgery, radiotherapy, and chemotherapy in all four cases), they all proved fatal within 5 weeks to 11 months.

Einhorn (1985) has reviewed the recent progress in the treatment of testicular cancer. The introduction of first cisplatin, then etoposide and ifosfamide as both primary and salvage treatment drugs has revolutionized the outcome of patients with testicular nonseminomatous germ cell tumors. It is now possible to cure as many as 90% of these patients with chemotherapy, sometimes followed by "mop-up" surgery of residual masses. There is no reason why this progress should not apply to primary germ cell tumors of the mediastinum. Obviously, it will be several years before this can be documented, owing to the extreme rarity of these lesions (the 56 patients reported by Knapp et al. in 1985 reflect the Mayo Clinic experience from 1930 to 1982). Kay et al. (1987) reported improved survival in 12 patients with nonseminomatous primary germ cell tumors of the mediastinum who received cisplatin, vinblastine (or etoposide) and bleomycin chemotherapy. However, these results, as well as those reported by Gooneratne et al. (1985) and Truong et al. (1986), seem to indicate that these tumors have a less favorable prognosis than their testicular counterparts for they are often bulky and invasive at the time of diagnosis.

References

Addis BJ, Isaacson PG (1986) Large cell lymphoma of the mediastinum: a B-cell tumor of probable thymic origin. Histopathology 10: 379-390

Allum WH, Watson DCT (1983) Recurrent thymoma with myasthenia gravis. Br Med J 286: 440

Appelqvist P, Kostiainen S, Franssila K, Mattila S, Groehn P (1982): Treatment and prognosis of thymoma: a review of 25 cases. J Surg Oncol 20: 265-268

Argubright KF, Mattox JH, Messer RH (1984): Thymoma in pregnancy. Obstet Gynecol Surv 39: 185-191

Arriagada R, Gerard-Marchant R, Tubiana M, Amiel JL, Hajj L (1981): Radiation therapy in the management of malignant thymic tumors. Acta Radiol [Oncol] 20: 167-172

Aygun C, Slawson RG, Bajaj K, Salazar OM (1984): Primary mediastinal seminoma. Urology 23: 109-117

Barnes RDS, O'Gorman (1962): Two cases of aplastic anaemia associated with tumors of the thymus. J Clin Pathol 15: 264-268

Benton C, Gerard P (1966): Thymolipoma in a patient with Graves' disease. J Thorac Cardiovasc Surg 51: 428-433

Bergh NP, Gatzinsky P, Larsson S, Lundin P, Ridell B (1978): Tumors of the thymus and thymic region. II. Clinicopathological studies on Hodgkin's disease of the thymus. Ann Thorac Surg 25: 99-106

Bernatz PE, Khonsari S, Harrison EG, Taylor WF (1973): Thymoma: factors influencing prognosis. Surg Clin North Am 53: 885-892

Boumghar M, Saegesser F (1982): Tumeurs granulomateuses prétendues pseudo-Hodgkiniennes de la loge thymique (lymphogranulosarcomes thymiques). Ann Chir Thorac Cardiovasc 36: 134-136

Chahinian AP, Bhardwaj S, Meyer RJ, Jaffrey IS, Kirschner PA, Holland JF (1981): Treatment of invasive or metastatic thymoma: report of 11 cases. Cancer 47: 1752-1761

Cohen DJ, Ronnigen LD, Graeber GM, Deshong JL, Jaffin J, Burge JR, Zajchuk R (1984): Management of patients with malignant thymoma. J Thorac Cardiovasc Surg 87: 301-307

Colby TV, Hoppe RT, Warnke RA (1982) Hodgkin's disease: a clinicopathologic study of 659 cases. Cancer 49: 1848-1858

Denayer M-A, Rao KR, Wirz D, McNally D (1986) Hepatic metastatic thymoma and myasthenia gravis 22 years after the apparent cure of an invasive thymoma: a case report and review of the literature. J Neurol Sci 76: 23-30

Einhorn LH (1985): Cancer of the testis: a new paradigm. Hosp Pract [Off] 21: 165-178

Engel FL, Kahana L (1963) Cushing's syndrome with malignant corticotropin-producing tumor: remission and relapse following subtotal adrenalectomy and tumor resection. Am J Med 34: 726-734

Fechner RE (1969) Recurrence of noninvasive thymomas: report of 4 cases and review of literature. Cancer 23: 1423-1427

Fujimura S, Kondo T, Handa M, Shiraishi Y, Tamahashi N, Nakada T (1987) Results of surgical treatment for thymoma based on 66 patients. J Thorac Cardiovasc Surg 93: 708-714

Gooneratne S, Keh P, Sreekanth S, Recant W, Talerman A (1985) Anterior mediastinal endodermal sinus (yolk sac) tumor in a female infant. Cancer 56: 1430-1433

Gray GF, Gutowski WT III (1979) Thymoma: a clinicopathological study of 54 cases. Am J Surg Pathol 3: 235-249

Guillan RA, Zelman S, Smalley RL, Iglesias PA (1971) Malignant thymoma associated with myasthenia gravis, and evidence of extrathoracic metastases: an analysis of published cases and report of a case. Cancer 27: 823-830

Havliček F, Rosai J (1984) A sarcoma of thymic stroma with features of liposarcoma. Am J Clin Pathol 82: 217-224

Hu E, Levine J (1986) Chemotherapy of malignant thymoma: case report and review of the literature. Cancer 57: 1101-1104

Hutchison GB (1984): Radiotherapy of stage I and II Hodgkin's disease: a collaborative study. Cancer 54: 1928-1942

Jose B, Yu AT, Morgan TF, Glicksman AS (1980) Malignant thymoma with extrathoracic metastasis: a case report and review of literature. J Surg Onol 15: 259-263

Kay PH, Wells FC, Goldstraw P (1987) A multidisciplinary approach to primary nonseminomatous germ cell tumors of the mediastinum. Ann Thorac Surg 44: 578-582

Keller AR, Castleman B (1974) Hodgkin's disease of the thymus gland. Cancer 33: 1615-1623

Knapp RH, Hurt RD, Payne WS, Farrow GM, Lewis BD, Hahn RG, Muhm JR, Earle JD (1985) Malignant germ cell tumors of the mediastinum. J Thorac Cardiovasc Surg 89: 82-89

Korhonen LK, Laustela E (1968) Thymolipoma: report of a case. Scand J Throac Cardiovasc Surg 2: 147-150

Kuzur ME, Cobleigh MA, Greco A, Einhorn LH, Oldham RK (1982) Endodermal sinus tumor of the mediastinum. Cancer 50: 766-774

Le Brigand H, Verley JM, Gharbi N (1979) Tumeurs du thymus, vol 2. Encycl Med Chir, poumon, Sect. 6047 D10

Le Brigand H, Levasseur P, Miranda AR, Gaud C, Wojakowski I (1980) Résultats du traitement chirurgical de la myasthenie (284 cas de thymectomies). Ann Chir 34: 169-172

Lee YM, Jackson SM (1985) Primary seminoma of the mediastinum: Cancer Control Agency of British Columbia experience. Cancer 55: 450-452

Lewis BD, Hurt RD, Payne S, Farrow GM, Knapp RH, Muhm JR (1983) Benign teratomas of the mediastinum. J Thorac Cardiovasc Surg 86: 727-731

Lewis JE, Wick MR, Scheithauer BW, Bernatz PE, Taylor WF (1987) Thymoma: a clinicopathologic review. Cancer 60: 2727-2743

Maggi G, Giaccone G, Donadio M, Ciuffreda L, Dalesio O, Leria G, Trifiletti G, Casadio C, Palestro G, Mancuso M, Calciati A (1986) Thymomas: a review of 169 cases, with particular reference to results of surgical treatment. Cancer 58: 765-776

Manivel C, Wick MR, Abenoza P, Rosai J (1986) The occurrence of sarcomatous componants in primary mediastinal germ cell tumors. Am J Surg Pathol 10: 711-717

Masaoka A, Monden Y, Nakahara K, Tanioka T (1981) Follow-up study of thymomas with special reference to their clinical stages. Cancer 48: 2485-2492

Mauch P, Hellman S (1984) Mediastinal Hodgkin's disease: significance of mediastinal involvement in early stage Hodgkin's disease. Hematol Oncol 2: 69-72

Menestrina F, Chilosi M, Bonetti F, Lestani M, Scarpa A, Novelli P, Doglioni C, Todeschini G, Ambrosetti A, Fiore-Donati L (1986) Mediastinal large-cell lymphoma of B-type, with sclerosis: histopathological and immunohistochemical study of 8 cases. Histopathology 10: 589-600

Miller JB, Variakojis D, Bitran JD, Sweet DL, Kinzie JJ, Golomb HM, Ultmann JE (1981) Diffuse hystiocytic lymphoma with sclerosis: a clinicopathologic entity frequently causing superior venacaval obstruction. Cancer 47: 748-756

Monden Y, Nakahara K, Kagotani K, Fujii Y, Masaoka A, Kawashima Y (1984) Myasthenia gravis with thymoma: analysis of and postoperative prognosis for 65 patients with thymomatous myasthenia gravis. Ann Thorac Surg 38: 46-52

Mulder DG, Herrmann C, Keesey J, Edwards H (1983) Thymectomy for myasthenia gravis. Am J Surg 146: 61-66

Mullen B, Richardson JD (1986) Primary anterior mediastinal tumors in children and adults. Ann Thorac Surg 42: 338-345

Nakahara K, Ohno K, Hashimoto J, Maeda H, Miyoshi S, Sakurai M, Monden Y, Kawashima Y (1988) Thymoma: results with complete resection and adjuvant postoperative irradiation in 141 consecutive patients. J Thorac Cardiovasc Surg 95: 1041-1047

Namba T, Brunner NG, Grob D (1978) Myasthenia gravis in patients with thymoma, with particular reference to onset after thymectomy. Medicine 57: 411-433

Nomori H, Horinouchi H, Kaseda S, Ishihara T, Torikata C (1988) Evaluation of the malignant grade of thymoma by morphometric analysis. Cancer 61: 982-988

North LB, Fuller LM, Sullivan-Halley JA, Hagemeister FB (1987) Regression of mediastinal Hodgkin's disease after therapy: evaluation of time interval. Radiology 164: 599-602

Otto HF, Loening TH, Lachenmayer L, Janzen RWC, Guertler KF, Fischer K (1982) Thymolipoma in association with myasthenia gravis. Cancer 50: 1623-1628

Papatestas AE, Genkins G, Kornfeld P, Eisenkraft JB, Fagerstrom RP, Pozner J, Aufses AH (1987a) Effects of thymectomy in myasthenia gravis. Ann Surg 206: 79-88

Papatestas AE, Pozner J, Genkins G, Kornfeld P, Matta RJ (1987b) Prognosis in occult thymomas in myasthenia gravis following transcervical thymectomy. Arch Surg 122: 1352-1356

Perrone T, Frizzera G, Rosai J (1986) Mediastinal diffuse large-cell lymphoma with sclerosis: a clinicopathologic study of 60 cases. Am J Surg Pathol 10: 176-191

Raghavan D, Barrett A (1980) Mediastinal seminomas. Cancer 46: 1187-1191

Reintgen D, Fetter BF, Roses A, McCarty KS (1978) Thymolipoma in association with myasthenia gravis. Arch Pathol Lab Med 102: 463-466

Ridell B, Larsson S (1980) Coexistence of a thymoma and Hodgkin's disease of the thymus: a case report. Acta Pathol Microbiol Scand [A] 88: 1-4

Rosai J (1981) Thymic tumors and tumor-like conditions. In: Ackerman's surgical pathology, vol 1, 6th edn. Mosby, St. Louis, p 311

Rosai J, Higa E (1972) Mediastinal endocrine neoplasm, of probable thymic origin, related to carcinoid tumor: clinicopathologic study of 8 cases. Cancer 29: 1061-1074

Rosai J, Levine GD (1976) Tumors of the thymus. In: Atlas of tumor pathology, fasc 13, ser 2. Armed Forces Institute of Pathology, Washington DC

Rosai J, Levine GD, Weber WR, Higa E (1976) Carcinoid tumors and oat cell carcinomas of the thymus. Pathol Annu 11: 201-226

Rosenberg M, Jauregui WO, Herrera MR, Roncoroni AJ, Rojas OR, Olmedo GSM (1986) Recurrence of thymic hyperplasia after trans-sternal thymectomy in myasthenia gravis. Chest 89: 888-889

Rosenow EC, Hurley BT (1984) Disorders of the thymus: a review. Arch Intern Med 144: 763-770

Rubush JL, Gardner IR, Boyd WC, Ehrenhaft JL (1973): Mediastinal tumors: review of 186 cases. J Thorac Cardiovasc Surg 65: 216-222

Saegesser F, Zoupanos G (1970) Thymolipomes. Schweiz Med Wochenschr 15: 657-662

Salyer WR, Eggleston JC (1976) Thymoma: a clinical and pathological study of 65 cases. Cancer 37: 229-249

Shamji F, Pearson FG, Todd TRJ, Ginsberg RJ, Ilves R, Cooper JD (1984) Results of surgical treatment for thymoma. J Thorac Cardiovasc Surg 87: 43-47

Shimosato Y, Kameya T, Nagai K, Suemasu K (1977) Squamous cell carcinoma of the thymus. An analysis of 8 cases. Am J Surg Pathol 1: 109-121

Snover DC, Levine GD, Rosai J (1982) Thymic carcinoma: five distinctive histological variants. Am J Surg Pathol 6: 451-470

Thomas CV, Manivel JC (1987) Thymic carcinoma and aplastic anemia: report of a previously undocumented association. Am J Hematol 25: 333-335

Trump DL, Mann RB (1982) Diffuse large cell and undifferentiated lymphomas with prominent mediastinal involvement: a poor prognostic subset of patients with non-Hodgkin's lymphoma. Cancer 50: 277-282

Truong LD, Harris L, Mattioli C, Hawkins E, Lee A, Wheeler T, Lane M (1986) Endodermal sinus tumor of the mediastinum: a report of 7 cases and review of the literature. Cancer 58: 730-739

Uematsu M, Kondo M (1986) A proposal for treatment of invasive thymoma. Cancer 58: 1979-1984

Ulbright TM, Loehrer PJ, Roth LM, Einhorn LH, Williams SD, Clark SA (1984) The development of non-germ cell malignancies within germ cell tumors: a clinicopathologic study of 11 cases. Cancer 54: 1824-1833

Verley JM, Hollmann KH (1985) Thymoma: a comparative study of clinical stages, histologic features, and survival in 200 cases. Cancer 55: 1074-1086

Vogelzang NJ, Raghaven D, Anderson RW, Rosai J, Levitt SH, Kennedy BJ (1982) Mediastinal nonseminomatous germ cell tumors: the role of combined modality therapy. Ann Thorac Surg 33: 333-339

Waldron JA, Farber LL, Cadman E (1984) Primary large cell lymphomas of the mediastinum: an analysis of 18 cases. Lab Invest 50: 64A

Wick MR, Scheithauer BW (1982) Oat-cell carcinoma of the thymus. Cancer 49: 1652-1657

Wick MR, Scott RE, Li C-Y, Carney JA (1980) Carcinoid tumor of the thymus: a clinicopathologic report of 7 cases with a review of the literature. Mayo Clin Proc 55: 246-254

Wick MR, Carney JA, Bernatz PE, Brown LR (1982a) Primary mediastinal carcinoid tumors. Am J Surg Pathol 6: 195-205

Wick MR, Scheithauer BW, Weiland LH, Bernatz PE (1982b) Primary thymic carcinomas. Am J Surg Pathol 6: 613-630

Wilkins EW, Castleman B (1979) Thymoma: a continuing survey at the Massachusetts General Hospital. Ann Thorac Surg 28: 252-256

Wychulis AR, Payne WS, Clagett OT, Woolner LB (1971) Surgical treatment of mediastinal tumors: a 40 year experience. J Thorac Cardiovasc Surg 62: 379-392

32 Effects of Thymectomy in Human Oncogenesis

Angelos E. Papatestas*

Relationship of Thymus to Oncogenesis

The function of the thymus in the immunologic interactions between tumors and the host remains obscure, but ample experimental and clinical evidence indicates that both the presence of thymic abnormalities and the removal of the thymus have a crucial role in the development of extrathymic tumors. Thymic pathology is often present in diseases with increased risk of neoplasia, while following experimental thymectomy there is a marked alteration in the growth of neoplasms. Of considerable interest, because of the potential for clinical application, are the reports indicating that thymectomy may have an inhibitory effect on the development of neoplasms.

Background

Evidence of Protective Effect of Thymectomy in Oncogenesis

In the immunological surveillance concept (Burnett 1962), the thymus, through its control of the immunological mechanisms, is considered to inhibit neoplastic growth with T cells that may eliminate neoplastic cells. Tumor cytolytic activity of T cells has been demonstrated in in vitro studies, but in vivo studies show that frequently, contrary to expectations, tumor growth is inhibited in thymectomized animals. Experimental thymectomy is followed by an alteration in the incidence of tumors and a reduced occurrence of neoplasms such as mammary tumors, lymphomas and leukemias (Allison and Taylor 1967; Martinez 1964; Yunis et al. 1969). It appears, therefore, that the thymus may have both an enhancing and an inhibiting effect on neoplastic growth. Since naturally occuring tumors have either weak or no cell-surface neoantigens, thymus-dependent recognition of neoplastic mutant cells may not occur, and the presence of the thymus may not have an inhibitory effect on these tumors. Furthermore, the observations that thymectomy is followed by a decreased incidence of certain neoplasms such as mammary cancer suggest the presence of the thymus may be necessary for the development of certain tumors. Persistent thymic abnormalities and the presence of thymoma have also been linked to an increased susceptibility to neoplasia (Moertel 1966).

The consistent observations indicating that thymectomy protects against neoplasms in some animal models support the suggestion (Reinisch et al. 1977) that the thymus, with its suppressor cell population, inhibits the activity of tumor-cytotoxic cells, and that thymectomy, by abolishing suppression, protects against neoplasia.

Olsson et al. (1980) who evaluated the influence of T-lymphocyte deprivation on AKR mice pointed out that thymus-derived lymphocyte cells have a cytolytic potential against malignant cells with cell surface neoantigens. The leukemia growth inhibition observed in AKR mice that underwent thymectomy seems to be mediated by cytotoxic, fetal antigen negative, lymphoid cells that can be inhibited in their activity by thymus-derived cells. Olsson et al. (1980) pointed out that thymectomy may be an important antineoplastic weapon, but that side effects such as autoimmune reactions may occur. Experience with thymectomy in patients with myasthenia gravis does not indicate that thymectomy is followed by an increased incidence of autoimmune phenomena. Indeed, thymectomy seems to protect against other autoimmune diseases (Yoshimatsu et al. 1979).

The early studies showing a protective effect of thymectomy against mammary tumors, lymphomas and leukemias (Allison and Taylor 1967) have been confirmed in subsequent reports with different tumors. Reinisch et al. (1977) reported that thymectomy in young adult life prevents murine sarcoma-induced tumors in aging mice. In their study, 25 of 30 sham thymectomized mice given murine sarcoma virus developed lymphoma by 10 months of age, but only four of the 30 mice that had undergone thymectomy and been given virus developed tumors. They suggest that thymectomy may have a protective effect either by removing suppressor cells, which results in enhanced cytolytic T-cell activity against syngeneic tumor cells, or by

* Deceased

removing a lymphoid organ known to be a site of viral replication.

Most of the studies on the effect of thymectomy on experimental neoplasms focus on the development of tumors subsequent to thymectomy. The available evidence indicates that experimental thymectomy in breast cancer not only decreases the risk of development of breast cancer but apparently affects the course of the disease following tumor appearance. Peer et al. (1980) have reported a prolongation of survival in C3H MTV^+ mice following thymectomy and tumorectomy, suggesting that thymectomy as an adjuvant to surgical ablation of tumors may have a therapeutic role.

While the role of the thymus and the effects of thymectomy in experimental oncogenesis have been extensively investigated and reported (Allison and Taylor 1967; Martinez 1964; Yunis et al. 1969), there is a remarkable paucity of such reports in relation to human oncogenesis (Papatestas et al. 1971). It appears, however, that the presence of thymic pathology is associated with an increased frequency of extrathymic neoplasms and that thymectomy is not associated with an increased risk of oncogenesis (Doll and Kinlen 1970; Vessey and Doll 1971). On the contrary, it appears that thymectomy may play a protective role, similar to that observed in experimental tumors (Papatestas et al. 1971).

Thymectomy performed following the development of neoplasms in humans have been reported for leukemia, and Hodgkin's disease (Dean et al. 1951; Patey 1971; Surkovich et al. 1969). Goldstein and Mackay (1969) suggest that thymectomy should be performed in diseases that precede the onset of lymphosarcoma and chronic lymphocytic leukemia.

Evidence of Enhancing Effect of Thymectomy in Oncogenesis

Several reports indicate that the effects of thymectomy on tumor growth are not uniform, and increases in tumor growth have been reported (Yohn et al. 1963). The requisite for neoantigens is fulfilled by tumors induced by chemicals, carcinogens or oncogenetic viruses. Carcinogen-induced transplantable tumors have been reported to increase following thymectomy. Hirota et al. (1980) reported that the incidence of primary fibrosarcomas 2-4 months after intramuscular injection of 7,12-dimethylbenz(a)anthrazine (DMBA) was increased in thymectomized chickens inoculated at 4 weeks of age. No increase was seen in those chickens inoculated at 1 week of age.

Hirokawa and Hayashi (1980) reported that female B6C3F1 mice thymectomized at 6 weeks of age developed reticulum cell sarcomas more frequently (Dunn's A type), but their controls were not genetically identical to their experimental group.

Factors Influencing Effect of Thymectomy on Neoplasms

1. The timing of thymectomy appears to influence tumor growth, resulting either in tumor suppression or tumor enhancement, as demonstrated by Yamasaki et al. (1982) and Nagaya (1973). Clear evidence that the thymus may have an enhancing as well as an inhibitory effect on neoplasia is provided by Nagaya's experiment. Early thymectomy in AKR mice reduced the risk of neoplastic growth. Transplantation of a "young" thymus following thymectomy at a late age had a similar effect. In contrast, transplantation of an "aged" thymus following thymectomy at an early age increased the risk of neoplastic growth. Nagaya's experiment (1973) indicates that changes occurring in the thymus with age may be crucial to the leukogenesis in these mice.
2. Neonatal thymectomy has a different effect on tumor growth than thymectomy in adult life. Since removal of the thymus in the neonatal period is also followed by immediate and profound immunodeficiency, it is difficult to determine whether its effect on tumor growth is secondary to the immunodeficiency. Adult thymectomy is not followed by an immunodeficiency, but immunomodulation is evident (Janeway 1975; Kappler et al. 1974; Kerbel and Eidinger 1972; Simpson and Cantor 1975). Age at operation and the interval prior to tumor appearance influence tumor growth even in the adult.
3. Thymectomy may interact with other immune-metabolic mechanisms influencing tumor growth. Wagner et al. (1982) reported an interaction of dietary fat and thymus in the induction of mammary tumors by DMBA in female Sprague-Dawley rats. Thymectomy at 35 days of age exerted a protective effect in rats fed low- or normal-fat diets, and this was not reversed by thymic fraction V. Indeed, tumor incidence was decreased even further with thymosin. In rats fed high-fat diets, tumors were increased compared to the low-fat and normal-fat groups and the protective effect of thymectomy was absent.
4. Surgical technique seems to influence results as well. Roubinian et al. (1976) reported that when female BALB CFC3H mice are subjected to continuous suction thymectomy, a procedure that results in retention of thymic remnants, the latent period before tumor development is significantly prolonged. In contrast, when the animals are thymectomized by control suction, a procedure which removes thymic

lobes completely, there is no effect on mammary tumorigenesis. The results of his experiment shows that incomplete T-cell depletion causes premature onset of non-T-cell cytotoxicity, an augmentation of T-cell cytotoxicity and an alteration in serum blocking activity to mammary tumor target cells as tested in the microcytotoxicity assay. Complete neonatal thymectomy effectively and completely abrogates immune response to mammary tumor target cells.

Possible Explanations for the Effect of Thymectomy on Neoplasia

1. The protective effect of thymectomy against tumor development has been attributed to either an enhanced generation of cytotoxic T-cells directed against syngeneic tumor cells or the removal of a lymphoid organ known to be a site of viral replication. This concept is supported by the demonstration of suppressor effect of thymus cells in adult animals and by evidence that thymectomy has an immunoregulating effect, possibly by altering the generation of suppressor cells (Takei et al. 1978). Adult thymectomy decreases suppressor T-cell activity while increasing helper cells and cytolytic T-cell activity. Evaluation of helper/suppressor ratios at various intervals following thymectomy for myasthenia gravis showed an increase in most patients immediately following thymectomy, but 6 and 12 months after thymectomy the ratios were decreased, and 2 years following surgery very low ratios were observed. It seems, therefore, that thymectomy, at least in myasthenic patients, leads to a gradual decrease of the T-helper subset of lymphocytes (Berrih et al. 1983). In another study evaluating patients with myasthenia gravis 5 years after removal of thymus, there were no significant differences in the percentages of T, B, non-B and non-T cells (Wijermans et al. 1980).
2. Although immunological mechanisms may be responsible for the effects of thymectomy on oncogenesis, its effect may be mediated through changes in the hormonal milieu or in metabolic activity (Franks et al. 1975). Nardell (1973) has pointed out that thymectomy increased the concentrations of saturated fatty acids and in many instances reduced the concentrations of polyunsaturated fatty acids.
3. Hirokawa and Hayashi (1980) pointed out that adult thymectomy decreases the weight of the pituitary and adrenals in experimental animals, while Welsh et al. (1970) reported increased incidence of mammary tumors in the female rat grafted with multiple pituitaries.

Protective Effect of Thymectomy Against Mammary Tumors

The most consistent observation of an inhibitory effect of thymectomy on neoplastic growth has been reported for mammary tumors. Both neonatal and adult thymectomy inhibits growth of mammary neoplasms, and an inhibitory effect is noted even after tumor development (Peer et al. 1980). Roubinian et al. (1976) suggested that mammary tumorigenesis may be influenced by a balance of thymic regulatory factors. Thymectomy decreases the incidence and delays the appearance of spontaneous virus-induced, chemically induced and transplantable mammary tumors (Martinez 1964; Yunis et al. 1969).

Analysis of the Effects of Thymectomy on Oncogenesis in Myasthenic Patients

Increased incidence of extrathymic neoplasms in patients with myasthenia gravis has been previously reported (Papatestas et al. 1971, 1977). In addition, several other reports suggest frequent coexistence of myasthenia gravis and extrathymic neoplasms, both benign and malignant (Ferguson 1962; Verdy et al. 1960; Vogel et al. 1977; Zoupanos and Saegesser 1971). A previous report which included 133 neoplasms observed among 1693 patients with myasthenia gravis treated at the Mount Sinai Medical Center showed that thymectomy resulted in a decreased risk of cancer development in people with this disease (Papatestas et al. 1977). Doll and Kinlen (1970) and Vessey and Doll (1971) have also reported no increase in extrathymic neoplasms in myasthenic patients who have undergone thymectomy.

An updated evaluation of the risk of cancer development following thymectomy in myasthenic patients continues to support the concept that thymectomy inhibits neoplastic growth. The number of patients with myasthenia gravis followed up at the Mount Sinai Medical Center up to the year 1988 is 2136, among whom 199 (9.3%) had developed malignant neoplasms. The 2136 patients did not include those with neonatal myasthenia gravis. Two or more primary sites of malignant neoplasms were noted in 25 patients (12.5%), more than double the 5.1% incidence of multiple primaries reported by Moertel (1966). The occurrence of multiple neoplasms was highest in women. Twenty-three (16.6%) of 120 myasthenic women who developed neoplasm had a second primary. For the purpose of evaluation of the effect of thymectomy on extrathymic neoplasms, only first primaries were considered in the current analysis. Eighty (42%) of these

Table 1. Patients with myasthenia gravis (MG) followed up at the Mount Sinai Medical Center

	All patients	All neoplasms		Neoplasms after onset of MG		Neoplasms after thymectomy	
		n	%	*n*	%	*n*	%*
Patients without thymoma							
Males, no thymectomy	486	41	8.4	39	8	–	–
Females, no thymectomy	568	73	12.8	53	9.3	–	–
Males, thymectomy	273	23	8.4	15	5.4	9	3.3
Females, thymectomy	508	33	5.8	25	4.4	14	2.4
Total	1890	170	8.9	132	6.9	23	2.70
Patients with thymoma							
Males, no thymectomy	17	1	5.8	1	5.8	–	–
Females, no thymectomy	32	7	21.2	5	15.6	–	–
Males, thymectomy	95	14	14.7	9	9.5	7	8.4
Females, thymectomy	102	7	6.3	6	5.8	5	4.9
Total	246	29	11.7	21	8.5	13	6.5

* The asterisk indicates the percent of patients with neoplasms who underwent thymectomy

Table 2. Diagnosis of neoplasm in relation to decade of onset of myasthenia gravis

All patients								Patients with thymectomy		
Age at diagnosis of MG (years)	Number of patients	Total cancers		Cancers before onset of MG		Cancers after onset of MG		Total patients with thymectomy	Cancers after thymectomy	
		n	%	*n*	%	*n*	%	*n*	*n*	%
0–10	63	0		0		0		27	0	0
10–20	253	5	1.9	0	0	5	1.2	172	2	1.1
20–30	404	17	4.2	1	0.2	16	3.9	252	5	1.9
30–40	324	28	8.6	6	1.8	22	6.7	173	5	2.8
40–50	303	31	10.2	7	2.3	25	8.2	140	8	5.7
50–60	336	48	14.2	9	2.6	39	11.6	126	9	7.1
60–70	278	43	15.4	18	6.4	25	8.9	97	4	4.1
70–80	138	22	15.9	4	2.8	18	13.0	34	3	8.8
80–90	17	3	17.6	1	5.8	2	11.7	3	0	0
Total	2121	198	9.3	46	2.1	152	7.1	1024	36	3.5

were noted among women who had not undergone thymectomy. Patients who had undergone thymectomy had associated neoplasms less frequently than did those who were treated without thymectomy. This was more obvious in patients without associated thymomas (Table 1). In 46 patients (2.1%), the appearance of the neoplasms preceded the onset of myasthenia gravis. In 153 patients (7.1%) the diagnosis of a malignancy followed the onset of the disease. In 36 of the 1024 patients with thymectomy (3.5%) the neoplasms appeared following thymectomy. The proportion of malignant neoplasms was lower in all age subgroups of patients who had undergone thymectomy when the age of onset of myasthenia gravis was considered (Table 2). The occurrence of associated neoplasms after the onset of myasthenia gravis in relation to age of onset in patients without thymomas is shown in Fig. 1. All neoplasms occurring after the onset of myasthenia gravis are included. Patients who did not have thymectomy had the highest proportion of associated neoplasms in all age groups. Among patients with thymectomy there were 23 with neoplasms that occurred before the removal of the thymus. These were included in the evaluation of neoplasms occurring in patients who had thymectomy. Despite this bias, it is obvious that there are fewer extrathymic neoplasms at all ages among the group that had thymectomy. When only neoplasms occurring following thymectomy were

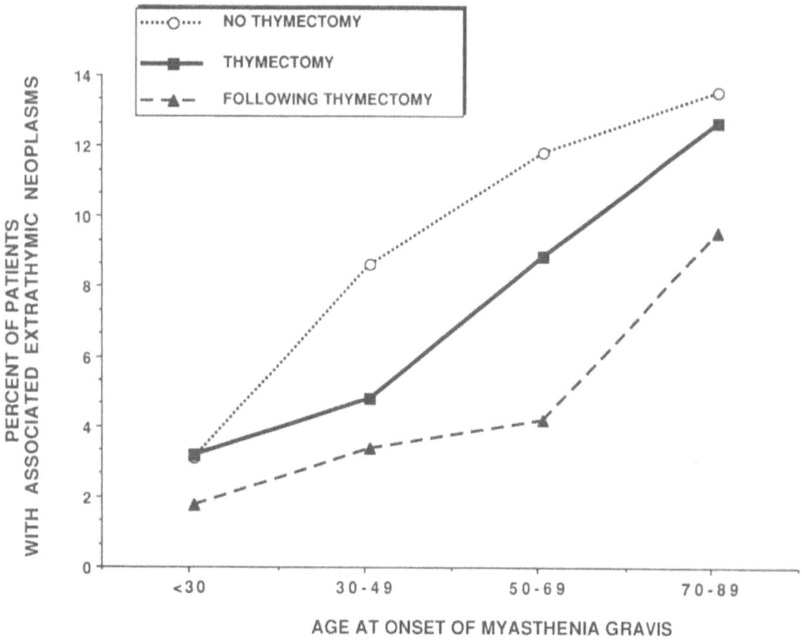

Fig. 1. Extrathymic neoplasms in patients without thymoma in relation to onset of disease. All neoplasms occurring following onset of myasthenia are included. *No thymectomy,* neoplasms in patients who did not have thymectomy; *thymectomy,* neoplasms in patients who had thymectomy, including the 23 tumors that preceded removal of the thymus; *following thymectomy,* neoplasms occurring following thymectomy

included in the group of patients who had thymectomy the differences became even more obvious.

Since a previous analysis indicated that the risk of neoplasia increases following the onset of myasthenia gravis, we evaluated what factors may contribute to the time of development of extrathymic neoplasms after the diagnosis of myasthenia gravis. The analysis was performed using a proportional hazards regression model (Cox 1985). Factors evaluated included presence/absence of thymoma, whether the patients had undergone thymectomy, age at the time of diagnosis of tumor or at last follow-up, sex, and presence/absence of remission. In order to establish the effect of thymectomy on development of extrathymic neoplasms without bias, three separate evaluations were performed. In the first, neoplasms developing after onset of disease but before thymectomy were considered as occurring in patients with thymectomy. The second analysis excluded such patients altogether, and the third analysis considered these neoplasms as having occurred in patients without thymectomy. This triple evaluation was carried out in order to investigate the possible bias introduced into the analysis by the group of neoplasms that occurred in patients prior to thymectomy.

In all three analyses (Tables 3 and 4) the results clearly indicated that the factors that contributed significantly to the early development of neoplasia were as follows:

1. *Age:* Older patients were at a higher risk.
2. *Presence of thymoma:* Myasthenic patients with coexistent thymic tumor were at a higher risk.
3. *Presence of thymus:* Myasthenic patients who underwent thymectomy showed a lower risk.
4. *Presence of remission:* Myasthenic patients who had reached remission had a lower risk.

These findings clearly demonstrate that thymectomy has a highly significant protective effect against extrathymic neoplasms in patients with myasthenia gravis.

Table 3. Factors influencing development of extrathymic neoplasms in patients with myasthenia gravis

Variable	Univariate p	Stepwise p	Coefficient/SE
Analysis 1: all patients = 1850, without neoplasm = 1726, with neoplasm = 124			
Age	0.0000	0.0006	3.4195
Thymoma	0.0042	0.0019	3.3545
No thymectomy	0.0003	0.0052	2.7452
Remission	0.0016	0.0228	−2.0884
Sex	0.0637	–	–
Analysis 2: all patients = 1843: without neoplasm = 1726, with neoplasm = 117			
No thymectomy	0.0000	0.0003	3.5327
Thymoma	0.0038	0.0007	3.6966
Age	0.0000	0.0023	3.0661
Remission	0.0005	0.0120	−2.2556
Sex	0.1405	–	–
Analysis 3: all patients = 1850: without neoplasm = 1726, with neoplasm = 124			
No thymectomy	0.0000	0.0000	4.3424
Thymoma	0.0042	0.0003	3.9434
Age	0.0000	0.0030	2.9689
Remission	0.0016	0.0423	−1.8777
Sex	0.0637	–	–

Table 4. Analysis in patients without thymoma

Variable	Univariate *p*	Stepwise *p*	Coefficient/SE
Analysis 1: all patients = 1643: without neoplasm = 1539, with neoplasm = 104			
Age	0.0000	0.0001	3.8149
No thymectomy	0.0000	0.0167	2.3269
Remission	0.0025	0.0267	−2.0196
Sex	0.0998	–	–
Analysis 2: all patients = 1637: without neoplasm = 1539, with neoplasm = 98			
Age	0.0000	0.0000	3.4143
No thymectomy	0.0000	0.0000	3.1227
Remission	0.0007	0.0013	−2.2142
Sex	0.1810	–	–
Analysis 3: all patients = 1643: without neoplasm = 1539, with neoplasm = 104			
No thymectomy	0.0000	0.0000	3.8818
Age	0.0000	0.0010	3.3016
Remission	0.0025	0.0501	−1.8027
Sex	0.0998	–	–

Table 5. Effect of surgical approach (all patients)

Variable	Univariate *p*	Stepwise *p*	Coefficient/SE
Excluding transcervical technique: all patients = 1215, without neoplasm = 1118, with neoplasm = 97			
Age	0.0002	0.0003	3.5945
Remission	0.0229	0.04546	−1.8079
Thymectomy	0,0631	–	–
Thymoma	0.0830	–	–
Sex	0.5241	–	–
Including transcervical technique: all patients = 1590: without neoplasm = 1488, with neoplasm = 102			
Thymectomy	0.0000	0.0003	3.3515
Age	0.0000	0.0010	3.3063
Remission	0.0002	–	–
Thymoma	0.0085	–	–
Sex	0.1735	–	–

Table 6. Effect of surgical approach (patients with thymomas)

Variable	Univariate *p*	Stepwise *p*	Coefficient/SE
Excluding transcervical technique: all patients = 1015: without neoplasm = 969, with neoplasm = 82			
Age	0.0001	0.0002	3.7220
Remission	0.0126	0.0268	−1.9409
Thymectomy	0.0081	–	–
Sex	0.4075	–	–
Including transcervical technique: all patients = 1506: without neoplasm = 1414, with neoplasm = 92			
Age	0.0000	0.0006	3.4564
Thymectomy	0.0000	0.0016	2.9412
Remission	0.0002	0.0042	−2.4274
Sex	0.1640	–	–

Indeed, in the third analysis it appears to be the strongest protective factor.

Since the presence of thymoma is a significant factor in the analysis, and thymectomy in patients with thymoma is not followed by the same results as those observed in patients without associated tumors, separate evaluations were carried out in patients with and without thymomas. The results indicate that thymectomy also has a protective effect against subsequent development of neoplasm in patients without thymoma (Table 4). In patients with associated thymomas no statistically significant protective effect of thymectomy was found. It should be noted that remission is less frequent in patients with associated thymomas than in those without thymomas and, as Saegesser and Zoupanos (1968) pointed out, immunologic abnormalities are not always corrected in patients with thymoma following removal of the tumor. These observations indicate that removal of the thymus in patients with thymoma may not have the same immunological effects as those observed in patients without associated thymic tumors.

Since the method of removal of thymus influences the effects of experimental thymectomy on tumor development, we evaluated the effects of thymectomy separately among patients undergoing operation via the transcervical and the transthoracic approach. The third type of analysis described above was employed. Tables 5 and 6 show that the protective effect of thymectomy is more evident among patients undergoing transcervical resection. Remission of symptoms of myasthenia remains an significant independent factor among patients undergoing thymectomy via approaches other than the transcervical.

We repeated the proportional hazards analysis among myasthenic women, focusing only on breast cancer following the onset of symptoms of myasthenia gravis. The purpose was to evaluate whether thymectomy has a specific protective effect against mammary tumors in myasthenia gravis. The analysis demonstrated such a protective effect.

Implications and Possible Clinical Applications

Most of the reports on the effect of thymectomy in oncogenesis deal with the protective effect of thymectomy against subsequent development of tumors. Thymectomy may have a protective effect against neoplasia even after the development of an extrathymic neoplasm, since Peer et al. (1980) reported that thymectomy combined with tumor excision in C3H mice with mammary tumors resulted in prolonged absolute survival, disease-free survival and survival following recurrence of tumor. Patey (1971) reported a benign clinical course in patients with Hodgkin's disease who underwent thymectomy.

The findings in the myasthenic patients strongly suggest that thymectomy in myasthenia gravis not only leads to a higher proportion of remissions than other treatments, but also inhibits neoplastic growth. Since thymectomy results in earlier remission of symptoms of myasthenia gravis when performed early in the course of the disease (Papatestas et al. 1975), and remission seems to be an independent factor having an inhibitory effect on the development of extrathymic malignant neoplasms, thymectomy should be the treatment of choice before there is progression of disease. There are reports that thymectomy arrests the development of symptoms of other autoimmune diseases besides myasthenia gravis. Yoshimatsu et al. (1979) reported good results with thymectomy in Behçet's disease, ulcerative colitis, chronic thyroiditis, systemic lupus erythematosus, autoimmune hemolytic anemia and Sjøgren's syndrome. In most of these autoimmune syndromes there is a high incidence of associated extrathymic neoplasms (Itoh and Maruchi 1975). The findings in myasthenic patients support the concept that thymectomy may have a similar effect in these diseases as well.

It is difficult to determine whether transcervical thymectomy has more of an inhibitory effect on the development of malignant tumors in myasthenic patients than transthoracic surgery. The strongest protective effect observed in our analysis, when patients were stratified into groups according to technique, supports the observation of Roubinian et al. (1976) that technique may play an important role in tumor inhibition.

References

Allison AC, Taylor RA (1967) Observations on thymectomy and carcinogenesis. Cancer Res 27: 703-707

Berrih S, Le Brigand H, Levasseur P, Gaud C, Bach JF (1983) Depletion of helper/inducer T cells after thymectomy in myasthenia patients. Clin Immunol Immunopathol 28 (2): 272-281

Burnett FM (1962) Role of the thymus and related organs in immunity. Br Med J 2: 807

Cox DR (1985) Regression models and life-tables. J R Stat Soc 34 (2): 187-220

Dean GO, Earle AM, Reilly WA (1951) Failure of thymectomy in lymphatic leukemia. AMA Arch Surg 63: 695-697

Doll R, Kinlen L (1970) Immunosurveillance and cancer: Epidemiological evidence. Br Med J iv: 420-422

Ferguson FR (1962) A critical review of the clinical features of myasthenia gravis. Proc R Soc Med 55: 49-52

Franks CR, Perkins RT, Bishop D (1975) The effect of sex hormones on the growth of HLA tumor nodules in male and female mice. Br J Cancer 31: 100-110

Goldstein G, Mackay IR (eds) (1969) The human thymus. Heinemann, London, p 304

Hirokawa K, Hayashi Y (1980) Effect of adult thymectomy on immune potentials, endocrine organs and tumor incidence in long-lived mice. Adv Exp Med Biol 129: 243-247

Hirota Y, Galton J, Lerman SP, Palladino MA, Thorbecke GJ (1980) Chemical carcinogen-induced transplantable fibrosarcomas in histocompatible chickens. II. Effect of age and thymectomy on tumor incidence. JNCI 65 (3): 595-601

Itoh K, Maruchi N (1975) Breast cancer in patients with Hashimoto's thyroiditis. Lancet ii: 1119-1121

Janeway CA Jr (1975) Cellular cooperation during in vivo antihapten antibody responses. III. The helper cell activity of activated thymocytes of spleen, cells treated with anti-theta serum, and of spleen cells from antithymocyte serum-treated or adult thymectomized donors. J Immunol 114: 1408-1414

Kappler JW, Hunter PC, Jacobs D, Lord E (1974) Functional heterogeneity among the T-derived lymphocytes of the mouse. I. Analysis by adult thymectomy. J Immunol 113: 27-38

Kerbel RS, Eidinger D (1972) Exhanced immune responsiveness to a thymus-independent antigen early after adult thymectomy: evidence for short-lived inhibitory thymus-derived cells. Eur J Immunol 2: 114-118

Martinez C (1964) Effect of early thymectomy on development of mammary tumors in mice. Nature 203: 1118

Moertel GG (1966) Multiple primary malignant neoplasms. Their incidence and significance. Springer, New York Berlin Heidelberg

Nagaya H (1973) Thymus function in spontaneous lymphoid leukemia: in vitro response of preleukemic and leukemic thymus cells to mitogens. J Immunol 111: 1052-1060

Nardell BE (1973) The effect of thymectomy on the fatty acid concentration of plasma, liver and fat pads. J Baltimore Coll Dent Surg 28 (1): 18-34

Olsson L, Ebbesen P, Hesse J (1980) Influence of T-lymphocyte deprivation on the antileukemic effect of bacillus Calmette-Guerin in vivo. Cancer Immunol Immunother 8 (4): 231-240

Papatestas AE, Osserman KE, Kark AE (1971) The relationship between thymus and oncogenesis. A study of the incidence of non-thymic malignancy in myasthenia gravis. Br J Cancer 25: 635-641

Papatestas AE, Genkins G, Kornfeld P, Horowitz S, Kark AE (1975) Transcervical thymectomy in myasthenia gravis. Surg Gynecol Obstet 140: 535-540

Papatestas AE, Kark AE, Genkins G, Aufses AH Jr (1977) Protective effect of thymectomy in a high cancer risk population. In: Nieburgs HE (ed) Prevention and detection of cancer. Part I: Prevention. Dekker, New York, pp 37-45

Patey DH (1971) A contribution to the study of Hodgkin's disease: late follow-up. Br J Surg 53: 387-389

Peer G, Papatestas AE, Tartter P, Bekesi G, Genkins G, Aufses AH Jr (1980) Effects of thymectomy on mammary tumor growth. J Surg Res 28: 348-355

Reinisch CL, Andrew SL, Schlossman SF (1977) Suppressor cell regulation of immune response to tumors: abrogation by adult thymectomy. Proc Natl Acad Sci 74: 2989-2992

Roubinian JR, Lane M, Slomich M, Blair PB (1976) Stimulation of immune mechanisms against mammary tumors in incomplete T cell depletion. J Immunol 117 (5): 1767-1773

Saegesser F, Zoupanos G (1968) Thymoma and acquired immunologic deficiency of immunoglobulins. Ann Chir Thorac Card 7: 535-541

Simpson E, Cantor H (1975) Regulation of the immune response by subclasses of T lymphocytes. II. The effect of adult thymectomy upon humoral and cellular responses in mice. Eur J Immunol 5: 337-343

Surkovich SV, Dolestkii SI, Dul'tsin MS, Kisliak NS, Makhonova LA, Koverzneva MM (1969) Thymectomy and X-ray of the thyroid gland in children with acute leukemia in the period of remission. Pediatriia 48 (5): 30-34

Takei F, Levy JG, Kilburn DG (1978) Effect of adult thymectomy on tumour immunity in mice. Br J Cancer 37: 723-731

Verdy M, Fauteux JP, Cadotte M, Cantin J, Boghes D (1960) Thyroid cancer and myasthenia gravis. Hum Pathol 11 (6): 690

Vessey MP, Doll R (1971) Thymectomy and cancer: a follow-up study. Br J Cancer 26: 53-58

Vogel JM, Kornfeld P, Forte FA, Jones RA, Genkins G, Papatestas AE, Horowitz SH (1977) Myasthenia gravis: association with chronic lymphocytic leukemia. NY State J Med (December) 2252-2256

Wagner DA, Naylor PH, Kim U, Shea W, Ip C, Ip MM (1982) Interaction of dietary fat and the thymus in the induction of mammary tumors by 7,12-dimethylbenz(a)antracene. Cancer Res 42: 1266-1273

Welsch CW, Jenkins TW, Meites J (1970) Increased incidence of mammary tumors in the female rat grafted with multiple pituitaries. Cancer Res 30: 1024-1029

Wijermans P, Oosterhuis HJ, Astaldi GC, Schellekens PT, Astaldi A (1980) Influence of adult thymectomy on immunocompetence in patients with myasthenia gravis. J Immunol 124 (4): 1977-1982

Yamasaki T, Tamashita J, Handa H, Namba Y, Nanaoka M (1982) Effects of adult thymectomy on the growth of 203-glioma - analysis of T-cell subpopulation in tumor immunology. No To Shinkei 34 (11): 1067-1075

Yohn DS, Funk CA, Kalnins VI, Grace JT (1963) Sex-related resistance in hamsters to adenovirus 12 oncogenesis. Influence of thymectomy at 3 weeks of age. J Natl Cancer Inst 35: 617-624

Yoshimatsu H, Ishikura Y, Murakami M, Kawahara H (1979) Clinical examinations of thymic abnormalities and significance of thymectomy in patients with myasthenia gravis and other autoimmune diseases. J Uoeh 1 (4): 487-505

Yunis EJH, Martinez EM, Smith J, Stutman I, Good RA (1969) Spontaneous mammary adenocarcinoma in mice: influence of thymectomy and reconstitution with thymus grafts or spleen cells. Cancer Res 29: 174-177

Zoupanos G, Saegesser F (1971) Thymic tumor, myasthenia, autoimmune thyroiditis, vesical papilloma. Two clinical case reports. Ann Chir Thorac Card 10: 191-196

Subject Index

MIX
Papier aus verantwortungsvollen Quellen
Paper from responsible sources
FSC® C105338

If you have any concerns about our products,
you can contact us on
ProductSafety@springernature.com

In case Publisher is established outside the EU,
the EU authorized representative is:
Springer Nature Customer Service Center GmbH
Europaplatz 3, 69115 Heidelberg, Germany

Printed by Libri Plureos GmbH
in Hamburg, Germany

family to work through, rather than react in maladaptive relational patterns, and promote healthier ones. However, it is important to remember that the clinician must always consult with the patient prior to involving any family members or friends (Jones et al., 2017). In the medical social worker's first meeting with Cynthia, she expressed that the change in responsibility of caring for their child was causing strain on her relationship with her partner. In addition, after trust had been established, Cynthia shared her personal history of an unreported sexual assault. A potential intervention for the social worker could be to support Cynthia with her immediate needs, which is to address not feeling heard and fear of sharing what she went through, and validation of her medical and trauma symptoms. As trust is formed, perhaps a referral to a trauma-informed mental health provider can be shared. One immediate intervention can be role-play with Cynthia to explore how she might discuss the change in roles with her partner, or, with permission, invite Cynthia and Victoria to meet with the social worker together to process the change in roles and what Cynthia is experiencing.

Chronic

Intrapersonal Most autoimmune diseases are considered chronic illnesses, meaning that the majority of individuals will remain in the chronic phase from diagnosis throughout the remainder of their lives. Moving from crisis into the chronic phase of an autoimmune illness, the medical social worker should continue to monitor and assess the client's mental well-being. Rheumatoid arthritis, MS, lupus, fibromyalgia, and other autoimmune diseases have a high prevalence of depression and anxiety (Bode & Taal, 2015; Dissanayake & Bertouch, 2010; Figueiredo-Braga et al., 2018). As we know from earlier in the chapter, emotional distress can induce flares, so attending to patients' psychological well-being over time can have significant impacts on their overall quality of life.

Dissanayake and Bertouch (2010) found that with RA, psychological factors consistently predicted more of the variance in an individual's level of physical functionality over time than did disease activity (Dissanayake & Bertouch, 2010). The intensity of negative affective states that is prevalent in individuals facing fibromyalgia has also been found to increase pain intensity, functional limitations, fatigue, cognitive deficits, and overall quality of life over time (Galvez-Sánchez et al., 2019). The medical social worker can play a significant role here by providing psychoeducation around the relationship between mental and physical health, as well as encouraging the individual to seek appropriate mental health care as needed.

Also in the chronic phase, the client is likely to experience cycles of symptom flares and potentially debilitating symptoms over a longer period. This means the person may experience a lower level of physical functionality and not be able to enjoy the same activities as they did pre-diagnosis. Decreased levels of functionality for those with autoimmune illnesses have been demonstrated to cause a decrease in self-esteem and negative body image perception (Galvez-Sánchez et al., 2019). Additionally, due to pain and fatigue, a person may not be able to work in the same capacity as they once did, or not be employed at all. Employment being a major component of life, this can have major ramifications on a person's perception of their self-efficacy and identity, as well as affecting a person's socioeconomic stability, ability to obtain health insurance, and, as a corollary, ability to pay for quality medical care. Furthermore, decreased physical ability typically leads to increased dependence on others. This further limits feelings of self-efficacy (Jones et al., 2017).

Interpersonal By the time a patient reaches the chronic phase of an autoimmune disease, it is likely that social roles of the client and their family and friends have shifted to adjust to the flares of pain, fatigue, and other symptoms. At times, this can cause tensions within the client's immediate social environment. Research has shown that the need to rely on a family member or friend for activities of daily living can have negative impacts on the relationship (Cowan et al., 2020). Over time, the need for caregiving can make a relationship feel unbalanced or one-directional, with one person primarily giving and another primarily receiving. For instance, romantic partnerships are ideally built on equitable shares of give and take, with both partners providing and receiving care and engaging in mutual activities together. However, if one romantic partner becomes a caregiver and the other a care receiver, the sense of mutuality becomes strained. The ability to share in enjoyable activities together can be lost, and with it, emotional closeness. The caregiver may feel resentment, and the care receiver may feel like a burden (Jones et al., 2017).

In a distinct but related problem, those in the chronic stage of an autoimmune disease may feel isolated. During flare-ups, the individual is likely to be unable to commit to plans with family and friends and may feel left out of once-enjoyed activities, a problem that can be more or less pronounced depending on their age and developmental stage. Young adults may be limited in their ability to go out with friends or start a family; parents may miss out on attending their child's sports game; older adults may not be able to spend quality time legacy building with their family. Chronic symptoms of autoimmune disorders may also adversely affect sexual health, which can put a strain on romantic relationships, further increasing feelings of isolation (Galvez-Sánchez et al., 2019).

Systems of Care Effective intervention within systems of care during the chronic phase of illness can have a significant impact on the individual's and family's quality of life. Due to the unpredictability of autoimmune diseases, the patient may have a length of time where they are doing relatively well, followed by a fluctuation in symptoms or progression of the illness. Flare-ups can lead to hospitalizations or trips to different medical professionals. Because flares often involve chronic, sporadic, widespread pain, and patients are at risk of being labeled and stigmatized as "drug seeking" within the healthcare system. The medical social worker should advocate for ongoing conversations around goals of care with the patient, support system, and care team as the disease progresses, to ensure everyone is on the same page regarding what is most important to the patient. Care coordination helps to avoid or exacerbate any medical trauma, i.e., frightening or life-threatening experiences brought on by missteps in care. It is also important that the interdisciplinary team are in frequent communication and actively listen to the patient's self-reports of symptoms and well-being. According to research by Bode and Taal (2015), the combination of pharmacological treatment for disease-specific activity, regular monitoring of self-reported symptoms, and ongoing mental health support is the most effective way to promote the highest quality of life for those with autoimmune diseases like rheumatoid arthritis (Bode & Taal, 2015). Thus, the medical social worker plays a pivotal role in providing the patient with or linking them to effective, ongoing mental healthcare, in addition to advocating for their voice to be heard in regular visits with medical providers.

Because treatment for autoimmune and rheumatic diseases is often both long term and determinative of progression, medical compliance can be both challenging and important to a person's health trajectory. Complicating life factors can interrupt adherence. A person who is pregnant with lupus, for instance, can discontinue medication before and during pregnancy and experience serious side effects as a result (CDC, 2018).

Medical compliance can be improved by close coordination of care, understanding of risk factors for noncompliance, and through open, frequent communication around the patient's goals for life, health, and care. A literature review on medication adherence in patients with autoimmune rheumatic diseases found that patient beliefs around medication necessity and increased knowledge of the disease were more significantly related to increased treatment adherence than specific economic or demographic factors (Anghel et al., 2018). Another study in the United Kingdom found that ethnicity explained a small amount of variance (with white patients having higher self-reported adherence than South Asian patients), though came to the conclusion that beliefs about treatment were more substantial in explaining nonadherence (Kumar et al., 2015). These findings identify a need for more research into the connection between beliefs about treatment and the impact of an individual's age, gender, ethnicity, or culture on those beliefs. Furthermore, they highlight the importance of obtaining a thorough assessment of the personal beliefs and health literacy from each patient.

There are several clinical interventions that can be utilized within the systems of care throughout the chronic stage of a client's autoimmune disease. In terms of therapeutic support, there is consistent evidence that cognitive behavioral therapy and mindfulness-based interventions are effective for those with rheumatoid arthritis and chronic pain (Dissanayake & Bertouch, 2010). Additionally, as highlighted previously in the chapter, those with autoimmune diseases who are experiencing frequent symptom flares may struggle with self-efficacy, self-esteem, and maintaining independence. Research has demonstrated that therapeutic interventions aimed at increasing a client's self-esteem may support positive self-efficacy, increase treatment adherence, and improve a client's adaptation to the illness experience (Galvez-Sánchez et al., 2019). By working with the client on their self-esteem and focusing on what is in their control, social workers may empower them to take action even as they struggle with feeling defeated or depressed. Another way to enhance adjustment is to integrate old and new self-conceptualizations, which can be done by encouraging the client to build awareness of the importance of socialization and some interpersonal relationships, and to maintain those pre-existing, meaningful social roles, and relationships that are possible now (Cowan et al., 2020). As an intervention, this can be done by exploring creative options for people to connect in a way that has as little variance from their life pre-diagnosis as possible. This could include planning less physically rigorous activities, scheduling social interactions around flares as much as possible, providing space to grieve what feels lost, and also encouraging self-compassion and grace when it is not possible.

Terminal

Intrapersonal Most autoimmune diseases are not terminal. However, in some instances, autoimmune diseases can progress to late stages, having detrimental effects on vital internal organs and causing other comorbidities that are themselves terminal. This may cause the client to face their mortality, which can induce feelings of fear, sadness, anger, grief, and loss. Exploring themes of spirituality and meaning may be of great importance for some patients at this stage of illness. If there are feelings of helplessness, despair, or loss of hope for an extended period, the individual may also experience demoralization. Due to the invisibility factor of these illnesses, although the patient is terminally ill, there also may still exist feelings of internalized stigma.

Interpersonal Caregiving needs are likely to increase exponentially as individual becomes significantly less able to care for themselves. It can be extremely difficult for friends and family to witness the person experiencing the suffering that can accompany terminal illness and end-of-life. Those close to the person may also experience anticipatory grief. Legacy work with clients and others in their world can promote healing and adaptability to the process if the patient is well enough to participate.

Systems of Care Due to the progressive effect on a patient's internal organs, that person may need to be in and out of inpatient care settings, such as nursing and rehabilitation centers, which can be disruptive to the patient's quality of life. Palliative care consultations are recommended when available, as palliative care's focus on symptom management and quality of life is consistent with autoimmune disease management. Palliative care consultations may not be made available as a matter of course with this group of illnesses, because autoimmune illnesses may not be properly understood as serious or life-threatening illnesses needing such services. However, if a patient's disease has progressed to the point of organ failure or another life-limiting diagnosis, palliative or even hospice care should definitely be considered. If not done already, goals of care and advanced care planning conversations are very important. Support from chaplain services can also be helpful if available and of interest.

Bereavement

Grief, loss, and bereavement are experiences that are woven throughout the lives of individuals and the systems in which they exist. Within the context of autoimmune diseases, grief is often experienced not simply in death, but also in a series of losses related to a patient's physical ability or role in society (Chancay et al., 2019; Cowan et al., 2020). The individual may incur many losses throughout the trajectory of their illness, which can often be disenfranchised due to the invisible nature of autoimmune diseases (Arora, 2013). These losses can also vary in tangibility and severity from person to person. For example, as the individual begins to lose their functionality, they may lose the ability to participate in activities of day-to-day life. Depending on age, developmental stage, and baseline level of activity, the loss of physical functionality can carry more weight for some than others. Loss of physical functioning due to pain or ability to utilize body parts affected by the disease can also lead to loss of ability to work, or role loss within the social environment (Chancay et al., 2019). With the nature of an autoimmune disease being that the body is attacking itself, and that bodily integrity is lost as a result, this creates difficulty for the client to trust themselves and their body.

Another loss that individuals with autoimmune diseases may grieve is the hope for a future that could have been. Due to the unpredictability of autoimmune diseases, specifically regarding the timing and course of disease progression and the degree of disability, patients and family and friends must also cope with a loss of clarity about what the future may hold and anticipate unknown future losses (Cowan et al., 2020). For example, research by Cowan et al. (2020) has found that many single adults facing MS do not actively seek a life partner, because MS has restricted their capacity to socialize and meet new people, creating a sense of lost opportunity (Cowan et al., 2020).

Caregivers, family, and friends may also experience feelings of loss as they bear witness to the individual who is facing the illness. Although they themselves are not experiencing the illness first hand, family, and friends may grieve for the person the patient once was. Depending on the specific illness and symptoms, the patient's mental health and/or affect may have changed significantly (Galvez-Sánchez et al., 2019; Figueiredo-Braga et al., 2018). In addition, with the loss of physical ability, their caregiver may not be able to participate physically in life like they once were able to, as the illness may limit traveling, shared hobbies, or sexual activity (Galvez-Sánchez et al., 2019).

If the person diagnosed with an autoimmune or rheumatological illness dies as a result of their illness, their caregivers, friends, and family will experience bereavement. The complexity of the bereavement experience will depend on several factors, including the relationship with the deceased and preparedness for death. Bereavement may be complicated by the stigma of invisibility surrounding rheumatological and autoimmune diseases, and the uncertainty of the progression of the illness. If the relationship is particularly close, or if other situational factors occur such as inability to be present at the time of death or uncertainty with the medical care provided, family and friends may be at higher risk of developing complicated grief (Shear, 2012), more recently defined as prolonged grief disorder (Prigerson et al., 2022).

For the medical social worker, it can be helpful to provide therapeutic support both throughout the illness trajectory and in bereavement (when applicable) from a grief lens. There may be times when the individuals and families facing an autoimmune illness may not have awareness that the emotions they are enduring throughout the series of losses can be identified as grief. If the medical social worker is able to seek clinical training in grief work and provide psychoeducation on grief and loss when appropriate, processing grief as it arises could be therapeutic for the patient and their friends and family. To limit disenfranchised loss and support patient well-being, it is important for an individual's experiences with loss to be supportively acknowledged without judgment (Arora, 2013). In addition, psychosocial support near end-of-life (when applicable) may lead to greater psychosocial outcomes for caregivers in bereavement. Increased communication between the caregiver and medical team, reduced sense of burden, and perceived preparedness for death are all factors that may positively impact the caregiver's bereavement process (Aoun et al., 2018). If the patient reaches the terminal stage of illness, medical social workers can focus on anticipatory loss with the patient and their family and friends.

Social Justice

There are known health disparities in incidence, severity, and course of some autoimmune diseases. Several autoimmune diseases disproportionately affect women and people of color (Amezcua et al., 2021; Office on Women's Health, 2019). The onset of certain autoimmune conditions such as rheumatoid arthritis has been associated with lower socioeconomic status (SES) (Parks et al., 2013). These are connected with environmental factors such as social determinants of health (SDOH). SDOHs are aspects of a client's social environment such as income, housing, neighborhood, food security, support system, level of education, and access to resources, which can have a significant impact on health outcomes. To use two examples of SDOH, geographic location and SES: A person with an autoimmune disease that requires regular visits to specialists such as rheumatologists and neurologists and who has a low income will more likely struggle to access equitable healthcare services and to remain "compliant" with care. Barriers such as distance from providers or lack of transportation make it difficult for a patient to be able to get to appointments and difficult to adhere to intensive treatment. This, in turn, will impact how a patient's disease progresses. To use access to nutritious food as another example: Patients with limited access to nutritious foods due to low socioeconomic status (SES), or who reside in food deserts, may be at higher risk for perpetuating an autoimmune condition, as research indicates the significant harmful impact of a diet rich in saturated fat and salts on some autoimmune conditions (e.g., Jörg et al., 2016).

Access to quality health insurance is another key component within the context of SDOH that can significantly impact a patient's experience with an autoimmune disease. As stated earlier, one of the keys to delaying progression and attaining remission is adherence to medical treatment. A patient with an autoimmune condition may need specific medications, equipment, or frequent medical appointments, depending on their disease and its impact. These aspects of care may not be attainable if a person does not have access to quality health insurance due to factors such as unemployment, low SES, or citizenship status. Without this access to care, the patient's disease may continue to progress. Stressors related to lack of resources may also contribute to or induce symptom flares, potentially causing more distress, and the patient can become stuck in a cycle of harm.

How does this appear in autoimmune disease? One study conducted by the University of Calgary showed how Indigenous individuals with arthritis tended to "tough out" their symptoms and connected this tendency with implicit racial bias leading to a harmful disconnect with providers (Hurd & Barnabe, 2018). It also suggested that several providers believed their Indigenous patients were somewhat responsible for their symptom flares and disease progression because they did not "buy into" arthritis care (Hurd & Barnabe, 2018). Such attitudes can perpetuate the disconnect between patients and their providers, especially if providers see only what they deem to be self-imposed barriers, and not the opportunity to work better with these patients.

Social justice being a core concept of social work values, the medical social worker's role can be pivotal when issues of healthcare inequality arise. Tackling systemic injustice may seem insurmountable, but the social work skills in advocacy and relationship building can be crucial to outcomes of the individual patients with whom we work. This looks like addressing bias as it occurs in the room and validating our patients' experiences. This also looks like joining with patients to advocate for them, while also empowering them to help themselves. There is still so much work to be done to dismantle the systems that create barriers for our patients in healthcare, and social workers play a major role in that journey.

Reflection Questions

1. How might the difficulty of early diagnosis impact a patient's trust in the healthcare system?
2. How might you introduce the idea of the losses experienced by the patient throughout the illness trajectory as something to grieve?
3. In what ways might patients of color experience an autoimmune disease differently than a white patient? How might you address this in your clinical work?

References

Amezcua, L., Rivera, V. M., Vazquez, T. C., Baezconde-Garbanati, L., & Langer-Gould, A. (2021). Health disparities, inequities, and social determinants of health in multiple sclerosis and related disorders in the US: A review. *JAMA Neurology, 78*(12), 1515–1524.

Anghel, L. A., Farcaş, A. M., & Oprean, R. N. (2018). Medication adherence and persistence in patients with autoimmune rheumatic diseases: A narrative review. *Patient Preference and Adherence, 12*, 1151–1166. https://doi.org/10.2147/PPA.S165101

Aoun, S. M., Ewing, G., Grande, G., Toye, C., & Bear, N. (2018). The impact of supporting family caregivers before bereavement on outcomes after bereavement: Adequacy of end-oflLife support and achievement of preferred place of death. *Journal of Pain and Symptom Management., 55*(2), 368–378. https://doi.org/10.1016/j.jpainsymman.2017.09.023

Arora, K. (2013). Spiritual direction as psychospiritual care for women with autoimmune diseases. In M. J. Stoltzfus, R. Green, & D. Schumm (Eds.), *Chronic illness, spirituality, and healing*. Palgrave Macmillan. https://doi.org/10.1057/9781137348456_3

Bidari, A., Ghavidel Parsa, B., & Ghalehbaghi, B. (2018). Challenges in fibromyalgia diagnosis: from meaning of symptoms to fibromyalgia labeling. *The Korean Journal of Pain, 31*(3), 147–154. https://doi.org/10.3344/kjp.2018.31.3.147

Bode, C., & Taal, E. (2015). Rheumatoid arthritis: Psychosocial aspects. Neil J. Smelser and Paul B. Baltes International encyclopedia of the social & behavioral sciences (2), 655-659 Elsevier.

Centers for Disease Control and Prevention (CDC). (2018, October 17). *Systemic Lupus Erythematosus (SLE)*. https://www.cdc.gov/lupus/facts/detailed.html

Chancay, M. G., Guendsechadze, S. N., & Blanco, I. (2019). Types of pain and their psychosocial impact in women with rheumatoid arthritis. Women's Midlife. *Health, 5*(3). https://doi.org/10.1186/s40695-019-0047-4

Chandrashekara, S. (2014). Current studies of biomarkers for the early diagnosis of rheumatoid arthritis. *Current Biomarker Findings, 4*, 107–119.

Cowan, C. K., Pierson, J. M., & Leggat, S. G. (2020). Psychosocial aspects of the lived experience of multiple sclerosis: Personal perspectives. *Disability and Rehabilitation, 42*(3), 349–359.

Dissanayake, R. K., & Bertouch, J. V. (2010). Psychosocial interventions as adjunct therapy for patients with rheumatoid arthritis: A systemic review. *International Journal of Rheumatic Diseases, 113*(4), 324–334.

Faurschou, M., Starklint, H., Halberg, P., & Jacobsen, S. (2006). Prognostic factors in lupus nephritis: Diagnostic and therapeutic delay increases the risk of terminal renal failure. *The Journal of Rheumatology, 33*(8), 1563–1569.

Figueiredo-Braga, M., Cornaby, C., Cortez, A., Bernardes, M., Terroso, G., Figueiredo, M., Dos Santos Mesquita, C., Costa, L., & Poole, B. D. (2018). Depression and anxiety in systemic lupus erythematosus. *Medicine (Baltimore), 97*(28).

Galvez-Sánchez, C. M., Duschek, S., & Reyes del Paso, G. A. (2019). Psychological impact of fibromyalgia: Current perspectives. *Psychology Research and Behavior Management, 12*, 117–127.

Hazes, J. M. W. (2003). Determinants of physical function in rheumatoid arthritis: Association with the disease process. *Rheumatology, 42*(Suppl.2), ii17-ii21.

Hurd, K., & Barnabe, C. (2018). Mortality causes and outcomes in Indigenous populations of Canada, the United States, and Australia with rheumatic disease: A systematic review. *Seminars in Arthritis and Rheumatism, 47*(4), 586–592.

Jones, B. J., Walsh, S., & Isaac, C. (2017). The relational impact of multiple sclerosis: An integrative review of the literature using a cognitive analytic framework. *Journal of Clinical Psychology in Medical Settings, 24*(3), 316–340.

Jörg, S., Grohme, D. A., Erzler, M., Binsfeld, M., Haghikia, A., Müller, D. N., Linker, R. A., & Kleinewietfeld, M. (2016). Environmental factors in autoimmune diseases and their role in multiple sclerosis. *Cellular and Molecular Life Sciences: CMLS, 73*(24), 4611–4622.

Kumar, K., Raza, K., Nightingale, P., Horne, R., Chapman, S., Greenfield, S., & Gill, P. (2015). Determinants of adherence to disease modifying anti-rheumatic drugs in White British and South Asian patients with rheumatoid arthritis: a cross sectional study. *BMC Musculoskeletal Disorders, 16*, 396. https://doi.org/10.1186/s12891-015-0831-8

MedlinePlus. (2021, March 31). *Autoimmune diseases*. U.S. National Library of Medicine. https://medlineplus.gov/autoimmunediseases.html

National Institute of Arthritis and Musculoskeletal and Skin Diseases (NIAMS). (2016, March). *Autoimmune diseases*. https://www.niams.nih.gov/health-topics/autoimmune-diseases#tab-overview

National Institute of Environmental Health Sciences (NIEHS). (2021, July 12). *Autoimmune diseases*. https://www.niehs.nih.gov/health/topics/conditions/autoimmune/index.cfm

National Institute of Neurological Disorders and Stroke (NINDS). (2019, August 5). *Multiple sclerosis information page*. https://www.ninds.nih.gov/Disorders/All-Disorders/Multiple-Sclerosis-Information-Page

Office on Women's Health. (2019, April 1). *Autoimmune diseases*. U.S. Department of Health & Human Services. https://www.womenshealth.gov/a-z-topics/autoimmune-diseases

Parks, C. G., D'Aloisio, A. A., DeRoo, L. A., Huiber, K., Rider, L. G., Miller, F. W., & Sandler, D. P. (2013). Childhood socioeconomic factors and perinatal characteristics influence development of rheumatoid arthritis in adulthood. *Annals of the Rheumatic Diseases, 72*(3), 350–356.

Prigerson, H. G., Shear, M. K., & Reynolds, C. F. (2022). Prolonged grief disorder diagnostic criteria—Helping those with naladaptive grief responses. *JAMA Psychiatry, 79*(4), 277–278. https://doi.org/10.1001/jamapsychiatry.2021.4201

Scott, D. L., Wolfe, F., & Huizinga, T. W. J. (2010). Rheumatoid arthritis. *Lancet, 376*, 1094–1108.

Shear, K. M. (2012). Grief and mourning gone awry: pathway and course of complicated grief. *Dialogues in Clinical Neuroscience, 14*(2), 119–128. https://doi.org/10.31887/DCNS.2012.14.2/mshear

Singh, G., & Hamid, A. (2021). Invalidation in fibromyalgia and rheumatoid arthritis and its effect on quality of life in Indian patients. *International Journal of Rheumatic Diseases, 24*, 1047–1052.

Young, A., Koduri, G., Batley, M., Kulinskaya, E., Gough, A., Norton, S., & Dixey, J. (2007). Mortality in rheumatoid arthritis. Increased in the early course of disease, in ischaemic heart disease and in pulmonary fibrosis. *Rheumatology, 46*, 350–357.

Chapter 2
Cancer and Oncology Social Work

Linda Mathew, Jacob Maier, and Annamma Abraham Kaba

Introduction

Cancer is a disease in which some of the cells in our body grow out of control and then spread to other areas of our body (NCI, 2021a). It is one of the leading causes of death worldwide, and the number of individuals diagnosed with cancer is growing. It is projected that almost 30 million individuals will be living with cancer by 2040 (Treanor, 2020). Cancer is a broad term that comprises dozens, if not hundreds, of diagnoses and illnesses (Fleishman & Messner, 2015). Diagnoses can be broken down into the categories of solid and liquid tumors. Patient experience varies vastly both within these two categories and between them. For example, the progression of a fast-growing solid tumor is different from the slow pace of chronic leukemia, which is a blood cancer and is considered a liquid tumor. Furthermore, the experience of a glioblastoma (GBM) brain tumor patient will probably be very different from the experience of a breast cancer patient, though both have solid tumor diagnoses.

As an oncology social worker (OSW), you will be working with patients and families either in the inpatient or outpatient (often called ambulatory) settings. Patients may be in acute emotional distress regarding their diagnosis, and/or they may be very concerned with how they will afford treatment while staying current on their mortgage and other bills. The wide range of patient and family experiences with cancer underscores the need for social workers to meet patients and caregivers where they are and provide empathic care throughout the treatment life cycle. It is crucial to remember that cancer is only part of a patient's identity, and often not the most important part.

L. Mathew (✉) · J. Maier · A. A. Kaba
Memorial Sloan Kettering Cancer Center, New York, NY, USA
e-mail: mathewl@mskcc.org; maierj@mskcc.org; abraham1@mskcc.org

M. Hemphill, A. Nathanson (eds.), *The Practice of Clinical Social Work in Healthcare*, Essential Clinical Social Work Series,
https://doi.org/10.1007/978-3-031-31650-0_2

Although the physical symptoms of cancer have long been studied, the psychological and social impacts of cancer have only become the subject of focused examination in the last 20 years (Holland, 2002). The subspecialty of psycho-oncology took shape in the mid-1970s, led by Dr. Jimmie Holland, to address the psychological social and behavioral factors that affect patients with cancer and their families. OSWs were the first to address the psychological and social problems of patients with cancer and they continue to be at the forefront of psycho-oncology care (Holland, 2002). The role of OSWs was shaped by evidence-based studies on distress management, caregiver burden, children's reaction to their parents' cancer diagnosis, and palliative care.

OSWs connect with patients and their caregivers at significant points of transition in the cancer trajectory, such as initial diagnosis, advanced or chronic disease, and end-of-life (EOL). The psychosocial tasks for patients with cancer vary depending on the diagnosis and whether the treatment is surgery, radiation, chemotherapy, immunotherapy, concurrent treatment, another type of therapy, or surveillance. Coping and adjustment to these tasks depend on multiple factors, such as health history, established coping strategies, and preexisting mental health issues. As you support patients, you may see them struggle with many emotional challenges, such as anxiety over the uncertainty of their diagnosis, depression related to a terminal prognosis, worry over the cost of treatment, anger regarding insensitive responses to the diagnosis by friends or family, or anger directed at themselves for the diagnosis, guilt over the inability to be a provider for their children, or something completely different altogether. Feelings of helplessness, uncertainty, and fear are also common patient experiences (Holland, 2002). This chapter will use case vignettes to highlight how social workers connect with patients with cancer and their caregivers during the initial, advanced disease, and end-of-life (EOL) phases.

Clinical Issues of Illness

Diagnosis

When a person is told "you have cancer," they often feel shocked, overwhelmed, or detached. A cancer diagnosis can precipitate a confrontation with the reality of one's mortality. The initial stage of the diagnosis brings stress about the risks and benefits of treatment; how to communicate with family members or children; how to negotiate work or school; and other uncertainties. Uncertainty, in fact, is a constant companion throughout all phases of the disease, and this often inflicts turmoil on everyday life. Many patients will approach their initial treatment with trepidation and fear, knowing little about the disease course, what they will be treated with, and how they will fare in treatment. Since there are so many unknowns, this initial stage can be overwhelming to absorb (Hartman, 2015).

As we consider these emotional stressors through a psycho-oncology lens, a case study may help to convey the emotional impact of cancer:

Mary was a 35-year-old, Latina, married woman and was diagnosed with stage IV endometrial cancer. She married her college sweetheart and they have a 4-year-old boy. She has four older siblings. She comes from a large close-knit extended family. Her mother died of the same cancer when Mary was a young child. Her mother had three older siblings and her death had a significant impact on the family. The similarities were understandably overwhelming for Mary as reminders of her mother's experience, especially given the advanced stage of the cancer. During her initial consultation with the OSW, Mary shared significant anxiety around starting treatment, especially with her family not being allowed to come into the chemotherapy suite with her due to COVID restrictions. The OSW connected with Mary by identifying and addressing the various sources of her fear, one of which was needle anxiety. The OSW used cognitive behavioral techniques to explore useful coping strategies with Mary. These included relaxation techniques and systematic desensitization that could be used when she came in for treatment. And, while Mary's sister was not allowed in the chemotherapy suite with her, the OSW encouraged Mary to have her sister on the phone while the needle was being placed and to let her sister's voice soothe her in these situations. The OSW and Mary also broke down the treatment day into manageable sections, with the OSW providing education on the pattern the schedule would follow, so that first appointments would not feel as overwhelming and she could focus on one hour at a time. The OSW would check in with Mary after each treatment to process how it went, what feelings came up, and if any adjustments might be helpful moving forward with her care.[1]

OSWs provide emotional support during the period following diagnosis by helping patients develop their support systems (internal and external), addressing barriers to care, and reviewing the information provided by the physician. OSWs can help patients adjust to the confusing oncological medical system and the language it employs. As time and treatment go on, OSWs can assess the patient's ability to retain and process complex medical information and work with the medical team to ensure patients fully comprehend their illness and all treatment options. OSWs can help patients process the anxiety, fear, and sadness that accompany the initial diagnosis and guide them through the decision-making process. They can meet with the patient and provide guidance on what to say to their children, family members, friends, or coworkers, and recommend tips that other patients found helpful during treatment. Psychosocial support during this initial phase of cancer treatment is critical, and so therefore is the OSW's role and availability to the patient (Hartman, 2015). In part, the support offered by the OSW amounts to empowerment, e.g., breathing or guided imagery techniques that may alleviate anxiety, insomnia,

[1] All names and other personal identifiers in the case are fictitious. Any similarity to actual persons, living or dead, or actual events is purely coincidental.

feelings of breathlessness, or nausea also serve to give patients a greater sense of control over themselves and the treatment process. OSWs provide crisis intervention to help strengthen existing coping strategies, cognitive behavioral therapy techniques to help reduce anxiety and fear, and problem-solve any practical concerns related to access to cancer care (e.g., financial resources, temporary housing, and transportation).

Advanced Disease

"Advanced disease" is defined as a phase of the disease trajectory in which disease is so extensive, and available effective treatments so limited, that a person cannot be cured, but in which the patient has not entered EOL (Harley et al., 2012). Advanced disease can be managed for months and even years with treatment, or may enter a repeating cycle of remission and recurrence (Boerger-Knowles & Ridley, 2014). Living with advanced cancer can bring about permanent changes in an individual's lifestyle and view of life, as they balance thoughts about their mortality with intentions to live their remaining life well, and/or efforts to live for many years with a good quality of life (Damaskos & Gerbino, 2014). The psychosocial impact of advanced disease may depend on treatment options available and prognosis (Boerger-Knowles & Ridley, 2014). For example, patients with advanced pancreatic cancer have fewer treatment options than those with metastatic breast cancer and may be expected to feel differently about their advanced disease as a result. Advanced disease will lead to EOL, at which point a patient may be referred, or self-refer, to hospice care. This case study highlights a patient's existential crisis while facing EOL, and how the OSW held this space as the patient and her husband processed their thoughts and feelings:

Kristine was a 56-year-old Black, cisgender woman, with advanced chondrosarcoma whose condition had sharply declined. Kristine had recently been told there were no further disease-modifying treatment options for her. After speaking with her family, Kristine determined that home hospice would be the best next step for her. Kristine had expressed concerns to her OSW about how her illness and death would affect her family, especially her two children, who were 20 and 17 years old. Kristine was a high-level executive and the primary breadwinner for her family and was still grieving the loss of her independence. She had recently lost the ability to move her legs and had been considering how the lack of mobility would impact her life going forward. Her husband, Dan, had concerns for his wife and children as well. He was curious and afraid about how Kristine would die. He felt the need to have as much information as possible but also found himself getting overwhelmed.

The OSW worked with Kristine, her husband, and her daughter, Olivia, on processing the feelings they had related to Kristine's decline. These discussions were aimed at addressing individual and familial responses to Kristine's death and strengthening coping for both the family unit and each individual. The OSW helped Dan to consider how he would feel about getting more information about his wife's decline. Kristine began exploring with her OSW the concepts of death and dying. She was hoping for some views on life and death that might resonate with her during this time of confusion, loss, and grief. The OSW provided psychoeducation about grief at EOL, normalizing it and explaining how grief may be experienced not only for the past but also for an imagined future that will not be. Additionally, Kristine and Dan worked on ways to build and share her legacy with their children.[1]

Helping patients and families cope with advanced disease is a frequent psychosocial support task for OSWs. This phase often includes a decline in physical functioning, which can create increased stress for families as they help the patient navigate activities of daily living. Empowering patients to ask for help when they need it, set healthy boundaries with friends and family, and communicate about their disease effectively and authentically are common tasks during this phase. As indicated in Kristine's situation, it is also important to remember that a patient and their caregiver may have different needs when it comes to psychosocial support. A patient may not want to know every detail related to their diagnosis and prognosis, while a caregiver may feel they need that information to feel more in control. Conversely, the patient may be the one eager to understand their medical situation in detail, or all parties may fall somewhere in between. While families do often act as a unit, it is important for the OSW to learn how each part of that unit functions, and how to support individuals separately. This intimate understanding of a family can help OSWs support the relationship between the patients, families, and a medical team.

For some patients, the progression of disease is even more stressful than the initial diagnosis. They can become discouraged about treatment failure, limited treatment options, and processing the reality that they will have to live henceforth within an ongoing cycle of treatments. Patients with advanced cancer have a unique understanding of their emotional or physical state, since they navigate constant challenges and burdens arising from their disease. Family and friends, however much they care, do not face the same burdens, and this chasm may increase tension and anxiety within the patient's support system.

Thanks to advancements in medical interventions, cancer is becoming a disease that can be managed over longer and longer periods. In the cases of many cancers, people are quite likely to live for years with advanced disease and to be in a position to live meaningful lives while undergoing episodic treatment and holding the knowledge that their lives are truncated. The ability to provide counseling to individuals living with advanced cancer is thus an increasing priority for OSWs. In supporting patients with advanced disease, OSWs must keep in mind the psychological, spiritual, and social concerns that distinguish this phase in the cancer journey, and be mindful that they are often the most difficult for patients and their support system.

In advanced disease, there is an opportunity to visualize and articulate a new vision of hope that embraces a time frame of day-to-day or month-to-month. There is some grief when hope for certain disease outcomes changes to hope for a meaningful life, however, shortened. Indeed, one-way OSWs can support patients with advanced cancer is by exploring what hope means to them. Hope can be a multidimensional concept that encompasses spirituality and existential issues, such as making meaning in the contemplation of their life. Research shows that living with hope helps people with advanced cancer adjust to their illness, can reduce their psychological distress, and can enhance their psychosocial well-being and quality of life (McClement & Chochinov, 2008; Kyngäs et al., 2001). Hope enables patients with cancer to cope with difficult situations and suffering. OSWs are in a unique position to foster hope during this time of suffering by giving information in an honest and compassionate way and letting patients know how others have coped through similar situations.

When EOL is reached, the need to integrate palliative care, which focuses on relieving physical symptoms and tries to achieve the best possible quality of life while addressing physical, psychological, and spiritual pain and suffering, is critical for patients and their intimate network of support (Altillo & Tropeano, 2015). Those with advanced disease may tap into their strengths through this process and will be reminded of how much knowledge, skill, and support they have already developed since their initial diagnosis.

Advanced cancer has the potential to strip away the sense of self that may have stabilized after a patient's initial cancer diagnosis and treatment (Ezra & Chi, 2015). This progression of cancer compels patients to revisit their mortality and find a sense of meaning and purpose in their lives. Meaning-Centered Psychotherapy (MCP), an existential psychotherapy with dozens of empirically supported adaptations, was developed to help patients with advanced cancer find a sense of meaning and purpose in their lives (Breitbart et al., 2010). The role of the OSW is *not* to *force* conversations that patients are not ready to have, but to assess what the patient understands about where they are in the disease trajectory and to help them find stability. OSWs honor the patient's thoughts to choose their own path by respecting their autonomy. This balance of hope and dealing with reality is essential.

Body Image

Many cancer treatments result in changes to a person's body. Surgical interventions can leave scars, remove body parts, and alter a person's appearance drastically. Breast cancer patients who undergo a mastectomy are challenged to cope with the loss of one or both breasts and the impact of this loss on their sense of identity and their self-esteem. Patients who must have portions of their colon removed must use colostomy bags to expel feces and urine and change these bags throughout the day. In cancers that involve the sexual organs, lifesaving procedures can drastically alter sexual functioning, or even result in the complete removal of internal/external sexual organs. These changes may be experienced as losses and can be accompanied by a grieving process, which is commonly seen in patients who experience alopecia (loss of hair) as a result of treatment (Dougherty, 2007). Such body changes are also visible reminders to patients of cancer and can therefore impact their psychological and social coping (Bahrami et al., 2017). OSWs can support patients through these changes by helping them reflect on what body image means to them and helping them develop a new sense of how they feel inside their body, not just their appearance. The practice of acceptance around these changes and the incorporation of "cancer" as part of one's identity, but not all of it, are major foci of psychosocial support around body image.

Psychosocial Interventions

A cancer diagnosis usually comes as a huge shock to patients and their families. With the help of family, friends, social support networks, and existing coping structures, most patients find equilibrium as they navigate living with cancer. However, some patients and families need more external psychosocial support than others. In one study, approximately 19% of patients with cancer have unmet psychosocial needs, while 9% of patients are currently utilizing psychosocial support services (Ernstmann et al., 2009). Another study looked at the racial disparities related to unmet needs and it revealed that African Americans and Hispanics expressed having unmet needs related to financial, practical, and emotional than whites (Sánchez-Díaz et al., 2021). Furthermore, the incidence of depression and anxiety is higher amongst patients with cancer than the general population (NCI, 2021b). Literature suggests that patients who are seeking support in coping with their diagnosis or treatment have a strong preference for counseling with an oncology social worker over a purely psychopharmacological intervention (Arch et al., 2018).

Utilizing a trauma-informed approach in the oncology field is crucial to support patients throughout their treatment. Because we are unaware of the trauma our patients experienced prior to their diagnosis, it is important to assess and explore the prior history of trauma that a cancer diagnosis can reactivate. By understanding our patients' past traumas, OSWs provide a sensitive, trauma-informed practice approach to their cancer care. Supportive counseling that facilitates reflection on past traumatic events, and how they relate to the cancer experience, will prevent re-traumatization of patients, while giving space to process trauma past and present (Lawson & Lawson, 2018).

There are many other interventions an OSW can use to help patients and families cope with cancer. Normalization and validation are two of the most basic and effective ways to provide emotional support. Patients and caregivers may feel that they are the only ones who feel the way they do. A simple, sincerely rendered statement of "you are not alone" or "that is a perfectly normal way to feel given what you have been through" can bring a patient tremendous relief. Cognitive behavioral therapy (CBT) and other cognitive therapies can help decrease fatigue and promote physical and emotional well-being across different cancer diagnoses (Daniels & Kissane, 2008). Mind-body interventions (which can include CBT, meditation, yoga, breathing exercises, etc.) were found to help reduce the fear of recurrence amongst survivors across diagnoses as well (Hall et al., 2018). MCP, which focuses on developing a sense of meaning and spiritual well-being, has also been proven to increase the quality of life amongst cancer patients (Breitbart et al., 2018). The common thread among all these interventions is the rapport that OSWs must build with patients and their caregivers, one based on trust and genuine empathy (Cameron, 2014). In a world where most people avoid conversations about illness or death, the ability to listen deeply and simply *be present* with a cancer patient offers much value.

Survivorship

Survivorship is a distinct phase with unique emotional, physical, and practical stressors (Damaskos & Parry, 2015). To the layperson, the idea of "surviving" cancer may suggest only positive thoughts, but the reality is very different. For example, a nearly universal emotional experience amongst cancer survivors is the fear of recurrence, anger and powerlessness that it happened at all, and grief for the self, life, and future plans that existed before cancer. The National Cancer Institute defines a cancer survivor as anyone who has been diagnosed with cancer, at any phase of treatment (NCI, 2021a). However, for the purposes of this chapter, survivorship can be refined to mean the period after active treatment has ended, when a patient is either deemed "cured" or remains on maintenance therapy.

Survivorship, by this definition, is becoming a more widespread reality: With the success of newer targeted therapies, we have seen an increased number of people living with cancer as a chronic illness (Damaskos & Parry, 2015). Fear of recurrence can be exacerbated by the sometimes sudden transition from active treatment to longer-term, maintenance care. During active treatment, patients may have multiple appointments in a week. Such a treatment schedule can be exhausting and onerous, but the frequent contact with the medical team often provides a level of comfort and reassurance. In the survivorship phase, a salient challenge is adjusting to less frequent testing and contact with the medical team.

During this process, the patient is regaining both physical and emotional wellness. The object is to accept their new level of functioning and reintegrate their sense of self while returning to life and community outside of the hospital. This is a dynamic process that involves reorganizing their self-concept, concurrent with reevaluating personal abilities (physical, cognitive, emotional, social, psychosocial, and spiritual) (Ore & Foli, 2020). This is often referred to as establishing a "new normal," rather than returning to the old "norms" of life.

Theresa was a 25-year-old, Asian American, non-binary person diagnosed with osteosarcoma. Theresa experienced several adolescent and young adult (AYA)-related concerns following their cancer diagnosis and start of treatment. Upon starting treatment, Theresa had to stop working in the career field they had recently entered and return to living with their parents for emotional and financial support. These changes brought up issues related to their cultural and religious communities, which impacted aspects of her identity and perception of their illness. During the treatment, Theresa expressed concerns related to body image and a diminished sense of self following changes in their physical appearance. The OSW working with Theresa provided emotional support and counseling around multiple areas of concern, including how disclosure of the diagnosis influenced their dating experience, especially within the context of their gender and cultural identities. Exploration and support were provided around sexual health and intimacy, as well as changing dynamics of peer relationships, and a growing sense of isolation. Along with supportive counseling with their OSW, Theresa benefited greatly from finding space to process their experience with other young adult patients through support groups and similar programs. They also established care with a staff psychologist to gain further support around the genetic component of their disease and long-term impacts.[1]

As illustrated in Theresa's story, OSWs can help cancer survivors and their families by enhancing coping skills to manage the uncertainty of this phase. By providing a space to vent frustrations and fears, OSWs can help normalize the confusing emotions that come with life after cancer. OSWs' role is to help survivors learn to live in the present and to sustain a balance between living in the here and now and comprehending an uncertain future (Damaskos & Parry, 2015). Population-specific support groups (e.g., by diagnosis, or demographic, such as AYA) can also be healing spaces, where patients and families are able to obtain support from others who understand their struggles intrinsically. Psychoeducational programs that offer guidance on how to navigate life after cancer are one of many interventions that cancer survivors find beneficial.

End-of-Life (EOL)

Understandably, the stage of EOL can cause significant distress in the patient and their immediate support system. The degree to which it does cause distress depends, in part, on the patient's preparation for it and acceptance of its approach. While palliative care can be involved at any point in the disease journey for the management of pain and discomfort, it is more common at this stage. Involvement of a palliative care team (that may have a social worker within it) can further help with decision-making about entering hospice or continuing with treatment, optimizing function and quality of life, and providing opportunities for personal growth. During this time, OSWs can support patients with cancer as they experience anticipatory loss, helping patients create a legacy activity that will remain with the family after they die.

James was a 37-year-old cisgender, Indian man with metastatic colorectal cancer. He and his life partner, Katie, had a daughter who was 5 years old. James had undergone several lines of treatment that failed and when he met with the OSW he was already connected to the palliative care team. James expressed his fears about dying and leaving his partner to raise their daughter. He reflected on the impact of his own mother's death when he was a teenager and the abandonment he felt. James wanted to leave knowing that his daughter would not feel abandoned. The OSW explored legacy planning with James and his partner. The OSW spent time helping James reflect on the process of leaving something for his daughter. The legacy projects included a video recording of him sharing his wishes for his daughter; a scrapbook of pictures; keepsakes; and a video montage of their memories together as a family. James spent the remainder of his time (approximately one and a half years) putting together a slideshow and a video of small family moments that both Katie and his daughter could hold on to. When he finished the legacy projects, he shared with the OSW that he felt a sense of completeness, and at peace with a confidence that his daughter would feel loved.

A life review explores a patient's value and contribution to their family and helps them process the reality of leaving behind people they care about; family focused grief work guides the patient's intimate network through their feelings of sadness, loss, and guilt (Kissane et al., 2006). When confronted with EOL, patients turn to OSWs to provide counsel, solace, and guidance. OSWs must keep in mind that caring for someone at EOL includes caring for their family and their intimate network of support. Another increasingly important concern for OSWs who care for patients at the EOL is their spiritual well-being and sense of meaning and purpose in life (Breitbart et al., 2010). OSWs are uniquely positioned to provide opportunities for sacred rituals that will impact both the patient and their support network. You can do this by exploring what rituals are important for the patient and family, how they want to say goodbye, and also whether they want a funeral or memorial service.

One intervention that oncology social workers can explore with cancer patients is Dignity therapy. Dignity therapy addresses existential distress among patients with advanced disease. It helps to alleviate suffering and create a sense of hope and purpose in patients with advanced cancer (McClement et al., 2007). It is a process in which a dying patient reflects on elements in their life that are important to them, and that they would most want family and friends to remember. The sessions are tape recorded and written out for the patient to give to their family and friends (McClement et al., 2007).

Caregivers have their own emotional responses to patients' diagnoses and prognoses, and they may require emotional support separate from that offered to patients (Mathew & Fulton, 2017). And, since cancer patients are living longer due to ever-improving treatments, the emotional implications of long-term caregiving are significant.

Caregivers' emotional responses can fluctuate in response to a patient's prognosis, stage of illness, and goals of care (GOC), as well as their own psychosocial and developmental stressors. The physical and emotional demands of caregiving often become more pronounced as the disease progresses to EOL. In the context of advanced illness, the caregiver must meet a new set of challenges in dealing with increasing functional limitations and dependence of the patient (Williams, 2014). Uncertainty about the future and disease trajectory can increase caregivers' anxiety and stress levels. There is often tremendous guilt for caregivers in acknowledging feelings of burden and need for individuation in caring for someone important to them, depending on cultural, age, and gender norms and the nature of the relationship with the patient. Not all caregivers will experience this role as a burden, but many will, at least in parts. Psychological and physical outcomes are mediated by the juxtaposition of the caregiver burden with the positive aspects of their role. These positive aspects can function as an opportunity for growth and satisfaction, as caregivers become more connected to the ones they are caring for. Between partners, it can be an opportunity for increased intimacy. The caregiving role can also provide an opportunity to repay care received earlier when roles were reversed, and often provides an increased sense of purpose or meaning in caregivers' lives (Mathew & Fulton, 2017).

To support caregivers, OSWs should assess the nature and quality of the preexisting patient–caregiver relationship. This will help to better understand communication patterns and mechanisms of mutual support. A history of ruptured attachment, or close enmeshment, in the relationship will impact how caregiving is experienced by both the caregiver and the patient. If the impact of caregiving is identified and assessed early in the treatment trajectory, effective interventions to meet the needs of caregivers can be recommended. These include (but are by no means limited to) caregiver-specific support groups, individual counseling for the caregiver, and couples counseling (Mathew & Fulton, 2017).

Bereavement

Each year approximately 600,000 people die from cancer in the United States (NCI, 2021a). Palliative care social workers, who may or may not be involved with EOL and bereavement, comprise the largest group of mental health professionals in hospice and palliative care (Blacker & Christ, 2011). Both suggest the need for OSWs to be versed in bereavement support. When a patient with cancer dies, it affects all those in their social support system, each of whom will cope differently. A bereaved person's attitude and reactions are shaped by cultural and spiritual values, as well as by their relationship with the person who died. It is important to remember that not every patient is automatically a "loved one" to their caregiver; that is to say, a history of trauma and/or conflict may be present in the relationships you encounter as an OSW.

It takes time for members of the bereaved support system to re-establish balance. Bereavement counseling has been shown to reduce the level of distress that mourners go through after the death of the patient (Blacker & Christ, 2011). Bereavement counseling (individual and support groups) may help the bereaved process their grief reactions, normalize them and, as a result, adjust to their new lives without the deceased. As bereavement support becomes an integral part of palliative cancer care, the adaptation of bereavement interventions with a focus on different cultures is crucial because it will increase the effectiveness of the intervention.

Social Justice

Cancer is a disease that affects us all, yet social disparities result in differences in cancer's impact, physically and emotionally. It is important to note too that even the studies that have been cited in this chapter suffer from a lack of representation of BIPOC, AAPI, Latinx, and LGBTQIA+ patients and families. Black Americans have some of the highest mortality rates and lowest survival rates for most types of cancer diagnoses (Abdalla et al., 2020; Chu Foy et al., 2018; Siegel et al., 2018; Wallace et al., 2020). In the Asian American Pacific Islanders (AAPI) community, cancer is the leading cause of death for women and men (Nguyen & Kagawa-Singer, 2008).

Culture, identity, and worldview shape how we think about a clinical encounter. When these differences cause clinician and patient interactions to go awry, it can generate distrust, anger, ambivalence, and overidentification issues that can significantly impact the therapeutic process and relationship (Bernstein, 2001). A history of cruelty and medical maltreatment toward communities of color in the United States has created a legacy of mistrust of the medical system. Conventional solutions to reducing disparities focus heavily on promoting access to care, yet fail to address underlying, persistent social injustices that lead to differences in outcomes. A few examples of solutions to reducing disparities include raising public and provider awareness of racial and ethnic disparities in care, increasing the knowledge base on causes and interventions to reduce disparities, and most importantly, treating patients with dignity and respect.

Factors that contribute to increased disparities in outcomes include: language and cultural barriers; discrimination related to class, race, and immigration status; health literacy; and challenges navigating and accessing the medical system. When care is only focused on individual behavior or lifestyle choices, it fails to address issues facing entire social and racial groups. An evaluation of institutional power and discrimination is crucial to broadening the scope of treatment options to excluded individuals and groups and, thus, to saving lives.

Supporting Black Indigenous People Of Color (BIPOC), Asian American Pacific Islander (AAPI), and Latinx Communities

There are many historic examples of the Western medical system manipulating the Black community (e.g., Marion Sims' experiments on enslaved African American women [Wall, 2006]; Tuskegee syphilis study [Scharff et al., 2010]). Today discrimination, including implicit bias, against BIPOC, AAPI, and Latinx patients continues (Floríndez et al., 2020; Godofredo, 2020). These atrocities and inequities lead many people of color to distrust the Western medical system, further exacerbated by the underrepresentation of certain groups among providers in the oncology care or medical setting. For instance, the Latinx community makes up 18% of the population of the United States, yet less than 1% of physicians are Latinx, while only about 3% of United States oncologists identify as Black or African American (Floríndez et al., 2020; Godofredo, 2020).

The context of medical racism and experimentation on vulnerable populations is crucial to understand as an OSW, especially because many cancer treatments are clinical trials, which are experimental in nature. Even when treatments are FDA approved, there is rarely certainty around how a treatment (radiation, chemotherapy, immunotherapy, etc.) will affect a patient or influence the course of their disease. As such, cancer treatments can be greeted with mistrust by BIPOC, AAPI, or Latinx communities that have historically been used as test subjects against their will. Compounding this, in clinical trials conducted for cancer drugs between 2014 and 2018, BIPOC/AAPI were underrepresented by nearly 70% (Al Hadidi et al., 2020). The underrepresentation of BIPOC in clinical trials, the disproportionate impact of poverty on BIPOC/AAPI families, the higher incidences of certain comorbid conditions in these communities, and the history of systemic medical racism all create barriers to members of these communities obtaining equitable oncological care (Al Hadidi et al., 2020; Siegel et al., 2018).

Members of the AAPI community are vulnerable to discrimination based on immigration status, lack of health insurance, inadequate language interpretation services, and more. One challenge in evaluating cancer programs in the AAPI community has to do with the wide range of racial categories that make up AAPI. The racial category of AAPI encompasses more than 50 diverse ethnic and language subgroups (Nguyen & Kagawa-Singer, 2008). One study conducted found that nearly 80% of the AAPI community who were cancer survivors had unmet needs, almost 5% higher than the general survivorship population (Le et al., 2017).

It is always important for OSWs who are working with BIPOC, AAPI, or Latinx patients to develop an understanding of their cultural and ethnic backgrounds, since these patients and families are not part of the dominant white, Eurocentric culture that the medical system is tailored to. Developing such an understanding can allow the OSW to provide better support throughout the treatment cycle and address systemic medical discrimination as it occurs. For example, a white OSW who works with a patient from an AAPI community would benefit from the awareness that person comes from a cultural background wherein the concept and value of the individual "self" are intrinsically tied to the health and welfare of the family. Decision-making is often a group process, which can clash with the Western model of individual autonomy. As a result, providers may make AAPI patients feel as though they are outsiders in the Western medical system (Quach et al., 2012). This othering contributes to an unfair internalization of responsibility for the patient–doctor relationship on the part of the patient. In some instances, AAPI patients who do not speak English as their first language may feel it is their fault that the medical team is not providing the information they need to make informed decisions (Quach et al., 2012). The OSW who is sensitive to these possible differences and unconscious biases will be better equipped to intervene as an advocate for their patient.

The importance of cultural understanding and linguistic support is apparent when OSWs support Latinx patients and families, too. Common values in the Latinx community such as "familismo" (valuing close/extended family support and involvement for care decisions), "respecto" (deference to elders/authority figures), and "personalismo" (friendliness) can all be misinterpreted by providers due to implicit bias (Floríndez et al., 2020). For instance, when Latinx families bring their children and extended family to appointments as an expression of familismo, providers may prejudge that the families are unable to afford childcare (Floríndez et al., 2020). Or providers, acting in some awareness of cultural norms such as "respecto and personalismo," may see that Latinx patients are less likely to complain when they receive small or less than adequate accommodations, and therefore be more likely to put those families in such places (Floríndez et al., 2020).

While much has been written about the distrust of the BIPOC community toward Western medicine, some recent literature has indicated that trust may be improving, providing impetus for the medical establishment to push for more inclusivity in research. One such study included rural populations and found that 75% of African American and Latinx patients surveyed trusted research conducted by their own physicians; however less than 10% had ever been asked to participate (Thetford et al., 2021). This finding highlights the double impact of living in a rural setting and facing discrimination against BIPOC and Latinx patients. Living outside of major metropolitan areas in and of itself can decrease access to oncology care: Patients travel an average of 51 min to reach an oncologist and 83 min to reach an academic medical center in rural areas (Charlton et al., 2015). Considering that over 1.6 million rural households do not own cars, it is clear that many rural patients will face serious obstacles to obtaining quality oncological care (Charlton et al., 2015). In the Rocky Mountain region, fewer than half of the hospitals have a formal pain or palliative care service, and fewer than ten percent of physicians in those hospitals reported having been trained in palliative care formally (Charlton et al., 2015). This points to a further disparity in care faced by people living in rural areas: lack of access to effective symptom management and comfort care.

Supporting Lesbian Gay Bisexual Transgender Queer Intersex Asexual+ (LGBTQIA+) Community

The medical system has for far too long failed to acknowledge the LGBTQIA+ community's existence and specific needs. Studies have shown that LGBTQIA+ patients are more likely to engage in care, are more satisfied with their care, and experience greater quality of care when their providers know their LGBTQIA+ status (Klitzman & Greenberg, 2002; Tamargo et al., 2017). Despite this statistic, in those studies, only a little over half of providers believed such information to be important, and only a third inquired about sexual orientation during intake. And while LGBTQIA+ disclosure is important to treatment, patients themselves are reluctant to make such disclosures on their own due to historical and ongoing stigma (Tamargo et al., 2017). If LGBTQIA+ status is not discussed, there can be deleterious impacts on health outcomes in oncology. Transgender men risk not being assessed for family history of breast cancer, or transgender women for prostate cancer (Damaskos et al., 2018). Gay and bisexual men risk not being screened appropriately for anal cancer, which occurs more among men who have sex with men (Stump-Sutliff et al., n.d.) And lesbian and bisexual women may not be screened adequately for potential increased risk of breast and gynecological cancers (Panganiban & O'Neil, 2021). Beyond health effects, the normalization of assessment of and discussion about LGBTQIA+ status and identity has positive psychological benefits in its acknowledgment of existence and communication of inclusiveness. As OSWs, we must support LGBTQIA+ patients by ensuring that their identities are seen as they wish to be seen and that they receive equitable and appropriate medical care.

Challenging Oppression and Recognizing Biases

It is the experience of these authors that BIPOC, AAPI, and Latinx patients are labeled "difficult" more often than white patients, whether for asking too many questions, declining a proposed treatment plan, or simply how they are expressing emotion. Security is called more quickly on these families than they are on white families as well, multiplying the emotional anguish of being treated for cancer. Aggression, insults, and racism are as commonplace in the medical field as they are in the rest of the world. As social workers, our Code of Ethics mandates that we seek to challenge oppression while empowering our patients (National Association of Social Workers, 2021). OSWs can help advocate for patients who are members of groups historically oppressed and marginalized as they navigate a medical system still rife with systemic racism. At the same time, we must be aware of our own social locations and biases, and affirmatively examine our assumptions about the patients we work with. As OSWs, it is imperative that we understand and address the correlation between racism and cancer. Empowering OSWs to advocate on behalf of BIPOC, AAPI, and Latinx patients and caregivers is essential to promoting anti-racism in cancer care.

Implications for Practice

Cancer covers a huge range of diseases and psychosocial scenarios. It is increasingly recognized that the diagnosis and treatment of cancer impact not just the individual but others they live and interact with, which can include biological as well as chosen families and larger spiritual communities. The evolving needs of patients and families at each of these treatment phases point to the continuity of care that OSWs must provide. OSWs are vital partners in the multidisciplinary team. Oncology social workers have a unique perspective, knowledge base, skill set, and commitment. They provide individual, family, and group counseling. As the chapter highlights, the OSW's role remains fluid as the patient moves through phases of their disease.

As in other areas of social work, stigma in seeking out psychological support can prevent patients and families from engaging in counseling, a truth that highlights the importance of discerning clinical skills to determine the specific needs of patients and families. For instance, not all patients who are referred to social work will need emotional support around their own diagnosis. Some may need help in addressing barriers to care (transportation, housing, and financial toxicity). It is also common for patients to be so focused on getting through the treatment process that they have difficulty accessing the emotional impact of the diagnosis until after treatment ends and they are in a posttreatment, survivorship phase.

Social justice, as in all aspects of social work, must be centered in the OSW's practice as they engage with cancer patients. We all hold multiple identities, some of which are unseen or unspoken, which means we should work hard to understand our inherent biases and learn to conduct assessments that respect an individual's full identity, encompassing race, class, and gender. If we are willing to listen deeply and acknowledge our own biases in the process, we can better empathize with and accompany patients and families on their journey. As OSWs, we must always be aware of who has been marginalized from the medical system and how cancer impacts patients and families differently based on that marginalization.

None of the interventions we employ can reverse a diagnosis or bring back a life. The OSW's role is to honor the person in the environment, a task that includes honoring psychological, social, somatic, spiritual, cultural, and economic aspects of an individual's experience. Not only do OSWS bear witness to the suffering of patients who feel they cannot share with anyone else, but they also provide supportive counseling, crisis intervention, psychoeducation, and cognitive behavioral interventions that are essential to managing cancer. By providing a space for patients and families to discuss their fears and anxieties, we create opportunities for hope to become possible again.

Authors' Reflections

"Your job is very hard and depressing, I don't know how you do it!" As the authors reflected on this common statement, we acknowledged that while the work is filled with grief and illness, it is our life's work to sit in the spaces of existential distress. We hold space for ambiguity as we walk alongside our patients and their families during the most difficult parts of their cancer journey, whatever the outcome. We share in their laughter and moments of joy, simultaneously allowing room for their fears and tears. It's incredible to witness how cancer patients and their families model courage and grace in the face of an often traumatic and life-changing experience. Our role as the oncology social worker is to provide a space for our patients to make meaningful connections both to their cancer journey and with their friends and families.

Reflection Questions

1. How might the experiences of a patient with a brain tumor and a patient with breast cancer differ? Why?
2. In what ways does your setting address the needs of LGBTQIA+ patients? Where might there be areas for improvement?
3. How might you intervene with a patient who is struggling with disease progression, feeling demoralized about the uncertainty and exhausted by the treatment?

References

Abdalla, E., Troy, R., Fall, S., Elhussin, I., Egiebor-Aiwan, O., & Nganwa, D. (2020). Racial differences in 5-year relative survival rates of cervical cancer by stage at diagnosis, between African American (black) and white women, living in the state of Alabama, USA. *BMC Cancer, 20*(1), 1–12. https://doi.org/10.1186/s12885-020-07338-7

Al Hadidi, S., Mims, M., Miller-Chism, C. N., & Kamble, R. (2020). Participation of African American persons in clinical trials supporting US Food and Drug Administration approval of cancer drugs. *Annals of Internal Medicine, 173*(4), 320–322. https://doi.org/10.7326/M20-0410

Altillo, T., & Tropeano, L. E. (2015). Pain and symptom management. In G. Christ, C. Messner, & L. Behar (Eds.), *Handbook of oncology social work: Psychosocial care of people with cancer* (pp. 239–246). Oxford University Press.

Arch, J. J., Vanderkruik, R., Kirk, A., & Carr, A. L. (2018). A closer lens: Cancer survivors' supportive intervention preferences and interventions received. *Psychooncology, 27*(5), 1434–1441. https://doi.org/10.1002/pon.4526

Bahrami, M., Mohamadirizi, M., Mohamadirizi, S., & Hosseini, S. A. (2017). Evaluation of body image in cancer patients and its association with clinical variables. *Journal of education and health promotion, 6*, 81. https://doi.org/10.4103/jehp.jehp_4_15

Bernstein, D. M. (2001). Therapist-patient relations and ethnic transference. In W.-S. Tseng & J. Streltzer (Eds.), *Culture and psychotherapy: A guide to clinical practice* (pp. 103–121). American Psychiatric Press.

Blacker, S., & Christ, G. H. (2011). Defining social work's role and leadership contributions in palliative care. In T. A. S. Otis-Green (Ed.), *Oxford textbook of palliative social work* (pp. 21–30). Oxford University Press.

Boerger-Knowles, K., & Ridley, T. (2014). Chronic cancer: Counseling the individual. *Social Work in Health Care, 53*(1), 11–30.

Breitbart, W., Rosenfeld, B., Gibson, C., Pessin, H., Poppito, S., Nelson, C., et al. (2010). Meaning-centered group psychotherapy for patients with advanced cancer: A pilot randomized controlled trial. *Psychooncology, 19*(1), 21–28. https://doi.org/10.1002/pon.1556

Breitbart, W., Pessin, H., Rosenfeld, B., Applebaum, A. J., Lichtenthal, W. G., Li, Y., et al. (2018). Individual meaning-centered psychotherapy for the treatment of psychological and existential distress: A randomized controlled trial in patients with advanced cancer. *Cancer, 124*(15), 3231–3239. https://doi.org/10.1002/cncr.31539

Cameron, M. (2014). This is common factors. *Clinical Social Work Journal, 42*(2), 151–160.

Charlton, M., Schlichting, J., Chioreso, C., Ward, M., & Vikas, P. (2015). Challenges of Rural Cancer Care in the United States. *Oncology (Williston Park, N.Y.), 29*(9), 633–640.

Chu Foy, K., Fisher, J. L., Lustberg, M. B., Gray, D. M., DeGraffinreid, C. R., & Paskett, E. D. (2018). Disparities in breast cancer tumor characteristics, treatment, time to treatment, and survival probability among African American and white women. *NPJ Breast Cancer, 4*(1), 1–6. https://doi.org/10.1038/s41523-018-0059-5

Damaskos, P., & Gerbino, S. (2014). Introduction to the special issue: Coping with chronic cancer: Clinical approaches for oncology social work practice. *Social Work in Health Care, 53*(1), 1–4.

Damaskos, P., & Parry, C. (2015). Cancer survivorship: Concepts, interventions, and research. In G. Christ, C. Messner, & L. Behar (Eds.), *Handbook of oncology social work: Psychosocial care of people with cancer* (pp. 57–64). Oxford University Press.

Damaskos, P., Amaya, B., Gordon, R., & Walters, C. B. (2018). Intersectionality and the LGBT cancer patient. *Seminars in Oncology Nursing, 34*(1), 30–36.

Daniels, J., & Kissane, D. W. (2008). Psychosocial interventions for cancer patients. *Current Opinion in Oncology, 20*(4), 367–371. https://doi.org/10.1097/CCO.0b013e3283021658

Dougherty, L. (2007). Using nursing diagnoses in prevention and management of chemotherapy-induced alopecia in the cancer patient. *International Journal of Nursing Terminologies and Classifications: The Official Journal of NANDA International, 18*(4), 142–149. https://doi.org/10.1111/j.1744-618X.2007.00069.x

Ernstmann, N., Neumann, M., Ommen, O., Galushko, M., Wirtz, M., Voltz, R., et al. (2009). Determinants and implications of cancer patients' psychosocial needs. *Supportive Care in Cancer, 17*(11), 1417–1423. https://doi.org/10.1007/s00520-009-0605-7

Ezra, E., & Chi, M. (2015). When the other shoe drops: Unique fears and challenges of recurrent disease. In G. Christ, C. Messner, & L. Behar (Eds.), *Handbook of oncology social work: Psychosocial care of people with cancer* (p. 107). Oxford University Press.

Fleishman, S. B., & Messner, C. (2015). Cancer in contemporary society: Grounding in oncology and psychosocial care. In G. Christ, C. Messner, & L. Behar (Eds.), *Handbook of oncology social work: Psychosocial care of people with cancer* (p. 1). Oxford University Press.

Floríndez, L. I., Floríndez, D. C., Como, D. H., Secola, R., & Duker, L. I. S. (2020). Differing interpretations of health care encounters: A qualitative study of non-Latinx health care providers' perceptions of Latinx patient behaviors. *Plos One, 15*(8), e0236706.

Godofredo, A. V. (2020). Racism, discrimination, and the practice of oncology. *Lancet, 395*, 1813.

Hall, D. L., Luberto, C. M., Philpotts, L. L., Song, R., Park, E. R., & Yeh, G. Y. (2018). Mind-body interventions for fear of cancer recurrence: A systematic review and meta-analysis. *Psychooncology, 27*(11), 2546–2558. https://doi.org/10.1002/pon.4757

Harley, C., Pini, S., Bartlett, Y. K., & Velikova, G. (2012). Defining chronic cancer: Patient experiences and self-management needs. *BMJ Supportive & Palliative Care, 2*(3), 248–255.

Hartman, K. K. (2015). Diagnosis and initiation of cancer treatment. In G. Christ, C. Messner, & L. Behar (Eds.), *Handbook of oncology social work: Psychosocial care of people with cancer* (pp. 43–50). Oxford University Press.

Holland, J. C. (2002). History of psycho-oncology: Overcoming attitudinal and conceptual barriers. *Psychosomatic Medicine, 64*(2), 206–221.

Kissane, D. W., McKenzie, M., Block, S., Moskowitz, C., McKenzie, D. P., & O'Neill, I. (2006). Family focused grief therapy: A randomized, controlled trial in palliative care and bereavement. *The American Journal of Psychiatry, 163*(7), 1208–1218.

Klitzman, R. L., & Greenberg, J. D. (2002). Patterns of communication between gay and lesbian patients and their health care providers. *Journal of Homosexuality, 42*(4), 65–75. https://doi.org/10.1300/J082v42n04_04

Kyngäs, H., Mikkonen, R., Nousiainen, E. M., Rytilahti, M., Seppänen, P., Vaattovaara, R., & Jämsä, T. (2001). Coping with the onset of cancer: Coping strategies and resources of young people with cancer. *European Journal of Cancer Care, 10*(1), 6–11.

Lawson, K. C., & Lawson, D. H. (2018). Insights into the psychology of trauma should inform the practice of oncology. *The Oncologist, 23*(7), 750.

Le, M. N., Nguyen, G. T., Pan, Z., Maglalang, D. D., Butt, F., Bautista, R., et al. (2017). Unmet needs of Asian American and Pacific Islander cancer survivors. *Journal of Cancer Education, 32*(2), 374–381. https://doi.org/10.1007/s13187-015-0952-7

Mathew, L., & Fulton, C. (2017). Chapter 12: Social isolation and caregiver burden. In B. Korc-Grodzicki & W. P. Tew (Eds.), *Handbook of geriatric oncology* (pp. 99–103). Demos Medical.
McClement, S. E., & Chochinov, H. M. (2008). Hope in advanced cancer patients. *European Journal of Cancer, 44*(8), 1169–1174. https://doi.org/10.1016/j.ejca.2008.02.031
McClement, S., Chochinov, H. M., Hack, T., Hassard, T., Kristjanson, L. J., & Harlos, M. (2007). Dignity therapy: Family member perspectives. *Journal of Palliative Medicine, 10*(5), 1076–1082.
National Association of Social Workers. (2021). *Code of ethics*. https://www.socialworkers.org/About/Ethics/Code-of-Ethics/Code-of-Ethics-English
National Cancer Institute. (2021a, May 5) *What is cancer?* https://www.cancer.gov/about-cancer/understanding/what-is-cancer
National Cancer Institute. (2021b, August 6). *Depression (PDQ)-Health professional version*. https://www.cancer.gov/about-cancer/coping/feelings/depression-hp-pdq
Nguyen, T. U. N., & Kagawa-Singer, M. (2008, November). Overcoming barriers to cancer care through health navigation programs. *Seminars in oncology nursing, 24*(4), 270–278.
Ore, M. L., & Foli, K. J. (2020). Reintegration for Post-treatment Cancer Survivors: A Concept Analysis. *Journal of holistic nursing: official journal of the American Holistic Nurses' Association, 38*(3), 300–317. https://doi.org/10.1177/0898010119883760
Panganiban, J. M., & O'Neil, J. (2021). Breast cancer and gynecologic risks in lesbian and bisexual women. *Nursing, 51*(3), 58–62.
Quach, T., Nuru-Jeter, A., Morris, P., Allen, L., Shema, S. J., Winters, J. K., et al. (2012). Experiences and perceptions of medical discrimination among a multiethnic sample of breast cancer patients in the Greater San Francisco Bay Area, California. *American Journal of Public Health, 102*(5), 1027–1034. https://doi.org/10.2105/AJPH.2011.300554
Sánchez-Díaz, C. T., Strayhorn, S., Tejeda, S., Vijayasiri, G., Rauscher, G. H., & Molina, Y. (2021). What mediates the racial/ethnic disparity in psychosocial stress among breast cancer patients? *Cancer Causes & Control, 32*(4), 357–367. https://doi.org/10.1007/s10552-021-01392-7
Scharff, D. P., Mathews, K. J., Jackson, P., Hoffsuemmer, J., Martin, E., & Edwards, D. (2010). More than Tuskegee: Understanding mistrust about research participation. *Journal of Health Care for the Poor and Underserved, 21*(3), 879. https://doi.org/10.1353/hpu.0.0323
Siegel, R. L., Miller, K. D., & Jemal, A. (2018). Cancer statistics, 2018. *CA: A Cancer Journal for Clinicians, 68*(1), 7–30. https://doi.org/10.3322/caac.21442
Stump-Sutliff, K., Watson, L. R., & Gersten, T. (n.d.). *Cancer risks for gay and bisexual men*. https://www.urmc.rochester.edu/encyclopedia/content.aspx?contenttypeid=134&contentid=131
Tamargo, C. L., Quinn, G. P., Sanchez, J. A., & Schabath, M. B. (2017). Cancer and the LGBTQ population: Quantitative and qualitative results from an oncology providers' survey on knowledge, attitudes, and practice behaviors. *Journal of Clinical Medicine, 6*(10), 93.
Thetford, K., Gillespie, T. W., Kim, Y.-I., Hansen, B., & Scarinci, I. C. (2021). Willingness of Latinx and African Americans to participate in non therapeutic trials: It depends on who runs the research. *Ethnicity & Disease, 31*(2), 263–272. https://doi.org/10.18865/ed.31.2.263
Treanor, C. J. (2020). Psychosocial support interventions for cancer caregivers: Reducing caregiver burden. *Current Opinion in Supportive and Palliative Care, 14*(3), 247–262.
Wall, L. L. (2006). The medical ethics of Dr J Marion Sims: A fresh look at the historical record. *Journal of Medical Ethics, 32*(6), 346–350. https://doi.org/10.1136/jme.2005.012559
Wallace, K., Li, H., Brazeal, J. G., Lewin, D. N., Sun, S., Ba, A., Paulos, C. M., Rachidi, S., Li, Z., & Alekseyenko, A. V. (2020). Platelet and hemoglobin count at diagnosis are associated with survival in African American and Caucasian patients with colorectal cancer. *Cancer Epidemiology, 67*. https://doi.org/10.1016/j.canep.2020.101746
Williams, I. (2014). Psychosocial burden of family caregivers to adults with cancer. In U. Goerling (Ed.), *Psycho-oncology. Recent results in cancer research* (Vol. 197, pp. 73–85). Springer. https://doi.org/10.1007/978-3-642-40187-9_6

Chapter 3
Cancer: Leukemia and Lymphoma

Eunju Lee and Madeline Rogers

Abbreviations

ACT	Acceptance and Commitment Therapy
ADL	Activities of Daily Living
AHM	Acute Hematologic Malignancies
AL	Acute Leukemia
ALL	Acute Lymphocytic Leukemia
AML	Acute Myeloid Leukemia
CLL	Chronic Lymphocytic Leukemia
CML	Chronic Myeloid Leukemia
DBT	Dialectical Behavior Therapy
DLBCL	Diffuse Large B Cell Lymphoma
DNR	Do Not Resuscitate
ECOG	Eastern Cooperative Oncology Group
EOL	End-of-Life
GVHD	Graft-Versus-Host-Disease
HL	Hodgkin's Lymphoma
HM	Hematological Malignancies
IADL	Instrumental Activities of Daily Living
ICU	Intensive Care Unit
JAMA	Journal of the American Medical Association
KPS	Karnofsky Performance Status
MCGT	Meaning-Centered Grief Therapy
MCP	Meaning-Centered Psychotherapy

E. Lee (✉)
New York University, New York City, NY, USA
e-mail: el1388@nyu.edu

M. Rogers
Weill Cornell Medicine, New York City, NY, USA
e-mail: madelinecrogers@gmail.com

M. Hemphill, A. Nathanson (eds.), *The Practice of Clinical Social Work in Healthcare*, Essential Clinical Social Work Series,
https://doi.org/10.1007/978-3-031-31650-0_3

MI	Motivational Interviewing
NHL	Non-Hodgkin's Lymphoma
PGD	Prolonged Grief Disorder
PTSD	Post-Traumatic Stress Disorder
SAMHSA	Substance Abuse and Mental Health Services Administration
SCT	Stem Cell Transplant
ST	Solid Tumors

Introduction

Leukemia and lymphoma belong to a group of cancers under the general category of blood cancers, also known as hematological malignancies (HM) or "liquid tumors," that vary in treatment, physical impact, and outcome. They are distinguished from other cancers (i.e., solid tumors) in that they begin in the bone marrow, where blood is produced. HM result from the growth of abnormal blood that spreads and interrupts the function of normal blood cells to fight infections and produce healthy new blood cells. Leukemia, a type of cancer found in the blood and bone marrow, is caused by the rapid production of abnormal white blood cells. The four main subtypes of leukemia are acute myeloid leukemia (AML), chronic myeloid leukemia (CML), acute lymphocytic leukemia (ALL), and chronic lymphocytic leukemia (CLL). As indicated by their names, leukemia can be both acute and chronic, which determines not only the management of the illness but also the psychosocial effects. Lymphoma affects the lymphatic system, which removes excess fluids from the body and produces lymphocytes, immune cells that fight infection. Abnormal lymphocytes transform into lymphoma cells that multiply and collect in the lymph nodes and other tissues, and over time impair the immune system. There are over 70 different subtypes of lymphoma, categorized into two broad groups: Non-Hodgkin's Lymphoma (NHL) and Hodgkin's Lymphoma (HL). Nearly 90% of patients with HL survive more than 5 years, making it one of the most treatable cancers (American Cancer Society, 2019, p. 14). Because leukemia and lymphoma are a highly diverse group of cancers with a range of subtypes that differ in their presentation, progression, and treatment (Bryant et al., 2016), it can be difficult to speak of these cancers or the experience of them as a monolith (Table 3.1).

There are, however, broad distinctions between HM and other types of cancer known as solid tumors (ST), and these differences impact the illness experience in a number of important ways. Although HM account for only 10% of all cancers in the United States (lls.org, 2021), advances in basic research and the development of new treatments in HM are disproportionately high (Chizuka et al., 2006), resulting in significant increases in the 5-year survival rate for many HM compared with advanced stage ST in the twenty-first century (Pulte et al., 2020). Many treatments for HM have curative intent, but they often require highly specialized, aggressive, intensive therapies that necessitate lengthy hospitalizations, mostly at large urban academic centers (Leblanc et al., 2016; McGrath & Holewa, 2007), and come with

Table 3.1 Disease specifications

	Lymphoma: Two main types		Leukemia: Four main types			
	HL	NHL[a]	ALL[b]	AML (31%)	CML (15%)	CLL (38%)
Expected new cases 2021	8830	81,560	5690	20,240	9110	21,250
Classifications based on World Health Organization (WHO)	2 main subtypes-Classic (95%) & Nodular; Classic subdivided to 4 types	> 61 subtypes (60% of cases are aggressive; 40% indolent)	2 main subtypes: B cell and T cell	11 subtypes based on genetic makeup	3 phases: chronic, accelerated, blast	2 main subtypes: B cell and T cell
Median age of dx	39	67	17	68	65	70
5-year survival rate (2011–2017)	88.3%	73.2%	38% > age 20; 89% < age 20	29.5%	70.6%	87.2%
Expected deaths 2021	960	20,720	1580	11,400	1220	4320
Median age at death	70	76	58	73	77	82

SEER (2020)
[a]7th most common cancer in the United States
[b]Primarily occurs in childhood, aged 2–5

significant toxicities and risks of mortality (El-Jawhri et al., 2020). Patients with HM have more unpredictable disease trajectories compared to patients with advanced ST (Verhoef et al., 2019), making prognostication difficult (Button et al., 2017) and deterioration rapid and unpredictable (McGrath & Holewa, 2007). The symptom burden that patients with HM experience is commonly related to the failure or suppression of bone marrow. Symptoms may include anemia, bleeding, and infection and often require hospitalization for treatment (Button et al., 2017). Despite high symptom burden, patients with HM are significantly less likely to receive specialist palliative care or hospice services compared to those with ST (Howell et al., 2011). They have higher utilization rates of emergency rooms and intensive care units (ICUs) and are more likely to receive aggressive cancer treatments in the last month of life compared to patients with ST (Hui et al., 2014). Data suggest that when compared to ST oncologists, hematologic oncologists are also more likely to equate palliative care with end-of-life (EOL) care and are more uncomfortable with death and dying, viewing it as a personal failing (Hui et al., 2015). Unsurprisingly, then, patients with HM admitted to hospice for EOL were generally sicker, had significantly shorter length of stay, and were more likely to die outside the home in an inpatient or other institutional setting (LeBlanc et al., 2015).

These unique characteristics of HM impact the way cancer is experienced by leukemia and lymphoma patients compared to patients with ST. So too does the specific subtype of cancer within the diverse collection of HM, each with different disease characteristics and disease progression (Hall et al., 2014). Some types of HM are acute and aggressive (e.g., ALL & AML), while others are asymptomatic or indolent (e.g., NHL), and others chronic, requiring constant surveillance with intermittent treatment (e.g., CLL & CML) (lls.org, 2021). Because HM are so varied and can occur across the lifespan, this chapter will focus on one broad classification – acute vs. chronic HM – and examine the psychosocial impact within the developmental stages of the adult life cycle (young, middle, and older adulthood) through three distinct but overlapping phases of illness: onset (diagnosis), course (treatment and/or surveillance), and outcome (death and bereavement) (Rolland, 1987). This matrix of phases of illness within the life cycle recognizes that illness occurs, is understood, and is accommodated differently within the unique developmental tasks in each stage of adult life (Rolland, 1987).

Clinical Issues of Illness

The following sections focus on distinguishing the possible impact of health and treatment on patients and associated clinical social work goals and interventions. For a summary of psychosocial issues and clinical interventions, see Table 3.2.

Hematological Malignancies

Acute Hematological Malignancies

Acute ALL and AML are acute and aggressive forms of leukemia, as is diffuse large B cell lymphoma (DLBCL), a particularly aggressive subtype of NHL and the most common subtype in adults. Though patients with these acute hematologic malignancies (AHM) can experience similar symptoms and treatment options, there are some differences in prevalence and prognosis. ALL is the most common type of childhood leukemia, while AML is the most common acute leukemia in adults. From 2009 to 2015, the 5-year overall survival rate for people with AML was 29.5% (SEER, 2020), making it the most lethal HM. The 5-year survival rate for patients with DLBCL is more optimistic, at 63.9% (SEER, 2020), but because of its aggressive nature, it must be treated as early as possible and the sooner a patient is diagnosed, the better their health outcome will be. Because AHM is often rapidly fatal without treatment, patients can feel "abducted by the illness" (Nissim et al., 2013, p. 498), where decisions regarding care must be made quickly after diagnosis within a short time frame, often with inadequate understanding of the illness or treatment (LeBlanc et al., 2016). Not yet having recovered from the initial traumatic shock of

Table 3.2 Psychosocial issues, clinical goals, and interventions

Acute hematologic malignancies			
Phase of illness	**Diagnosis/onset**	**Acute and chronic**	**Terminal and bereavement**
Possible challenges	Shock Fear Immediate treatment Sudden hospitalization	Intense induction chemo Possible SCT and GVHD Prolonged hospitalization Symptom burden from treatment Frequent follow-up and monitoring	Continued aggressive treatment Possibility of new clinical trials Uncertainty of being at EOL Likelihood of ICU admission Absence of palliative care support Likelihood of hospital death
Possible interventions	Disease education, esp. around what to expect Assessment of logistical support in preparation for treatment, incl. psychosocial and financial resources Mindfulness to cope with "fight-flight" response, and focus on here and now Fertility and family planning for young adults Advance directives conversations Values and goals of care clarification MI to address ambivalence re: Treatment	Body image and role identity preservation Resource support: Housing, transportation, caregiver needs ACT to build acceptance and psychological flexibility Life review for the older adult MCP to build resilience and meaning Digital support to reduce isolation Trauma-informed care	Advance directives conversations Clarification of goals of care and EOL life preferences, incl. DNR and hospice Advocacy for palliative care support Dignity therapy to support generativity, control, and continuity of self in face of psycho/physical distress Reframe binary from "fight vs. giving up" narrative to holding uncertainty MCGT to address PGD from traumatic, unprepared death
Chronic hematologic malignancies			
Phase of illness	**Diagnosis/onset**	**Chronic and treatment**	**Terminal and bereavement**
Possible challenges	Older age onset with comorbidities and/or debilities "Wait and watch" anxiety Uncertain treatment plan	Slow progression: Anxiety connected with "waiting for the other shoe to drop" Symptom burden and resultant care needs	Continued aggressive treatment Possibility of new clinical trials Uncertainty of being at EOL Likelihood of ICU admission Absence of palliative care support Likelihood of hospital death

(continued)

Table 3.2 (continued)

Possible interventions	Disease education and translation of medical info in layman terms Advance directives conversations Values and goals of care clarification ACT to build acceptance and psychological flexibility MCP to address effects of increased physical dependence	Mindfulness, meditation, and breathing techniques to manage anxiety of uncertainty Resource support, incl. caregiving needs DBT for distress tolerance Existential therapy to identify areas of control; find meaning in face of anxiety Narrative and MCP to make sense of and identify meaning of illness Logotherapy to engage in sources of meaning: play, work, relationships	Advance directives conversations Clarification of goals of care and EOL life preferences, incl. DNR and hospice Advocacy for palliative care support Dignity therapy to support generativity, control, and continuity of self in face of psycho/physical distress Reframe binary "fight vs. giving up" narrative to holding uncertainty MCGT to address PGD-risk from traumatic, unexpected death

learning their diagnosis, the patient is encouraged to suppress their natural reactions of fear and disbelief and to feign reason and control outwardly while experiencing inwardly psychic and emotional unraveling. When chosen, treatment comes quickly, causing sudden disruption and suspension of the patient's pre-diagnosis life and catapulting patients into a highly medicalized world, all under the specter of an uncertain prognosis (Amonoo et al., 2021). Fear of recurrence, the unpredictable nature of the illness, and the chronic and late effects of treatment (Jones et al., 2015) mark a disquieting maintenance period. Death of patients with AHM, like diagnosis, is also often sudden and unexpected, without the benefit of hospice or palliative care interventions, which can serve as protective factors against complicated grief (Mason et al., 2020), now known as prolonged grief disorder (PGD), where grief is intense, prolonged, and manifests in cognitive, emotional, and behavioral symptoms that impair social, occupational, and other important areas of functioning for more than a year after the loss.

Crisis The experience of being diagnosed with AHM has been described as being "like getting hit by a truck that you didn't see coming" (Nissim et al., 2013, p. 497). Because there are often no major symptoms, this life-threatening diagnosis often comes after a prolonged but mundane cold, or unexplained fatigue. The news may be delivered after a "routine" blood test, sometimes from an urgent care or emergency department physician who is unfamiliar to the patient, thus amplifying a sense of shock and devastation (Nissim et al., 2013). Because of the acute nature of the disease, treatment often comes immediately after diagnosis, suddenly removing patients from all aspects of their known life into an isolated, sterilized, and unfamiliar inpatient setting where one loses all sense of personal control and predictability.

Not only is treatment urgent and abrupt, it is also intensive and highly toxic, beginning with inpatient induction chemotherapy. Severed from the known world and cast into a medical abyss, one patient with AHM described the experience by stating, "It wasn't induction [chemotherapy]. It was an abduction" (Nissim et al., 2013, p. 498).

Among other factors such as socioeconomic status (which will be addressed later in this chapter), the psychosocial impact of this abduction is shaped by the patient's stage of adult development. In young adulthood, several important developmental milestones await, such as completing education, establishing autonomy, creating an identity, forming romantic relationships, pursuing gainful employment and financial independence, and having children (Husson et al., 2018). An acute leukemia (AL) diagnosis not only disrupts the unfolding of these psychosocial events but also, like many sudden and unexpected losses, challenges the "assumptive world" (Lethborg et al., 2006, p. 28) and leaves the future in question. As the young AML survivor Suleika Jaouad (2021) writes, "The future had once seemed infinite with possibility. Now it was shrouded in doom, a dark space ahead filled only with the promise of more poisonous treatments and terrifying unknowns" (p. 199). The primary psychosocial tasks in the aftermath of diagnosis then will be to assess symptoms of traumatic response, moderating its impact with grounding exercises aimed at staying in the present, and eschewing future-oriented catastrophic thinking. The goal is to increase the distress tolerance of the newly diagnosed so that they can access the ability to plan and engage in rational and thoughtful decision-making regarding their treatment. Activities within one's control such as diet, physical activity as tolerated, and engagement in sources of social and spiritual connection such as social media, music, poetry, and the arts should be encouraged as reminders of agency and continued meaning making and growth.

The intensive, prolonged, and isolating treatment of AHM is "life interrupted," wherein the young adult reverts back to parental care for material support such as housing and transportation as well as physical care, placing them at risk for feelings of being infantilized. It can disrupt the development of one's identity, self-worth, social cognition, and emotional regulation (Husson et al., 2018), alienating them from their active, healthy peers. The effects of toxic treatments and side effects (e.g., hairlessness, steroid-induced swelling, and weight loss) can also bring about negative body image, affecting the ability to develop and/or maintain intimate relationships. An estimated 75% of childless young adults express a desire for future progeny (Husson et al., 2018), prompting pursuit of fertility treatments, which may need to be weighed against the risk of delaying life-saving treatment. The cost of fertility treatment, which is often not covered by health insurance, adds yet another financial burden to the young adult, who may also be facing loss of employment and with it, associated health insurance. Emotionally, the prospect of leaving a legacy in the form of a next generation may serve as a beacon of forward-looking hope for someone with a serious illness, but simultaneously it may evoke anguish at the thought of possibly not being part of that future. Additionally, though there is little difference in live births from IVF treatments between women with or without cancer histories, the overall success rate remains low, at about 30% (Cardozo et al., 2015). Having just come out of a cloud of uncertainty regarding treatment outcome, the stress of managing yet another unknown may be determined untenable. All these factors might explain why rates of psychological distress among young adults with cancer are significantly higher than among older adults (Sansom-Daly & Wakefield, 2013). Recognizing the specific and often neglected needs particular to the young adult population, large cancer hospitals have launched young adult programs, composed of interdisciplinary teams often led by oncology social workers, dedicated to working exclusively with this population. Additionally, social media platforms may provide easily accessible forms of mutual support and education for this population comfortable in the virtual space.

In middle adulthood, a HM diagnosis means social, family, and work responsibilities are sidelined at a time when they are likely to be most consuming. At a stage marked by Erikson's (1950) tension between generativity versus stagnation, life is suddenly halted and stagnation is forced by illness. Most pronounced may be a loss of roles: roles of parent, partner, wage earner, caregiver of aging parent(s), and professional. Even the most established adult might find themselves in a crisis of identity, made worse by the high symptom burdens of treatment, including increased vulnerability to infections, decreased cognitive and physical vitality, and fatigue (Allart-Vorelli et al., 2015), which can disrupt role resumption. Although patients with cancer regardless of whether ST or HM face common challenges of loss of control, agency, and uncertainty, patients with HM are reported to experience a higher prevalence of psychosocial distress, anxiety, and depression, possibly related to higher levels of post-traumatic stress disorder (PTSD) symptoms and poorer quality of life (Bryant et al., 2016). Without timely and focused psychosocial intervention, such distress may lead to painful existential suffering marked by loss of meaning, death anxiety, and demoralization (Vehling & Kissane, 2018). A focus on strength-based assessments and interventions will enable the clinician to strategize with the patient ways to reinforce and enhance existing sources of meaning, rebuild connections to sources that the patient has become disconnected from, and create connections to new sources. Meaning-centered psychotherapy (MCP) (Breitbart et al., 2010) may have particular salience in facilitating this process.

The family system of the middle-adult patient must realign with role changes that affect all its members. Financial, household, and parental responsibilities shift to the healthy parent who must also take on the additional role of partner caregiver through a prolonged period of treatment and recovery that can last many months or years. Minor-aged children will likely be required to rely more heavily on professional or extended family caregivers, with varying degrees of understanding the cause of their disrupted lives or the fate of their AHM parent and the family unit. Recognizing such systemic effects of serious illness, it seems important to define the patient and family as one unit of care (as in hospice care), but this is challenged by the fact that so much of the AHM patient's care takes place for a prolonged period within the hospital walls and visitation by family members, especially young children, is likely to be limited due to the patient's highly immunocompromised state. Fortunately, the pervasiveness of cellphones and video platforms has increased contact between sequestered patients and friends and family. Maintaining consistent social connections with family and friends during this challenging period may provide protective factors against the despair that often accompanies prolonged isolation and uncertainty.

For the older adult, an AHM diagnosis comes with a bleak survival rate compared to their younger counterparts, due to the likelihood of frailty and comorbidities, and physicians' disinclination to utilize aggressive treatments because of the expectation that older adults are less likely to benefit from intensive therapies (Oran & Weisdorf, 2012). This conventional wisdom of "less is more" for older adults is being debated, however, so that the optimal approach to the treatment of this AHM patient population is less clear (Solomon et al., 2018). In fact, the American Society of Hematology in its 2020 guidelines for treating newly diagnosed AML in older adults recommends more-intensive therapy over less-intensive therapy "when deemed tolerable… [with] ongoing discussions between clinicians and patients, continuously addressing goals of care and the relative risk-benefit balance of treatment" (Sekeres et al., 2020, p. 1).

Ideally, all treatment decisions are made collaboratively between the healthcare provider and patient, where the patient's understanding of their illness, treatment options, and associated risks and benefits are verified and confirmed. Ongoing discussions ensure a dynamic process where the patient is allowed the opportunity to reassess and readdress decisions at various junctures in the treatment course. Open conversations regarding the patient's values and preferences help elucidate the goals of care, such as when the burden of treatment is deemed to outweigh the potential benefits and when the desire for quality of life supersedes quantity. Such practices can dispel ambiguity and empower the patient to become actively engaged in their care. The older patient can only be a part of this dyad of care if they possess or are gently guided in medical literacy that yields an informed and realistic understanding of treatment risks and benefits. Additionally, in order for the patient to articulate clear goals of care that align with their worldview and values, trust in their care provider and their judgment is imperative. When these conditions are met, the patient may feel equipped to adequately manage the wishes and recommendations of friends and family, even if they conflict with the patient's own preferences. Increased physical frailty that is common with aging may make the older patient more vulnerable, a vulnerability that only increases with waning social roles and responsibilities, and/or diminished material and social resources strained further by a cancer diagnosis.

The role of the oncology social worker with this population is essential, not only in assisting the patient with access to resources but in helping to navigate complex health information and systems. Most importantly, the social worker can facilitate conversations about patients' goals and values, execute advance directives, and clarify treatment options with a unique appreciation of the complex psychosocial inner life of the older adult straddling a choice between quality or quantity of a mortal, aging life. Techniques such as motivational interviewing (MI) may be particularly useful in sorting through the understandable ambivalence patients feel about undergoing intensive medical care. For the older adult, regardless of the outcome of medical intervention, an AL diagnosis will doubtlessly usher in thoughts of mortality: a heightened awareness that life ends, and with this, the task of coming to terms with the entirety of one's life; reflecting on and appraising it in the context of the eighth stage of Erikson's (1950) developmental tasks – whether life was well lived (integration) or one of the regrets (despair). When such life review extracts despair and regret, acceptance and commitment therapy (ACT) may be a useful intervention in supporting the patient to come to terms with the past, mindfully make space for uncomfortable emotions with acceptance of their presence, and build their capacity for psychological flexibility, while helping illuminate the patient's values and behaviors consistent with them (Hayes et al., 2013).

Chronic For patients with AHM who undergo intensive induction chemotherapy followed by a successful stem cell transplant (SCT), the 100 days has special significance as a milestone when the patient has passed the period of greatest risk for critical side effects and when stem cells have engrafted and begun making new blood cells. Although circled on the calendar and duly celebrated, it marks only the beginning. The first-year post-transplant is akin to the first year of an infant's life when patients remain at high risk for infection, having decimated the immune system to aide in engraftment and in cases of allogenic (donor) SCT, modulate the effects of potential graft-versus-host disease (GVHD). GVHD occurs when the donor's cells attack the patient's healthy cells because it is perceived as foreign and primarily affects the skin, gastrointestinal tract, and liver. GVHD occurs in about 40–60% of matched and unmatched allogeneic SCT, respectively (Gooptu & Koreth, 2017), and can be chronic or acute with acute GVHD being a leading cause of post-SCT morbidity and mortality (Yu et al., 2020). Less critical short-term effects of AHM therapies were identified as nausea/vomiting, diarrhea, hair loss, mouth sores, and rash (Crossnohere et al., 2019), and the most concerning long-term effects were organ dysfunction, "chemobrain" (cancer treatment–related cognitive impairment), fatigue, and neuropathy, the most prevalent of these being fatigue, or lack of vitality and energy (Allart-Vorelli et al., 2015). Such a high ongoing symptom burden is among the reasons patients with HM report poorer quality of life compared to the general public in psychological, social, professional, and financial domains (Allart-Vorelli et al., 2015).

Normalizing these symptoms and reminding patients of their transitory nature will likely serve to reassure and mitigate their emotional impact. Another common negative effect on quality of life is the pervasive sense of uncertainty regarding recurrence and death. This living in a liminal space is often met with heightened anxiety and pernicious ruminations, which the clinician can help patients manage with mindfulness practices aimed at grounding them in the present moment. Integrating mindfulness as part of daily life will prove invaluable to patients with HM because though mortality rates improve dramatically during the first 5 years post-SCT, it remains an estimated four to nine times higher than in the general population for at least 25 years thereafter, which translates to an estimated 30% lower life expectancy (Martin et al., 2010). The major causes of these deaths include recurrent disease, second malignancies, infections, GVHD, and respiratory and cardiovascular diseases (Martin et al., 2010).

The specter of recurrence and/or life-threatening effects of treatment is met by constant vigilance on the part of many survivors of HM. For those who have experienced sudden and intensive treatment such as induction therapy and SCT, this vigilance may transform into hypervigilance, a hallmark symptom of PTSD, along with intrusive thoughts, dissociation, avoidance, and others. One study of patients with AML reported greater than 28% of participants met criteria for clinically significant PTSD (Amonoo et al., 2021). Rodin et al. (2018) reported one-third of their participants with AL met full or partial diagnostic criteria for acute stress disorder. Depicting the traumatic experiences of diagnosis, abrupt and prolonged hospitalization, and immediate intensive treatment of patients with AL, Nissim et al. (2013) elucidate on the psychological coping responses to the trauma, which is informative for the social work clinician. Patients with AHM noted protective factors of (1) trust and reassurance – finding safety in the trusting relationship with the medical team; (2) surrendering control – conceding that the complicated nature of the illness and treatment requires "handing over control" to the experts and focusing on compliance, which is the only sphere of patients' control; (3) preference for limited information to manage feelings of being overwhelmed; and, (4) present-oriented agenda in order to focus on the immediate task and manage anxiety about an uncertain future (Nissim et al., 2013). These coping strategies align with the principles of trauma-informed care as outlined by the Substance Abuse and Mental Health Services Administration (SAMHSA): safety, trustworthiness and transparency, collaboration and mutuality, and empowerment and choice (samhsa.gov). It offers guidance for social work intervention strategies on how best to assist patients with AHM with PTSD. Only when the hyperarousal symptoms of PTSD are tended to can the patient engage in thoughtful reflection about the illness that can be incorporated into a wider meaning-making narrative. The work of making meaning is a task that confronts anyone with a serious, potentially life-limiting illness. It is a unifying element regardless of the specific HM. Despite the heterogeneity of HM – from urgent and acute to slow and chronic with differing trajectories of the illness experience – the terminal phase for patients with advanced HM shares similar complexities and dilemmas.

Chronic Hematological Malignancies

Acute The most common chronic subtypes of leukemia are chronic lymphocytic leukemia (CLL) and chronic myeloid leukemia (CML). These leukemias are nearly exclusive to adults, in particular men, with the onset typically occurring late in life. The majority of those diagnosed with CML are in adults aged 65 years and for CLL adults aged 70 years and older (Davis et al., 2014). Recognizing disease onset in older adults can be complicated by expected changes in physical health at this stage of life, like fatigue and changes in appetite, thus impeding the recognition of HM symptoms and the diagnostic process. Additionally, CLL and CML may not have early symptoms, with 50% of patients with CLL and patients with CML asymptomatic at the time of diagnosis (Thompson et al., 2015). Given the chronic nature of

CML and CLL, their course can be conceptualized as constant and slow developing, yet with a looming potential for quick progression. The treatment approach therefore is often to "wait and watch" (also referred to as active surveillance) for those who are asymptomatic or to focus on symptom management and disease control, often via oral pills for those who are symptomatic and in a later stage of the disease (Shawver et al., 2002). While the "wait and watch" approach may be medically sound, it can be met with unease by the patient whose need for control over the illness demands immediate action to not only manage the illness but to vigorously work toward a cure. Interventions aimed at increasing distress tolerance such as those in dialectical behavioral therapy (DBT) might be helpful during this stage. Conversely, a patient who is asymptomatic and whose illness has not impinged on their quality of life may be tempted to ignore the diagnosis altogether and disregard recommendations for medical monitoring and follow-up. For these patients, the role of family caregivers will prove to be particularly essential. Of the two groups of lymphoma, HL is much rarer than NHL. HL has a gradual onset, is slow developing, and is typically diagnosed in young adults aged 15–40 or adults aged 60 and over. By contrast, NHL is more likely to occur in older adults (Table 3.1), can have an acute or gradual onset, and may be indolent or aggressive, with a treatment plan dependent on the stage of the cancer. Treatment options for NHL and HL include active surveillance, chemotherapy, radiation, and more newly developed targeted therapies.

When thinking about the degree of incapacitation for patients with these diagnoses, it is important to keep in mind the chronic nature of the illness and the typically older age of onset. If the onset of illness is gradual with low symptom burden and is supported by an active surveillance approach for treatment, the patient may experience only relatively mild levels of incapacitation throughout the disease trajectory. The older adult with ow symptom burden may feel more discomfort with other physical ailments typical of aging than from cancer or cancer treatment. When treatment is required, the side effects from treatment may be a larger contributor to incapacitation than the cancer itself as older adults are especially vulnerable to short- and long-term treatment toxicities due to more preexisting chronic diseases, impaired physical and cognitive function, and decreased physiologic reserve (Kadambi, 2020). As with patients with AHM, treatment may include long hospitalizations, increasing the risk of impairment in their ability to carry out activities of daily living (ADLs) and instrumental activities of daily living (IADLs). For the older patient, concrete service needs to assist them in their ADLs and IADLs may supersede psychoaffective support needs, but it is important to remember that patient distress is significantly associated with increased care needs (Kadambi, 2020), thus making it necessary for the social work clinician to provide complimentary emotional support, utilizing interventions such as ACT and MCP.

Crisis Diagnosis is a major component of the crisis phase for these chronic HM subtypes. Receiving the diagnosis may provoke a variety of reactions and present a complex clinical picture. There might be initial relief in having gained understanding of the etiology of various low-level symptoms or shock of receiving a diagnosis of cancer when feeling healthy otherwise. Simultaneously, the requirement to understand the intricacy of liquid tumors, which demands high health literacy, can feel overwhelming. Furthermore, the acute crisis of having received a diagnosis of CLL, CML, HL, or indolent NHL is often then contrasted with the "wait and watch" treatment approach that is so common with these chronic, slowly progressing cancers. As indicated earlier, for many, when receiving a cancer diagnosis, there can be a sense of satisfaction and mastery gained from the tasks of treatment planning and for those prescribed a "wait and watch" regimen, they are largely denied this instrument of perceived control. This early point in a chronic cancer journey may be characterized by certainty in diagnosis, and yet uncertainty and ambiguity about disease trajectory, treatment, and prognosis. Increasing the patient's capacity to tolerate ambiguity and uncertainty, and focusing on the present without succumbing to learned helplessness and/or anxiety-provoking thoughts about the possibility of a disastrous future, will be important clinical goals of the oncology social worker when working with patients with these chronic HMs.

Chronic Due to the slow progression of chronic HM, and its lower likelihood of needing initial treatment, the patient's greatest challenge in such cases is usually adjusting to and accommodating the reality of a new chronic illness. There may be a struggle to try to return to pre-diagnosis normality as they balance their hope for a continued low level of disease with fear and preparation for potential progression. This fear and preparation may take the form of the person with cancer investing deeply in their own active surveillance, developing a keen readiness to detect signs of cancer progression, and becoming overall anxious and "on edge," a stark illustration of a "fight" survival response in action. At worst, the patient may be so consumed by hypervigilance and monitoring of their illness that they severely restrict important aspects of their life including social, creative, and physical activities that could increase their sense of well-being. This psychological state is similar to that of the experience of survivorship, wherein those in remission balance relief in having successfully treated their cancer with an intense fear of recurrence. A fear of the progression of illness is likely to cause peaks of anxiety in periods leading up to and during appointments with their oncologist, as they consider the possibility of hearing that the cancer has progressed. Importantly, this anxiety can negatively affect their prognostic understanding (Derry et al., 2019). Given the detrimental effects of anxiety, interventions to address maladaptive anxiety – including guided meditation, deep breathing exercises, mindfulness, and other somatic-based therapies – may be particularly useful.

When active treatment is required for these subtypes, the chronic phase of illness may resemble what is commonly experienced by patients with ST, and the toll of the disease on daily life can become more apparent. The person with cancer may need to stay at the hospital for extended periods for management of overwhelming acute side effects from treatment that exceed the present symptom burden of the cancer itself. Or, an acute event can trigger the beginning of a gradual-but-perceptible, progressive decline in overall functioning. Confronting cancer at a stage of life in which they are already experiencing the inevitable biological effects of aging, older adults are more likely to have comorbid conditions than younger patients, and tolerating treatment may be particularly arduous (Trevino et al., 2021). Changes in the patient's performance status (measured by such tools as the Eastern Cooperative Oncology Group (ECOG) and Karnofsky performance status (KPS) scales), combined with the inevitability of physical decline with aging, may cause the older adult to struggle with challenges to their sense of agency, control, independence, and meaning. In working with this population, it may be beneficial to allow space for the patient to reflect on these changes and grieve their losses, while also exploring and accentuating ways in which they are able to maintain their sense of self-worth and continue to live a valuable and meaningful life. ACT can be an effective intervention when focusing on balancing acknowledgment and acceptance of the grief with an effort to highlight the older patient's strengths, values, and history of resilience. DBT can help to increase distress tolerance, manage potential emotional dysregulation, and maintain focus on the present. Brief narrative, existential, logo, and/or meaning-centered therapies can facilitate constructing a meaningful narrative of the illness journey and underscoring where meaning and committed action are present currently. Recovering from treatment is a difficult process for older adults living alone or with a similarly aged partner, as supplemental caregiving may be warranted. This might require the adult child(ren) to adjust their daily lives to accommodate caregiving for the parent with HM or to hire professional help, depending on the availability of financial resources. As these recommendations suggest, in addition to the intra-psychic needs of the older patient with HM, social supports have been identified as having an important and direct role in buffering the stressful effects of illness (Kadambi, 2020). To mitigate the isolation and loneliness often encountered by an older adult whose social and work roles have diminished with age, a number of social support interventions may be offered. The use of social media platforms, Internet-based support groups, peer support, patient navigation programs, and collaboration with healthcare and community-based geriatric programs are some of the possible interventions aimed at expanding social support (Kadambi, 2020). The task of accepting one's frailty and need for additional care and support may feel demoralizing for the older cancer patient and necessitate a difficult adjustment for the previously independent person, especially given our modern Western culture's propensity to idealize individual autonomy and self-sufficiency.

Terminal

Despite the variation in illness trajectories and treatment plans among patients with various forms of HM, they can be said to experience the terminal phase of their illness differently than their ST counterparts. Because of the unpredictability of illness course and the possibility of curative therapies even in the most advanced and refractory HM (El-Jawahri et al., 2020), the transition between the curative and palliative phases of illness is difficult to discern for both patients with HM and for clinicians. Thus, patients with HM often receive intensive interventions in the EOL phase. They experience high rates of hospitalizations, urgent care visits, ICU admissions, chemotherapy, and life-sustaining blood product administration (Hui et al., 2014). Indeed, prognostic uncertainty defines HM, with up to 50% of HM patients surviving and recovering after ICU admissions (El-Jawahri et al., 2020). With ever-expanding options and clinical trials for patients with HM, oncologists may continue to opt for more treatment even as the patient's clinical status worsens. Taking the lead from their hematologic oncologist, patients and families may be unprepared for or slow to acknowledge the reality that the patient has entered the terminal phase of their cancer. In such cases, it is more difficult to make appropriate medical decisions regarding the goals of care. This may explain why patients with HM have a higher likelihood of dying in the hospital and lower rates of hospice referrals, being more than twice as likely to die in inpatient settings as those with ST (El-Jawahri et al., 2020). It is also a strong argument for early integration of palliative care services in the care of HM patients and the need for early and frequent conversations around advanced care planning.

There are other implications of an unpredictable disease trajectory and ambiguous EOL phase for patients with HM and their families. First, patients with advanced cancer who lack accurate prognostic understanding are less likely to have advanced directives in place at EOL, including a healthcare Proxy, Living Will, and Do Not Resuscitate (DNR) order, or to have considered their preferences around code status (Epstein et al., 2016). Accurate prognostic awareness may be particularly challenging for the young adult patient whose foray into death and mortality may be limited to intellectual speculation about a vague future. Prognostic incertitude has been shown to decrease the likelihood of the person with cancer receiving their preferred EOL care and to increase the likelihood of their receiving life-sustaining measures that are statistically unlikely to be effective, for example, CPR, which frequently resuscitates a patient only for that patient to require intubation and encounter various related, life-threatening complications; the rate of survival resulting in hospital discharge following CPR is only 13% for cancer patients with ST and a mere 7% for those with HM (Giza et al., 2018). A second consequence of an unclear terminal phase is the absence of crucial conversations on EOL wishes with friends and family, who may be called upon to make critical surrogate medical decisions. Lacking guidance from the patient, the surrogate decision maker may be overwhelmed with doubt, indecision about "doing the right thing," and fear of future regret, while simultaneously grieving the potential death of the patient. If the choice pertains to the withdrawal of life-sustaining treatment with relatively low burden, such as continued infusion of blood products or iv antibiotics, then the decision may be even more psychologically fraught, especially for parents of young adult patients. Studies have shown that EOL conversations are not only associated with patients' reporting preferences for less aggressive care, but that they can also reduce psychological distress of the bereaved family (Wright et al., 2008), as families have the opportunity to engage in important tasks of relationship closure (Byock, 2014). Bereft of EOL conversations, patients with minor-aged children are robbed of the opportunity to pursue important legacy work; the older adult, meanwhile, may face their death amid psychological and physical turmoil, deprived of the benefit of meaning-making interventions such as Chochinov's Dignity Therapy (2011). Additionally, when death is unexpected and characterized by aggressive care in an ICU or hospital setting, people closest to the patient are more likely to perceive the experience of death as traumatic, which has the potential to negatively affect bereavement and the integration of the loss (Anderson et al., 2008). Finally, because palliative care clinicians and/or hospice services are rarely involved, patients with HM are noted to experience substantial physical and psychological symptom burden at EOL (El-Jawahri et al., 2020). Unrealistic expectations by both patients and oncologists, the inability of hospice programs to provide transfusion support, and rapid and unpredictable trajectory of decline at EOL have been cited, respectively, as system-based, cultural, and illness-specific barriers to timely palliative care use in patients with HM (El-Jawahri et al., 2020). Without focused attention by palliative care specialists on symptom management, both psychological and physical, the patient with HM is at higher risk of suffering throughout the trajectory of their illness, and friends and family are at higher risk for difficult bereavement. Cognizant of the unique barriers to palliative care experienced by patients with HM, social work clinicians working with leukemia and lymphoma services may be able to close the gap of unmet psychosocial needs by helping members of the team as well as the patient to dispel rigid binary thinking about "fighting" or "giving up"; and to understand and welcome the complementary role of palliative care – or, as it is often described, to "hope for the best while preparing for the worst."

Bereavement

The uncertain timing of the terminal phase for a patient with HM and the barriers to recognizing it may complicate bereavement for family and friends. Post-loss, friends and family may find themselves in a state of shock, asking, "How did we get here?" As friends and family attempt to make sense of the ambiguity of the disease process, feelings of guilt and regret for missed opportunities to advocate for different EOL care and to say goodbye may be identified only retrospectively. As alluded to earlier, caregivers of patients who died in the ICU are at an increased risk of developing PTSD when compared to caregivers of patients who died at home with hospice care. Compared to caregivers of patients who died at home with hospice care (Wright et al., 2010), they are also at higher risk for PGD, where bereavement difficulties persist or worsen rather than diminish with time (Prigerson et al., 2021). Given that bereaved caregivers with PGD underutilize mental health services, and that bereavement interventions can be provided both pre- and post-loss, it may be particularly important to connect family members of patients with HM with clinical social workers prior to the patient's death (Lichtenthal et al., 2011). Post-death, Jordan and Litz (2014) recommend treatments that center on cognitive-behavioral principles and therapeutic techniques of exposure, behavioral activation, and cognitive restructuring that aim at increasing the bereaved person's engagement with the outside world and encouraging social reintegration.

Life cycle and relational dynamics also play an important role in bereavement. Family members of an older adult who dies may be better able to integrate the death as natural and expected than families who have lost a child or young adult. Part of the bereavement experience for family members "left behind," besides the residual challenges of understanding the disease process itself, is informed by the life cycle of the deceased. Consideration of the deceased patient's life stage and that of the family member can help guide intervention appropriateness, as well as screening for risk and assessing if intervention is indicated (Roberts et al., 2017). For example, if the patient was a young adult, a meaning-centered approach may be particularly beneficial for bereaved parents who are confronted with grief over their child's "unfinished business" and the loss of an anticipated future. One such intervention is meaning-centered grief therapy (MCGT), a structured, evidence-based intervention developed for parents who have lost a child to cancer which supports the parents in, among other things, reflecting on and connecting with their child's legacy and exploring ways in which they might carry it forward (Lichtenthal et al., 2019).

Bereavement care is not standardized and there is variability across institutions, or even within an institution, dependent on factors like resource availability and professional training. When a patient dies, the family often experiences a sudden loss of contact with the care team and/or receives impersonal and insufficient outreach. Continuity of care, including bereavement support, is vital for caregivers of patients with HM, who likely have not received the benefits of palliative or hospice care (which follows the bereaved for 13 months post-death). Bereavement may be further complicated if the care of a person with HM was perceived as suboptimal. In cases where pervasive inequities in healthcare contributed to poor care and outcome, no amount of bereavement intervention can adequately address the sense of injustice, which is more aptly addressed at the structural level.

Social Justice

Consistent with numerous reports citing significant inequities in health-related incidences and outcomes in communities of color, racial/ethnic disparities in incidence and survival for patients diagnosed with HM have likewise been noted (Kirtane & Lee, 2017). Among the most troubling statistic is that the probability of death for Black and Hispanic patients with ALL was about 45% and 46% higher, respectively, than for white patients; Black and Hispanic adolescent and young adult patients have a 62% and 35% higher risk of HL deaths, respectively; and Blacks are 49% less likely to receive SCT than whites (Kirtane & Lee, 2017). Speculating on the causes of these disparities, Kirtane and Lee (2017) posited the following factors: structural barriers to care, variable access to care, (non) "compliance" with therapies, and overall disease heterogeneity.

Barriers to quality healthcare for communities of color have been well documented, with research noting that Black Americans not only have lower rates of health insurance coverage but grapple with distrust of the healthcare system stemming from awareness of historic abuse and mistreatment by the medical system as well as ongoing racism and discrimination. These factors drive disparities in health access and also account for lower quality of care and outcome (Hamel et al., 2020; Mahajan et al., 2021). In 2018, an estimated 18% of all Hispanics and 10% of all Blacks were uninsured, compared to 5.4% of non-Hispanic whites, and this factor was noted as a common barrier to access and utilization of medical care, leading to delayed diagnosis, delayed treatment initiation, and disparities in outcomes (Williams et al., 2020). Disparities in outcome are likely due to more than the issue of access. Glance et al. (2013) cite numerous studies that reveal continued racial segregation of the healthcare system, noting that 25% of hospitals in the United States care for almost 90% of Black older adults; hospitals serving disproportionately high concentrations of non-white patients tend to be lower quality institutions, and patients admitted to these hospitals are less likely to receive recommended care and more likely to experience complications and die. This is a reminder of the history of racial segregation in medicine, and of how recent that history is: hospitals were desegregated less than two generations ago, when they were threatened with the loss of federal funds from the Medicaid and Medicare programs enacted in 1966.

Rural patients are likewise affected by their zip codes. Although one in five people in the United States lives in rural communities, the percentage of oncologists practicing in rural areas in 2019 was a mere 7.4%; this small percentage was in itself an incremental increase from the 5.5% of the period between 2014 and 2019 (Levit et al., 2020). Patients with cancer in rural areas face limited access to oncology providers and have high rates of cancer-related mortality and other negative treatment outcomes (Levit et al., 2020). This may be particularly true for patients with HM because the highly technical and specialized nature of the disease makes it difficult for patients to be treated at local hospitals and they may be required to travel hours from their homes to large urban, academic centers (LeBlanc et al., 2016).

The racial and geographic gap in healthcare has long been recognized, and various strategies have been aimed at raising public and provider awareness, expanding health insurance coverage, mitigating the financial toxicity of care, expanding the capacity and number of providers in underserved communities, opening avenues to clinical trial participation, and creating partnerships between providers and community leaders. Despite these varied efforts at local and national levels, the *New York Times* recently reported that, according to a 2021 special issue of the *Journal of American Medical Association* (JAMA) on health inequities, "the racial health gap did not significantly narrow from 1999 to 2018" (Rabin, 2021, p. 16). This article quoted Dr. Harlan Krumholz, one of the JAMA study's senior authors: "We're failing. If our national goals are to improve the population's health and promote more health equity, then we have to admit that whatever we're doing now is not doing the trick" (Rabin, 2021, p. 16).

The persistence of health inequities into the twenty-first century may be explained in part by America's long history of medical abuse and mistreatment of non-white populations, which has left an indelible legacy of distrust, if not aversion, of the medical system, especially among Black and Indigenous communities. For patients with HM, especially AL, trust in the healthcare system and providers is crucial, as patients are confronted with a "dizzying array of treatment risks and benefits" (LeBlanc et al., 2016, p. 2064) that are technical and complex, making processing information difficult, even for the most "health literate." Intimidated by highly technical medical information, patients may be overwhelmed and opt for more passive decision-making (LeBlanc et al., 2016), counterintuitive though this may be given the patients' lack of trust in the healthcare system and provider. This passivity is likely to engender the patient's anger and regret if the outcome is poor.

Though much depends on the communication skills of the physician, the task of digesting and discerning risks and benefits of treatment is especially daunting for those with lower levels of education, those who carry trauma histories, and/or who come from adverse community environments, including structures of racism. For patients who have experienced racism throughout their lives, access to healthcare means something more than mere access and availability. In order for efficacious utilization of health care by historically marginalized communities of color; institutions must take into consideration and accommodate for the cognitive and psychological work involved in deciding whether to avail oneself of a potential healthcare resource. The decision to seek care and to maintain "compliance" may be hampered by fear, distrust, and even anger.

Access to optimal healthcare encompasses more than the availability of medical facilities and providers, requiring also a set of infrastructural provisions, including lodging and transportation, that make consistent long-term treatment and surveillance possible. These logistics amplify the financial burden of cancer care, as does the cost of treatment itself, especially where treatment requires prolonged hospitalizations, intensive chemotherapies, innovative treatment protocols, and close symptom management that may include frequent and expensive blood and platelet transfusions. The wealth gap between the average white and Black American may explain why one study of Black breast cancer patients found that these patients more frequently reported distress over material concerns (such as housing) than their white counterparts (Hinyard et al., 2017). Further exacerbating the economic stress of Black patients with HM, among all cancer diagnoses, hematological oncology patients significantly scored the lowest on workability scores at 6, 12, and 18 months following their first sick day leave (de Boer et al., 2008), deferring their reentry into financially viable livelihoods.

Access to material resources and social support, critical to any successful cancer treatment and outcome, is not commonly recognized as contributing factors to "non-compliance." Non-adherence is usually viewed in terms of individual, not structural failing; it is seen as stemming from the ignorance or unwillingness of the patient to comply with medical recommendations. Often attributed to patients of color, this depiction belies a more troubling implicit racial bias. It fails to recognize that compliance requires access to resources, medical, and social; it implies that factors hampering a patient's ability to practice treatment compliance do not, in fact, exist. Confronted with perceived insurmountable obstacles to care, treatment can be seen by some people with HM as an impossibility. Moreover, the question of whether compliance contributes significantly to differences in outcomes for patients of color is disputed (Kirtane & Lee, 2017).

Less disputed is the scarcity of matching unrelated bone marrow donors for African Americans, who are able to find a match donor 25% of the time, while their white counterparts are successful about 75% of the time (Institute for Justice, 2020). The importance of match donors in mitigating the prevalence of GVHD in patients with SCT has been noted earlier and is critical to a positive treatment outcome. Compared to ST, there are more advances in innovative therapies and clinical trials in the field of HM. However, recruitment and enrollment of Black and other communities of color in clinical trials is low compared with white patients (Williams et al., 2020), and racial demographic data for many of the trials involving immunotherapy for hematologic malignancies are not reported (Kirtane & Lee, 2017), making it hard to even begin to assess the breadth of this problem. Underrepresentation in clinical trials for cancer may be a result of several factors, including lack of racially sensitive education and disregard for the fraught history of medical experimentation on Black and other communities of color. Spurred by the painful reality of stark disparities in deaths caused by the novel coronavirus COVID-19, the social determinants of health have become part of the larger conversation on race in America, in which care of the patient with HM must be included.

Authors' Reflections

During Susan Sontag's treatment for her breast cancer, she wrote in her *Illness as Metaphor* (1978, p. 3), "Illness is the night-side of life, a more onerous citizenship. Everyone who is born holds dual citizenship, in the kingdom of the well and in the kingdom of the sick. Although we all prefer to use only the good passport, sooner or later each of us is obliged, at least for a spell, to identify ourselves as citizens of that other place." For patients with the unique passports of HM, arrival into the "kingdom of illness" is by way of an abrupt airdrop and then being greeted, in one patient's words, with "a fire hose of information." Barely able to catch one's breath, they have landed on rough and uncertain terrain, where stretches of flat, steady ground can suddenly shift to reveal plummeting precipices, and roadmaps are written in complicated foreign "medicalese." Patients with HM are not short-term visitors, as treatment and surveillance can last many years. Because treatments for HM often have curative intent, the hope for returning to the kingdom of the well is omnipresent even as one is cut, poked, bruised, and wrecked by the potentially life-saving treatment. All of this speaks to the unique and enormous burden of HM on one's body and psyche. As Suleika Jaouad (2021) writes, "Worse are the psychological imprints of illness, largely invisible to others and devoid of easy fixes. Depression descends like a demon… Anxiety surges…. Panic overtakes…. Grief continues to haunt …." (pp. 212–213). One of the greatest challenges in working with this population is to stay where the patient is; to not assume or impart prior knowledge of a roadmap of an illness, but to understand that all journeys of illness are uniquely individual and can only be known by walking it. We, as supportive guides, must walk with them, which means we are also likely to get distressed, tired, disheartened, and lost. Working with HM patients, it is especially challenging to know that the road of treatment will be extremely treacherous, uncertain if the patients will even make it to the other side, and yet our job is to encourage them forward. In doing so, are we sometimes forced to feign bluster to try to keep them going, if only because they can't go back? Even when we see road signs of danger that they do not?

Anyone who has traveled knows that leaving home can be uncomfortable. We are required to adapt, to resist our desire to cling to the comfort of the known; to trust strangers and the experience even when everything around us unbalances us. A long foray into the kingdom of the ill does more than just unbalance; it changes us by creating a void of the self where we no longer know who we are because we have been away from home so long. Patients with HM who undergo SCT are literally no longer themselves, even in molecular terms. More than any other psychological turmoil, this emptiness of the self seems most terrifying. Our social identities accord us with many garbs of self, and when these are lost so markedly and for so long, we stand naked. And the only thing within our reach is the blanket of illness that at least hides everything that has been lost, even if the blanket is scratchy and uncomfortable, and gives no warmth. We work to remind our patients of the whole persons they are but when they feel everything has been taken away from them, do reminders of who they were (are?) bring them solace or anguish? What does it mean to "validate and normalize" our patients' loss and grief without accepting the comprehensive ways in which illness consumes them? And how do we give hope without invalidating or minimizing the depth of their losses? Holding these complexities can lead to inaction, being afraid of saying or doing the wrong thing. And if our own fears of competency become primary, what then of our patients? How can we stay present and open to what is needed from us? Is it possible that what is required from us is paradoxically a similar nakedness?

As healthcare social workers, we focus on our patients as they undergo treatment: guiding them and their friends and family, interpreting "medicalese," providing concrete resources, and offering supportive counseling, interventions, and compassionate human support. We are good at crisis management, at getting patients through the rough times. But we may think less about what happens after the crisis subsides and patients are thrust back into the kingdom of the well. This is when they realize that they are no longer like the others; that they will forever be dual citizens. Delving deeper into the experience of patients with HM has made vivid a gap in our care: that survivorship is poorly labeled, and life post-cancer has to be about more than mere survival. Surviving is about engaging in the arduous task of releasing, reworking, reconceiving, and reclaiming a life forever changed by cancer. In grief and trauma literature, there is an idea of transformative growth borne out of such nakedness, of being "broken open." It is a relentlessly optimistic view of human potential, which we, as a profession that believes in the possibilities of change, understandably gravitate toward. But, such transformations are usually known only in retrospect; if it happens, it happens after the crises of illness have abated, outside of our clinical interactions. The goal of our relationships with our HM patients, then, is merely to have shone a glimmer ray of light on an opening toward a life renewed and reclaimed. Our larger hope for our patients is that they claim a new citizenship altogether, beyond the kingdoms of the well and the sick.

In cases where patients do not survive their illness, the family is similarly confronted with the task of survival. They had been the unwitting companions of their beloved through the kingdom of the sick, and now find themselves in yet another altogether foreign land, that of grief and loss. They grieve not only their beloved but also their own identity, which had been shaped and defined through that relationship. A new undertaking awaits the bereft: to grieve these losses and find their way in this new world, and ultimately, through the integration of the loss, to find the deceased in that world. They, too, now carry a more onerous citizenship.

Reflection Questions

1. How might the nature of having an invisible cancer impact a patient's experience of it?
2. How might you address a patient's concerns that they might miss signs of cancer recurrence in survivorship, when the initial symptoms were vague or found by accident? How might your clinical work differ in working with patients with recurrence?
3. How might you address barriers to quality care for patients of color, in your role?

References

Allart-Vorelli, P., Porro, B., Baguet, F., Michel, A., & Cousson-Gélie, F. (2015). Hematological cancer and quality of life: A systematic literature review. *Blood Cancer Journal, 5*(4), e305. https://doi.org/10.1038/bcj.2015.29

American Cancer Society. (2019). *Cancer treatment & survivorship facts & figures 2019–2021*. American Cancer Society.

Amonoo, H. L., Leblanc, T. W., Kavanaugh, A. R., Webb, J. A., Traeger, L. N., Jagielo, A. D., et al. (2021). Posttraumatic stress disorder (PTSD) symptoms in patients with acute myeloid leukemia (AML). *Cancer, 127*, 2500. https://doi.org/10.1002/cncr.33524

Anderson, W. G., Arnold, R. M., Angus, D. C., & Bryce, C. L. (2008). Posttraumatic stress and complicated grief in family members of patients in the intensive care unit. *Journal of General Internal Medicine, 23*(11), 1871–1876.

Breitbart, W., Rosenfeld, B., Gibson, C., Pessin, H., Poppito, S., Nelson, C., et al. (2010). Meaning-centered group psychotherapy for patients with advanced cancer: A pilot randomized controlled trial. *Psycho-Oncology, 19*(1), 21–28. https://doi.org/10.1002/pon.1556

Bryant, J., Mansfield, E., Hall, A., Waller, A., Boyes, A., Jayakody, A., … Sanson-Fisher, R. (2016, February 27). *The psychosocial outcomes of individuals with haematological cancers: Are we doing enough high quality research, and what is it telling us?* https://www.sciencedirect.com/science/article/pii/S1040842816300403

Button, E., Chan, R. J., Chambers, S., Butler, J., & Yates, P. (2017). A systematic review of prognostic factors at the end of life for people with a hematological malignancy. *BMC Cancer, 17*(1), 213. https://doi.org/10.1186/s12885-017-3207-7

Byock, I. (2014). *Four things that matter most: A book about living* (10th Anniversary ed.). Atria Books.

Cardozo, E. R., Thomson, A. P., Karmon, A. E., Dickinson, K. A., Wright, D. L., & Sabatini, M. E. (2015). Ovarian stimulation and in-vitro fertilization outcomes of cancer patients undergoing fertility preservation compared to age matched controls: A 17-year experience. *Journal of Assisted Reproduction and Genetics, 32*(4), 587–596. https://doi.org/10.1007/s10815-015-0428-z

Chizuka, A., Suda, M., Shibata, T., Kusumi, E., Hori, A., Hamaki, T., ... Kami, M. (2006, September 21). *Difference between hematological malignancy and solid tumor research articles published in four major medical journals.* https://www.nature.com/articles/2404369

Crossnohere, N. L., Richardson, D. R., Reinhart, C., O'Donoghue, B., Love, S. M., Smith, B. D., & Bridges, J. (2019). Side effects from acute myeloid leukemia treatment: Results from a national survey. *Current Medical Research and Opinion, 35*(11), 1965–1970. https://doi.org/10.1080/03007995.2019.1631149

Davis, A., Viera, A. J., & Mead, M. D. (2014). Leukemia: An overview for primary care. *American Family Physician, 89*(9), 731–738.

de Boer, A. G., Verbeek, J. H., Spelten, E. R., Uitterhoeve, A. L., Ansink, A. C., de Reijke, T. M., Kammeijer, M., Sprangers, M. A., & van Dijk, F. J. (2008). Work ability and return-to-work in cancer patients. *British Journal of Cancer, 98*(8), 1342–1347. https://doi.org/10.1038/sj.bjc.6604302

Derry, H. M., Maciejewski, P. K., Epstein, A. S., Shah, M. A., LeBlanc, T. W., Reyna, V., & Prigerson, H. G. (2019). Associations between anxiety, poor prognosis, and accurate understanding of scan results among advanced cancer patients. *Journal of Palliative Medicine, 22*(8), 961–965.

El-Jawahri, A., Nelson, A. M., Gray, T. F., Lee, S. J., & Leblanc, T. W. (2020). Palliative and end-of-life care for patients with hematologic malignancies. *Journal of Clinical Oncology, 38*(9), 944–953. https://doi.org/10.1200/jco.18.02386

Erikson, E. H. (1950). *Childhood and society.* Norton.

Epstein, A. S., Prigerson, H. G., O'Reilly, E. M., & Maciejewski, P. K. (2016). Discussions of Life Expectancy and Changes in Illness Understanding in Patients With Advanced Cancer. *Journal of Clinical Oncology: Official Journal of the American Society of Clinical Oncology, 34*(20), 2398–2403. https://doi.org/10.1200/JCO.2015.63.6696

Giza, D. E., Rodrigo, M., Crommett, J., Botz, G., Ewer, M. S., Iliescu, G., et al. (2018). Impact of cardiopulmonary resuscitation (CPR) on the survival of patients with cancer: DNR before or after cardiac arrest? *Journal of Clinical Oncology, 36*(34), 71. https://doi.org/10.1200/jco.2018.36.34_suppl.71

Glance, L. G., Osler, T. M., Mukamel, D. B., Meredith, J. W., Li, Y., Qian, F., & Dick, A. W. (2013). Trends in racial disparities for injured patients admitted to trauma centers. *Health Services Research, 48*(5), 1684–1703. https://doi.org/10.1111/1475-6773.12064

Gooptu, M., & Koreth, J. (2017). Better acute graft-*versus*-host disease outcomes for allogeneic transplant recipients in the modern era: A tacrolimus effect? *Haematologica, 102*(5), 806–808. https://doi.org/10.3324/haematol.2017.165266

Hall, A., D'Este, C., Tzelepis, F., Lynagh, M., & Sanson-Fisher, R. (2014). Factors associated with haematological cancer survivors experiencing a high level of unmet need across multiple items of supportive care: A cross-sectional survey study. *Supportive Care in Cancer, 22*(11), 2899–2909. https://doi.org/10.1007/s00520-014-2264-6

Hamel, L., Lopes, L., Munana, C., Artiga, S., & Brodie, M. (2020, October). *KFF/the undefeated survey on race and health (Rep.).* https://files.kff.org/attachment/Report-Race-Health-and-COVID-19-The-Views-and-Experiences-of-Black-Americans.pdf

Hayes, S. C., Levin, M. E., Plumb-Vilardaga, J., Villatte, J. L., & Pistorello, J. (2013). Acceptance and commitment therapy and contextual behavioral science: Examining the progress of a distinctive model of behavioral and cognitive therapy. *Behavior Therapy, 44*(2), 180–198. https://doi.org/10.1016/j.beth.2009.08.002

Hinyard, L., Schwartz, T., & Keller, J. (2017). Differences in psychosocial stressors between black and white cancer patients. *Journal of Community and Supportive Oncology, 15*, e314–e320. https://doi.org/10.12788/jcso.0366

Howell, D. A., Shellens, R., Roman, E., Garry, A. C., Patmore, R., & Howard, M. R. (2011). Haematological malignancy: Are patients appropriately referred for specialist palliative and hospice care? A systematic review and meta-analysis of published data. *Palliative Medicine, 25*(6), 630–641. https://doi.org/10.1177/0269216310391692

Hui, D., Didwaniya, N., Vidal, M., Shin, S. H., Chisholm, G., Roquemore, J., & Bruera, E. (2014). Quality of end-of-life care in patients with hematologic malignancies: A retrospective cohort study. *Cancer, 120*(10), 1572–1578. https://doi.org/10.1002/cncr.28614

Hui, D., Bansal, S., Park, M., Reddy, A., Cortes, J., Fossella, F., & Bruera, E. (2015). Differences in attitudes and beliefs toward end-of-life care between hematologic and solid tumor oncology specialists. *Annals of Oncology, 26*(7), 1440–1446. https://doi.org/10.1093/annonc/mdv028

Husson, O., Huijgens, P. C., & van der Graaf, W. (2018). Psychosocial challenges and health-related quality of life of adolescents and young adults with hematologic malignancies. *Blood, 132*(4), 385–392. https://doi.org/10.1182/blood-2017-11-778555

Institute for Justice. (2020, August 10). *Bone marrow statistics*. https://ij.org/bonemarrowstatistics/

Jaouad, S. (2021). *Between two kingdoms: What almost dying taught me about living*. Bantam Press.

Jones, W. C., Parry, C., Devine, S., Main, D. S., & Okuyama, S. (2015). Understanding distress in posttreatment adult leukemia and lymphoma survivors: A lifespan perspective. *Journal of Psychosocial Oncology, 33*(2), 142–162. https://doi.org/10.1080/07347332.2014.1002658

Jordan, A. H., & Litz, B. T. (2014). Prolonged grief disorder: Diagnostic, assessment, and treatment considerations. *Professional Psychology: Research and Practice, 45*, 180–187.

Kadambi, S., Soto-Perez-de-Celis, E., Garg, T., Loh, K. P., Krok-Schoen, J. L., Battisti, N., Moffat, G. T., Gil-Jr, L. A., Mohile, S., & Hsu, T. (2020). Social support for older adults with cancer: Young International Society of Geriatric Oncology review paper. *Journal of Geriatric Oncology, 11*(2), 217–224. https://doi.org/10.1016/j.jgo.2019.09.005

Kirtane, K., & Lee, S. J. (2017). Racial and ethnic disparities in hematologic malignancies. *Blood, 130*(15), 1699–1705. https://doi.org/10.1182/blood-2017-04-778225

Leblanc, T. W., Abernethy, A. P., & Casarett, D. J. (2015). What is different about patients with hematologic malignancies? A retrospective cohort study of cancer patients referred to a hospice research network. *Journal of Pain and Symptom Management, 49*(3), 505–512. https://doi.org/10.1016/j.jpainsymman.2014.07.003

Leblanc, T. W., Fish, L. J., Bloom, C. T., El-Jawahri, A., Davis, D. M., Locke, S. C., et al. (2016). Patient experiences of acute myeloid leukemia: A qualitative study about diagnosis, illness understanding, and treatment decision-making. *Psycho-Oncology, 26*(12), 2063–2068. https://doi.org/10.1002/pon.4309

Lethborg, C., Aranda, S., Bloch, S., & Kissane, D. (2006). The role of meaning in advanced cancer–integrating the constructs of assumptive world, sense of coherence and meaning-based coping. *Journal of Psychosocial Oncology, 24*(1), 27–42. https://doi.org/10.1300/J077v24n01_03

Levit, L. A., Byatt, L., Lyss, A. P., Paskett, E. D., Levit, K., Kirkwood, K., Schenkel, C., & Schilsky, R. L. (2020). Closing the rural cancer care gap: Three institutional approaches. *JCO Oncology Practice, 16*(7), 422–430. https://doi.org/10.1200/op.20.00174

Lichtenthal, W. G., Nilsson, M., Kissane, D. W., Breitbart, W., Kacel, E., Jones, E. C., & Prigerson, H. G. (2011). Underutilization of mental health services among bereaved caregivers with prolonged grief disorder. *Psychiatric Services, 62*(10), 1225–1229.

Lichtenthal, W. G., Catarozoli, C., Masterson, M., Slivjak, E., Schofield, E., Roberts, K. E., Neimeyer, R. A., Wiener, L., Prigerson, H. G., Kissane, D. W., Li, Y., & Breitbart, W. (2019). An open trial of meaning-centered grief therapy: Rationale and preliminary evaluation. *Palliative & Supportive Care, 17*(1), 2–12. https://doi.org/10.1017/S1478951518000925

Mahajan, S., Caraballo, C., Lu, Y., Valero-Elizondo, J., Massey, D., Annapureddy, A. R., Roy, B., Riley, C., Murugiah, K., Onuma, O., Nunez-Smith, M., Forman, H. P., Nasir, K., Herrin, J., & Krumholz, H. M. (2021). Trends in differences in health status and Health Care Access and affordability by race and ethnicity in the United States, 1999-2018. *The Journal of the American Medical Association, 326*(7), 637. https://doi.org/10.1001/jama.2021.9907

Martin, P. J., Counts, G. W., Jr., Appelbaum, F. R., Lee, S. J., Sanders, J. E., Deeg, H. J., Flowers, M. E., Syrjala, K. L., Hansen, J. A., Storb, R. F., & Storer, B. E. (2010). Life expectancy in patients surviving more than 5 years after hematopoietic cell transplantation. *Journal of Clinical Oncology, 28*(6), 1011–1016. https://doi.org/10.1200/JCO.2009.25.6693

Mason, T. M., Tofthagen, C. S., & Buck, H. G. (2020). Complicated grief: Risk factors, protective factors, and interventions. *Journal of Social Work in End-of-Life & Palliative Care, 16*(2), 151–174. https://doi.org/10.1080/15524256.2020.1745726

Mcgrath, P., & Holewa, H. (2007). Special considerations for haematology patients in relation to end-of-life care: Australian findings. *European Journal of Cancer Care, 16*(2), 164–171. https://doi.org/10.1111/j.1365-2354.2006.00745.x

Nissim, R., Zimmermann, C., Minden, M., Rydall, A., Yuen, D., Mischitelle, A., et al. (2013). Abducted by the illness: A qualitative study of traumatic stress in individuals with acute leukemia. *Leukemia Research, 37*(5), 496–502. https://doi.org/10.1016/j.leukres.2012.12.007

Oran, B., & Weisdorf, D. J. (2012). Survival for older patients with acute myeloid leukemia: A population-based study. *Haematologica, 97*(12), 1916–1924. https://doi.org/10.3324/haematol.2012.066100

Prigerson, H. G., Kakarala, S., Gang, J., & Maciejewski, P. K. (2021). History and status of prolonged grief disorder as a psychiatric diagnosis. *Annual Review of Clinical Psychology, 17*, 109–126.

Pulte, D., Jansen, L., & Brenner, H. (2020). Changes in long term survival after diagnosis with common hematologic malignancies in the early 21st century. *Blood Cancer Journal, 10*(5). https://doi.org/10.1038/s41408-020-0323-4

Rabin, R. C. (2021, August 18). Despite efforts to improve access to care, a racial health gap persists. *New York Times*.

Roberts, K., Holland, J., Prigerson, H. G., Sweeney, C., Corner, G., Breitbart, W., & Lichtenthal, W. G. (2017). Development of the bereavement risk inventory and screening questionnaire (BRISQ): Item generation and expert panel feedback. *Palliative & Supportive Care, 15*(1), 57–66. https://doi.org/10.1017/S1478951516000626

Rodin, G., Deckert, A., Tong, E., Le, L. W., Rydall, A., Schimmer, A., Marmar, C. R., Lo, C., & Zimmermann, C. (2018). Traumatic stress in patients with acute leukemia: A prospective cohort study. *Psycho-Oncology, 27*(2), 515–523. https://doi.org/10.1002/pon.4488

Rolland, J. S. (1987). Chronic illness and the life cycle: A conceptual framework. *Family Process, 26*(2), 203–221. https://doi.org/10.1111/j.1545-5300.1987.00203.x

Sansom-Daly, U. M., & Wakefield, C. E. (2013). Distress and adjustment among adolescents and young adults with cancer: An empirical and conceptual review. *Translational Pediatrics, 2*(4), 167–197. https://doi.org/10.3978/j.issn.2224-4336.2013.10.06

SEER. (2020). *Seer cancer stat facts*. https://seer.cancer.gov/statfacts/

Sekeres, M. A., Guyatt, G., Abel, G., Alibhai, S., Altman, J. K., Buckstein, R., Choe, H., Desai, P., Erba, H., Hourigan, C. S., LeBlanc, T. W., Litzow, M., MacEachern, J., Michaelis, L. C., Mukherjee, S., O'Dwyer, K., Rosko, A., Stone, R., Agarwal, A., Colunga-Lozano, L. E., et al. (2020). American Society of Hematology 2020 guidelines for treating newly diagnosed acute myeloid leukemia in older adults. *Blood Advances, 4*(15), 3528–3549. https://doi.org/10.1182/bloodadvances.2020001920

Shawver, L. K., Slamon, D., & Ullrich, A. (2002). Smart drugs: Tyrosine kinase inhibitors in cancer therapy. *Cancer Cell, 1*(2), 117–123.

Solomon, S. R., Jackson, K. C., Zhang, X., Solh, M., Bashey, A., Holland, H. K., & Morris, L. E. (2018). Treatment patterns and outcomes of unselected elderly Acute Myeloid Leukemia (AML) patients referred to a combined Acute Leukemia and Hematopoietic Stem Cell Transplant (HSCT) program. *Blood, 132*(Supplement 1), 2675–2675. https://doi.org/10.1182/blood-2018-99-111048

Sontang, S. (1978). *Illness as metaphor*. Farrar, Straus and Giroux.

Thompson, P. A., Kantarjian, H. M., & Cortes, J. E. (2015). Diagnosis and treatment of chronic myeloid leukemia in 2015. *Mayo Clinic Proceedings, 90*(10), 1440–1454. https://doi.org/10.1016/j.mayocp.2015.08.010

Trevino, K. M., Saracino, R. M., & Roth, A. J. (2021). Symptomatology, assessment, and treatment of anxiety in older adults with cancer. *Journal of Geriatric Oncology, 12*(2), 316–319.
Vehling, S., & Kissane, D. W. (2018). Existential distress in cancer: Alleviating suffering from fundamental loss and change. *Psycho-Oncology, 27*(11), 2525–2530. https://doi.org/10.1002/pon.4872
Verhoef, M., Nijs, E. J., Ootjers, C. S., Fiocco, M., Fogteloo, A. J., Heringhaus, C., et al. (2019). End-of-Life trajectories of patients with hematological malignancies and patients with advanced solid tumors visiting the emergency department: The need for a proactive integrated care approach. *American Journal of Hospice and Palliative Medicine, 37*(9), 692–700. https://doi.org/10.1177/1049909119896533
Williams, S., Ayers, A., Hildebrandt, M., McNeill, L., & Flowers, C. (2020). Strategies for overcoming disparities for patients with hematologic malignancies and for improving enrollment on clinical trials. *Oncology, 34*(06), 10.46883/onc.3406.0216.
Wright, A. A., Zhang, B., Ray, A., Mack, J. W., Trice, E., Balboni, T., Mitchell, S. L., Jackson, V. A., Block, S. D., Maciejewski, P. K., & Prigerson, H. G. (2008). Associations between end-of-life discussions, patient mental health, medical care near death, and caregiver bereavement adjustment. *The Journal of the American Medical Association, 300*(14), 1665–1673. https://doi.org/10.1001/jama.300.14.1665
Wright, A. A., Keating, N. L., Balboni, T. A., Matulonis, U. A., Block, S. D., & Prigerson, H. G. (2010). Place of death: Correlations with quality of life of patients with cancer and predictors of bereaved caregivers' mental health. *Journal of Clinical Oncology, 28*(29), 4457–4464. https://doi.org/10.1200/JCO.2009.26.3863
Yu, J., Judy, J. T., Parasuraman, S., Sinha, M., & Weisdorf, D. (2020). Inpatient healthcare resource utilization, costs, and mortality in adult patients with acute graft-versus-host disease, including steroid-refractory or high-risk disease, following allogeneic hematopoietic cell transplantation. *Biology of Blood and Marrow Transplantation, 26*(3), 600–605. https://doi.org/10.1016/j.bbmt.2019.10.028

Chapter 4
Communicable Diseases

Adam Schoenfarber and Sheila Langan

Introduction

The lingering suspicion that something is wrong—off. The worry that one might catch a cold. A coworker at the office has the sniffles and was out today. The person who sneezed on the bus did not cover their nose and they just looked *ill.*

The first symptom people experience of a communicable disease is often fear, not only from getting the disease and experiencing its physical effects. The fear of infection fuels a process by which individuals, perceived as potentially or actually ill, are "disqualified from full social acceptance" (Pantelic et al., 2019, p. 1). People in this situation face real and perceived barriers, either externally—in discriminatory, enacted stigma—or internally. Self-stigma, also referred to as "spoiled identity," can have profound effects on how people pursue care, treat their own disease, and live with illness (Pantelic et al., 2019). As Isabel Wilkerson writes in *Caste: The Origins of Our Discontents* (2020):

> The virus brought the interconnectedness of the planet into vivid, terrifying relief. Distance and geography could contain Ebola for a time, but Ebola did not recognize race or color or caste or national origin. A human being was a human being and a prospective new host to a frighteningly efficient virus. The contagion had initially not been seen as the global human crisis it was. Those suffering were West Africans with ill-equipped health systems, a hemi-

A. Schoenfarber (✉)
Westchester Medical Center, Valhalla, NY, USA

Fordham University, New York City, NY, USA
e-mail: aschoenfarber@fordham.edu

S. Langan
Memorial Sloan Kettering Cancer Center, New York City, NY, USA
e-mail: SL1586@nyu.edu

M. Hemphill, A. Nathanson (eds.), *The Practice of Clinical Social Work in Healthcare*, Essential Clinical Social Work Series,
https://doi.org/10.1007/978-3-031-31650-0_4

> sphere away. But Ebola, and potentially planet-wide catastrophes like it, as the world would discover beyond imagining six years later, have a way of reminding human beings that we are all indeed one species, all interwoven, more alike than different, more interdependent on one another than we might otherwise want to believe. (p. 201)

People fear not only disease and the effect of disease on the body but also the effects of the story that they, and the societal and cultural systems surrounding them, tell about themselves, and how they exist in relation to others, and receive care, based on that story.

This chapter introduces the psychosocial issues and clinical goals relevant to communicable diseases (Table 4.1) and discusses the critical role that healthcare social workers play in the emotional and psychological health of people with communicable diseases and their families. Healthcare social workers occupy a unique space in the healthcare system as a result of their application of concepts of relational care and systems-thinking, conducting interventions at micro-, meso-, and macro system levels with impacted (or potentially impacted) individuals and groups. Healthcare social workers can help prevent the potential spread of disease through community education and individual empowerment. They can attend to the initial anxiety of symptoms experienced before diagnosis and the trauma of ruptured identity at the time of diagnosis. They can assist in the learning and adjustment to life with the illness that happens to people with communicable diseases and support those people if their disease becomes terminal who experience anticipatory grief. Healthcare social workers may also provide support for those without communicable diseases too, whose lives are nonetheless shaped by the myriad complex emotions and experiences of existing in a world in which communicable diseases are prevalent and possible.

Table 4.1 Psychosocial issues, clinical goals, and interventions

Phase	Psychosocial issues	Clinical goals and interventions
Acute/crisis	Stigma Anxiety (including death anxiety) Depression Fear Depersonalization Isolation	Affirm humanity and dignity Co-construct meaning and narrative Cognitive restructuring Interpersonal connection Psychoeducation
Chronic	Internalizing new identities Post-traumatic stress Demoralization Hopelessness Helplessness	Meaning-centered work Resolve ambivalence Focus on grit and resilience Modeling and mentorship
Terminal	Feelings of being a burden Isolation Anxiety Fear of destruction of personhood	Reconciliation Legacy work Anticipatory bereavement support

Illness Overview

Communicable diseases refer specifically to infections from an outside source, which are transmitted through person-to-person contact. This may occur through inhaled respiratory droplets, fluid transmission (blood, semen, mucus, sputum, and waste), or mother-to-child (pregnancy, the birthing process, or breastfeeding). These differ from noncommunicable infectious diseases (NCD), such as tetanus or food poisoning, which are not communicable person-to-person but rather transmitted from exposure to natural or inanimate sources (Correl, 2021).

There are hundreds of communicable diseases which represent huge threats to the population. Some communicable diseases are more common and more dangerous. Pneumonia, for instance, whether bacterial or viral, is an infection of the lungs transmitted through inhaled fluid droplets. It is difficult to identify how many new infections of pneumonia occur annually. However, in 2018, the CDC identified 1.5 million visits to hospital emergency departments with a primary diagnosis of pneumonia (National Center for Health Statistics [NCHS], 2021).

Rates of communicable diseases disproportionately affect Black Americans, the Latinx population, and sexual minorities and people of the LGBTQIA community (Jeremiah et al., 2020). The causes for this are multivariate and intersectional, including, but not limited to: restricted access to healthcare services; poor sexual health literacy; population growth; urbanization; economic development; climate change; worldwide dismantling of public health systems; international travel, tourism, and commerce; microbial resistance due to indiscriminate use of anotics; an increasingly older population; and more complex issues such as socioeconomic inequalities, power discrepancies, poverty, and the language used in the discourse around disease (Gorin, 2002; Jeremiah et al., 2020; Mabhala et al., 2020; NCHS, 2021).

Language

Social workers intentionally use person-first or person-centered language that is affirming, inclusive, and empowering. This model was first used in the 1970s as part of an advocacy effort by Americans living with disabilities to destigmatize and normalize health conditions (Crocker & Smith, 2019).

To model this linguistic shift, we refer not to "HIV patients" but to people living with HIV/AIDS (PLWHA). Rather than refer to "victims of COVID-19" or "pneumonia sufferers," we refer to people who survive COVID-19 infection and people undergoing treatment for pneumonia. We use "people experiencing homelessness" as opposed to "homeless people." We try to avoid exacerbating stigmatization through the use of deficit-oriented language.

In the spirit of inclusivity and affirmative, anti-racist care, we elect to intentionally capitalize the B in Black and Brown to reflect the unique shared sense of identity and culture among Black Americans. To include all groups who fall under the LGBTQIA umbrella, we use LGBTQIA to acknowledge people who are two-spirit, pansexual, asexual, nonbinary, and many other identities. References to families should be understood to be inclusive of both consanguineous families of origin and families of choice.

Illness Onset, Course, and Degree of Incapacitation

For all of the many communicable diseases that exist, there are many more courses and experiences of illness, varying both between diseases and within the same disease category. The onset of illness from a communicable disease can be acute and rapid after exposure—such as with influenza, COVID-19, or Ebola—or delayed and gradual, such as with human immunodeficiency virus (HIV), hepatitis B, and Epstein–Barr.

The course of illness can be progressive, as with meningitis; constant; or relapsing/episodic with periods of latency, such as with HIV or herpes. Even within one disease, the projected course can change depending on the individual's response and how science and medical knowledge grow and adapt.

Outcomes, too, vary significantly both depending on disease and among individuals who contract the same disease. Outcomes are also heavily dependent on the resources available to an individual and community. For example, respiratory infections, HIV/AIDS, and tuberculosis are significantly more deadly in poorer countries, where preventative measures and treatment are inaccessible to much of the population. The World Health Organization (WHO) therefore considers them to be "diseases of poverty" because the burden and impact are linked to socioeconomic status (2012).

The degree of incapacitation resulting from an infectious disease can range from a runny nose or fatigue from the common cold to paralysis from polio. One of the most pervasive incapacitating factors in communicable disease is social stigma. Fear, lack of knowledge, and the disproportional impact of social determinants of health drive scapegoating, discrimination, societal stigma, and self-stigma (Barrett & Brown, 2008). These in turn impact individuals' safety, mental health, coping, and sense of self, in addition to their willingness to get tested, receive treatment, and disclose their status (Ma et al., 2019; France et al., 2015).

Given the vast range of communicable diseases, we will focus in-depth throughout this chapter on two examples social workers in a medical setting in the United States are likely to encounter: HIV and COVID-19.

HIV

HIV has a gradual onset, with flu-like symptoms appearing in approximately two-thirds of people anywhere from 2 to 4 weeks post-infection (About HIV & AIDS, 2021). This first stage, the acute HIV infection, can last a few days or a few weeks. In the second stage, known as clinical latency or chronic HIV infection, the virus multiplies at lower levels, so people may experience no symptoms or mild symptoms. According to the CDC (2021), it is possible to remain in this stage for 10–15 years without treatment, though some people progress through it faster. Without treatment, the body's immune system grows weaker and eventually progresses to the final stage of HIV, acquired immunodeficiency syndrome (AIDS). If AIDS develops and goes untreated, incapacitation becomes progressively more severe and the prognosis is terminal, with common symptoms including fevers, rashes and sores, significant weight loss/wasting, HIV-associated dementia, pneumonia, Kaposi sarcoma (cancer), and high vulnerability to other infections.

Whereas in the first decades of the AIDS epidemic, HIV was considered a terminal diagnosis, it has since become a chronic, long-term condition, manageable with the advent and improvement of antiretroviral therapy (ART) for those with enough access to care (Deeks et al., 2013). If one has access to and can consistently take ART, it can suppress the viral load to the point that the virus does not progress and becomes undetectable. If the virus is undetectable, it also becomes non-transmissible to intimate partners—this is referred to as U = U (McKeon & Goldstein, 2020). Regular care and follow-ups, to manage ART side effects and test for viral load, are important.

COVID-19

The COVID-19 virus has an acute onset, with symptoms typically developing within 5 days of exposure, though symptoms have been reported to develop anywhere from 2 to 8 days postexposure. Some infected individuals are asymptomatic; some have mild courses, with cold or flu-like symptoms and/or sensory losses in taste and smell; and others experience severe symptoms requiring hospitalization, such as high fever, confusion, hypoxia, acute respiratory distress syndrome, COVID-19-associated pneumonia, sepsis, and other inflammatory responses. Depending on the severity of the case, hospitalization can entail minimally invasive supports such as medication, fluids, and oxygen via a nasal cannula or critical care interventions such as intubation, sedation, and pressors to stabilize blood pressure. The infection-fatality risk for patients hospitalized primarily for COVID-19 in the United States has decreased, dropping from 15.1% during the months when the Delta variant was dominant (July–October 2021) to 4.9% during the later Omicron phase of April–July 2022, with patients over age 65 or with more than three underlying medical conditions at highest risk (Adjei et al., 2022). As is the case with many aspects of COVID-19, the long-term effects are still emerging and vary greatly. Some reported "long-haul" symptoms after recovery include: shortness of breath, fatigue, anxiety, brain fog, joint pain, and ongoing loss of smell or taste (Rubin, 2020).

Clinical Issues

As onset, course, outcomes, and incapacitation vary among the greater than 80 communicable diseases identified by World Health Organization (WHO), so too do the time phases of illness. While the longitudinal course of illness has "certain universal, practical illness-related tasks" (Rolland, 1987, p. 4), patient experience throughout the illness is elastic and variable, depending on the significance of symptom burden, perception of morbidity, and public understanding of the disease. For example, the crisis phase of minor influenza is often vastly less dramatic than a new diagnosis of COVID-19.

Prior to diagnosis, people who have the possibility of infection often face the psychological distress not only of the possibility of illness but also the probability of being stigmatized. For people who consider being tested for HIV, stigma, shame, and blame may be anticipated and may serve as a barrier to testing and disclosure. Likewise, stigma in a pandemic can perpetuate the spread of a virus, as people become reluctant to get tested, especially when they only have mild symptoms, or to share information about their contacts prior to receiving a diagnosis (Villa et al., 2020).

The threat of COVID-19 infection affects individuals and groups psychosocially to varying degrees today. In the face of vaccine advancements, changing public guidance about precautions, and discord over mandates, some experience fatigue while others remain vigilant to the threat of disease. We are all impacted by its constantly shifting landscape, and our futures as individuals, groups, and societies are touched by uncertainty, threatening in a manner that may constitute as traumatic or, rather, a shared trauma of having survived thus far, recovering and yet still not free of the threat of infection. The unpredictable nature of pandemics and epidemics can also challenge our sense of order and expectations around certain life stages and/or planning for our lives (whether the disease is liable to affect people across age groups, as with HIV, or whether it brings heightened anxiety for those in certain vulnerable age groups, as with COVID-19). Whether or not one has had or has the disease or virus, one is part of a world in which one's everyday decisions and larger life choices are shaped, to varying degrees, by its existence.

For all those newly diagnosed with a communicable disease, stress and anxiety can be high, as patients wonder what is ahead for them—especially if they have high-risk factors for severe infection—and whether they may have infected others. People who are waiting for results of an HIV test or are newly diagnosed with HIV are known to grapple with emotional distress, self-esteem, anxiety, and fear around selective disclosure of serostatus (Heijnders & Van Der Meij, 2006). With HIV diagnosis, there may also be fear associated with HIV's recent history as a rapidly progressing terminal illness. In this case, the dissemination of information on recent medical treatments and the assurance of such information being understood is critically important to overcoming such fear, recognizing the strong possibility of living a long life, minimally impacted by HIV-related symptoms, and adjusting to a new diagnosis.

The existence of stigma around certain communicable diseases intensifies negative feelings and experiences for individuals and groups who are blamed for their spread. During the COVID-19 pandemic, the Asian community was targeted for hate crimes following public messaging that laid blame for the virus early on (Villa et al., 2020). Essential workers, who were not able to adhere to physical distancing practices by nature of their work, were also initially reacted to with fear. At onset and throughout the course of HIV illness, stigma has been a significantly incapacitating factor, particularly for those with multiple intersecting marginalized identities, such as LGBTQIA people of color (Nydegger & Hill, 2020). A person living with HIV's sense of self and ability to cope with news of having the disease and who belongs to a minority group (in race, ethnicity, sexuality, and gender) may be particularly challenged by the message from the dominant culture about the diagnosis that, at best, is *othering* (as a situation that *happens to you, not me*) and, at worst, is deeply prejudiced and perpetuating of systemic oppression.

Those who have it and have internal narratives of individualized risk factors (e.g., age and the presence of other chronic illnesses) and perceived vulnerability, physically, emotionally, and otherwise can feel highly distressed by diagnosis. For instance, people with young children who worked might have felt particular pressure to not get sick with COVID-19—for fear of lost income, lost childcare (who would care for their children if they became ill too?), and an inability to function well enough.

Throughout the course of an illness, healthcare social workers monitor for biopsychosocial suffering that may accompany a communicable disease. By helping patients to co-construct meaning and place the illness within a narrative of their life, social workers can help patients to develop new resiliency factors to navigate the full course of the illness. Table 4.1 summarizes psychosocial issues that occur throughout different stages of the illness, as well as clinical goals and interventions social workers and patients may consider (see Table 4.1).

Crisis

Intrapersonal The crisis stage of communicable illness emerges before confirmation of diagnosis, and sometimes even before contagion. Due to the social reputation of a disease and the perception of those who carry the disease, stigma is often the first pre-diagnosis symptom of a communicable disease. Stigma may be enacted or experienced by the person with the disease, anticipated, or perceived based on the behavior that they have witnessed or engaged in, or internalized based upon their own views of an illness. Many diseases begin with patients experiencing influenza-like symptoms such as congestion, changes in respiratory status, and changes in digestion. If public perception and stigma explain the disease as rooted in behaviors and personal responsibility or immorality, a person with that diagnosis and their families may feel distress and low self-esteem. A social worker may assist with these experiences through practical interventions to help them through the crisis and through psychosocial interventions, focused on co-constructing a different, more neutral, or positive meaning and narrative surrounding the situation. A social worker could facilitate a shift in narrative and cognitive focus—from how it occurred (i.e., "I did this to myself"), to self-care and compassion for having it (i.e., "I deserve self-compassion and it will help me feel at my emotional best in face of this physical challenge").

In some cases, those presumed to have the disease are classified as undesirable due to racism, xenophobia, homophobia, or any number of prejudices. Their humanity and personhood are called into question, and they are seen by society and by themselves as one and the same with their disease, instead of as a whole person (Ma et al., 2019). This depersonalization can be internalized. As a result, a person may feel differently about themselves (*less than they were*), and feel the need to hide their struggle related to health fears and coping with physical difficulties (so that others will not see them one-dimensionally—as *their disease/lesser than before*). To avoid stigma, a person can also avoid diagnosis, medication management, and care, which can not only worsen their own prognosis but also increase their likelihood of being a disease vector within their community.

Kunzler et al. (2021) note that psychological distress due to fear of destruction of personhood and lack of understanding of the disease is common in the early stages of highly contagious events, such as the COVID-19, SARS, and Ebola outbreaks. As one experiences physical symptoms, the distress and knowledge of potential for impending illness can impact the disease process and worsen the presentation of symptoms, creating an anxiety-symptom cycle. A patient with a confirmed new diagnosis begins to grapple with personal death awareness, and abstract understanding that their life may never be the same.

Social workers can utilize various approaches and modalities to counteract such harmful psychosocial effects. Meaning-centered care, which assumes that humans naturally search for and ascribe meaning to help cope with the burden of illness, can be incorporated to prevent suffering from developing into a deeper despair. Frankl (1985) argues that despair is suffering without meaning; applied here, his theory suggests that searching or building meaning connected with life with illness can counteract despair. Cognitive behavioral therapy (CBT), an evidence-based intervention, can be used to identify and monitor automatic thoughts associated with illness, and work to shift, question and restructure negative, and unhelpful thoughts that negatively impact self-image and core identity. The plethora of modalities recommended speak to the many challenges that may arise while supporting patients.

Social workers can also address intersectional stigma. Nydegger and Hill (2020) observe that intersectional identities such as race, ethnicity, gender presentation, and sexual orientation also intersect with disease status, contagion, and risk, as well as compounding factors such as poverty and access to health systems to create a kind of intersectional stigma. Social workers pay special attention to practices within minority groups and communities of color to offer culturally humble, antiracist, and culturally affirmative care.

Interpersonal Family and social reactions will likely vary depending on the route of transmission of disease (contact, respiratory droplet, fluid exchange, or mother–child). As mentioned earlier, the term "families" in this context may refer to families of origin (the families into which we are born), and/or families of choice, the people to whom we gravitate in adulthood who may replace or supplement families of origin. While families of origin may be consanguineous and share history, religion, and important childhood experiences, families of choice may reflect people who closely share our values, beliefs, and hopes for the future. LGBTQIA people have long created families of choice after losing access to or setting safe boundaries with families of origin due to homophobia or beliefs that denigrate the humanity of LGBTQIA people. In the case of communicable illness associated with stigmatized behavior, separation from families of origin is common. It is not unusual for communities to feel anger, outrage, and fear, usually around internalized anxiety about being infected with the disease, and the latency period between potential exposure and confirmation of diagnosis. Communities direct these emotions toward an attributable source to reduce societal feelings of helplessness and panic (Saeed et al., 2020). These feelings can emerge and crystalize as anti-immigrant violence, as seen in the rise of anti-Chinese and more broadly anti-Asian sentiment during COVID-19; as homophobic and racist neglect of patients and caregivers during the HIV/AIDS epidemic; or as anti-Italian sentiment prevalent during the smallpox outbreaks of the early 1900s (Saeed et al., 2020).

Isolation is a common theme across the spectrum of communicable diseases. This includes not only self-isolation to protect others from infection, but also ostracization, loss of employment, rejection, blaming, and verbal and physical abuse due to perceived immoral acts associated with fluid transmitted—and highly stigmatized—diseases such as HIV or Hepatitis C (Ma et al., 2019). Through a review of the literature, Ma et al. (2019) found that psychoeducation, social support programs, psychotherapeutic intervention using acceptance and commitment therapy–based groups, and narrative intervention improved self-stigma and community connection among PLWHA. They also noted that psychoeducational groups involving family–child dyads had positive results addressing isolation and stigma within the family unit (2019). Psychoeducation topics relevant to myriad communicable diseases can be offered throughout the phases of an illness and can be categorized into biopsychosocial categories. Table 4.2 summarizes the psychoeducation topics relevant throughout each phase of the illness. In the crisis phase of an illness psychoeducation topics may focus on biological and physical processes, including how the disease is transmitted, how patients might monitor for changes in their symptoms, disease progression, and how best to intervene in symptom management from curative and palliative perspectives. Psychological aspects include: recognizing

Table 4.2 Psychoeducation topics

Crisis	Chronic	Terminal
Method of transmission Symptom monitoring Self-disclosure Psychological support resources Recognizing ambivalence Mindful breathing for anxiety	Self-managing chronic health news Navigating healthcare Accessing resources Modeling and reciprocity	Signs and symptoms of disease course Symptom interventions Hospice benefit and end-of-life care resources

Caption: A table listing psychoeducation topics identified as relevant through multiple phases of communicable diseases

ambivalence in decision-making; anxiety reduction techniques; self-management; reception of chronic health news; and support around anticipatory bereavement and personal death anxiety. Social aspects of the disease include disclosure to friends and family; navigating the social safety net and healthcare generally; and modeling and acting as disease ambassador for others in crisis phases of the disease.

Systems of Care Interaction with the public health system and safety net is critical at the crisis stage, as persons may engage in reckless behavior out of hopelessness or denial of the severity of their disease. However, equal effort must be made to support healthcare social workers and healthcare professionals more broadly, due to increased risk of exposure to people who may be contagious, and increased exposure to the vicarious trauma of the disease in question. In a scoping review, Kunzler et al. (2021) examined the use of mental health and psychological support during highly contagious disease outbreaks to support healthcare workers. They identified psychological first aid (PFA) to equip volunteers as having mixed results compared to safety training containing stress management components and support groups for stress management and self-efficacy. Kunzler et al. (2021) also note that pre-incident stress inoculation training (including education in developing a personal resilience plan, and self-monitoring of stressors) had strong results in preventing post-traumatic stress disorder (PTSD) among healthcare social workers.

Institutional mistrust goes hand-in-hand with intersectional stigma. Because healthcare social workers are affiliated with healthcare institutions and are aligned with social work's mission toward social justice, they need to prove themselves trustworthy to the community they serve before expecting trust and rapport from clients and their systems of support.

One way social workers can do this on the micro level is intentional use of person-centered language. Such language choices suggest that the social worker has the desire and capacity to hold the full experience of a person and is, therefore, able to bear witness to the aftermath of discrimination and trauma that their patients may have faced. This can lead to multiple positive outcomes, including empowerment, greater self-assertiveness, and receipt of understanding, empathy, and validation. It can also lead to non-avoidance in engaging with healthcare (particularly if trauma and discrimination were experienced in the process of receiving care for illness).

Given that patients who identify as LGBTQIA are more likely to report past experiences of medical mismanagement and are six times more likely to feel reluctant to seek help from the healthcare system in the future (Human Rights Watch, 2018), such an approach may be particularly helpful to the pursuit of treatment adherence if in ill health of any kind.

Chronic

Intrapersonal Patients continue to cope with anxiety of the unknown, fear of chronic ill health, and even death, if their communicable disease has ongoing symptoms, becoming chronic. The course of disease may be over days or weeks, in the case of highly infectious diseases with rapid disease trajectories such as COVID-19, or over years for PLWHA.

People moving into the chronic phase of an illness face changes in everyday functioning and independence, employment rates, and instrumental activities of daily living (Moore et al., 2018). They also grapple with changes in physical appearance and demoralization, hopelessness, and helplessness (Myers, 1991). However, these feelings and outlooks may be mitigated, partially through the development of a co-constructed narrative of personal control and competence. The case study below provides an example of this work, as the social worker supports Aline to shape a new story and identity about her ability to care for her partner, Paul. The development of grit, the "perseverance and passion for long-term goals, with an emphasis on stamina and maintenance of effort despite adversity" (Moore et al., 2018, p. 3214) and ambition are other key internal coping mechanisms, providing goals related to illness and helping to weather challenges in their way. Motivational interviewing can amplify ambition, grit, and future orientation through lifestyle changes. In this work, patient resistance is understood as rational behavior that sustains perceived homeostasis; it reframes resistance as ambivalence around sustaining harmful behaviors (Miller and Rollnick, 2013).

Applied to patients with COVID-19 and PLWHA, motivational interviewing can be used to affirm the efforts that patients have already made connections with healthy lifestyle choices and build motivation for change for yet more related changes. CBT and Acceptance and Commitment Therapy (ACT) can also be used to assist in the shift of personal perception, reframing the illness approach. With PLWHA, for instance, cognitive restructuring can lead to a cognitive shift away from treating HIV as an illness that can be addressed when symptoms to a chronic physical condition that requires ongoing treatment regardless of symptomatology.

Interpersonal Social support may buffer the effects of isolation for those experiencing a communicable disease. As one moves from the acute crisis phase into a chronic one, their symptom burden and risk for transmission are better understood and more controllable. This opens additional opportunities for socialization to reduce stigma and improve community connections and meaning-centered care through reciprocity, mentorship, and role modeling. Reciprocity in this context refers to equal distribution and recognition of effort and care. Mentorship and role modeling become critical factors to demonstrate to those in the crisis phase of the illness that not only survival, but meaningful life, is possible in future states of the disease process. Such support may have additional indirect benefits; for example, Logie et al. (2016) suggest that social support groups tailored toward recent LGBTQIA immigrants from African and Caribbean countries also improved community structural supports, such as access to housing employment and healthcare.

Family members' experience and relationship closeness may oscillate, improving when risk of transmission is minimized or when education is offered to reduce stigma around caregiving roles. This inconsistency can induce feelings of guilt, disappointment, abandonment, and regret among family members. To reinforce positive caregiving roles, clinicians may incorporate caregivers into group and family treatment modalities (Ma et al., 2019; Myers, 1991).

Those who survive the crisis stage and illness and live into the chronic stage may face additional interpersonal challenges. For example, people living long term with a communicable disease such as HIV or long-haul COVID-19 may experience either guilt or anger in contemplating those who did not survive the crisis phase of the illness (Hansen et al., 2006).

Paul is a 50-year-old white Protestant Christian man who, prior to illness, regularly ran marathons with his wife, Aline, and took his teenage son, Mateo, to the beach. Paul is in the chronic phase of COVID-19 infection and is no longer contagious. He spent 3 months on an extracorporeal membrane oxygenation (ECMO) machine in an isolation room in the medical intensive care unit (MICU) and was given a tracheostomy. As a result of the tracheostomy, Paul is temporarily non-verbal but can communicate through head nodding and responds to simple commands. He is too debilitated to use his hands to write. His prognosis is not good, but a significant protective factor is that he is only in single-organ failure (lungs) and might be a good candidate for a lung transplant.

Aline's involvement in Paul's care can help to improve outcomes. However, Aline has a hard time visiting Paul. Although no longer contagious, hospital protocol mandated that personal protective equipment (PPE)—gloves, gown, N95 mask, hair covering, and face shield—be worn and, with it, she could go into Paul's room for 4 h each day. She comes to the window of his room daily but is displaying somatic signs of anxiety, breathing hard and becoming flushed any time someone encourages her to enter the room to hold Paul's hand and support him to participate in physical therapy.

Through careful rapport building, the social worker creates a safe space in which Aline can disclose that she is transgender, and her last hospital experience was at her own gender affirmation surgery. The clinical work with Aline becomes a dual process of acknowledging real fears of discrimination due to her gender identity and presentation in an unfamiliar setting, and exploring maladaptive coping which presents as fear, shame, feeling alone, and helpless. Through use of CBT techniques, Aline is able to identify that her primary anxiety is based in automatic negative thoughts. Some are realistic, but catastrophizing: that she could catch COVID-19 and no one would be able to care for Mateo. That she might be blamed for Paul's illness by staff with homophobic bias and that he would receive worse care due to their association. Some are based on projective identification: that Paul will suffer if he sees Aline because he is sick, and she is not. Others are based in dissociation and traumatic experiences of the body, including intrusive thoughts of her own fretful experience on a ventilator as a patient recovering from her gender affirmation surgery. Cognitive restructuring can assist in reframing maladaptive thoughts through identification, interrogation of the thought, and reframing it in a healthier way. In this case, the thought "I might get COVID-19" can be substituted based on rational observation: "I am vaccinated and following medical advice, Paul is no longer contagious, and I have sufficient protection."

Psychoeducation around the mind-body connection can also help to soothe Aline's anxiety. Mindfulness and biofeedback can help Aline to identify somatic symptoms brought on by her thoughts and feelings. By engaging in slow, steady breathing and grounding techniques, Aline can trigger her parasympathetic nervous system to cause a physical reaction in her brain to help calm her body and prevent panic.[1]

Systems of Care Chronic illness has an especially negative impact on those whose socioeconomic stability is already tenuous (Kunzler et al., 2021; Logie et al., 2016; Moore et al., 2018; Nydegger & Hill, 2020). People may be more likely to lose their jobs due to recurrent absence or require Social Security Disability benefits due to long-term effects of disease. People living with chronic communicable diseases may have dual and triple diagnoses. The complication of substance use disorders and more severe mental health issues may mean patients may consider an institutional setting such as skilled nursing, assisted living, or transitional or supportive housing, as available to meet their needs. Housing is a critical resource, since homelessness has been linked to the loss of ability to work due to health status (Lombardi et al., 2020).

Successful intervention in the chronic phase of an illness relies on consistent, well-trained case managers to help patients navigate social safety net services. Case managers provide important follow-up, advocacy, and general support for patients through the myriad concrete tasks of navigating the healthcare system. For example, they can partner with patients to coordinate care, link patients to services, and support patients in executing care plans. Care managers also improve levels of consistency in medication and care follow-up, contributing to more favorable sequelae such as improved labs, patient safety, and patient satisfaction. Patients can benefit from guidance from case managers as they move through the progression and stabilization of their illness (Hines & Mercury, 2013).

[1]All names and other personal identifiers in the case are fictitious. Any similarity to actual persons, living or dead, or actual events is purely coincidental.

End-of-Life

Intrapersonal The terminal stages of a communicable illness may co-occur with the acute crisis phase of the disease or come many years later, following a latency of the chronic phase of the illness. Additionally, the terminal phase of any illness may in fact be compounded by the acute phase of a new illness, such as pneumonia due to a weakened immune system from a long-standing chronic illness. No matter how a patient finds themselves in the terminal phase of disease, one can expect increased symptom burden, increased psychological distress, and suffering due to the loss of meaning. Patients also experience a shift in internalized identity: from that of a stable, if sick, person, to that of a person who is dying.

Terminal stages may involve significant acute needs that cannot be managed outside of hospital settings. Patients may be medically sedated to prevent effects of decline-related agitation. Due to the risk of contagion, especially in the early period of any new disease, patients are more likely to die in a preventive isolation (Williams, 2020). Prior to death, patients may grapple with feelings of abandonment by family and medical professionals. In the case of HIV, due to public stigma in the early days of the epidemic, medical professionals often refused care to patients. Lack of access led to unsupported deaths in settings that were under-resourced and staffed by volunteers (Adams, 1989). In COVID-19, death in isolation may be mitigated by use of digital technology. In later phases of public awareness of communicable disease, people living through chronic phases of the illness may experience survivor's guilt and feel that death is inevitable after seeing many of their cohort die decades earlier (Hansen et al., 2006). Survivors often struggle to make sense and meaning out of how and why they lived through an illness that claimed other lives, especially the lives of those close to them and bear the burden of long-term side effects. Social workers can aid survivors by creating space for them to process their own illness experience and to form a community through support groups.

Anthony was a 38-year-old Black, heterosexual, single man, admitted to the hospital with altered mental status, AIDS-related wasting, and secondary pneumonia. He had first been diagnosed with HIV 15 years earlier, however, he had never been able to accept this diagnosis, often wondering if he might have some other condition that was impacting his white blood cell counts. Anthony felt such intense shame at the idea of having HIV that he could not bring himself to take ART every day, since this meant incorporating his diagnosis into his daily life.

His symptoms had worsened in the previous 2 years, requiring him to go on disability leave from his job, and he had become increasingly estranged from his family. Anthony was surprised when the medical team recommended hospice care, stating that he was too young for it. He still declined to take ART, stating that he did not need it.

Social workers initially engaged with Anthony by not discussing his diagnosis but instead focusing on him as a person—his story and his values. This helped to reassure Anthony that the team saw him as more than his medical condition. He gave the social workers permission to speak with his family, who expressed their concern over their estrangement and explained that they were not ashamed of his diagnosis but frustrated with his seeming refusal to take care of himself.

Over the course of his hospitalization, Anthony was able to reconnect with family, accepting visits from and speaking on the phone with relatives he had not seen in years, which was meaningful for everyone involved. Because his hospitalization took place during the COVID-19 pandemic, only local family members were allowed to visit, which was distressing for his father, who had traveled from another state to see him. Anthony's condition worsened and he died after 2 weeks in the hospital. Throughout this time, social workers provided support to both Anthony and his family members, acknowledging the power of stigma and blame at play and the additional layer of sadness and frustration attributable to the COVID-19 pandemic.[1]

Interpersonal Communicable diseases present unique challenges due to the infectious nature of the illness. Depending on the severity and ease of transmission, some degree of precaution will likely be needed at end-of-life that may make care more complex. This may be as simple as the use of appropriate protective equipment such as gloves, masks, eye protection, and gowns. This equipment can feel burdensome for lay people and create a perceived barrier that separates them physically and psychologically from providing meaningful contact at end-of-life. Meaningful contact might be as simple as skin-to-skin contact, like placing a hand on someone's cheek to wipe away a tear, or as complex as personal care involving cleaning of sensitive body areas. Social workers can help patients and families reframe any method of intentional connection as meaningful.

In the early stages of new diseases, when little is known about the illness, end-of-life may be a very solitary experience. Before it is fully understood what contact can or cannot transmit disease, precautions can be introduced that entirely bar in-person contact. Use of electronic tablets and video visits during the COVID-19 epidemic exemplified that while telehealth and telemedicine are emerging tools, they do not fully satiate our need for connection at end-of-life (Calton et al., 2021). Families often find meaning, closure, and the bridge to bereavement in the involved care of a person important to you at end-of-life. The inability to provide this may mean the families will grapple with complex bereavement due to lack of final communication.

Psychological distress during and after the terminal phase of an illness can be addressed by social workers through individual and group intervention. Interventions that focus on mindful awareness of current adaptive and maladaptive coping strategies can help patients to identify short- and long-term goals related to coping. Healthcare social workers can help families to establish feelings of control and predictability; express and manage emotions; address feelings of guilt and shame; develop a sense of self-mastery; and explore the changing nature of relationships (Hansen et al., 2006).

Systems of Care In the terminal phase of illness, providers and healthcare systems can feel the strain of care, particularly during seasonal presentation of recurrent communicable diseases such as influenza, or during epidemics of communicable diseases, and care needs can become acute, requiring unexpected, intensive interventions in intensive care units. During the early phases of newly identified communicable diseases, as the medical community is still in the process of understanding treatment needs, people are less likely to have access to palliative and hospice services. Patients and their families may face the additional stress and distress of waiting for care and receiving it within institutions with limited resources, developing protocols, long waits, and uncertain courses and outcomes for patients with communicable diseases who need urgent and intensive care. Traumatic response is understandable for people and their families who face life-threatening health conditions *and* healthcare provision problems simultaneously.

Healthcare workers who are in direct contact with people in the terminal phase of a communicable illness face their own unique challenges. Healthcare workers are susceptible to infection by illnesses that are easily transmitted through respiratory droplets, and in some cases exposure to sputum, mucus, blood, and waste. This carries increased risks of anxiety over safety in a work setting, as well as potential pressure from family members who have concerns about the healthcare workers' safety. Moral distress is a person's experience of feeling constrained or unable to act in the way they believe is most appropriate; in a healthcare worker's case, it may be due to the policies of an institution or the scarcity of resources with which to serve a patient properly. The risk to healthcare workers for depression, anxiety, insomnia, vicarious trauma, moral distress, and demoralization is greater still. It can lead to feelings of burnout and compassion fatigue, both of which are linked to professionals leaving their field of practice prematurely. Early studies of healthcare workers in China revealed that healthcare workers caring for people diagnosed with COVID-19 had higher incidence of depression, anxiety, insomnia, and psychological distress than those working with people not diagnosed with COVID-19 (Anderson-Shaw & Zair, 2020). While all diseases carry risk for psychological effects on healthcare professionals, such as vicarious trauma, communicable diseases carry the very real possibility of physical transmission of the disease, which, in turn, compounds psychological effects.

For palliative care and hospice social workers working with people with communicable diseases, there are critical challenges. When Gergerich et al. (2020) surveyed social workers in hospice and palliative care during the summer of 2020, they found that social workers in hospice and palliative care experienced challenges regarding isolation, barriers in communication, disruptions of the healthcare systems, and issues related to grieving. The hospice social workers experienced feeling "non-essential" in the face of praise for "essential workers" in hospital and curative-focused care settings. This sense of being nonessential was substantiated by factors like scarcity of resources (including critical PPE) and the expectation that they would take on new interventions and roles due to colleagues becoming ill themselves or working from home. However, Gergerich et al. (2020) also note themes of strength and resiliency among hospice and palliative care social workers, including interdisciplinary team and family support, the ability to adapt to a rapidly changing healthcare landscape, and new perspectives on life and death with a serious communicable disease, which increased a sense of meaning and purpose. Social workers have the distinct opportunity to bear witness and be present with people through deeply challenging experiences.

Bereavement

Bereavement following a death due to communicable disease is deeply complicated by the unpredictability of disease course; by the potential for blame, shame, and guilt of transmission; and by societal stigma. For example, a couple who are sick with the same illness may have vastly different trajectories, and if one of them dies the survivor may be wracked with guilt about potentially having transmitted the illness to their partner and living through it. In families with differing views on reasonable precautions for diseases such as COVID-19, bereavement can be particularly complex. In public health crises especially, the stigma and sheer volume of loss can eclipse the deeply personal nature of grief and the individual identities of those who die.

Death may be a shocking, unexpected event. During the height of the AIDS epidemic in the USA, some patients deteriorated rapidly, heightening the trauma of their deaths for both the important people in their lives and for their medical providers. Due to policies governing quarantine and social distancing during COVID-19, many hospitals implemented visitor restrictions, meaning that the last time some people saw someone close to them was right before they entered the hospital. This, combined with the strain on funeral resources, created an atmosphere rife with ambiguous loss—the unresolved grief that comes from someone being either physically present but psychologically absent, or as is more relevant here, physically absent but psychologically present (Scheinfeld et al., 2021). The lack of opportunity to engage in rituals of mourning, such as sitting shiva or having a funeral Mass or a wake, furthered the ambiguous, unresolved nature of these losses.

The inability to mourn publicly and receive social support can also contribute to disenfranchised grief, in which one's grief experience is unsanctioned or unacknowledged by society (Doka, 1999). Disenfranchised grief is strongly associated with deaths from HIV/AIDS (Mallinson, 2013). LGBTQIA relationships have a long and traumatic history of being recognized neither legally nor by wider society as valid in the same way as heterosexual partnerships, and the gay community was largely abandoned by the public health system during the first decade of the AIDS epidemic, making it especially difficult for friends, families, and loved ones of those who died to mourn in any widely supported way. Any estrangement that follows a family's refusal to accept an individual's sexual orientation or gender identity also complicates grief. This type of grief does not resolve but worsens over time, as do the stigma and feelings attached to it (Mallinson, 2013).

Because communicable diseases spread from person to person, a person who believes that they have transmitted to another (or others) may experience intense guilt. The possibility of transmission to family, friends, and intimate partners, especially when some carriers can be asymptomatic, creates an environment of blame—either directed at oneself or at others—and questioning (Cavalera, 2020). Tension may build in personal, family, and work communities around what constitutes reasonable precautions, which makes closeness fraught and fearful. Survivor's guilt also weighs heavy for those who did not get as sick as someone close to them, or who also were sick but survived.

Potential interventions include bereavement groups centered around specific types of loss or common relationships, which help survivors to process the loss in supportive, affirming company, and meaning-making rituals to honor the deceased, such as community memorials or involvement in advocacy work. Trauma-informed guilt reduction therapy can address guilt, shame, and moral injury by supporting the bereaved in appraising their role in the deceased's illness and examining cognitions linked to guilt and shame (Haller et al., 2020). Other perspectives suggest that guilt may be something that the bereaved learns how to live with in a meaningful way. The continuing bonds model of grief can aid individuals in understanding and cherishing their ongoing relationship to the deceased, including the larger community, cultural, and political contexts at play (Klass, 2006).

Social Justice

Social justice and injustice are deeply interwoven with communicable diseases, intersecting with risk factors, access to resources, stigma, and public health response. Social determinants of health such as lower income, lack of access to health insurance and healthcare, and medical mistrust are significant risk factors. COVID-19 has had a documented, disproportionate impact on communities of color and of lower socioeconomic status (Abrams & Szefler, 2020). At the same time, it is important not to frame risk factors as a question of certain communities or demographics inherently being at a higher risk, but to examine the structural factors that place them at a higher risk. For at-risk groups should not be treated as risk factors in and of themselves; rather, the possible factors in incidence rates should be understood more fully, and attention and resources should be devoted to them, in order to mitigate risk. While Black men who have sex with men (MSM) are less likely to achieve viral suppression with HIV, they are no more likely to engage in risky behaviors than other MSM (Matthews et al., 2016). Social workers or other providers understanding this will not necessarily focus interventions and approaches on the supposed risky behaviors of this group. Social workers working with people who have communicable diseases have a perspective oriented to social justice that may be particularly efficacious. They know that identifying a group or community as more susceptible to an illness may increase their marginalization and vulnerability, and know how to balance this awareness with assessment for social determinants of health, advocacy for equitable access to care, and exploration of prior experiences with healthcare that inform patients' perspectives (Nydegger & Hill, 2020).

Access to resources, including levels and quality of care, health insurance, geographic location, and financial stability greatly impact one's ability to navigate an illness. Beyond stratified availability of care, clinicians' awareness of implicit personal and institutional bias will be critical should rationing of medical care and equipment become necessary in a pandemic or emergency context. In addition, living with a chronic infectious disease can preclude individuals from receiving certain treatments. For example, people living with HIV are significantly less likely to receive organ transplants or become organ donors, despite studies that have proven both to be successful for PLWHA (Botha et al., 2019).

Stigma in communicable disease is perpetuated by scapegoating, discrimination, and public health messaging—or lack thereof. Rooted in historical, societal, and cultural contexts, stigma brings a person's humanity into question and leads to disempowerment, isolation, and barriers to effective disease management (Ma et al., 2019; France et al., 2015). There are many types of stigmas, the most prevalent being enacted stigma (i.e., the experience of being discriminated against), perceived stigma (i.e., an individual recognizes or anticipates stigmatization), and self-stigma (i.e., negative self-judgments that settle into internalized blame, shame, and worthlessness) (Ma et al., 2019; France et al., 2015). Social workers should call attention to stigma when it is at play both within patient narratives and in interdisciplinary conversation, advocate against it, and be aware of how racism, homophobia, and other forms of discrimination intersect with disease experience. Clinicians should also be especially attuned to the prevalence and impact of self-stigma and utilize modalities such as CBT, psychoeducation, support groups, psychotherapy, and community interventions.

Communicable diseases pose a threat to public health and safety and are therefore met with public health responses of varying impact and efficacy, in which social injustice and stigma are often perpetuated by messaging. Initial public health discourse around COVID-19 included conflicted messaging regarding effective protective measures and was infused with hateful rhetoric against China (Ransing et al., 2020; Villa et al., 2020). During the AIDS epidemic, the Centers for Disease Control initially released public campaigns naming "homosexuals, heroin users, hemophiliacs, and Haitians," referred to as the 4Hs, as high-risk groups for HIV, resulting in heavy stigmatization for these communities (Matthews et al., 2016, p. 5). This othering also led to public officials ignoring or downplaying the severity of the crisis, with President Reagan famously not uttering the word AIDS publicly until 1985, 4 years and over 8000 deaths after it had first been identified in 1981. In the early years of the AIDS epidemic, many states created criminal exposure laws for HIV, both criminalizing potentially exposing another person and increasing sentences for other crimes if the individual was shown to have HIV (CDC, 2021). Despite the fact that these laws have not been shown to reduce transmission—rather, they increase stigma and reluctance to be tested—as of 2022, 35 states still have laws criminalizing HIV.

Because communicable diseases cannot be separated from the larger community and societal systems, in considering them it is important to expand Rolland's (1987) three interwoven threads of illness, individual, and family life cycles to include meso- and macro systems. Communicable diseases impact the entire public health-care system, from individual to local to global levels. In addition, public reaction to infectious disease deeply colors the individual experience of being sick or living through a pandemic and any shame or trauma that endures. Murray Bowen, the founder of Bowenian family systems theory, conceptualizes society as a family system in and of itself, providing a bridge between public health and Rolland's framework. For Bowen, when a family experiences high levels of stress and anxiety, it regresses to a lower level of functioning. Society mirrors this in a process, in a phenomenon called societal regression (Haefner, 2014).

How has society recently demonstrated societal regression? The crisis phase of a pandemic exerts both stress and an insular pull on societies, leading to Rolland's (1987) concepts of isolation and entropy, as seen in hoarding of resources, discriminatory quarantining and travel restrictions, othering, scapegoating, and widespread injustice. A pandemic forces society into a state in which illness and death must be accommodated on a broad scale, prompting societal transition, change, and upheaval. Public health crises do not happen in a vacuum; rather, they build upon and are worsened by existing inequity. This was the case with the COVID-19 pandemic in the United States, in which public safety measures such as mask-wearing and physical distancing became intensely politicized, and the structural racism that has been part of American society was more plainly exposed. Transition phases such as this are times of great vulnerability, when the illness, individual, family, and society life structures are reconsidered in the face of ongoing change (Rolland, 1987).

Authors' Reflections

The threat and experience of communicable diseases represent both the frailty of our physical structure and our shared humanity. We are susceptible to the natural, unseen dangers of the world in which we live. Be it a poorly timed breath, an unlucky open wound, or an unprotected moment of physical intimacy, we are susceptible. The natural response to this level of inherent threat may be panic, but it does not need to be. Social workers can help reframe our exposure as vulnerability. We can help clients to understand that dying in the world is the cost of living in the world.

No one of us is entirely immune; no one of us is entirely free of risk. The comfort that many humans take in diseases that have limited transmissibility is a cold, false one that often is driven by and drives harmful prejudices about *otherized* groups. The error of assuming that we are safe because we are not part of a certain group, or do not engage in a specific behavior, is one that deprives standing, care, and empathy to those who came first; those who suffered from an illness without a name or died from a germ that those in power refused to acknowledge. The world is opening its eyes to our shared frailty and vulnerability. United States Vice President Kamala

Harris reflected on the COVID-19 pandemic as a "stark warning" and a "wake-up call for all of us" as she pledged to monitor and identify gaps in global preparedness for the next pandemic (C-SPAN, 2021). We as social workers must continue to reframe our shared vulnerability from a panic-inducing fear of susceptibility to an opportunity to unite behind the banner of science, progress, and empathy for one another. We are not immune to loving those who die of communicable diseases; to the memories of suffering; to the urge to connect, even when proximal connection is in essence proximal danger. As humans, we must embrace our vulnerability as an inextricable component of love, memory, and connection.

The vast range of communicable diseases and the shared vulnerability we experience make this area of healthcare social work especially complex and personal. The work can be rife with feelings of countertransference and frustrations with systemic injustice, particularly when working with patients who are stigmatized or face an illness that could have been prevented through more equitable access to care. Supporting patients and families through moments of uncertainty such as the early days of the COVID pandemic, when we ourselves might be just as scared and unsure, necessitates humility and self-compassion. Connecting with patients through isolation restrictions or layers of PPE requires us to pay even more careful attention to our body language and voices as tools, and to explore creative ways of ensuring patients are not isolated from their support networks. The terrain of communicable diseases, the lived experiences of our patients, and our place in the work shifts constantly with larger societal forces. It demands a careful balance of grounding ourselves in a person-centered approach while remaining highly attuned to mezzo and macro factors. It is hard work but well worth it. In connecting with our clients, we connect with, and reinforce, our shared humanity, our frailties, and our hopes for a future where we and our families can thrive.

Reflection Questions

1. How might a shared experience of the COVID-19 pandemic impact your work with a patient who is experiencing fear of catching it?
2. How might the experience of communities of color in healthcare as a whole impact an individual's experience of a communicable disease?
3. In what ways is a macro social work lens crucial in working with people with communicable diseases?

References

About HIV & AIDS. (2021, April 8). *About HIV & AIDS: Symptoms of HIV*. HIV.gov. https://www.hiv.gov/hiv-basics/overview/about-hiv-and-aids/symptoms-of-hiv

Abrams, E. M., & Szefler, S. J. (2020). COVID-19 and the impact of social determinants of health. *The Lancet Respiratory Medicine, 8*(7), 659–661. https://doi.org/10.1016/s2213-2600(20)30234-4

Adams, J. M. (1989). Life and death on ward 5. *The Washington Post,* F12.

Adjei, S., Hong, K., Molinari, N. M., et al. (2022). Mortality risk among patients hospitalized primarily for COVID-19 during the Omicron and Delta variant pandemic periods—United States,

April 2020–June 2022. *Morbidity and Mortality Weekly Report, 71*(37), 1182–1189. https://doi.org/10.15585/mmwr.mm7137a4
Anderson-Shaw, L. K., & Zar, F. A. (2020). COVID-19, moral conflict, distress, and dying alone. *Journal of Bioethical Inquiry, 17*, 777–782
Barrett, R., & Brown, P. (2008). Stigma in the time of influenza: Social and institutional responses to pandemic emergencies. *The Journal of Infectious Diseases, 197*(s1), S34–S37. https://doi.org/10.1086/524986
Botha, J., Fabian, J., Etheredge, H., Conradie, F., & Tiemessen, C. T. (2019). HIV and solid organ transplantation: Where are we now? *Current HIV/AIDS Reports, 16*(5), 404–413. https://doi.org/10.1007/s11904-019-00460-7
Calton, B. A., Bischoff, K., & Pantilat, S. Z. (2021). "I just need to hold his hand": Telemedicine is powerful, but not perfect. *Journal of Palliative Medicine, 24*(2), 166–167. https://doi.org/10.1089/jpm.2020.0573
Cavalera, C. (2020). COVID-19 psychological implications: The role of shame and guilt. *Frontiers in Psychology, 11*. https://doi.org/10.3389/fpsyg.2020.571828
Centers for Disease Control. (2021, December 2). *HIV and STD criminalization laws*. CDC.gov. https://www.cdc.gov/hiv/policies/law/states/exposure.html
Correl, R. (2021). *Differences between communicable and infectious diseases: It's more than just semantics*. VeryWell Health. https://www.verywellhealth.com/the-difference-between-communicable-and-infectious-diseases-4151985
Crocker, A. F., & Smith, S. N. (2019). Person-first language: Are we practicing what we preach? *Journal of Multidisciplinary Healthcare, 12*, 125–129. https://doi.org/10.2147/JMDH.S140067
C-SPAN. (2021, September 22). *Vice President Harris remarks at Covid-19 virtual summit* [Video File]. https://www.c-span.org/video/?c4978162/vice-president-harris-us-contribute-250-million-global-pandemic-preparedness-fund
Deeks, S. G., Lewin, S. R., & Havlir, D. V. (2013). *The end of AIDS: HIV infection as a chronic disease*. Lancet. https://doi.org/10.1016/S0140-6736(13)61809-7
Doka, K. J. (1999). Disenfranchised grief. *Bereavement Care, 18*(3), 37–39. https://doi.org/10.1080/02682629908657467
France, N. F., Mcdonald, S. H., Conroy, R. R., Byrne, E., Mallouris, C., Hodgson, I., & Larkan, F. N. (2015). An unspoken world of unspoken things: A study identifying and exploring core beliefs underlying self-stigma among people living with HIV and AIDS in Ireland. *Swiss Medical Weekly, 145*, w14113. https://doi.org/10.4414/smw.2015.14113
Frankl, V. E. (1985). *The unconscious God*. Washington Square Press.
Gergerich, E., Mallonee, J., Gherardi, S., Kale-Cheever, M., & Duga, F. (2020). Strengths and struggles for families involved in hospice care during the COVID-19 pandemic. *Journal of Social Work in End-of-Life & Palliative Care*, 1–20. https://doi.org/10.1080/15524256.2020.1845907
Gorin, S. H. (2002). The crisis of public health revisited: Implications for social work. *Health & Social Work, 27*(1), 56–60. https://doi.org/10.1093/hsw/27.1.56
Haefner, J. (2014). An application of Bowen family systems theory. *Issues in Mental Health Nursing, 35*(11), 835–841. https://doi.org/10.3109/01612840.2014.921257
Haller, M., Norman, S. B., Davis, B. C., Capone, C., Browne, K., & Allard, C. B. (2020). A model for treating COVID-19-related guilt, shame, and moral injury. *Psychological Trauma: Theory, Research, Practice and Policy, 12*(S1), S174–S176. https://doi.org/10.1037/tra0000742
Hansen, N. B., Tarakeshwar, N., Ghebremichael, M., Zhang, H., Kochman, A., & Sikkema, K. J. (2006). Longitudinal effects of coping on outcome in a randomized controlled trial of a group intervention for HIV-positive adults with AIDS-related bereavement. *Death Studies, 30*(7), 609–636. https://doi.org/10.1080/07481180600776002
Heijnders, M., & Van Der Meij, S. (2006). The fight against stigma: An overview of stigma-reduction strategies and interventions. *Psychology, Health & Medicine, 11*(3), 353–363. https://doi-org.avoserv2.library.fordham.edu/10.1080/13548500600595327
Hines, P., & Mercury, M. (2013). Designing the role of the embedded care manager. *Professional Case Management, 18*(4), 182–187.

Jeremiah, R., Taylor, B., Castillo, A., & Garcia, V. (2020). A qualitative community assessment of racial/ethnic sexual gender minority young adults: Principles for strategies to motivate action(s) for realistic tasks (SMART Thinking). Addressing HIV/AIDS, Viral Hepatitis, mental health, and substance abuse. *American. Journal of Men's Health, 14*(5). https://doi.org/10.1177/1557988320966230

Klass, D. (2006). Continuing conversation about continuing bonds. *Death Studies, 30*(9), 843–858. https://doi.org/10.1080/07481180600886959

Kunzler, A. M., Stoffers-Winterling, J., Stoll, M., Mancini, A. L., Lehmann, S., Blessin, M., Gilan, D., Helmreich, I., Hufert, F., & Lieb, K. (2021). Mental health and psychosocial support strategies in highly contagious emerging disease outbreaks of substantial public concern: A systematic scoping review. *PLoS One, 16*(2). https://doi.org/10.1371/journal.pone.0244748

Logie, C. H., Lacombe-Duncan, A., Lee-Foon, N., Ryan, S., & Ramsay, H. (2016). It's for us - newcomers, LGBTQ persons, and HIV-positive persons. You feel free to be: a qualitative study exploring social support group participation among African and Caribbean lesbian, gay, bisexual and transgender newcomers and refugees in Toronto, Canada. *BMC International Health and Human Rights, 16*(1), 18. https://doi.org/10.1186/s12914-016-0092-0.

Lombardi, K., Pines, J. M., Mazer-Amirshahi, M., & Pourmand, A. (2020). Findings of a national dataset analysis on the visits of homeless patients to US emergency departments during 2005–2015. *Public Health, 178*, 82–89. https://doi-org.avoserv2.library.fordham.edu/10.1016/j.puhe.2019.09.003

Ma, P. H. X., Chan, Z. C. Y., & Loke, A. Y. (2019). Self-stigma reduction interventions for people living with HIV/AIDS and their families: A systematic review. *AIDS and Behavior, 23*(3), 707. https://doi-org.avoserv2.library.fordham.edu/10.1007/s10461-018-2304-1

Mallinson, K. R. (2013). Grief in the context of HIV: Recommendations for practice. *Journal of the Association of Nurses in AIDS Care, 24*(Supplement 1), S61–S71. https://doi.org/10.1016/j.jana.2012.08.012

Matthews, D. D., Smith, J. C., Brown, A. L., & Malebranche, D. J. (2016). Reconciling epidemiology and social justice in the public health discourse around the sexual networks of black men who have sex with men. *American Journal of Public Health, 106*(5), 808–814. https://doi.org/10.2105/AJPH.2015.303031

Mabhala, M. A., Yohannes, A., Massey, A., & Reid, J. A. (2020). Mind your Language: Discursive Practices Produce Unequal Power and Control Over Infectious Disease: A Critical Discourse Analysis. *International Journal of Preventive Medicine, 11*, 37. https://doi.org/10.4103/ijpvm.IJPVM_431_17.

McKeon Olson, R., & Goldstein, R. (2020, April 22). *Ending stigma and empowering people living with HIV.* Harvard Health Publishing. https://www.health.harvard.edu/blog/uu-ending-stigma-and-empowering-people-living-with-hiv-2020042219583

Miller, W. R., & Rollnick, S. (2013). *Motivational interviewing: Helping people change* (3rd ed.). Guilford Press.

Moore, R. C., Hussain, M. A., Watson, C. W.-M., Fazeli, P. L., Marquine, M. J., Yarns, B. C., Jeste, D. V., & Moore, D. J. (2018). Grit and ambition are associated with better neurocognitive and everyday functioning among adults living with HIV. *AIDS and Behavior, 22*(10), 3214–3225.

Myers, T. (1991). Psychosocial issues in AIDS/ESRD. *Loss, Grief & Care, 5*(1–2), 205–209.

National Center for Health Statistics. (2021). *Health, United States, 2019.* https://doi.org/10.15620/cdc:100685

Nydegger, L. A., & Hill, M. J. (2020). Examining COVID-19 and HIV: The impact of intersectional stigma on short- and long-term health outcomes among African Americans. *International Social Work, 63*(5), 655–659. https://doi.org/10.1177/0020872820940017

Pantelic, M., Steinert, J. I., Park, J., Mellors, S., & Murau, F. (2019). Management of a spoiled identity: Systematic review of interventions to address self-stigma among people living with and affected by HIV. *BMJ Globalization and Health, 4*(2), e001285. https://doi.org/10.1136/bmjgh-2018-001285

Ransing, R., Ramalho, R., de Filippis, R., Ojeahere, M. I., Karaliuniene, R., Orsolini, L., Pinto Da Costa, M., Ullah, I., Grandinetti, P., Gashi Bytyçi, D., Grigo, O., Mhamunkar, A., el Hayek, S., Essam, L., Larnaout, A., Shalbafan, M., Nofal, M., Soler-Vidal, J., Pereira-Sanchez, V., & Adiukwu, F. (2020). Infectious disease outbreak related stigma and discrimination during the COVID-19 pandemic: Drivers, facilitators, manifestations, and outcomes across the world. *Brain, Behavior, and Immunity, 89*, 555–558. https://doi.org/10.1016/j.bbi.2020.07.033

Rolland, J. S. (1987). Chronic illness and the life cycle: A conceptual framework. *Family Process, 26*(2), 203–221.

Rubin, R. (2020). As their numbers grow, COVID-19 "long haulers" stump experts. *The Journal of the American Medical Association, 324*(14), 1381.

Scheinfeld, E., Gangi, K., Nelson, E. C., & Sinardi, C. C. (2021). Please scream inside your heart: Compounded loss and coping during the COVID-19 pandemic. *Health Communication, 37*, 1–13.

Saeed, F., Mihan, R., Mousavi, S. Z., Reniers, R. L., Bateni, F. S., Alikhani, R., & Mousavi, S. B. (2020). A Narrative Review of Stigma Related to Infectious Disease Outbreaks: What Can Be Learned in the Face of the Covid-19 Pandemic?. *Frontiers in Psychiatry, 11*, 565919. https://doi.org/10.3389/fpsyt.2020.565919.

Villa, S., Jaramillo, E., Mangioni, D., Bandera, A., Gori, A., & Raviglione, M. C. (2020). Stigma at the time of the COVID-19 pandemic. *Clinical Microbiology and Infection, 26*(11), 1450–1452. https://doi.org/10.1016/j.cmi.2020.08.001

Wilkerson, I. (2020). *Caste: The origins of our discontents*. Random House.

Williams, J. P. (2020, April 29). *For those who've lived both, COVID-19 carries echoes of the early AIDS crisis*. The US News and World Report. https://www.usnews.com/news/healthiest-communities/articles/2020-04-29/hiv-and-the-coronavirus-pandemic-carries-echoes-of-early-aids-crisis

Chapter 5
Dementia and Neurodegenerative Diseases

Kaila N. Robertson and Abigail Nathanson

Introduction

Dementia, a broad term that equates with Mild and Major Neurocognitive Disorders (NCDs) in the DSM-5 (American Psychiatric Association, 2013), refers to progressive impairment in cognitive functioning, specifically judgment, mood, speech, and memory (Stark, 2019). Dementia is a grouping of symptoms, such as apathy, memory loss, or personality changes, with different underlying medical causes (Rolland, 2017; Nathanson & Latimer, 2021). Underlying medical causes range from strokes, neurodegenerative diseases like Alzheimer's disease or Parkinson's disease, and HIV/AIDS to traumatic brain injuries and other medical conditions (Stark, 2019). It is estimated that 10% of adults over 65 and 50% of those over 85 are affected by dementia (Rolland, 2017). Relatedly, the Centers for Disease Control and Prevention (CDC, 2020) estimates that the number of people living with Alzheimer's disease alone will nearly triple by 2060, from 5.8 million to 14 million. These demographic shifts underscore the need for competent social work practice with this growing population.

NCDs can be thought of as vascular, which means they came from loss of blood to the brain such as from a stroke, or nonvascular, meaning they developed as a result of an underlying disease process. Some forms of dementia may be reversible, such as cognitive impairment resulting from a traumatic brain injury or substance

K. N. Robertson (✉)
Westchester Medical Center, Valhalla, NY, USA
e-mail: knr233@nyu.edu

A. Nathanson
Silver School of Social Work, New York University, New York, NY, USA
e-mail: an768@nyu.edu

M. Hemphill, A. Nathanson (eds.), *The Practice of Clinical Social Work in Healthcare*, Essential Clinical Social Work Series,
https://doi.org/10.1007/978-3-031-31650-0_5

abuse (Stark, 2019), or from medication interactions, thyroid and endocrine conditions, or vitamin deficiencies. For the purposes of this chapter, we will focus on the psychosocial impact of nonreversible causes of dementia and will cover both vascular and nonvascular impacts. A person with dementia will be referred to as PWD; persons with dementia will be referred to as "PWDs."

The most common cause of dementia is Alzheimer's disease (Alzheimer's Association, 2021), accounting for 60–80% of NCDs (Rolland, 2017). Alzheimer's disease, a nonvascular form of dementia, is a terminal diagnosis distinct from the normal aging process. PWDs with Alzheimer's disease have a decline spanning an average of 7–20 years (Nathanson & Latimer, 2021). Early symptoms often present subtly and include memory loss that disrupts daily life, difficulty completing familiar tasks or solving problems, confusion with time and place, changes in mood and personality including withdrawal from social relationships, and problems with speaking, writing, and judgment (Alzheimer's Association, 2009). People often have Alzheimer's disease and vascular dementia concurrently, complicating any ability to prognosticate or anticipate decline. Other common nonvascular causes of dementia include Parkinson's disease and Lewy Body dementia, both of which have symptoms similar to Alzheimer's disease (Stark, 2019). Lewy Body dementia generally includes psychotic features. Parkinson's disease is a complex neurodegenerative disease that progressively impairs motor skills and often produces cognitive symptoms like dementia (Gonzalez-Ramos et al., 2019).

Vascular dementia, the second most common cause of NCD, is caused by a lack of blood flow to certain parts of the brain, often after a sudden event such as a stroke (Alzheimer's Association, 2021). The onset of this type of dementia is acute, unlike most nonvascular causes which gradually increase over time (Rolland, 2017). Symptoms depend on which part of the brain was impacted and may include decline in executive functioning, rigidity or motor control issues, language difficulty, and changes in behavior (Korczyn et al., 2012). Vascular dementia tends to be constant after the first six months, rather than progressive as with Alzheimer's disease (Rolland, 2017), meaning that the person's symptoms will not get better, nor will they get much worse unless another vascular event occurs. That said, as with nonvascular dementia, the course of vascular dementia is unpredictable, though typically marked by a slower decline than Alzheimer's disease (Korczyn et al., 2012).

Vascular dementia can cause physical disfigurement and disability early in the course of illness, depending on the region of the brain affected (Korczyn et al., 2012). Diagnosis is somewhat more certain than nonvascular dementias, especially in younger PWDs, but differentiating between vascular dementia and Alzheimer's disease can be difficult (American Psychiatric Association [APA], 2013), particularly as many people with Alzheimer's disease also have vascular damage and dementia.

Table 5.1 Psychosocial issues, clinical goals, and interventions

Phase	Psychosocial issues	Clinical goals and interventions
Acute	Social stigma Care planning Trauma Anticipatory loss	Psychoeducation on disease progression Facilitation of advance care planning, wills, and funerals Integration of trauma history into intake and care planning Normalization of feelings of anticipatory loss
Chronic	High caregiving burden Ambiguous loss Uncertain trajectory Long-term care facilities	Referral to community resources and lessons on therapeutic tools such as breathing and relaxation to reduce caregiver burden Psychoeducation on ambiguous loss; recognizing and normalizing losses with caregiver Facilitation of conversations on level of care needed, incl. Possibility of long-term care
Terminal	Caregiver exhaustion Ambiguous loss and closure Chemical restraint Complex medical decisions	Coordination of care where necessary; referral to home health aide services and advocacy to increase hours Advocacy for PWD and education on how systems of care impact use of chemical restraint Educational resources for healthcare decision-makers; facilitation of conversations on what the PWD would have wanted for their care if advance care planning is not in place

Clinical Issues in Dementia

Due to the degenerative nature of the illness, the clinical issues of dementia are best understood in three temporal phases: acute (including the initial symptom onset and diagnostic phases), chronic (which may last for a decade or more), and terminal. Table 5.1 describes common psychosocial issues that manifest at each stage of illness, alongside related clinical goals and interventions.

Acute

The acute phase of NCD is a crucial time for communication between PWDs, families or other caregivers, and the treatment team. Caregivers can be understood to be formal, in terms of paid aides or healthcare team members, or informal, such as family of choice, family of origin (both referred to here as "family" with equal weight), friends, partners, and community members. It may refer to people who physically provide care for a person's bodily needs, or to people who coordinate and make decisions around care, or to people who provide emotional support and social stimulation. Given the long-term trajectory of NCDs, it is important that the PWD and caregivers understand the typical course of illness and begin to plan accordingly for caregiving needs (Rolland, 2017).

Intrapersonal In the acute phase of NCD, common intrapersonal themes include adjustment to the diagnosis and the influence of early attachment paradigms on the PWD's view of the diagnosis.

The acute or crisis phase may look different depending on the individual, their support system, and their diagnosis. PWDs report a range of reactions upon receiving a diagnosis of NCD—shocked, embarrassed, relieved to understand what is happening to them, or denial (Hagan, 2020). It can be difficult to establish if a PWD's inability to "accept" their diagnosis is due to expected emotional shock or is itself evidence of cognitive decline.

At onset of symptoms, PWD may try to hide or deny their dementia symptoms due to associated social stigma (Rolland, 2017; Birt et al., 2019) or fears of dependence. With the onset of memory loss, recall difficulty, and apathy, PWDs may also struggle to maintain previous levels of social connections (Birt et al., 2019). Isolation is especially concerning, as social interaction is protective against cognitive decline (Birt et al., 2019) and a subjective experience of loneliness is associated with greater symptom burden (Abedini et al., 2020).

For the persons with progressive dementia, a diagnosis can signal the loss of self and the loss of autonomy (Karlawish, 2021). When there is insecurity in the PWD's attachment style, the fear of being dependent on another person and the vulnerability inherent in such an illness can be intensely dysregulating (Nelis et al., 2014). A person's usual ability to navigate closeness and distance to maintain their own sense of safety (how we understand attachment) is compromised when the PWD realizes they will be completely dependent upon others as their illness progresses. A history of mental illness, trauma experience, and other factors greatly impact how a person deals with feeling powerless, vulnerable, or dependent on others.

Interpersonal Key issues for PWDs and their caregivers in the acute phase are care planning, meaning-making, anticipation of more losses to come (anticipatory grief) (Rubin et al., 2019), and grief for the losses already experienced.

Clear communication and understanding during the acute phase, before the PWD develops more severe impairment, can enable the PWD and caregivers to develop advance care directives that honor and support the PWD's personhood (Rolland et al., 2017). At this stage, it is important for social workers to identify who the PWD's family and caregivers are. Systems of oppression, such as homophobia, misogyny, transphobia, and racism, may result in social workers and other hospital staff excluding chosen family, partners, and extended family who may be key players in care (Acquaviva, 2017), or in assumptions that the primary responsibility of care is with someone who appears female, like a daughter or wife. In addition to advance care directives, PWDs and families benefit from open and honest discussions which facilitate planning for the PWD's decline from financial, legal, caregiving, and coping perspectives (Rolland et al., 2017).

Particularly given that dementia diagnoses are uncertain, it is important for social workers to understand what the diagnosis means to the PWD and their caregivers (Rolland, 2017). Where the uncertainty of the diagnosis and trajectory of illness can instill feelings of helplessness or being out of control, meaning-making can help PWD and their caregivers reclaim a sense of autonomy. They cannot control the illness, but they have agency in how they navigate the illness. For example, PWD and caregivers might choose to focus on spending time together, or a PWD might write down important memories to share with future generations.

Rolland (2012) refers to a "framing event" (p. 461) that characterizes the PWD and their family's experience or shapes the meaning of the illness. For some, this may be receiving a diagnosis of NCD, or the recognition of distressing symptoms. For others, it could be a hospitalization for a health crisis, or a change to the living situation which brings out or worsens symptoms. Berzoff (2004) asserts that for many PWDs with progressive diseases like ALS, there can be many crises throughout the course of illness. During the acute phase of dementia, the framing event can provide a starting point for PWD, caregivers, and their social workers to begin a collaborative process of meaning-making early in the illness.

Marisa is a 65-year-old cisgender woman caring for her 93-year-old mother, Sara, who is also a cisgender woman, who has a formal diagnosis of unspecified dementia. Six months prior, Sara was hospitalized for uncontrolled leg pain. Marisa noticed a marked decline in her mother's functioning after she returned home from the hospital. This followed many years of Sara being relatively stable despite her diagnosis of NCD, and Marisa blamed herself for Sara's rapid decline now, since Marisa was the one who took Sara to the hospital. In this case example, Marisa and Sara's first framing event or crisis may have been the original diagnosis. However, Sara's hospitalization later became the new frame through which Marisa viewed her mother's illness, as it supplanted the original crisis of a diagnosis. In this example, the meaning Marisa gave to her mother's disease process created feelings of guilt and anger. Together with her social worker, Marisa identified other possible interpretations of her mother's hospitalization: that it showed how Marisa cared deeply for her mother and that Marisa, far from being a source of Sara's decline, was a strong advocate for Sara's wellbeing.[1]

Especially with progressive NCDs like Alzheimer's disease, caregivers may experience anticipatory grief and ambiguous loss (Boss, 2011). Anticipatory grief, or grieving before the actual loss takes place (Rubin et al., 2019), may begin as soon as the diagnosis is made and may continue throughout the illness. For example, caregivers might grieve the impending loss of the PWD, or grieve the impending loss of the person they knew as dementia symptoms progress (Rubin et al., 2019). Caregivers may experience ambiguous loss throughout the disease trajectory, where they feel they are losing the PWD psychologically long before physical decline or death (Paun et al., 2022). During the acute phase, the loss of established roles and relationships, an extension of the psychological losses, is often a focus for PWDs and caregivers, even when the PWD's health and physical functioning are still relatively intact (Rubin et al., 2019).

[1]All names and other personal identifiers in the case are fictitious. Any similarity to actual persons, living or dead, or actual events is purely coincidental.

Further, nonvascular dementia has a gradual onset, with many PWDs displaying symptoms for two to three years before seeking diagnosis, where vascular dementia tends to have an acute onset like a stroke (Rolland, 2017). In cases of nonvascular dementia, families may feel guilt for not noticing symptoms sooner, for not pushing the PWD to get a diagnostic workup, or for losing time while trying to find the right medical team (Nathanson & Latimer, 2021). With the benefit of hindsight, they may look back and more clearly see how signs of dementia were emerging long before diagnosis. Again, it is important for social workers to understand what the illness means to the PWD and the caregivers in order to best serve their needs. For example, a diagnosis of NCD in the PWD means that biological relatives may now be at an increased risk of developing NCD themselves, potentially creating a new family legacy around dementia and sparking anticipatory grief in family members (Rolland, 2017).

Systems of Care Systems of care can provide support for important interpersonal tasks, particularly communication and care planning. Two additional points of focus for this phase are the involvement of palliative care and helping families to determine the appropriate level of care for the PWD at this stage in their NCD.

Students and new social workers should be aware that, because common dementia diagnoses like Alzheimer's disease are terminal and incurable (Keogh et al., 2019), doctors and PWDs alike can experience heightened anxiety when discussing diagnosis (Hagan, 2020). The distress associated with diagnosis can lead to lower-quality conversations between doctors and PWDs (2020) or may even prompt the doctor to disclose the diagnosis to a caregiver rather than the PWD (Rolland, 2017). Therefore, it is important to facilitate adequate communication when it seems families may not be clear about what to expect with the diagnosis (2017).

It can be a challenge for families and healthcare systems to include PWDs in their own decision-making (Nathanson & Latimer, 2021). PWDs may have difficulty making decisions related to healthcare and advance care directives (Chang & Bourgeois, 2020). Limiting the use of hypothetical scenarios and using visual aids where possible may help PWDs better understand and participate in decision-making (2020). Despite the challenges, including PWDs in conversations about goals of care (GOC), advance care directives, and caregiving plans—and encouraging family members to include them—can increase PWDs' sense of autonomy, a powerful psychological step in face of increased dependence and loss of freedom (Bonds et al., 2020). It may also be helpful for the social worker to consider a patient's and family's culture when handling these questions of communication. This may include being mindful of cultures where older family members play significant roles in decision-making and overall family structure (2020), or of whether the culture's decision-making processes tend to be more individualistic or collectivist in approach.

The palliative care model, with its emphasis on advance care planning and comfort care, attends to the challenges presented by dementia's degenerative and unpredictable course. In fact, Reinhardt et al. (2014) argue that palliative care is essential to dementia caregiving and increases positive outcomes for both the PWD and family. Timmons et al. (2022), too, argue that palliative care services are useful from the crisis phase of dementia onwards, as these services allow the PWD to define their needs, participate in their care decisions before their mental capacity diminishes, and receive spiritual and emotional support needed in the acute phase of illness. Across all illnesses, palliative care services and GOC conversations lower the risk of aggressive intervention and death in the hospital for terminal patients (Saracino et al., 2018). Social workers can play a significant role by providing education on hospice and palliative care services, referring PWDs and families to these services, and encouraging discussions on advance care directives and care planning early in illness.

After diagnosis, if impairment is mild, PWDs may be able to maintain their independence (Rubin et al., 2019) without significant changes to their system of care for a period of time. However, PWDs with vascular dementia or rapidly progressing dementia may require additional or professional care sooner than others. Engaging home care or arranging admission to a residential facility is an especially momentous decision that, as well as bringing major changes to routines, may affect the PWD's self-esteem and induce feelings of guilt and distress for the caregiver (Wilson, 2020).

Social Work Intervention

Social work interventions during the acute phase must take into account the newness of symptoms for the PWD and for family members, as family systems have likely not yet fully adapted to their "new normal." While there are many interventions available to social workers during this phase, trauma assessment, psychoeducation, and care planning will be discussed in this section.

Social workers should be mindful of assessing for evidence of traumatic response patterns in PWDs. From the outset, it is critical to be aware of the PWD's trauma history and to recognize that some trauma experiences cannot always be named from the outside. As PWDs decline, their memories go back to older times and experiences; if those times included trauma, PWDs can end up re-living these experiences in the present, with no context to orient them. Further complicating matters, as dementia progresses, a PWD may continue to react to old traumas after having forgotten their previous coping strategies to deal with those traumas (Wilson, 2020). Unfortunately, from the outside looking in, it can be hard to distinguish between trauma reactions and behavioral changes when dementia or delirium is present (Ganzel, 2018).

As not everyone readily names the traumas in their lives, social workers should look for signs that a person has survived trauma: Difficulty trusting people; signs of fight/flight/freeze; tendencies toward dissociation; etc. Long-standing traumas, such as interpersonal and developmental traumas, also may not be named or known by the people around the PWD during a routine assessment for traumatic history.

PWDs may respond with terror or fight/flight/freeze responses to events that seem neutral to the outside observer.

Some traumas are readily named and identified. For example, a 96-year-old Holocaust survivor with vascular dementia, who was usually relaxed and trusting pre-dementia, had sudden episodes of aggressive behavior ("fight" response) toward his home health aides. Upon further investigation, it was revealed that he only exhibited aggressive behavior in the bathroom. Eventually, clinicians realized that disrobing in the bathroom reminded him of an earlier time where the fear of being killed in the gas showers of the concentration camps was real and omnipresent. Considerations of his sense of physical autonomy, gender differences with the aides providing personal care, and ways of managing temperature changes from being unclothed were also assessed.

In addition to taking a trauma history, social workers can intervene by providing critical psychoeducation during the acute phase of illness. In instances where the PWD is unable to acknowledge their dementia symptoms, social workers can provide psychoeducation to caregivers, letting them know that this inability on the part of the PWD is a common reaction, often due to social stigma or denial (Timmons et al., 2022). Some family members may benefit from psychoeducation about the struggles they face, whether these struggles are characterized by overwhelm, fear, anger, guilt, or sadness. Helping caregivers feel more "normal" and less alone is critical. Furthermore, social workers are well-positioned to help caregivers address the health and mental health consequences of caregiving through psychoeducation and therapeutic support. Rolland (2017) suggests inquiring about caregivers' access to healthcare, teaching stress reduction techniques, and connecting caregivers to local caregiving resources as ways to empower them during this arduous chronic phase of dementia.

Finally, during the acute phase, the social worker can assist in care planning for the PWD. Specifically, the social worker can suggest that the PWD and family discuss caregiving roles and help them anticipate future care needs like where the PWD will live, where care will take place, and how the family feels about institutional placement (Nathanson & Latimer, 2021). Where culturally appropriate, encouragement and assistance should be offered in planning the funeral, discussing the will, and preparing for any memorial. Addressing these items early in the disease trajectory can greatly reduce family conflict in the terminal and bereavement phases (Rolland, 2017).

Chronic

The chronic phase of dementia varies widely and often lasts years, leaving PWDs and caregivers unsure of what to expect (Melis et al., 2019). In addition to uncertain trajectories, progressive decline in communication and functioning are characteristic of the chronic phase of NCDs (Rolland, 2017). While the longevity of the chronic phase may exhaust caregiving networks and necessitate ongoing adjustments and new supports, it may also present opportunities for reconciliation between family members (Nathanson & Latimer, 2021), optimism for the time that the PWD has left (Rolland, 2017), and integration of ongoing ambiguous loss, which in the case of dementia is the psychological loss of someone who is physically present (Boss, 2016).

Intrapersonal The chronic phase of NCD presents ongoing intrapersonal challenges for the PWD, often related to self-esteem, coping, communication, and connection.

PWDs must continually adapt to growing cognitive deficits during the chronic phase, which can have a negative impact on their self-esteem (Rolland, 2017). Many people develop depression with vascular dementia, for both physiological and psychological reasons; in turn, depression itself may be a significant risk factor for the development of dementia (Korczyn et al., 2012). The loss of coping mechanisms, self-esteem, personality changes, and even simple changes in roles or routines speaks to the loss of identity that Rolland (2017) notes as common in people with mild NCD. As the disease progresses, the PWD's attachment style may affect the probability of certain behaviors occurring. For example, insecure attachment may be associated with wandering at night, delusions, and depression (Nelis et al., 2014). Those with insecure attachment styles, Nelis et al. (2014) point out, view the self as unworthy or others as unreliable, and generally exhibit lower psychological well-being. From this data, we can extrapolate that PWDs with an insecure attachment style may be seeking comfort or connection outside of themselves and their caregiving system as their surroundings become unfamiliar and uncertain.

At its core, dementia attacks a person's ability to communicate (Alzheimer's Association, 2009) or even to be aware of their internal state. This makes it difficult for the PWD, particularly those with moderate to severe NCD, to know and express their needs, wishes, and desires. This challenge has worsened in face of pandemic conditions. Personal protective equipment (PPE), specifically surgical and N95 masks, must be worn by clinicians and caregivers to slow the spread of the virus, but these make it harder for a PWD to understand and communicate their needs. Family members have not been able to visit PWDs in facilities as often due to social distancing requirements. These restrictions and safety guidelines can produce feelings of abandonment and confusion in PWD. Oyinlola and Olusa (2020) noted that PWDs commonly exhibited feelings of frustration and isolation with regard to masking mandates and social distancing because they were unable to understand or remember the external circumstances that necessitated these public health guidelines.

Interpersonal Interpersonal dynamics during the chronic phase of NCD vary widely, but generally include loss, grief, and the opportunity for meaning-making as the illness progresses.

Just as the PWD is losing part of their former identity during the chronic phase, family and caregivers are often losing the person as they knew them. Paun et al. (2022) and Nathanson and Rogers (2020) describe the series of relational ruptures to which the caregivers must adjust during the chronic phase, often without being able to fully recognize or grieve each successive loss. This manifests differently depending on the relationship and each individual. The attachment relationship between the caregiver and the PWD can affect the health and mental health of both parties, with a secure attachment relationship tending to improve outcomes (Nelis et al., 2014). Children whose parents have dementia go through a "role reversal" wherein the child must care for the parent in the way the parent may have once cared for them or in the way the child may have wished to be cared for (Nathanson & Latimer, 2021). Some cultures view hands-on caregiving for parents as more normative than others (Nathanson & Rogers, 2020). It is important, as always, for social workers to be attuned to the individual and family identities, and their culturally ascribed differences. For spouses and significant others, as the relationship shifts from mutual support to a caregiving dyad, the caregiving spouse stands to lose the emotional and logistical support they once received from their partner (Daniels et al., 2007).

In addition to the ambiguous and anticipatory loss of the PWD, caregivers may also suffer caregiving-related losses during the chronic phase of illness, such as a loss of finances, control over their time, or a job (Noyes et al., 2010). Overall, nearly one in four caregivers in America reported that their own health suffered while caregiving, and almost half said they experienced at least one financial impact (National Alliance on Caregiving [NAC] & American Association of Retired Persons [AARP], 2020). Furthermore, unaddressed ambiguous losses that tend to occur during the chronic phase of illness, such as loss of role, identity, free time, and expected future, may lead to worse mental health outcomes (Nathanson & Rogers, 2020).

Despite the possibility for negative feelings toward caregiving to develop, it is also possible for positive emotions and bonding to increase between the PWD and their caregivers during this time (Rubin et al., 2019). According to Noyes et al. (2010), the family and caregivers' ability to make meaning of the illness experience may help them cope in both the near and long term. Some caregivers may make meaning out of the act of caregiving itself, either as an expression of an internal value or a sense of duty to the PWD. Others may have a strong spiritual or religious background and lead to a larger sense of meaning or purpose within the context of the illness. Social workers can build on the family's meaning-making by validating and encouraging further exploration.

Systems of Care Systems of care have a significant impact on the chronic phase of NCD, playing a role in safety, long-term care placement, and assessment of disease progression.

Most care for PWDs takes place in the home, which provides increased opportunity to personally tailor activities and care to the person's life, unique characteristics, and culture (Alzheimer's Association, 2009). NCD entails significant safety risks, such as wandering at night or leaving on kitchen appliances, which can necessitate the professional assistance of home health aides or placement in a long-term facility, often referred to colloquially as "placement." Placement is often a stressful decision for the PWD and family. It can upend routines (Wilson, 2020), increase financial burden, and engender feelings of guilt in caregivers (Rolland, 2017). At the same time, placement allows family members to function more as supportive or loving relatives rather than full-time caregivers, mitigates safety risks, and provides social stimulation and community for the PWD when the facility is well-equipped to deal with the needs of a PWD. Still, the stigma of placement in a facility, whether due to personal experience with poorly equipped facilities, or societal mores, can weigh heavily on all involved.

Social workers can be a valuable resource to families as they navigate this decision. Importantly, social workers may help families navigate the emotional and practical aspects of decision-making at this critical point in care. From a practical perspective, social workers may provide psychoeducation on the family's options, such as home health aides or placement in a facility, and help them navigate insurance. Emotionally, social workers can discuss with the family common psychosocial benefits and challenges of long-term facilities. Additionally, social workers can provide psychoeducation on the macro dimension of dementia care. Perhaps the family would like to keep the PWD at home but, due to socioeconomic or logistical factors or insurance coverage, do not have access to 24/7 care by home health aides. Social workers can also validate that the family has reached their capacity to handle the care needs of the PWD on their own, depending on the specific family situation (Rolland, 2017).

Within the system of care, social workers can watch for changes in functioning and presentation, as well as symptoms of pain or distress, and relay observations to the care team and family; this is especially important as common health problems like urinary tract infections may mimic the symptoms of worsening dementia (Nathanson & Latimer, 2021). As the disease progresses through the chronic stage, social workers can also periodically check in with the PWD and family about advance directives and healthcare decisions, as preferences can change over time (Rolland, 2017).

An 84-year-old Latinx cisgender woman, Maria, with vascular dementia resulting from a stroke, was admitted to hospice care with orders for full cardiopulmonary resuscitation. She and her daughter, Beatriz,—a 41-year-old cisgender woman who was her mother's healthcare agent—both wished for resuscitation to be performed in the event that Maria stopped breathing or her heart stopped beating. After several months in hospice, Maria had not regained any cognitive or mobility functioning after her stroke. She was still able to speak, but lacked the ability to engage in meaningful conversations. Previously a busy, extraverted woman who walked up and down the halls of her building chatting with neighbors up until the day before her stroke, Maria was now bedridden and socially isolated.

When Maria developed a respiratory infection, Beatriz asked to meet with the nurse and social worker to revisit goals of care (GOC) and advance care directives, as she considered her mother's values in life to encompass wanting to live as a fairly able-bodied, cognizant person, and to die naturally (without extensive medical intervention). Beatriz tried to reconcile those values with the life Maria was currently living. Initially, Beatriz had expected Maria to return to full functioning, and therefore documented wishes for resuscitation and the use of antibiotics. As Maria's condition deteriorated, however, and significant recovery became unlikely, Beatriz gave primary weight to the pain of her mother's downward trajectory. "She would be mortified to know that people were seeing her like this," Beatriz remarked. Together, Beatriz and the care team amended Maria's advance care directives to include a Do-Not-Resuscitate (DNR) order, which Beatriz felt was the right decision at this point in Maria's care.[1]

Social Work Intervention

During the chronic phase, social workers can advocate for the PWD's comfort and overall well-being by diligently observing PWD behavior, collaborating with the interdisciplinary care team, and imparting communication skills to caregivers.

Social workers play a role by observing patterns of behavior in the PWD and clarifying potential causes of the behavior. They can do this by borrowing from the Alzheimer's Association's (2009) view, which urges caregivers to consider alternative explanations for challenging behavior. This organization encourages caregivers to translate patient actions. In the absence of typical communication skills, refusing to eat may indicate that the person's taste has changed, and they no longer want to eat a specific food, or that they are having trouble swallowing; refusing to get dressed may mean that the person is in pain (Alzheimer's Association, 2009). By becoming familiar with nonverbal pain scales, social workers will be able to advocate for the PWD who is experiencing pain in coordination with the care team.

Once a pattern of behavior is identified, social workers can suggest different ways to care for the PWD. This is an opportunity to collaborate with music or recreation therapists on the care team to provide meaningful activities for the PWD. For example, Steward (2021) found that small adjustments to a PWD's environment, such as turning a person's bed or chair to face a window, or learning to better anticipate their care needs, may help calm restlessness. Further, social workers can assist families and systems of care by offering ways to involve the PWD in their own care. Asking the PWD for help with tasks that fall within their current abilities may alleviate helplessness. Engaging a PWD may activate their long-term memories through life review and can help renew their sense of purpose in life. These activities can be crucial in helping the PWD to feel supported.

Additionally, it may be helpful to provide communication tips to caregivers and the larger care team. The Alzheimer's Association (2009) states that using short sentences, leaving adequate time for the PWD to respond, focusing on feelings and not facts, mitigating environmental distractions like music or TV, and watching body language are all helpful when communicating with a PWD. Thus, verbal communication can stay intact as much as possible for as long as possible.

Terminal

In the terminal stage of dementia, PWDs are usually bedbound and nonverbal. At this time, the PWD may lose their long-term memory, which often remains intact until the late stage of the disease (Rolland, 2017). PWDs in the terminal phase of dementia and their healthcare providers must rely on caregivers and appointed decision-makers to navigate healthcare decisions at this point in the disease progression. This underscores the importance of having early and ongoing conversations with PWD and their caregivers about advance care directives (Rolland, 2017; Nathanson & Latimer, 2021).

Intrapersonal and Interpersonal Despite the PWD's limited functioning and communication in the terminal phase, there remain opportunities for connection. This section will highlight such opportunities and their effect, which is to create comfort and closeness. Additionally, it will discuss the increased complexity of caregiving during the terminal phase.

While tremendous gains have been made in better understanding the nonverbal pain cues and symptom management needs of people in the end stages of dementia, it may be difficult to discern a person's internal experience at this stage, as they often have limited ability to communicate verbally. Still, even as PWDs become nonverbal and bedbound, they might still enjoy moments of connection with their environment and with others (Hospice Foundation of America [HFA], 2011). Focus on informed and carefully titrated sensory stimulation, environmental interventions, and pain and symptom management are primary. Hospice organizations encourage caregivers to employ soft music, light touch, flowers, or pictures of people close to them, provisions assumed to bring peace and connection to the PWD.

By the time a PWD enters the terminal stage of illness, caregivers may be deeply entrenched in their role and even derive a sense of mastery from caring for the PWD (Nathanson & Rogers, 2020). At the same time, caregiving for a PWD is a high-intensity task (Noyes et al., 2010) over a prolonged period of time, and caregivers may feel exhausted physically and emotionally (NAC & AARP, 2020). During the terminal phase, caregivers continue to suffer pre-death losses related to the PWD's decline in functioning. Noyes et al. (2010) term these "primary losses." Significant primary losses include the loss of the ability to communicate with the PWD and the loss of intimacy or relationship with the PWD due to decline (Noyes et al., 2010). Dupuis (2008) found that this "psychological death" occurring with PWD can create emotional turmoil for caregivers during the terminal phase.

Moreover, caregivers can be faced with complex medical decisions for PWDs at the end of life (EOL), especially if there are not adequate advance care directives in place. For example, it is common for PWDs with end-stage Alzheimer's disease to lose their ability to swallow (Alzheimer's Association, 2016). It can be very difficult for caregivers and families to decline to pursue artificial nutrition, despite research showing that feeding tubes do little to improve either quantity or quality of life for people with terminal dementia (Dunn, 2016) and can increase the risk of bedsores (Reinhardt et al., 2014), infections, and aspirations, while decreasing care options.

On the other hand, Walters (2022) explores the ethical tension that can arise when thorough advance care directives are in place. Some states allow a PWD to sign an order stating they prefer not to be hand-fed when they are no longer able to feed themselves. In practice, this creates a conflict between the wishes of the "former self," or the PWD before their symptoms progressed, and the "present self," the PWD today, who might enjoy being hand-fed (Walters, 2022, p. 14). Walters (2022) underscores the importance of the PWD and their caregivers discussing the values behind such advance care directives in order to help reduce distress when later carrying out these wishes.

Rubin et al. (2019) point out that dialogue and closure are less possible for families and caregivers of PWD as compared to families dealing with other illnesses, like cancer. EOL is normally a time for life review, relationship review, and sometimes reconciliation (Gerbino & Henderson, 2004), whereas the nonverbal PWD often does not have the ability to participate in these end-of-life rituals and closure activities. Thus, caregivers and families can also suffer the loss of the possibility that a tenuous or complicated relationship might be repaired, in a way similar to that of adult children grieving a parent from whom they were estranged and who died before reconciliation could take place.

Systems of Care There are several ways that the nature of a PWD's decline is affected by the environment of care, and the systems that sustain that environment. This section will focus on utilization of hospice services and the management of PWD behavior in different settings.

The caregivers of PWDs have historically underutilized hospice and palliative care services, though numbers of PWD on hospice are now growing (Sloane et al., 2008). There are several reasons for this. One, whether a PWD's family will be offered hospice or palliative care service often depends on the specific care team's familiarity with services. Underutilization can also result from PWDs' inability to advocate for themselves at EOL, while caregivers potentially miss the signs that they are declining (2008). PWD frequently die of a secondary illness, such as pneumonia, resulting in a quick decline that makes availing of hospice services less likely (2008). Still, the utilization of hospice services can be highly beneficial in the terminal phase of NCD. Changes in routine and environment can be very upsetting to PWDs (Wilson, 2020), making the risk of hospitalization a great concern for the system of care. Hospice services, though not always available or feasible, ideally help to limit hospitalization by providing necessary care where the patient resides.

PWDs are more likely to be chemically restrained compared to those dying of cancer or other diseases (Sloane et al., 2008). "Chemical restraint" refers to the use of medication to control behavior, often to the point of a PWD being nearly or totally bed-bound when they would otherwise be ambulatory. PWDs in the terminal phase, and even in the chronic phase, who are living in long-term care facilities often display behaviors that are difficult to manage and control in any setting, but particularly in congregate care. The question of what makes dementia behaviors "problematic," however, is an ethical gray area. For example, a PWD who takes themselves for a walk does not see their behavior as a problem. If they are in a safe setting it may be good to be able to exercise, but in a facility with low staff-to-patient ratios and strict safety protocols, staff may consider the risk of wandering, unattended falls, and other dangerous situations as primary concerns. While there is extensive research on managing physical safety and emotional distress with the use of carefully titrated medications, PWDs are at risk for overmedication, which can be an infringement on civil liberties and a health risk. Chemical restraint and hospitalization is a particular risk for PWDs with Parkinson's disease or Lewy Body dementia who experience psychosis as a symptom (Stark, 2019). A last-resort intervention, chemical restraints are carefully regulated by laws and policy (Robins et al., 2021).

Social Work Intervention

Given the challenges of the terminal phase, social workers can be a crucial resource to PWDs and caregivers during this time. Specifically, this section will focus on the social worker's role in providing psychoeducation, advocacy, and grief interventions during the terminal phase.

Social workers presented with a terminal phase PWD should be aware of the risk of chemical restraint and hospitalization in their efforts to advocate for PWD. They can provide psychoeducation to caregivers about these risks, as well as other options for symptom management such as geriatric psychiatrists, geriatricians, neuropsychiatrists, and hospice and palliative care services, as appropriate.

As caregivers and families navigate the terminal phase, social workers can help them to process their grief. Since the PWD may be physically present and psychologically absent, Nathanson and Latimer (2021) suggest that social workers help caregivers work to integrate the loss of the person they once knew with the person who remains. Naming and normalizing this type of ambiguous loss can be helpful for caregivers (Nathanson & Rogers, 2020).

Continuing bonds, a concept from grief literature, refers to the ongoing relationships that people have with people or things that are gone (Currier et al., 2015). Relatedly, Rubin et al. (2019) underscore the importance of continuing bonds in caregiver coping even before the PWD dies. Social workers can encourage caregivers and families to foster continuing bonds during the terminal phase of dementia by accessing memories of the PWD before their decline (Rubin et al., 2019), telling stories, reminiscing, and pursuing activities to honor the person (Currier et al., 2015).

Bereavement

Grieving for a person who has died from dementia starts long before death. Just as the trajectory of illness in NCD is heterogeneous and uncertain, grief and losses may manifest differently in each caregiver. Anticipatory grief can begin as early as the time of diagnosis in the acute phase of the illness (Rolland, 2017), or when mild cognitive impairments become apparent (Rubin et al., 2019). On the other hand, grief may not be present initially at diagnosis or death, as the slow decline of NCD can make it unclear when the losses are happening or have happened. Key issues presented in this section include attachment, disenfranchised grief, ambiguous grief, and caregiving-related losses.

Attachment to the PWD and overall attachment style of the bereaved can also influence the grieving process. Insecure attachment has been linked to symptoms of complicated grief, a process in which the grief process becomes stuck and the emotions, outlook, and behaviors linked to grieving worsen (Currier et al., 2015). Secure attachment to a higher power has been found to moderate grief symptoms in the bereaved (Kelley & Chan, 2012). In dementia caregivers, spouses who reported feeling close to the PWD, a measure for secure attachment, reported higher levels of life satisfaction and lower levels of anticipatory grief (Pote & Wright, 2018). Thus, social workers can inquire about the nature of the relationship with the PWD as a means to better understand their grieving process.

Given how unique the bereavement process is for caregivers of PWDs, there are many ways in which their grief may be disenfranchised, from ambiguous losses that go unrecognized during the disease process to the relief some caregivers may feel when the PWD dies (Nathanson & Rogers, 2020).

As the illness progresses, caregivers often experience many ambiguous losses which they are not able to fully grieve in the moment (Paun et al., 2022). The model of dementia grief proposed by Blandin and Pepin (2017) lays out three stages that caregivers and families move through: separation, liminality, and re-emergence. In separation, the person suffers a loss but the loss is not yet acknowledged. Liminality refers to the state after the loss has occurred, when a new status quo is beginning to take hold, as is often the case in dementia. The ability to tolerate difficult emotions in the liminal state is what moves caregivers into the final step, re-emergence, when the loss is acknowledged and processed. When re-emergence has not occurred, one of the main tasks of grieving caregivers is to name, acknowledge, and process each of these losses (Nathanson & Rogers, 2020). For dementia grievers, these losses might include moments when it became clear the PWD was no longer able to walk, or able to recognize family members.

The caregiver may also have suffered caregiving-related losses that they were not able to grieve while the PWD was alive (Noyes et al., 2010), including the loss of a job, health, finances, or even trips they planned to take before the PWD was diagnosed. Rubin et al. (2019) describe this as the two-track model of dementia grief. The first track is the impact of caregiving on the caregiver's overall functioning, similar to Noyes et al. (2010)'s concept of caregiving-related losses. The second track is the caregiver's integration of the loss, even before the PWD dies (Rubin et al., 2019). Their ability to cope after the loss may depend on their ability to make meaning from the totality of their losses, not just the loss of the PWD (Noyes et al., 2010).

Some caregivers may view the death of the PWD as a relief after the long duration and intense burden of caregiving (Stahl & Schulz, 2019). Other caregivers may experience yet another devastating sense of loss after the PWD dies—the loss of their role as a caregiver (Nathanson & Rogers, 2020). This can be the case with caregivers who view caregiving as a normative and expected part of the family process. Taking into account how the individual caregiver views the loss, social workers can assist grieving caregivers by encouraging them to access social support (through friends and family or bereavement groups), find meaning in their caregiving experience, and develop new rituals after the person has died (Nathanson & Latimer, 2021).

Social Justice

This section will focus on the role of disparities in incidence of NCD, caregiving for PWDs, and disenfranchisement. It suggests an unequal incidence and burden of illness, which makes the psychosocial challenges described earlier in this chapter all the more difficult to bear.

Black Americans are twice as likely to develop Alzheimer's disease, the most common form of dementia (Rolland, 2017), as their white counterparts. They are also on average diagnosed later than white Americans are, resulting in higher morbidity rates after initial diagnosis (Bonds et al., 2020). Additionally, education level and gender are risk factors for developing dementia in general, with those who have lower levels of education and women carrying a greater risk (Stark, 2019). This is likely due to life-long stress and unequal access to healthcare (Rolland, 2017). Exposure to trauma in adulthood may also increase the risk of dementia (Ganzel, 2018).

Coinciding with the higher risk of developing dementia among disenfranchised populations, PWDs themselves are often further disenfranchised throughout the disease process. PWDs are often excluded from making their own care decisions even when they still have the capacity to do so (Nathanson & Latimer, 2021). Fortunately, literature on dementia is moving away from speaking to caregivers alone, in favor of speaking to the PWD-caregiver dyad (Bonds et al., 2020). Yet dementia symptoms, such as agitation or memory loss, remain highly stigmatized and likely to lead to isolation of the PWD (Birt et al., 2019; Rolland, 2017). This stigma may also show up when social workers, healthcare professionals, and caregivers assume that a particular behavior is a symptom of dementia, though the Alzheimer's Association (2009) indicates that many such behaviors may be methods of nonverbal communication.

In fact, PWD and their caregivers are largely disenfranchised in research as a group, overall. Gaugler et al. (2019) point out that researchers tend to operate from a deficit-oriented perspective and select psychosocial outcomes without asking PWDs and families what they want out of interventions. Keogh et al. (2019) add that psychosocial interventions largely focus on the PWD, the caregiver, or the PWD-caregiver dyad, leaving out the role of the care team. Similarly, Rolland (2017) states that interventions tend not to target family dynamics. Not only does this represent a gap in research but a potential segment of the population whose needs are being ignored. For instance, Bonds et al. (2020) emphasize the role of family centered decision-making in African-American families. However, research may be focused on PWD-caregiver dyads, overlooking the role of culture in decision-making. Specifically, Bonds et al. (2020) explain "Given the importance of decision-making involvement of [PWDs] and the interdependent nature of African American families, understanding patterns... can highlight strategies to improve decision-making for care planning while caregiving" (p. 384). Similarly, understanding family dynamics in decision-making might inform culturally congruent social work interventions and improve overall outcomes.

As with all illnesses, there are disparities in caregiving responsibilities and stress, particularly for women and people of color. In general, over two-thirds of family caregivers for chronically ill PWDs are women (NAC & AARP, 2020). This is also true of dementia care, where women provide the majority of unpaid family caregiving (Rolland, 2017). As is the case with most facets of American life, financial caregiving burdens are experienced unequally across racial lines. Black Americans making over $50,000 experience more financial burden than their white, Asian, and LatinX counterparts, while all races making less than $50,000 experience similar, but more significant, financial impacts (NAC & AARP, 2020). Relatedly, Hooyman and Gonyea (1999) indicate that work disruptions and economic burdens such as these are significant predictors of stress for female caregivers. Women have been historically oppressed in the labor market and continue to be underpaid compared to men, while economic and social structures rely on women to do the informal, unpaid labor of caregiving (Hooyman & Gonyea, 1999). In this context, an economic burden may cause greater overall disruption, and therefore more stress, to women. Taken together, this means that Black women and women of any race making less than $50,000 are at particular risk for increased financial and emotional stress. Furthermore, it is important to note that caregiving costs, be it monetary, physical, or psychological, are all heightened in high-intensity caregiving situations (NAC & AARP, 2020).

Caregivers for PWDs have higher health and mental health morbidity (Rolland, 2017). By 2034, the percentage of United States households headed by someone over the age of 65 will grow to 34%, up from 26% in 2018 (JCHS, 2019). In addition to the growing numbers of older adults in the United States, the federal government has decentralized care of vulnerable populations to state and local governments, resulting in the care burden falling on families (Hooyman & Gonyea, 1999). As the United States population continues to age, more informal caregivers will likely take on the role of caregiver for PWDs, and they will need additional support in the form of paid time off, access to healthcare, psychosocial support, and more.

Author's Reflections

Before I came to social work, I was a marketer at a magazine. After a difficult year, the head of the publication came in to give a speech. "Do you remember sine curves from school?" he asked. This was not what I expected to hear. He went on to explain that sine curves are a wave function that goes up and down, up and down, on and on forever. That's life, he told us—the curve will always turn. When you're at the top, have humility because you will be at the bottom again. When you're at the bottom, have faith and optimism, knowing that the curve will bring you back to the top.

I think about this speech when it comes to EOL care, especially as it pertains to dementia. Many of us new social workers and social work students are symbolically at the top of the curve. Our cognitive functioning is such that we can study, work, and carry on with our lives. That said, the curve always turns. We were once babies without the ability to understand language or make decisions, and we could very well end up back in that vulnerable and reliant position.

What do we do with that knowledge that we will certainly die, and alongside that, the awareness that we may be so vulnerable at EOL? I try to have humility and keep in mind that I do not know what is or is not going on inside the mind of someone with dementia. I try not to assume what they are capable of, or not. I ask PWDs questions I am genuinely interested in hearing the answer to—such as their favorite memories, their parents, and their children—rather than sticking to comfortable topics like the weather. At the same time, I try to validate their family members who may be at their limit, exhausted by caregiving or by visiting, or who love caregiving and are not ready to "let" the person go.

Working with PWDs and their caregivers, I am also reminded of how much the little things matter. Life can be worth living just to see the sunshine come in the window in the morning. I have seen caregivers who are in immense pain, having cared for their partner or parent for years, nonetheless able to feel elation because their loved one with dementia smiled at them. I have also seen an exhausted caregiver and nurse burst into a fit of laughter after a PWD called the caregiver stupid. "That's Mom! She's in there!" PWD and caregivers may be at the bottom of the curve, so to speak, but they give me so much hope. In these little moments, the bottom doesn't look so bad. –K.N.R

Reflection Questions

1. How might you work with a caregiver to process the many losses experienced during caregiving with PWD?
2. What might some best practices be for interdisciplinary teams working with families of color?
3. In what ways can you continue to maintain personhood for people with dementia throughout the trajectory of the illness?

References

Abedini, N. C., Choi, H., Wei, M. Y., Langa, K. M., & Chopra, V. (2020). The relationship of loneliness to end-of-life experience in older Americans: A cohort study. *Journal of the American Geriatrics Society, 68*(5), 1064–1071.

Acquaviva, K. D. (2017). *LGBTQ-inclusive hospice and palliative care: A practical guide to transforming professional practice*. Columbia University Press.

Alzheimer's Association. (2009). *Dementia care practice recommendations for professionals working in home setting*. https://www.alz.org/national/documents/phase_4_home_care_recs.pdf

Alzheimer's Association. (2016). *End of life decisions: Honoring the wishes of a person with Alzheimer's disease*. https://www.alz.org/national/documents/brochure_endoflifedecisions.pdf

Alzheimer's Association. (2021). Alzheimer's disease facts and figures. *Alzheimer's Dementia, 17*(3). https://www.alz.org/media/documents/alzheimers-facts-and-figures.pdf

American Psychiatric Association. (2013). *Diagnostic and statistical manual of mental disorders* (5th ed.). https://doi.org/10.1176/appi.books.9780890425596

Berzoff, J. (2004). The symptom is stillness. In J. Berzoff & P. Silverman (Eds.), *Living with dying*. Columbia University Press.

Birt, L., Griffiths, R., Charlesworth, G., Higgs, P., Orrell, M., Phuong, L., & Poland, F. (2019). Maintaining social connections in dementia: A qualitative synthesis. *Qualitative Health Research, 30*(1), 23–42.

Blandin, K., & Pepin, R. (2017). Dementia grief: A theoretical model of a unique grief experience. *Dementia, 16*(1), 67–78.

Bonds, K., MinKyoung, S., Whitlach, C. J., Lyons, K. S., Kaye, J. A., & Lee, C. S. (2020). Patterns of dyadic appraisal of decision-making involvement of African American persons living with dementia. *Gerontologist, 61*(3), 383–391.

Boss, P. (2011). *Loving someone who has dementia*. Jossey-Bass.

Boss, P. (2016). The context and process of theory development: The story of ambiguous *loss*. *Journal of Family Theory and Review, 8*(3), 269–286. https://doi.org/10.1111/jftr.12152

Centers for Disease Control and Prevention. (2020). *Alzheimer's disease and related dementias*. https://www.cdc.gov/aging/aginginfo/alzheimers.htm

Chang, W. D., & Bourgeois, M. S. (2020). Effects of visual aids for end-of-life care on decisional capacity of people with dementia. *American Journal of Speech-Language Pathology, 29*, 185–200.

Currier, J. M., Irish, J. E. F., Neimeyer, R. A., & Foster, J. D. (2015). Attachment, continuing bonds, and complicated grief following violent loss: Testing a moderated model. *Death Studies, 39*(4), 201–210. https://doi.org/10.1080/07481187.2014.975869

Daniels, K. J., Lamson, A. L., & Hodgson, J. (2007). An exploration of the marital relationship and Alzheimer's disease: One couple's story. *Families, Systems & Health, 25*(2), 162–177.

Dunn, H. (2016). *Hard choices for loving people: CPR, feeding tubes, palliative care, comfort measures and the patient with a serious illness* (6th ed.). Quality of Life Publishing Company.

Dupuis, S. L. (2008). Understanding ambiguous loss in the context of dementia care. *Adult Children's Perspectives, 37*(2), 93–115. https://doi.org/10.1300/J083v37n02_08

Ganzel, B. L. (2018). Trauma-informed hospice and palliative care. *The Gerontologist, 58*(3), 409–419. https://doi.org/10.1093/geront/gnw146

Gaugler, J. E., Bain, L. J., Mitchell, L., Finally, J., Fazio, S., & Jutkowitz, E. (2019). Reconsidering frameworks of Alzheimer's dementia when assessing psychosocial outcomes. *Alzheimer's & Dementia: Translation Research & Clinical Interventions, 5*, 388–397.

Gerbino, S., & Henderson, S. (2004). End of life bioethics in clinical social work practice. In J. Berzoff & P. Silverman (Eds.), *Living with dying*. Columbia University Press.

Gonzalez-Ramos, G., Cohen, E. V., Luce, V., & Gonzalez, M. J. (2019). Clinical social work in the care of Parkinson's disease: Role, functions and opportunities in integrated health care. *Social Work in Health Care, 58*(1), 108–125.

Hagan, R. J. (2020). What next? Experiences of social support and signposting after a diagnosis of dementia. *Health and Social Care in the Community, 28*, 1170–1179.

Hooyman, N., & Gonyea, J. (1999). A feminist model of family care: Practice and policy directions. *Journal of Women and Aging, 11*(2–3), 149–170.

Hospice Foundation of America. (2011). *Caregiver's guide to the dying process*. https://hospicefoundation.org/HFA-Products/Caregiver-s-Guide-to-the-Dying-Process

Joint Center for Housing Studies of Harvard University. (2019). *Housing America's older adults: A supplement to the state of the Nation's housing report*. Harvard University. https://www.jchs.harvard.edu/sites/default/files/Harvard_JCHS_Housing_Americas_Older_Adults_2019.pdf?fbclid=IwAR2zCi2HWJkUKaN9lnqi2zypDlNbWIFFHwvQzbQZPnQG9K8iYR9SIe9nBoI

Karlawish, J. (2021). *The problem of Alzheimer's: How science, culture and politics turned a rare disease into a crisis and what we can do about it*. St. Martin's Press.

Kelley, M., & Chan, K. T. (2012). Assessing the role of attachment to god, meaning and religious coping as mediators in the grief experience. *Death Studies, 36*(3), 199–227.

Keogh, F., Mountain, G., Joddrell, P., & Lord, K. (2019). Psychosocial interventions for community-dwelling people following diagnosis of mild to moderate dementia: Findings of a systemic scoping review. *American Journal of Geriatric Psychiatry, 27*(6), 641–651.

Korczyn, A. D., Vakhapova, V., & Grinberg, L. T. (2012). Vascular dementia. *Journal of Neurological Sciences, 322*(1–2), 2–10. https://doi.org/10.1016/j.jns.2012.03.027

Melis, R. J. F., Haaksma, M. L., & Muniz-Terrera, G. (2019). Understanding and predicting longitudinal course of dementia. *Current Opinion in Psychiatry, 32*(2), 123–129. https://doi.org/10.1097/YCO.0000000000000482

Nathanson, A., & Latimer, A. (2021). Dementia: Challenges and opportunities across the trajectory of care. In T. Altilio, J. Cagle, & S. Otis-Green (Eds.), *The Oxford textbook of palliative social work*. Oxford University Press.

Nathanson, A., & Rogers, M. (2020). When ambiguous loss becomes ambiguous grief: Clinical work with bereaved dementia caregivers. *Health and Social Work., 45*, 268. https://doi.org/10.1093/hsw/hlaa026

National Alliance for Caregiving and American Association of Retired Persons. (2020). *Report: Caregiving in the US*. https://www.caregiving.org/caregiving-in-the-us-2020/

Nelis, S. M., Clare, L., & Whitaker, C. J. (2014). Attachment in people with dementia and their caregivers: A systematic review. *Dementia, 13*(6), 747–767.

Noyes, B. B., Hill, R. D., Hicken, B. L., Luptak, M., Rupper, R., Dailey, N. K., & Bair, B. D. (2010). The role of grief in dementia caregiving. *American Journal of Alzheimer's Disease & Other Dementias, 25*(1), 9–17. https://doi.org/10.1177/1533317509333902

Oyinlola, O., & Olusa, O. (2020). Social work with older persons living with dementia in Nigeria: COVID-19. *Journal of Gerontological Social Work, 63*(6–7), 638–641.

Paun, O., Loukissa, D., Chirica, M. G., & Nowell, H. M. (2022). Loss and grief in the context of dementia caregiving. *Journal of Psychosocial Nursing, 60*(10), 7–10.

Pote, S., & Wright, S. (2018). Evaluating anticipatory grief as a moderator of life and marital satisfaction for spousal caregivers of individuals with dementia. *Educational Gerontology, 44*(2–3), 196–207.
Reinhardt, J. P., Chichin, E., Posner, L., & Kassabian, S. (2014). Vital conversations with family in the nursing home: Preparation for end-stage dementia care. *Journal of Social Work in Palliative and End of Life Care, 10*, 112–116. https://doi.org/10.1080/15524256.2014.906371
Robins, L. M., Lee, D. A., Bell, J. S., Srikanth, V., Mohler, R., Hill, K. D., & Haines, T. P. (2021). Definition and measurement of physical and chemical restraint in long-term care: A systematic review. *International Journal of Environmental Research and Public Health, 18*(3639). https://doi.org/10.3390/ijerph18073639
Rolland, J. S. (2012). Mastering family challenges in serious illness and disability. In F. Walsh (Ed.), *Normal family processes* (4th ed., pp. 452–482). Guilford Press.
Rolland, J. S. (2017). Neurocognitive impairment: Addressing couple and family challenges. *Family Process, 56*(4), 799–818.
Rolland, J. S., Emanuel, L., & Torke, A. (2017). Applying a family systems lens to proxy decision making in clinical practice and research. *Families, Systems & Health, 35*(1), 7–18.
Rubin, S. S., Manevich, A., & Doron, I. I. (2019). The two-track model of dementia grief (TTM-DG): The theoretical and clinical significance of the continuing bond in sickness and in death. *Death Studies, 45*, 755. https://doi.org/10.1080/07481187.2019.1688014
Saracino, R. M., Bai, M., Blatt, L., Solomon, L., & McCorkle, R. (2018). Geriatric palliative care: Meeting the needs of a growing population. *Geriatric Nursing, 39*(2), 225–229.
Sloane, P. D., Zimmerman, S., Williams, C. S., & Hanson, L. C. (2008). Dying with dementia in long term care. *The Gerontologist, 48*(6), 741–751. https://doi.org/10.1093/geront/48.6.741
Stahl, S. T., & Schulz, R. (2019). Feeling relieved after the death of a family member with dementia: Associations with post bereavement adjustment. *The American Journal of Geriatric Psychiatry, 27*(4), 408–416.
Stark, S. W. (2019). *Psychology of dementia*. Salem Press Encyclopedia of Health.
Steward, A. (2021). Applying person-centered activities for dementia caregivers and activity professionals: A review of creative engagement from a social work perspective. *Journal of Gerontological Social Work, 64*(3), 334–337.
Timmons, S., Fox, S., Drennan, J., Guerin, S., & Kernohan, G. W. (2022). Palliative care for older people with dementia – We need a paradigm shift in our approach. *Age and Aging, 51*(3), 1–4.
Walters, W. (2022). Ethical considerations in palliative care. In T. Altilio, J. Cagle, & S. Otis-Green (Eds.), *The Oxford textbook of palliative social work* (2nd ed.). Oxford University Press.
Wilson, H. (2020). Social work assessments for people with advanced dementia in "the new normal". *Working with Older People, 24*(4), 293–297.

Chapter 6
Diabetes

Diana M. Cory and Peter (Tse Jen) Chu

Illness Overview

The two types of diabetes we will discuss vary in etiology, onset, and progression. Type I diabetes is caused when an individual's pancreas does not produce the insulin hormone that is needed for their body to turn the glucose that food supplies into energy. It is often diagnosed early in life. However, it can also be diagnosed in adulthood and is usually preceded by a triggering event such as the flu or a cold (Cowap, 2015). Typically, the consequences are a somewhat shortened lifespan and an increased risk of heart disease, kidney failure, and blindness, which are heavily dependent on how well (or poorly) the disease is managed. Type I diabetes is most commonly managed by diet and insulin therapy that is administered by injection or insulin pump, along with a glucometer and a continuous glucose monitor.

Type II diabetes is caused by the pancreas producing an insufficient amount of insulin to support healthy bodily function. Unlike Type 1 diabetes, where the pancreas does not produce any insulin, with Type II diabetes the pancreas is able to produce some insulin, just not enough for a person's body to sustain healthy functioning. Type II diabetes is usually first diagnosed in early adulthood; however, the rising number of younger people with obesity is contributing to increasing diagnoses in younger people (Colosia et al., 2013), as the pancreas cannot make enough insulin to support an increased body mass. Type II diabetes is primarily managed by

D. M. Cory (✉)
Columbia University Department of Pediatrics, New York, NY, USA
e-mail: dmc2226@cumc.columbia.edu

P. (T. J). Chu
Coalition of Asian-American Independent Practice Associations, New York, NY, USA
e-mail: chejenchu@gmail.com

M. Hemphill, A. Nathanson (eds.), *The Practice of Clinical Social Work in Healthcare*, Essential Clinical Social Work Series,
https://doi.org/10.1007/978-3-031-31650-0_6

a change in the diet, sometimes oral medication, or insulin therapy and the monitoring of glucose.

The social worker's role with patients who have diabetes can vary based on the context in which these patients are seen. As a social worker, you might find yourself in a diabetes clinic, a general medical clinic, or an inpatient unit in a hospital. You may also find yourself in a setting where diabetes is not considered the "primary" concern and there is another specialty or social service focus. Regardless of the setting, it is essential to remember that diabetes is not *who* the person is. Although the individual may have to spend an inordinate amount of time managing their diabetes, the disease represents only a small part of their life and complexity as a human being. Addressing the whole person is an essential component in the social work practice of psychosocial assessment and is reflected in the concept of patient-centered care (Hudon et al., 2012). Hudon et al. (2012) highlight the importance of recognizing the patient's perception of disease, their life context, and the uncertainty of diagnosis, as well as acknowledging "patient expertise" (p. 174) with regard to their own lives and recognizing that care and treatment must be realistically achievable, while keeping in mind the patient's strengths (as well as limitations). This approach emphasizes the multitude of psychosocial factors that can impact an individual living with diabetes and their ability to care for themselves.

Individuals with diabetes often struggle with the hypervigilance required to maintain their diabetes care every day. Their daily routine requires checking their blood sugar approximately 10 times daily, including before every meal and snack and before and after exercise (and sometimes more). They must count the carbohydrates in everything they eat and drink, so that they know how much insulin their body needs to process what they are ingesting. Monitoring their diet involves opting for nutritious foods that are less likely to induce blood sugar spikes and making sure they eat at regular intervals so that their blood sugar does not drop. Modifying their diet can also include staying away from processed foods and sugary drinks that can wreak havoc on their blood sugar levels, causing low or high blood sugar. They must always carry a glucose monitor, test strips, and a lancing device (and lancets) to draw blood from their fingers for blood sugar checks, as their blood sugar can change from moment to moment. Additionally, they must carry insulin (for regular care, and fast-acting insulin for high blood sugar); glucagon (injection) for quickly raising blood sugar in an emergency when someone is severely hypoglycemic; and something to treat non-emergency low blood sugar (e.g., fruit gummies).

When it comes to treating their diabetes each day, some individuals choose a removable insulin pump and/or a continuous glucose monitor (CGM) attached to their body to both monitor and provide insulin. Others choose to use individual injections when their body needs insulin and rely on intermittent blood sugar checks alone. Still others may choose to use individual injections and a CGM. Regardless of the method of treatment, each person with diabetes will need to know how to calculate their insulin needs, requiring basic math knowledge and literacy. They will also need to know the signs of low and high blood sugar so that they know when and how to address their symptoms. Diabetes symptoms can include: frequent urination; feeling very thirsty; feeling very hungry (even though you are eating or have just eaten); extreme fatigue; blurry vision; cuts/bruises that are slow to heal; weight loss (even though you are eating more, Type 1); and tingling, pain, or numbness in hands/feet (Type 2) (American Diabetes Association [ADA], 2022a, b, c).

Each person with diabetes must confront the knowledge that they may experience medical complications at some point in their life. There can be damage to their eyes, heart, blood vessels, nervous system, teeth, gums, feet, skin, and/or kidneys. Keeping their symptoms controlled can make a big difference between early complications (e.g., losing a toe at age 20) and delaying long-term side effects, or even preventing serious side effects from taking root in their bodies (ADA, 2022a, b, c).

Individuals have to come to terms with the likelihood that their disease will be with them throughout their life. No matter a person's age, adjusting to living with diabetes can be a life-long journey, a process of constant adaptation to the ebb and flow that the disease brings. Diabetes changes a person's relationship with food, eating, culture, travel, friends/partners/family members, and activities, and how they participate in education/school and the world of work. The social worker's challenge is to support the individual in navigating the many complexities of their life while dealing with diabetes (ADA, 2019; Coleman & Caswell, 2020). It is an endeavor that requires the individual's and the social worker's constant assessment of their physical, mental, and emotional health in order to ensure their overall well-being.

When we consider these elements through a psychosocial lens, examining a specific individual's circumstances can illustrate and clarify the complexities of life with diabetes.

Henry is a 30 year-old who identifies as cisgender man of Dominican ancestry diagnosed with Type I diabetes in childhood. He has lived his entire life in the Washington Heights neighborhood of New York City. He lives with his mother and father, and sometimes his 5-year-old niece, and has a dog named "Jax" who is a white Siberian husky. His income is through Supplemental Security Income (SSI) for his mental health and learning challenges. Henry has cognitive delays and poor coping skills and suffers from anxiety and depression which are inconsistently treated due to his reluctance to participate in group and individual therapy. He frequently uses unprescribed drugs (marijuana and ecstasy) to self-medicate. He is also a tobacco smoker. Henry was never able to acquire the skills needed to safely manage his diabetes, as his cognitive challenges have gotten in the way. Henry has had an inconsistent parental presence in his life and is frequently offered foods, drinks, and snacks that offer little to no nutritional value to him and can adversely affect his glucose level. His family appears to "ignore" his condition and assume that he is "taking care of it" without the acknowledgment of what it actually takes to do so. Henry often feels isolated and misunderstood. He struggles with consistently checking his blood sugar and maintaining the supplies needed to do so. His poor executive functioning contributes to his inability to make progress in this area. He was in a specialized education program to address his learning challenges for most of his education and did not graduate from high school. Henry acknowledges the control of his diabetes is poor. He does not want to insult his mother by not eating what she makes and does not have the skills to acquire and retain what is needed to "carb count" for his insulin dosing. He often runs out of lancets, insulin, glucose testing strips, and needles and is unable to rectify this often until he has been without or "rationing" for some time. Henry states that he has no one he can depend on and wishes he had friends, but mostly wants a girlfriend.[1]

While not everyone with diabetes has the multiple challenges that Henry does, many face conflicted feelings about their diabetes and how it negatively impacts their life. For the social worker, working with someone with Henry's challenges, it is crucial to be patient with him and to provide a space where he feels heard. Individuals with diabetes talk of just wanting to be "normal" and at times almost "pretend" that they do not have diabetes, becoming reckless in their self-care. Their recklessness can impact their ability to think clearly and accomplish necessary daily tasks to maintain their quality of life. Poor control can negatively affect their moods causing discord in their relationships with others (Naicker et al., 2017; Roy & Lloyd, 2012). Many adults blame themselves for their diabetes and carry shame and fear with them as well as baseline anxiety around managing their life in conjunction with their disease. Still others live in the fantasy world that "if only" they could get a pancreatic transplant, everything would be okay. It is essential that the social worker, as part of the medical team, is part of the conversation with the nurse practitioners, nurses, diabetes educators, and doctors about each person's own set of circumstances unique to them. These circumstances can cause them to take good care of their diabetes or not, and it is important to withhold judgment. The providers have not "walked in their shoes" and must listen empathically so as to better understand their patients' experiences. Individuals rarely look far ahead to consider the long-term impact of mismanaging their disease, as it is often too abstract or too frightening to consider. Some are so often present-focused on coping and surviving now that it is hard for them to imagine the future ahead. Their struggle is complicated, as there is a multitude of social and emotional factors that can affect their daily lives. It is our job as social workers to recognize the psychosocial challenges that arise and support individuals to address and overcome them. Social workers working with this population must consider what interventions can be most effective in assisting patients to find some level of control over their disease.

Clinical Issues in Diabetes

When an individual receives a new diagnosis, it is not only they who are affected. The ramifications of this diagnosis reverberate among those close to the individual, as they anticipate what it will mean for the person with diabetes to have this disease

[1] All names and other personal identifiers in the case are fictitious. Any similarity to actual persons, living or dead, or actual events is purely coincidental.

permeate every area of their life (Didericksen & Das, 2019). It can elicit fear, uncertainty, guilt, shame, and any number of other emotions. Your patient might exhibit anger, despair, poor adherence to self-care, lack of acceptance/questioning the diagnosis, and/or self-blame. It is important to assess how and when the individual learned of their diagnosis, and how their belief system affects their perception of what health is and the myths and stories they have learned about diabetes and health (Gonzalez et al., 2016). Their adjustment to this new information depends greatly on their ability to process their emotions, and on the necessary and imminent changes to their daily life.

The social worker can utilize the family systems framework to help the person recognize and strengthen the support they have within their parent–child, sibling, and extended family relationships (Bowen Center, 2021). These support systems facilitate adjustment to new diagnosis, necessary lifestyle changes and self-care. Whether these family relationships are strong or weak, the person often benefits additionally from support outside their family system in the form of a therapeutic group, individual therapy, or a community support program. Eliciting the person's assessment of their current circumstances, and what they see as supportive and helpful, assists the social worker in determining the interventions they might use, as well as gives the individual an opportunity to take ownership of their care. Listening with empathy as they sort through their adjusted expectations for the future, the social worker can assist them with problem-solving any barriers to successful self-care in this new context. Psychoeducation with regard to diabetes care and tools to manage their risk of depression and anxiety can also markedly improve their general well-being.

The social worker can help patients recognize the thoughts and feelings that can negatively influence their self-perceptions and overall mood. A negative self-perception for a person with diabetes may include such thoughts as: "I am less able, less of a person than I once was or imagined I would be; there is something wrong with me; I'm a bad person;" or, "This is all my fault." Utilizing motivational interviewing, solution-focused therapy, meditation, mindfulness, and other techniques can promote a sense of control over their circumstances (Ni et al., 2020; Redman, 2012). Additionally, encouraging them to participate in the diabetes community (clinic support groups, online chats, diabetes-focused applications, peer-to-peer interactions, etc.) can help to ease some of the sense of isolation and lessen feelings of self-pity and hopelessness. There is also considerable evidence in the literature that support from one's peer group creates a sense of belonging that can enhance one's ability to sustain self-care (Pienaar & Reid, 2020).

When considering your role and the appropriate interventions in your particular setting, you have the opportunity to think creatively and "outside the box" to find innovative ways to assist those with whom you work.

You might be able to:

- Provide regular counseling on coping with chronic illness
- Refer them to a group/online page for coping with diabetes

- Assist them in educating those closest to them with regard to how to care for their disease
- Address lifestyle/cultural concerns they might have
- Problem-solve possible solutions with them

If you are a community health worker, you are likely to be able to visit the person at home and assess for needs that may not otherwise be evident. The social worker's assessment and subsequent interventions are often dependent on listening and observing what is realistic for the patient and, to borrow a phrase from the harm reduction movement, meeting them "where they are" (McVinney, 2003).

Identifying barriers to effective self-care and brainstorming possible solutions can help individuals feel empowered and allow them to experience a sense of agency, which is important in the face of the disempowering nature of diabetes symptoms and care. When assessing the whole person, recognizing what kind of learner they are and how they like to receive information can help you identify and target the best strategies to help them. For example, providing graphic organizers or images may convey the details of diabetes care (i.e., where to inject insulin on the body; how to rotate sites; how to test blood sugar; how to count carbohydrates; etc.). Using the "teach-back method" can also serve to gauge patient understanding of the education provided (Oh et al., 2021). Providing materials in a patient's preferred language and using an interpreter when needed can also make a big difference in their ability to trust the information they are receiving. Communicating in the way that the individual can best understand will help emphasize that you are truly there to support them in getting the information they need to make the best decisions for themselves.

Financial Aspects of Care

Individuals with diabetes may struggle with financial concerns, particularly when uninsured or inadequately insured to pay for the medication and supplies needed to manage their disease. The cost of supplies (for the insurance company and the individual combined) continues to rise, driven by the increasing price of insulin: "The mean annual cost of T1D care increased from $11,178 in 2012 to $17,060 in 2016, driven primarily by growth in the cost of insulin ($3,285 to $6,255) and the cost of diabetes technology ($1,747 to $4,581)" (Crossen et al., 2020, p. 644). The increased cost of insulin pumps and continuous glucose monitors (CGM), and the limitations that insurance companies put on the amount of supplies an individual can access, create additional challenges that lead some to neglect their care or ration supplies. At times, it can be difficult for someone to admit their financial circumstances and how they are handling those issues, and it might take some relationship building before you are able to learn that finances are a worry. A national study of adults with diabetes and congenital heart disease found that nearly one in seven reported financial barriers to healthcare (Parikh et al., 2014). You might suggest options to alleviate this situation when resources are available. Such resources can come in the form of chronic illness programs and foundations that will assist with costs for prescriptions, medical equipment, supplies, etc. The challenge with some of these organizations becomes evident when the individual is required to provide financial evidence of need and they do not have it, or the application process is only in the English language and their primary language is different. These potential hurdles to accessing health resources can be addressed and, if done effectively, can open doors for many people on the periphery of the medical system to get the care they want and need (Billimek & August, 2014).

Environmental Factors

An individual's housing insecurity can negatively impact their ability to adhere to their care. They might live in a housing situation where they have little autonomy or personal space. They may have limited access to refrigeration for insulin and fresh foods; they might have roommates who eat their healthy food or who buy inappropriate foods without sensitivity to their special medical needs. Other individuals with diabetes may be homeless, not knowing where they will sleep from one night to the next. Their private space might be limited or virtually non-existent, and they might be at the mercy of the landlord or the friend/acquaintance with whom they are staying. Many high-risk individuals have unstable housing or tenuous immigration status, and fear any system that collects their personal information, as it could be used to harm or deport them. They might live in a shelter where they cannot have anything sharp and must keep their supplies, needed frequently for the care they require, in a location that is not easily accessible. As Berkowitz et al. (2018) suggest, there is a strong correlation between housing instability and increased diabetes-related emergencies and inpatient hospitalization. The social worker may find themselves writing advocacy letters for the individual and connecting them with pro bono legal services to address housing issues and discrimination in the interest of avoiding unnecessary diabetic emergencies and maintaining their health.

Throughout the ongoing assessment of the individual, it is critical to consider what basic needs are or are not being met, and the implications for adherence to care. It is important to ask yourself as a social worker whether this person has a history of, or is currently experiencing:

- Trauma
- Food insecurity
- Mental illness
- Family and/or community violence
- Abandonment
- Neglect
- Addiction
- Unstable housing/homelessness
- Medical comorbidities

These are just some of the factors that can contribute to an individual's ability or inability to fully adhere to their diabetes care (Tareen & Tareen, 2017). Understanding such factors can assist the social worker with seeing and addressing the wider challenges to an individual's successful self-care.

Lifestyle Changes

Patients diagnosed with Type II diabetes can find themselves having to make changes to prevent premature loss of function, much like those with Type I. Some struggle to accept that their lifestyle could be harming their health as they have been "fine" until this point in their life. They might discover their illness as a result of a medical event like a heart attack, stroke, or seizure. They may end up in the hospital after an accident, where testing confirms their diagnosis of Type II diabetes. Their potential mistrust of the medical system can cause them to doubt their test results and it might take them some time to connect with the diabetes clinic. The hospital or the outpatient clinic is often where they begin to learn about Type II diabetes care and about food options that can support good health. They are frequently introduced to a care team consisting of an educator/nutritionist, an endocrinologist, and sometimes, but not always, a social worker. A connection to a comprehensive diabetes center can help limit future hospitalization and risk of severe disability or death (Rubin, 2015).

For many, changing the way they eat is an overwhelming, seemingly impossible task. Individuals can have strong connections to the foods they eat, as food is often a way we are nurtured by the ones who care for us growing up. Family and cultural identity is frequently wrapped up in the foods we make and share, and thus the desire to connect with loved ones can impede the individual's efforts to adhere to specific dietary restrictions or changes. Barriers can appear in the form of lack of health-promoting food options in the home, or having limited food options in their community (Mezuk et al., 2016). The "convenience" of the convenience store can make choosing something nutrient rich a difficult task. Tiwari and Ambinakudige (2021) quote the Neighborhood Food Insecurity Index (NFII): "about 43 million (13.14%) people in the United States live in neighborhoods with high food vulnerability" (Section 4.4). Nearly one in six Americans may have limited access to healthy foods (Tiwari & Ambinakudige, 2021).

Alongside difficulties adhering to the diet, many patients find that adding or increasing exercise in their lives is daunting. They might not have a park or area to exercise nearby or may live in a household where exercise is not a regular part of daily life or not valued. Family members and friends may consciously or unconsciously sabotage the individual's efforts to improve their health by keeping sugary drinks and snacks in the house or providing a lot of packaged foods for meals and snacking. In these instances, drastic changes in lifestyle can be counterproductive. Prioritizing a person's sense of autonomy and confidence about managing their health may lead to more long-term adherence.

Using something akin to harm reduction can assist an individual with slowly implementing new, healthier choices so that they can make progress toward better health (Hawk et al., 2017). The harm reduction approach encourages celebrating improvements rather than punishing regressive behavior (by using criticism, harsh blame, guilt, and threats) and holds that this allows the individual to gain confidence in their ability to keep themselves healthy. Individuals often require tremendous support over many years from their multidisciplinary team as well as their friends and those closest to them in order to tackle the challenge of managing their diabetes successfully. Recognizing the real barriers for an individual requires that social workers continuously and holistically assess the individual in their environment to provide support for their ever-changing needs.

Rita is a 45-year-old European American who identifies as a cisgender woman with Type II diabetes and has worked for the city bus company for the past 20 years. She graduated from high school and did a two-year associate degree in mechanics. She now works repairing the buses at the busyard. She gets two breaks of 15 minutes each, and gets 30 minutes at 12 pm to eat her lunch. She works five days per week. Legally she is supposed to receive accommodations to care for her diabetes while at work; however, leaving her post to check her blood sugar or have a snack when needed is frowned upon. Most of her colleagues are male and tease her for needing more breaks than others because she's "a woman." While she tries to remain unaffected by such comments, they make her feel isolated from her coworkers, fatigued, and sad as well as pressured to continue to work despite her medical needs. Rita has three teenage children at home and her husband works nights as an electrician for the city. Her mother and father live with them and both have Type II diabetes. Her mother does most of the cooking for the household and has kidney disease and peripheral neuropathy. Her mother tends to cook traditional family recipes that are often high in fat and carbohydrates. Rita's mother continues to purchase sugary snacks for her grandchildren.[2]

The difficulties of managing life with diabetes are evident in the multiple challenges Rita faces each day. It is important for the social worker supporting Rita to acknowledge her strengths and help her to use them to problem-solve her work difficulties when it comes to self-care. Individuals with Type II diabetes can have many of the same symptoms as those with Type I; however, symptoms of Type II tend to develop over time. An individual can be diagnosed with prediabetes, often giving them the opportunity to prevent the disease from developing by making health-promoting lifestyle choices such as improving sleep, losing weight, adjusting eating habits, and exercising regularly. The social worker can help the individual understand how diabetes can affect their daily life and their future and help them work toward accepting their diagnosis while learning how to manage their disease. The social worker's role on the multidisciplinary team can be not only to assist the

[2] All names and other personal identifiers in the case are fictitious. Any similarity to actual persons, living or dead, or actual events is purely coincidental.

patient in identifying what is beneficial and realistic in terms of self-care but also to support them as they explore how to structure their life to improve their health (Sebire et al., 2018). Additionally, the social worker is in a unique position to provide reminders to the team that caring for individuals with diabetes requires practitioners to be sensitive to patients' questions and concerns (both spoken and unspoken), acknowledging the patients' expertise about what is important for their well-being. Reminding team members that the complexities of each human being are unique and require active listening to leave room for patients and their families to contribute to their overall care.

Social Stigma

Depending on the individual's bond with family and friends, they may experience different levels of acceptance, support, or criticism related to the way they manage their illness. When family members and friends put stock in various myths about diabetes, or make assumptions about individuals with diabetes, this has ramifications for their interactions with the patient (Himmelstein & Puhl, 2021). The individual with diabetes may also harbor various feelings about how involved they want their family members and friends to be with their support and care. They may be experiencing anger, shame, frustration, and fear for the future. Those on the outside looking in might have limited knowledge about diabetes and offer unhelpful advice or commentary, e.g., expressing skepticism about the number of times someone has to test their blood sugar over the course of a day or week and make a judgment about whether or not this is necessary based on limited knowledge.

Other individuals with diabetes might have trouble coming to terms with the dietary and lifestyle changes that are part of diabetes management and care. While insulin pumps have become more and more efficiently designed, those who choose to use them as their insulin source still have to wear them outside of their body. They are subject to stares and strange comments from others who do not understand, and this can be difficult to manage over time. A family member might want to make a favorite dessert for a special occasion and be disappointed and hurt when the individual with diabetes cannot eat it. Yet another family member or friend may want to be too involved with the person's diabetes care and become pushy, e.g., asking to do their finger sticks or injections or to share diabetes-friendly recipes. Others may blame the individual for their illness and say judgmental things to them, while still others may have diabetes themselves and not done anything to address it. They may have heart problems, kidney disease, missing extremities, or any number of other medical issues that can be caused by poor diabetes control, a distressing thing for a fellow person with diabetes to witness. In all of these scenarios and others, individuals with diabetes can feel overwhelmed by the behavior of those close to them, and sometimes choose not to share their health-related concerns with them as a result, potentially leading to feelings of isolation, disability, and decreased mobility (McCaffery et al., 2020).

Impact on Caregivers

Witnessing the prolonged suffering and deterioration of an individual with diabetes can take a toll on their family members, friends, and care team. Stressed and overwhelmed, people who care for individuals with diabetes can find themselves complaining about how patients are "resistant" to lifestyle modification, not adherent with prescribed therapy, and insistent on some unreasonable demands. Lynch et al. (2018) found that most caregivers of individuals with chronic illness reported compassion fatigue that impairs their physical, mental, emotional, and social functioning. Unlike healthcare professionals, who do not know the patient personally, family and friends in their role as caregivers tend to become emotionally and physically invested in looking after someone close to them. This experience can be traumatic and manifest as feelings of emotional and physical exhaustion, coupled with a sense of powerlessness and frustration. Especially when individuals with diabetes receive lower extremity amputation as a treatment for a foot ulcer, a common complication of poorly managed diabetes, the level of caregivers' physical, emotional, social, and financial burden can greatly increase (Costa et al., 2018; Çamur et al., 2020). The caregiver may have to accompany the patient to recommended physical therapies, appeal a prosthetic coverage denial or cancellation of insurance policy, and be available to collaborate with the care team. Even with everything done correctly, there is still a high risk of postoperative mortality among patients with diabetes who undergo amputation (Gurney et al., 2018). If exhausted caregivers do not get the help they need to process the feelings of helplessness, guilt, and emotional detachment, they may develop health issues or symptoms of post-traumatic stress disorder.

End-of-Life and Bereavement

Anticipatory grief and chronic sorrow are dominant themes when working with individuals with late-stage diabetes complications. As distinguished from grief about the passing of another person, anticipatory grief is triggered by witnessing the long-term suffering of a close friend or family member with a chronic or terminal illness, or by the anticipation of one's own future suffering and incapacitation. Chronic sorrow can be experienced by anyone, as it is fueled by a sense of "ongoing loss" (Hayes, 2001), particularly the loss of the ability to meet typical cultural and developmental milestones due to illness or loss. Anticipatory grief and chronic sorrow may be caused by a progressing disease that will lead to future loss, whether it be a specific and tangible loss such as the loss of a limb, or a symbolic one, e.g., unfulfilled expectations (Varga & Gallagher, 2020). Hayes (2001) asserts that individuals with Type 1 diabetes experience the negative impact of symptoms consistent with themes of chronic sorrow including: fear of an uncertain future; unhelpful attitudes of others; regrets; and difficulty managing their disease. Patients with diabetes must often navigate the loss of normative life, such as being told by doctors to minimize their intake of traditional food and eat food that seems unfamiliar. For many cultures, food is an important way to show affection and connection to one's heritage. Sudden and radical changes to eating habits may have a negative impact on patients' social relationships and make them feel a large part of their self-identity has been ripped away (Beverly et al., 2018).

When diabetes gets worse over time, it will have an impact on multiple physiological systems and may cause complications that affect almost every part of the body. There may be no visible impairment or deformity, but patients in the late or advanced stages of diabetes often suffer from myocardial infarctions (heart attacks), strokes, nerve damage, blindness, lower-extremity amputations, and end-stage renal disease (see chapter on *Kidney and Liver Disease*). Certain psychiatric illnesses may be comorbid with diabetes. One study shows that neuropathic pain in the lower limbs is prevalent among Type II diabetes patients, and the intensity of pain with neuropathic characteristics has a positive correlation with depressive symptoms (de Lima et al., 2019).

It is necessary for social workers to understand how diabetes patients affected with complications can exhibit symptoms of grief and loss for their dreams, and for life expectations unfulfilled. Patients' diminished health can have a deep psychological impact on them. For example, a 55-year-old mother received hemodialysis three times per week for two years, lost several toes, and required surgical removal of part of her right leg. Feeling depressed and alone in the hospital, she refused to engage in discussion about the impending amputation and asked her adult children to make every medical decision for her. For the care team, this patient may seem to be in disbelief or denial of the severity of her complications.[3] However, it is easy to overlook the complex psychological and emotional impact of diabetes, as studies have shown that depressive symptoms and less-than-optimal diabetes self-management are closely related (Schmitt et al., 2021). It is essential to identify the influences of mood comorbidity that may be causing suboptimal self-management and glycemic outcomes.

Caregivers' emotional responses to the intensity of care and the patient's death can vary dramatically depending on multiple factors, such as their relationships with the deceased, cultural values and beliefs, and perception of the patient's responsibility for their own health. A caregiving Asian American adult daughter reported symptoms of prolonged grief and post-traumatic stress after taking care of her 60-year-old mother for three years before she died from multiple organ failure due to sepsis, a potential complication from her long-standing diabetes. Witnessing her mother's prolonged suffering, including proximal amputations, constant fatigue from dialysis, and multiple falls due to strokes, the daughter felt powerless and depressed for not being able to prevent her mother's condition from getting worse. Days before her mother died, the daughter chose to have "full code status" for lifesaving measures and declined to sign Do Not Resuscitate (DNR), Do Not Intubate (DNI), or Allow Natural Death (AND) orders on her mother's

[3] All names and other personal identifiers in the case are fictitious. Any similarity to actual persons, living or dead, or actual events is purely coincidental.

behalf. For the daughter, sending her mother to hospice care was not an option as it would mean to her that she lacked gratitude for the sacrifices her mother made to give her a good life.[4] While social workers can offer culturally sensitive counseling services to family caregivers on dealing with decisions about end-of-life care, it is crucial that all members of the team participate in widespread interdisciplinary education to prevent cross-cultural misunderstanding and distress (He & van Heugten, 2020).

When social workers work with the bereaved, assessing for any immediate safety issues, including the need for food, clothing, shelter, and medications and the level of suicide risk, is essential. Additional assessment might include exploration of other urgent needs, such as planning a funeral, sorting out the deceased's affairs, and handling financial matters. When (or as) basic safety needs are assured, emotional and spiritual needs must be assessed and addressed. While helping the bereaved person, it is important for the social worker to ask themselves: What does healing mean and look like for this individual?

A fundamental understanding of the nature and norms of grief may be helpful to social workers who encounter and support the bereaved of diabetes patients. As Stroebe et al. (2017) point out, there is no "normal" reaction to loss, no typical grief stages, or orderly mourning progression. Psychiatrist Elisabeth Kübler-Ross (1969) introduced the now well-known five stages of grief: denial, anger, bargaining, depression, and acceptance. Today, Kübler-Ross's five stages are not really viewed as "stages" in the sense of a sequential pattern, but rather a description of various common responses to grief and loss; what grief looks like can vary greatly from person to person. Through compassionate listening, social workers can draw out strengths and healing from family narratives as family members strive to make sense of their grief. For example, after a 75-year-old cisgender Hispanic woman with Type II diabetes died from cardiac arrest, her daughter, who was her live-in caregiver, expressed relief after finding boxes of chocolates under the mother's bed. The daughter had been feeling responsible for not taking "good enough" care of her mother's condition. Realizing that her mother's inadequate diabetes care was not her sole responsibility relieved some of these feelings of guilt, in relation to her mother's death and in relation to the sense of relief she was experiencing no longer needing to be her caregiver.

The vigilance required for diabetes care transfers to the caregiver when the individual is no longer able to test their blood sugar or give themselves an injection, for example. This can further impact the relationship of caregiver and patient, as well as the ability or inability of each to provide or accept care. Social workers may use narrative therapy to assist the bereaved in exploring their feelings and perceptions of the deceased, continuing the conversation about decision regret, and working together to uncover their personal sense of meaning drawn from the loss event (Peri et al., 2016). Ultimately, much of the healing work will rest with the bereaved as they reinvent their relationship with the deceased and rework their worldview.

---

[4] All names and other personal identifiers in the case are fictitious. Any similarity to actual persons, living or dead, or actual events is purely coincidental.

Social Justice

Issues of social justice are woven through narratives of living with diabetes, with major implications for the support and interventions that the social work community can provide. The layers of injustice are at times formidable and demoralizing. Institutional and societal racism and classism, persecution (overt or covert) along with limited access to comprehensive diabetes care and resources, perpetuate rife inequality in the healthcare system particularly for people of color. As noted by Subica and Brown (2020), "health disparities are the concrete manifestation of detrimental social factors such as racism, discrimination and stigma that segregate individuals into disadvantaged communities...where they are systematically denied access to health-protective resources" (p. 166).

Individuals with diabetes can find themselves living in socioeconomically disadvantaged areas, where it is more likely their access to comprehensive diabetes care will be limited (Barnard-Kelly & Cherñavvsky, 2020). They may feel limited to their local primary care doctor (due to barriers to transportation access, e.g., or lack of access to technological infrastructure for telehealth), who knows little about comprehensive diabetes care resulting in suboptimal care. Suboptimal care can lead to premature complications, with consequences for an individual's quality of life and life span. A patient may make efforts to access care in a more specialized setting (traveling outside their community and spending much-needed money on transport to do so), only to find that their insurance does not cover the transport or the appointment, which deters the patient from returning to that setting. Often patients are referred to diabetes specialists without regard to whether the practitioner is covered by the individual's insurance, creating a roadblock to specialized care. For some, the overwhelming financial and logistical burden of obtaining supplies needed to properly care for their disease is exacerbated by their limited or lack of insurance coverage often linked to the high cost of these supplies. As a result, those with poor insurance coverage or no insurance coverage often present with poor health outcomes. On top of all this, the societal and social stigma associated with diabetes, often based on myths and misinformation, can cause individuals to hesitate to access proper treatment.

Institutional and structural racism contributes to and sustains lack of access and discriminatory practices both explicit and implicit (Hu et al., 2014; Meng et al., 2016). Historical marginalization and the othering of non-white populations continues to breed mistrust and avoidance of mainstream medicine in many communities. Frequently, the medical system's implicit expectation is that those who speak another language, lack technological savvy, have limited financial resources, or other life challenges have to try harder, navigate better, and advocate more for themselves and those closest to them just to get their basic medical needs met (Fernandez et al., 2011). This continued implicit "epidemic of disempowerment" (Marmot, 2017, p. 543) keeps individuals with multiple healthcare needs, including diabetes, on the periphery, with little to no access to much-needed care. According to the Centers for Disease Control and Prevention (2022a, b), the prevalence of adults with diabetes by race and ethnicity in the United States based on 2018–2019 data is 14.5% American Indian/Alaskan Native; 12.1% Black, non-Hispanic; 11.8% Hispanic; 9.5% of Asian, non-Hispanic; and 7.4% of white, non-Hispanic, further emphasizing the impact of marginalization of specific populations by the historically white power structure of the healthcare system. Additionally, diabetes is disproportionately present in adults with less formal education: 13.4% with less than a high school education; 9.2% with high school education; and 7.1% with more than a high school education (CDC, 2022a, b) increasing the gap between individuals with diabetes and their access to care. Those who hold the power and the money lack the awareness or the will to acknowledge that needs differ across cultural and biopsychosocial structures and require taking the time to listen and truly hear the perspectives of others in order to provide appropriately accessible care. The healthcare system's attempt to provide more readily available care is frequently flawed, as it minimizes the importance of earning community trust. It tends to neglect the idea that an equitable plan to provide comprehensive healthcare for diabetes populations must include time for the plan to take hold and include the voices and languages of affected communities in its development. As it stands now, the ability of an individual with diabetes to self-manage is likely to be influenced by prevailing economic conditions, cultural norms and expectations, and the underpinning logic of the healthcare system (Hinder & Greenhalgh, 2012), which has consistently sent the message that individuals must compromise their sense of autonomy and identity in order to get their needs met.

The healthcare system's *accessible care plans* are frequently based on studies and data that are inherently biased due to the limitations of the research data and a lack of effort invested in making the studies themselves equitable in their administration and execution. Often these studies are hampered by lack of staff, especially multilingual staff, and by budget constraints. The healthcare system is badly in need of an overhaul to refocus on human beings, rather than on money and crude data, if the barriers between medical providers and individuals seeking care are to be dissolved (Bailey et al., 2017). Without such a transformation, individuals with chronic conditions like diabetes that involve long-term, multifaceted care are likely to receive subpar treatment that misses crucial opportunities to reverse or stabilize sickness.

Access to comprehensive care and resources is generally limited, or available only if one is already aware of the options that exist and knows how to request, or demand, them. According to the National Academies of Science, Engineering and Medicine (2017), "the effect of interpersonal, institutional, and systemic biases in policies and practices (structural inequities) is the 'sorting' of people into resource-rich or resource-poor neighborhoods" (p. 101). Some geographical locations have inadequate transportation options, limited availability of competent language translation, and poor funding of local, available care and programs. Combined with all this, individuals from these areas tend to face unconscious judgment from healthcare professionals. Comprehensive care centers are often built around universities in large cities, which limits access for those in rural and under-resourced communities. Additionally, care centers are frequently rife with institutional racism that is difficult for organizations to acknowledge or address, as it has long been embedded in their systems. While the implementation of telehealth has improved this somewhat, lack of technological infrastructure in both urban and rural settings, including multilingual resources, continues to stymie the ability of many to access care on a comprehensive scale (Ray et al., 2017).

In instances where the technology is available to a patient with diabetes, apps that center on managing diabetes can provide individuals with information about their disease and symptoms as well as meal planning, self-management tools, and resources outlining the impact of the disease on their overall health. Introducing apps, online chat groups, and other forms of community building can help individuals shift their perspective and support them in improving their quality of life. There are, however, barriers to utilizing and benefiting from these supports. Crossen et al. (2020) assert that "the cost of T1D care is now driven by mounting insulin prices and growing utilization and cost of Diabetes technology" (p. 644), and individuals' ability to utilize interventions can be reduced by high costs. Other salient barriers to adequate care and self-care include literacy; trauma; conflicting cultural and religious belief systems; mistrust of the medical establishment; and language. All of these must be considered with comprehensive care in the context of diabetes as potential limitations on an individual's ability to understand their disease and successfully care for themselves.

However, the fact is that people with poor blood sugar control often understand their disease and their responsibilities quite well (Greenfield et al., 2011). It is often their own interpretation of what is expected to manage their diabetes that influences what they do (or do not do) to adhere to the "recommended" care routine. Some may have chronic exposure to external stressors, such as job strain, early life adversity, lack of safety at home or in their neighborhood, and poor interpersonal skills. It is important for the social worker to understand that individuals are often ambivalent about prioritizing diabetes in their day-to-day life, as they are addressing the daily challenges of living. The social worker should consider counseling techniques that take into account the individual as a whole person in order to make their intervention(s) more efficacious and motivating, and the outcomes sustainable for the individual living with diabetes. Diabetes is a lifelong challenge to manage and live with. It is important for the social worker to remind themselves that self-care with this disease does not get easier, but may become a bit more manageable.

Authors' Reflections

While the impact of this disease is different for each person, the struggle to be healthy each and every day can be a heavy burden and consistent success managing their disease is virtually impossible to attain for most. As social workers, we have to remember to be patient and kind as their disease is not going to go away. There is no cure. Empathically listening and reinforcing that we are not there to judge them is the most caring thing we can do. Helping them to take small steps toward taking better care of themselves and emphasizing how brave they are for seeking help assists in giving them hope for the future. Diabetes is a roller coaster through periods of stability and times of instability all throughout the individuals' life stages bringing different challenges along the way. Working with this population of people can be formidable given the intensity with which they need to focus on their self-care. The individual who lives with diabetes can suffer alone with their feelings of frustration, anger, inadequacy, and at times hopelessness. They can dismiss the need for extra support or guidance in an effort to be "okay" and seemingly independent. As social workers, it is our job to listen with compassion and empathy so that they know they have a safe place to land when they are ready to accept support. Helping them to feel a sense of agency in when and how they accept support and what kind can help to carve out space where they can express their worries openly and honestly. The constant challenge of maintaining a proper diet and managing insulin needs can sometimes make them "give up" for a time. At times, they will care for themselves minimally, so as not to end up in the hospital, but still causing considerable harm to their bodies over time. Some have never learned how to take care of themselves and struggle to integrate a new way of living when they are diagnosed later in life, and others adapt feeling empowered by the ability to "do something". Working with individuals with diabetes requires suspension of judgment and understanding that the care is complex and ever changing making it difficult to master.

We have spent considerable time counseling individuals with diabetes to support them in finding ways past their personal barriers to be able to care for themselves. Those who continue to struggle can respond well to "small victories" on their road to competent self-care and it is essential for social workers to point out these successes in order to instill hope. We who have historically had supportive home lives and communities are often more successful keeping ourselves on track and quickly recovering when we go off track. Others can continue to be conflicted due to mixed messages from their support systems and/or comorbidities (e.g., depression, hypertension, retinopathy, thyroid disease, dyslipidemia, non-alcohol-related fatty liver disease, kidney disease, and obesity). In recent years, individuals open to technology have learned how to integrate various management apps and glucose monitors to make handling their condition more realistic for them. In the diabetes clinic, helping individuals to master injections, insulin pumps, and healthy, affordable food choices allows them to gain confidence in their ability to self-care. While some of these tools make diabetes easier to manage, the intense focus on self-care is still there and is necessary for stable health. The social work role has always been to think creatively and problem-solve with individuals to assist them in using their strengths and personal motivation to take control of their diabetes. Helping individuals sustain their motivation is frequently dependent on leveraging their coping skills and available support systems. Assisting them in finding their inner strength and fortitude can help individuals with diabetes move toward successful self-care.

Reflection Questions

1. In what ways does the prevalence of diabetes make it more complicated to treat psychosocially?
2. How do the experiences of marginalized communities differ in their ability to manage diabetes, from communities with more resources and social capital?
3. How might you help a patient who expresses ambivalence about making lifestyle changes to better address diabetes?

References

American Diabetes Association. (2019). *Your health care team*. http://archives.diabetes.org/living-with-diabetes/treatment-and-care/whos-on-your-health-care-team.html

American Diabetes Association. (2022a). *Type 1 overview*. https://diabetes.org/diabetes/type-1/symptoms

American Diabetes Association. (2022b). *Type 2 overview*. https://diabetes.org/diabetes/type-2/symptoms

American Diabetes Association. (2022c). *Complications*. https://diabetes.org/search?keywords=COMPLICATIONS&page=0

Bailey, Z. D., Krieger, N., Agénor, M., Graves, J., Linos, N., & Bassett, M. T. (2017). Structural racism and health inequities in the USA: Evidence and interventions. *Lancet, 389*(10077), 1453–1463. https://doi.org/10.1016/S0140-6736(17)30569-X

Barnard-Kelly, K. D., & Cherñavvsky, D. (2020). Social inequality and diabetes: A commentary. *Diabetes Therapy, 11*, 803–811. https://doi.org/10.1007/s13300-020-00791-4

Berkowitz, S. A., Kalkhoran, S., Edwards, S. T., Essien, U. R., & Baggett, T. P. (2018). Unstable housing and diabetes-related emergency department visits and hospitalization: A nationally representative study of safety-net clinic patients. *Diabetes Care, 41*(5), 933–939.

Beverly, E. A., Ritholz, M. D., Wray, L. A., Chiu, C. J., & Suhl, E. (2018). Understanding the meaning of food in people with type 2 diabetes living in northern Appalachia. *Diabetes Spectrum: A Publication of the American Diabetes Association, 31*(1), 14–24. https://doi.org/10.2337/ds16-0059

Billimek, J., & August, K. J. (2014). Costs and beliefs: Understanding individual- and neighborhood-level correlates of medication nonadherence among Mexican Americans with type 2 diabetes. *Health Psychology, 33*(12), 1602–1605. https://doi-org.avoserv2.library.fordham.edu/10.1037/hea0000020

Bowen Center. (2021). *The Bowen Center for the study of the family*. https://thebowencenter.org

Camur, S., Batibay, S. G., & Bayram, S. (2020). Effect of lower extremity amputation on caregiving burden in caregivers of patients with diabetic foot: Prospective cohort study. *International Wound Journal, 17*(4), 890.

Centers for Disease Control and Prevention. (2022a). *By the numbers: Diabetes in America*. https://www.cdc.gov/diabetes/health-equity/diabetes-by-the-numbers.html

Centers for Disease Control and Prevention. (2022b). *Prevalence of diagnosed diabetes*. https://www.cdc.gov/diabetes/data/statistics-report/diagnosed-diabetes.html

Coleman, S. E., & Caswell, N. (2020). Diabetes and eating disorders: an exploration of "Diabulimia." *BMC Psychology, 1*. https://doi.org/10.1186/s40359-020-00468-4

Colosia, A. D., Palencia, R., & Khan, S. (2013). Prevalence of hypertension and obesity in patients with type 2 diabetes mellitus in observational studies: A systematic literature review. *Diabetes, Metabolic Syndrome and Obesity: Targets and Therapy, 2013*, 327–338. https://doi.org/10.2147/DMSO.S51325

Costa, M. S. A., Machado, J. C., & Pereira, M. G. (2018). Burden changes in caregivers of patients with type 2 diabetes: A longitudinal study. *Journal of Advanced Nursing, 74*(10), 2322–2330. https://doi.org/10.1111/jan.13728

Cowap, N. (2015). Diabetes. *Mercury Learning & Information, 2–4*. http://search.ebscohost.com/login.aspx?direct=true&site=eds-live&db=e000xww&AN=1809105

Crossen, S., Xing, G., & Hoch, J. S. (2020). Changing costs of type 1 diabetes care among US children and adolescents. *Pediatric Diabetes, 21*(4), 644–648.

de Lima, L. R., Stival, M. M., Funghetto, S. S., Volpe, C. R. G., Rehem, T. C. M. S. B., Santos, W. S., & Funez, M. I. (2019). Lower quality of life, lower limb pain with neuropathic characteristics, female sex, and ineffective metabolic control are predictors of depressive symptoms in patients with type 2 diabetes mellitus treated in primary care. *International Journal of Diabetes in Developing Countries: Incorporating Diabetes Bulletin, 39*(3), 463. https://doi.org/10.1007/s13410-018-0667-5

Didericksen, K. W., & Das, B. M. (2019). Type 2 diabetes as a familial illness: Findings from a focus group study. *Families, Systems & Health, 37*(3). https://doi.org/10.1037/fsh0000436

Fernandez, A., Schillinger, D., Warton, E. M., Adler, N., Moffet, H. H., Schenker, Y., Salgado, M. V., Ahmed, A., & Karter, A. J. (2011). Language barriers, physician-patient language concordance, and glycemic control among insured Latinos with diabetes: The diabetes study of northern California (DISTANCE). *Journal of General Internal Medicine, 26*(2), 170–176. https://doi.org/10.1007/s11606-010-1507-6

Gonzalez, J. S., Tanenbaum, M. L., & Commissariat, P. V. (2016). Psychosocial factors in medication adherence and diabetes self-management: Implications for research and practice. *The American Psychologist, 71*(7).

Greenfield, C., Gilles, M., Porter, C., Shaw, P., & Willis, K. (2011). It's not just about the HbA1c, Doc! Understanding the psychosocial is also important in managing diabetes? *Australian Journal of Rural Health, 19*(1), 15–19.

Gurney, J. K., Stanley, J., Sarfati, D., Rumball-Smith, J., & York, S. (2018). Postoperative death after lower-limb amputation in a national prevalent cohort of patients with diabetes. *Diabetes Care, 41*(6), 1204–1211. https://doi.org/10.2337/dc17-2557

Hawk, M., Coulter, R. W. S., Egan, J. E., Fisk, S., Friedman, M. R., Tula, M., & Kinsky, S. (2017). Harm reduction principles for healthcare settings. *Harm Reduction Journal, 14*, 1–9. https://doi.org/10.1186/s12954-017-0196-4

Hayes, M. (2001). A phenomenological study of chronic sorrow in people with type 1 diabetes. *Practical Diabetes International, 18*(2), 65–69.

He, L., & van Heugten, K. (2020). Chinese migrant workers' care experiences: A model of the mediating roles of filial piety. *Qualitative Health Research, 30*(11), 1749–1761. https://doi.org/10.1177/1049732320925420

Himmelstein, M. S., & Puhl, R. M. (2021). At multiple fronts: Diabetes stigma and weight stigma in adults with type 2 diabetes. *Diabetic Medicine, 38*(1), e14387.

Hinder, S., & Greenhalgh, T. (2012). "This does my head in". Ethnographic study of self-management by people with diabetes. *BMC Health Services Research, 12*(1), 83. https://doi.org/10.1186/1472-6963-12-83

Hu, R., Shi, L., Rane, S., Zhu, J., & Chen, C. C. (2014). Insurance, racial/ethnic, SES-related disparities in quality of care among US adults with diabetes. *Journal of Immigrant and Minority Health, 16*(4), 565.

Hudon, C., Fortin, M., Haggerty, J., Loignon, C., Lambert, M., & Poitras, M.-E. (2012). Patient-centered care in chronic disease management: A thematic analysis of the literature in family medicine. *Patient Education and Counseling, 88*, 170–176.

Kübler-Ross, E. (1969). *On Death and Dying*. Macmillan.

Lynch, S. H., Shuster, G., & Lobo, M. L. (2018). The family caregiver experience – Examining the positive and negative aspects of compassion satisfaction and compassion fatigue as caregiving outcomes. *Aging & Mental Health, 22*(11), 1424–1431.

Marmot, M. (2017). Social justice, epidemiology and health inequalities. *European Journal of Epidemiology, 32*, 537–546. https://doi.org/10.1007/s10654-017-0286-3

McCaffery, J. M., Anderson, A., Coday, M., Espeland, M. A., Gorin, A. A., Johnson, K. C., Knowler, W. C., Myers, C. A., Rejeski, W. J., Steinberg, H. O., Steptoe, A., & Wing, R. R. (2020). Loneliness relates to functional mobility in older adults with type 2 diabetes: The look AHEAD study. *Journal of Aging Research.*

McVinney, D. (2003). Meeting clients "where they are". BP's David Pratt speaks with Don McVinney of the Harm Reduction Coalition. *The Body Positive, 16*(1), 10–14. https://www.thebodypro.com/article/meeting-clients-where-are

Meng, Y. Y., Diamant, A., Jones, J., Lin, W., Chen, X., Wu, S. H., Pourat, N., Roby, D., & Kominski, G. F. (2016). Racial and ethnic disparities in diabetes care and impact of vendor-based disease management programs. *Diabetes Care, 39*(5), 743–749.

Mezuk, B., Li, X., Cederin, K., Rice, K., Sundquist, J., & Sundquist, K. (2016). Beyond access: Characteristics of the food environment and risk of diabetes. *American Journal of Epidemiology, 183*(12), 1129–1137. https://doi.org/10.1093/aje/kwv318

Naicker, K., Johnson, J. A., Skogen, J. C., Manuel, D., Øverland, S., Sivertsen, B., & Colman, I. (2017, March). Type 2 diabetes and comorbid symptoms of depression and anxiety: Longitudinal associations with mortality risk. *Diabetes Care, 40*(3), 352–358. https://doi.org/10.2337/dc16-2018

National Academies of Sciences, Engineering, and Medicine. (2017). *Communities in action: Pathways to health equity*. The National Academies Press.

Ni, Y., Ma, L., & Li, J. (2020). Effects of mindfulness-based stress reduction and mindfulness-based cognitive therapy in people with diabetes: A systematic review and meta-analysis. *Journal of Nursing Scholarship: An Official Publication of Sigma Theta Tau International Honor Society of Nursing, 52*(4), 379–388. https://doi.org/10.1111/jnu.12560

Oh, E. G., Lee, H. J., Yang, Y. L., & Kim, Y. M. (2021). Effectiveness of discharge education with the teach-back method on 30-day readmission: A systematic review. *Journal of Patient Safety, 17*(4), 305–310. https://doi.org/10.1097/PTS.0000000000000596

Parikh, P. B., Yang, J., Leigh, S., Dorjee, K., Parikh, R., Sakellarios, N., Meng, H., & Brown, D. L. (2014). The impact of financial barriers on access to care, quality of care and vascular morbidity among patients with diabetes and coronary heart disease. *Journal of General Internal Medicine, 29*(1), 76. https://doi-org.avoserv2.library.fordham.edu/10.1007/s11606-013-2635-6

Peri, T., Hasson-Ohayon, I., Garber, S., Tuval-Mashiach, R., & Boelen, P. A. (2016). Narrative reconstruction therapy for prolonged grief disorder – Rationale and case study. *European Journal of Psychotraumatology, 7*, 1–N.PAG. https://doi-org.avoserv2.library.fordham.edu/10.3402/ejpt.v7.30687

Pienaar, M., & Reid, M. (2020). Self-management in face-to-face peer support for adults with type 2 diabetes living in low- or middle-income countries: A systematic review. *BMC Public Health, 20*(1). https://bmcpublichealth.biomedcentral.com/articles/10.1186/s12889-020-09954-1

Ray, R., Sewell, A. A., Gilbert, K. L., & Roberts, J. D. (2017). Missed opportunity? Leveraging mobile technology to reduce racial health disparities. *Journal of Health Politics, Policy and Law, 42*(5), 901–924. https://doi.org/10.1215/03616878-3940477

Redman, B. K. (2012). Best practices in PSM preparation and support. In *Advanced practice nursing ethics in chronic disease self-management*. Springer.

Roy, T., & Lloyd, C. E. (2012). Epidemiology of depression and diabetes: A systematic review. *Journal of Affective Disorders, 142*(Supplement), S8–S21. https://doi.org/10.1016/S0165-0327(12)70004-6

Rubin, D. J. (2015). Hospital readmission of patients with diabetes. *Current Diabetes Reports, 15*, 17. https://doi.org/10.1007/s11892-015-0584-7

Schmitt, A., Bendig, E., Baumeister, H., Hermanns, N., & Kulzer, B. (2021). Associations of depression and diabetes distress with self-management behavior and glycemic control. *Health Psychology, 40*(2), 113–124. https://doi.org/10.1037/hea0001037

Sebire, S. J., Toumpakari, Z., Turner, K. M., et al. (2018). "I've made this my lifestyle now": A prospective qualitative study of motivation for lifestyle change among people with newly diagnosed type two diabetes mellitus. *BMC Public Health, 18.* https://doi.org/10.1186/s12889-018-5114-5

Stroebe, M., Schut, H., & Boerner, K. (2017). Cautioning health-care professionals: Bereaved persons are misguided through the stages of grief. *Omega: Journal of Death & Dying, 74*(4), 455–473.

Subica, A. M., & Brown, B. J. (2020). Addressing health disparities through deliberative methods: Citizens' panels for health equity. *American Journal of Public Health, 110*(2), 166–173. https://doi.org/10.2105/AJPH.2019.305450

Tareen, R. S., & Tareen, K. (2017). Psychosocial aspects of diabetes management: Dilemma of diabetes distress. *Translational Pediatrics, 6*(4), 383–396. https://doi.org/10.21037/tp.2017.10.04

Tiwari, S., & Ambinakudige, S. (2021). Neighborhood food insecurity index to identify food vulnerability and food deserts in the United States. *Journal of Food Security, 9*(4), 148–159. https://doi.org/10.12691/jfs-9-4-2

Varga, S., & Gallagher, S. (2020). Anticipatory-vicarious grief: The anatomy of a moral emotion. *The Monist, 103*(2), 176–189. https://doi.org/10.1093/monist/onz034

Chapter 7
Heart and Lung Failure

Abigail L. Latimer and Caitlin Mayton

Illness Overview

Any condition that affects the lungs' ability to move air in or out, or the heart's ability to move blood and oxygen, can contribute to illness and failure. Many conditions affecting the heart and lungs are chronic, progressive, and episodic, like heart failure and chronic obstructive pulmonary disease (COPD) (Christ & Diwan, 2008; NIH, n.d.-a, b; Rolland, 1987). This means the patient experiences some good lung or heart functioning and an overall slow progression of illness with moments of emergent increased symptomatology that worsens their previous baseline (Barker & Schrer, 2016). Some patients will experience a more stable condition with a steep worsening of symptoms before death, similar to typical patterns of congenital illnesses, cancers, and severe infections (Barker & Schrer, 2016). Depending on the nature of the disease, behavioral modifications can be one way to reduce risk and symptom exacerbation. There are a variety of advanced medical treatments that can improve symptoms (e.g., oxygen, medications, and therapies), are curative, or can delay progression to death (e.g., ventricular assist devices and implantable cardioverter defibrillator) (NIH, n.d.-a, b).

The patient's physical trajectory or speed of decline usually influences their emotional well-being and ability to adjust to their new heart or lung diagnosis. For example, if a patient has a gradual physical decline, this allows the patient to partner with their social worker to form a strong social support, and the social worker to

A. L. Latimer (✉)
University of Kentucky, Lexington, KY, USA
e-mail: Abbie.latimer@uky.edu

C. Mayton
Virginia Commonwealth University, Richmond, VA, USA
e-mail: maytonch@vcu.edu

M. Hemphill, A. Nathanson (eds.), *The Practice of Clinical Social Work in Healthcare*, Essential Clinical Social Work Series,
https://doi.org/10.1007/978-3-031-31650-0_7

assist the patient in adjusting to their evolving "new normal." If a patient has a quick decline, on the other hand, the social worker, in partnership with the patient, will create goals to best support their emotional well-being and sense of self, whether that is providing brief counseling or assisting the patient in end-of-life goals. Regardless of the physical progression, the social worker must continue to promote a patient's emotional well-being and sense of self throughout their illness trajectory.

Prognosticating and predicting trajectories can be challenging, and this level of uncertainty can compromise the quality of life and psychological well-being for both patients and caregivers (Cagle et al., 2017; Christ & Diwan, 2008; Hopp et al., 2015; Rolland, 1987). It is reasonable to expect that the better a patient's quality of life and the less their uncertainty surrounding prognosis, the better the average patient will do psychologically in adjustment to life with physical impairment and limitations caused by heart and lung disease or failure. That does not guarantee that patients will be better adjusted to their illness if they are fully informed, however, since the degree to which their illness intrudes on their physical well-being will also determine their experience.

Life expectancy will be dependent on the nature of the illness (e.g., acute, chronic, and acute-on-chronic) and the presence of comorbidities (e.g., diabetes, dementia, etc.). For acute causes, such as severe infections like pneumonia or COVID-19, severity requiring intensive critical care may set the stage for imminent death. However, if patients recover from these infections or have a more gradual onset of heart or respiratory failure, death may seem far off or unlikely. In both cases, prognosis can change suddenly and alter a patient's psychological state.

The symptomatic nature of heart and respiratory failure creates the most considerable impact on quality of life and incapacitation. Symptoms can be exacerbated by age and comorbidities (National Institutes of Health [NIH], n.d.-a, b). Older patients experience a greater symptom burden and have a poorer quality of life than younger patients (Cagle et al., 2017). An older patient who is, e.g., simultaneously experiencing shortness of breath and dizziness is likely unable to pick up their grandchildren, grocery shop, or even climb their own stairs. Early shortness of breath and difficulty breathing can be present for failures in either organ, reflecting the interdependent relationship discussed previously (NIH, n.d.-a, b). Not having enough oxygen can cause irritability, confusion, and somnolence (NIH, n.d.-a, b). Patients may be misdiagnosed given that irritability, anxiety, and confusion are often incorrectly presumed to be either normal parts of aging, dementia, or mental health illness (Checa et al., 2020). The build-up of fluid when the heart cannot pump blood and oxygen efficiently can cause fatigue and swelling (NIH, n.d.-a, b). These combined symptoms contribute to individuals losing their independence, control, and ability to engage in activities of daily living (ADLs). Conversely, a 20-year-old patient arriving at the clinic with new symptoms of severe fatigue and shortness of breath is likely experiencing isolation stemming from the inability to partake in milestones such as finishing college, starting a career, or continuing their hobbies, and it is important for the clinician to remember their developmental life stage. Working with this patient will look vastly different than working with a retired patient who has mobility issues.

Clinical Issues for Patients and Family

Throughout the illness trajectory, patients and families will face a myriad of issues related to caregiving demands, navigating healthcare systems, adjusting to health behaviors and activities of daily living (ADLs), and psychological, emotional, and spiritual well-being (Cagle et al., 2017; Christ & Diwan, 2008). The differing courses of illness contribute to various uncertainties: the patient can have a rapid, unexpected onset with an uncertain recovery, or an expected decline but uncertainty about how or when it will happen. Capacitation can fluctuate with illness progression, requiring patients and families to adjust accordingly (NIH, n.d.-a, b; Rolland, 1987). As patients and families adjust to psychological and symptom burdens, coping with changes and loss is necessary for overall health and well-being. Social workers will meet patients in various healthcare settings (e.g., hospitals, acute or long-term care facilities, primary care offices, community programs, and hospices). Social work interventions in each differ, guided by the common psychosocial impacts of the physical symptoms and issues commonly seen with those settings, as well as by the time limitations and resource constraints of each.

Crisis

Intrapersonal Social workers will have an important role in facilitating information dissemination and helping patients and their families understand their illness throughout each stage, but this is especially true at points when patients receive a new diagnosis or experience exacerbation of symptoms. Limited health literacy and jargon used by clinicians can complicate patients' understanding of their illness and contribute to distress, or diminish their ability to cope and acknowledge the life-limiting nature of their illness (Checa et al., 2020; May et al., 2016). Some patients may have understood the meaning of their symptoms differently, normalizing and dismissing them for some time (Checa et al., 2020). An improvement of understanding of what medical reports and recommendations mean requires awareness of and adjustment to such possible sources of misunderstanding, as well as to cultural differences in information delivery (between provider and patient). This may result in making informed choices about treatment options or improved treatment and care compliance (i.e., using medications regularly and as prescribed). Many will need guidance on dealing with their symptoms, treatment options, use of medication, and use of oxygen or other breathing devices (e.g., Bipaps, CPAPS, nebulizers, etc.), which social workers or case managers can provide as they order such equipment or medical services at home (Gardener et al., 2018).

To be equipped to have such conversations, social workers must, themselves, have an understanding about medical diagnoses, treatments, and prognoses. Social workers will need knowledge regarding a patient's specific stage and available treatment options to help guide conversations, facilitate support and resources, and provide education on self-management behaviors (e.g., taking medication, smoking cessation, exercise, basic nutritional information, etc.). Social workers can meet with a patient after a physician has provided a new medical regimen to further explain or translate medical jargon (from unrelated "facts" to information that is relevant and meaningful to the patient and their caregivers). This can be done using the "teach-back method," an intervention where the patient or caregivers repeat back, in their own words, what was discussed (Yen & Leasure, 2019). The teach-back method is widely used in healthcare at various stages in disease and treatment, helping to increase the patient's health knowledge.

Regardless of medical course and outcome, the effort to communicate better with patients about their health can have another psychological and emotional benefit. It can feel assuring and anxiety reducing to have previously incomprehensible information explained to people who may, otherwise, feel unsure of their medical team's attentiveness to them and their needs. It can assist with the psychological adjustment to the news of diagnosis and prognosis. Without such an intervention, patients and their caregivers may exit a medical appointment without understanding their health, unprepared to come to a decision, or unable to follow medical advice. Uncertainty, in other words, may continue for the patient and caregiver(s), despite the appearance otherwise.

As patients grapple with receiving a new diagnosis or wait to receive information about their condition, they also manage symptoms that can be debilitating. Symptom burden (e.g., shortness of breath, irritability, and fatigue) makes maintaining overall well-being and implementing new self-care strategies challenging (Burton et al., 2012; Cagle et al., 2017; Zakrisson et al., 2019). Social workers can engage in health promotion education and encourage behaviors intended to minimize illness impact, promote treatment effects, and improve self-efficacy (i.e., medication adherence, diet, smoking cessation, and exercise) (Christ & Diwan, 2008). This is an especially important role given that patients may resist implementing these desired behaviors. For instance, they may not want to take certain medications because of unwanted side effects, or not want to eat certain foods because of taste. Social workers can provide general health promotion education by creating and disseminating lists of relevant resources or by referring to smoking cessation or weight loss or healthy lifestyles programs.

Patients may adopt an external locus of control, feeling like their illness has been caused by factors that are beyond their power, further contributing to a sense of diminished self-efficacy that, in turn, lessens interest in engaging in self-management behaviors (Checa et al., 2020). Social workers can utilize clinical therapeutic techniques such as motivational interviewing and cognitive behavioral therapy to help patients reconstruct internal narratives that are negative in outlook or negative to self. They can help reduce distress and cultivate empowerment (Rzadkiewicz & Nasiłowski, 2019). In face of the possibility of decline in heart and lung failure, cognitive restructuring toward a narrative that is accepting of one's health and focuses intentionally on what is helpful to one to optimize health can be of critical value to a person's mood and sense of control over their future. Social workers can normalize patients' engaging in some avoidant strategies (e.g., positive thinking, focusing on relationships, and keeping routine) as a healthy short-term mechanism to cope with the realization of their diagnosis or while waiting on diagnosis (Checa et al., 2020). A full psychosocial and spiritual assessment is necessary to identify strengths and opportunities to promote adaptive functioning. *What is important to you?* and *Where do you find meaning now?* are questions that can help a person focus and reflect on what matters to them now and engage in a process of cultivating it even in illness. Additionally, depending on prognosis, activities such as yoga and breathing exercises can further help to improve physical and mental health, especially since anxiety and shortness of breath are interconnected experiences (Rzadkiewicz & Nasiłowski, 2019), and chaplains may be utilized for advanced spiritual interventions.

The emotional weight of this stage of illness will also be dependent on the lived experiences up to this time, as well as on the patient's prognosis and understanding of that prognosis (May et al., 2016). Patients may have been experiencing debility for some time and may already feel depressed, lonely, and anxious, all symptoms that can be magnified by the breathlessness associated with their illness (Checa et al., 2020; Hopp et al., 2015). Patients may worry about being a burden or may already feel burdensome, which may worsen if they will require more from their caregivers and support networks (Checa et al., 2020). Grief and anticipatory grief reactions are expected over intangible and tangible losses (e.g., identity, activities, roles, and home). Patients may have feelings of fear and uncertainty over whether treatments will be available, will be effective, and/or what will be required of them (May et al., 2016). A social support system is crucial to help with managing these intense emotions and reducing the sense of isolation. Social workers may need to help patients identify emotionally and instrumentally helpful persons in their lives, remember that one person may not possess both qualities, and seek help versus isolation (May et al., 2016). This means within a patient's support team, the patient may identify their partner as the emotional support, i.e., someone with whom they can be vulnerable; a neighbor as someone who can provide logistical support in the form of transportation, and a sibling as the best person to reiterate the new medical regimen discussed at the last physician appointment. Each patient's support team may look different, and as social workers, our role, at times, is to be creative in empowering the patient to identify a strong support team, regardless of the number of people identified. The patient's support plan may change over time, and it is important to check in with the patient and medical team regarding support needs.

Interpersonal While social workers attend to the emotional needs of patients, we must remember that patients do not exist in vacuums, and the family or support system will, too, need assessment and intervention. Even if the patients do not identify with any support systems, social workers may need to involve additional healthcare or community organizations to support them as they adjust to their illness. The process of adjusting to a diagnosis or illness progression may thrust family systems into a crisis requiring adjustments to daily life, roles, and relationships (Rolland, 1987). As the patient develops self-efficacy in their self-management behaviors, caregivers may also be navigating new carer roles and responsibilities. They, too, grieve losses of identity and of their life before diagnosis or before the exacerbation of symptoms (Rolland, 1987). If symptoms have been present for a long time, many adjustments may have already been made. Still, if symptoms are new or worsened, support persons must prepare for how to help the patient and make plans for the future amid great uncertainty as to when another physical decline or symptom exacerbation will occur to jeopardize that future (Hopp et al., 2015).

Social workers can normalize a patient's feelings and experiences through psychoeducation, similar to their education-focused strategies with patients. Caregivers seek competency and a sense of control over the illness, as well as competence navigating healthcare and community resource systems (May et al., 2016). Social workers can alleviate burden by facilitating resources, education, identification and normalization of feelings, and guidance in adjusting to day-to-day activities. Further, social workers can engage caregivers in maintaining their well-being and encourage the implementation of self-care (e.g., eating, showering, daily medications, social support, etc.) (Burton et al., 2012).

Systems of Care Patients, families, and support systems are particularly vulnerable to poor care coordination and delivery as they seek to understand the illness, what will be expected of them, and how they may support the patient (May et al., 2016). Symptoms can evolve quickly in some cases, which can be especially frightening. Centuries of mistrust with healthcare systems may be especially burdensome and challenging for patients of color and their carers. Past dysfunctional or non-transparent relationships with healthcare providers may also emerge as a barrier for patients of color seeking care and information, further complicating their understanding and processing of their diagnoses. Available treatment options will depend on a myriad of medical factors; what is possible may change suddenly, and intensive support may be required. For all of these reasons, emphasis on establishing trusting relationships among the patient, caregiver, healthcare providers, and the social worker is crucial (Checa et al., 2020). These trusting relationships will enable the social worker and healthcare team to facilitate decision-making around whether available treatment options are congruent with patients' values and care goals (Christ & Diwan, 2008; Hopp et al., 2015). While referrals to palliative and hospice agencies are low in heart and lung patients (May et al., 2016), these specialized services can be helpful as an added layer of support.

Some patients may be motivated and ready to discuss the future, and completing a healthcare power of attorney (HCPOA) or advance directive may be desired. Speaking to a patient about these choices during medical stability may feel premature; however, holding space to discuss this early can empower a patient to thoughtfully decide on a range of issues, from who they want to be their medical decision maker, to if they want a ventilator or artificial nutrition/hydration. Normalizing these conversations is important. No one wants to think about completing an HCPOA at any age; however, clinical social workers are able to provide patients with the ability to ensure their wishes are being carried out during all stages of their care. Other healthcare providers may be reluctant to engage in future planning due to uncertainty in illness trajectory or the reality that death may occur suddenly (May et al., 2016). How much information patients want to know about their illness or the future (e.g., life expectancy and the evolution of symptoms) will vary based on personality, experiences, beliefs, and culture, so determining information preferences is complex and will need to be determined on an individual basis after meeting with a patient to hear their wishes (Gardener et al., 2018).

Regardless of the setting, an essential role for social workers during the crisis phase, and subsequent stages of illness, is facilitating communication with healthcare providers and leading care coordination (Cagle et al., 2017). This role can be challenging but ultimately assists patients in understanding their diagnosis, setting realistic expectations, and supporting caregivers (Hopp et al., 2015). Facilitating care coordination is especially important if the patient is older, where they may be experiencing multiple comorbidities complicating their illness trajectory and have a need of multiple healthcare providers (Christ & Diwan, 2008).

If establishing a diagnosis or treatment plan, or treating symptom exacerbation, become prolonged processes, patients and their support systems can experience additional stress from financial burden and extended hospitalization. Furthermore, for those employed, issues around time off and insurance will inform decisions to continue treatment. Interventions may require the wearing of oxygen or other continuous medications. Conducting full assessments of patients' socioeconomic resources (e.g., income, insurance, social standing, etc.) and environmental factors (e.g., abuse or neglect, living conditions, transportation, etc.) that may pose risk to illness progression or treatment efficacy is necessary (May et al., 2016).

Chronic

Intrapersonal The chronic stage of illness is a cycle of stability, exacerbation, and recovery, which can be mentally exhausting for the medical care team, patient, and caregivers. Patients may initially deal with the chronic phase optimistically, which can be a helpful coping response and promote resilience (Checa et al., 2020). However, feelings of optimism can oscillate with demoralization as their symptoms worsen, their condition is prolonged, and they lose independence and autonomy. Furthermore, as patients face continued physical deterioration, they will rely on those close to them and caregivers for support and assistance more while transitioning into a new identity resulting in increased vulnerability (May et al., 2016).

The continued uncertain illness trajectory means predicting acute crises is challenging, which further complicates medical decision-making and planning for the future (Hopp et al., 2015). Patients must now learn how to manage their life-limiting illness at home and can no longer rely on their medical team to alleviate symptom burden (May et al., 2016). This means patients and support persons must attempt to maintain a sense of normality while integrating self-management skills, monitoring their new medical devices, coping with symptom burden, and attending numerous medical appointments, in addition to attempting to work and maintain a social and family life. The daily requirements it takes to manage and live with a chronic illness can leave patients feeling overwhelmed, anxious, and depressed, further deterring them from effectively engaging in self-management behaviors (Checa et al., 2020; May et al., 2016).

If a patient can manage the above successfully, this increases their resiliency and decreases their feelings of being overwhelmed by allowing the patient to control some aspects of their illness (May et al., 2016). Unfortunately, when a patient struggles to maintain their new self-management regimen, it can have negative repercussions for their self-esteem and self-identity. This can lead to increased self-isolation (May et al., 2016). This isolation, combined with a fear of increased symptom burden (e.g., breathlessness, edema, fatigue), leads to further avoiding self-management prescribed by the medical care team (e.g., diet, medications, exercise, cardiac, or pulmonary rehabilitation). Poor self-management can tip the stability scale and create a crisis episode that leads to illness exacerbation and continues disease progression. For instance, patients who have increased symptoms of breathlessness or recently received a shock from their pacemaker may experience fear and anxiety (i.e., racing heart, fatigue, fainting, or chest pain). These are also symptoms of heart and lung failure.

Studies have reported that patients with heart disease are 15 times more likely to have anxiety and panic disorders than the general population (Foldes-Busque et al., 2021). Social workers have an opportunity to intervene with patients who consistently report frustration over how to cope with anxiety and fear of symptom flare-ups. Potential retraumatization is a serious concern for patients struggling with heart and lung failure. Social workers can provide support by actively listening to the patient's concerns and routinely following up with both the patient and support persons to identify appropriate support resources (Weingarten, 2013).

As patients experience life-limiting symptoms, they can feel more isolated, especially when there are access-to-care challenges and support system disruptions (Hopp et al., 2015). Patients who experience breathlessness and fatigue have limited mobility and may be experiencing symptoms of trauma, such as hypervigilance, dissociation, powerlessness, and fear, factors that can increase isolation (Hopp et al., 2015). Psychological symptoms can hamper self-management and precipitate job, hobby, and relationship loss, which in turn can reduce a patient's social network and sense of purpose or identity, as well as belonging. In addition, patients may be unable to afford medications as job loss often results in loss of insurance, which can lead to missing cardiac rehabilitation appointments and losing resources. Social workers may need to assist patients in tasks associated with daily life, such as applying for health insurance, medication assistance programs, or other financial assistance.

Intangible grief related to the loss of familiar places and persons and a general sense of normality is inherent and recurs at each decline in status. As social support is crucial in offering relief and strength, social workers may need to be creative when identifying ways to connect patients to others (Checa et al., 2020). For example, social workers may need to facilitate social support for patients by leveraging existing sources of support for more time or instrumental assistance, modifying existing activities to make them more tolerable, and referring patients to support groups, both online and in person. These interventions can have the added benefit of increasing the patient's self-efficacy, encouraging engaging in more social activities, and increasing self-management behaviors (Zakrisson et al., 2019).

Completing a thorough psychosocial assessment, regardless of setting, allows a social worker to learn the patient's perception of the internal and external resources at their disposal and their understanding of their medical regimen. As discussed earlier, social workers need to note both the patient and support person's mental health, as psychological distress is significant during this phase. A social worker may provide, or refer a patient to, cognitive behavioral therapy, somatic trauma therapy, or encourage a patient and family unit to try meditation or mindfulness. Engaging patients in mindfulness, e.g., can lower anxiety and thereby increase emotional and physical quality of life (Rechenberg et al., 2020).

Social workers will serve as advocates for patients to communicate to the rest of the medical team and can provide informal and formal support resources (May et al., 2016). Other tasks may include problem-solving on logistical issues such as who can provide transportation for the patient or respite opportunities for support persons. Social workers may also need to provide education on managing IV medications at home.

Unfortunately, social workers are rarely available to provide consistent long-term care to patients and their caregivers due to differing expectations of clinical settings (Christ & Diwan, 2008). For example, if a social worker is in the hospital, that person may be limited to completing tasks directly associated with discharge planning, an essential component of care transition and promoting quality of life, so it may not be feasible to conduct psychological or psychosocial interventions. If additional interventions are needed during discharge, a social worker may refer a patient to a licensed provider in the community. For heart and lung failure, which are highly chronic and often involve multiple care transitions, these structural limitations of the social work role can severely impact buy-in to self-management and treatment adherence.

Interpersonal The quality of existing support person relationships may be affected as the individual becomes more dependent on the caregiver. Caregivers may experience loss of their former identity as they take on the new identity and often-consuming responsibilities of being a caregiver (Rolland, 1987). Caregivers experience considerable stress and may struggle with a lack of confidence or have depressive symptoms associated with witnessing deterioration of the patient and an increasing task burden (Cagle et al., 2017). Caring for a person with chronic illness is difficult for many reasons. Caregivers may feel anxiety from not knowing how to help, not being able to access the patient during hospitalizations, and not dealing with potential safety issues at home when the patient is unable to ambulate, dress, or bathe (Hopp et al., 2015).

It is not uncommon for patients to be admitted to the intensive care unit (ICU) for stabilization or ongoing support of symptoms to prolong life. However, this admission is costly, leading to cumulative emotional strain (Rolland, 1987). The emotional toll on the family unit can range from feelings of hopelessness on the part of both the patient and carer to concerns regarding mortality, the continuing deterioration of the patient's baseline, and decreasing quality of life. Furthermore, ICU care and outcomes may be experienced differently depending on the patient's race or ethnicity (McGowan et al., 2022). Black patients, compared to white patients, may be offered more intensive treatment at end of life, have poorer quality of death experiences, and have greater financial strain during an ICU admission (McGowan et al., 2022). Social workers can be mindful of this reality, not only as it impacts patients during the admission, but also how past ICU admissions impact future care perceptions and decision-making.

These undulating symptoms and hospitalizations can put more pressure on caregivers and support persons, particularly in acute medical settings where the focus is on the patient's symptoms. In addition, due to potential communication breakdowns that may occur between the medical team, patient, and caregivers, caregivers often do not know how or when to ask for help from providers (Cagle et al., 2017). Disruptions and gaps in care can perpetuate a sense of isolation for caregivers, where they continue to feel insulated in caring for the patient. Social workers may provide an extra layer of support by partnering with the multidisciplinary team and serving as a communication conduit between the family on new caregiving expectations and medical regimens. Additionally, social workers can offer compassionate check-ins with careers and support persons on their affective state, and implement coping and respite strategies.

As patients and caregivers become more proficient in self-management of the disease and can successfully maneuver within healthcare systems, they feel empowered to continue their support. This resultant confidence enables both the patient and carer to cope when unexpected crises occur (May et al., 2016). Additionally, a social worker can assist the support person in recognizing what symptoms are normal or expected. Normalizing possible progression of care, symptom burden, and self-management strategies can increase the carer and patient's ability to adapt. The more positive reinforcement patients and caregivers receive, the more successful they will be at managing symptom deterioration (May et al., 2016). Social support is important because it provides the opportunity for social work collaboration to assist with changing identity negotiations between the patient and their support unit (Weingarten, 2013).

Systems of Care and Social Justice During the chronic stage, discussions can focus on symptom management, curative options for patients, or how to manage new medical technologies. They rarely focus on end-of-life care as it relates to a patient's quality of life (Checa et al., 2020; May et al., 2016). Medical providers in acute medical settings may feel unsure how to discuss illness progression with patients and families due to the inherent uncertainty of illness and the reality of needing to focus on the present because physical deterioration can be sudden and fatal (Checa et al., 2020; May et al., 2016). Patients and caregivers consistently report a desire to be fully educated and express that they feel unprepared for what to expect after being diagnosed.

Grief from the loss of previous life and identity compounded by inadequate medical information about their diagnosis and prognosis can delay end-of-life decision-making (Checa et al., 2020). Patients seek meaning and value in life, and social workers can serve a vital role in exploring and expressing spiritual connectedness and religious practice as a means of coping (Cagle et al., 2017; Checa et al., 2020).

In heart and lung failure, with so much uncertainty of progression and high symptom burden, unspoken hierarchies within multidisciplinary teams are present and may result in siloed care. Social workers have the expertise to prevent fragmented care by encouraging and gathering important information to communicate to the patient and their care team, and potentially by intervening from one team or department to another. This could mean contacting the hospital chaplain to speak to a patient who has expressed interest in religious or spiritual discussion and is nervous prior to a procedure. The social worker may also assist the family in completing Family Medical Leave Act (FMLA) paperwork or providing a Social Security disability application if the patient's physical symptoms preclude them from continuing work. In such cases, a lack of income can change the support team's ability to provide support to the patient. Outreach from the hospital social worker to the patient's primary care office social worker can patch together a new caregiving team, strengthen the existing caregiving team, and assist in completing/following up on FMLA and SSA, in addition to providing mental health support. Social workers, inpatient and outpatient, can also ask to be involved in medical teams' meetings to ensure that they are aware of patient issues and not reliant on that team's referral to social work according to its assessment of need. As social workers intervene with patients on any related matter, they may initiate further discussion with the medical team about whether the patient needs a higher level of care or additional resources. In each of these ways, social workers have the opportunity to help alleviate the communication frustration that many patients and caregivers identify as a barrier to care (May et al., 2016).

Heart and lung failure, by the nature of the illness and decline, may leave patients particularly psychologically vulnerable. Social workers have the opportunity to work with the medical team, patient, and support persons to assess and treat psychosocial barriers, provide a consistent level of coordination between the medical team, and continue to help the patient manage situational depression that is likely to increase with disease progression (Hopp et al., 2015). Depression may lead a patient to withdrawal from care and isolate, a reaction that could have serious negative health as well as mental health consequences. In these challenging circumstances, social workers are positioned to identify what is meaningful for them as it relates to their life and health, access care that is in-line with those values, and maintain a sense of autonomy and control in their lives in the exercise of their right to choose their treatment and care. If clinically appropriate, and in conjunction with the medical team, social workers can empower the patient and carer to critically engage and participate in their treatment with a view to breaking the cycle of unnecessary and undesired re-hospitalization. In addition, social workers can lead the transition to end-of-life care focused on alleviating symptoms and away from life-prolonging interventions by facilitating conversations about available hospice services (Hopp et al., 2015). The affirming sense that arises thus may combat depression and may continue even in face of health decline.

Social workers can increase the effectiveness of the multidisciplinary team by encouraging palliative and hospice care to be a part of a patient's treatment plan if indicated for pain and symptom management and end-of-life care. Hospice care is overwhelmingly underutilized (Hopp et al., 2015). This is alarming for all patient populations; for people dying from organ failure without such intervention, it suggests that significant pain and difficult symptoms and the associated anxiety, depression, and spiritual and social burdens are left inadequately addressed. Consider the lung failure patient: without anti-anxiety or adequate pain medication during their final days, this person may experience more distressing breathing difficulties as their lungs continue to fail. This can feel traumatic for the patient and their caregivers; it can also lead to undesired hospital visits and unnecessary suffering.

Patients have a better prognosis and quality of life if they possess structural and interactional advantages, and structural resilience (May et al., 2016). *Structural advantage* relates to socioeconomic status, proximity to a medical center, living environment, and quality of care current medical providers provide. *Interactional advantage* is defined by cognitive ability, health literacy, and quality of interactions. *Structural resilience* is coping with illness, the ability to self-manage medical expectations, and the ability to partner with a caregiver (May et al., 2016).

A patient's socioeconomic status, race, and gender all impact disease progression and quality of life. To apply to an existing outcome disparity: Being black is not the variable that leads to a poorer outcome with lung or heart disease. It is all the surrounding factors, such as racism, white supremacy, medicalizing race as a biological variable, and exposure to more pollution than other racial groups (Dubbin et al., 2017; May et al., 2016), that produce poorer outcomes. Furthermore, poorer patients, disproportionately black patients, may have poorer quality of facility care due to sociopolitical issues such as Medicaid underfunding (Wachterman & Sommers, 2021). Access to quality care is also particularly challenging for rural patients. As a social worker, it is important to provide resources and interventions that support patients when systems get in the way of patients successfully maneuvering through the complex prescribed medical regimens and healthcare systems.

End-of-Life

Symptoms leading to death can occur suddenly—at the time of diagnosis, or during a symptom exacerbation—or may come on more gradually in heart and lung failure. The dying experience is influenced by the availability and timing of possible treatment as well as the history of engaging in self-management behaviors (Olano-Lizarraga et al., 2016). In other words, a person in heart or lung failure may experience end-of-life as the result of a situation that was preventable (i.e., the unavailability of a treatment or engaging in risky health behaviors). Similar to other phases, social workers will adjust their assessments and interventions to individual experiences, taking into account patients' specific illness trajectory and available resources.

Intrapersonal When dying is sudden or unexpected, patients may hold on to hope that there will be a curative treatment or reversal of their illness, especially if they do not have a clear understanding of their illness, if factors make prognostication difficult, or if there are barriers to communicating about end-of-life (Olano-Lizarraga et al., 2016). If a patient has experienced a chronic and progressive decline with their illness, involving frequent hospitalizations, it may be difficult to believe that this latest hospitalization will result in their death. Furthermore, accepting death may be particularly hard if a patient has used positive coping strategies to view themselves as living with a chronic illness versus dying from a chronic illness (Gardener et al., 2018). Assessing a patient's understanding of their prognosis with questions like, "What have the doctors told you about your illness?" and "What are you hoping for from this hospitalization?" can be neutral ways to determine whether the patient is expecting to recover. When a patient is able to participate in counseling, it is important to continue discussing hope, which "helps individuals rise above, but not ignore, suffering" (Hemphill Ruden, 2019, pp. 300–301). Hope will look different at this stage, and go from hope of a cure to hoping to discharge to hospice, complete HCPOA, or manage pain adequately, in full and realistic understanding of the patient's health status.

It is important that social workers communicate with the medical team to stay abreast of the patient's prognosis in terms of anticipated life expectancy and status changes. This communication allows social workers to identify appropriate interventions that are dependent on the patient's anticipated time of death. If death is imminent (hours to weeks), patients may or may not have the consciousness to participate in assessments and interventions. Furthermore, there may be intensive medical treatments where the patient may be unable to communicate (e.g., sedation, loss of consciousness) or be nonvocal (e.g., mechanical ventilation). Social workers will want to fully assess the patient's ability and desire to communicate and be conscientious about having conversations in front of patients when they are unable to actively participate. Utilizing communication devices (e.g., pen and paper, communication boards) and seeking the patient's permission to have family members speak for them can be helpful.

Social workers have a crucial role in mitigating distress and demoralization that patients may experience as they anticipate death. Engaging patients in life review can help acknowledge and restore a person's identity, which may have been lost during the illness. An individual's life story is more than their illness; however, the integration of identity with the chronic illness may have been necessary to survive and function from day to day. Social workers can help patients search for meaning, cognizant that meaning found now may differ from the sense they had established earlier in the illness. Confronting mortality can be terrifying, and patients may feel a sense of hopelessness and demoralization (Rodin, 2020). Social workers can allow patients a space to openly discuss, reflect on their thoughts and feelings, and alleviate distress by allowing it to be there and understanding it better (Rodin, 2020). This process can be complicated by the patient's pain, commonly associated with end-of-life stage organ failure. A social worker should anticipate meeting with a patient frequently for short amounts of time to honor the patient's pain management regimen, which may leave the patient with limited capacity for lucid interactions (Hemphill Ruden, 2019). Even with short interactions, the possibility for such reflective and processing work may yet be present—albeit in a way that may strike the social worker, who is more conscious and alert, as fragmented.

Interpersonal Families and caregivers also experience an uncertain and challenging transition to the terminal phase of illness (Waldrop et al., 2005). The realization that the patient is dying may depend on communication and information received by providers and their observations of the patient's physical decline and personality changes. Family members and caregivers will also want to make meaning by identifying strength and resilience, changing relationships or life perspectives, and renewing spirituality. Many of the same strategies social workers implement with patients can be appropriate for caregivers, as they are also searching for meaning and balancing identity. Caregiving consumes so many of the roles and responsibilities in daily life that, after years of functioning as a caregiver and making great sacrifices, caregivers can struggle to know what to do when that space is no longer filled with the effort and tasks required to care for the person who is ill. Caregivers may anticipate the death of the patient and grieve their death while also feeling conflicting emotions of relief and guilt. They may experience anticipatory grief and the loss of caregiver identity, role, and purpose, which may need ongoing exploration and additional counseling interventions post-death.

Patients' symptoms may come on suddenly or gradually, but one of the most challenging aspects of anticipated death for caregivers may be witnessing perceived suffering (Waldrop et al., 2005). When death is imminent (hours to days, days to weeks), instrumental caregiving expands further as the patient loses more of the capacity to care for one's self. End-of-life caregiving may include efforts to keep the patient clean, warm, and dry, and all other household duties as well, since the patient will no longer be able to participate in these. As death nears and incapacitation worsens, demands of caregiving can further strain relationships, employment, and financial responsibilities, thrusting the family system into another stage of transition, possibly after a period of stability (Rolland, 1987).

Symptom severity and caregiving resources may require a change in the level of care (to a facility or hospital). Caregivers and families can feel unprepared for such transitions but have a strong desire to uphold patient wishes (Waldrop et al., 2005). Social workers may be uniquely positioned to help caregivers identify their needs and capabilities while incorporating patients' goals and values. While providing end-of-life care at home can be desired, the reality of the intense nature of symptoms associated with heart and lung failure can make this impossible. Hospitalization or at least an additional support service, such as hospice, may be required to allow comfort and alleviate symptoms at the end-of-life.

Systems of Care and Social Justice When the social worker addresses the family's worry over perceived suffering, it may warrant further medical decision-making about when to remove treatments that have prolonged life without benefit to the quality of life. This decision can be complex, as the patient may be dependent on interventions to sustain life (e.g., mechanical ventilation, extracorporeal membrane oxygenation, ventricular assist devices, and inotropic medications). Families and healthcare providers may disagree about deactivation or removal interventions. Social workers may experience moral distress by witnessing these disagreements, wanting to preserve patient autonomy and self-determination, and feeling participatory in prolonging suffering (Fantus et al., 2017). Open dialogue about these ethical constraints and dilemmas with supervisors, medical teams, and bioethical teams may help resolve conflicts and reduce moral distress intensity.

Social workers may further experience moral distress by witnessing a lack of adequate care and services related to socioeconomic status (Fantus et al., 2017). While palliative and hospice care can improve quality of life at the end-of-life (Cagle et al., 2017), available and affordable palliative care services are absent for those with low income and by payor source (Wachterman & Sommers, 2021). Depending on the patient's payor source, patients may be denied long-term care and medications. Furthermore, access to palliative and hospice care is often inadequate or absent for indigenous peoples, people who live in rural areas, those who live or practice in tribes or tribal cultures, and those without cancer diagnoses (Wachterman & Sommers, 2021). Despite patients receiving hospice benefits, significant symptom burden may warrant frequent hospitalizations, and social workers may be between two administrative systems, the hospital, and hospice (Hopp et al., 2015). Practicing caution when discussing the delivery and experience of palliative and hospice services will support their dual roles as patient advocate and hospital worker. They can benefit from being educated in primary palliative care skills and the dying process, as this will help them to advocate for patient needs.

Reginald is a 73-year-old Black cisgender man diagnosed with advanced heart failure three years ago. He is divorced and has no children. The social worker (SWer) meets him in the hospital with his ex-wife, where he was admitted for the fifth time in two months for shortness of breath and swelling in his legs. He lives alone, but his ex-wife, Gloria, lives next door and visits daily. He no longer works and he receives social security, but he does not always have enough money for food and medications at the end of the month. Reginald tells the hospital SWer he wants to get better, but has not demonstrated any engagement in self-management behaviors. The medical team treats him with a continuous inotropic medication infusion and considers him for a left ventricular assist device (LVAD). The SWer shares concerns with the medical team about him managing a complicated medical treatment plan given his limited resources and support system, but Reginald seeks and accepts help, encouragement, and support from Gloria. The

SWer uses motivational interviewing techniques to build trust and rapport while engaging Reginald in self-management behaviors. The hospital SW discusses his treatment plan with Reginald and Gloria, and facilitates resources in the community to ensure he can manage the medication, have transportation, and be safe at home.

Reginald and Gloria attend the first few clinic appointments and establish a relationship with the outpatient SWer. Over the last several months, the outpatient SWer focused on reinforcing self-management strategies, providing psychoeducation about chronic illness, and identifying unmet day-to-day needs. Unfortunately, the patient missed his most recent appointment and did not call to cancel. The SWer called Reginald, who sounded distracted and dismissive, and reported that he did not need a follow-up visit. Shortly after, Gloria called, sounding tearful, and informed the SWer that Reginald is working part-time to help pay for his medications; however, his work is leaving him with an increased symptom burden, especially swelling in his legs. She is also concerned he is not taking good care of his medication peripherally inserted central catheter (PICC) line, risking infection. Gloria expressed feeling overwhelmed, frustrated, and worried that Reginald will not get an LVAD. The SW provided active and reflective listening and validated her concerns. The SWer provided psychoeducation about how caregiving impacts physical and mental health and explored ways Gloria cares for herself. Gloria also received a referral to a mental health therapist to help her identify adaptive coping strategies and behaviors to help her manage her distress. Gloria also received information about a local support group for caregivers of patients with heart failure for additional social support.

Over the next 18 months, Reginald continues to withdraw from Gloria and the treatment team. He attends appointments irregularly and is hospitalized several times. The outpatient SWer tries to connect with Reginald via phone calls, but he is reluctant to discuss his concerns or express his needs openly. As a result, the medical team has decided not to give him an LVAD.

In the subsequent hospitalization, the hospital SWer coordinates with the medical team and finds out his current medication regimen is no longer as effective. Still, they cannot predict when it will stop working. The SWer discusses the team's decision with Reginald and he shares confusion and frustration as he believes he has been working hard to get the LVAD. The SW explores with Reginald what he thinks it means if he does not have an LVAD, and he confirms he knows he will die without it. The SWer facilitates a discussion about the use of hospice services, but Reginald refuses and insists he wants to keep trying to be considered for an LVAD.

Reginald is discharged again, still on continuous inotropic medication, and readmitted within the next month. This admission, his symptoms have worsened, and he is scared he is dying. The SWer provides active and reflective listening, allowing Reginald to discuss his fears, mainly not being able to breathe. Together with the medical team, they talk to Reginald and Gloria about using hospice to transi-

tion off the medication while addressing symptoms. He is agreeable and admitted to hospice, where he dies two weeks later.[1]

Authors' Reflections

The chronic and unpredictable nature of most heart and lung illnesses can lead to clinicians and providers feeling exhausted. It is easy for our countertransference to spill out into our language with each other and with patients and families (Katz & Johnson, 2016). When we feel frustration or grief when patients do not adhere to a prescribed regimen or decline to participate in a therapy that could save their life, we can resort to blame language. We may hear other providers label patients as "non-compliant" or "difficult" and use such language ourselves. Social workers will need to look for the presence and development of these types of biases and try to empathize with and understand the patient's perspective of how challenging it is to manage a list of requirements, often with minimal resources, minimal understanding of their illness, and possible medical mistrust. Another way to promote personhood is by focusing on the disease as an obstacle, rather than the person as failing or problematic (Kelemen et al., 2016). For example, Kelemen et al. (2016) suggest referring to "the heart failure getting worse" as opposed to saying the "person is getting worse" (p. 1781), which helps prevent the patient being or feeling defined by the disease. Rooting our language in person-centered care is another means of educating colleagues and teammates, as well as promoting personhood.

Reflection Questions

1. What are some of the biggest challenges in working with people with heart failure?
2. How might the experiences of patients of color be different than white patients in dealing with heart failure? How may it be different for the caregivers of these two patient groups?
3. List some of the losses that might occur as a result of heart failure. How might you address the grief inherent in these losses?

[1] All names and other personal identifiers in the case are fictitious. Any similarity to actual persons, living or dead, or actual events is purely coincidental.

References

Burton, A. M., Sautter, J. M., Tulsky, J. A., Lindquist, J. H., Hays, J. C., Olsen, M. K., Zimmerman, S. I., & Steinhauser, K. E. (2012). Burden and well-being among a diverse sample of cancer, congestive heart failure, and chronic obstructive pulmonary disease caregivers. *Journal of Pain and Symptom Management, 44*(3), 410–420. https://doi.org/10.1016/j.jpainsymman.2011.09.018

Barker, P. C. & Scherer, J. S. (2016). *Fast facts and concepts #326 illness trajectories: Description and clinical use*. Palliative Care Network of Wisconsin.

Cagle, J. G., Bunting, M., Kelemen, A., Lee, J., Terry, D., & Harris, R. (2017). Psychosocial needs and interventions for heart failure patients and families receiving palliative care support: A systematic review. *Heart Failure Reviews, 22*(5), 565–580.

Checa, C., Medina-Perucha, L., Muñoz, M. Á., Verdú-Rotellar, J. M., & Berenguera, A. (2020). Living with advanced heart failure: A qualitative study. *Plos One, 15*(12), e0243974.

Christ, G., & Diwan, S. (2008). *The role of social work in managing chronic illness care*. Council for Social Work Education.

Dubbin, L., McLemore, M., & Shim, J. K. (2017). Illness narratives of African Americans living with coronary heart disease: A critical interactionist analysis. *Qualitative Health Research, 27*(4), 497–508. https://doi.org/10.1177/1049732316645319

Fantus, S., Greenberg, R. A., Muskat, B., & Katz, D. (2017). Exploring moral distress for hospital social workers. *British Journal of Social Work, 47*(8), 2273–2290.

Foldes-Busque, G., Dionne, C. E., Turcotte, S., Tully, P. J., Tremblay, M. A., Poirier, P., & Denis, I. (2021). Epidemiology and prognostic implications of panic disorder and generalized anxiety disorder in patients with coronary artery disease: rationale and design for a longitudinal cohort study. *BMC Cardiovascular Disorders, 21*(1), 26. https://doi.org/10.1186/s12872-021-01848-3. PMID: 33435888; PMCID: PMC7801787.

Gardener, A. C., Ewing, G., Kuhn, I., & Farquhar, M. (2018). Support needs of patients with COPD: A systematic literature search and narrative review. *International Journal of Chronic Obstructive Pulmonary Disease, 13*, 1021–1035. https://doi.org/10.2147/COPD.S155622

Hemphill Ruden, M. (2019). A call for hope-centered work: A preliminary study of oncology social workers' perceptions of the role and value of hope at end-of-life. *Clinical Social Work Journal, 47*, 300–307. https://doi.org/10.1007/s10615-019-00715-1

Hopp, F. P., Camp, J. K., & Perry, T. E. (2015). Addressing heart failure challenges through illness-informed social work. *Health & Social Work, 40*(30), 201–208.

Katz, R., & Johnson, T. A. (2016). *When professionals weep: Emotional and countertransference responses in palliative and end-of-life care*. Routledge.

Kelemen, A. M., Ruiz, G., & Groninger, H. (2016). Choosing words wisely in communication with patients with heart failure and families. *American Journal of Cardiology, 117*, 1779–1782. https://doi.org/10.1016/j.amjcard.2016.03.003

May, C. R., Cummings, A., Myall, M., Harvey, J., Pope, C., Griffiths, P., Roderick, P., Arber, M., Boehmer, K., Mair, F. S., & Richardson, A. (2016). Experiences of long-term life-limiting conditions among patients and carers: what can we learn from a meta-review of systematic reviews of qualitative studies of chronic heart failure, chronic obstructive pulmonary disease and chronic kidney disease? *BMJ Open, 6*(10), e011694.

McGowan, S. K., Sarigiannis, K. A., Fox, S. C., Gottlieb, M. A., & Chen, E. (2022). Racial disparities in ICU outcomes: A systematic review. *Critical Care Medicine, 50*(1), 1–20. https://doi.org/10.1097/CCM.0000000000005269

National Institutes of Health. (n.d.-a). *Heart failure*. https://www.nhlbi.nih.gov/health-topics/heart-failure

National Institutes of Health. (n.d.-b). *Respiratory failure*. https://www.nhlbi.nih.gov/health-topics/respiratory-failure

Olano-Lizarraga, M., Oroviogoicoechea, C., Errasti-Ibarrondo, B., & Saracíbar-Razquin, M. (2016). The personal experience of living with chronic heart failure: a qualitative meta-synthesis of the literature. *Journal of Clinical Nursing, 25*(17–18), 2413–2429.

Rolland, J. S. (1987). Family illness paradigms: Evolution and significance. *Family Systems Medicine, 5*(4), 482–503. https://doi.org/10.1037/h0089735
Rechenberg, K., Cousin, L., & Redwine, L. (2020). Mindfulness, anxiety symptoms, and quality of life in heart failure. *The Journal of Cardiovascular Nursing, 35*(4), 358–363.
Rzadkiewicz, M., & Nasiłowski, J. (2019). Psychosocial interventions for patients with severe COPD-An up-to-date literature review. *Medicina (Kaunas), 55*(9), 597. https://doi.org/10.3390/medicina55090597. PMID: 31527553; PMCID: PMC6780939.
Wachterman, M. W., & Sommers, B. D. (2021). Dying poor in the US- disparities in end-of-life care. *Journal of the American Medical Association, 325*(5), 423–424.
Waldrop, D. P., Kramer, B. J., Skretny, J. A., Milch, R. A., & Finn, W. (2005). Final transitions: Family caregiving at the end of life. *Journal of Palliative Medicine, 8*(3), 623–638.
Weingarten, K. (2013). The "cruel radiance of what is": Helping couples live with chronic illness. *Journal of Family Process, 52*(1), 83–101. https://doi.org/10.1111/famp.12017
Yen, P. H., & Leasure, A. R. (2019). Use and effectiveness of the teach-back method in patient education and health outcomes. *Federal Practitioner, 36*(6), 284–289.
Zakrisson, A. B., Arne, M., Hasselgren, M., Lisspers, K., Ställberg, B., & Theander, K. (2019). A complex intervention of self-management for patients with COPD or CHF in primary care improved performance and satisfaction with regard to own selected activities; A longitudinal follow-up. *Journal of Advanced Nursing, 75*(1), 175–186. https://doi.org/10.1111/jan.13899. Epub 2018 Nov 27. PMID: 30375028.

Chapter 8
Heart Attack and Stroke

Andy Schlesinger

Introduction

Among the disease courses represented in this book, heart attack and stroke are most distinguished by the suddenness of their onset. About 800,000 Americans each year will experience a heart attack, and another 800,000 will experience a stroke (CDC, 2021; Virani et al., 2021). These sudden acute events can make patients feel uncertain and fearful of a recurrence, which can be distressing and make it difficult to plan for the future. Some of these patients may have to cope with long-term changes to their physical function. For all these reasons, these patients are at high risk for depression within a year after the acute event (McCarthy, 2011; Murphy, 2020).

Heart attack and stroke are also distinguished by the concomitant risk of sudden death. Of the 1.6 million people each year who experience either a heart attack or stroke in the United States, about 30% of them will die from the acute event (Mayer et al., 2013; Virani et al., 2021). This can be distressing for the family in ways that can complicate and prolong their grief. And because the event can be sudden and unexpected, the hospital course for these patients might be complicated by a lack of advance directives, making it more difficult for families and providers alike to make appropriate decisions about end-of-life (EOL) care.

That statistic also means that more than two-thirds of those who experience these events each year will survive them. All social workers in healthcare will likely work with patients and families who have experienced the psychosocial impacts of a heart attack or stroke. Social workers can intervene, educate, support, and connect patients to resources and services, whether during inpatient hospital stays or rehabilitation,

A. Schlesinger (✉)
Callen-Lorde Community Health Center, New York, NY, USA
e-mail: aschlesinger@callen-lorde.org

M. Hemphill, A. Nathanson (eds.), *The Practice of Clinical Social Work in Healthcare*, Essential Clinical Social Work Series,
https://doi.org/10.1007/978-3-031-31650-0_8

while patients are connected with other outpatient or community services, or in the context of psychotherapy or bereavement counseling. These interventions may have the greatest effect when they are strength-based, trauma-informed, transdisciplinary, and values-oriented and target the family as the unit receiving care.

During the crisis phase, social workers may consider helping patients and families navigate the hospital system and communicate when the event has impaired a patient's ability to speak and understand. During the chronic phase after the acute event, patients may experience long-term residual deficits in their physical function, including impaired mobility, aphasia, and loss of cognitive or executive function. They are at risk for developing post-stroke depression, as well as ongoing anxiety about their health, that can negatively impact their cognitive schema and exacerbate underlying cognitive impairment caused by the acute event. Effective social work interventions might include practical interventions like promoting lifestyle changes, as well as integrated modalities involving psychotherapy in conjunction with occupational therapy, physical therapy, music therapy, and support groups that encourage social support.

For those patients who die from the acute event, families may be at risk for developing complications in their grieving because of the sudden, unexpected nature of the loss. Effective interventions with these families may include traditional bereavement therapy, support groups, and specialized interventions such as existential psychotherapies.

Illness Overview

While heart attacks and strokes are fundamentally different medical events, there are some similarities that align their psychosocial impacts. Both happen suddenly. Both involve a lack of blood flow to a critical part of the body, and the residual effects largely result from tissue damage from the time period that blood flow to that organ was inhibited. For the purposes of this chapter, heart attack and stroke will be referred to collectively as "acute events."

Most heart attacks will occur inside the home, with the majority of the rest happening either in public or in a nursing care facility (Virani et al., 2021). Thousands of others will experience a heart attack while already admitted to the hospital. Where the acute event happens, whether it's a heart attack or a stroke, can affect whether and how long it takes for a patient to receive life-saving care, the severity of residual deficits, and how patients and families alike make meaning of the acute event.

While patients and families may have once expected a heart attack or stroke to be a death sentence, more and more people are surviving these acute events, thanks in part to improvements in treatments. For example, an estimated 7.6 million Americans over the age of 20 self-report having survived a stroke (Virani et al., 2021).

Greater survivability also means that more people are living with residual deficits to their physical and cognitive function following an acute event than ever before.

Post-stroke residual deficits include pain syndromes, cognitive impairment and dementia, gait instability, epilepsy, falls and fractures, and anxiety and depression (Virani et al., 2021). All these can manifest significant long-term psychosocial consequences for patients and families.

More people survive heart attacks, too, and most of them are able to return to work within the first 12 months post-event (Virani et al., 2021) and experience fewer physical impairments than stroke survivors. Yet many of them will still live with residual deficits, especially cognitive deficits that impact executive function and impair consciousness (Virani et al., 2021). And despite improved survival rates, the risk of sudden death from heart attack is substantial and increases exponentially with age (Virani et al., 2021).

Almost 325,000 and 150,000 people each year will die from heart attack and stroke, respectively (Mayer et al., 2013; Virani et al., 2021). That means that hundreds of thousands of families each year share the grueling task of integrating the sudden loss of a family member. That suddenness may be traumatizing for many grieving families, making trauma-informed care an indispensable framework for affirmative bereavement interventions.

A patient's sex, race, age, socioeconomic status, and other social identifiers also have a significant impact on their health outcomes. Regardless of underlying genetic or biological determinants of risk, social conditions are a fundamental determinant of disease (Link, 1995). These conditions impact whether a person is recommended appropriate preventive regimens before the acute event, how long it takes them to be seen if they receive emergency care, and whether they receive appropriate and medically necessary rehabilitation after the acute event.

Clinical Issues in the Crisis Phase

Many people who experience heart attack or stroke will not receive emergency medical care, either because the event was so mild that they did not seek it or because they died before they could get it. For those who do receive emergency medical care, social workers are most likely to encounter them in an institutional setting, like a hospital or a rehabilitation facility. On average, patients who are admitted to the hospital for a stroke or heart attack will stay in the hospital for about a week (Virani et al., 2021; Wegiel, 2018).

Psychosocial impacts on patients and families during the crisis phase of the acute event can vary widely depending on the severity of the event, ranging from a mild event with little physical change to an extreme event that results in death. Those impacts also depend on an individual's current and past mental and physical health, their support systems, their access to resources, and social determinants that might affect their ability to access care.

The hospital course may have been preceded by uncertainty about which symptoms are subacute and which require emergency care. In heart attack, patients may experience chest pain, upper back or neck pain, indigestion, heartburn, nausea or vomiting, extreme fatigue, dizziness, or shortness of breath, among other symptoms (American Heart Association, 2015); in stroke, they may experience numbness, confusion, trouble seeing, trouble walking, or severe headache (American Stroke Association, n.d.). The severity of symptoms doesn't always correspond with the seriousness of the hospital course, and they can manifest differently in men versus women.

Patients who receive emergency care may feel shock at the unexpected, sudden acute event. That shock may impact whether and how patients and families accept medical and social work interventions while the patient is in the hospital. Families may also feel hypervigilance about related symptoms and the risk of having an acute event or guilt or shame if they thought the symptoms were innocuous, but they actually led to sudden death.

For these reasons, social workers should assess patients' and families' understanding of the acute event early in the hospital course to identify how the family functions, existing coping mechanisms, and strengths and vulnerabilities (O'Donnell et al., 2020). This assessment can guide education about what inpatient experiences they may encounter, including by identifying which family members can tolerate information sharing, helping manage strong emotions within the family system, and collaborating about post-discharge care. Correcting misunderstandings about the likelihood of rehabilitation and recovery may also be helpful.

For the majority of the 1.6 million people in the United States who experience a heart attack or stroke each year, the acute event may be the first time they are receiving inpatient care at a hospital. They may be unfamiliar with hospital disciplines and may be encountering all of them for the first time at once. This can be overwhelming, even beyond the distress of the event itself.

Heightened negative emotion can interfere with attention and inhibition control (Harle, 2013). Social workers can provide education multiple times and in different ways so patients and families are better able to absorb that information (Mayer et al., 2013). They can also expect patients and families to react strongly and automatically to new, unfamiliar information about the patient's condition and prognosis. That heightened emotion can impair information processing, and they may pay closer attention to the delivery of news than the attendant information (Tulsky, 2005), so an empathetic, collaborative approach may make these conversations more effective. And social workers can be an important conduit between and among families and treatment teams, translating complex, unfamiliar medical and hospital jargon into language they can understand and act on (O'Donnell et al., 2020).

Depending on the severity of the acute event, functional change may be minimal or may be severe and instantaneous, or it may result in death.

Mild Events After Crisis

For patients whose acute event is mild, hospital stays may be short. They may require minimally invasive procedures, such as stent or shunt placements, to assist in long-term recovery. These procedures are generally low risk but may be distressing for the patient and family. They also may be learning for the first time about underlying diseases that led to the acute event, and this can lead to a wide range of feelings, from relief that they survived a close call to embarrassment and stigma that they had the acute event.

Social workers can normalize the distress patients and families are experiencing and help answer some questions about health maintenance that can prepare these patients to adapt to and accept functional and psychosocial changes. They can also be prepared to connect patients and families with outpatient resources such as legal and counseling services that may restore a sense of control in an otherwise unpredictable time.

Hospital social workers may also help families to channel distress and uncertainty into advance care planning. These conversations "elicit a patient's goals, values, cultural influences, and preferences for care is an integral part of providing goal concordant care" (O'Donnell et al., 2020, p. 5). These conversations can help patients and families make meaning from the acute event. For those patients who feel distressed or paralyzed by the lack of actionable steps to integrate the mild event into their cognitive schema, developing advance directives might channel that energy into a tangible, objective action item.

Severe Events After Crisis

Patients who recover from a serious acute event may experience distressing changes in function during the hospital course. These patients may require a higher level of care and be placed in the medical intensive care unit (MICU), which can be distressing to patient and family alike. Patients may not understand what is happening to them and be uncomfortable or in pain. Families may feel shock and distress at seeing the patient connected to machines.

Patients' responsiveness during the hospital course may vary greatly depending on the severity of the acute event. Aphasia, residual confusion, or amnesia secondary to a severe stroke may be present. The patient may be sedated or intubated in the MICU and unable to respond. Patients may also experience other immediate impacts to their function, such as hemiparesis. These changes may improve during the hospital course and through rehabilitation, but many patients will live with long-term residual deficits. During the hospital course, patients may feel anxiety and distress about which physical changes are temporary and which are permanent, and families may feel distress at seeing them compromised from their pre-event level of function.

Social workers can facilitate communication among family members in these situations and thereby ease distress. This may involve becoming more attuned to gestures and body language through which patients communicate nonverbally, e.g., expressions of pain like wincing or grimacing. This may also involve simple tools, such as pen and paper or erasable whiteboards, for those patients who may be intubated but able to read and write, or picture boards that patients and providers can point to and can be easily carried around. Depending on available technologies, tools could also include high-tech options, such as speech-generating devices for aphasia. Social workers can educate families who are struggling to communicate with patients about these alternative strategies.

As patients and families anticipate long-term adjustments to their lives, they may benefit from resource counseling about home care, skilled nursing, and other support services. They may need education on equipment that can help the patient live independently with residual deficits. And they may be wondering what structural changes they may need to make their homes accessible to the patient with long-term physical deficits.

Acute Events After Crisis

For some patients whose acute event leads to death, the entire illness course is compressed into days or weeks. Patients and families are likely to feel trauma responses such as dissociation, hyperarousal, intense anxiety, emotional paralysis, and horror. Because the acute event is usually sudden and unexpected, these families may need to make EOL decisions for patients in the absence of advance directives that could mitigate families' uncertainty and distress. (For more on the absence of advance directives and the psychosocial impacts after an acute event that leads to sudden death, see *Clinical Issues in the Terminal Phase*.)

Social workers have an opportunity to model trauma-informed care to improve family experiences: that approach can signal that the medical team understands and empathizes with their suffering, and it can help build a trusting environment to promote further interventions as they come (Fischer, 2019).

Clinical Issues in the Chronic Phase After a Mild Event

As mentioned in the *Crisis* section, patients who survive the acute event can experience a wide range of long-term changes. For some, the acute events will be mild with few, if any, noticeable physical changes; yet even for those patients, adjusting to life after the acute event can cause significant psychosocial impact.

These patients may be encouraged to follow up more regularly with specialty providers that require more frequent and substantial visits to medical offices. That can strain family systems and change roles and dynamics. Patients may feel uncertain, anxious, powerless, isolated, embarrassed, ashamed, stigmatized, and like the world that was previously inherently safe is now threatening or dangerous – all feelings that can worsen health outcomes after the acute event (Claiborne, 2006).

Uncertainty can make it difficult for these patients to plan for the future (Lawson & McHenry, 2011) and lead to avoidance that can be associated with complications after the acute event (Moser, 1996). For example, a patient who survived a mild heart attack may limit activities such as walking that may exacerbate loss of function rather than protect the heart from strain. Patients whose social avoidance leads to isolation may be less adherent to their medical regimens and have higher readmission rates and increased morbidity (O'Donnell et al., 2020).

Not all patients struggle after the acute event; some experience post-traumatic growth, a well-demonstrated outcome of life-threatening conditions for some people (Hefferon et al., 2008; Peng & Wan, 2018). Patients who survive an acute event may feel like they had a close call and reorient their relationship to their health and bodies for the better; Petrie et al. (1999) found that 58% of study respondents reported positive life changes after a heart attack, with the majority of those changes related to healthier lifestyles. The acute event may also help them clarify their values and priorities and find motivation to achieve new things – i.e., find "new possibilities" and "appreciation of life" (Tedeschi & Calhoun, 1996, p. 459).

Interventions and Approaches After a Mild Event

Effective social work interventions and approaches with patients and families after a mild acute event include treating the family as the unit of care, care coordination, and behavioral modification that promotes lifestyle changes.

Interventions during the chronic phase are most effective when the social worker treats the family, not just the patient, as the unit receiving care (McCarthy, 2011). While patients may experience the direct impacts of the acute event, family members are also adapting to those changes themselves. Good communication also facilitates optimal care, provides the patient with the opportunity to reach his maximum functional potential (Zorowitz et al., 2002), and improves mental quality of life for those patients (Claiborne, 2006). This can involve helping patients and families integrate residual deficits after the acute event into the patient's life, identifying safety concerns, and coming up with cooperative solutions for those deficits.

These approaches are fundamental to consistent, compassionate care coordination. Care coordination "prevents patient decline, facilitates patient access to resources supporting adherence to medical treatment, enhances restorative efforts, and achieves efficient integrated care" (Claiborne, 2006, p. 88).

Stroke survivors who receive care coordination may be less depressed, have improved psychological well-being, and have better cognitive functioning (Claiborne, 2006). Similarly, Huffman et al. (2014) found that collaborative care between mental health and primary care providers improved the mental health-related quality of life for patients with recent cardiac events, including reduced depression and anxiety. This is in part because patients receiving collaborative care also may have significantly improved self-care practices, e.g., adherence to treatment (Claiborne, 2006).

Social workers can help patients improve self-care by brainstorming questions for providers and strategizing about lifestyle changes, as well as addressing barriers to adherence like transportation and remembering medications (Claiborne, 2006). This approach can promote a feeling of intimacy with the social worker, which can enhance the patient's feeling of social integration and protect against the isolation that can worsen health outcomes after the acute event (Claiborne, 2006).

Social workers working with patients who are in the chronic phase may want to familiarize themselves with the sorts of lifestyle changes medical providers are likely to recommend, which include quitting tobacco, increasing physical activity, eating more fruits and vegetables while eating less fat and salt, and limiting alcohol consumption (Lee et al., 2016). Motivational interviewing may also help make behavioral modification and lifestyle change more effective, although a meta-analysis conducted by Lee et al. (2016) was inconclusive.

Clinical Issues in the Chronic Phase After a Severe Event

The chronic phase after a severe event can be characterized by adjustment to a new level of function that includes deficits to the patient's ability to perform their activities of daily living (ADLs) and cognitive changes that impact their ability to understand and communicate. Patients may also need to start new medication regimens, which can be costly and challenging to adhere to. These changes can cause lasting negative psychosocial impacts.

Immediately after the crisis phase, patients may experience debility due to deconditioning after being in the hospital for an extended period. They may need to adapt to ongoing pain and a loss of physical control. Patients may also need durable medical equipment at home, such as supplemental oxygen and adaptive equipment for eating, or even implanted devices they need to maintain and tolerate. Their homes may need to be changed to allow accessibility, including by adding ramps or widening doorways to accommodate wheelchairs – or families may need to move. These all can be costly, distressing symbolic reminders of the acute event.

Looking ahead, the first 6 to 12 months after the acute event are critical to recovery (Virani et al., 2021), so assistance in selecting formal inpatient or outpatient rehabilitation for those patients who need it can be especially impactful in facilitating long-term improvement. Families may face significant challenges to securing needed care, e.g., paying for ongoing care, adapting to family changes, and securing childcare and work accommodations. Advocating for patient needs with insurance providers and connecting families with low-cost resources can improve health outcomes for these families (McCarthy, 2011).

After about 6 to 12 months, the majority of these patients' functional improvements will have occurred (Claiborne, 2006). More than half of patients will have regained functional independence after that time, but as many as 30% of stroke survivors will have permanent impairments (Zorowitz et al., 2002) and 20% of heart attack survivors who were admitted to the hospital will have some impaired neurological function after discharge (Virani et al., 2021). Collectively, physical and cognitive deficits are associated with reduced function, reduced quality of life, and shortened life span (Virani et al., 2021).

Some of these patients will receive home care services, through which social workers have additional opportunities to assess patients in their home environments. Still others will be so compromised by the acute event that they will be unable to care for themselves independently or even with the help of family members and home health workers. These patients will need to move into nursing care facilities.

Interpersonal Changes

Adapting to residual deficits may cause significant role adjustments in the family system that can degrade a patient's social and family functioning (McCarthy, 2011). Significantly, these patients face an increased risk of unemployment (McCarthy, 2011), whether because of residual deficits or other psychosocial impacts. In circumstances where the patient was a primary earner, members of the family may need to adapt to a different role in the family. All of these changes can cause feelings of powerlessness and loss of control amid the financial demands of recovery.

Family members may also need to reduce or stop work in order to become caregivers. Their comfort with and adaptiveness to providing this kind of intimate care, such as assistance with bathing and toileting, can depend on the nature of their relationship with the patient (e.g., spouse, parent-child, neighbors). Some may have little experience in the practical aspects of caregiving, like bed transfers and bathing, and may benefit from practical training so they can effectively provide care. For patients who experience cognitive and psychological changes, caregivers may need to adapt to new, challenging behaviors like yelling, physical resistance, or catatonia and learn behavior management skills (McCarthy, 2011).

Conversely, families might avoid the patient with residual deficits, which can exacerbate the patient's social isolation and integration and worsen health outcomes. The patient might be a reminder that their lifestyle choices are dangerous (e.g., a smoker whose smoker mother had a heart attack) or might provoke anxiety and fear about the genetic determinants of the acute event, wondering whether they may be at risk themselves. They may also simply feel embarrassed or uncomfortable when interacting with a patient who has suffered noticeable and significant physical changes, like being wheelchair-bound or managing significant aphasia.

Physical Changes

After an initial period of recovery, the patient may need to come to terms with long-term residual deficits that defy their expectations – i.e., adjust to a "new normal." Physical impairments are more common in stroke survivors than heart attack survivors, but both groups experience deficits that can affect their daily living.

More than half of heart attack survivors will experience severe fatigue after the event (American Heart Association, 2015). Many of these patients report less engagement in activities they enjoyed prior to the acute event, which can exacerbate the anger, guilt, irritation, and fear they likely already feel (Claiborne, 2006) and increase the likelihood of post-event depression. Reduced physical activity is also a risk factor for recurrence (Virani et al., 2021). Social workers may want to explore fatigue to help determine what changes can be made to maximize their ability to enjoy premorbid hobbies.

Stroke is one of the leading causes of physical disability in the United States (Virani et al., 2021). Post-stroke deficits include compromised mobility, restricted range of motion, numbness, paralysis, and fatigue (Zorowitz et al., 2002) that can compromise a patient's ability to perform ADLs. They also include pain syndromes and gait instability, with higher risk for falls and fractures (Virani et al., 2021). Adapting to all these changes can be intimidating and time-consuming.

Patients may feel demoralized without clearly defined goals and well-managed expectations around improvement after the initial recovery phase. Adjustment may not be linear and can go on for years. Survivors may see their function, cognition, and quality of life worsen, even in the absence of recurrence, in ways that might accelerate natural age-related functional decline (Virani et al., 2021).

A year after his stroke, John, a 56-year-old single white man living in New York City, had recovered to the point where he was able to live alone again and return to work. He had residual left-side hemiparesis (partial paralysis), mostly affecting his hand and arm, but its effect on his daily living was limited because John is right-handed and he received some adaptive equipment from the rehabilitation center. Although his occupational therapy was long over, he had diligently stuck to his home exercise plan and was satisfied with his level of function. His neighbors didn't even know that he had had a stroke – and he didn't want to tell them.

One hot summer afternoon, John got a craving for ice cream. He consistently followed his nutritionist's recommendations, so he hadn't had that treat in a while. But John wanted to celebrate. There were times during rehab where he wasn't sure whether he could live independently like this anymore. John stuffed his keys into his pocket, exited into the hot midday sun, and headed to his favorite ice cream shop.

It wasn't until he got back to his apartment door that he had a sinking realization: With the ice cream cone in his right hand, he couldn't reach into his pocket to grab his keys. It was another reminder of the long tail of his stroke and another pang of grief. He was also stuck with a painful choice: either abandon the ice cream that symbolized his return to independence to get inside or eat his ice cream awkwardly in the sweltering hallway in full view of his neighbors.[1]

As patients and families adapt in real time, they cannot know whether the changes they encounter will be temporary or permanent. This uncertainty can interfere with recovery and increase the likelihood of anxiety and depression. Patients may be resistant to interventions, thinking either that changes are temporary and will go away on their own or that they're immutable, making rehabilitation pointless. Families may also be reluctant to make adaptations to the home, which can exacerbate the physical burden of those physical changes on patients.

Cognitive and Psychological Changes

As previously mentioned, heart attack survivors are more likely to experience impaired consciousness and cognitive deficits than physical deficits (Virani et al., 2021). Similarly, strokes impact brain health, i.e., the ability to function adaptively in one's environment (Gorelick, 2017). Deficits can also include loss of executive function and dementia (McCarthy, 2011).

Stroke survivors are especially at risk for developing long-term aphasia, "an acquired communication disorder caused by brain damage that impairs a person's ability to understand, produce, and use language" (LaPointe, 2005, p. 2). As many as 38% of stroke survivors will develop aphasia after recovery (Berthier, 2005), and between one and two million Americans are currently living with aphasia (Greenfield & Ganzfried, 2016).

As Greenfield and Ganzfried (2016) observe, post-stroke aphasia can significantly limit a patient's ability to communicate with family members and providers because it's hard to find and form words during conversation (i.e., expressive aphasia) or understand jokes (i.e., receptive aphasia). They may avoid noisy environments or using the telephone and find it difficult to read road signs or count money, limiting their ability to engage in daily activities. And they may be unable to fill out forms, adding additional challenges to accessing recovery services. These difficulties can exacerbate negative feelings and magnify fear that they won't be able to cope with the unexpected when they go out, creating a negative feedback loop of avoidance.

This avoidance might also have negative physical consequences. For example, a patient with residual urinary incontinence following a stroke may limit their water intake to avoid having an accident but then be too dehydrated to give blood for routine health checkups. Social workers can notice when the avoidance in response to functional impairments is worsening a patient's quality of life and brainstorm alternative strategies to cope with those changes.

---

[1] All names and other personal identifiers in the case are fictitious. Any similarity to actual persons, living or dead, or actual events is purely coincidental.

Patients who survive a heart attack or stroke can experience a range of other negative psychological effects from the acute event and in adapting to residual deficits, including anger, anxiety, guilt, irritation, and fear (Claiborne, 2006). These feelings can culminate in depression, a psychological condition that is correlated with poorer engagement in rehabilitation, long-term social function, and increased mortality (McCarthy, 2011).

Depression

Recent data suggest post-stroke depression affects about a third of stroke survivors, primarily in the first year after the acute event (Virani et al., 2021), and stroke survivors who have more severe residual impairments are at higher risk of developing post-stroke depression (McCarthy, 2011). Depression in heart attack survivors occurs at a comparable rate to stroke survivors, although without the same relationship between depression and post-event function (Murphy, 2020). Symptoms and medication side effects can also mask depression and grief, making them difficult to diagnose.

Post-event depression is correlated with poor health outcomes. It is associated with a higher risk of recurrence, worsening function over the first year post-stroke, and higher likelihood of having a fatal stroke (Virani et al., 2021), which is similar in heart attack survivors (Murphy, 2020). Post-stroke depression is associated with a range of other poor indicators, such as poor engagement in rehabilitation, worse compliance with their medical regimen, longer hospital inpatient periods, higher readmission rates, and impaired social and family functioning (McCarthy, 2011; Murphy, 2020; O'Donnell et al., 2020; Patel et al., 2003).

Beyond its physical impacts, depression can rob a person of their interest and motivation to engage in activities that used to bring them pleasure, lessen their quality of sleep and energy throughout the day, and make it harder to make decisions or engage in activities that require concentration, such as work. Depression and cognitive impairment related to depression also interfere with relationships, including with caregivers, and reduce patients' ability to cope with disability (Patel et al., 2003).

Family caregivers are likely to experience some of the same negative psychosocial impacts that patients do. They may experience difficulty returning to work, stress due to the high costs of home healthcare, and unmet instrumental needs (McCarthy, 2011), factors that can engender fear, anxiety, depression, and sense of powerlessness (Virani et al., 2021). Social workers can explore these feelings with family caregivers – especially without the patient present, which may encourage them to more freely express negative feelings – and recommend counseling or other referrals when appropriate.

Interventions and Approaches

Effective social work interventions during the chronic phase after an acute event include patient education, counseling on helpful communication practices, depression screening tools, and psychotherapeutic modalities like cognitive behavioral therapy (CBT).

Because rehabilitation is oriented around deficits and how to compensate for them, it is particularly helpful for social work interventions to emphasize strengths, which patients themselves may not even recognize. Setting achievable goals for and celebrating progress during rehabilitation emphasizes how patients can achieve pre-event function with new strategies and adaptive equipment. Strength-based efforts also include connecting with environmental strengths like supportive family relationships and community resources, and treating the patient as an expert in their personal recovery. These interventions are even better when they are values-based, e.g., if a patient values connectedness with family, social workers may want to focus on strengthening new communication strategies such as drawing their thoughts on paper.

Social workers can also encourage helpful practices around post-stroke aphasia: ensure you have the person's attention before you speak, minimize background noise, keep communication simple but appropriately adult, confirm understanding with yes or no questions, give the person time to speak and resist the urge to finish sentences or offer words, and consider alternate forms of communication, like drawings, gestures, and facial expressions (Greenfield & Ganzfried, 2016).

For social workers without specialized training in uncovering post-event depression, the Beck Depression Inventory may serve as a rapid, accurate assessment tool that's simple to implement (Salter et al., 2007). The Hospital Anxiety and Depression Scale (HADS) is another effective tool that can help discern depression through physical and somatic symptoms in the hospital setting (Bjelland et al., 2002). Social workers may also track themes that emerged in a Williams et al. (2005) study of stroke survivors to aid in identifying depression: Nondepressed survivors reflected facing adversity through strength, finding meaning in setback, and hope for the future; depressed survivors reflected battling a new reality and preparing for the worst.

Effective psychotherapeutic interventions for post-event depression include CBT and other short-term psychotherapies, as well as increased physical activity, especially for older patients (Murphy, 2020).

Clinical Issues in the Terminal Phase

In some instances, death results from underlying disease or complications in recovery. For other patients whose acute event is so severe that it causes sudden death, the illness course can be compressed into a span of days or weeks.

During that time, families may struggle to understand and accept the prognosis and disagree about care. The hospital course may be complicated by significant functional impairments that limit communication and loss of decision-making capacity. Families may need to make childcare or work arrangements to spend time at the hospital with the patient, which can exacerbate distress. And they may be put into EOL situations without advance directives.

When patients are significantly compromised, patient histories, decisions about care, and updates may need to be communicated by and with family members instead of patients themselves. Social workers should remember that these families may be overwhelmed and disoriented by being in an unexpected life-threatening situation, which can reduce attention span and inhibition control and degrade information processing (Harle, 2013; Tulsky, 2005).

Because the acute event may be sudden and occur before the patient or family is aware of the underlying disease, patients may not have advance directives that could mitigate the uncertainty and distress. Although the effects of written advance directives on the quality of EOL care may be controversial, they can improve family members' communication with hospital providers and can be correlated with more realistic expectations (Teno, 2007).

Without those directives, families may have internal disagreements over what the patients' EOL wishes would have been, which may lead to worse health outcomes (Tulsky, 2005). No matter their care decisions, family members may feel guilt that persists and magnifies in grieving. Patients without advance directives may lack other EOL documents, such as wills or plans for funeral arrangements, which can perpetuate disagreements for months and years. Families may channel that distress into distrust of or dissatisfaction with the treatment team.

Social workers have a unique opportunity to lead and shape family meetings that support the family as they cope with this terminal phase. "As key members of interprofessional palliative care teams, social workers provide team-based leadership in areas of social, psychological, and cultural aspects of care" and deploy frameworks like "the social ecological model and family systems theory" to understand psychosocial dynamics that other hospital disciplines might not (O'Donnell et al., 2020, p. 3).

These family meetings are best when the treatment team has shared information and coordinated their purposes in advance and when they work collaboratively to create a trusting environment that helps families accept treatment recommendations (Tulsky, 2005). This is especially germane during an acute event, where family members are likely meeting providers for the first time and may have little experience with hospitals. They are also best when the treatment team acknowledges intense uncertainty – not just in family members' decision-making, but in "the ambiguity that at times may cloud medical practice" (Tulsky, 2005 p. 362).

Bereavement

Nearly two-thirds of stroke deaths each year occur outside the setting of an acute care facility, and only about a quarter of heart attacks that occur outside that setting survive to reach acute care (Virani et al., 2021). In the majority of sudden deaths from stroke or heart attack, families may first interact with a social worker in the context of bereavement.

These families may just be beginning to make meaning of the fatal acute event, and that meaning may be negative. The patient's belongings in situ may be a symbolic reminder of the sudden loss. They may have not gotten effective information (or any information at all) about the factors that led to the fatal event, which could result in confusion or disbelief.

For those who died of the acute event in an institutional setting, families may face different challenges in processing loss. It may have been extremely distressing for families to see the patient die while surrounded by machines. They may have had to make EOL care decisions that they regret or over which they have had disagreements with other family members. The experience may also have provoked distrust in healthcare workers.

No matter the setting or circumstance of death, family members may struggle with shock at its suddenness, especially when the underlying disease was not known. That suddenness may limit families' abilities to mobilize resources to influence the outcome (Mayer et al., 2013). Families may feel unprepared to make the immediate decisions necessary to keep the family system functioning, such as financial issues and childcare.

Family and friends of patients who died of heart attack are also at elevated risk themselves of having a heart attack shortly after the death – as much as 21 times more likely in the first 24 h (Mostofsky, 2012). Social workers interacting with families within the first week after sudden cardiac death may want to introduce distress tolerance and emotion regulation skills and tools to them.

Physiological risk factors aside, unexpected deaths radically alter the family system, and families may struggle to incorporate the loss into their lives and adapt to a profoundly changed reality (Mayer et al., 2013). Death can profoundly affect family members' cognitive schema about the world (Mayer et al., 2013), e.g., from a fundamental assumption that the world is safe to a fear that tragedy is just around the corner.

Ying is a 40-year-old Hmong woman who flew back to her small Minnesota hometown when her father had his first heart attack in 2019. Because the event was mild, Ying's father was only hospitalized for a few days and then discharged to outpatient cardiac rehab for 2 months. Ying's father didn't regain all his strength, but he was able to perform all his ADLs without assistance, and Ying's mother helped out with household tasks and accompanying him to appointments.

Eighteen months later, Ying's father was working in his garden when he had another heart attack, this time severe. Emergency services were slow to arrive because it occurred at the height of the COVID-19 pandemic, but there was an ICU bed for him that afternoon – where the family was not able to visit him due to newly implemented protocols. When Ying arrived by plane the next day, her family was extremely distressed. As an Animist family, they believed that Ying's father was sick because his soul had wandered away from his body in search of something he needed. They wanted to call his soul back – i.e., give offerings to the spirits of the land to make his soul happy and bring it back to his body (Her-Xiong & Schroepfer, 2018). But they could not evade COVID-19 visitor restrictions, even after pleading with hospital staff. Two days later, Ying's father died; to Ying and her family, his soul was fated to wander the Earth forever.

Ying decided to relocate to her hometown after his death to help her family cope and grieve. During the days, she cooked for her family and watched her nieces and nephews – but at night, she felt anxious and empty. After a few months, a non-Hmong friend noticed her sadness and encouraged her to start psychotherapy, and Ying agreed. But it was difficult for her to find a provider to whom she didn't have to explain Hmong culture, so she struggled with motivation to stay in treatment and dropped out after five sessions.[2]

Because families may experience the sudden death as traumatic, bereavement interventions with them should be culturally appropriate and trauma-informed. Social workers are also uniquely positioned to help interpret difficult medical issues into language families can understand, sit with uncertainty and discomfort with families, and address unanswered questions that can limit the family's ability to make meaning after the loss (Mayer et al., 2013).

Practical interventions, including problem-solving and brainstorming about tasks such as obtaining death certificates and planning ceremonies where appropriate, may be invaluable right after the death. Ceremonies, funerals, memorials, or informal rituals and gatherings can be an effective way to create meaning and can protect against the prolonged grief and post-traumatic symptoms that may otherwise characterize bereavement after a sudden death (Hegarty et al., 2020; Mayer et al., 2013).

Acknowledging the family's subjective experience of the death may also be key to successfully intervening in their bereavement (Tang, 2017). Effective cognitive appraisal cautions against assuming that family members will experience "complicated" bereavement after a sudden death. Some may experience post-traumatic growth at having to adapt to the loss, reinforcing their resilience and personal strength, and some also may sublimate their feelings as a new desire to help others (Mayer et al., 2013).

Meaning-based existential therapies may also promote better bereavement outcomes. Whenever a death results in feelings of powerlessness or challenges a basic belief that the world is benevolent and just, exploration of one's struggle to find meaning that "emphasizes people's need to impose meaning on their life experiences" may be beneficial (Neimeyer et al., 2011, p. 71). These meaning-based

[2] All names and other personal identifiers in the case are fictitious. Any similarity to actual persons, living or dead, or actual events is purely coincidental.

interventions include narrative retelling, wherein the bereft family member can reiterate the story of the death in safety; therapeutic writing, which creates an alternate space for meaning reconstruction; metaphoric visualization, which permits a different kind of understanding of and relationship with the death; and taking a pro-symptom position, which invites the bereft family member to draw closer to their feelings of sadness and pain instead of resisting those feelings (Neimeyer et al., 2011).

Sharing stories of loss and grief in social contexts is often perceived as unacceptable, and "survivors after sudden deaths are often neglected by healthcare professionals, who quickly move on to care for their next client" (Mayer et al., 2013). This may be because those providers are occupied by their next patient and family or because those providers feel discomfort in sitting with the consequences of the sudden death that leads to avoidance. So social workers have a unique opportunity to create trusting spaces with families to explore these stories and feelings.

Social Justice

Race and Ethnicity

Race and ethnicity can have a significant impact on the incidence and treatment of heart attacks and strokes in ways that suggest that hospital providers, including social workers, need to find more effective ways to communicate with people of color, anticipate barriers to accepting referrals and care, and educate communities.

Black and Latinx people are more likely to experience stroke, have poorer functional status after rehabilitation, and are more likely to develop dementia 5 years after the acute event than white people or their other counterparts of color (Virani et al., 2021). Black people are also more likely to have more severe strokes, be less independent, and have a recurrence within 1 year and die from that recurrence. And Latinx stroke survivors perform worse on neurological, functional, and cognitive outcomes than their white counterparts (Virani et al., 2021).

Despite these disparities, Black and Latinx people are also more likely to be discharged home versus to a nursing care facility or other inpatient setting than their white counterparts (Virani et al., 2021) and are significantly less likely to receive appropriate procedures and therapies when receiving acute care after a heart attack (Geiger, 2003). This is true regardless of the race of the provider.

Social workers may extrapolate that long-term functional status for Black and Latinx people depends in part on whether hospital providers believe their conditions warrant further institutional care. Geiger (2003) suggests a likely cause is "institutional racism" driven by "unconscious negative stereotyping" (van Ryn, 2001; van Ryn & Burke, 2000), i.e., "there may be something in the process of medical education, professional acculturation, or practice experience that subtly biases" (p. 431) physicians regardless of that physician's own race.

These unconscious processes may go both ways: Black and Latinx people have historically been harmed, not helped, by medical institutions, which may cause them to resist inpatient rehabilitation placements or other interventions that might improve health outcomes. This may also result from a lack of effective education about stroke warning signs and risk factors (Virani et al., 2021), which may point less to a genetic component than it does to poor outreach to Latinx communities with the wrong messengers.

One effective intervention may be educating hospital providers, especially emergency department clinicians, about trauma-informed care. Trauma-informed care can dispel some of the biases that affect treatment protocols (Agboola et al., 2021).

Gender

Women suffer more heart attacks and strokes and are more likely to develop long-term residual deficits and experience negative psychosocial impacts than men. While some of these factors may be attributable to genetic and demographic factors – e.g., there are more older women than older men in the United States – it may also be a result of bias in treatment.

For example, women are more likely to experience delays in appropriate medical care during the acute event (Geiger, 2003). They experience longer wait times before receiving care when arriving at emergency departments. And they are less likely to get guideline-recommended treatment during, and medications after, the acute event (Geiger, 2003).

Not surprisingly, women also experience significant differences in disability and recovery post-stroke, in mortality rates, and in post-stroke depression (Persky, 2010). They are more likely to have residual deficits after rehabilitation, and those deficits are more likely to be severe, and they are more likely to die from the acute event. Post-stroke depression is also more common in female stroke survivors and their families (McCarthy, 2011).

Some of these disparities may be explained in part by gender differences in the symptoms that precipitate heart attacks, leading women to underestimate the significance of those symptoms and not seek care. But this cannot be the sole, or even primary, determinant. Delays in care might be related to unconscious bias in how hospital providers perceive the risk and urgency of women who present in emergency departments with heart attacks and strokes.

Economic Disadvantage

At every stage of treatment, payor status is a powerful predictor of whether the patient will receive appropriate treatment. Socioeconomic status is inextricably linked with racial background, gender, and other social identifiers.

Patients with lower income and educational attainment are more likely to experience severe stroke symptoms and to die from a stroke than economically advantaged patients (Virani et al., 2021). Lower-income patients are also more likely to experience sudden cardiac death (Virani et al., 2021). And financial strain is closely correlated with the development of post-event depression (Murphy, 2020).

Lower-income patients may have fewer resources with which to access services like rehabilitation or home care – and because the first 6 to 12 months after the event are so important to recovery, prognosis for these patients is likely worse. These patients and their family caregivers are more likely to be hourly wage earners, so they lose proportionately more income from the demands of recovery, which may also lead to worse treatment adherence. And recovery for these patients can be complicated by housing and food insecurity.

This may result from lack of effective education; "stroke knowledge is lowest for those living in communities with greater economic need and sociodemographic distress," and poor knowledge about heart attacks and strokes contribute to higher risk for recurrence (Virani et al., 2021, p. 511). Social workers can anticipate gaps in education and consider different education styles that can promote better health outcomes, including education about payor options like Medicaid and other state programs.

Age

Although stroke and heart attack largely affect older adults, recent data suggest that the rate of stroke is increasing among young adults, even as it has been diminishing in adults over 55 (Virani et al., 2021). Social workers may therefore find themselves working with younger patients with heart attack and stroke.

These young people may feel invisible in the rehabilitation process and chronic phase after the acute event (Roding, 2003). They may also feel that having a stroke is asynchronous with the stage of their life cycle they are in, which can cause them additional distress and put them at risk of developing post-stroke depression (McCarthy, 2011; Murphy, 2020).

Families who experience unexpected and untimely deaths may be more prone to experiencing complications in their grief (Neimeyer et al., 2011), so families of young people may be especially vulnerable. In a cross-sectional survey of surviving family members in Australia, Ingles et al. (2016) found that one in two family members of young people who suffered sudden cardiac death reported significant psychological distress, especially symptoms associated with prolonged grief and post-traumatic stress. Effective social work interventions should anticipate these vulnerabilities, including through trauma-informed care.

Author's Reflection: Seeking Out the Wisdom of Survivors

Heart attacks and strokes can fundamentally alter the cognitive schema of patients and families by virtue of their suddenness. The world that may have once felt inherently safe prior to the acute event may now feel inherently and unpredictably dangerous. Those who struggle to integrate the meaning of that acute event into their lives may feel uncertain about the future and worry that something life-changing is around each corner. They may avoid activities that previously seemed innocuous out of fear of provoking a recurrence or fear that they would not be able to cope because of new functional impairments.

Hospital social workers, through repeated secondary exposure to these events, can wrestle with those same fundamental questions of uncertainty and control. How do we make sense of the world, knowing that people's lives can fundamentally and dramatically change in an instant? We may see families on the cusp of happiness change course after sudden death, young patients experience acute events tragically and asynchronously with their stage of life, and so on. To work with these patients fully and openly is to accept morbid unpredictability ourselves.

Unsurprisingly, that acceptance can be fraught. And rather than integrating that perspective constructively, we can instead experience it as secondary trauma, wherein clinicians experience a traumatic reaction in witnessing and interacting with situations perceived as traumatic to others.

That secondary trauma might show up as hypervigilance. We may panic when we aren't able to reach a family member, wondering whether they've experienced an incapacitating acute event. We may feel a surge of dread each time we see an incoming phone call, wondering whether we're going to get life-altering news. We may pore obsessively over our own health information and make preemptive lifestyle changes, no matter how extreme or unproven.

It might also show up as disconnectedness. Rather than take on that lack of control, we might distance ourselves from it. We may righteously blame our patients for causing their acute events and feel anger toward them. We may put less effort into relationships with our vulnerable family and friends. We may stop engaging in the activities we once found pleasurable or keep our children and older parents away from such activities. All of this is an effort to reclaim control from the grips of uncertainty; all this is resistance, rather than acceptance.

What can hospital social workers do to integrate the inexorable truth of uncertainty without disconnecting from our compassion? Without trying to wrest control where there is none to be had?

First, we might remember that our experiences as hospital social workers are skewed toward the acutely medically vulnerable. In our work, the majority of people we see are actively experiencing or recovering from medical crises. Even more precarious, we have just enough information (e.g., from chart review, clinical observation, transdisciplinary team meetings) to fully appreciate the fragility of life, but not enough information (e.g., if we provided hands-on medical care like the doctors and nurses we work with) to feel empowered to do something about it. It may help to step back and remember that we are interacting with a small, unrepresentative portion of the population – i.e., that the vast majority of people are not experiencing acute events like this in any given year.

Second, we may apply that ubiquitous strength-based perspective to reframe our relationships with these patients. What if, in addition to seeing these patients as medically vulnerable, we can also see them as repositories of a special kind of wisdom? Those patients that survive the acute event are navigating territory that few truly understand or relate to. They may be creating new neural passageways through damaged brain tissue that defy explanation or even imagination. They may be achieving extraordinary human feats of resilience, even when they themselves feel demoralized. And they may have powerful, unspoken strengths helping them cope and recover that they themselves may not even be aware of. As clinicians, do we dare feel awed and inspired by them?

Attempting that perspective shift can accomplish a few things. First, it repositions the patient as the expert of their own experience and recovery. At a time when that patient might feel powerless, it uplifts their dignity and inherent human power. That shift can improve the social worker's therapeutic bond with the patient, leveling the power dynamic. It can also reorient therapeutic engagement with patients, so that our questions and interventions promote strengths and solutions over deficits and problems. This approach may not be appropriate for every patient in every circumstance, but those for whom it resonates may be empowered by that reframe.

For clinicians, too, that shift may soothe our own preoccupations with control and uncertainty. Regarding our patients as resilient reminds us that we, too, could be resilient in the face of similar adversity. Instead of simply treating and intervening, we may learn from our fellow humans – identify unexpected tips and strategies to persist against myriad challenges that help us as much as they help our patients when we emphasize them. All of that might nurture gratitude that we are connected to each other, even in moments of suffering, and help us draw closer to the great uncertainty that is the human experience.

Reflection Questions

1. How does the suddenness of the onset of heart attacks and strokes impact how people cope with them? In what way is coping different for patients and caregivers?
2. How might you work with a heart attack survivor who is fearful of recurrence?
3. What are some of the biggest challenges in working with this population?

References

Agboola, I. K., Coupet, E., & Wong, A. H. (2021). "The coats that we can take off and the ones we Can't": The role of trauma-informed care on race and bias during agitation in the emergency department. *Annals of Emergency Medicine, 77*(5), 493–498. https://doi.org/10.1016/j.annemergmed.2020.11.021

American Heart Association. (2015, July 31). Lifestyle changes for heart attack prevention. https://www.heart.org/en/health-topics/heart-attack/life-after-a-heart-attack/lifestyle-changes-for-heart-attack-prevention

American Stroke Association. (n.d.). Stroke symptoms. https://www.stroke.org/en/about-stroke/stroke-symptoms

Berthier, M. L. (2005). Poststroke aphasia: Epidemiology, pathophysiology and treatment. *Drugs and Aging, 22*(2), 163–182.

Bjelland, I., Dahl, A. A., Haug, T. T., & Neckelmann, D. (2002). The validity of the hospital anxiety and depression scale. *Journal of Psychosomatic Research, 52*(2), 69–77. https://doi.org/10.1016/s0022-3999(01)00296-3

Centers for Disease Control and Prevention. (2021, May 25). Stroke facts. https://www.cdc.gov/stroke/facts.htm

Claiborne, N. (2006). Effectiveness of a care coordination model for stroke survivors: A randomized study. *Health & Social Work, 31*(2), 87–96.

Fischer, K. R., Bakes, K. M., Corbin, T. J., Fein, J. A., Harris, E. J., James, T. L., & Melzer-Lange, M. D. (2019). Trauma-informed care for violently injured patients in the emergency department. *Annals of Emergency Medicine, 73*(2), 193–202. https://doi.org/10.1016/j.annemergmed.2018.10.018

Geiger, H. J. (2003). Racial and ethnic disparities in diagnosis and treatment: A review of the evidence and a consideration of causes. In B. D. Smedley, A. Y. Stith, & A. R. Nelson (Eds.), *Unequal treatment: Confronting racial and ethnic disparities in health care* (pp. 417–454). The National Academies Press.

Gorelick, P. B., Furie, K. L., Iadecola, C., Smith, E. E., Waddy, S. P., Lloyd-Jones, D. M., Bae, H. J., Bauman, M. A., Dichgans, M., Duncan, P. W., Girgus, M., Howard, V. J., Lazar, R. M., Seshandri, S., Testai, F. D., van Gaal, S., Yaffe, K., Wasiak, H., & Zerna, C. (2017). Defining optimal brain health in adults: A presidential advisory from the american heart association/american stroke association. *Stroke, 48*(10), e284–e303. https://doi.org/10.1161/STR.0000000000000148

Greenfield, M., & Ganzfried, E. S. (2016). *The word escapes me: Voices of aphasia*. Balboa Press.

Harle, K. M., Shenoy, P., & Paulus, M. P. (2013). The influence of emotions on cognitive control: Feelings and beliefs–where do they meet? *Frontiers in Human Neuroscience, 7*(508).

Hefferon, K., Grealy, M., & Mutrie, N. (2008). Post-traumatic growth and life threatening physical illness: A systematic review of the qualitative literature. *British Journal of Health Psychology, 14*(2), 343–378. https://doi.org/10.1348/135910708X332936

Hegarty, G., Storey, L., Dempster, M., & Rogers, D. (2020). Correlates of post-traumatic growth following a myocardial infarction: A systematic review. *Journal of Clinical Psychology in Medical Settings, 28*(1), 394–404. https://doi.org/10.1007/s10880-020-09727-3

Her-Xiong, Y., & Schroepfer, T. (2018). Walking in two worlds: Hmong end of life beliefs & rituals. *Journal of Social Work in End-of-life and Palliative Care, 14*(4), 291–314. https://doi.org/10.1080/15524256.2018.1522288

Huffman, J. C., Mastromauro, C. A., Beach, S. R., Celano, C. M., DuBois, C. M., Healy, B. C., et al. (2014). Collaborative care for depression and anxiety disorders in patients with recent cardiac events: The Management of Sadness and Anxiety in Cardiology (MOSAIC) randomized clinical trial. *JAMA Internal Medicine, 174*(6), 927–935. https://doi.org/10.1001/jamainternmed.2014.739

Ingles, J., Spinks, C., Yeates, J., McGeechan, K., Kasparian, N., & Semsarian, C. (2016). Posttraumatic stress and prolonged grief after the sudden cardiac death of a young relative. *JAMA Internal Medicine, 176*(3), 402–405.

LaPointe, L. L. (2005). Foundations: Adaptation, accommodation, aristos. In L. L. LaPointe (Ed.), *Aphasia and related neurogenic language disorders* (pp. 1–18). Thieme.

Lawson, R. R., & McHenry, K. M. (2011). Emerging opportunities for palliative social workers. In T. Altilio & S. Otis-Green (Eds.), *Oxford textbook of palliative social work* (pp. 351–358). Oxford University Press. https://doi.org/10.1093/med/9780199739110.003.0032

Lee, W. W. M., Choi, K. C., Yum, R. W. Y., Yu, D. S. F., & Chair, S. Y. (2016). Effectiveness of motivational interviewing on lifestyle modification and health outcomes of clients at risk or diagnosed with cardiovascular diseases: A systematic review. *International Journal of Nursing Studies, 53*, 331–341. https://doi.org/10.1016/j.ijnurstu.2015.09.010

Link, B. G., & Phelan, J. (1995). Social conditions as fundamental causes of disease. *Journal of Health and Social Behavior, 35*, 80–94.

Mayer, D. D. M., Rosenfeld, A. G., & Gilbert, K. (2013). Lives forever changed: Family bereavement experiences after sudden cardiac death. *Applied Nursing Research, 26*(4), 168–173.

McCarthy, M. J., Powers, L. E., & Lyons, K. S. (2011). Poststroke depression: Social workers' role in addressing an Underrecognized psychological problem for couples who have experienced stroke. *Health & Social Work, 36*(2), 139–148.

Moser, D. K., & Dracup, K. (1996). Is anxiety early after myocardial infarction associated with subsequent ischemic and arrhythmic events? *Psychosomatic Medicine, 58*(5), 395–401.

Mostofsky, E., Maclure, M., Sherwood, J. B., Tofler, G. H., Muller, J. E., & Mittleman, M. A. (2012). Risk of acute myocardial infarction after death of a significant person in one's life: The determinants of MI onset study. *Circulation, 125*(3), 491–496.

Murphy, B., Le Grande, M., Alvarenga, M., Worcester, M., & Jackson, A. (2020). Anxiety and depression after a cardiac event: Prevalence and predictors. *Frontiers in Psychology, 10*, 3010.

Neimeyer, R. A., Burke, L. A., McKay, M. M., & van Dyke Stringer, J. G. (2011). Grief therapy and the reconstruction of meaning: From principles to practice. *Journal of Contemporary Psychotherapy, 40*(2), 73–83. https://doi.org/10.1007/s10879-009-9135-3

O'Donnell, A., Gonyea, J. G., & Leff, V. (2020). Social work involvement in palliative care heart failure research: A review of recent literature. *Current Opinion in Supportive and Palliative Care, 14*(1), 3–8. https://doi.org/10.1097/SPC.0000000000000482

Patel, M., Coshall, C., Rudd, A. G., & Wolfe, C. D. A. (2003). Natural history of cognitive impairment after stroke and factors associated with its recovery. *Clinical Rehabilitation, 17*(2), 158–166. https://doi.org/10.1191/0269215503cr596oa

Peng, Z., & Wan, L. (2018). Posttraumatic growth of stroke survivors and its correlation with rumination and social support. *Journal of Neuroscience Nursing, 50*(4), 252–257. https://doi.org/10.1097/JNN.0000000000000371

Persky, R. W., Turtzo, L. C., & McCullough, L. D. (2010). Stroke in women: Disparities and outcomes. *Current Cardiology Reports, 12*(1), 6–13. https://doi.org/10.1007/s11886-009-0080-2

Petrie, K. J., Buick, D. L., Weinman, J., & Booth, R. J. (1999). Positive effects of illness reported by myocardial infarction and breast cancer patients. *Journal of Psychosomatic Research, 47*(6), 537–543.

Roding, J., Lindstrom, B., Malm, J., & Ohman, A. (2003). Frustrated and invisible – Younger stroke patients' experiences of the rehabilitation process. *Disability and Rehabilitation, 25*(15), 867–874. https://doi.org/10.1080/0963828031000122276

Salter, K., Bhogal, S. K., Foley, N., Jutai, J., & Teasell, R. (2007). The assessment of poststroke depression. *Topics in Stroke Rehabilitation, 14*(3), 1–24. https://doi.org/10.1310/tsr1403-1

Tang, S., & Chow, A. Y. M. (2017). Subjective and objective traumatic death: Distinct roles in developing complicated grief and depression among older adults in Hong Kong. *International Psychogeriatrics, 29*(3), 409–417. https://doi.org/10.1017/S1041610216001873

Tedeschi, R. G., & Calhoun, L. G. (1996). The posttraumatic growth inventory: Measuring the positive legacy of trauma. *Journal of Traumatic Stress, 9*(3), 455–471. https://doi.org/10.1002/jts.2490090305

Teno, J. M., Gruneir, A., Schwartz, Z., Nanda, A., & Wetle, T. (2007). Association between advance directives and quality of end-of-life care: A National Study. *Journal of the American Geriatrics Society, 55*(2), 189–194. https://doi.org/10.1111/j.1532-5415.2007.01045.x

Tulsky, J. A. (2005). Beyond advance directives: Importance of communication skills at the end of life. *JAMA, 294*(3), 359–365. https://doi.org/10.1001/jama.294.3.359

van Ryn, M. (2001). The implications of social cognition research and theory for the provider contribution to race/ethnicity disparities in health care. In *Physicians for human rights committee on racial and ethnic disparities in diagnosis and treatment in the U.S. health care system.* Physicians for Human Rights.

van Ryn, M., & Burke, J. (2000). The effect of patient race and socio-economic status on physician's perceptions of patients. *Social Science and Medicine, 50*(6), 813–828. https://doi.org/10.1016/s0277-9536(99)00338-x

Virani, S. S., Alonso, A., Benjamin, E. J., Bittencourt, M. S., Callaway, C. W., Carson, A. P., Chamberlain, A. M., Chang, A. R., Cheng, S., Delling, F. N., Djousse, L., Elkind, M. S. V., Ferguson, J. F., Fornage, M., Khan, S. S., Kissela, B. M., Knutson, K. L., Kwan, T. W., Lackland, D., et al. (2021). Heart disease and stroke statistics—2020 update: A report from the American Heart Association. *Circulation, 141*, e139–e596. https://doi.org/10.1161/CIR.0000000000000757

Węgiel, M., Dziewierz, A., Wojtasik-Bakalarz, J., Sorysz, D., Surdacki, A., Bartuś, S., Dudek, D., & Rakowski, T. (2018). Hospitalization length after myocardial infarction: Risk-assessment-based time of hospital discharge vs. real life practice. *Journal of Clinical Medicine, 7*(12), 564. https://doi.org/10.3390/jcm7120564

Williams, C. L., Rittman, M. R., Boylstein, C., Faircloth, C., & Haijing, Q. (2005). Qualitative and quantitative measurement of depression in veterans recovering from stroke. *Journal of Rehabilitation Research and Development, 42*(3), 277–290. https://doi.org/10.1682/jrrd.2004.02.0017

Zorowitz, R. D., Gross, E., & Polinski, D. M. (2002). The stroke survivor. *Disability and rehabilitation, 24*(13), 666–679. https://doi.org/10.1080/09638280110109291

Chapter 9
Liver and Kidney Diseases

Maya Joyandeh and Michelle Willoughby

Introduction

In this chapter, kidney and liver diseases are presented together in an effort to move away from separate medical descriptions of illnesses to a psychosocial understanding with common trajectories of both diseases. According to the National Kidney Foundation (2017), kidney disease, which is when the kidneys stop working enough to sustain a healthy life, may be caused by hypertension, diabetes, and a family history of kidney failure. Poor glucose control in diabetics and non-compliance with medications and diet can contribute greatly to an individual's risk of kidney disease diagnosis.

Liver disease has more variety in cause, though similar psychosocial experiences. There are more than 100 types of liver disease. Common types include hepatitis C, alcohol-related liver disease, non-alcoholic fatty liver disease, and liver cancers. End-stage liver disease (ESLD) can lead to a liver transplant or end of life (EOL). The American Liver Foundation (2017) listed risk factors for liver disease as obesity, heavy alcohol use, diabetes, needle use, genetics, and chemical exposure. Common medications such as acetaminophen, statins, or Vicodin can negatively impact liver functioning. Chronic liver disease can also be caused by substance use disorder. There is a strong correlation, for example, between intravenous drug use and hepatitis C (Patel et al., 2018). Most chronic liver disease results in cirrhosis, which is scarring of the liver, leaving it unable to function well enough to sustain

M. Joyandeh (✉)
Teaneck, NJ, USA
e-mail: Maya.Joyandeh@gmail.com

M. Willoughby
New York University, New York, NY, USA
e-mail: mw1983@nyu.edu

M. Hemphill, A. Nathanson (eds.), *The Practice of Clinical Social Work in Healthcare*, Essential Clinical Social Work Series,
https://doi.org/10.1007/978-3-031-31650-0_9

good health. Medical complications of cirrhosis may include ascites, abdominal fluid buildup causing abdominal swelling, and hepatic encephalopathy, which involves declining brain function and changes in mental status for patients with advanced liver disease (Volk, 2020).

In considering the common psychosocial experiences of people with kidney and liver diseases, it is important to acknowledge how variable the impact of diagnosis is. For some, it is arrived at with relatively few symptoms, and the focus is on prevention of progression outside of the care facility. For others, it is arrived at with many symptoms and pressure to make medical decisions *now*; understandably, patients in this situation may feel particularly psychologically overwhelmed.

Variations in the circumstances that led to disease can also mean differences in feelings and reactions to being treated for kidney or liver disease. Both illnesses can, but not always, be related to lifestyle factors, such as drinking alcohol excessively, obesity, and smoking tobacco. For those who feel responsible for causing their illness, even if inaccurately, there can be feelings associated with internalized stigma: guilt, depression, and withdrawal or feelings of being deserving of ill health (Schomerus et al., 2022; O'Hare et al., 2018). If people have developed these diseases as a result of other health risks (i.e., diabetes, genetic predispositions, or autoimmune hepatitis), they may feel other negative feelings (such as anger, connected with asking: *Why me?*) connected to having or managing disease (O'Hare et al., 2018).

Social workers serving individuals affected by kidney or liver disease are commonly found in hospitals, outpatient medical clinics, dialysis centers, substance use treatment centers, and organ transplant programs. Social workers working and encountering patients in hospitals typically do not continue to see these patients into the community, and patients are referred to social work assistance at the most appropriate outpatient clinic. This discontinuity may have significant ramifications for an individual's ability to cope, make sustained lifestyle changes, and adhere to a treatment regimen (Ufere et al., 2020; Adisa et al., 2018). A social worker working at a dialysis center or a transplant program, by contrast, could provide support to patients and caregivers over weeks to years, covering a range of interventions and approaches designed to support this specific population.

Kidney and liver diseases are more prevalent in communities with a lower socioeconomic status and in certain ethnic groups (Norton et al., 2016; Kardashian et al., 2021). Black Americans are disproportionately affected by kidney disease (Tucker, 2021). Hispanic Americans have higher rates of non-alcoholic fatty liver disease when compared to the national average (Kardashian et al., 2021). Social workers must be attuned to the social and political factors contributing to these health disparities.

Illness: Onset, Course, and Degree of Incapacitation

Liver and kidney failure can present as either an acute injury or a gradual-onset disease process. In acute kidney injury (AKI) or acute liver injury (ALI), the organs suffer a sudden failure, usually within a few days. This most commonly occurs as a side effect from medication, or as a complication of surgery, and the patient most likely has already been hospitalized, sometimes requiring a stay in an intensive care unit (ICU). A gradual-onset disease process may start with non-life-threatening symptoms such as fatigue, pain, changes in urination, skin or mentation, or changes in blood work. The outcome and course of liver and kidney diseases is uncertain, unless it is end-stage liver disease (ESLD) or end-stage renal disease (ESRD).

When first meeting with a patient who is newly diagnosed, the social worker should consider the emotional shock of diagnosis and be aware that trauma reactions, in addition to feeling overwhelmed and confused, can manifest. These reactions may look like shock and dissociation or like intense anxiety, irritability, mistrust, and agitation. Many patients have never heard of these illnesses, even as others may know enough about them to understand what an impact the diagnosis can have on their lives. A patient may experience anxiety and confusion, which can lead to information-seeking, or to shutting down, if they are unable or unwilling to process the information being given to them.

According to the American Liver Foundation (2017), patients can live for years with liver disease and may have few or no symptoms. This experience is different from an AKI or ALI. When kidney and liver diseases progress gradually, over months or years, and the disease is already diagnosed, then individuals may already be speaking with a specialist regarding their symptoms, risks, and how to avoid further progression. Treatment may include medications, diet, exercise, and close monitoring. In this situation, a social worker's active role may be contingent on referral or invitation by a specialist or patient.

The course of kidney and liver diseases can vary widely. Liver disease can be progressive, constant, or episodic, depending on the diagnosis. Kidney disease progresses through five stages. In the first stage, there is normal kidney function; however, urine tests or blood work can detect abnormalities that point to kidney disease. Recommended treatment at this time would include observation, medications, and a change in diet. The second and third stages occur as the kidney's functioning worsens. By the fourth stage, discussions about dialysis and kidney transplant take place. Hemodialysis, or "dialysis," is a medical intervention often involving several hours-long visits to a clinic every week with regular intravenous access to a machine, which takes the blood from a patient's body, cleans it in a machine to help clear toxins, and returns it to the patient. At the fifth stage, dialysis will have begun, and other options like transplant may be explored if appropriate (American Kidney Fund, 2021) (see Organ Transplant chapter).

If these diseases are left untreated, a person can die within a few days to a few weeks, depending on the functioning of the liver and kidneys. With treatment, the prognosis can change dramatically. In kidney disease, people live 5–10 years, on average, when undergoing hemodialysis treatment. Many can even survive 20–30 years (American Kidney Fund, 2021). In liver disease, a person can live a few days or weeks to even years without treatment, depending on the severity of the disease (American Liver Foundation, 2017).

Due to the short time frame of survival with advanced, untreated disease, it can be challenging under such circumstances to make decisions among remaining options for care. The patient is left to decide within hours to days of terminal diagnosis whether to begin treatment such as disease-modifying interventions and/or palliative care or to pursue hospice. According to Bansal and Schell (2018), it is essential for patients with ESRD to focus specifically on advance care planning early on. When approaching end of life, patients' decision-making capabilities may be compromised, and they may no longer be able to voice their wishes regarding their medical care.

If a patient decides to move forward with disease-modifying treatment, it is important to ensure that the patient has fully absorbed the likely efficacy and outcomes of treatments and is not just responding, in their shock, with unreasonable expectations for what treatment is and is not likely to accomplish. It is essential for the social worker to provide education on the options of care, including modifying care goals to symptom management, and to facilitate the patient's comprehension of, and comprehensive thinking through, those options.

For patients pursuing disease-modifying treatment, social workers may assist in finding a dialysis unit, making a referral for kidney or liver transplant, and supporting a healthy lifestyle moving forward. At this juncture, social workers should be looking for clues to determine the risk and protective factors of this new treatment plan.

- Is there family or social support?
- Can the patient pay for medications?
- Is transportation available for treatments?
- Is the patient able to commit to a healthier lifestyle?

If the social worker finds gaps in these areas, those gaps would be starting points in working with the patient to ensure better outcomes. Gaps in these areas are often reflective of larger socioeconomic disparities in society, reflective of larger struggles with racism and anti-immigration policies.

The degree of incapacitation can vary, depending on the progression of the disease and how it manifests in each individual. Various symptoms of disease may occur that affect one's cognition, movement, and energy and can cause disfigurement. In both kidney and liver diseases, cognitive deficits may occur. Many patients report a feeling of fogginess and can have difficulty retaining information. Hepatic encephalopathy can cause mental status changes and confusion, which may consequently require 24-h care for the patient. Care needs for patients with hepatic encephalopathy can be likened to those of a patient with Alzheimer's disease (Bajaj et al., 2011). Considering these cognitive effects, social workers can work with family members or others in the patient's support system to ensure that medical information is adequately understood and retained.

Sudden changes in health and functioning can be frustrating and frightening for someone facing kidney or liver disease, especially in younger populations. Younger patients can be particularly shocked to learn that they are in ill health and requiring treatment, forced to adjust expectations for themselves and their lives quickly. Social workers must consistently assess cognitive changes and cannot assume low health literacy, or a permanent deficit, as an explanation for difficulties with comprehension or retention of medical information. For many, mental fogginess can dissipate; the medical team should be aware of any shift from the patient's baseline, including mental and cognitive changes, and consider these changes compared against typical effects of patients' physical conditions.

Physical changes, such as muscle weakness, paresthesia, cramping, and muscle pain, can occur in kidney disease (National Kidney Foundation, 2017). Itchy skin may also occur in both kidney and liver diseases (National Kidney Foundation, 2017; American Liver Foundation, 2017). A change in diet or medication may alleviate this symptom. In kidney disease, a catheter is commonly inserted into the chest to administer dialysis treatment. For long-term treatment, a fistula may be placed in the arm (National Kidney Foundation, 2006). Both types of dialysis access sites can cause disfigurement, which can commonly be a source of embarrassment or induce a negative body image in patients.

In liver disease, buildup of ascites, or excess abdominal fluid, can impede movement. Liver disease can also cause chronic fatigue, vomiting, weight loss, or jaundice (American Liver Foundation, 2017). Abdominal swelling and jaundice can negatively affect a patient's self- image, as well as their physical well-being. Individuals who have certain liver diseases caused by alcohol use disorder may, unfortunately, face stigma, lack of empathy, and judgment. Such stigmatizing can have a disastrous impact on care and well-being. Patients with cirrhosis and depression may not adhere to treatment due to this stigma, feeling demotivated and perhaps even deserving of ill health (Vaughn-Sandler et al., 2014).

When left untreated, both kidney and liver diseases can cause body swelling. Liver disease can cause abdominal swelling and kidney disease can cause swelling in the feet and ankles. Many patients may exhibit fatigue due to the buildup of toxins in the blood. Fatigue is a common symptom in liver and kidney diseases (American Liver Foundation, 2017; Davey et al., 2019). For a once-active individual, this can be life-altering, inhibiting the ability to participate in social functions, recreational activities, and work.

Treatment itself can limit one's freedom of movement, as it can be frequent, last for long periods, and make outside life activities difficult to maintain. When approaching a patient undergoing dialysis, it is imperative for the social worker to understand and explore how these changes are affecting the individual.

- Is the patient in the workforce?
- Is the patient the primary financial or caregiving support for their family or community?
- How does lack of exercise affect identity?
- How does one's absence from social gatherings impact social standing?

Providing information on local support groups may give patients access to a source of comfort. Not only can support groups give someone struggling with these diseases a sense of community, but the other members may have information or feedback on how to further explore other aspects of one's own identity and find new areas of enjoyment and fulfillment. Feelings of isolation can be quickly extinguished once the person feels others can relate and engage with them in a process of discovering a "new normal." A social worker can provide support on what this new normal life can look like.

Social stigma is a salient concern for those suffering from these specific diseases. In kidney disease, the appearance of a fistula or central venous catheter, a tube typically placed on the neck or upper chest, can cause stares. People may judge someone based on the appearance of abdominal swelling or a change in skin tone. The general public could make assumptions that the patient is appearing this way due to an unhealthy lifestyle or that these health problems are due to medical non-adherence. Diabetes can be a cause of kidney disease, which may lead some people to falsely assume that poor diet choices led the patient to this health crisis. Lack of access to healthy and affordable foods can be a significant factor in developing these illnesses. Food insecurity disproportionately affects Black and Hispanic Americans when compared to the national average (Tucker, 2021). Since some liver diseases are caused by substance misuse, many people with liver disease experience stigma, regardless of substance use history.

Clinical Impacts of Illness

Crisis

In the crisis stage, the patient may be hospitalized or waiting at home for important test results. When symptoms do not require hospitalization but possibly need follow-up, some people will spend time waiting at home or at work for their nephrologist to confirm the absence or presence of a health issue that requires immediate treatment or hospitalization. Feelings and reactions during this period of waiting range from denial, or refusing to accept the potential existence of severe health concerns, to significant emotional distress.

Some individuals may choose to keep emotional distress, if present, to themselves during this time of uncertainty, and their family and friends may be unaware of it. When walking the tightrope between health and illness, a patient may experience loneliness and isolation, intentional (through private coping with disease) or unintentional (family and friends are unaware, even though "signs" are there and openly shared). Some may not feel distress because they do not identify with the "diagnosed club," anticipating instead positive news from the physician. Others may not identify as part of this group even once they have an established diagnosis. In these cases, their deteriorating health demonstrates a continuation of the past problematic behavioral patterns that are linked to acknowledgment and addressing of health limitations and issues.

Patients may already be in the intensive care unit (ICU), experiencing painful and frightening symptoms such as edema, cardiac arrest, or sepsis. During this period, patients and their caregivers may be experiencing worry, anxiety, and depression and may be going through a psychological trauma in response to the sudden and/or shocking shift to a life-threatening situation. This time period may trigger depression and anxiety (Abdul Halain et al., 2022; Boehm et al., 2021). Patients and caregivers are at risk for ICU-related post-traumatic stress disorder, which can have more detrimental long-term effects (Noyes & Schlesinger, 2017). A past history of or co-occurring mental health disorder is likely to add complexity to the patient's outlook on their physical health, on their emotional well-being, and on their coping in the face of medical stressors.

When depression is diagnosed by a clinician, it is important to consider the types of depression. Major depressive disorder, a diagnosis determined by the presence of multiple behavioral, cognitive, and emotional states, and situational depression and adjustment disorder, a dysphoric episode developed in response to external life stressors, are most relevant due to the traumatic nature of being diagnosed with a life-threatening illness. Patients who are suffering from major depressive disorder may respond to talk therapy, cognitive behavioral therapy (CBT), somatic trauma therapy, motivational interviewing, or acceptance and commitment therapy, with or without medication (such as antidepressants) (Kroll, 2022; Anderson et al., 2018). Through consultation with a mental health professional, patients can learn coping strategies and process their emotions to adapt to a new normal (Kroll, 2022). Involving family members in the therapeutic process through family therapy may be effective as well (Carr, 2019).

In response to a crisis, caregivers may experience anger toward the patient, assigning blame for perceived bad habits, such as substance misuse or poor diet. They may also feel embarrassment. These feelings of shame and embarrassment may prevent discussions from taking place regarding the emotional toll of diagnosis and treatment planning. Family members may be in a state of shock or worry, especially if symptoms exhibit quickly and unexpectedly. Some caregivers may be trying to plan for possible outcomes, researching treatment, speaking to experts and professionals in the field, or setting up care in the home if needed. Patients, in turn, may feel shame (associated with the feelings described) or anger in being misunderstood or less emotionally supported than they need and deserve (Schomerus et al., 2022; Adelman et al., 2014).

Education and engagement are crucial for patients and their families during this time. The medical team is responsible for providing information on treatment options, lifestyle changes, and emotional support services. Clinicians can use motivational interviewing techniques to discuss lifestyle changes such as smoking cessation and the positive effects of exercise for patients with chronic kidney disease (Choi et al., 2019). Marlow et al. (2016) recommended that individuals with ESRD learn adaptive coping skills. In this study, social workers identified those patients in denial of their kidney disease and referred them to acceptance and commitment therapy, with the goal of acceptance. Saleh et al. (2021) found that there is insufficient research on current educational strategies for patients with cirrhosis and their caregivers. Using a patient empowerment approach in education is always recommended.

A diagnosis can be overwhelming, and this makes it imperative that specialists discuss patients' situations with them in detail, including the likely course of the disease, the need to consider advanced care planning, and information on transplant candidacy or rehabilitation services, as culturally and cognitively appropriate. Some patients can exhibit low health literacy, lack of foresight, and lack of preparation for life ahead with kidney or liver disease. Within a matter of days to weeks, patients with kidney disease can go from hospitalization to being transported to an outpatient dialysis unit 3 days per week.

Chronic

Once in the chronic stage of disease, patients have most likely chosen a path of treatment, management, or end-of-life planning. Treatment and management can include dialysis of kidney disease, rehabilitation for alcoholism for liver disease, and changes in diet and lifestyle (Choi et al., 2019; Verma et al., 2019). While treatment may extend one's life for months to years, the initial shock of diagnosis, and the drastic modification of diet and habits, can be overwhelming. Patients may face a loss of independence and can be faced with reliance on caregivers and a large interdisciplinary medical team with whom they now have regular, compulsory interactions.

It can be a struggle to adjust to this new dynamic and patients may have a range of responses, including withdrawal and lashing out (O'Hare et al., 2018). Some may feel anxious and defer decision-making to the medical team, a reliance that may help to relieve anxiety. Chronic kidney and liver diseases are often accompanied by financial concerns, too: the diseases can cause fatigue, making it difficult to continue to work. Social workers can address financial assistance options such as applying for Social Security Disability Insurance and can help patients and families check eligibility for state programs (Caplan et al., 2017). Such steps, by relieving financial stress, allow a patient more peace of mind in the face of financial losses resulting from illness, treatment, and care.

For those individuals with liver disease associated with substance use, continued outpatient substance misuse treatment and commitment to abstinence is essential. About one third of cirrhosis cases are caused by heavy alcohol use (Patel et al., 2018), but it is equally important to note that this means two thirds of cirrhosis cases are not caused by heavy alcohol use. Middle-aged males are the demographic most represented in cirrhosis (D'amico et al., 2006).

Some individuals who were using substances at baseline may continue to use substances as a way to cope with the illness. Ongoing substance use and misuse needs to be addressed by the medical team with this in mind. Continued professional support and education are of vital importance to maintain or encourage abstinence from substances, if such intervention is indicated as needed (Shrestha et al., 2020). Such intervention addresses the fact that co-occurring mental health and substance use disorders affect patient health outcomes (Patel et al., 2018).

Common psychological issues in the chronic phase include negative thinking about self-worth and treatment outcomes, self-blame, emotional distress, and low and depressed mood (Kondo et al., 2020; Choi et al., 2019). The involvement of clinical professionals, like social workers and psychiatrists, among others, is principal to identifying, diagnosing, and treating these symptoms. In some instances, psychotropic medications may be necessary to alleviate and manage these common yet disruptive emotions.

Depression is common among patients with chronic liver disease and kidney disease (Kondo et al., 2020; Patel et al., 2018). Due to the nature of these diseases, many patients experience symptoms that are related to the diagnosis but manifest as depressive symptoms, such as fatigue, memory impairment, and poor appetite (Kondo et al., 2020). Patients with chronic liver disease and depression often face poorer outcomes and higher mortality rates than those patients with chronic liver disease without depression (Russ et al., 2015). Depression, alcohol use disorder, and substance use contribute to a decreased quality of life in patients with chronic liver disease (Verma et al., 2019). Verma et al. (2019) studied the effects on quality of life for patients with liver disease after participating in programming on chronic liver disease, depression, and substance use disorder using a Screening, Brief Intervention, and Referral to Treatment (SBIRT) model. This study found that patients with depression reported a better quality of life after participation in this treatment program. This, and research that supports the routine screening of patients (i.e., Volk, 2020), suggests the value of mental health assessment and intervention for patients in this population. Nair et al. (2021) found that individuals with advanced chronic kidney disease cited their spirituality as a way to cope. Assessments of patients and caregivers should include spirituality. Recommended therapeutic interventions include meaning-centered therapy (MCP) and acceptance and commitment therapy (ACT).

End-of-life (EOL) planning can include execution of advance directives (i.e., Health Care Proxy, Do Not Resuscitate order, Do Not Intubate order, MOLST/POLST forms), removal of extensive disease-modifying treatment, palliative or hospice care, and funeral planning. The patient may indicate their wishes regarding medical care in writing, in the form of specific directives about who should make decisions for them if they cannot (i.e., advance directives), or broader guidelines for care and elucidation of priorities for EOL experience (i.e., *Five Wishes*). Social workers providing education on EOL planning and encouragement to have discourse about EOL wishes, as well as facilitating those discussions, can helpfully guide patients and their families in their decision-making and emotional processing of what could lie ahead. Social workers can also help to empower patients by normalizing a discussion around if/when treatment does not work or if/when disease progresses more.

On a practical and emotional level, a delay in such discussions gives caregivers less time to prepare for EOL, less time to know the patient's preferences, and less time for any work needed to realize those preferences. EOL wishes may include withholding extensive disease-modifying treatment, or life-sustaining treatment, such as artificial nutrition or ventilators, under specific circumstances in the progression of the illness. In the case where a patient has decided not to pursue disease-modifying treatment or has started treatment and then made the choice to end such treatment, education on hospice care can be instrumental for the patient and the caregiver. This helps both patient and caregiver understand the shift from active treatment to comfort measures, pain management, and management of other physical symptoms. This shift in care aligns with and facilitates a psychological shift toward preparation for death and living the remaining span of life as well as possible.

It is important to note that making the informed and thoughtful decision to cease treatment in the context of serious and terminal illness should not be confused with suicidal behavior. Managing depressive symptoms, which are a risk factor for suicide, should not be confused with avoiding frank assessment of quality of life in determining which disease-modifying treatments to continue or discontinue (Salvatore, 2020). People suffering from kidney and liver diseases are vulnerable to suicidal ideation and have easy access to means of hastening death by passive suicide; for example, death can occur as a result of missing dialysis treatments or reverting back to unhealthy habits (Salvatore, 2020; Le Strat et al., 2015). More on this issue will be discussed in the Terminal section of this chapter.

The involvement of family (whether families of origin or choice) is critical in cases where there is chronic illness treatment and should be facilitated wherever possible. Families can support the patient in many ways; they, too, can be educated about the patient's disease and treatment, new medications and treatment modalities, and transitions in care. Conversely, when families are uninvolved, social work intervention becomes particularly crucial. Transportation to and from treatment can become a financial burden, especially when a wheelchair or stretcher is medically necessary. To reduce out-of-pocket costs, the family may take on the responsibility of transporting the patient to appointments and treatments, which may have a financial impact on the family's ability to work and manage other roles. Dialysis treatment is typically three times a week, sometimes beginning very early in the morning, and medical appointments for both diseases are frequent, impacting the patient's ability to work or engage in community roles. The social worker should provide resources on transportation options through insurance, if applicable, as well as exploring local paratransit, and transportation services from local community centers or foundations.

Individuals diagnosed with kidney or liver disease may be in the workforce and could be the primary earner in their household. It is challenging to remain in the workforce despite the impacts of chronic illness, but the patient's inability to work may represent a major financial burden for the family. There will most likely be a new normal, which may include adjusting to reduced income with the additional challenge of having to pay medical bills. Other family members may need to enter the workforce, causing disruption in the family constellation and caregiving and possibly feelings of shame, blame, and new stress that can negatively affect relationships and the family as a whole.

Family members may experience worry over the effects of having reduced income, such as the possibility of losing their home or managing childcare, delaying education or their own health needs, and other concerns. Social workers, typically from the hospital or treatment center, may be able to provide family therapy and assistance with concrete services, such as financial aid, food delivery through the county, and discount cards for prescription medications. Lessening financial burden when possible can be an immeasurable relief to caregivers, other family members, and the patient as they struggle with the costs of continued commitment to care.

If the patient is medically eligible to receive a kidney or liver transplant, additional psychosocial issues may arise. As a relative is more likely to be a good match for an organ donation than a stranger, dynamics within the family around transplant may be complex: Feelings of burden and guilt can occur when the relative is not willing to donate or when the relative is willing, but not a viable match. Patients and families may have questions and anxiety around the possibility and timing of a transplant. (Please see Transplant chapter for a more in-depth discussion on the social justice and systemic racism issues related to organ transplantation in the United States.) Craig et al. (2016) found that participants in a coping skills group for patients waiting for liver or kidney transplant had lowered depression and anxiety scores after participation. Coping skills groups may also decrease caregiver burden.

The caregivers of undocumented immigrants with end-stage kidney disease receiving emergency dialysis face unique challenges including concerns for healthcare coverage and immigration issues. Family life can be disrupted with children missing school, and parentification of the child can occur. Caregivers are at risk for financial hardship and psychosocial distress (Cervantes et al., 2020).

Nguyen et al. (2015) found that current alcohol use in patients with chronic liver disease led to higher caregiver burden. Nguyen et al. (2015) found that caregivers of patients with cirrhosis reported lower mental health scores compared to the general population. Frequent hospitalizations, alcohol use, history of hepatic encephalopathy, and low income were identified as predictors of high caregiver burden. Identifying additional support, so that the burden is shared among a few people, and creating a "team" to care for the patient rather than exhausting one person, is an important tactic to address with caregivers. Hansen et al. (2021) recommended that medical team members examine the impact of ESLD on the quality of life of both patients and caregivers as parts of one unit.

Support groups for caregivers can be a space of empathy and social support. Social workers can address financial concerns, teach coping skills, and provide mental health support and resources to them (Bajaj et al., 2011). Social workers can encourage self-care practices with caregivers and help to identify backup caregivers. Caregivers may also benefit from educational resources on how to be a caregiver (Volk, 2020).

Medical and mental health professionals in treatment centers and hospitals can carry their own biases and beliefs on what constitutes optimal treatment for patients. Projecting their own values regarding treatment, medical professionals can heavily encourage certain types of treatment over others (in such a way that the patient's own goals of treatment are not fully explored, expressed, or supported). The availability of treatment resources differs in different countries, reflecting the common values and purview of patient care in those places. In the United States, in-center hemodialysis is considered the first step of dialysis treatment. In other countries, such as China or Thailand, peritoneal dialysis, which is done through a catheter in the abdomen as opposed to a needle in the arm, is the first treatment offered before going to a center for treatment and is cost-effective (Li et al., 2017). Peritoneal dialysis does not require medical professionals, so the patient is easily able to perform this in the comfort of his own home.

The standard treatment options available to patients in the United States – i.e., going to outpatient centers – can overwhelm or frustrate patients who feel overly managed by medical professionals. This can lead a patient to feel out of control and uncomfortably dependent on others. It can also offer benefits, however. Patients have access to a range of mental health professionals, like social workers, who can meet with patients during treatment and provide supportive counseling and concrete services while working to build motivation and understanding of the importance of healthy lifestyle choices. The social worker can help to create a sense of safety and protection by building and maintaining a knowledgeable, open-minded, and non-judgmental zone of care.

Greater support and involvement can potentially help with treatment compliance and, in turn, better health outcomes. Due to the nature of kidney and liver diseases, some patients are non-adherent with their medical care, and therefore, it is common for them to miss important medical appointments or not to schedule them at all. With a team of professionals checking in on the patient at treatment, the patient is more likely to become more compliant at keeping these appointments and adhering to a new, healthier lifestyle. Goals of care can and should be continued to be discussed and modified, so that the patient is continually engaged in treatment choices. Motivational interviewing also can help toward continued engagement. It is a common tool used to help the patient identify their motivations for change, to express empathy through reflective listening, and to help further develop the patient's goals (Anderson et al., 2018).

Terminal

In the terminal stage of kidney and liver diseases, the patient and family are faced with the reality that there is no chance for recovery, and death due to the illness is inevitable. In kidney and liver diseases, once disease-modifying treatment has ended, death can occur from within a few days to within a few weeks. Death can also be acute, such as from cardiac arrest or pneumonia, within the context of a chronic illness decline.

The patient may have lost the ability to perform activities of daily living (ADLs), experience symptoms more intensely, and frequent the Emergency Department to manage their symptoms more often than earlier in the disease process (Rakoski et al., 2012; Ufere et al., 2020). Ufere et al. (2020) found that after diagnosis of end-stage liver disease, patients and caregivers reported emotional turmoil, delayed illness understanding, caregiver burnout, inability or reduced ability to work, and financial strain. Participants of the study reported that mental health resources, financial hardship resources, a hospital discharge checklist, online resources, and caregiver support all had the potential to ease burden and bring a better quality of life. End-of-life counseling and documenting care wishes is vitally important at this stage of the disease process and may involve the patient if they are cognitively intact enough to participate. If they are not, decisions may be based on their prior stated and/or written wishes or the input of their designated healthcare decision-maker. It is important for the social worker to consider the role of culture, spirituality, and individual patient wishes when engaging the patient and caregiver.

Healthcare providers cannot solely focus on the patient but must also address caregiver needs. Families need education as well, including on the long-term effects and complications that may occur from disease and treatment, as well as in their bereavement. New medications and treatment modalities can be further explored with families or perhaps the cessation of disease-modifying treatment and what that would entail. It is important to evaluate whether the caregiver can provide or make arrangements for necessary care at the end of life and what resources are available. According to the Cleveland Clinic (2019), "Caregiver burnout is a state of physical, emotional and mental exhaustion. Stressed caregivers may experience fatigue, anxiety and depression. Some ways to prevent burnout include joining a caregiver support group and using respite care services" (paras. 1). Burnout can be caused by the emotional demands of caregiving and is often reduced when caregiving is shared with other family members, friends, or hired assistance. Depression among caregivers is also an issue that may be underdiagnosed – perhaps because the caregiver focuses on support of the patient, not themselves.

Terminal stages in kidney and liver diseases can be highly symptomatic and difficult to manage due to the physical consequences of having a kidney or liver shut down. At this stage in the disease process, if outpatient treatment is no longer an option and the patient can no longer live at home, an inpatient hospital or institutional setting may be necessary to manage rapidly shifting and changing symptoms at end of life. Education for the patient and the family must continue, so that they are faced with the available options to move forward in care.

Bereavement

Several factors influence the experience of bereavement when a person with kidney or liver disease dies. The nature of the illness itself (chronic and unpredictable or a sudden crisis) may partially determine how well a family absorbs the reality of what has happened. How much time a patient and their family have to absorb news that they are at the terminal phase of disease also shapes the intensity, complexity, and narrative of bereavement. A study of physicians who provide care to individuals with end-stage liver disease reported that these individuals often receive information on hospice care late in the process, such as during an acute hospitalization or when death is imminent, as opposed to during an earlier period of relative stability (Ufere et al., 2019). More action is needed to provide education and support to patients and caregivers earlier in the disease processes, when it is easier to have meaningful, carefully considered conversations.

When death is sudden, or occurs in an otherwise "shocking" manner, the bereaved may struggle to accept the reality of the loss more. A death may be experienced as shocking when it occurs to a person who seems too young to die; patients with liver disease may face end of life in middle age, when most of their peers are healthy and expecting to live for decades more. The death can cause mental distress, as well as financial hardship for the families involved. This response may be complicated if the patient was suffering from substance use disorder or if the death was hastened due to medical non-adherence, as the bereaved may struggle with feelings of blame and guilt for "why" the death happened. The patient may still have young children, and the impact on the child(ren) must be considered (see Chapter on *Helping Children Cope* for more information). The social worker may provide psychoeducation and resources to families on how to engage with their children about end of life/death.

Social Justice

Social workers should consider in their assessment, advocacy, and intervention strategies the social determinants of health that disproportionately impact marginalized community members (Barcelos Winchester, 2019; Ross & de Saxe Zerden, 2020). Social determinants of health include healthcare access and quality, education access and quality, economic stability, neighborhood and built environment, and social and community context (Brown & Elliott, 2021).

There are health disparities in rates of chronic kidney disease and outcomes when comparing Black and white Americans (Norton et al., 2016). Black Americans are at greater risk for chronic kidney disease due to higher rates of hypertension and diabetes, which have both genetic and socioeconomic causes. Black patients are less likely to be identified as kidney transplant candidates, to be referred to transplant evaluation, to complete such evaluation, and to be placed on a waitlist at a transplant center. These patients even wait longer for a kidney and are less likely to receive a deceased donor kidney. People of color are also less likely to receive a living donor transplant, such as from a family member or close friend (Brown, 2021). To reduce these disparities, social workers may advocate for patients who may be unfairly excluded from transplant consideration; they can provide education to medical teams on *differences* that might otherwise be seen as barriers to successful care and for greater equality of access to, and availability of, resources and supports for patients (see Organ Transplant chapter).

Communities of color and communities with low socioeconomic status disproportionately experience chronic liver disease. Native Americans experience higher mortality rates from alcohol-related liver disease when compared to other ethnic groups. Lack of access to medical care, food insecurity, insecure housing, and poverty play a role in these kinds of health disparities (Kardashian et al., 2021). Disparities in telehealth disproportionately impact older adults and Black adults with liver disease (Wegerman et al., 2022). Hispanic adults have the highest prevalence of non-alcoholic fatty liver disease in the US Education on diet and nutrition and discussions exploring patient access to healthy foods are recommended. Patients should be screened for social determinants of health, provided with substance use and mental health resources if applicable, and offered information on coping skills. Social workers can advocate for more equitable policies on local, state, and federal levels to address social determinants of health (Kardashian et al., 2021). The impact of cost is a factor that must be taken into account. Social workers can help patients utilize benefits provided on a local or national level or through organizations specific to these diseases.

There is a stigma surrounding the connection between substance use and patients affected by liver disease. Patients are sometimes viewed as undeserving of care and blamed for their own health issues. Resistance to understanding substance use disorder as a medical condition persists, with many instead seeing it as an issue of willpower despite the extensive research documenting the intense difficulty of sustaining sobriety even with specialized treatment. This stigma may lead patients and caregivers to be less open in talking about the health issues they are facing. Patients may internalize the judgments of others (Schomerus et al., 2022). Collaboration with a multidisciplinary team and utilizing a flexible, person-centered approach are key for effective engagement (Winder et al., 2020). The ability to pay for services, networking to access services, and social status also play an important role in these dynamics (Barcelos Winchester, 2019).

Patient with Liver Disease

A 52-year-old, Spanish-speaking, Dominican cisgender married male with two young children has presented to the hospital with abdominal pain, after previously being diagnosed with cirrhosis. Upon meeting with the family, the social worker was able to address concerns that were expressed, including the patient's continued alcohol use. In this case, the social worker had assistance from an interpreter. She assessed the patient's current usage, his understanding of the effects of drinking, and his willingness to abstain. Once she ascertained that he was increasingly aware of the costs of his alcohol use, she worked to build his motivation to change by exploring medical and non-medical benefits that mattered to the patient. He said he wanted to stop drinking to have a chance to see his children grow up. She provided handouts in Spanish on substance use treatment and psychoeducation about what to expect. She also provided psychoeducation on mindfulness and grounding techniques to help manage the distress that may arise when ceasing alcohol use. The social worker also provided the man's spouse with information on Al-Anon, a support group meeting for family members and friends of those struggling with addiction.

During the interaction, the patient reported symptoms of depression congruent with his cultural and gender expression, including anger and irritability. The social worker assessed suicidality. He denied suicidal ideation, and no signs or symptoms were observed. The social worker engaged in an exploration of the patient's depressive thoughts and behaviors in reaction to them. After validating his experience and normalizing typical responses to illness, and exploring his history with depressive thoughts and adversity, and internalized views, they began to engage in a plan to shift cognitions and behaviors toward mood-elevating thoughts and activities.

In a separate discussion with the patient's spouse that explored their biggest stressors associated with the patient's illness and care, the social worker learned that they had difficulty securing transportation to appointments and that she was working longer hours because the patient was unable to work. The social worker researched transportation options and benefits; she also explored with the patient's spouse how she was managing her multiple "jobs" and how she could minimize her work or create breaks for herself. Psychoeducation on caregiver burnout was provided as a motivational and preventive measure, to encourage the patient's spouse to prioritize caring for herself as well.[1]

Patient with Kidney Disease

A 63-year-old Caucasian married cisgender woman is diagnosed with end-stage renal disease and encouraged by her nephrologist to continue in-center hemodialysis and pursue transplant candidacy, as this is her best chance of survival. The transplant center determined that this patient is a candidate for kidney transplant. The waitlist for receiving a deceased-donor kidney is several years in this location, and therefore the social worker discusses the option of living-donor kidney donation, with the patient's husband and son as the top choices for a living donor. It can be a challenge involving family in discussions about life expectancy, as there can be a wide range of emotions and reactions to this topic. The patient's son appeared to have the understanding that transplant was his mother's best chance at survival and was willing to begin testing to determine compatibility. The social worker utilized family phone conferences and discussions with the physician to engage and involve the whole family, as well as the medical team, to determine possible outcomes for various options. The social worker also encouraged the patient to take more control of her transplant testing and medical

[1]All names and other personal identifiers in the case are fictitious. Any similarity to actual persons, living or dead, or actual events is purely coincidental.

care, explaining that ultimately it will be up to the patient whether she continues to exhibit compliance with her medication regimen and renal diet, even post-transplant. The patient's son completed the testing, and the center found him to be a proper match for his mother for transplant. After more thought, the patient decided that she could not take her son's kidney, as the guilt was too much for her to carry. The social worker then continued individual therapy with the patient, with a focus on accepting her illness to allow her to grieve the loss of the kidney she had chosen not to accept while also accepting her inevitable future as a dialysis patient.[2]

Authors' Reflections

The diversity of backgrounds and disease experiences make it difficult to adequately prepare a patient with kidney or liver disease to face their challenges. Yet more work can be done to create educational materials and engage with individuals in this disease group. Many patients seem to lose a sense of what to do when faced with the crisis of kidney disease and the different forms of treatments. Education and support are also imperative for patients and families dealing with liver disease. A more comprehensive approach is needed for education on liver disease and kidney disease during hospitalizations and in the outpatient setting. Healthcare providers must reinforce education on the disease process and its effects throughout a patient's course. It may be helpful for patients and families to reflect on what they heard in a medical discussion to ensure that they understand what is being said. Information on mental health providers, behavioral health programs, support groups for patients and caregivers, and organ affiliated associations should be presented to patients and families so they are aware of the different kinds of support available. The caregiver aspect of care should always be addressed in hospital and clinic visits, because caregiver support is an integral component of a patient's medical course. The emotional toll on patients and caregivers can be severe and more structural support in the healthcare system is needed. From a clinician's perspective, the need to continuously educate the patient and families can feel repetitive and, at times, disheartening if the patient does not seem to be absorbing the information or adapting to the newly ordered lifestyle change. Because recovery can be greatly affected by the patient's own self-motivation to improve one's personal health, clinicians in this field may feel a sense of failure or anger toward patients if they do not comply. Additionally, while some patients are experiencing anger and frustration, they may release those emotions onto the social worker or other staff that care for them. While there are difficulties in this field, experiencing the relief and joy after a successful transplant

[2] All names and other personal identifiers in the case are fictitious. Any similarity to actual persons, living or dead, or actual events is purely coincidental.

or recovery of the kidney or liver is what gives the clinicians the hope that their work is meaningful and that change can truly happen for these patients.

Reflection Questions

1. How might patients of color experience kidney and liver diseases differently than white patients? How might this inform your work?
2. How might you respond to a patient who chose to forgo available disease-modifying or managing treatments and instead chose to plan for end of life?
3. What are the biggest challenges in working with this population?

References

Abdul Halain, A., Tang, L. Y., Chong, M. C., Ibrahim, N. A., & Abdullah, K. L. (2022). Psychological distress among the family members of Intensive Care Unit (ICU) patients: A scoping review. *Journal of Clinical Nursing, 31*(5–6), 497–507.

Adelman, R. D., Tmanova, L. L., Delgado, D., Dion, S., & Lachs, M. S. (2014). Caregiver burden: A clinical review. *JAMA, 311*(10), 1052–1060. https://doi.org/10.1001/jama.2014.304

Adisa, O., Jaar, B. G., Masud, T., Sahlie, A., Obadina, C., Ang, J., Lea, J. P., & Plantinga, L. C. (2018). Association of social worker-assessed psychosocial factors with 30-day hospital readmissions among hemodialysis patients. *BMC Nephrology, 19*(1), 360. https://doi-org.proxy.library.nyu.edu/10.1186/s12882-018-1162-4

American Kidney Fund. (2021). *Stages of chronic kidney disease.* https://www.kidneyfund.org/kidney-disease/chronic-kidney-disease-ckd/stages-of-chronic-kidney-diesease/#what-do-the-stages-of-chronic-kidney-disease-ckd-refer-to

American Liver Foundation. (2017). *The progression of liver disease.* https://liverfoundation.org/for-patients/about-the-liver/the-progression-of-liver-disease/#hepatitis-inflammation

Anderson, E., Aldous, A., & Lupu, D. (2018). Make your wishes about you (MY WAY): Using motivational interviewing to foster advance care planning for patients with chronic kidney disease. *Nephrology Nursing Journal, 45*(5), 411–421.

Bajaj, J. S., Wade, J. B., Gibson, D. P., Heuman, D. M., Thacker, L. R., Sterling, R. K., Stravitz, R. T., Luketic, V., Fuchs, M., White, M. B., Bell, D. E., Gilles, H., Morton, K., Noble, N., Puri, P., & Sanyal, A. J. (2011). The multi-dimensional burden of cirrhosis and hepatic encephalopathy on patients and caregivers. *The American Journal of Gastroenterology, 106*(9), 1646–1653. https://doi.org/10.1038/ajg.2011.157. Epub 2011 May 10. PMID: 21556040; PMCID: PMC3989143.

Bansal, A. D., & Schell, J. O. (2018). A practical guide for the care of patients with end-stage renal disease near the end of life. *Seminars in Dialysis, 31*, 170–176.

Barcelos Winchester, S. (2019). Social determinants of health assessment tool: Implications for healthcare practice. *Social Work in Public Health, 34*(5), 395–408. https://doi-org.proxy.library.nyu.edu/10.1080/19371918.2019.1614507

Boehm, L. M., Jones, A. C., Selim, A. A., Virdun, C., Garrard, C. F., Walden, R. L., Wesley Ely, E., & Hosie, A. (2021). Delirium-related distress in the ICU: A qualitative meta-synthesis of patient and family perspectives and experiences. *International Journal of Nursing Studies, 122*, N.PAG. https://doi-org.proxy.library.nyu.edu/10.1016/j.ijnurstu.2021.104030

Brown, J. S. (2021). Addressing the issue: Health disparities and social determinants of health among Blacks/African Americans in comparison to non-minorities with chronic kidney disease. *Nephrology Nursing Journal, 48*(5), 489–492. https://doi.org/10.37526/1526-744X.2021.48.5.489

Brown, J. S., & Elliott, R. W. (2021). Social determinants of health: Understanding the basics and their impact on chronic kidney disease. *Nephrology Nursing Journal, 48*(2), 131–145.

Caplan, M. A., Washington, T. R., & Swanner, L. (2017). Beyond income: A social justice approach to assessing poverty among older adults with chronic kidney disease. *Journal of Gerontological Social Work, 60*(6–7), 553–568. https://doi.org/10.1080/01634372.2017.1344174

Carr, A. (2019). Couple therapy, family therapy and systemic interventions for adult focused problems: The current evidence base. *Journal of Family Therapy, 41*(4), 492–536. https://doi-org.proxy.library.nyu.edu/10.1111/1467-6427.12225

Cervantes, L., Carr, A. L., Welles, C. C., Zoucha, J., Steiner, J. F., Johnson, T., Earnest, M., Camacho, C., Suresh, K., & Hasnain-Wynia, R. (2020). The experience of primary caregivers of undocumented immigrants with end-stage kidney disease that rely on emergency-only hemodialysis. *Journal of General Internal Medicine, 35*(8), 2389–2397. https://doi.org/10.1007/s11606-020-05696-3

Choi, N. G., Sullivan, J. E., DiNitto, D. M., & Kunik, M. (2019). Associations between psychological distress and health-related behaviors among adults with chronic kidney disease. *Preventive Medicine, 126*, 1–7.

Cleveland Clinic. (2019). *Caregiver burnout.* https://my.clevelandclinic.org/health/diseases/9225-caregiver-burnout

Craig, J. A., Miner, D., Remtulla, T., Miller, J., & Zanussi, L. W. (2016). Piloting a coping skills group intervention to reduce depression and anxiety symptoms in patients awaiting kidney or liver transplant. *Health & Social Work, 42*(1), 44–52.

D'amico, C., Garcia-Tsao, G., & Pagliaro, L. (2006). Natural history and prognostic indicators of survival in cirrhosis: A systematic review of 118 studies. *Journal of Hepatology, 44*(1), 217–231. https://doi.org/10.1016/j.jhep.2005.10.013

Davey, C. H., Webel, A. R., Sehgal, A. R., Voss, J. G., & Huml, A. M. (2019). Fatigue in individuals with end stage renal disease. *Nephrology Nursing Journal, 46*(5), 497–508.

Hansen, L., Chang, M. F., Lee, C. S., Hiatt, S., Firsicki, E. J., Dieckmann, N. F., & Lyons, K. S. (2021). Physical and mental quality of life in patients with end-stage liver disease and their informal caregivers. *Clinical Gastroenterology and Hepatology, 19*, 155–161.

Kardashian, A., Wilder, J., Terrault, N. A., & Price, J. C. (2021). Addressing social determinants of liver disease during the COVID-19 pandemic and beyond: A call to action. *Hepatology, 73*, 811–820. https://doi.org/10.1002/hep.31605

Kondo, K., Antick, J. R., Ayers, C. K., Kansagara, D., & Chopra, P. (2020). Depression screening tools for patients with kidney failure. *Clinical Journal of the American Society of Nephrology, 15*(12), 1785–1795. https://doi.org/10.2215/CJN.05540420

Kroll, D. S. (2022). *Caring for patients with depression in primary care.* Springer. https://doi.org/10.1007/978-3-031-08495-9_2

Le Strat, Y., Dubertret, C., & Le Foll, B. (2015). Major depression and suicide attempts in patients with liver disease in the United States. *Liver International, 35*(7), 1910–1916. https://doi-org.proxy.library.nyu.edu/10.1111/liv.12612

Li, P. K., Chow, K. M., Van de Luijtgaarden, M. W., Johnson, D. W., Jager, K. J., Mehrotra, R., Naicker, S., Pecoits-Filho, R., Yu, X. Q., & Lameire, N. (2017). Changes in the worldwide epidemiology of peritoneal dialysis. *Nature Reviews Nephrology, 13*(2), 90–103.

Marlow, N. M., Simpson, K. N., Kazley, A. S., Balliet, W. E., Chavin, K. D., & Baliga, P. K. (2016). Variations in coping stages for individuals with chronic kidney disease: Results from an exploratory study with patient navigators. *Journal of Health Psychology, 21*(7), 1299–1310.

Nair, D., Bonnet, K., Wild, M. G., Umeukeje, E. M., Fissell, R. B., Faulkner, M. L., Bahri, N. S., Bruce, M. A., Schlundt, D. G., Wallston, K. A., & Cavanaugh, K. L. (2021). Psychological adaptation to serious illness: A qualitative study of culturally diverse patients with advanced chronic kidney disease. *Journal of Pain and Symptom Management, 61*(1), 32–41.e2. https://doi.org/10.1016/j.jpainsymman.2020.07.014

National Kidney Foundation. (2006). *Hemodialysis access: What you need to know.* https://www.kidney.org/sites/default/files/11-50-0216_va.pdf

National Kidney Foundation. (2017). *Chronic kidney disease symptoms and causes.* https://www.kidney.org/atoz/content/about-chronic-kidney-disease

Nguyen, D. L., Chao, D., Ma, G., & Morgan, T. (2015). Quality of life and factors predictive of burden among primary caregivers of chronic liver disease patients. *Annals of Gastroenterology, 28*, 124–129.

Norton, J. M., Moxey-Mims, M. M., Eggers, P. W., Narva, A. S., Star, R. A., Kimmel, P. L., & Rodgers, G. P. (2016). Social determinants of racial disparities in CKD. *Journal of the American Society of Nephrology, 27*(9), 2576–2595. https://doi.org/10.1681/ASN.2016010027

Noyes, E. M., & Schlesinger, J. J. (2017). ICU-related PTSD – A review of PTSD and the potential effects of collaborative songwriting therapy. *Journal of Critical Care, 42*, 78–84. https://doi-org.proxy.library.nyu.edu/10.1016/j.jcrc.2017.06.014

O'Hare, A. M., Richards, C., Szarka, J., McFarland, L. V., Showalter, W., Vig, E. K., Sudore, R. L., Crowley, S. T., Trivedi, R., & Taylor, J. S. (2018). Emotional impact of illness and care on patients with advanced kidney disease. *Clinical Journal of the American Society of Nephrology: CJASN, 13*(7), 1022–1029. https://doi.org/10.2215/CJN.14261217

Patel, K., Maguire, E., Chartier, M., Akpan, I., & Rogal, S. (2018). Integrating care for patients with chronic liver disease and mental health and substance use disorders. *Federal Practitioner: For the Health Care Professionals of the VA, DoD, and PHS, 35*(Suppl 2), S14–S23.

Rakoski, M. O., McCammon, R. J., Piette, J. D., Iwashyna, T. J., Marrero, J. A., Lok, A. S., Langa, K. M., & Volk, M. L. (2012). Burden of cirrhosis on older Americans and their families: Analysis of the health and retirement study. *Journal of Hepatology, 55*(1), 184–191. https://doi.org/10.1002/hep.24616

Ross, A. M., & de Saxe Zerden, L. (2020). Prevention, health promotion, and social work: Aligning health and human service systems through a workforce for health. *American Journal of Public Health, 110*, S186–S190. https://doi-org.proxy.library.nyu.edu/10.2105/AJPH.2020.305690

Russ, T. C., Kivimaki, M., Morling, J. R., Starr, J. M., Stamatakis, E., & Batty, G. D. (2015). Association between psychological distress and liver disease mortality: A meta-analysis of individual study participants. *Gastroenterology, 148*(5), 958–966. https://doi.org/10.1053/j.gastro.2015.02.004

Saleh, Z. M., Bloom, P. P., Grzyb, K., & Tapper, E. B. (2021). How do patients with cirrhosis and their caregivers learn about and manage their health? A review and qualitative study. *Hepatology Communications, 5*(2), 168–176.

Salvatore, T. (2020). Self-directed death by ESRD patients: Suicide vs. voluntary termination of hemodialysis. *Public Safety Journal, 2*(1), 10–14.

Schomerus, G., Leonhard, A., Manthey, J., Morris, J., Neufeld, M., Kilian, C., et al. (2022). The stigma of alcohol-related liver disease and its impact on healthcare. *Journal of Hepatology, 77*, 516–524.

Shrestha, D., Rathi, A., Grover, A., Taneja, S., Duseja, A., Chawla, Y., & Dhiman, R. K. (2020). Factors affecting psychological burden on the information caregiver of patients with cirrhosis: Looking beyond the patient. *Journal of Clinical and Experimental Hepatology, 10*(1), 9–16.

Tucker, J. K. (2021). Social justice as a tool to eliminate inequities in kidney disease. *Seminars in Nephrology, 41*(3), 203–210. https://doi.org/10.1016/j.semnephrol.2021.05.001

Ufere, N. N., Donlan, J., Waldman, L., Dienstag, J. L., Friedman, L. S., Corey, K. E., Hashemi, N., Carolan, P., Mullen, A. C., Thiim, M., Bhan, I., Nipp, R., Greer, J. A., Temel, J. S., Chung, R. T., & El-Jawahri, A. (2019). Barriers to use of palliative care and advance care planning discussions for patients with end-stage liver disease. *Clinical Gastroenterology and Hepatology, 17*(12), 2592–2599. https://doi-org.proxy.library.nyu.edu/10.1016/j.cgh.2019.03.022

Ufere, N. N., Donlan, J., Indrioli, T., Richter, J., Thompson, R., Jackson, V., Volandes, A., Chung, R., Traeger, L., & El-Jawahri, A. (2020). Burdensome transitions of care for patients with end-stage liver disease and their caregivers. *Digestive Diseases and Sciences, 66*(9), 2942–2955.

Vaughn-Sandler, V., Sherman, C., & Aronsohn, A. (2014). Consequences of perceived stigma among patients with cirrhosis. *Digestive Diseases and Sciences, 59*, 681–686.

Verma, A., Horrow, J., & Navarro, V. (2019). A behavioral health program for alcohol use disorder, substance abuse, and depression in chronic liver disease. *Hepatology Communications, 3*(5), 646–655.

Volk, M. L. (2020). Burden of cirrhosis on patients and caregivers. *Hepatology Communications, 4*(8), 1107–1111.

Wegermann, K., Wilder, J. M., Parish, A., Niedzwiecki, D., Gellad, Z. F., Muir, A. J., & Patel, Y. A. (2022). Racial and socioeconomic disparities in utilization of telehealth in patients with liver disease during COVID-19. *Digestive Diseases and Sciences, 67*(1), 93–99. https://doi.org/10.1007/s10620-021-06842-5

Winder, G. S., Fernandez, A. C., Klevering, K., & Mellinger, J. L. (2020). Confronting the crisis of comorbid alcohol use disorder and alcohol-related liver disease with a novel multidisciplinary clinic. *Psychosomatics, 61*(3), 238–253. https://doi-org.proxy.library.nyu.edu/10.1016/j.psym.2019.12.004

Chapter 10
Organ Transplant

Marsha Clarke and Chelsea K. Brown

Introduction

The common illness trajectory of organ failure is impacted by the ways in which inequality endangers historically marginalized groups, particularly Black patients in need of life-saving transplantation. Organ transplant is marked by crisis moments, uncertainty and hardship in recovery, and ongoing care post-transplant. Disparities in care and treatment in organ transplantation further challenge patients of color, jeopardizing not only their very survival but also their emotional and psychological welfare. Black people make up 13% of the US population and are overrepresented with end-stage organ diseases. They are less likely to be referred for pre-transplant evaluation, placed on a waitlist, and/or receive a donor organ, yet they account for approximately 30% of candidates for organ transplantation (Russell et al., 2012; Siminoff et al., 2006). Spurred by the disproportionate rates of COVID-19 infections and deaths among Black, Latinx, and other minority groups, experts have sought to engage in more robust critical analysis about the ways in which various social determinants of health affect transplant candidacy, morbidity, and mortality (Purnell et al., 2021). This chapter will share research and literature that supports the need for such analysis and urgent efforts to change the disparities in organ transplant programs.

Critical race theory (CRT) is an academic framework that seeks to critically assess systems and strategize ways of changing institutional policies and practices

M. Clarke (✉)
Emory University Healthcare Hospital, Atlanta, GA, USA
e-mail: Clarkem851@gmail.com

C. K. Brown
Division of Palliative Medicine, University of California, San Francisco, CA, USA
e-mail: Chels5690@gmail.com

M. Hemphill, A. Nathanson (eds.), *The Practice of Clinical Social Work in Healthcare*, Essential Clinical Social Work Series,
https://doi.org/10.1007/978-3-031-31650-0_10

that perpetuate racial disparities (Kolivoski et al., 2014). Social work practice and CRT share similar principles, which include promoting social justice and social change with, and on behalf of, those affected by injustice. Social Work Code of Ethics and its principles need to be applied within transplant practice. It seeks to empower social workers to shift their assessments and interventions toward understanding the nuances of social determinants of health, an essential perspective when presenting psychosocial concerns to larger transplant teams.

The aim of this chapter is to enhance social workers' commitment to social justice in organ transplant with the overall welfare of patients of color in mind, as well as to furnish a better understanding of the psychosocial impacts of the organ transplantation process on all patients. It strives to widen social workers' understanding of healthcare inequities, patient and family distress, the transplant process, and its impact on the overall welfare of individual patients and patient groups of various racial backgrounds. It also discusses the use of evidence-informed social work assessment and intervention tools while encouraging transplant social workers to respond to, and educate about, racial and ethnic inequities in the transplantation community and to engage in dialogue about the difficult ethical and moral dilemmas involved in having to make choices of who is deserving of a limited supply of organ resources. Importantly, social workers can acknowledge and empower other clinicians to recognize that any such scarcity of resources does not exonerate healthcare professionals from accountability in the area of equality and social justice.

Illness: Onset, Course, and Degree of Incapacitation

End-stage organ diseases are among the leading causes of death in the United States, and organ transplants often offer the best possible outcomes. In 2019, more than 106,300 patients were listed on the national transplant waiting list. Of this number, it is estimated that 17 patients die each day while waiting for organ transplantation (HRSA, Organ Donation Statistics, 2019). While organ transplantation offers life extension with the hope for improved quality of life, it is not a cure; even so, it is considered a successful form of alternative treatment that may help patients live 10, 15, or sometimes 20 years longer. Nonetheless, due to the high demand and low supply of organs, candidates often die while waiting for transplant (Wright et al., 2007). With this understanding, it is unsurprising that social workers are called to intervene with a range of psychosocial and existential concerns with this population – from diagnosis through end of life. Social workers support patients facing depression, spiritual distress, and anxiety that comes from seeing oneself as becoming a burden to others (Sher & Maldonado, 2019).

The need for organ transplant can stem from a variety of illness onsets, depending on the specific type of organ failure. Whether the heart, lung, kidney, or liver, the patient's need for organ transplant could be a result of either an acute trauma or a progressive chronic disease. In the acute setting, many patients will be considered for urgent transplant following a cardiac arrest, a motor vehicle accident, or traumatic injury. Conversely, there are various chronic diseases with gradual onset, such as interstitial lung disease, pulmonary hypertension, cirrhosis, or heart failure, which progress over time, eventually leading to the need for transplantation.

Regardless of the onset of organ failure, once a patient has reached this stage of illness, they may be referred by a physician, or self-refer, for transplant consideration (Kuntz et al., 2015). Unfortunately, upon diagnosis of organ failure, not all patient populations are equally likely to be offered the option of organ transplant. For example, Boulware et al. (2021) examined how Black individuals are less likely than white individuals to be referred for kidney transplant. Instead, Black patients experienced biased estimates of their kidney function based on factors such as missed or delayed nephrology care and suboptimal communication with their medical providers, which further impacts their access to transplant.

Organ failure can have an unpredictable course (Wentlandt et al., 2017) and is dependent on several factors: the type of organ injury, whether a patient eventually qualifies for an organ transplant, and whether the patient's body survives with the new organ in the post-transplant setting. Typical examples of progressive organ failure requiring transplant may include heart failure, end-stage renal disease, or pulmonary hypertension, all of which become progressively worse over time. These serious illnesses often reach a point where they no longer respond to daily medication management, and organ transplant then becomes the only remaining life-saving procedure. The waitlist for a transplant is often quite long, sometimes years, and many patients die before an organ is available to them. Organ failure in these patients may quickly progress to a terminal phase (Annema et al., 2017).

Alternatively, if a patient in organ failure is approved for transplant and survives surgery, their life with a new organ transplant may be described as a "constant" course of illness, wherein their organ function has stabilized, and the patient may have many years of acceptable quality of life and low symptom burden, despite the ongoing presence of a serious medical condition. Lastly, even when a patient survives transplant surgery, there are risks of ongoing post-transplant complications, such as "rejection" of their new organ or the inability to tolerate immunosuppressive medications (Wentlandt et al., 2017). The latter course of illness may be categorized as a "relapsing" or "episodic" course of illness, with many ups and downs for the patient and family.

Outcomes following successful transplantation are often inconsistent. Wendtlandt et al. (2017) noted that "transplant introduces risks including perioperative death and other sequelae such as organ rejection, infection, renal insufficiency, and malignancy" (p. 3008). Additionally, cognitive dysfunction and delirium pre- and post-transplant are common and adversely impact post-transplant outcomes. Fatigue, chronic pain, jaundice, edema, and respiratory failure are all typical symptom pictures resulting from suboptimal organ function following a transplant procedure (Sher & Maldonado, 2019). However, when a patient's body can adequately adjust to life with the new organ, symptoms that were bothersome before surgery may resolve, and patients may note that their overall quality of life has improved significantly. It is important to note that even in the setting of a successful transplant, the patient's energy often remains low. The risk of recurrent infections may remain high due to immunosuppressive medications that are used to protect the new organ in the body (Sher & Maldonado, 2019). This immunosuppressed state is particularly noteworthy for its medical and psychosocial aspects in the context of a pandemic like COVID-19.

Clinical Issues of Illness

Crisis

Intrapersonal When a patient first learns that they are at an "end stage" in their organ failure, they may feel shocked and anxious as they contemplate that organ transplant is the only available next step for treatment and survival. Perhaps more frightening is the realization that even with an organ transplant, life-threatening medical complications can ensue. At this stage and severity of illness, patients may experience feelings of guilt around perceived "failure" of previous attempted medical management of their chronic illness, such as oral or intravenous medications, or abandonment due to lack of more available treatment options. Additionally, many patients need an organ transplant in the setting of a diagnosed substance use disorder, and there may be intense feelings of guilt and shame around this life experience. Patients at this stage of organ failure have often already experienced significant loss of physical function and independence, loss of employment, and increasing dependence on others for their care (Annema et al., 2017). In preparing to counsel the patient regarding the option of organ transplant, social workers should begin to build rapport with their patients, explore and align with their patient's experience of the healthcare system thus far, and begin to think about areas of psychosocial concern for transplant candidacy. The social worker should provide counseling around loss of independence and psychoeducation around what it will be like to adjust to life with transplant, as well as formally evaluate the patient's psychosocial readiness for transplantation, if appropriate.

While this period of transplant consideration can be one filled with hope, determining whether a patient is a transplant candidate may also elicit feelings connected with being intruded upon, scrutinized, and personally judged as "appropriateness" for transplant is assessed. Sher and Maldonado (2019) explain:

> The main purpose of pre-transplant psychosocial evaluations is to assess for the presence of psychosocial vulnerabilities that may contribute to treatment nonadherence and diminish post-transplant quality of life and use objective screening tools to identify patients in need of help with psychosocial problems in order to increase the odds of maximizing good outcomes after transplantation… Perhaps most importantly, transplant teams have recognized that there is evidence that multiple psychosocial vulnerabilities or the "additive effect" of concerns has a "predictive value" of post-transplant complications, "which may then affect the patient's quality of life and the ultimate graft survival." (p. 23)

Common psychosocial assessment tools used by transplant social workers include the Transplant Evaluation and Rating Scale (TERS), the Psychosocial Assessment of Candidates for Transplantation (PACT), and most recently, the Stanford Integrated Psychosocial Assessment for Transplantation (SIPAT) (Kuntz et al., 2015). The specific psychosocial assessment tool used by the social worker is determined by the transplant program in question. Though the assessment tools vary, they all include assessment of the patient's cultural, spiritual, and ethnic background, mental health and substance use history, social support structure, financial picture, and understanding of illness. Although Sher and Maldonado (2019) describe transplant assessment tools as "objective" determinants of transplant candidacy (p. 23), additional scholars have recently raised concerns regarding this objectivity. For example, Boulware et al. (2021) provide evidence that both the medical and psychosocial evaluations used for the kidney transplant work-up process disadvantage Black patients. In particular, this disadvantage is driven by the use of racialized eGFR equations and "strict socio-contextual criteria for assessing transplant suitability" that are "compounded by overarching structural inequities, including Black individuals' limited access to healthcare…inadequate decision support, financial barriers, and logistical challenges to completing transplant evaluations" (p. 2). Bui et al. (2019) have also highlighted that despite attempts for standardized tools to introduce objectivity, transplant evaluations are inherently subjective, in that the interviewer is not immune to unconscious biases regarding patient behaviors and life experiences.

The social worker should keep social determinants of health and internal biases in mind when concluding their evaluation of psychosocial "readiness" for transplant, as well as providing clinical recommendations for steps that the patient and caregivers can take to improve readiness for transplant. In the process of completing a psychosocial evaluation, patients often struggle to identify barriers to managing their care or determining their level of readiness for life with a transplant.

In these circumstances, it is crucial that the transplant social worker be versed in motivational interviewing techniques to determine readiness for transplant, as well as to identify strategies to address barriers to, and facilitators for engagement with, medical care (Kuntz et al., 2015). Motivational interviewing, though initially developed for assessing and intervening with substance use behaviors, has also been adapted as a brief intervention or "communication style" to address ambivalence toward various types of behavior change (Sher & Maldonado, 2019). Utilizing motivational interviewing skills including open-ended questions, affirmations, reflective listening, and summarizing – sometimes referred to as "OARS" – allows the social worker to identify areas of resistance to engagement with care, generate motivation for transplant, and formulate a plan of action for change (Sher & Maldonado, 2019).

After all transplant clinicians have completed their respective evaluations of the patient, a committee of various disciplines (physicians, social workers, nurses, pharmacists, and financial counselors) come together to determine whether the patient is a candidate for organ transplant; this group of providers is often called a Transplant Selection Committee (Sher & Maldonado, 2019). When patients are being evaluated by this committee, their candidacy is often categorized as "approved," "deferred," or "denied." To reach a decision regarding candidacy, transplant clinicians often categorize patient behaviors within the healthcare system as "adherent," "nonadherent," or "non-compliant." If a Black patient receives a label such as "non-compliant," this typically results in an identified "psychosocial barrier" to transplant candidacy.

In response to this designation, it is important for the social worker to recognize and advocate for awareness that these labeled "behaviors" are highly stigmatizing and often lack nuance regarding the psychological, environmental, or structural barriers to participation in care that can stem from social determinants of health. It is the social worker's responsibility to advocate to their Transplant Selection Committee about the impact of these environmental, cultural, and social circumstances and to raise awareness about where there might be space for the social work clinician to work closely with the patient to reduce these barriers and improve candidacy. During this evaluation period, the social worker's role is crucial for supportive counseling, psychoeducation, and optimizing physical, emotional, and mental well-being of patients in preparation for transplant candidacy. The social worker's interventions should be targeted to reducing psychosocial barriers, identifying strengths and protective factors for coping and participation in care, and improving candidacy wherever possible.

Certain psychosocial issues that frequently present as barriers to transplant candidacy require social work support and intervention. For example, a patient who has end-stage alcohol-related cirrhosis with ongoing alcohol use would be immediately declined for transplant candidacy, given risk of continued injury to the transplanted liver. In this situation, the social worker's response to the team should include (1) completing a full substance use assessment, (2) assessing motivation for cessation, and (3) outlining steps to improve candidacy, such as specific expectations for participation in cessation treatments for a period prior to re-evaluation for transplant (e.g., 6 months of no alcohol consumption, biweekly toxicology screens, and weekly participation in a culturally congruent treatment program, such as Alcoholics Anonymous meetings).

Interpersonal Caregivers who are already providing extensive support and care are often stressed further by the short- and long-term demands of transplant. It's important to note that the social support and caregiving requirements for transplant candidacy generally place a much greater burden on families experiencing poverty and limited community resources (Purnell et al., 2021). For example, requiring a 24/7 caregiver post-transplant and attendance at regular medical follow-ups necessitates caregivers taking significant time off work and enjoying a certain level of financial security. Additionally, some transplant programs require the patient and their designated caregiver to relocate within a certain distance of the transplant center for a specific period of time. This can prove difficult for families with limited resources and multigenerational caregiving responsibilities (Yagelniski et al., 2020). Transplant social workers can pair families with appropriate peer support groups, help families navigate and address the need for time off of work, assist with accessing childcare resources, and identify local lodging options for immediate post-transplant caregiving needs, all functions that help alleviate disproportionate burden (Yagelniski et al., 2020).

During the transplant evaluation process, the social worker is often the "go-to" clinician for counseling on the importance of self-care for caregivers, particularly when caregiver fatigue is noted (Kuntz et al., 2015). As family system concerns arise during the transplant evaluation, it is the social worker's responsibility to identify, counsel, and offer resources to maximize patient transplant candidacy and minimize family distress. One of the crucial social work interventions during this crisis phase is providing psychoeducation to patients and families about the transplantation process and post-transplant caregiving requirements (Sher & Maldonado, 2019). Providing this education and guidance empowers the patient and caregiving unit to be better prepared to meet the requirements, request time off work for caregiving, and equip the home to aid physical recovery and overall healing for a physically and emotionally arduous process.

Systems of Care Unfortunately, despite universal recognition of the importance of optimizing pre-transplant psychosocial conditions for patients with end-stage organ failure, there are no national standards for psychosocial assessment and social work assessment tools continue to vary by individual transplant program (Kuntz et al., 2015). The lack of standardization and internal bias of clinicians completing psychosocial assessments has led to "a high degree of variability among transplant programs across the United States" (Sher & Maldonado, 2019, p. 19). As our field of social work is acutely aware, with variability and inconsistency often comes risk for increased healthcare disparity. For example, a 2021 study found that "Black individuals were 25% less likely to be waitlisted [than white individuals], even after adjusting for medical factors and social determinants of health" (Wesselman et al., 2021, p. 262). Transplant experts have highlighted that, overall, Black patients are disproportionately harmed by being less likely to be urgently referred to transplant specialists for evaluation and, eventually, less likely to be thought of as "appropriate" transplant candidates (Boulware et al., 2021).

It is incumbent upon transplant social workers to recognize interpersonal and structural racism, xenophobia, and discrimination that prevents patients with various intersectional identities from being considered for a life-saving transplant. For example, social workers have the training and expertise to complete careful assessments that recognize the environmental and socioeconomic conditions that limit a patient's ability to attend medical appointments successfully – a criterion that often influences a patient's transplant candidacy – and should strive to address them thoroughly with the patient, team, and institutional representatives. Transplant social workers can work with the patient to ensure that appointment attendance is feasible; they can rectify misconceptions and biases within their evaluation teams and aim to schedule appointments with the patient's life circumstances in mind; they can advocate at policy and national levels to analyze, evaluate, and improve our approach to determining whether a patient is "psychosocially appropriate" for organ transplant. Social workers can also advocate for transplant programmatic training that includes cultural humility, as well as trauma-informed care at all levels of the transplant evaluation process (Kuntz et al., 2015).

The following case study highlights how implicit biases may impact a patient's evaluation outcomes for liver transplant candidacy. Please note the names and patient demographics in the case vignettes are changed to protect their privacy.

Shiye is a 32-year-old cisgender, a straight man with a history of hepatic cirrhosis and major depressive disorder (MDD). He is alert and oriented to person, place, and time with no impairments in mental functioning. He identifies as Dakota Sioux and lives with his father and siblings. Shiye was recently informed that his liver disease has advanced to end stage and that the only remaining life-prolonging intervention is to pursue a liver transplant. The hepatologist refers Shiye to the University Hospital's Liver Transplant Center so that he can begin the "work-up" process for transplant.

After learning about the risks and benefits of transplant surgery, Shiye consents to move forward with being evaluated for candidacy. Over the next 2 weeks, he is scheduled to meet with a transplant coordinator, a transplant surgeon, a financial counselor, a dietician, and a social worker. Although Shiye is quickly approved for transplant from a medical perspective, he feels worried that certain members of the transplant team may think that he is not "psychologically ready" for transplant. His social worker, Meredith, raises concern for his history of MDD, highlighting that the transplant and recovery process can be invasive and overwhelming at times, which could trigger a difficult depressive episode. Meredith recommends that Shiye meet with the transplant psychiatrist for additional evaluation.

Shiye's visit with the transplant psychiatrist felt frustrating. Though it was clear that the psychiatrist was competent in understanding Shiye's history of MDD, he did not agree with the psychiatrist's recommendations to initiate psychotherapy or consider anti-depression medication. Shiye then learned from the transplant coordinator that if he did not demonstrate an effort to engage in psychotherapy, he may be disqualified as a transplant candidate. Shiye immediately requested to speak with the transplant social worker to voice his frustration.

As Meredith and Shiye spoke, he was able to explain that he had his own spiritual and communal approach to managing his depressive symptoms. He spoke about his reliance on prayer to his ancestors, smudging, and participating in purification rituals or "sweating." He described feeling well-supported by his family and Dakota Sioux community with these practices. He noted that these rituals had helped to decrease his symptoms of depression. Shiye emphasized that he did not wish to discuss his emotions with a therapist and stated that he felt strongly that this was a "white person's preference." He expressed concern that this preference could disqualify him from transplant; he also expressed anger that the psychiatrist did not engage him in a fuller exploration of intervention options, which made him inaccurately appear resistant to any intervention at all.

The following week, Meredith prepared to attend the weekly Transplant Selection Committee meeting where Shiye's candidacy would be determined. As Shiye's case was discussed, several physicians and the psychiatrist emphasized their discomfort with approving Shiye for transplant unless he was willing to engage in mental health treatment. Meredith was able to use her advocacy and psychoeducation skills to talk with her colleagues about assumptions and biases that the group may be holding when defining "appropriate" and "effective" mental health treatment. She reminded her team that their conception of this should be congruent with the patient's cultural, racial, and spiritual background. She was able to articulate how Shiye's Dakota Sioux communal and spiritual practices had led to a significant decrease in his depressive symptoms. Although the Transplant Selection Committee was initially hesitant to approve Shiye out of concern for his post-transplant coping, most providers eventually voiced their recognition of Shiye's motivation to address mental health issues and readiness for transplant, as well as his strengths and protective factors (such as his current spiritual and communal mental health practices) that could mitigate the possible barrier of increased depression in the post-transplant setting. Meredith was also able to serve as a mediator between Shiye's cultural preferences and the Transplant Selection Committee's concerns, offering to meet again with Shiye to establish a plan for management of depressive symptoms that is aligned with his communal and spiritual practices. With Shiye's permission, Meredith was able to connect with a spiritual leader from Shiye's community to establish a supportive care plan for his post-transplant recovery. Over the next 2 weeks, Meredith was able to report back to her transplant team that Shiye had agreed to: (1) meet biweekly with his community leader for support around adjustment to life with transplant, as well as continued discussion regarding effectiveness of his spiritual and communal practices for coping and (2) join the organ transplant support group, which met once a month, for ongoing support.[1]

Chronic

Intrapersonal Once a patient has begun the recovery process post-transplant, they begin to adjust to their life with a new organ. Issues such as anticipatory anxiety related to rejection of the new organ are common; more specifically, patients living with transplant may experience a sense of "burnout" from the need to attend frequent medical appointments and observe strict medication regimens to maintain the new organ's function in the body. Even when the body is well-adjusted to life with a transplanted organ, there can be fear and anxiety around the potential side effects from immunosuppressive medications, such as risk for cancer (Sher & Maldonado, 2019). In addition to coping with a chronic condition, patients often find their identity and relationships with friends and family are affected by the demands of chronic

[1] All names and other personal identifiers in the case are fictitious. Any similarity to actual persons, living or dead, or actual events is purely coincidental.

illness, including limited time to socialize without consideration of appointments, diet restrictions, and medication regimes. The net effect of these experiences can be a feeling of being "over-medicalized" and more like a "patient" than a "person" (Michaud et al., 2019).

Although all patients may struggle with challenges around medication adherence, or anxiety related to rejection or graft failure, young adults may face additional challenges associated with the individuating self and reaching specific milestones – graduating school, moving out of their childhood home, and achieving other symbolic and actual markers of independence. In thinking about how to address the psychosocial needs of adolescents and young adults living with transplant, Michaud et al. (2019) studied how to maximize adherence and quality of life in the post-transplant setting. They hypothesized that increased opportunity for autonomy, a sense of competence, and relating to others were key to maintaining motivation for adherence and optimal functioning following transplant for young adults (Michaud et al., 2019).

Social workers often play an important role in supporting adolescents and young adults living with transplant, particularly when they are transitioning out of pediatric care toward adult transplant clinics. The transplant social worker is key to providing guidance to newly adult patients about the differences between pediatric and adult clinics, including reduced frequency of visits, reduced reminders for lab tests and medication refills, and in many cases, fewer internal resources for psychosocial and spiritual support (Michaud et al., 2019). This transition from a pediatric clinic to an adult clinic requires increased autonomy and independence with managing care; the social worker can empower young adult patients during this time of transition by providing counseling and education around how to independently navigate issues such as employment, intimacy, and mental health management. These are issues that all young adults must journey through, but that can be particularly challenging in the setting of living with chronic disease for many years.

For patients of all ages, receiving support, psychoeducation, and therapeutic connection from a clinical social worker makes an essential difference. Within the post-transplant clinic, social workers can assist with a variety of issues, such as access to medication, assessing and intervening with ongoing motivation for adherence to treatment plans after transplant, mental health concerns, and addressing barriers to care that may arise, such as financial concerns or loss of insurance. For patients who do experience feelings of depression, anxiety, and/or loss of identity, social workers can provide therapeutic interventions, including general counseling services that promote emotional catharsis and cognitive examination and challenging, referrals to psychotherapy, or coaching on mind-body relaxation techniques (Kuntz et al., 2015).

Interpersonal The lifelong commitment of caring for an organ transplant has a profound impact not only on the patient but also on their caregiver system. In the immediate post-transplant period, caregivers are needed for 24/7 support with medication management, activities of daily living, and frequent medical appointments. Understandably, these intense care requirements may lead to what has been described as "caregiver strain" or "caregiver burnout," which may include experiences of fatigue, feelings of overwhelm or depression, and issues related to chronic financial insecurity that extend beyond transplant surgery and depend on the patient's ability to recover (Yagelniski et al., 2020). The social worker can help alleviate this burden by providing psychoeducation on essential self-care practices and resources on caregiver support groups, counseling services, and psychotherapy resources when needed.

Systems of Care One of the reasons living with transplant can be so strenuous is that patients and their caregivers must interface with multiple (often fragmented) systems. Living with transplant requires close follow-up with insurance companies, employers, and multiple healthcare specialists. Because of the unpredictable medical course of organ failure and transplantation, patients' functional status and symptom burden may vacillate between disabled and able-bodied. These fluctuations in well-being can lead to confusion around sources of income and, in some situations, loss of insurance. As such, patients and caregivers must learn to be attuned to the nuances of employment, insurance, and changes to benefits. Both hospital and clinic social workers can assist patients and families with navigating these various systems. Social workers are skilled at understanding and accessing multiple services, such as employment and insurance benefits, prescription assistance, and community resources that may aid in managing long-term care needs.

Purnell et al. (2021) have asserted that the fragmented nature of these systems is particularly amplified for Black patients and families. Researchers have identified racial disparities in the transplant community that disproportionately affect Black individuals with regard to employment, access to health insurance, access to specialty care coordination, and access to culturally and linguistically appropriate treatment decision support. For the most part, there are also likely similar rates and experiences for other groups such as Latinx and Native American populations (Purnell et al., 2021; Kuntz et al., 2015). These issues can engender feelings of mistrust toward the healthcare system, reduce ability to participate in follow-up care, and ultimately increase medical complications and poorer health outcomes (Purnell et al., 2021). Social workers should consider systemic and policy advocacy efforts that can be implemented to address transplant inequities across system levels. These efforts may include involvement in quality or process improvement within their own healthcare system, legislative and lobbying efforts for barriers to employment and benefit access, and education to colleagues, teammates, and healthcare institutions about these inequities and the impact on healthcare outcomes.

Terminal

In 2019, over 106,300 patients were listed on the national transplant waiting list, with at least 17 patients dying each day (Health Resources and Services Administration [HRSA], Organ Donation Statistics, 2019). Many of these patients died waiting for transplant and without having goals of care communication with their physician (Santivasi et al., 2017). Medical decline is often rapid, with multi-system organ failures and impaired decision-making becoming a factor. Caregivers are often placed in the difficult position of having to make substitute judgments about aggressive treatment versus comfort-focused care in the setting of medical futility. The social worker's role includes being sensitive to the emotional, spiritual, physical, and psychological trauma associated with impending death. The proactive social worker engages, explores, and actively listens to patients' and caregivers' existential concerns and provides psychosocial support. This support seeks to humanize the patient's existential suffering. Social workers collaborate and coordinate goals of care interdisciplinary meetings to ensure that patient/caregiver voices and care preferences are central to the plan of care. Social workers' facilitation of a patient-centered approach affirms the patient's dignity particularly during the dying phase. Such end-of-life (EOL) interventions and care decisions may help to facilitate a "good death" for terminally ill patients. According to the American Institute of Medicine's definition, a good death is free from avoidable distress and suffering, for patients, family members, and healthcare providers, is in general accordance with patient and family members' wishes, and is reasonably consistent with clinical, cultural, and ethical standards.

It is important that healthcare practitioners initiate early communication with patients about their EOL care preference, preferably at the time of placement on the transplant list. Early EOL care communication is viewed as significant to the patient's overall treatment management (Wright et al., 2007).

Intrapersonal The journey to transplantation is often fraught with dread related to psychosocial challenges and quality-of-life concerns. This dread can be the foundation of psychosocial stress and stressors caused by deterioration in health. Psychosocial stressors may include, but are not limited to, death anxiety, anticipatory grief, financial hardship, shifts in roles, interpersonal struggles with relationship changes, and loss of dignity and identity through diminishing ability to participate in life as one once did. Social workers' command of the biopsychosocial assessment and applications of evidence-informed practices are essential to bolstering patients', and their caregivers', healthy coping. Social workers utilize core clinical modalities, such as individual, group, family, psychoeducation, and cognitive behavioral techniques to help patients and their caregivers manage intense feelings of anxiety, fear, sadness, and helplessness, thus restoring a return of their homeostasis and/or a move from denial of being at EOL to acceptance (Sher & Maldonado, 2019). Social workers should also be able to assess for and intervene with trauma responses that are triggered at this stage, such as feelings of horror, powerlessness, dissociation, and hyperarousal.

When goals of care communications are patient-centered, patients are helped toward preserving a sense of dignity at EOL. Noteworthy for the transplant social worker is Harvey Chochinov's work on Dignity Therapy, which focuses on facilitating terminally ill patients' self-reflection to promote a sense of generativity instead of stagnation, a sense of meaning instead of crisis and loss alone. Dignity Therapy may help patients to address unfinished business and help patients preserve their personhood, which may be eroded through the indignities of illness. These struggles may be especially numerous and marked for the transplant patient who has undergone arduous treatment and surgery without successful outcome. Existential distress or psychosocial concerns are common experiences for patients, even more so than physical symptoms and pain (Chochinov et al., 2005), which are unfortunately common for transplant patients with failing organs. Poor communication around goals of care is believed to contribute to more suffering for patients and their caregivers. To prevent this for the transplant patient, social workers may act as mediators and translators in goals of care discussions, ensuring that communications are clear and understood. Good "bedside manner," which comes with self-awareness and sensitivity to patient/caregiver reactions, can also be encouraged among the medical team by the social worker.

Patients'/caregivers' angst about whether they will live until a transplant becomes available is often distressing. The degree to which patients can cope with such uncertainty can correlate with their resilience and mental health overall. Efforts should be made to link patients and caregivers with appropriate treatment and preventative resources if serious mental health disturbances emerge at this time.

Interpersonal Patients awaiting transplant can be called on at a moment's notice. As such, they are encouraged to live close to the hospital, a medical imperative that brings with it disruption and added financial burden. Other psychological stressors include patients/caregivers being aware that someone has to die in order for them to receive an organ. Such a reality is difficult to reconcile with one's overall sense of self and can induce guilt. *How can I, a caring person, wish for an accident to happen?* Patients/caregivers may be aware that receiving a transplant is necessary and life-saving, an awareness that can bring with it angst from simultaneously *wanting* and *not wanting* an organ to be available.

Social work perspectives and approaches offer much for patients/caregivers grappling with treatment ambivalence and the indignities of transplantation. Social work's assessment of practical needs and working knowledge of hospital and community resources helps a person overcome barriers to care associated with lack of resources. In addition, social work can help overcome ambivalence by identifying patient values and care preferences and counseling people facing emotional hardship and difficulty adjusting to, and coping with, failing health.

Systems of Care Goals of care communication may be difficult for the provider, who may not be comfortable discussing related topics with the patient, feel afraid to unwittingly cause harm to the patient, or struggle with facing the failure of care. Patients and caregivers, meanwhile, may show resistance or welcome to discourse around EOL, depending on various factors including treatment and illness history and family cohesion and closeness. For all these reasons, goals of care communication can be complicated, rife with fear and strong emotion, and incomplete or unsuccessful in putting patients' and caregivers' minds at ease with clear instructions and guidelines around important items like execution of wills, making funeral arrangements, and closing bank accounts. Psychological and emotional well-being can also be promoted by EOL discussions directed by the social worker that focus on self-reflection, life review, explorations of meaning and purpose, experiences of self-love and love of others, emotional closure with family/friends, and reconciling with the past or developing an integrated narrative about the past (Byock, 1996).

Bereavement

It is important that social workers have a healthy attitude toward death and dying, especially their own, and a strong grasp of the sociocultural context of death and dying, as well as the bereavement process and stages of grief. Rando (1984) notes that grief is defined as a psychological, social, and somatic response to a perceived loss. Social workers' understanding and recognition of the elements of grief allow for thoughtful assessment and appropriate interventions to support bereaved families. The death of a patient can be disruptive to caregivers' homeostasis, as they have lost not only the person they cared for but also their work, normal routine, identity as a caregiver, and more. The grief process often begins with a sense of shock and disbelief, a stunned and incredulous reaction that may be an attempt to self-protect from overwhelming feelings of loss and pain. It is often followed by awareness of the reality of death, which may be especially difficult to face in transplant, as *what if* questions dominate: *What if he had stopped drinking earlier? What if he had agreed to be assessed for transplant earlier? What if there was a better match available?*

The unpredictable nature of the transplantation process may make grief both difficult to anticipate and difficult to reconcile. Efforts toward anticipatory preparation for loss may be challenged by the acute-on-chronic (acute decline after long-term chronic disease) nature of decline. It is important that social workers understand the psychological impact of the circumstances of the illness and resulting death and dying on caregivers of deceased transplant patients. This includes the deceased donor and the living donor caregivers and the need to extend bereavement services to them. Death and dying in transplantation can be complicated for caregivers of the deceased donor as well, as they may re-experience the trauma of the patient's death for a second time. Caregivers of a deceased donor often consent to donation hoping the patient will live on. As such, bereavement support can be very helpful with mitigating such re-traumatization caused by the death. Bereavement support may also be necessary to some of these families as they work through complicated grief and find meaning through their loss (Wright et al., 2007).

Social Justice

To maintain a commitment to social justice, the social worker must navigate between a dual allegiance to their code of ethics and their position with a social services organization or healthcare facility. The code of ethics emphasizes the importance of social workers' advocacy role against social injustice and discriminatory practices and policies. It advocates the social worker's respect and value for every individual and their cultural context. Institutional and systemic racism is a formidable force that may prevent social workers from being adequately and ethically able to do their jobs. Critical race theory (CRT) provides a framework that concretizes this commitment, providing a lens through which to recognize, analyze, and change power dynamics that maintain institutional racism and reinforce racial inequality.

Social services organizations may demonstrate, in their daily operations, connections between institutional racism and internalized/interpersonal racism, apparent in their hiring and retention practices and through the focus and limits of their work and practice. Examples include discriminatory staffing patterns and policies toward patients and theoretical biases that pathologize patients, families, and communities (which may, in the case of transplant patients, result in exclusion from transplant candidacy and a chance to survive). It is the responsibility and obligation of social workers to document patterns of discrimination in their place of employment, present the findings to their supervisors, and advocate for individual patients and for policy change when disparity and injustice are seen. Only through sustained and intentional efforts to become an anti-racist organization can social services go beyond token or symbolic measures to disrupt racism (Miller & Garran, 2009).

Transparency and the ethical promotion of equity and fairness in transplantation are crucial to promoting wellness for all patients. Currently, Black patients have less chance of getting well from organ failure than their white counterparts. Despite the clear need for greater equity, it has remained elusive. While there continue to be advances in reducing overt racism and discrimination (such as increased focus on *access to care* for patients), covert and institutional policies and practices continue to systematically reflect racial inequalities in healthcare delivery to Black people. Black people and other minority transplant candidates continue to suffer the painful indignities, and sometimes deadly consequences, of medical neglect (Kolivoski et al., 2014).

"We Are Done Dying" is the title of a national campaign of coordinated efforts to redress historical and current social injustices imposed on Black people. The campaign's contract demands include calls for access to quality healthcare and solutions for the challenging economic realities that sustain social determinants that trap many Black people in an often inescapable cycle of poverty and poor health. How does this appear in transplant? The answer: with skewed assessments and unchecked, subjective determinations of transplant candidacy, as well as in a lack of support that can result in racial disparities in mortality rates and health-related quality-of-life concerns for Black people and other minority groups. This is part of a substantial history of incidents of medical abuse of Black people (Purnell et al., 2021).

Black people's distrust of the healthcare system is caused by well-documented disparity and abuse. Wells and Gowda's (2020) Legacy of Distrust article discussed level of education to be a predictor of such distrust, i.e., it is particularly an issue among Black people with high school education or less; they are less supportive of organ donation and less likely to consent to organ donation. However, even when controlling for education level, being Black remains a predictor of distrust. The literature has also identified some of the underlying contributing factors that may be related to discriminatory care practices. They include, but are not limited to, distrust and poor communication between white medical professionals and Black patients. Trust facilitates care-seeking behavior and promotes patient transparency and adherence to treatment. Distrust of the healthcare system impedes care-seeking behavior, which compromises access to medical care. In a cyclical way, this puts Black patients and other marginalized groups at further risk of receiving lower-quality care (Wells & Gowda, 2020).

Because of Black patients' lived experiences, they may present with a lack of awareness about the transplant process, unaddressed religious myths and misperceptions about donation, distrust of the medical community, fear of premature declaration of their death for donations, and racism that justifies exclusion from needed treatment. A CRT framework exposes the cyclical nature of racism in healthcare and advocates for care to be equitable across racial groups. Social determinants of health are created by limited resources and the systematic racism that causes them; ill health restricts Black people and other minority groups from fully participating in all aspects of society (education, income, housing, and access to adequate healthcare) and perpetuates gaps in opportunity and resources. Social work practice in transplant, as in anywhere in the field, requires cultural sensitivity, humility, and responsiveness and acknowledgment and understanding of cultural identity, the unique history of enslavement, and the continuing impact of living in an environment of oppression, racism, and gross inequalities. Social workers must embrace a strength-based approach that seeks to empower individuals in seeking solutions to existential concerns and issues. Social workers must sustain and access support systems of import, such as a family's places of worship, schools, and community programs. At the macro level, social workers seek to intervene in policy planning, advocacy, and administration (Logan, 2009). Social workers must strive to continually assess interpersonal and internalized values and conceptualize racism's impact on our patients' or clients' access to quality healthcare. It is not enough to just observe the racial inequalities in healthcare. Social workers have to be ready to make calls to action, promoting anti-racist discussion and policy changes in line with equitable care (Purnell et al., 2021).

Author's Reflections

The psychology of illness is universal, but the emotional and physical burden of it is often greater for Black patients. Social workers' perspectives, supported by the NASW's code of ethics, show that it is imperative to address racial health disparities for Black people and other minority groups. They face numerous prejudicial challenges that compound the overwhelming feelings accompanying the diagnostic process. Barriers to care include the spectrum of social determinants of health and distrust of the healthcare system based on its historical practices of medical abuse/neglect of Black people and other minority groups. These practices include the perpetuation of systemic structural and institutional racism through policy and practices that pathologize and covertly exclude Black people and other minority groups from quality healthcare access. Black people typically have the worst medical outcomes, regardless of whether their disease is early or advanced at diagnosis. As a clinician of color, I have experience, too many well-intended practitioners including social workers acquiesce to problematic and biased mandates from the institution they work for, which might support their own unrecognized bias. As social workers, we need to reflect on our interpersonal and internalized values and practices in the context of race to ensure no unintentional harm is done to patients. We must consistently document and advocate for policy changes that recognize equity and equality for racially marginalized patients. Our code of ethics affords us a great guide in which we can re-read and ensure our personal and professional values are aligned with it. Advocating against social injustice, such as structural and institutional racism, is complex. We can start with one person, and that person is ourselves, as we seek to empower and enhance patients and their caregivers' quality of life – M. C.

Reflection Questions

1. How might you work with a patient experiencing the uncertainty and anxiety of waiting for an organ transplant?
2. In what ways do social determinants of health (SDOH) impact the experience of organ transplant?
3. What would be the biggest challenges for you in working with this population?

References

Annema, C., Roodbol, P. F., Van den Heuvel, E. R., Metselaar, H. J., Van Hoek, B., Porte, R. J., & Ranchor, A. V. (2017). Trajectories of anxiety and depression in liver transplant candidates during the waiting-list period. *British Journal of Health Psychology, 22*, 481–501.

Boulware, L. E., Purnell, T. S., & Mohottige, D. (2021). Systemic kidney transplant inequities for black individuals: Examining the contribution of racialized kidney function estimating equations. *JAMA Network Open*. https://doi.org/10.1001/jamanetworkopen.2020.34630

Bui, Q. M., Allen, L. A., LeMond, L., Brambatti, M., & Adler, E. (2019). Psychosocial evaluation of candidates for heart transplant and ventricular assist devices. *Circulation. Heart Failure*. https://doi.org/10.1161/circheartfailure.119.006058

Byock, I. R. (1996). The nature of suffering and the nature of opportunity at the end of life. *Clinics in Geriatric Medicine, 12*(2), 237–251.

Chochinov, H. M., Hack, T., Kristjanson, L. J., McClemont, S., & Harlos, M. (2005). Dignity therapy: A novel psychotherapeutic intervention for patients near the end of life. *Journal of Clinical Oncology, 23*(24), 5520–5525.

Health Resources and Services Administration, Organ Donation Statistics. (2019). www.organdonor.gov

Kolivoski, K. M., Weaver, A., & Constance-Huggins, M. (2014). Critical race theory: Opportunities for application in social work practice and policy. *Families in Society: The Journal of Contemporary Social Services, 95*(4), 269–276.

Kuntz, K., Weinland, S. R., & Butt, Z. (2015). Psychosocial challenges in solid organ transplantation. *Journal of Clinical Psychology in Medical Settings, 22*, 122–135.

Logan, S. M. L. (2009). Social work practice with African Americans. In A. R. Roberts & G. J. Green (Eds.), *Social worker's desk reference* (2nd ed., p. 963). Oxford University Press.
Michaud, V., Achille, M., Chainey, F., Phan, V., Girardin, C., & Clermont, M. J. (2019). Mixed-methods evaluation of a transition and young adult clinic for kidney transplant recipients. *Pediatric Transplantation, 23*, 1–14.
Miller, J., & Garran, A. M. (2009). The legacy of racism for social work practice today and what to do about it. In A. R. Roberts & G. J. Greene (Eds.), *Social worker's desk reference* (2nd ed., pp. 928–933). Oxford University Press.
Purnell, T. S., Simpson, D. C., Callender, C. O., & Boulware, L. E. (2021). Dismantling structural racism as a root cause of racial disparities in COVID-19 and transplantation. *American Journal of Transplantation, 21*(7), 2327–2332.
Rando, T. A. (1984). Grief, dying and death: Clinical interventions for caregivers. Champaign, IL: Research Press Co. *Journal of Community Health, 37*(1), 3740–3747.
Russell, E., Robinson, D. H. Z., Thompson, N. J., Perryman, J. P., & Arriola, K. R. J. (2012). Distrust in Healthcare system and organ donation intentions among African Americans. *Journal of Community Health, 37*, 40–47.
Santivasi, W. L., Strand, J. J., Mueller, P. S., & Beckman, T. J. (2017). The organ transplant imperative. *Mayo Clinic Proceedings, 92*(6), 940–946.
Sher, Y., & Maldonado, J. R. (2019). *Psychosocial care of end-stage organ disease and transplant patients*. Springer.
Siminoff, L. A., Burant, C. J., & Ibrahim, S. A. (2006). Racial disparities in preferences and perceptions regarding organ donations. *Journal of General Internal Medicine, 21*(9), 995–1000.
Wells, L., & Gowda, A. (2020). Legacy of mistrust: African Americans and the US healthcare system. *Proceedings of UCLA Health, 24*, 1–3.
Wentlandt, K., Weiss, A., O'Connor, E., & Kaya, E. (2017). Palliative and end of life care in solid organ transplantation. *American Journal of Transplantation, 17*, 3008–3019.
Wesselman, H., Ford, C. G., Leyva, Y., Li, X., Chang, C. C. H., Dew, M. A., Kendall, K., Croswell, E., Pleis, J. R., Ng, Y. H., Unruh, M. L., Shapiro, R., & Myaskovsky, L. (2021). Social determinants of health and race disparities in kidney transplant. *Clinical Journal of the American Society of Nephrology, 16*, 262–274.
Wright, L., Pape, D., Ross, K., Campbell, M., & Bowman, K. (2007). Approaching end of life care in organ transplantation: The impact of transplant patients' death and dying. *Progress in Transplantation, 17*(1), 57–61.
Yagelniski, A., Rosaasen, B. S. P., Cardinal, L., Fenton, M. E., Tam, J., & Mansell, H. (2020). A qualitative study to explore the needs of lung transplant caregivers. *Progress in Transplantation, 30*(3), 243–248.

Chapter 11
Traumatic Injury and Traumatic Brain Injury

Richard Wenthen and Zoe A. Landers

Introduction

The psychosocial effects of severe injury, including physical trauma and traumatic brain injury (TBI), are broadly distinguishable from what would be considered "illness" in how they are incurred and experienced and as such produce a distinct impact on the individual and their social support system. At approximately 4.4% of all hospital discharges in the United States and at an annual expense of more than $4.2 trillion in medical costs and lost productivity, physical trauma is a serious injury to the body that requires medical intervention and is a leading cause of death and disability (DiMaggio et al., 2016; Centers for Disease Control and Prevention [CDC], 2021a). Equally prevalent in female and male patients, the epidemiology of inpatient traumatic physical injury in the United States is evolving to include increasingly older, more severely injured patients with preexisting comorbid conditions and subsequently elevated mortality risk (DiMaggio et al., 2016). Though serious physical trauma covers a wide range of injury types, racial and ethnic minority patients in the United States (people of color and Hispanic people) are at greater risk for inpatient mortality and adverse outcomes than patients who are white/non-Hispanic given similar presenting factors (Hicks et al., 2014; Richie et al., 2021). We will explore in greater detail how certain identities and communities, particularly those that are marginalized, may be differently affected as the result of traumatic injury in the *Social Justice* section.

R. Wenthen (✉)
Northwell Health, Manhasset, NY, USA
e-mail: richardwenthen@gmail.com

Z. A. Landers
New York, NY, USA
e-mail: zoe.landers.lcsw@gmail.com

M. Hemphill, A. Nathanson (eds.), *The Practice of Clinical Social Work in Healthcare*, Essential Clinical Social Work Series,
https://doi.org/10.1007/978-3-031-31650-0_11

Generally, physical trauma results from blunt force trauma (where a force or object strikes the body causing TBI, broken bones, deep cuts, concussions), penetrating trauma (where an object pierces the body or skin creating an open wound), burns, or controlled injury (planned injury to the body from surgery) (National Institute of General Medical Sciences, 2018). Traumatic physical injury may occur from falls, motor vehicle accidents, violent assault, sporting accidents, amputations, natural disasters, and workplace accidents. Some examples of physical trauma include fractures, stab or gunshot wounds, crushing injuries, TBI and concussions, burns, dislocations, amputations, and severe internal organ, nerve, or extremity injury (DiMaggio et al., 2016).

The unique aspects of the onset of injury, the rehabilitation period, and chronic effects will be explored as recovery from traumatic injury presents various tasks of psychological adaptation for patients and their caregivers. They must navigate the different phases of injury, acclimate to changes in the patient's physical and psychological agency, and adjust to evolving identities and roles within their relational and global meaning systems. This chapter discusses ideas for how social workers may attune to the diverse challenges faced by adult patients and their caregivers as they all consider the gravity and phases of traumatic injury. Note that we use the word *trauma* in two ways: as the medical descriptor of grievous physical injury and to discuss the psychological and behavioral response to a situation or series of events that overwhelm the individual's ability to cope (Kleber, 2019).

Illness Onset, Course, and Degree of Incapacitation

Traumatic injury, as is implied by its name, has an acute onset. These injuries are not associated with degenerative or progressive disease—rather, they are the result of sudden and often unexpected experiences that may leave the person vulnerable to systemic shock (University of Florida Health, 2016). Here we see the dual meaning of *trauma* is already at play, as the event causing the physically traumatic injury may also result in posttraumatic psychological sequelae, or consequences, for the patient and their social system. Sometimes, depending on the severity of injury, a patient may die in the immediacy of the event or shortly thereafter. If not, the course of a traumatic injury will include a recovery process, the trajectory and experience of which may be varied.

Throughout this course, a patient's functional progress will be related to the severity of their physical trauma and influenced by multiple biopsychosocial factors: family and personal medical history, psychological and cognitive functioning, access to medical and rehabilitative services, insurance coverage, socioeconomic resources, sociodemographics, etc. (Kempen et al., 2001; Schemitsch & Nauth, 2020; Truong et al., 2020). Recovery is tracked compared to baseline, which can be perceived both medically and socially. Medically, a baseline is established by taking measurement of, or collecting data on, a patient's condition at an early stage. Ideally, this would be done prior to the variation that has now presented. Similarly, a social worker will assess a patient's social baseline: This is an understanding of a patient's ability to complete activities of daily living (ADLs) and engage socially and cognitively, prior to the variation created by the presenting problem (Davis et al., 2020).

In the case of traumatic injury, baseline refers to the patient's way of navigating the world prior to the injury event. Following medical stabilization, the patient may either gradually return to baseline, decline, or remain functionally unchanged. Should the patient be unable to return to baseline functioning, the injury may lead to long-term disability and/or require constant care throughout the patient's lifetime.

In the case of TBI the course may be even more unpredictable as cognitive function will be impaired. In severe cases, this may include coma, disturbed consciousness, posttraumatic agitation and amnesia, and ultimately a recovery process in attempt to regain pre-injury levels of functioning which may sometimes result in chronic or worsening impairment (Oberholzer & Müri, 2019). Notably, the highest rates of TBI hospitalizations recorded in the United States are experienced by people aged 75 and older, followed by those aged 65–74, and then aged 55–64; the most common mechanism of the incident is an accidental fall (CDC, 2021b). As with other traumatic injury, the increasingly older demographic of TBI injury increases the medical, functional, and psychological complexity of patient recovery (DiMaggio et al., 2016). Should return to pre-injury baseline not be possible the patient will attempt to establish a new baseline, a process that will include variable subjective degrees of success and rates of progression medically, functionally, and psychologically.

The outcome of a traumatic injury and/or TBI can be difficult to assess at onset. Depending on the nature of the physical trauma and variables like comorbidities and age, death may seem either imminent or unlikely following initial medical acuity and stabilization. Patients may be significantly incapacitated at onset of injury and for a short time thereafter but eventually regain functioning that comes near, if not entirely attaining, pre-injury levels. In some cases, this will require introduction of new devices and equipment, as well as adaptation to accommodate the effects of the injury. For instance, a 45-year-old Black cisgender man who required a below-the-knee amputation following traumatic injury was eventually able to re-engage with the world as he once had, returning to competitive marathoning with the use of a prosthesis following a physical rehabilitation journey over a year.[1]

Conversely, an injury may be more global, involving major organ damage and failure or TBI with an unpredictable trajectory and result. In severe cases, patients will die while medically acute; others may be medically stable but remain in a coma with minimal neurological activity or experience permanent deficits that ultimately contribute to death. For example, a 23-year-old white cisgender woman who presumed her worsening headache to be alcohol related was brought to the emergency room after being found unconscious. Scans revealed that the intracranial pressure caused by a brain bleed induced a pontine stroke, resulting in irreparable brain damage. Once medically stabilized following neurosurgical intervention, the patient was left permanently ventilator dependent and unable to follow commands. Later,

[1] All names and other personal identifiers in the case are fictitious. Any similarity to actual persons, living or dead, or actual events is purely coincidental.

in a long-term care facility, the patient developed an infection that led to her death. When attempting to prognosticate outcomes of traumatic injuries, it is again necessary to account for related biopsychosocial factors. In the case of a TBI, age can be vital given that brain health, developmental stage, and neuroplasticity factor in the recovery journey, enabling or inhibiting the brain's ability to reconstruct pathways required to more closely return to prior levels of functioning both cognitively and physically (Sophie Su et al., 2016).

A person's degree of incapacitation may change throughout the course of a traumatic injury. Cognitive impairment is a primary concern in the wake of TBI, and there are various ways this could present: memory loss, inability to recognize familiar things, difficulty exercising appropriate judgment, altered moods or behaviors, difficulty planning or completing tasks and communicating, etc. (CDC, 2011). The three main types of TBI are mild (i.e., concussion), moderate, and severe. Mild TBI may result in mild cognitive effects that eventually resolve; moderate to severe TBI is often a progressive disorder with worsening symptoms through the chronic stages (Changoor et al., 2020). Long-term consequences are still being studied, though there seems to be a correlation between TBI and neurodegenerative disease (Bramlett & Dietrich, 2015), as well as increased risk for posttraumatic anxiety as people age, particularly in women (Rauen et al., 2021).

Ability to feel sensation may become impaired with a traumatic injury, or new, worsening, or episodic pain may begin. Motor function and the way one has become accustomed to moving through the world may be impaired temporarily or permanently. Traumatic physical injury may result in disfigurement, scarring, or amputation. Social stigmatization and ostracization may be experienced by people who are no longer able to participate in the world as expected or as they once did, who are noticeably disabled, or who may require assistive devices. The physical effects and psychosocial ramifications of traumatic injury can be myriad, with one aspect potentially informing or exacerbating the other. Although there may be similarities found in types of traumatic injury or in recovery journeys, each individual will process, cope, and grieve in their own unique way. As such, beneficial supports and interventions will be similarly personalized and varied.

Clinical Issues of Illness

Crisis

Intrapersonal How the patient is received, involved, and reassured by medical professionals and caregivers in the crisis phase of illness may foster psychological resiliency, or the ability to adapt well under stress (American Psychological Association, 2020), and mitigate the development of injury-related distress (IRD) and/or posttraumatic psychological disorders (Victorson et al., 2005). Familiarity with the details of the patient's entry into the medical system will help guide social work understanding of whether the patient is feeling supported or isolated as they navigate recovery from a catastrophic, life-bifurcating event. With some traumatic injuries, there may be multiple crisis points where medical teams need to make decisions in the patient's best interests, e.g., if they are unconscious, inebriated, or too cognitively impaired to consent to medical care or when there is no surrogate decision-maker. Even mild cognitive impairment may impact the ability to retain and process information at the pace required to make high-stakes and time-sensitive medical decisions. In turn, this may increase patient, caregiver, and provider distress around acute medical decision-making.

Many patients feel overwhelmed by the shock, abrupt change in situation, physical pain, and stress of medical and logistical decision-making. If conscious, a patient may be consumed by pain, fear, insecurity, and thoughts of responsibility and/or guilt for the events that occurred. They may be experiencing beliefs such as "I am going to die"; "I'm never going to be okay again"; "It's all my fault"; "Who will provide for my family?"; or "Will I ever be okay again?" For those who entered the medical system unconscious, the visceral shock of awakening in an acute medical care setting surrounded by unknown care providers often evokes feelings of sadness, confusion, and curiosity (Ringdal et al., 2008).

Unsurprisingly, traumatic physical injury is strongly associated with subsequent mental health problems demonstrated in at least five domains: acute stress disorder, posttraumatic stress disorder (PTSD), anxiety, depression, and patient subjective experiences of their traumatic injury (Wiseman et al., 2013). Dependence upon others, pain, and a sense of having lost control may further compound patient IRD and impair self-esteem as they become increasingly aware of the chronicity of their new physical baseline and limited potential for recovery of baseline functioning (Ringdal et al., 2008).

Trauma-informed care is especially important (see Chap. 13: *Trauma-Informed Approaches and Interventions in Serious Illness*). The incidence of PTSD for survivors of traumatic injury may range from 30% to 93% compared with a prevalence of approximately 8% within the general US population (Wiseman et al., 2013). The impact of PTSD following traumatic injury may be more pronounced for people of color and/or people living in poverty who may experience mistrust of the medical system and difficulties accessing consistent quality care as the result of systemic oppression (Beiter et al., 2022).

Due to the cataclysmic onset and life-altering nature of traumatic injury, patients are often overwhelmed not only by the suddenness of the change in their physical and medical circumstances but also by the psychological impact of the incident that caused their traumatic injury. With patients and caregivers alike, social workers should consider modeling their interventions on the principles of psychological first aid that specifically address how to communicate with people in acute psychological distress or shock and that are aligned with the social work principles of safety, dignity, and human rights (World Health Organization [WHO] et al., 2011). This further includes conveying hope and evidence-based reassurance for patients to help facilitate psychological stabilization.

As patients are likely to experience some degree of posttraumatic stress, consider implementing in each interaction the trauma-informed care principles of establishing safety, collaboration, choice, empowerment, and trustworthiness (Kusmaul,

2018) to help re-establish a sense of self-efficacy, trust, and agency. Social workers with specific advanced training in the provision of trauma-informed care may provide psychoeducation on coping skills, IRD, and relaxation techniques combined with exposure exercises that may be helpful in improving acute and long-term coping post-injury (Victorson et al., 2005). Repeating and reviewing information ensures accurate communication and comprehension (WHO et al., 2011). Fostering connection with loved ones and friends, and where appropriate, fellowship between patients, may bolster psychological resilience (Ringdal et al., 2008). While some patients benefit from retelling the story of the traumatic injury as part of ascribing and making meaning of what happened, persistent emotional rumination and venting may actually increase IRD (Peter et al., 2012; Victorson et al., 2005). It is for this reason that social workers without advanced trauma training should not attempt to re-process a trauma with patients. Depending upon the degree of cognitive impairment, social work intervention may focus less on direct communication with the patient and more on supporting the caregivers and facilitating resource access.

Interpersonal The moment of injury is a precise psychological and physiological demarcation; a patient's life thereafter tends to be defined as belonging to the time either before or after traumatic injury. The same rupture and life-changing impact often extend to the patient's caregivers and social circle (Geard et al., 2020; Ringdal et al., 2008). Caregivers shoulder not only the psychological shock of learning that someone they care about has been traumatically injured but also the simultaneous burden of contending with the uncertainty of immediate and ultimate outcomes and their effects on the caregiver system. Most caregivers will experience emotional reactions including grief, anxiety, distress, and depression as they negotiate this disruption of social/professional/familial life, the physical strain of caregiving, communication challenges, and the process of recalibrating their identity (Degeneffe, 2001; Geard et al., 2020). Subsequent to injury, there is often an immediate mobilization of the caregiving system where key members pivot from focusing on day-to-day life to providing support and care for the patient. In most cases, there is also a noticeable impact on one or more of the following caregiver resources: financial, temporal, emotional, physical, relational, and spiritual (Geard et al., 2020). Members of the extended caregiving network may temporarily adjust their lives to provide peripheral support for primary caregivers by taking on some responsibilities of daily life. Other primary caregivers may not have access to extended networks of concrete, emotional, and/or spiritual support, possibly reinforcing posttraumatic psychological distress risk factors of feeling alone and overwhelmed during a traumatic life event (Kleber, 2019).

As with the patient, caregiver shock and fear may impair executive functioning, assimilation of information, capacity for emotional regulation, self-care, and self-efficacy. In providing support, be aware of how the entire caregiving system may be juggling multiple logistical stressors and how this may impede their ability to provide adequate care for the patient (Azman et al., 2019). To mitigate burnout and facilitate adaptation to the current life circumstances, caregivers may benefit from mobilizing existing strategies or being connected to resources in the following areas: caregiving responsibilities of the patient or the caregiver (childcare, animal care, elder care), professional responsibilities (income generation, job security, employment benefits), personal responsibilities (home upkeep, payment of bills, management of mail, social and community roles), and planning for patient caregiving (information about the illness, treatments, costs, home care, and patient needs). Some caregivers may need support balancing caregiving needs with personal autonomy; respite as self-care is paramount to effective longer-term adaptation (AARP, 2020; Geard et al., 2020). For instance, a social worker may refer a client to, or facilitate, a caregiver support group where members can find companionship and share practical tips. This can mitigate feelings of isolation and normalize the complicated emotions often associated with caregiving, including anger, sadness, guilt, burnout, and resentment. To address concrete needs, a social worker may link a caregiver client with available financial programming or community resources that can provide respite homecare services or offer assistance navigating social systems that can provide affordable long-term care (e.g., Medicaid) or supplies. Respite home care allows the caregiver to take time to rest, recharge, and engage in activities that they enjoy outside of their caregiving role. Alleviating some of the financial burden associated with caregiving can address a major source of stress and ensure the care recipient has their needs well met.

Systems of Care First responders play a critical role in the immediate stabilization and triage of traumatic injury. Transport to an equipped medical facility may involve prolonged or multiple modes of transport. Ability to stabilize injury may directly play a role in a patient's survival and their physical and psychological outcomes, as does ease of access to specialists and Level 1 Trauma Centers, which are comprehensive regional medical facilities equipped to provide the highest levels of surgical and rehabilitative care to critically injured persons (Brazinova et al., 2015; CDC, 2021b). Expert medical practitioners specializing in orthopedics, otolaryngology, plastic surgery, neurosurgery, neurology, anesthesiology, radiology, and trauma surgery who are supported by a skilled nursing staff and have access to a well-equipped operating theater, emergency room, and intensive care unit will best be able to address the potentially myriad needs of the patient who is traumatically injured (Brazinova et al., 2015).

Quality and consistency of care by medical healthcare professionals influence patient mental health outcomes. For instance, biased and insulting comments about patient disabilities or patients being placed in necessary but uncaring situations (such as when clothes have to be cut or discarded without patient consent or awareness to provide access to vital areas of the patient's body) may contribute to feelings of worthlessness, shame, loss of identity, and insecurity. Delays in pain alleviation or in meeting requests for care may contribute to feelings of abandonment, worthlessness, and irrelevance as a disabled human being and, thus, of being a burden (Peter et al., 2012; Ringdal et al., 2008). Culturally attuned services, language interpreter services, and support from a chaplain or other religious support may ease the experience.

Where appropriate, social workers should identify concrete services, including assistance with medical insurance and financial aid, that may benefit patients and facilitate resource access. Issues of immediate and ongoing patient safety may arise that require interdisciplinary consultation if the patient's traumatic injuries resulted from assault or negligence. In some cases, government protective services may need to be consulted to preserve patient safety and guide healthcare system assessment of ongoing perpetrator involvement in the patient's medical care, visitations, and discharge planning. This may be complicated not only by psychological and financial dependence on the perpetrator but also by other factors that compromise independence including socioeconomic standing, immigration status, the existence of dependents, and more. This may require connecting the patient to legal resources or organizations supporting those affected by intimate partner violence (IPV), elder abuse, labor trafficking, or similar issues.

Chronic

Intrapersonal Recovery and rehabilitation may be an arduous process that involves a significant investment of physical and emotional resources for both patient and caregivers. Continued uncertainty about when, how, or if the patient may return to baseline functioning in one or more areas, and/or whether the patient will adapt to new baselines, may extend beyond weeks into years. Issues of impact differ and evolve with time; what is a predominant concern in the short term may no longer be pivotal in the long term as the patient and caregiving systems become increasingly practiced in care provision or as patient functioning improves (Conti et al., 2019).

For some, the process of adjusting to life with impairment or disability from injury and/or the associated chronic pain becomes the central activity of their psychological process—at times to the exclusion of prior interests and supportive relationships. The psychological bifurcation of life "before" and "after" traumatic injury deepens: This may include adjusting to variable or static levels of impairment and deciphering actual versus perceived vulnerability and safety in the world. Disfigurement and scarring from the traumatic injury may trigger IRD or be the source of questions, comments, stares, and jokes. In response to these and to the patient's own internalized judgments about their post-injury self-image, some patients may reclaim a sense of physical empowerment by choosing to undergo cosmetic surgery to mask scarring or elective amputation to address functional debility.

For instance, a 20-year-old Latinx cisgender woman residing in a tropical climate developed severe and prominent keloid scarring on her shoulders, arm, and neck. These had required extensive surgical and neurological repair following a near-fatal car accident. Cosmetic surgery and decorative tattoos vastly improved her self-image, her sense of ownership over her traumatically injured limb, and her comfort in wearing climate-appropriate clothing while significantly reducing her fear of being taunted, pursued, and mocked in public.[2]

TBI may impact the patient's ability to modulate and process emotions, control their behaviors or bodily functions, communicate effectively, or adaptively negotiate what is likely a cataclysmic change in their life and reintegrate into life at home (Degeneffe, 2001). Overreliance on behavioral disengagement, emotional rumination and venting, self-blame, denial, and self-medication may increase IRD and impede mobilization of more effective coping mechanisms (Victorson et al., 2005). As highlighted in the following case example, regular assessment of psychological functioning, IRD, and health-related quality of life (QoL) is imperative as the patient negotiates arriving home to a reality where they may find themselves in their own "No Man's Land," dependent and seeing themselves as a burden to those they care about (Ringdal et al., 2008; Rauen et al., 2021).

A 32-year-old queer Asian-American cisgender woman surgeon was in a car accident that resulted in her fiancée's death, the facial disfigurement of her sibling, and the permanent paralysis of her own dominant hand, along with mild TBI impairing her cognitive processing. Her career as a surgeon, through which she had hoped to provide for her financially insecure family, was irrevocably terminated by her injuries. Returning home accentuated grappling with intense IRD, survivor's guilt, grief, loss of identity, shame, PTSD, and major depression that was further amplified seeing her sibling's facial disfigurement daily. The perception and certitude of being a burden on her resource-stretched family prevented her from owning her needs for support and psychological care.

Eight months post-injury, during a routine orthopedic appointment, in conjunction with a detailed assessment of general social and mental health functioning that specifically asked about IRD, posttraumatic stress, anxiety, and depression, the patient completed psychological questionnaires including a suicide risk assessment. For the first time since injury, she disclosed persistent suicide ideation, secretive use of alcohol to numb chronic pain, and the extent of her psychological distress, including flashbacks, nightmares, and survivor's guilt.

The social worker validated, contextualized, and normalized the patient's many posttraumatic reactions: IRD, survivor's guilt, complicated grief from the loss of her fiancée and her career, her coping utilizing alcohol to decrease her shame, her sense of powerlessness over her responses to the trauma, and her sense of isolation. Drawing upon the principles of psychological first aid and trauma-informed care, the social worker provided psychoeducation about psychological symptoms and specific information on how trauma-focused mental health treatment and community-based supports would improve the patient's psychological recovery.

To help build and support patient affect regulation, the social worker identified and practiced several practical, mindfulness-based skills with the patient and collaboratively developed a detailed safety plan to address suicide risk. The social worker helped the patient identify how her thoughts were influencing her behav-

[2] All names and other personal identifiers in the case are fictitious. Any similarity to actual persons, living or dead, or actual events is purely coincidental.

iors and emotions, thus compounding IRD. Subsequently they identified how the patient's preconceived notions of living with chronic traumatic injury were limiting her ability to determine positive future outcomes and alternative ways of creating and fostering connection within her social system. This helped the patient begin to actively integrate thoughts of a more hopeful future. Furthermore, the social worker connected the patient to mental health support services in her community with providers skilled in the treatment of psychological trauma.

In a future appointment, the patient credited her conversation with the social worker with planting the seed that she could change how she was approaching life post-injury. Beginning to see that possibility instilled hope that she could develop a meaningful life as a person with chronic traumatic injury. Ongoing counseling and community support groups helped her regain a renewed sense of agency and self-efficacy as she learned how to share and accept her needs for support while finding new ways to meaningfully interact with and participate in her community.[3]

The patient's perceptions about how others will receive them may compound their feelings of isolation and self-blame. This may impede patient comfort in accessing the full support of their community, which subsequently intensifies IRD (Victorson et al., 2005). The degree of shame and stigma related to the injury narrative influences psychological burden and recovery. Patients who sustained traumatic injury from a sporting or motor vehicle accident may feel more comfortable accessing the support of their community and subsequently experience less social estrangement than a patient injured as the result of a violent crime, sex, and illicit or criminal activity. This might be particularly delicate if the patient's actions contributed to the demise or injury of another. Return to life in the community would highlight not only the change in the patient's functioning and agency but also feelings of blame and being blamed for the death of the other. In such a case, the patient may experience compounding feelings of culpability, guilt, moral injury, and survivor's guilt.

Almost a quarter of traumatic injury patients report chronic pain 3 years out from serious injury and more than a third endorse moderate pain-related disability (Holmes et al., 2013). Likelihood of chronic pain is increased by socioeconomic disadvantage, greater injury severity, and higher initial pain. Problem-solving skills and higher ratings of self-efficacy may improve pain outcomes. Chronic pain increases overall psychological distress, perception of impairment, and social isolation.

As noted with the above case example, these effects can be compounded as demoralization and decreased mental health functioning may negatively influence adherence to medical treatment, medication compliance, and consistent utilization of rehabilitation services. Those with preexisting psychiatric conditions and/or alcohol or substance use disorders may be at further elevated risk for suicide, for developing mood and/or posttraumatic psychological disorders, or for neuropsychological deficits in the case of TBI. Furthermore, they may be at heightened risk for abusing alcohol, other substances, and/or prescription medication in the attempt

[3] All names and other personal identifiers in the case are fictitious. Any similarity to actual persons, living or dead, or actual events is purely coincidental.

to modulate pain and/or the psychological impact of their injury (Oliverio et al., 2020; Victorson et al., 2005).

Social workers are uniquely suited to help patients move from loss to acceptance and adaptation to current functioning and capabilities. Exploring what is successful recovery for the patient, ascertaining how they may increase self-efficacy in their healthcare or pain management, evoking curiosity about adaptations that may be implemented, and identifying how to reintegrate within the community in a meaningful way are all means of bolstering self-efficacy and self-esteem (Peter et al., 2012). Increased self-efficacy and self-esteem in turn improve overall mental health, acceptance of the traumatic injury with fewer cognitive distortions, and perception of injury manageability. Additional protective factors include having positive social support, a sense of purpose and community (including spiritual practice), and working toward achieving greater autonomy. An ability to return to work, personal pursuits, and activities within the community further help with regaining a sense of psychological equilibrium and improvement in QoL.

Interpersonal Families are increasingly recognized as the primary caregivers responsible for long-term patient care following acute rehabilitation, which translates to an intricate link between patient outcomes to the overall well-being and functioning of the caregiver system (Azman et al., 2019; Degeneffe, 2001). Conti et al. (2019) write that most who assume caregiving responsibilities experience a reduction in overall life satisfaction and endorse feeling mentally strained by caregiving, a decline in cognitive function, and increased social isolation and stigmatization. Like patients, caregivers experience an increased incidence of psychological disorders such as depression, anxiety, and posttraumatic distress, and 36% of family caregivers identify their situations as highly stressful (AARP, 2020). Caregiver neglect of their own health (physical, mental, social, professional) not only impacts caregiver morale and relationship with the patient but also over time may reduce the quality and consistency of the support provided for patient functioning (Azman et al., 2019; Conti et al., 2019).

Provision of long-term care in the home requires constant commitment to highly complex tasks that involve some medical and nursing knowledge such as continence care, medication management, behavioral interventions, and addressing secondary physical conditions (Azman et al., 2019; Conti et al., 2019). Some patients with TBI may exhibit challenging behavior, socially inappropriate sexual expression, and communication barriers requiring significant adjustment as caregivers become fully responsible for an adult person who is now functionally dependent (Degeneffe, 2001). Despite this, some aspects of caregiving may be emotionally gratifying: notably, improved emotional connection with the patient and the sense of well-being born from mutual coping (Conti et al., 2019).

Social work can play a direct role in improving coping and resilience by helping caregivers manage expectations, obtain relevant financial and other resources, identify the signs of caregiver burnout and vicarious traumatization, and develop an action plan to address ongoing caregiver health (AARP, 2020; Azman et al., 2019). Facilitating access to treatment information and practical skills education for patient physical care—specifically to minimize secondary medical conditions, which thus reduces caregiver burden—improves caregiver functioning and patient long-term outcomes (Azman et al., 2019; Geard et al., 2020; Conti et al., 2019). Promoting opportunities for caregivers to make sense of and bestow spiritual or subjective meaning on the changes in life following a critical situation may be assistive to their long-term adjustment (Geard et al., 2020). For instance, some caregivers may come to view the traumatic injury as a catalyst for bringing them closer to the patient and healing prior relational wounds. Psychoeducational and support groups have been shown to be an effective tool for improving caregiver efficacy, mitigating caregiver burnout, and reducing social isolation while providing a venue for families to exchange experiences of care in helping the patient recover (AARP, 2020; Azman et al., 2019; Petersen & Sanders, 2015).

Systems of Care In the chronic phase of treatment, common barriers with systems of care may include accessing follow-up care with qualified medical and rehabilitation specialists, receiving injury-specific homecare services and case management, or acquiring assistive devices. Changes in insurance coverage, limited availability of services, financial barriers, impaired cognition and/or physical mobility, and lack of information about long-term care needs, along with poor care coordination, present considerable challenges to accessing care systems. The lack of provider knowledge, poor willingness to learn, or lack of empathy for traumatic injury impacts patient willingness to seek ongoing medical care. Environmental accommodations (e.g., appointment reminders, sufficient appointment time, office layout, written information) that take into account the cognitive and physical impairments of patients help facilitate care access and adherence (Dams-O'Connor et al., 2018).

Patient, caregiver, and family access to therapy, support groups, ongoing education about traumatic injury, care advances, and prevention of secondary medical issues are important considerations for recovery outcomes (Azman et al., 2019; Conti et al., 2019). Assessing mental health functioning of patients and caregivers at regular intervals increases the likelihood of immediate support and intervention with improved psychological outcomes (Wiseman et al., 2013). However, many psychological questionnaires are not designed with traumatic injury in mind, and a clinical diagnostic interview may be required to distinguish between situationally contingent depressed mood and persistent adjustment disorder (Post & van Leeuwan, 2012) or other posttraumatic psychological disorders. As access to systems may change over time, alongside patient needs, the ability of patients and caregivers to identify, access, and utilize new systems of care will become increasingly important.

Terminal

Traumatic physical injury and TBI are vast in their scope, and therefore termination of life may not follow a predictable progression. Demographic and identifying factors (such as age, race, ethnicity, socioeconomic status, and employment), reduced agency and cognitive functioning, secondary or comorbid medical conditions, lifestyle factors, and access to care may impact the progression of death (Dams-O'Connor et al., 2018). This is particularly important for older patients, especially those with frailty and serious illness, as critical traumatic injury is often a fatal diagnosis: 80% die or become seriously impaired within 1 year of severe TBI (Lilley et al., 2018). Sudden death and/or rapid decline in functioning may mean palliative and hospice care options are underutilized, or logistical and psychological preparation for end of life (EOL) is overall lacking. As Lilley et al. (2018) write:

> This group of patients is unique in that their sudden critical illness and cognitive impairment results in major, immediate medical decisions being made by surrogates with physicians who are typically meeting these patients for the first time. Currently, in-hospital mortality… does not account for the value some patients place on access to palliative care, avoidance of high-intensity treatments, or appropriate enrollment in hospice. (p. 45)

Thus, trauma surgeons are increasingly responsible for providing EOL care for this population. Multidisciplinary teams may commence discussions with caregivers and/or legal representatives about whether and when to withdraw or withhold life-saving measures for patients with TBI in very poor prognostic conditions. Once decisions are made regarding which life-saving measures will be withdrawn or withheld, and at what time, palliative therapy is often initiated (van Veen et al., 2020).

Particularly with this population and their caregivers, underlying posttraumatic stress may complicate care as common EOL emotions (fear, despair, guilt, anger, anxiety), sensations (such as pain, difficulty breathing, and paralysis), and thoughts ("I am going to die" or "I am powerless") may evoke memories of the patient and/or caregiver's underlying psychological and/or medical traumas. Reactivated posttraumatic stress responses may heighten patient and/or caregiver distrust and reluctance to communicate openly with providers or follow treatment recommendations, leading to the patient and/or caregivers being perceived as oppositional or noncompliant. Patients and/or their caregivers may be mislabeled as "problematic," and subsequently, opportunities to help patients and/or their caregivers re-regulate their psychologically traumatized systems and address possible other symptoms of suicidal ideation, depression, respiratory or digestive distress, and somaticized pain may be missed (Janssen, n.d.). For instance, a Holocaust survivor fell while showering and hit their head, sustaining a severe TBI. The patient underwent neurosurgical intervention but remained unresponsive with poor prognosis due to comorbidities and postoperative complications. The multidisciplinary team recommended cessation of curative treatment and pursuit of hospice care. During a family meeting to clarify goals of care, the patient's Orthodox family expressed unwillingness to stop curative treatment. While this resistance might not have been immediately understandable to an outside observer, in reality underlying historical posttraumatic stress for the caregivers was reactivated by feeling trapped and powerless over patient outcomes combined with a religious belief in continuation of life and cultural mistrust of the healthcare system. Subsequently, the patient's family became distrustful of and combative toward the providing team and resistant to treatment recommendations. As a result of the heightened stress, the patient's spouse began to experience severe migraines and gastrointestinal complications, further depleting the family's psychological and caretaking resources.[4]

A prolonged decline may lead to emotional and physical exhaustion for patients and caregivers. Protracted deterioration of a patient's condition logistically and emotionally increases the caregiving burden and may further drain system resources. If the patient transitions to inpatient care, caregivers may feel simultaneously relieved, guilty for not having done enough, and disoriented as their role in active care substantively changes. A temporary decline in caregiver functioning may occur once the patient is transitioned, as they process the full psychological weight and physical exhaustion of the long and all-encompassing caregiving experience. Patients and caregivers may be relieved once EOL occurs.

Bereavement

Traumatic injury carries a potential litany of losses along a spectrum of magnitude in various areas of life. Bereavement occurs from the moment of injury until after death. The pre-death losses may be particularly challenging to identify and grieve. Patients and their social systems may grieve more concrete, tangible losses (e.g., life, limb, specific abilities), and they may be faced with more symbolic, intangible losses (e.g., sense of self, personal identity, feeling of independence, perceived level of autonomy). Due to the often unpredictable nature of the deficits and long-term outcomes of some traumatic injuries (especially TBI), losses may be perceived as nonfinite, and the possibly unknown future level of functioning may be felt as a composite of ambiguous losses when compared to the patient's former baseline. Chronic sorrow may be felt by patients and caregivers as time goes on and deficits potentially persist; the patient may be limited in ongoing and/or unforeseen ways; typical developmental or other life milestones may become unobtainable (Harris & Winokuer, 2019).

Patients may be living day-to-day with ongoing reminders of newly presented deficits (e.g., limited physical dexterity, long- or short-term memory loss, speech impairment, compromised ambulation requiring an assistive device, etc.). In these cases, patients may not feel that a single event is to be grieved; rather, a new level of flexibility and adaptation may be required to accommodate new needs that may concurrently serve as a constant reminder of what has been lost. In this way, the results of a traumatic injury may be experienced as living losses (Harris & Winokuer, 2019).

There are many ways these new deficits may permeate across aspects of the individual's life. For example, the felt experience of new disfigurement or noticeable deficit may affect preexisting romantic relationship dynamics, drastically alter the individual's sense of self in relation to new potential partners, or negatively impact the patient's confidence across social arenas due to intrapsychic and extrinsic

---

[4]All names and other personal identifiers in the case are fictitious. Any similarity to actual persons, living or dead, or actual events is purely coincidental.

factors. Patient vulnerability to stigmatization may increase as they re-engage with larger social systems. This may result in intangible losses of comfort, confidence, and the way the patient formerly perceived themselves in relation to others. Deeply felt nonfinite losses may seep into various aspects of life and affect the individual in subtle and overt ways, potentially acting as lifelong reminders of everything of which the individual is no longer capable. This, in turn, can lead the individual to reevaluate how they fit within a larger context, likely altering their sense of self. This can also be considered a redefining of the patient's assumptive world or how the self/others/the world are subjectively perceived and presumed to be.

It is paramount that social workers account for how caregivers, both preexisting and newly established, may also be grieving. In the event of death in the immediate wake of a traumatic injury, those closest to the patient may be bereaved. However, as many continue to live with traumatic injury and TBI, there is nuance in how caregivers experience ongoing grief and losses. Since older adults with functional decline are most at risk for TBI, the patient may have already been receiving support from an informal caregiver. Additionally, some newly impaired individuals may have been caregivers prior to injury. Traumatic injury can shake the foundation of subjective realities for those to whom the individual provided care, as well as those who relied upon that individual's assistance.

A 70-year-old Black heterosexual cisgender man fell down a flight of stairs, was found unresponsive, and was immediately intubated upon arrival at a hospital. CT revealed a subarachnoid hematoma; he was scheduled for surgery and his recovery was uncertain. Upon conducting psychosocial assessment with the patient's 63-year-old spouse, it was found that the patient was fully independent prior to admission (PTA) and was the primary caregiver for a 38-year-old son with a developmental disability. The spouse explained that she is still working and the family relies on her income and the informal support provided to the son by the patient. Pertinent questions the social worker would seek to answer include:

- *How will the son be cared for, either temporarily or permanently?*
- *If the patient will newly require a caregiver, who will be able to provide this assistance?*
- *What areas of their lives may be affected (*e.g., *finances, time, career, routine,* etc.*)?*
- *Through all this change, what may be lost for the family unit as a whole, as well as individually (patient, spouse, and son)?*
- *What are some intangible losses experienced?*

While in the hospital, the social worker normalized the spouse's feelings as she processed the complexity of the situation and helped prioritize tasks by order of urgency. As the patient was receiving medical care, the social worker focused on the well-being of the patient's son. Through further discussion, the social worker helped the spouse identify how she could rebalance professional obligations in order to provide additional assistance to her son and coordinate the patient's care. The social worker further assisted the spouse in identifying informal social supports to provide care for her son, so that she would have time to coordinate care for her family. The social worker provided the spouse with city-based resources for adults with developmental disabilities, including affordable day programs. The social worker also referred the spouse to a community-based caregiver program through which she was linked with a care coordinator that provided access to ongoing individual counseling, support groups, educational programming, and legal services. The social worker remained available to the family to offer psycho-emotional support and continued to facilitate access to available social programming to mitigate the disruptive repercussions of the patient's injury on the family system.[5]

Ambiguous loss can be broken down into two categorical types: when someone is perceived as psychologically present but physically absent (e.g., lost in war/catastrophe, kidnapped/missing or absent familial figure) and, oppositely, when someone is perceived as physically present but psychologically absent (e.g., degenerative cognitive conditions, severe mental illness, addiction) (Boss, 1999). As these losses are not clear cut, they can be more complicated to name, process, and grieve. When physical impairments prevent the same kind of engagement as was standard for the patient at baseline, or when TBI results in prolonged altered cognitive functioning, the latter type of ambiguous loss may be felt. Though the individual who experienced the injury will remain physically present, certain aspects of their identity may be lost, complicating the grieving process. As long-term outcomes can be difficult to predict, this potentially ongoing, unending sense of loss is what generates feelings of chronic sorrow.

As the very nature of traumatic injury occurrence can be quite random, the ability to process the associated losses in real time can be challenging. This is especially true when the patient dies. When death is immediate or shortly after the incident occurs, the patient's social system experiences the shock of the sudden removal of that person. The bereavement processes of those close to the patient will be affected by the suddenness of death. In the aftermath of sudden death from traumatic injury, it can be helpful to provide emotional support and validation as caregivers grieve and come to a meaningful understanding of the loss and their role in the patient's life (Neimeyer et al., 2010).

When the patient lives for some time following the injury but is left with deficits that ultimately contribute to death, the patient and social system have more time to integrate losses into a bereavement period. This may be accompanied by feelings of anticipatory grief as death becomes imminent (Nielsen et al., 2016). The ambiguity of the associated losses and the complicated trajectory leading to the patient's death may leave the patient and social supports without a sense of closure or acceptance of the perceived injustice that this has happened to them (Boss, 2022; Scott et al., 2016). Table 11.1 describes concepts that may be helpful in guiding how the social worker legitimizes evolving and enduring experiences of loss along the spectrum of treatment for patients and caregivers.

---

[5]All names and other personal identifiers in the case are fictitious. Any similarity to actual persons, living or dead, or actual events is purely coincidental.

Table 11.1 Psychosocial issues, clinical goals, and interventions

Phase	Psychosocial issues	Clinical goals and interventions
Acute/ crisis	Adjustment to injury, loss of agency, and pain Psychological shock and overwhelm, injury-related distress, acute and posttraumatic stress disorder, anxiety, depression Caregiving, impact on resources Communication challenges Recalibration of identity	Employ psychological first aid and trauma-informed care principles Re-establish sense of self-efficacy, trust, and agency Establish clear communication Provide psychoeducation on traumatic injury and coping skills Foster psychological resilience, hope, and treatment adherence Offer tangible resources to mitigate stress Mental health assessment Mobilize existing informal support networks
Chronic	Long-term adjustment to life with impairment from injury and/or chronic pain, burden to others Alcohol and substance abuse Suicide risk, self-harm risk Psychological bifurcation of life before and after traumatic injury Loss of safety in the world Disfigurement and scarring, post-injury self-image, shame and stigma Concerns around reintegrating into home and community Decreased caregiver overall life satisfaction, increased mental strain, declining cognitive function, increased social isolation and stigmatization Increased incidence of psychological disorders (depression, anxiety, and posttraumatic distress and stress)	Validate, contextualize, and normalize emotional experiences Utilize meaning-making exercises Connect patient/caregiver with ongoing mental health treatment Access community-based resources Employ mindfulness and embodiment-oriented techniques Redirect damaging coping mechanisms toward more sustainable options Instill hope Empower patient/caregiver to share and accept their needs Explore new ways to engage with the world Manage expectations Develop an action plan to address caregiver burnout Provide education and training resources for patient and caregiver Access support groups Assess for mental health, suicide risk, alcohol and substance use, self-harm, isolation, chronic pain, and health-related quality of life
Terminal	Posttraumatic stress amplifying common end-of-life emotions, sensations, and thoughts Communication of end-of-life care preferences Suicidal ideation, depression, respiratory or digestive distress, and somaticized pain Emotional and physical exhaustion, burnout Relief, guilt for not having done enough, role change	Further utilization of meaning-making modalities Normalize conflicting and complicated feelings surrounding death (resentment, relief, joy, despair, guilt, etc.) Provide emotional support and validation Assist investigation of closure or acceptance and how that may be achieved/perceived Assess mental health, including posttraumatic stress symptoms

Social Justice

As traumatic injury may be broadly defined and encompasses a wide breadth of injury occurrences and presentations, information outlining traumatic injury health outcome disparities is in consideration of a particular kind of traumatic injury. For instance, data specific to TBI in the United States reveal disparate outcomes related to different demographic and identifying factors—Table 11.2 outlines these data. The disparities presented here, though collected in particular consideration of TBI, can be utilized and extrapolated to infer how the experience of traumatic injury of any kind will be influenced by an individual's personal identities and participation in certain communities in relation to the social systems in which we participate.

Demographic and identifying factors that put members of these communities at increased risk of TBI may likewise increase their risk of incurring traumatic injury of any kind. Ultimately, inequity and disparity are inevitable byproducts of the privatized structure of healthcare in the context of the systemic power structures that compose the United States.

Specifically in regard to traumatic injury, access to rehabilitative services can be key to facilitating functional recovery. People who are uninsured may not be able to access inpatient or outpatient rehabilitative services following an acute hospital stay. This may prevent uninsured people from availing of the post-acute level of medical care and/or attaining the frequency of rehabilitative therapies recommended for them by the hospital team, resulting in barriers to experiencing the best possible recovery process. Eligible US citizens may be able to be enrolled in Medicaid while in the hospital if appropriate documentation is provided, and this may enable access to some rehabilitation facilities and services upon discharge.

People who are undocumented may have inpatient emergency medical services covered by Emergency Medicaid offered on a city or state level, but this may not extend to cover any rehabilitation services beyond the initial hospital admission. If "charity" admission to inpatient rehab is not available, the patient's social system will have to be involved in the discharge planning process and assessed for ability to care for the patient appropriately. This may mean the patient is to be medically and functionally optimized in the hospital for discharge with family/social supports, and inpatient rehabilitation may not be an option (unless paid for privately).

People who are undomiciled may not have a physical place to which they are able to go and receive care, and not everyone will have informal support systems capable of providing care. This situation is a major deficit in the American healthcare model by which a lack of appropriate social healthcare programming and infrastructure burdens people who are undocumented, uninsured, and/or undomiciled with additional strain that affects the patient, their social system (if present), and the hospital. Social workers' unique understanding of systems issues and consequent societal ramifications provides a powerful perspective that allows us as a profession to actively advocate for increased access to appropriate care.

It is imperative that the social worker be mindful of the diversity of potential relationship types and family/social structures and consider how healthcare and

Table 11.2 Health disparities and TBI

American Indian/Alaska Native people	Higher chance of hospitalization or death compared to other racial or ethnic groups Contributing factors include higher rates of: Motor vehicle accidents Substance use Suicide attempts Increased difficulty in accessing appropriate healthcare
Hispanic and non-Hispanic Black people	Less likely to receive follow-up care and/or rehabilitation treatment More likely to experience poor functional, psychosocial, and employment-related outcomes
Military service members and veterans	From 2000 and 2019, 400,000+ US service members were diagnosed with a TBI About 80% of these cases are attributed to accidents incurred while the individual was not deployed This population may: Experience ongoing symptoms Have co-occurring conditions, e.g., PTSD or depression Have difficulty accessing necessary physical and mental healthcare services Be likely to report suicidal ideation
People in correctional or detention facilities	Though specifics are not known, aggregate data suggests approximately 46% of the people in these facilities have a history of TBI. Correlations are found with: Mental health problems, e.g., depression and anxiety Substance use disorder Difficulty regulating expressions of anger Suicidal ideation/attempts
People who experience homelessness	When compared to the general population, these people are: Two to four times more likely to have a history of any type of TBI Up to ten times more likely to have a history of moderate to severe TBI When they have a history of TBI, they are more likely to report: Experiencing trauma/violence during childhood Substance use Suicidal ideation/attempts
Survivors of IPV	Those who have experienced a TBI due to assault are more likely to be diagnosed with PTSD, insomnia, and depression and to report worse overall health
Low income, uninsured, or undocumented peoples	Less likely to receive neurosurgical intervention Less likely to receive inpatient services, including inpatient rehabilitation services More likely to die in hospital
People living in rural areas	Greater risk of dying from a TBI. Some reasons include: The additional time needed for travel to emergency medical care Less access to facilities able to provide the appropriate level of care Difficulty accessing specialized care

Note. Adapted from "Health Disparities and TBI," by CDC (2021c)

legal systems are primarily designed from the perspective of a dominant culture and around an assumptive norm. The legislation regarding surrogate decision-makers and guardianship can vary significantly by state, and the social worker should be aware of best legal and ethical practices in their location.

Queer people, people in nontraditional relationship structures, people who have no or limited contact with biologically close relatives, people with communal family structures, and other culturally diverse social systems may not have their wishes accurately reflected by this default structure. Consider that some people may have no informal support system available to them at all and may be marginalized by the healthcare system if they do not have substantial financial assets and/or insurance coverage to compensate. The long-term care plan following a traumatic injury often takes the availability of family and informal support for granted, and this can be problematic for those without such resources. It is necessary to be aware of the laws concerning surrogate decision-making in your area, as ultimately legality will take precedence; bioethicists and legal teams may be available to assist in navigating these situations and advocating for patients and their families.

Authors' Reflections

My personal experience as a social worker in healthcare has spanned the micro-macro spectrum. I worked as a medical social worker at Lenox Hill Hospital in Manhattan for years, including through the coronavirus (COVID-19) pandemic, before transitioning into the Community and Population Health department at Northwell Health where we utilize social determinant of health data to create and implement programming to mitigate social deficits in access to healthcare and promote overall wellness throughout New York.

My time at bedside was primarily on neurosurgical ICU and telemetry units with a high percentage of TBI and other traumatic injury occurrences. I found that my ability to remain a clear and consistent presence for my patients and families who were experiencing sudden, extreme change was paramount. There is no shying away from reality in these moments. Sitting in it, rather, and holding space to allow patients and families to feel the totality of their experience sometimes calls for a boundlessness on the part of the social worker. I believe this is often the most profound task and one the social worker is uniquely poised to undertake.

The inherent inequities of our healthcare system are often highlighted by traumatic injury as those affected are understandably less prepared for the possibility of an unpredictable and devastating event. For those without exorbitant socioeconomic means, this presents a seemingly insurmountable dilemma as patients and caregivers scramble to access newly and immediately necessary supportive services that often take months to coordinate, a process in which the social worker participates intimately. For me, these inequities and the task of trying to navigate them are the most frustrating aspect of the work, and it bolstered my desire to continue a pathway into macro social work in healthcare. It can be disheartening when what would best serve the patient and family is evident, but due to systemic factors, these services are unobtainable regardless of the best efforts of the social worker.

I have found that along the totality of the healthcare micro-macro spectrum—from the chaos of the hospital setting in the wake of an event that is often both physically and psychologically traumatic to the broader scope of addressing and amending systemic deficits—that social work skills and our perspective can be incredibly meaningful to those we serve. Our particular lens complements the other clinical disciplines in the hospital where we can be a grounding force by demonstrating consistent understanding, respect, and advocacy for each patient as a whole, unique person—at times, this can be one of the most relevant interventions to employ. Social workers are also adept at utilizing a systems perspective with a finely honed understanding of social justice practice relative to ingrained systemic marginalizing power structures—this prowess should be elevated and our perspective reinforced as we endeavor to realize justice in healthcare. -R.W.

Psychologically traumatizing events irrevocably alter our sense of self, as any extreme sense of powerlessness and loss of control over a situation not only disrupts our beliefs and expectations of how the world operates but also demolishes our basic assumptions of safety, self-efficacy, trust, spirituality, and invulnerability (Kleber, 2019). With traumatic injury and TBI, whether the injury is temporary or chronic, the sudden loss of agency in one's world that is compounded by a complete change in identity and perception of self in the world ushers in new and often significant psychological stress, not only on the patient but also on their extended caregiving network, as the patient becomes inherently vulnerable to and dependent upon others. In parallel, all parties grapple over time to adjust to an altered sense of personal agency in the "new normal" of life as a patient or the caregiver of a patient (Petersen & Saunders, 2015).

Working with this population as a mental health provider requires holding space for witnessing considerable suffering and sensations of feeling trapped within a considerably transformed experience where former rubrics of coping may now feel insufficient and inadequate for not only the patient but also their loved ones and their team of providers. In this context, suicidal ideation commonly becomes a space of comfort as patients imagine an end to their seemingly interminable present-moment experience. While providing mental health services to patients suffering from severe brachial plexus injuries, I encountered numerous patients whose lives were irrevocably and catastrophically changed. Over a third of those patients sought solace in fantasies of suicide (Landers et al., 2018), which elicited an expanse of feelings for me as a provider, fellow human, and spiritual being. I still recall a patient who relayed to me how every night he prayed to not wake up in the morning, and each morning he lamented not having died on scene despite being actively engaged in both his family and professional life. Holding that patient's experience and the medical team's emotions in learning how much this popular and outwardly jovial patient desired to terminate his life led me to examine many of my own beliefs around the value of life, the medical system's insistence on preserving life at all costs, and of living in a dramatically altered experience of self and body in the world.

Ultimately this patient, along with many others who experience such despair, moved beyond that experience; being guided to discover his ability to pivot, accept, and adapt to the new normal helped him reignite a sense of self-efficacy, self-worth, and self-esteem and achieve long-term adjustment. Patients will cycle through questions of "Who am I now?", "Who am I in this new body/mind?", "Who am I to others?", "Am I safe in the world?", and "How can I live or do things with this (emotional and physical) pain?" In processing these questions and related emotions across the phases of recovery, patients come to a different understanding and acceptance of self whereby they find new space to operate in the world as they are. As social workers, we may play a privileged and prominent role in helping patients and their caregivers bridge from the depths of personal darkness to the discovery of a new light and life within the context of their experience while we examine our own values, morals, and biases around what it means to live a good or worthwhile life. – Z.L.

Reflection Questions

1. What might be the biggest challenges for you in working with this population?
2. How might the experiences of people in marginalized populations impact their access and utilization of healthcare systems and their perspective on traumatic injury, treatment, and recovery?
3. How might you work with a patient struggling to adjust to the suddenness of their losses and changes?
4. What are some of the biases and fears you may harbor in working with this population and specifically with people in marginalized populations who are likely to experience mistrust or issues of access within the healthcare system?

References

AARP. (2020, May 14). *Caregiver burnout: Steps for coping with stress*. https://www.aarp.org/caregiving/life-balance/info-2019/caregiver-stress-burnout.html?intcmp=AE-CAR-CRC-LL

American Psychological Association. (2020, February 1). *Building your resilience*. https://www.apa.org/topics/resilience

Azman, A., Jali, N. A., Singh, P. S. J., Abdullah, J. M., & Ibrahim, H. (2019). Family roles, challenges and needs in caring for Traumatic Brain Injury (TBI) family members: A systematic review. *Journal of Health Research, 34*(6), 495–504.

Beiter, K., Danos, D., Conrad, D., Broyles, S., Zabaleta, J., Mussel, J., & Philippi, S. (2022). PTSD treatment reduces risk of trauma recidivism in a diverse community at a safety-net hospital: A propensity score analysis of data from a level one trauma center. *Injury, 53*(7), 2493–2500.

Boss, P. (1999). *Ambiguous loss: Learning to live with unresolved grief*. Harvard University Press.

Boss, P. (2022). *The myth of closure: Ambiguous loss in a time of pandemic and change*. W.W. Norton et Company.

Bramlett, H. M., & Dietrich, W. D. (2015). Long-term consequences of traumatic brain injury: Current status of potential mechanisms of injury and neurological outcomes. *Journal of Neurotrauma, 32*(23), 1834–1848. https://doi.org/10.1089/neu.2014.3352

Brazinova, A., Majdan, M., Leitgeb, J., et al. (2015). Factors that may improve outcomes of early traumatic brain injury care: Prospective multicenter study in Austria. *Scandinavian Journal of Trauma, Resuscitation, and Emergency Medicine, 23*, 1–11.

Centers for Disease Control and Prevention. (2011). *Cognitive impairment: A call for action, now!* United States Department of Health and Human Services. https://www.cdc.gov/aging/pdf/cognitive_impairment/cogimp_poilicy_final.pdf

Centers for Disease Control and Prevention. (2021a). *Cost of injury data.* https://www.cdc.gov/injury/wisqars/cost/index.html#print

Centers for Disease Control and Prevention. (2021b). *Surveillance report of traumatic brain injury-related hospitalizations and deaths by age group, sex, and mechanism of injury—United States, 2016 and 2017.* https://www.cdc.gov/traumaticbraininjury/pdf/TBI-surveillance-report-2016-2017-508.pdf

Centers for Disease Control and Prevention. (2021c). *Health disparities and TBI.* https://www.cdc.gov/traumaticbraininjury/health-disparities-tbi.html

Changoor, A., Colella, B., Monette, G., & Green, R. (2020). Moderate-severe TBI as a progressive disorder: Cognitive declines in the chronic stages of injury. *Neurology, 94*(15), 5035.

Conti, A., Clari, M., Nolan, M., Wallace, E., Tommasini, M., Mozzone, S., & Campagna, S. (2019). The relationship between psychological and physical secondary conditions and family caregiver burden in spinal cord injury: A correlational study. *Top Spinal Cord Injury and Rehabilitation, 25*(4), 271–280.

Dams-O'Connor, K., Landau, A., Hoffman, J., & St De Lore, J. (2018). Patient perspectives on quality and access to healthcare after brain injury. *Brain Injury, 32*(4), 431–441.

Davis, M., Graf, G., Hoefer, R., LaBrenz, C., Lee, K., Mitschke, D., Murphy, E. R., Padilla-Medina, D., Robinson, S. R., Slater, H., Troutman, B., Schrag, R. V., Xu, L., & Mauldin, R. L. (2020). *11.2 single-subjects design.* Foundations of Social Work Research. https://uta.pressbooks.pub/foundationsofsocialworkresearch/chapter/11-2-single-subjects-design/#:~:text=The%20baseline%20stage%20is%20the,drinking%20during%20the%20work%20week

Degeneffe, C. E. (2001). Family caregiving and traumatic brain injury. *Health & Social Work, 26*(4), 257–268. https://doi.org/10.1093/hsw/26.4.257

DiMaggio, C., Ayoung-Chee, P., ShinSeki, M., Wilson, C., Marshall, G., Lee, D. C., Wall, S., Maulana, S., Pachter, H. L., & Frangos, S. (2016). Traumatic injury in the United States: In-patient epidemiology 2000-2011. *Injury, 47*(7), 1393–1403.

Geard, A., Kirkevold, M., Løvstad, M., & Schanke, A. K. (2020). How do family members of individuals with spinal cord and acquired brain injuries make sense of their experiences: A qualitative study of meaning making processes. *Health Psychology Open, 7*, 1–13.

Harris, D. & Winokuer, H. (2019). *Principles and Practice of Grief Counseling.* Springer Publishing Company.

Hicks, C. W., Hashmi, Z. G., Velopulos, C., et al. (2014). Association between race and age in survival after trauma. *JAMA Surgery, 149*(7), 642–647.

Holmes, A., Williamson, O., Hogg, M., Arnold, C., & O'Donnell, M. (2013). Determinants of chronic pain 3 years after moderate or serious injury. *Pain Medicine, 14*, 336–344.

Janssen, J. S. (n.d.). Trauma informed end-of-life care. *Social Work Today.* https://www.socialworktoday.com/news/enews_0616_1.shtml

Kempen, G. I., Scaf-Klomp, W., Ranchor, A. V., Sanderman, R., & Ormel, J. (2001). Social predictors of recovery in late middle-aged and older persons after injury to the extremities: A prospective study. *The Journals of Gerontology Series B: Psychological Sciences and Social Sciences, 56*(4), S229. https://doi.org/10.1093/geronb/56.4.s229

Kleber, R. J. (2019). Trauma and public mental health: A focused review. *Frontiers in Psychiatry, 10*, 1–6.

Kusmaul, N. (2018). Trauma informed hospice and end-of-life care. *SWHPN Voice.* https://39k5cm1a9u1968hg74aj3x51-wpengine.netdna-ssl.com/wp-content/uploads/2019/06/Trauma_Informed_End_of_Life_Care_Kusmaul.pdf

Landers, Z., Jethanandani, R., Lee, S. K., Mancuso, C. A., Seehaus, M., & Wolfe, S. W. (2018). The psychological impact of adult brachial plexus injury. *The Journal of Hand Surgery of America, 43*(10), 950.

Lilley, E. J., Scott, J. W., & Weissman, J. S. (2018). End-of-life care in older patients after serious or severe traumatic brain injury in low-mortality hospitals compared with all other hospitals. *JAMA Surgery, 153*(1), 44–50.

National Institute of General Medical Sciences. (2018). *Physical trauma.* https://www.nigms.nih.gov/education/fact-sheets/Pages/physical-trauma.aspx

Neimeyer, R. A., Burke, L. A., Mackay, M. M., & van Dyke Stringer, J. G. (2010). Grief therapy and the reconstruction of meaning: From principles to practice. *Journal of Contemporary Psychotherapy, 40*(2), 73–83.

Nielsen, M. K., Neergaard, M. A., Jensen, A. B., Bro, F., & Guldin, M. (2016). Do we need to change our understanding of anticipatory grief in caregivers? A systematic review of caregiver studies during end-of-life caregiving and bereavement. *Clinical Psychology Review, 44*, 75–93. https://doi.org/10.1016/j.cpr.2016.01.002

Oberholzer, M., & Müri, R. M. (2019). Neurorehabilitation of Traumatic Brain Injury (TBI): A clinical review. *Medical Sciences (Basel, Switzerland), 7*(3), 47.

Oliverio, R., Karelina, K., & Weil, Z. M. (2020). Sex, drugs, and TBI: The role of sex in substance abuse related to traumatic brain injuries. *Frontiers in Neurology, 11*, 1–5.

Peter, C., Müller, R., Cieza, A., & Geyh, S. (2012). Psychological resources in spinal cord injury: A systematic literature review. *Spinal Cord, 50*, 188–201.

Petersen, H., & Sanders, S. (2015). Caregiving and traumatic brain injury: Coping with grief and loss. *Health & Social Work, 40*(4), 325–328.

Post, M. W. M., & van Leeuwan, C. M. C. (2012). Psychosocial issues in spinal cord injury: A review. *Spinal Cord, 50*, 382–389.

Rauen, K., Späni, C. B., Tartaglia, M. C., Ferretti, M. T., Reichelt, L., Probst, P., Schäpers, B., Müller, F., Jahn, K., & Plesnila, N. (2021). Quality of life after brain injury: A cross-sectional analysis uncovers age- and sex-related differences over the adult life span. *GeroScience, 43*, 263–278.

Richie, E. A., Nugent, J. G., & Raslan, A. M. (2021). Racial and ethnic inequities in mortality during hospitalization for traumatic brain injury: A call to action. *Frontiers in Surgery.* https://www.frontiersin.org/articles/10.3389/fsurg.2021.690971/full

Ringdal, M., Plos, K., & Bergbom, I. (2008). Memories of being injured and patients' care trajectory after physical trauma. *BMC Nursing, 7*(8), 1–12.

Schemitsch, C., & Nauth, A. (2020). Psychological factors and recovery from trauma. *Injury, 51*, S64. https://doi.org/10.1016/j.injury.2019.10.081

Scott, W., McEvoy, A., Garland, R., Bernier, E., Milioto, M., Trost, Z., & Sullivan, M. (2016). Sources of injustice among individuals with persistent pain following musculoskeletal injury. *Psychological Injury and Law, 9*(1), 6–15. https://doi.org/10.1007/s12207-015-9249-8

Sophie Su, Y. R., Veeravagu, A., & Grant, G. (2016). Neuroplasticity after Traumatic Brain Injury. In D. Laskowitz & G. Grant (Eds.), *Translational research in traumatic brain injury*. CRC Press/Taylor and Francis Group.

Truong, L. K., Mosewich, A. D., Holt, C. J., Le, C. Y., Miciak, M., & Whittaker, J. L. (2020). Psychological, social and contextual factors across recovery stages following a sport-related knee injury: A scoping review. *British Journal of Sports Medicine, 54*(19), 1149–1156. https://doi.org/10.1136/bjsports-2019-101206

University of Florida Health. (2016, October 12). *Traumatic injury*. https://ufhealth.org/traumatic-injury#:~:text=Traumatic%20injury%20is%20a%20term,to%20save%20life%20and%20limb

van Veen, E., van der Jagt, M., Citerio, G., Stocchetti, N., Epker, J. L., Gommers, D., Burdorf, L., Menon, D. K., Maas, A. I. R., Lingsma, H. F., & Kompanje, E. J. O. (2020). End-of-life practices in traumatic brain injury patients: Report of a questionnaire from the CENTER-TBI study. *Journal of Critical Care, 58*, 78–88. https://www.sciencedirect.com/science/article/pii/S0883944120305438

Victorson, D., Farmer, L., Burnett, K., Ouellette, A., & Barocas, J. (2005). Maladaptive coping strategies and injury-related distress following traumatic physical injury. *Rehabilitation Psychology, 50*(4), 408–415.

Wiseman, T., Foster, K., & Curtis, K. (2013). Mental health following traumatic physical injury: An integrative literature review. *Injury, 44*(11), 1383–1390.

World Health Organization, War Trauma Foundation and World Vision International. (2011, October 2). *Psychological first aid: Guide for field workers*. https://www.who.int/publications/i/item/9789241548205

Chapter 12
Communicating with Children About an Adult's Illness

Nancy F. Cincotta and Rachel Rusch

Introduction

In many situations in which an adult faces a serious illness, there is a young person who is affected: child, grandchild, niece or nephew, student, or friend. Healthcare providers who have devoted their lives to working with adults facing illness frequently perceive themselves as lacking the expertise to work with children or younger individuals in the patient's circle. This chapter aims to help clinicians to develop a framework for thinking about the needs of children, adolescents, and young adults within the network of the adult patient they have in front of them. In some cases, it will be the purview of the social worker to directly engage children in their practice. More often, they will be called upon to offer guidance to the adults regarding the children in the patient's life, offering advice on how to communicate, share medical information, and create a safe space for children to understand and cope with the experience of an adult in their lives' illness. In this chapter, the term "loved one" will be used in deference to the existent literature on child development, and "family" refers to all adults and children in a child's immediate sphere of influence.

Children, by virtue of their cognitive ability, their size, and their place in the family, may be overlooked and underserved. Yet the reality is that children facing the serious illness and death of a loved one have the longest time to live after the illness experience and thus may feel the ramifications of that illness for their lifetime.

N. F. Cincotta (✉)
Columbia University School of Social Work, New York, NY, USA
e-mail: nfc1@columbia.edu

R. Rusch
Children's Hospital Los Angeles, Los Angeles, CA, USA
e-mail: rachelruschlcsw@gmail.com

M. Hemphill, A. Nathanson (eds.), *The Practice of Clinical Social Work in Healthcare*, Essential Clinical Social Work Series,
https://doi.org/10.1007/978-3-031-31650-0_12

A child's experience witnessing serious illness can also be influenced by access to care, or lack thereof, for both adult and child. Social workers are in a position to serve as leaders in shaping the systems of care to ensure that all who are in need have the opportunity to receive readily available, culturally responsive, supportive care (Patneaude & Kett, 2020). If this area is not a typical part of one's clinical practice, what skills does one possess that may provide a foundation for continued, ongoing, and effective communication with children and their families?

Communicating with Children, Adolescents, and Young Adults

Entering into communication with a child or an adolescent/young adult (AYA is defined here to include ages 13–29) about the serious illness and mortality of a parent or caregiver can feel like invading a sensitive and vulnerable space. Families often look to psychosocial clinicians in such instances for extra support, which looks different for each family and person based on their individual cognitive and emotional development. For some, it may entail offering language to a parent or other family members as they prepare to talk with their child about treatment. For others, it may be partnering with family members to lead conversations with children or AYAs about death and bereavement. In working with young people over time, much has been learned about supportive spaces and intentional therapeutic intervention and their benefits (Quillen et al., 2021). Social workers are uniquely positioned as experts in advanced communication to promote open and accessible dialogue through a system-based perspective for children and AYAs whose lives are affected by an adult's serious illness.

The following Table 12.1 provides useful ideas and practical guidance for clinicians who are working in this area:

Table 12.1 Practical ideas for helping children with the illness experience

Work toward giving a child control and gaining mastery in the situation
Normalize their experience
Offer guidance to the adults in the situation
Identify someone in advance who can be responsible for the child during difficult times (i.e., hospital visits, wake, funeral, memorial service)
Have items that will provide comfort and familiarity available to the child (e.g., headphones, expressive arts supplies, journaling materials, books)
Keep the language and conceptualization of the situation consistent with the child's age and development
Offer the child options in situations where choices are possible
Create legacy activities that will serve as therapeutic activities in the present while also providing significant meaning in the future (e.g., making a handprint collage—The more family members' hands, the better!)

The Role of the Social Worker

Social work skills and perspective are useful in many different ways across medical settings. Social workers advocate for involvement of social work support for children and AYAs who are navigating the illness and/or death of a loved one can have a great and positive impact on present and future coping for all those involved. They utilize system-based perspectives to determine what may already be understood by a child or AYA and how best to offer them continued support. Such assessment can provide a foundation for further therapeutic intervention, engagement of community resources, and strengthened communication among all members of the family and the medical care team.

A child's community may include their family, school, sports, neighborhood, and religious groups. Each of these communities exists within a larger societal context with particular stressors or privileges. A child whose greater communities are impacted by marginalization, systemic racism, and historic social injustice requires supportive care that is informed by these considerations (Elk & Gazaway, 2021). Social workers must incorporate these social work tenets in their work to avoid generalization, to inform a continual process of evaluating biases in ourselves and in colleagues, and to advocate for individualized assessment. They must offer care with humility, continue to educate themselves with regard to the communities they serve, and allow their practice to evolve continuously over time.

The social work psychosocial assessment can provide key information with regard to the systems within which a child functions (see Table 12.2). A typical psychosocial assessment can be adapted to aid in promoting supportive communication for a child whose loved one is facing a serious illness. Depending on the cognitive and emotional ability of the child, these questions can be asked of a

Table 12.2 Child-focused assessment questions

What is the relationship between the child and the individual receiving treatment?
Who is the child's primary caregiver?
Who are the others in their family system?
Who lives with the child at home? (including pets)
What is the child's/AYA's current understanding of what is happening for their loved one?
Do they have a community or individuals they look to for support at difficult times?
Is there a spiritual or faith tradition that provides the family with tools in their ongoing coping?
What grade is the child in at school, and is school a place where the child is well connected and supported?
Has the child experienced the illness or death of a loved one before (whether a person, a pet, etc.)? What were these experiences like for them?
How have they dealt with stressful situations in the past, and on whom or what have they relied for support?
What are the child's/AYA's favorite activities?
What questions do they have at this moment? Are there things the child has heard a family member say that they are wondering about? *(The child should be explicitly told that all questions are okay to ask!)*

parent, of the child or AYA directly, or in partnership with the child and their family members. Before beginning such an inquiry, a social worker may introduce themselves and their role as extra support in the care of their family member.

A social worker can promote a safe and healing space by ensuring that a child and their family members understand they are free to share as much or as little information as they would like. Although work within families can be kept confidential and children are encouraged to trust professionals, clinicians are mandated reporters of the suspicion of child abuse and neglect and as such are obligated to contact child protective services should there be a concern about such. Similarly, if a child discloses information about actual or potential harm to themselves or others, such information must be disclosed. These limits to confidentiality should always be shared with children and families prior to the start of individualized treatment and at the time of any disclosure that requires escalated supportive services (Workers, 2008).

Such inquiry can be helpful both for information gathering and to begin to assess possible areas for additional communication, clarification, and support. These questions can be interspersed within rapport-building reflections and engagement. As play is often the medium through which young children express themselves and gain understanding of the world, providing avenues for expression (drawing supplies, games, small toys, or books) to utilize during conversation can be helpful. Such engagement can provide a foundation from which to partner with additional family members, clinicians, and community support. For additional ideas on supplies and play interventions, please see Kaduson and Schaefer's work (2001).

Communication with Children

Children, adolescents, and young adults have shared that having a safe space for open and honest communication is helpful in their future coping and ongoing grief process (Fearnley & Bowland, 2019). Prognostic uncertainty and emotional distress can be perceived as difficult barriers to overcome for the loved one who is ill, and engaging in open and honest communication with respect for the child's level of development can set the stage for continued therapeutic intervention and adaptive coping and growth within the child's relationship with the patient (Park et al., 2021). Children tend to sense that their family may be moving through difficult times, knowledge that in turn can be difficult for the child to manage on their own. Individual and thoughtful communication can be aided by an attuned care team (Eklund et al., 2021; Stein et al., 2019). Social workers are well situated to lead this advanced communication from a person-centered and system-informed perspective.

Developmental Considerations: What Children Understand

What children know and how they understand it is a product of the intersection between their cognitive and physical development, family and cultural environments, and their lived experience of the medical situation. Throughout childhood, children are in a "learning trajectory" over the course of which they gain knowledge and learn to cope with life, to formulate a concept of themselves and their peers, and to harness the boundless emotions they experience. Trying to make sense of an adult loved one's illness or death occurs within that normal volatility of childhood. Understanding cognitive development, the way children think, and the successive increments of emotional growth allows the practitioner to help family members put the illness in a context a child can comprehend.

Much has been explored with regard to the cognitive and emotional developmental stages for typically developing children (Piaget, 1953; Stern, 1985). Awareness and familiarity of these stages of development may be useful when working with a child who is experiencing the illness of an adult (Christ & Christ, 2006). For example, in conceptualizing how children come to understand emotions, Harter and Buddin (1987) explore the notion of multidimensional thought in a unidimensional mind. This concept can help adults understand a child's inability to think beyond their cognitive ability. For instance, a typically developing 4-year-old may not be able to express joy while experiencing sadness. For the adolescent who may feel immortal, the threat of loss of a parent may not seem like a reality until it occurs, which may impede valuable end-of-life experiences (Christ et al., 2002).

Framework for Conceptualizing Illness

Conceptualizing illness through the eyes of the child requires envisioning the child's experience of the world throughout different periods of development. For instance, a young child may be able to conceptualize treatment as helping good cells fight the bad cells. An older child may understand that steroids are a medication that can help people feel better or stronger and be able to distinguish between symptoms of the underlying illness and adverse effects of medications. Young adults may appreciate the concrete issues and language surrounding illness, but may not have yet developed coping skills to address their feelings. As an illness trajectory changes and a child matures, additional information should be provided accordingly.

When an ill parent or adult family member seems less available, sleeps more, eats differently, or takes part in different activities, these changes will be noticed by children of all ages, who will need help in understanding the impact of the illness and its treatment. Children may mistakenly assume that they are less loved by the individual who is ill or perceive that they might have done something wrong that alienated the ill person from them. Actively engaging and soliciting the child's conceptualization and experience over time can aid in alleviating these concerns while offering avenues for deepened communication. Additional experiences that may require explanation are the visible effects of treatment, such as puffy cheeks from steroids or hair loss from chemotherapy, as well as the invisible effects of the illness, such as exhaustion, pain, or confusion.

Language of Illness

Children need explanations in developmentally appropriate language, clarification of the words they hear, and an opportunity to ask questions about any information they are being given. Their level of comprehension needs to be understood, recognized, and respected. At times, children can appear to understand a surprising amount, especially as they learn to repeat new information that they have heard frequently. However, they may not grasp the meaning of what they hear. For instance, words with two meanings (homonyms) can be complicated for young children. Being informed that their dad was *getting fired* could be a frightening concept for the child who envisions their parent being placed in a fire. Blood, a naturally frightening thing for children, is the subject of many medical conversations employing terminology that may be unfamiliar and figures of speech that may raise confusion and questions in children's minds. Some examples include "drawing blood" (the 5-year-old may ask, *Do you have to be an artist to draw blood?*) and taking blood (the 7-year-old may wonder, *Where do you take it? How do you take it? Do you take all of it? What happens if you take all of someone's blood?*). When someone talks of a blood drive, a child may envision blood in a car somehow interacting with the steering wheel.

It becomes important to think about the meaning and the context of language when working with children who are experiencing the serious illness of a loved one. Euphemisms may be intended by adults to explain difficult concepts with gentleness but may in fact have the opposite effect when processed by a child's literal-minded consciousness. For example, the thought of being *put to sleep* for a procedure can alarm children, causing them to worry about what happens when they sleep at night. When someone dies, suggesting that they are *lost* may cause a child to believe that the person is missing and may one day return. Other concepts may simply be difficult to understand, such as *withdrawing care*. One child was confused when they learned that the family was *stopping treatment* for a loved one. They did not know that treatment was being discontinued because it was ineffective; instead, they believed that their family had opted to intentionally cause the death of their relative.

The course of an illness may seem foreign to a child. Choosing the right language to help a child conceptualize the illness can aid in supporting the child's experience and understanding. For example, use of the word "cure" is only helpful if the condition is not life-limiting. There are other words a child might hear that require explanation, such as control, remission, and relapse. Similarly, use of the words "death" and "dying" can provide a more clear and helpful space for a child to gain understanding, as opposed to euphemisms such as "losing" someone or having them "pass away" or "go to sleep."

Perceptions and Misperceptions

While a social worker may be able to anticipate reactions to certain words with some degree of accuracy, they will need to be attuned to the child's reactions and questions and be willing to engage accordingly. Among the more complicated challenges for practitioners working with children is *understanding what they understand*, both in language and in nuance of the situation. Medical information can be difficult for even the most highly educated adults to comprehend; for children there are layers of emotional and developmental complexity that may inhibit their understanding. It is easy for a child to misperceive information and for adults not to recognize that a child needs further clarification. This is concerning in part because, if a child does not understand the reality or the gravity of the situation, they can feel unloved and unimportant during the course of illness and angry and hurt in retrospect. If additional medical information should emerge later from other sources, it may erode trust in the primary caregivers and influence future relationships.

Helpful Hints

It is important to review what has been understood by the child in language and in context. When giving medical information to a child, find ways to have the child reflect back to you what they heard. For instance, a social worker might ask the child: *If your teacher at school asked what was happening with your mom, what would you say?; So tell me, what is going on with your mom?; What do you understand about your dad's illness?*; *Do you know the name of his illness?*; *What do you know about the treatment for his illness?*; *and What do you say when your friends ask you about your Mom?* When asking such questions, it can be helpful to reiterate that there are no "right" or "wrong" answers. Your goal in speaking with the child is to:

- *Learn* what the child understood and their response
- *Help* children learn communication skills
- *Rehearse* with the child how to ask and respond to questions
- *Assess* for misperceptions
- *Clarify* information (when appropriate)
- *Create a safe space* for future conversations

The following table (12.3 CATPAWS) provides social workers with a framework to help adults understand what children may be thinking when navigating serious illness in their family. These questions may be different for every child, depending

Table 12.3 CATPAWS: a framework for the types of questions children may ask

Causality	Did I do something to cause this? Did they? Why did this happen?
Anticipation	What is going to happen next?
Transmission	Am I or others going to catch it?
Panic	Are they going to die? Am I going to die?
Assurance	Assurance that the ill person continues to care (even as some things may seem as though they have changed because of the demands the illness places on the individual). Assurance that the child is safe and supported.
Worries	What else is going to happen? Who will take care of me? Will I get cancer too?
Self-interest	How does this affect me? How will my life change? Will I be able to continue my activities? Will you still be able to play with me?

on their individual development and their family's circumstance. These considerations may also be helpful to be aware of when working with any aged child or AYAs.

Young children may ask the same questions repeatedly as they seek a fuller understanding of the situation. They might share their understanding in unexpected places—e.g., telling the grocery store clerk, "My daddy has cancer." This is an expected part of processing new information in a developing brain. Conversely, AYAs depending on their personal style and level of comfort with the situation may not ask anything at all. In these circumstances, it can be helpful to offer a safe environment for posing questions as they arise, reiterating that they can be in control of the conversation in whatever way feels most comfortable.

Children come to understand illness through their own developmental lens and therefore need help understanding the illness and its ramifications not just at diagnosis but, ongoingly, as they mature and as the illness changes. Harter and Buddin's (1987) concept of multidimensional thought in a unidimensional mind explains how children understand information and express emotions within their own cognitive framework. Depending on their age and level of development, it may not be possible for them to understand and experience more than one emotion at a time. For example, when a young child connects electronically with someone who is ill whom they cannot visit, they may be unhappy because they miss in-person interactions with that person, and, in this situation, they likely cannot express more positive emotions connected with seeing that person. This developmental characteristic may lead to confusion between children and their adult caregivers and may even compromise well-intended communications. It is important that adults' expectations of the child's ability to communicate do not exceed the child's cognitive and emotional ability.

Parental and Caregiver Guidance

A primary role for social workers working with those who are ill is aiding them in communicating with their children about their illness. By enabling adults to find developmentally appropriate language, they can feel empowered and encouraged to move forward with emotionally difficult conversations.

An important goal during the course of illness for parents and other caregivers is maintaining their roles as supports and guides for their children. When certain activities cannot be overseen by a parent due to illness, planning for other adults to assume this role helps the adult who is ailing to fulfill their emotional need to be in charge of their child's care while at the same time facilitating continuity in the child's physical experience. Thinking through activities in which they can be involved, and making plans for their children's care as necessary, can create meaningful, stabilizing opportunities for family life in the course of a serious illness and at the end of life. Learning to delegate tasks, yet remaining emotionally present, helps to foster positive bonds.

Engaging in individual work with a child, outside of family work with the adult involved, needs to be approached with the consideration and permission of the child's parent/caregiver. Debilitating illness may make certain things more difficult to achieve from a parental perspective. Patients may need assistance in assessing what they can and cannot do, but even the exercise of making this assessment helps keep control of the process of parenting in the patient's hands for as long as possible, in whatever ways remain feasible.

The following table (12.4) provides social workers with tools to offer parents and caregivers who are supporting children and AYAs who are navigating serious illness within their family:

Family Communication Styles

It is useful to ascertain the communication styles of the adults and children involved in the serious illness of a loved one. From our practice experience, we have learned that if presented with a parent who is shy or very private and reticent to open discussion, it would be inappropriate to give the child more information than the adult has sought, knows, or is willing to discuss. If an adult engages in very open and explicit conversation, the family will have to determine the level of dialogue with their child/children. It is the adult's prerogative to limit what is shared.

Each family has a communication style, and children learn and take their cues from the adults with whom they live and interact. There may be multigenerational or intergenerational aspects to a child's family and community system that have informed family communication over time. Communication patterns after diagnosis will generally mirror the styles that existed prior to the onset of the illness. The ways that families have dealt with previous crises or difficult times will likely be

Table 12.4 Guidance for parents and caregivers regarding children, adolescents, and young adults

Developmental insight/ common assumptions	Parental/caregiver guidance/important considerations
Trust serves as the foundation for relationships and instills faith in the relationship	Be honest, in a developmentally appropriate way, during the course of your illness.
Children see and hear everything; they understand the climate in their household	Give children, adolescents, and young adults as much information as they seek and can understand.
Adults often conceptualize and worry about many components of the illness and its future trajectory	It is not necessary to present everything you are thinking or worrying about in each moment. Respond to the questions that are asked and give information that addresses current concerns and questions.
Children of all ages rely on their parents or caretakers throughout their lives	Ensure that the child understands that they can always come to you for information or with questions. Identify another adult who can be available in this role should a crisis occur.
Children may move quickly between subjects… and that's okay	Children can help themselves navigate big concepts and emotions by moving in between new topics and familiar topics. Don't be alarmed if a child asks a difficult question about illness in one moment and then about what they are having for dinner the next. They are helping themselves integrate new and significant information in a way that feels comfortable and is consistent with their capacity.
Adults teach children their patterns of communication	Recognize that children will follow your lead, often mirroring your behavior.
Think about who needs what from whom (and when) related to your illness	Parents know their children better than anyone else. Provide information at a pace and style that works for you and works for them.
Every family is different, as is every individual	Work within your communication style and with what you know works for your child.
How information is transmitted publicly can be as important as what is said	Be wary of posting information on social media that younger family members have not heard directly from the adults in the family. See communication with children as the priority.
Feeling like an integral part of what is happening during the illness, regardless of phase, will help a child with the experience	Excluding children can make them feel unwanted or disconnected at an important time in the life of the family. Include children in what is happening in a developmentally appropriate way over time.
Often the things a child can produce in their imagination are more powerful and frightening than what truth and open dialogue can provide	Note any wariness or fear when communicating with children. Trust in your connection and your ability to provide a safe and supportive space.
Family life is important in a child's ability to cope	Make space for fun. Find new ways of creating meaning and memory-making that may be required due to changes in the course of the illness.

replicated throughout the illness trajectory. Being aware of the individual's and family's style of communication is an important part of one's assessment and influences the treatment plan. While open and developmentally attuned communication has been shown to lessen a child's anxiety and increase feelings of safety over time, there may be times when cultural or individual needs may call for adaptations in communication (Stein et al., 2019). While respecting the family system, social workers can influence the clarity of communication while balancing and respecting a family's personal culture and values.

Defining the illness, as well as necessary procedures and medications, will aid in clarifying misperceptions and will enable the child to conceptualize the process. When explaining the illness, it is helpful to break it down into components that can be recognized by the child. Did it have an acute or gradual onset? How has it affected how the adult feels? What are the treatments the child can understand? Explaining a particular condition to a child can begin with what they may have recognized about the illness.

Communication with children follows a continuum, starting at diagnosis, through the course of treatment, during illness progression or remission and through bereavement. Whether the illness trajectory is constant, episodic, relapsing, or progressive, all will require ongoing explanations as the child's knowledge base grows and cognitive development evolves. It is essential to continue the assessment process and work with the family system throughout the different stages of the loved one's illness, particularly with regard to coping, communication, and understanding. Supporting children through the continuum of an adult's advanced serious illness and end of life will help the child learn to live with illness and loss in their lifetime.

Considerations Regarding Limiting Communication

There may be circumstances in which more limited communication with children is what the family desires or the situation warrants. Adults have the right to choose the manner in which they share information about their illness and how it is communicated to the children, adolescents, and young adults in their lives. As professionals focused on helping others communicate, social workers working with families typically seek to establish an environment conducive to disclosing developmentally appropriate information. Professionals cannot expect patients to have conversations with their children that they may not feel able or ready to have with themselves. In rare circumstances, an adult may opt not to know all the medical information about their own condition, and in these cases, disclosure to children will need to be mitigated. Even within these situations, social workers can be a source of connectivity and can foster loving moments between the adult and the child, outside of explicit illness dialogues.

In some cases, the illness and its manifestations may be so unanticipated and progress so quickly that there is no time to bring a child into conversations. In such situations, continued therapeutic engagement can ensure supportive communication. At times, a family may feel uncomfortable or uncertain about what the child may be able to cope with and express their desire to not discuss the illness with them. This may be informed by a family's personal culture, previous experience with serious illness, religious beliefs, etc. With this in mind, each family should be assessed anew for their individual needs (Cincotta et al., in press).

A clinician may then be able to join with family members to further assess the child's understanding and facilitate the answering of any questions or worries that they may have. Sometimes questions left unaddressed may be more frightening in a child's imagination. Clinicians can often provide psychotherapeutic education in a compassionate way while continuing to respect the family's autonomy, wisdom, and culture.

There are certain genetic conditions, such as sickle cell anemia, breast cancer, or Huntington's disease, that present clinical scenarios that a child might have to navigate themselves in the future. In such circumstances, it may be reasonable to wait until the child is of a certain age to learn about the condition and make decisions about their future with the support of their family and primary care team.

Partnering with Colleagues Who Specialize in Working with Children

Some social workers may feel less comfortable working with children and may find it difficult to imagine communicating with a child about serious illness. When possible, interprofessional colleagues with expertise in working with children might be invited to join in the work. Such partnership can aid in comfort and education for all involved. Children often appreciate being invited to ask questions of a medical team member in association with psychosocial support. Clinicians who may be available to consult with and provide education and support to families include (but are not limited to) social workers with expertise in general pediatrics and pediatric palliative care, child life specialists, expressive and creative arts therapists, child psychologists, and pediatricians. When children have spiritual and religious identities, additional support may be available through hospital-based spiritual care services or community support as well.

Social workers can partner with community systems to provide comprehensive support for a child. Such partnerships complement efforts toward social justice and social change and can provide additional avenues for therapeutic intervention in support of a child's grief process (Jonas et al., 2018). For example, a social worker may seek the permission of a parent to speak with a counselor or teacher at a child's school to provide insight into the child's current stressors and to partner in providing support within the child's school environment. As children spend much of their time in the school setting, Stylianou and Zembylas (2018) argue that additional support within that environment can augment a child's coping in the moment and in face of future stressors. If a child is in need of specialized additional support, referrals to other organizations for services may be warranted. If a parent lacks the mental capacity to care for the child, whether by medically related delirium or dementia, the adult who is the caretaker for the child would be the person with whom service would need to be coordinated.

Communicating at End of Life and in Bereavement

It is not expected that social workers in the adult arena will often find themselves providing ongoing treatment to a child facing the advanced illness or death of a loved one. In such situations, it behooves social workers to maintain a referral list of those in the community or the hospital who can provide assistance. It may be necessary to initiate additional therapeutic support until connection to such services can be made (Table 12.5).

Often when a family member dies, the focus moves away from the needs of children as family members prepare for rituals and navigate logistics of the loss. For this reason, the following suggestions can guide clinicians as they help families during this transitional time.

The following Table 12.6 speaks to the potential needs of children at the time of death of their family member:

In the following situation, the inpatient social worker helped a child's father deal with the child's needs, at the time of his wife's illness and death and in the days thereafter, by providing books and language to help the pair communicate.

At the time of referral, a 7-year-old boy of Asian descent was having new issues with bedwetting. His mother had received an advanced cancer diagnosis, underwent surgery, moved rapidly to treatment during the same hospitalization, and then died unexpectedly. She was never able to return home.

The child was not allowed to visit his mother in the hospital. He was not at an age where talking was his preferred communication or processing modality, but he was eager to "play hospital." At each session he would meticulously set up a hospital room, with a woman in a bed and a toy child who he would literally throw out of the room. He did this for several visits.

The child gained a sense of control over the situation through this form of play, desensitizing himself to the feeling of being "thrown out" of his mother's hospital room. The unexpected diagnosis, the rapid change in his mother's health, and her ultimate death metaphorically became the object of his play. The toy child in the play scenes was repeatedly prevented from being able to get into the space where the mother was. While the play was happening, the backstory of the woman in the bed (his mother) emerged. The child had given his mother his small blanket for support when she entered the hospital. The blanket was lost during a room transfer. He wished to find the blanket, but he was never allowed to look for it. The blanket was not found in the play scenes either, but ultimately the boy in the play scenes could begin to talk about the mysterious loss of the blanket and the unexpected nature of his mother's absence. The bedwetting stopped as the child became more comfortable playing out his mother's end-of-life scenario.

Table 12.5 Needs of children at the end of life of a loved one

Experiences and visitation at the end of life may be meaningful or may make a child uncomfortable; including or not including a child at these moments is the purview of the family
Someone who knows the child well (and understands the child's personality) can be instrumental in deciding how much or how little to involve a particular child
At difficult times it is helpful for the child to feel that adults are in control, even if the child does not agree with all the decisions that are made
Explain the choices being made in connection to the person who is at the end of life
Work toward a feeling of inclusion for the child in an appropriate manner: virtually, physically, or emotionally
Be creative about communication; afford the child an opportunity to express their own voice
On critical days in the life of the family, allow the child choices in attending school or not
Have a significant person accompany a child during visits, funerals, and memorial events, so that the child's needs can be met and the child feels physically and emotionally attended to

Table 12.6 Needs of children at the time of death and immediately thereafter

Invite the child to make something for the person who is ill or perhaps to put in the coffin or go with the body during cremation
Prepare the child about what to expect before more public moments: funerals, memorial services, and other rituals
Acknowledge children in eulogies, obituaries, and in any other public venues
Explain the choices being made in connection to the person who is at the end of life
Plan a time to talk or create an activity about the life of the deceased and their connection to the child
Create age-appropriate activities over the course of time after a meaningful person has died, affording the child the message that it is appropriate to remember, feel sad, express joy, and think about the person who has died. Children will not always bring forward what they are feeling; they will need the "grownups" to raise and discuss feelings.

Ultimately the social worker made a referral for additional services to help the child further understand and manage his feelings about his mother's death. The initial social work connection established trust for the little boy to meet with a pediatric social worker trained in supporting children facing serious illness and death in their families.[1] A brief look at that work is represented below.

Suggested Tools and Activities for Parents, Caregivers, and Professionals

Parents/caregivers: Go for a walk with the child outdoors. Along the way, each person can look for a special stone. When they are found, the stones can be traded between adult and child and then kept in pockets or by the bedside. When

[1] All names and other personal identifiers in the case are fictitious. Any similarity to actual persons, living or dead, or actual events is purely coincidental.

the child sees or holds the stone, it can be a reminder that they are loved and connected to their loved one, who can do the same with their own stone. Such an activity can help reinforce bonds even when loved ones are apart from one another. (If the family cannot go for a walk, each of them can draw a picture together, representing their relationship, and trade the picture with a similar intention.)

Professionals: Many children communicate best when either at play or in an activity (Ceballos et al., 2021). With permission from the adults who care for the child, taking the child for a walk around the hospital unit or around the hallways of a clinic space can be a helpful, welcoming way for a child to feel engaged.

Letter writing: It is often easier to express oneself in a letter, and when someone is in the hospital or otherwise away from home, letter writing becomes convenient as well (Boles & Jones, 2021). Even if the individual is no longer alive, the letter can serve as a vehicle of communication. If a child is too young to write a letter, they can dictate it to a trusted adult. This need not be a written document; it could be a drawing. The tradition of allowing a child to place a letter in the coffin of a deceased person, or having it placed for them, has become a tradition in some bereavement communities.

Journaling: A book can be shared between parent and older child. One writes their entry and then it goes to the other to read, and then the authors rotate. It allows the adult and the child a protected time to share personal thoughts and feelings with each other, whether they are in the same location or not.

Bibliotherapy (reading together and reading with others): Bibliotherapy, or using books to help children cope with illness and death, can be one of the most powerful interventions to help families during the course of an illness. Publications specifically addressing bibliotherapy (Cincotta & Moore, 2021; Rusch et al., 2020) can help the practitioner develop a useful library in their office or hospital waiting areas that will help educate and support children living through the illness of a loved one.

The following table (12.7) outlines the potential benefit of utilizing bibliotherapy in this setting:

Bibliotherapy and COVID-19

With 140,000 children in the USA having had a parent or grandparent die of COVID-19, and hundreds of thousands more experiencing someone in their family having had the disease, it has become apparent that helping children understand and learn to cope with COVID-19 is essential (Hillis et al., 2021).

The COVID-19 pandemic and attendant lifestyle changes were something most could not imagine. Working from home, remote learning, not seeing loved ones and friends, the use of masks, and fear of a contagious illness were global changes that children, parents, and society experienced simultaneously. Having a way to explain

Table 12.7 What books can do

Provide comfort within a familiar medium
Reaffirm and clarify information that children have heard in other places
Educate children beyond the knowledge they have been given by adults or healthcare providers
Become an avenue for mastery over a situation (particularly as they can be read over and over again)
Allow children to be connected with others who have felt what they are feeling and lived through what they are living through
Alternatively, allow a child to escape to a place away from the illness
Open a dialogue between caregiver and child
Provide language to carry on the dialogue
Be available at all hours of the day, in any location
Be a tool for a professional to use with a child
Help a child identify and address feelings
Provide support around new and difficult feelings
Allow parents and caregivers space to communicate about these feelings and emotions

and help children adjust to the pandemic became important. Books specifically addressing COVID-19 emerged quickly, highlighting how natural bibliotherapy is as an educational and coping tool.

Authors' Reflections

We all have memories from growing up that center on a standout moment, a moment when something greatly moved us or became very clear to us. It may be useful to draw on those moments from our own memories to better connect with the children we serve.

One little boy whose father had died wanted to know, "How do you know that you can help me?" In another situation, a child, while walking around the nurse's station, bounced back and forth in conversation between talk of illness and death and talk of ice cream flavors and unicorns. Conversations with children and adolescents may not always be linear and may not stay focused on the difficult or sad experience of the situation. Being willing to enter the child's space, to be present for the range of their emotions, is essential. It means recognizing that children, even in times of grief or great distress, will be children and need childlike activities and interventions. Honoring this reality is the essence of the social work doctrine of meeting the client where the client is at. The striking honesty and openness of children can be daunting at first but also rather enlightening.

In one case, an 8-year-old's family had a viewing when his father died, but the coffin remained closed. The child wanted to see the body but did not see a way to make this clear to the adults present. He walked up and down and around the closed coffin, even lingered there, but no one picked up on his cue, although he thought his intention was obvious. Children may not always express their emotions and reluctant adults may not always recognize a child's overture.

The impact on the child of a beloved adult's journey of illness needs to be recognized: how it changes their lives and challenges their ability to cope. Children of all ages may know much more than the adults around them perceive and have extremely good "radar" as to the emotional climate in their environment. To talk about what is going on, they often require little more than a simple invitation to enter a dialogue and circumstances that support their questions. The work for the significant adults in the world of the child is to plan and enable happy and fulfilling moments while dealing with the difficult ones. At the end of the day, every child wants and needs to know that they will be taken care of and that they are integral to their family, regardless of the illness experience or its outcome.

Reflection Questions

1. What might be the most challenging part of working with children around illness and loss for you?
2. How do age and developmental milestones impact clinical assessment and intervention?
3. In what ways does work with children differ from work with adults?

Illness, Grief, and Bereavement Resources

National Websites: Developmentally Appropriate Materials and Programs

Bo's Place www.bosplace.org
Dougy Center: The National Center for Grieving Children and Families www.dougy.org
Experience Camps experiencecamps.org
Judi's House/JAG Institute judishouse.org
National Alliance for Grieving Children www.childrengrieve.org
Sesame Street in Communities: Helping Children Grieve sesamestreetincommunities.org/topics/grief/
Apart of Me: Helping Young People Cope with Grief Apartofme.app

Books to Assist Children Related to COVID-19

Edwards, D., Tomu, T., & Fernandez, N. L. (2020). *The Unwelcome Stranger*. Pangea Publishing. (*education and dealing with uncertainty*).

Gratias, M. (2020). *Captain Corona & the 19 COVID Warriors*. Progress Not Perfection, LLC. https://mailchi.mp/melissagratias/captaincorona (*focus on "we are in this together"*).

Growe, R., Burch, J. M., & Garofoli, V. (2020). *A Kid's Guide to Coronavirus*. American Psychological Association – Magination Press. https://www.apa.org/pubs/magination/kids-guide-coronavirus-ebook.pdf (*self-help and managing anxiety*).

Horne, K., Albers, N., & Shields, E. (2020). *Careless Corny: A Cautionary Tale*. Children's Hospital Los Angeles.

Ross, M., & Iradukunda, B. (2020). *I Love You*. Nabu Press. www.nabu.org/wp-content/uploads/2020/04/COVID19_003_I-Love-You_Portrait _EnglishOnly.pdf (*dealing with isolation from relatives and global-worldwide view*)

Thompson, L. S., & Thompson, J. (2020). *Lucy's Mask*. Independently published. (*reassurance and comfort*).
Tuchel, T. (2020). *Wearing A Mask: A Social Narrative for Children*. Autism Little Learners. https://www.yai.org/sites/default/files/wearing_a_mask_social_story_1.pdf
Zucker, B. (2020). *Unstuck! 10 Things to Do to Stay Safe and Sane During the Pandemic*. American Psychological Association – Magination Press. https://www.apa.org/pubs/magination/unstuck-ebook.pdf (*education and safety*).

References

Boles, J. C., & Jones, M. T. (2021). Legacy perceptions and interventions for adults and children receiving palliative care: A systematic review. *Palliative Medicine, 35*(3), 529–551.
Ceballos, P. L., Post, P., & Rodríguez, M. (2021). Practicing child-centered play therapy from a multicultural and social justice framework. In E. Gil & A. A. Drewes (Eds.), *Cultural issues in play therapy* (pp. 13–31). The Guilford Press.
Christ, G. H., & Christ, A. E. (2006). Current approaches to helping children cope with a parent's terminal illness. *CA: A Cancer Journal for Clinicians, 56*(4), 197–212.
Christ, G. H., Siegel, K., & Christ, A. E. (2002). Adolescent grief: "It never really hit me… until it actually happened". *JAMA, 288*(10), 1269–1278.
Cincotta, N. F., & Moore, T. (2021). Bibliotherapy. In T. Alitilio, S. Otis-Green, & J. Cagle (Eds.), *Oxford textbook of palliative social work* (2nd ed.). Oxford University Press.
Cincotta, N., Paul, S., & Patneaude, A. (in press). Chapter 19: Children, teens, and young adults with cancer. In S. Hedlund, B. Miller, G. Christ, & C. Messner (Eds.), *Oncology and palliative social work: Psychosocial care for people coping with cancer*. Oxford University Press.
Eklund, R., Lövgren, M., Alvariza, A., Kreicbergs, U., & Udo, C. (2021). Talking about death when a parent with dependent children dies of cancer: A pilot study of the Family Talk Intervention in palliative care. *Death Studies*, 1–11. https://doi-org.ezproxy.cul.columbia.edu/10.1080/07481187.2021.1947415
Elk, R., & Gazaway, S. (2021). Engaging social justice methods to create palliative care programs that reflect the cultural values of African American patients with serious illness and their families: A path towards health equity. *The Journal of Law, Medicine & Ethics, 49*(2), 222–230.
Fearnley, R., & Boland, J. W. (2019). Parental life-limiting illness: What do we tell the children? *Healthcare, 7*(1), 47.
Harter, S., & Buddin, B. J. (1987). Children's understanding of the simultaneity of two emotions: A five-stage developmental acquisition sequence. *Developmental Psychology, 23*(3), 388–399. https://doi.org/10.1037/0012-1649.23.3.388
Hillis, S. D., Blenkinsop, A., Villaveces, A., Annor, F. B., Liburd, L., Massetti, G. M., Demissie, Z., Mercy, J. A., Nelson, C. A., Cluver, L., Flaxman, S., Sherr, L., Donnelly, C. A., Ratmann, O., & Unwin, H. J. T. (2021). COVID-19-associated orphanhood and caregiver death in the United States. *Pediatrics*, Article e2021053760. https://doi.org/10.1542/peds.2021-053760
Jonas, D., Scanlon, C., Rusch, R., Ito, J., & Joselow, M. (2018). Bereavement after a child's death. *Child and Adolescent Psychiatric Clinics of North America, 27*(4), 579–590.
Kaduson, H., & Schaefer, C. (Eds.). (2001). *101 Favorite play therapy techniques* (Vol. 111). Jason Aronson.
Park, E. M., Jensen, C., Song, M. K., Yopp, J. M., Deal, A. M., Rauch, P. K., Greer, J. A., & Rosenstein, D. L. (2021). Talking with children about prognosis: The decisions and experiences of mothers with metastatic cancer. *JCO Oncology Practice, 17*(6), e840–e847.
Patneaude, A., & Kett, J. (2020). Cultural responsiveness and palliative care during the COVID-19 pandemic. *Palliative Medicine Reports, 1*(1), 171–173.

Piaget, J. (1953). *The origins of intelligence in children*. Routledge/Keagan Paul.
Quillen, L. J., Borstelmann, N. A., Stanton, K. E., Nelson, C. A., Chien, S. A., Bowers, S. M., Swift, C. L., Gonzalez, Y., Yi, S. M., & Park, E. M. (2021). Addressing the needs of parents with advanced cancer: Attitudes, practice behaviors, and training experiences of oncology social workers. *Palliative & Supportive Care, 19*(3), 329–334.
Rusch, R., Greenman, J., Scanlon, C., Horne, K., & Jonas, D. F. (2020). Bibliotherapy and bereavement: Harnessing the power of reading to enhance family coping in pediatric palliative care. *Journal of Social Work in End-of-Life & Palliative Care, 16*(2), 85–98.
Stein, A., Dalton, L., Rapa, E., Bluebond-Langner, M., Hanington, L., Stein, K. F., Ziebland, S., Rochat, T., Harrop, E., Kelly, B., Bland, R., & Communication Expert Group. (2019). Communication with children and adolescents about the diagnosis of their own life-threatening condition. *Lancet, 393*(10176), 1150–1163.
Stern, D. N. (1985). *The interpersonal world of the infant: A view from psychoanalysis and developmental psychology*. Basic Books.
Stylianou, P., & Zembylas, M. (2018). Dealing with the concepts of "grief" and "grieving" in the classroom: Children's perceptions, emotions, and behavior. *Omega, 77*(3), 240–266.
Workers, N. A. (2008). *NASW code of ethics (guide to the everyday professional conduct of social workers)*. NASW.

Chapter 13
Trauma-Informed Approaches and Interventions in Serious Illness

Jennifer DiBiase and Abigail Nathanson

Introduction

From Person to Patient

Our relationships to our bodies are complex, often informed by sociopolitical identities within our communities. Whether our bodies feel safe and strong, damaged and unlovable, cared for by the people around us, or objectified, they hold the history of what we have been through in our lives. When serious illness occurs, it does so in the context of our previous experiences with healthcare, times when we have felt unsafe in our bodies, and how we physically, emotionally, and spiritually embody the experiences of our families and communities.

Upon diagnosis of a serious illness, patients may choose more frequent and consistent engagement with a healthcare system. These encounters are likely to include physical contact with providers and clinicians, including hands-on physical examination, diagnostic procedures, and treatments that may feel invasive, uncomfortable, or painful. Serious illness or injury brings extensive uncertainty, fear of physical pain or death, and sensations of powerlessness. These experiences may be evocative, consciously or unconsciously, of earlier trauma (Levenson, 2020; Raja et al., 2015; Reeves, 2015).

J. DiBiase (✉)
Mount Sinai Beth Israel, New York, NY, USA
e-mail: Jennifer.DiBiase@mountsinai.org

A. Nathanson
Silver School of Social Work, New York University, New York, NY, USA
e-mail: an768@nyu.edu

M. Hemphill, A. Nathanson (eds.), *The Practice of Clinical Social Work in Healthcare*, Essential Clinical Social Work Series,
https://doi.org/10.1007/978-3-031-31650-0_13

In this highly charged context, patients are asked to make decisions about the future that can feel overwhelming. They must also learn, or remember, how to navigate a healthcare system that has its own culture, language, norms, and power hierarchy. This type of engagement activates coping strategies that may have helped the patient in the past to learn, acculturate, tolerate stress, and survive both physically and emotionally. In these ways, illness elicits a stress response that amplifies both strengths and vulnerabilities in our preexisting coping styles.

When people experience illness, they may make the challenging journey from "person" to "patient." From a trauma-informed lens, this transition is noteworthy and denotes a definition of self defined by one role (a patient) in relation to others (a healthcare system). People who have experienced trauma often have learned ways to feel safe in the world that involve avoiding dependence on others or any reminders of their own vulnerability; in the patient role, such avoidance becomes nearly impossible. For those with a history of abuse and trauma, whether physical, emotional, psychological, financial, relational, racial, sexual, or other, the need to lean on others may feel unsafe, while uncertainty about how one will fare may feel particularly threatening, exacerbating symptoms of past traumatic experiences (Levenson, 2020).

The patient who is dealing with limited income and healthcare benefits, inadequate housing, food insecurity, or caregiver responsibilities throughout treatment and care may feel especially vulnerable. For patients with trauma histories, adjusting to the experience of the illness coupled with new demands of trusting others to provide care, and perhaps growing awareness of physical, financial, and relational limitations, can make navigating the healthcare system extraordinarily difficult. Oriented by a biomedical approach to personhood, the US healthcare system is often ill-equipped to engage with these relational and psychosocial complexities in order to co-create an environment that resists re-traumatization and fosters healing.

Social workers are educated in a person-in-environment perspective and take a holistic view of a patient presenting to a healthcare setting (Dubus & Howard, 2016). Social workers are also uniquely trained to understand the impact of trauma experienced by individuals as a result of childhood and adult adversity and systemic discrimination (Larkin et al., 2014). In the medical setting, we observe the ways in which trauma can impact the patient's experience of serious illness. It can affect their engagement with preventative care and medical evaluation when symptoms first present; it can affect coping with rigorous treatment schedules and medical follow-up, right through end of life. We also observe how experiences with illness become folded into the family and community narrative in ways consequential to relationships with the healthcare system for generations to come.

In this chapter, we will explore trauma-informed care and how healthcare may be experienced by a person with a history of trauma, from the single clinical encounter to processes at the healthcare system level. We will examine how providers and systems can be more accommodating and responsive to meet patients' needs.

Understanding Trauma in Serious Illness

Trauma may be conceptualized as single, repeated, and/or prolonged exposure to heightened states of fear that overwhelm our existing coping strategies, threaten our sense of agency and control, and influence our view of ourselves, others, and the world (APA, 2013). The nervous system, through the fight/flight/freeze response, works to protect us in these moments of intense physical and psychological distress by helping us reach a place of safety. In most cases, our bodies' coping strategies reactivate, we can recognize the threat has passed, and we can return to a calm, responsive baseline. In some cases, during intense single-incident or repeated traumas, our nervous systems can become "stuck" in these safety-seeking modes, interpreting the outside world as a threatening place, the self as vulnerable, and other people as harmful. From these states, a challenging new relationship with our bodies and with the world around us can emerge.

When intrusive thoughts, re-experiencing of the event(s), heightened arousal and reactivity, depersonalization, derealization, and changes in mood and cognition occur for weeks to months after the event(s), our nervous systems may be unable to "reset," leading to a prolonged stress response (APA, 2013). When we begin to reorganize our lives, such as our routines and relationships, to avoid the feelings, thoughts, and physiological sensations associated with the traumatic event, it is a signal that our nervous systems are no longer able to help us survive and regulate in response to the stressors we engage on a daily basis. When such symptoms present within the time frame immediately following to 1 month after the event, in diagnostic terms, this is referred to as acute stress disorder (ASD) (APA, 2013). When symptoms persist beyond 1 month, this is referred to as post-traumatic stress disorder (PTSD) (APA, 2013).

Complex post-traumatic stress disorder (CPTSD) is a response to repeated or prolonged exposure to trauma, when a person feels stuck in a pathological environment and unable to escape (Herman, 1992). Attachment to caregivers (in childhood) or important people in one's life (such as a romantic partner in adulthood) is often disrupted, which makes it extraordinarily difficult for healthy social engagement to occur and for a person to be able to be soothed when stressed (Knight, 2015). A survivor's sense of self is also distorted, often causing them to lose connection with their values, beliefs, and physical connection to their own body (Knight, 2015). The tools one used for survival in the past, such as avoidance or a heightened need for closeness, may be ill-fit for the here and now, creating new challenges for survivors of trauma as they reach for stability and safety (Cloitre et al., 2019; Herman, 1992).

How we approach the idea of a formal psychiatric diagnosis can also be understood with a trauma-informed lens. Conceptualizing traumatic stress disorders through diagnoses helps to give structure for therapeutic interventions and important validation for patients, families, and their communities. However, the diagnosis itself offers only a limited view of an individual and should be used merely as a jumping-off point from which we explore what a patient experiences in their thoughts, their relationships, and their bodies. Diagnoses and other labels related to trauma can inadvertently trigger stigmatization of patients and should be utilized thoughtfully in our dialogue within treatment teams and in the medical record.

As providers and clinicians, understanding the symptoms of trauma and knowing how to respond in a clinical encounter can help build trust and prevent re-traumatization. When appropriate, assessing and integrating an individual's history of trauma into their care plan for chronic and serious illness helps us to better understand their internal and external resources for coping with stress (Feldman, 2017; Hamberger et al., 2019; Raja et al., 2015). It can also open a dialogue on how we can be most supportive when we notice there is activation or reactivation of the nervous system's "survival mode" over the course of treatment. When a trauma-informed framework is applied to our systems and practices within the healthcare environment, we are also able to be more responsive to the needs of the patient's support system and to one another as healthcare professionals. We grow more aware of the environment and more attentive to the range of stress responses that we may experience or observe in one another (SAMHSA, 2014).

Trauma from a Population Health Perspective

As a result of the adverse childhood experiences (ACEs) study in the United States in the 1990s and increased global attention to social determinants of health, healthcare providers are becoming more aware of healthcare needs that arise across the lifespan in response to trauma and how trauma impacts the way an individual interacts with healthcare systems (Felitti et al., 1998; Larkin et al., 2014). We are also increasingly acknowledging that relational and developmental traumas are pervasive among USA and indeed world populations. The ACEs study established a correlation between self-reported childhood exposure to emotional, physical, or sexual abuse; household dysfunction; and health risk behaviors and diseases with high mortality in adulthood (Felitti et al., 1998). The higher the number of exposures to ACEs (such as witnessing domestic violence, enduring abuse or neglect, or parental separation and divorce), the higher the ACE score. Higher ACE scores were strongly correlated with greater risk of disease and death in adulthood, even when not accompanied by high health risk behaviors such as drug and alcohol use.

The results called attention to the risk of exposure to even one adverse childhood experience and its long-lasting impact on physical health. While research in ACEs has led to the initiation of public health efforts such as preventative screening in childhood in California, we should not discount the benefit of screening across the lifespan, even after chronic diseases have developed. A high ACE score, whether discovered in childhood or adulthood, gives us as healthcare providers the crucial understanding that some of the coping responses we see in patients now at one point served to assist in emotional regulation and survival. We also need to be mindful that the screening tool for ACEs is deficit-focused and be attentive to an individual's protective factors that may be corrective (Kelly-Irving & Delpierre, 2019). The ACEs data suggests that in care for chronically or seriously ill adults, taking a broad system approach that *anticipates* pervasive trauma can be an important first step toward nurturing overall well-being.

In response to the strong correlation between serious and chronic illness and childhood adversity, there have been efforts to integrate behavioral health into primary care. Screening tools and case management are utilized to help identify psychosocial barriers to accessing preventative care (Ramanuj et al., 2019; Vanderlip et al., 2016). A growing social work and case manager presence in primary and specialty medical clinics is a positive shift in medical culture, although these changes have been introduced primarily to lower costs for the facility and insurer (Rowe et al., 2017). The case finding, assessments, and interventions are primarily reactive rather than proactive or preventative, with patients often being identified for support only when they are experiencing a psychosocial or emotional crisis that may impact healthcare utilization costs. Social work, case manager, and care coordinator positions are often under-resourced relative to the needs of the community (Peikes et al., 2014).

There are few incentives in preventative medical care to reward providers for basic screening for mental health concerns, exploration of a patient's perceptions and goals for their health over time, or the creation of an environment where an individual can feel safe to explore their psychosocial concerns in any depth. The US healthcare system maintains a largely siloed approach to treating mental health and physical health concerns, and this is a barrier to addressing illness from a biopsychosocial-spiritual perspective (de Saxe Zerden et al., 2020). In this way, illness continues to be dissociated from the person who embodies it, perpetuating a sense of disconnect for individuals and their treatment teams.

Even when people with trauma histories are able to access the care they need, the act of receiving care can be deeply triggering (Raja et al., 2015; Reeves, 2015). Relating to and engaging with others can be extraordinarily stressful when one must seek assistance from individuals and systems that are consciously or unconsciously seen as contributing to the underlying trauma (Levenson, 2020). In a medical, educational, or legal setting, providers and clinicians often observe the use of coping strategies or behaviors at play when an individual struggles to regulate their emotions, such as strong expressions of anger, mistrust, irritability, or anxiety. Providers and clinicians are often so conditioned within these systems that they are unable to identify, or are desensitized to, the stressful or traumatic stimuli that may lead to a patient to feeling unsafe or threatened. Simple and broad changes to these environments that are trauma-informed can accommodate a greater range of experiences and stress responses (Hamberger et al., 2019). Service providers trained in identifying these adaptations to trauma can aim to co-regulate instead of responding negatively and authoritatively to strong emotional reactions.

Trauma-Related Responses in the Medical Setting

Identifying, understanding, and attending to a patient's response when they become emotionally dysregulated, in a clinical encounter or at any time throughout the course of medical treatment, is critical to the efficacy of our social work interventions. These responses may appear as ruptures in the clinical relationship, since disengagement or disagreement about the treatment plan may feel uncomfortable and overwhelming for both patient and provider (Raja et al., 2015; Reeves, 2015). However, these responses also serve as opportunities, signaling as they do moments where the patient might have felt unsafe. Provider and patient may find it difficult or impossible to identify the exact stimulus for the traumatic response, since the stimulus could be a very subtle, unconscious reminder of an earlier trauma experienced by the patient. But we can nonetheless respond in a way that helps the patient regulate and return to a place of safety, providing an opportunity for repair within the relationship that may begin to slowly reshape a patient's experience in the healthcare system and within their own bodies.

Physical sensations and symptoms that result from serious illness may challenge coping strategies that patients have previously relied upon in times of stress, such as exercise, dissociation from the body, or stimulus management. Those with a history of trauma may find it feels unfamiliar and distressing to turn their attention to areas of the body where pain or discomfort is located, being reminded that the body can be a source of pain and threat can cause recall of many different traumas (Bosco et al., 2013). This can be even more distressing if the illness draws attention to locations on the body where trauma occurred.

Trauma can also have implications for our customary dependence on the patient's self-assessment of symptoms and response to different treatments as a way of navigating care (Porcelli et al., 2013). This practice assumes the patient has a level of familiarity and comfort with their body that allows for overall body awareness. However, if a patient has relied upon the coping mechanism of dissociation, whether from their physical body or from their thoughts and feelings, providers and clinicians might be confused by the way a patient reports their symptoms (Bosco et al., 2013). There could be dissonance, for example, between what the patient reports verbally and other ways they're communicating, such as nonverbally or through behavioral actions. Patients may also struggle to put words to their bodily sensations. A patient's mood, affect, or attunement with the provider might shift after a physical exam that includes touch, especially if this results in discomfort (Raja et al., 2015). Providers may also sometimes be surprised that a patient did not seek medical care earlier, when symptoms first arose. Although there are many possible reasons for this, it is important to consider that a history of trauma may be one. And even when we correctly identify a trauma-related response in our patient, we must remember that they may not have a similar awareness of this disconnect or dissociation with their body.

Patients who have experienced trauma may also be accustomed to maintaining a level of hypervigilance within and outside of their body in order to foster a sense of safety. It may feel normal for them to constantly scan their inner experience and the physical environment to sustain emotional regulation and a sense of well-being, even if they do so without conscious awareness. When experiencing a serious illness, the patient may become overwhelmed by their own, or their medical team's, increased attention on their body. Bringing the unconscious into the conscious and sharing with a provider may be experienced as threatening and disruptive to their baseline coping strategies. Under this perceived threat, patients may experience changes in their mood, affect, reduced tolerance to physical discomfort, and impaired capacity to relate to others, including their medical team (Porcelli et al., 2013).

With patients who struggle to attend to and communicate around bodily sensations, it is important to note that this kind of response may be multifactorial (Sirri et al., 2013). While assessing or screening for symptoms of trauma, it is essential for providers to demonstrate cultural humility, acknowledging that one's relationship with their body is partially determined by their family and community norms. Elements of this relationship may include the degree to which the body is expected to look according to the dominant value system, the degree to which pain and suffering are seen as inevitable (this may vary by sex and gender, such as responses to menstrual pain and bloat), and the degree to which it is acceptable to ask for care to be given to one's body. Family, community, and religious narratives around pain, illness, suffering, and how one communicates with medical professionals all have a role to play. Providers and clinicians should remain curious and listen for individual, family, and collective beliefs around serious illness and symptom management to build trust and rapport and develop an individualized plan of care.

Interdisciplinary medical teams may find themselves faced with the challenge of not only pain management but also treating shortness of breath, anxiety, sleep disturbance, and depressive symptoms, which are often experienced as a composite of emotional, physical, and spiritual pain, especially for those with histories of trauma. It can be difficult for providers and their patients to parse these symptoms for treatment, as each individual may hold emotional and physical discomfort in their body in their own unique way. When care is offered in a siloed rather than interdisciplinary team approach and the patient does not respond to treatment, providers and clinicians are more likely to be unsure of how to move forward and offer the patient relief (Clark, 1999). The patient, meanwhile, may then experience the same sensation of powerlessness and violation within each silo, further reinforcing their own traumatic state.

Serious and chronic illness inherently invokes an awareness of one's mortality and fragility, feelings that were likely present while a patient was experiencing trauma. In response, a patient may become stuck in a traumatic fight, flight, or freeze response and struggle with accessing the higher cognitive and executive functioning that is needed for medical decision-making and treatment planning, such as attention and recall. This is often exhibited as ambivalence and indecision or trouble expressing their needs and preferences (Ganzel, 2018; Hamberger et al., 2019; Sirri et al., 2013). It can also look like a disconnect between a patient's stated healthcare goals and their related actions. For example, a patient without any barriers to accessing care may be inconsistent with their radiation treatments, despite verbalizing a goal for interventions that can extend life and relieve symptoms and after repeatedly voicing agreement with the plan. Providers are likely to respond with their own confusion, frustration, and powerlessness. If they hold a rigid understanding of their patient's presentation, they may deem their patients illogical or "in denial" and these patients may be further marginalized by the team.

Illness places a demand on patients to tolerate uncertainty and change; much is outside of the patient's control. With serious illness, there is typically some level of uncertainty about the exact course of the disease, leaving the patient and their support system destabilized, unable to fully adjust to a new baseline because of the ongoing fear of sudden change (Ganzel, 2018; Hamberger et al., 2019; Sirri et al., 2013). The lack of a sense of control and agency might serve as reminders of traumatic events or prolonged experiences of trauma. For those with a history of trauma, routine may be a primary means of coping, offering structure, stability, and safety. Yet routine is elusive: Frequent medical appointments, procedures, and treatments, as well as time needed for rest and recovery, disrupt the routines of both the patient and the family. Rigorous treatment schedules often present logistical challenges with regard to childcare or adult caregiving and employment and burden on finances, all of which require the patient to be flexible and depend on others for support. The need to be adaptable might challenge patients who derive security through routine. The delays and hiccups that patients experience within the healthcare system might destabilize a trauma survivor even more than the average patient, leading to a strong emotional response that is unexpected for clinic staff.

Other coping strategies may be seen in patients with serious illness who are also survivors of trauma. For some, substance use may be employed as a tool for regulating painful thoughts, feelings, and psychosocial challenges that are sequelae of trauma (Brady & Back, 2012). For others, impacts on eating, exercise, spending, and sexual habits may be evident, as may self-harm behaviors. In our care for patients with current or prior substance use disorder, it is important to work toward an accurate substance use assessment to ensure the patient's safety as they begin new medications and treatments. It is also important to explore whether illness challenges the coping strategies that a patient has relied upon to refrain from substance use. Encouraging a nonjudgmental, open dialogue with the patient (for instance, "Would you feel comfortable telling me about your relationship to drugs and alcohol" vs. "How much do you use drugs and alcohol?") allows for opportunities to discuss substance use openly and without judgment, offer psychoeducation, and proactively co-create a plan for treatment or for the patient to identify and access their internal and external resources for coping with triggers. While it is unlikely that those who care for patients with serious illness are also addiction specialists, it is important to recognize the overlap between trauma, serious illness, and substance use and acquire basic communication skills and resources for referral to attend to the patient's needs (Jones et al., 2022). It is also important to recognize that people with a history of long-term opioid use may require levels of pain medication that would trigger lethal dose concerns in opiate-naive populations; while we are never the prescribers or recommenders of such medications, recognizing the stigmatization of labeling patients as "drug seeking" when they have both an opiate use history and illness-related pain may be a meaningful opportunity for staff psychoeducation.

If misidentified, manifestations of traumatic stress as a patient navigates serious illness may be interpreted by medical staff as the patient being "difficult," "resistant," or "challenging" (Levenson, 2017). These kinds of labels can be stigmatizing and lead to bias throughout the clinical team or as the patient moves through the healthcare system. An understanding of trauma and trauma-informed interventions can reframe what we observe and experience in relation to our patients and help identify a path forward in their care.

When Healthcare is the Trauma

There are many ways in which the process of receiving medical care can be the primary trigger of a traumatic stress response, regardless of the patient's trauma history. The way in which the diagnosis is delivered can create an emotional response that completely overwhelms a patient's coping strategies. They may be alone and feeling physically unwell, which can exacerbate feelings of vulnerability and fear. The communication of treatment options can be experienced by patients in a similar way. Although a few alternatives may be offered, patients may still feel a lack of control or agency. This feeling of a lack of control, when experienced as highly distressing, is at the very core of what makes an adverse experience into a traumatic one.

Diagnostic interventions, procedures, treatments, and surgeries are most often invasive and uncomfortable and can be experienced as threats within our bodies. Hemodialysis, critical care, and treatment for end-stage cancer are examples of medical experiences that can lead to traumatic stress (Ganzel, 2018). The informed consent process for procedures, treatments, and medications aims to communicate how the intervention will impact the body so that the patient (or their decision-maker) cognitively understands the risks, benefits, and process related to a specific medical intervention on the body. Without psychoeducation, too, the patient may be unprepared for the impact it might have on their sense of self, their ability to feel safe in the world, and its long-term impact on the way our body copes with stress.

Patients may also become dependent on life-prolonging treatments in ways that disrupt daily life and cause ongoing, uncomfortable symptoms that are difficult to tolerate (Ganzel, 2018). The critical care environment and the life-sustaining treatments provided there often contribute to delirium, which can cause emotional distress and disorientation for patients that may linger for weeks or months. These interventions may also impair the patient's ability to talk or move voluntarily and to communicate their basic needs and preferences to care teams. Patients may be restrained (physically or chemically) in order to continue these life-sustaining treatments safely without risk of accidental removal, and such restraints may be experienced as traumatic for both patient and family.

Symptoms may be difficult to control at times, even with medications and other interventions. For those with serious illness, symptoms include acute and/or chronic pain, shortness of breath, nausea, vomiting, weight changes, fatigue, cognitive changes, depression, and anxiety. This sustained physical distress can be difficult to tolerate. Many patients lose hope of feeling well enough to engage in life in a way that feels meaningful for them. Even when symptoms are treated holistically, patients may continue to live with some level of discomfort over the course of their illness trajectory.

Procedures and surgeries over the course of serious illness may alter one's physical appearance. This is often a difficult adjustment for patients as they see the external manifestation of illness and must work to cognitively, emotionally, and physically integrate these changes into their understanding of the self – changes that affect how a patient moves through the world and relates to others and that challenge their premorbid views and values regarding appearance and ability.

Caregiving and Trauma

Family, friends, and others in the patient's support system may carry their own histories of trauma into the medical setting and, like the patients they care for, are challenged by complex medical decision-making, changes in routine, lack of control, and uncertainty. The increased emotional and physical stress that is experienced as a caregiver is likely to test and strain existing coping strategies. In cases where an otherwise important person's relationship to the patient is not legally recognized, such as in the case of a friend or romantic partner, they may feel marginalized by the care team. Memories associated with traumatic loss often come to the fore when someone close is ill, and thus members of the support system may re-experience strong grief reactions from the past (Wilson et al., 2021). Being in the medical environment and observing the patient receiving medical care may activate their own fight, flight, or freeze response (Davidson et al., 2012). This becomes particularly relevant whenever we depend on the caregiver to engage in medical decision-making on the patient's behalf or when we are collaborating on a safe hospital discharge plan.

The witnessing of the patient's medical experience or trauma can also be embodied as trauma by the caregiver, whether they are providing emotional or logistical care. Observing a patient coping with symptoms of serious illness such as confusion, pain, shortness of breath, changes in the physical body such as weight loss or amputation, or a loss of ability to communicate can cause the caregiver to feel helplessness, overwhelmed, anger, and fear. This may be exacerbated if the caregiver feels unable to advocate effectively with the care team on the patient's behalf, whether on account of a cultural or language barriers, lack of familiarity with medical language, difficulty navigating the healthcare system, or if their own history of trauma that makes them feel "stuck" in a traumatic stress response. One example of this is postintensive care syndrome-family, or PICS-F, which highlights the depressive and traumatic stress that can result when a family member spends time supporting a patient in the intensive care unit (Davidson et al., 2012). The fear and uncertainty experienced as they witness critical care interventions often alarming to behold may be so overwhelming to the caregiver's coping strategies as to lead to acute stress disorder or even post-traumatic stress disorder (Davidson et al., 2012).

Assessment of the family system's communication preferences and active efforts to align the delivery of medical updates and treatment planning with these preferences are examples of trauma-informed practices that can help the caregiver to self- or co-regulate during these stressful conversations. Efforts to engage caregivers in hands-on, nonmedical care when appropriate (clipping fingernails, applying lotion, brushing hair, etc.) can help increase connection with the patient and soothe and comfort the caregiver while also affirming their place as an important member of the care team (Davidson et al., 2012).

Part of recognizing the uniqueness of each family system is being aware of the potential for relational trauma within the family system, trauma that can be re-experienced as families struggle to maintain homeostasis in the face of serious illness and loss. Friends and families may have difficulty reorganizing their roles within the family system or community to accommodate the patient's inability to participate in a predictable way. Additionally, if relational, domestic, intimate partner, developmental, or child abuse has been present within the relationship, this may result in a wide range of emotional responses to the patient's disability or death, the possible reactions including sadness, anger, relief, fear, guilt, or grief. Each family system or community has its own rich psychosocial structure and intergenerational norms that allow it to survive. In most medical settings, our job is not to unpack this history and strive for comprehensive understanding of the family's or community's dynamic relational processes; rarely would most health social workers have the specialized training or bandwidth to do this with integrity. Instead, we focus on the recognition of traumatic responses, providing opportunities for regulation and safety and advocating for care delivery that is less likely to re-traumatize the patient. This allows us to create structures and practices in the care setting that can support and contain the many manifestations of emotional, behavioral, and physical stress that are likely to arise and that affect delivery of care to the patient.

The challenges that caregivers face during serious illness may increase risk of a prolonged grief response or prolonged grief disorder (PGD). PGD refers to a grief response that persists for more than a year and causes the individual to become significantly destabilized and disoriented. Sufferers of PGD may lose a sense of their identity and their place in relationships or have difficulty believing and processing that the loss has occurred (Prigerson et al., 2021). As clinicians, we may interact with the caregiver before, during, and for a short time after the loss of the patient we are caring for. A trauma-informed approach to patient care must also consider the impact of medical care on the caregiver, friend, and community member who carries the legacy of the care experience forward. Integrating an assessment of bereavement risk into the patient's care plan can help the caregiver identify coping strategies in advance of the loss. Trauma-informed care also creates a structure of support that can respond to the caregiver's stress and grief response, however it may present, in a way that promotes healing and connection.

As providers and clinicians in the medical setting, we may observe strong emotional, behavioral, and physical stress-related responses from caregivers. In some cases such responses may feel unexpected and even become disruptive to care planning. This could look like withdrawing and becoming unreachable by medical teams for treatment planning, being unable to regulate emotions in care planning discussions, having difficulty recalling aspects of the treatment plan, or becoming physically injured or ill. It is important to keep in mind that caregivers may have their own traumatic experiences related to their bodies and to their relationships, including their relationships with healthcare and with systems that have perpetuated racism or oppression for themselves, their families, and their communities.

Trauma-Informed Medical Care

Trauma-informed care adapts the healthcare environment to the specific needs of those who have experienced trauma. Those with histories of recurrent physical, emotional, or sexual abuse and/or exposure to domestic violence or disruptions in primary attachment relationships may have complex relationships with their bodies. Confronting this in a medical setting when experiencing a physical exam, invasive procedures, or simply recounting symptoms may reactivate memories and physical sensations from the original trauma. The provider is seen to be in a position of authority and dictating the agenda and flow of the appointment, creating additional vulnerability. By becoming trauma-sensitive at all levels of healthcare delivery, the system may begin to accommodate a wider range of patient reactions and responses.

Raja et al. (2015) discuss universal trauma-informed practices in a medical setting that begin with sharing control over the appointment and environment with the patient. Employing communication and behavioral techniques before, during, and between appointments, the provider can reimagine themselves as being in partnership with the patient, and this can transform the patient's perception, too.

1. Patients can be encouraged to bring a support person with them as they need and be given the option of bringing them into the exam or consultation room.
2. Patients should be informed of possible insurance or payment concerns ahead of the time of billing, to help them manage expectations and give them opportunity to troubleshoot any issues.
3. The provider or clinician can invite the patient to create an agenda for the appointment and inform them of the estimated length of time for the visit. The provider should encourage the patient to share their goals for each health condition, and let these goals inform next steps and the overall treatment plan.
4. Choices should be offered throughout the appointment, such as leaving the door ajar or choosing to be examined while sitting rather than lying down.
5. If an exam or procedure is indicated, the provider should verbalize each action in advance and offer the patient the opportunity to pause or stop, if possible, at any time.
6. The provider should indicate a clear plan for follow-up and explore any barriers for the patient to accomplish these next steps. Symptom logs distributed to patients, e.g., sleep diaries or pain records, should include an option for self-assessment of mood. Indications or expressions of ambivalence or hesitation throughout treatment present opportunities for further exploration.

7. Patients should be encouraged to call the provider or their team after the visit as they need with questions or concerns. This gesture allows for the possibility that strong emotions, even when not observable by the provider, may hijack cognitive processes for those with a history of trauma and prevent patients from optimal communication at the time of the appointment (Levenson, 2020; Hamberger et al., 2019; Raja et al., 2015; SAMHSA, 2014).

Each of these provider-driven interventions is designed to build trust. The provider becomes curious and responsive to their patients' reactions rather than pathologizing an emotional, cognitive, or behavioral response that feels challenging for them.

Outside of the treatment room, clinic or hospital staff should be trained in basic communication techniques that focus on de-escalation when a patient is experiencing heightened stress. There should be a balance between offering flexibility and choice and a stable structure with healthy boundaries that encourage an empathetic and safe holding environment (Hamberger et al., 2019; SAMHSA, 2014). Providers and staff need to be mindful of power dynamics inherent in the provider-patient relationship, as well as their role and position in a system that perpetuates health disparities. This relationship may remind patients of experiences in which abuse of power was central to interpersonal violence or system-level oppression. Clinic staff at all levels also need to be aware of their power dynamic with patients, as they often appear as gatekeepers to services, benefits, and care through tasks of scheduling, verifying insurance, and collecting co-pays. It is imperative that providers and clinicians seek to understand the individual's and family's experience within these systems of power and identify where oppression has occurred and how it is carried forward in the provision of care (Brown et al., 2020). There must be an active push against the status quo in order to promote equity, enhance feelings of safety in clinical encounters, assist individuals in meeting their unique healthcare goals, and help to change the narrative around medical care that can persist for generations. Social workers, with their training and commitment to social justice, are uniquely positioned within the medical system to apply this biopsychosocial perspective to assessment and treatment plans within their interdisciplinary teams.

In a hospital setting, patients often have limited choice, control, or privacy. Patients admitted to the hospital are most often experiencing a crisis, which can strain their existing coping strategies. Feeling physically unwell can increase feelings of vulnerability and uncertainty. They are subjected to the routines and timetables of the facility, even if incongruous to their normal routines and bodily needs and, thus, potentially disorienting. They are typically cared for by providers with whom they do not have a previous relationship. Patients are often dressed in a hospital gown and in a lying position, with teams of fully dressed providers standing above them, rotating in and out of the room throughout the day, even when the patient may be compromised by sleep or medication. This may create or re-awaken feelings of dehumanization and disempowerment. Medical teams are often composed of multiple medical doctors and health professionals at different levels of training who rotate on and off service, resulting in a repetitive cycle of patient self-disclosure, relationship building, and termination. Conversations with treatment teams can be overheard by a roommate or visitor despite efforts to respect privacy. The environment is often loud, with shifting noise levels from patients, staff conversations, or normal operations on the unit. It is fast-paced, and there is an expectation for complex medical decisions to be made quickly. While language interpreters are available, staff may try to save time and attempt communication in basic English (Diamond et al., 2010) or by using bilingual family members as interpreters. Patients often report experiencing overt discrimination or microaggressions because of their race, gender, class, sexual orientation, age, or disability (Diop et al., 2021). In many ways, the hospital setting is not conducive to healing in the way that is needed to treat a person holistically.

Trauma-informed care in the acute care setting aims to enhance choice, control, privacy, and safety for all patients during the provision of care, in the context of the realistic limitations of the American healthcare environment. The table below offers some suggestions on how to do so and to create flexibility in the hospital environment (Table 13.1).

We know from data on ACEs and social determinants of health that those with chronic medical conditions or cancer have a heightened statistical likelihood of having experienced trauma early in their lives. Patients with high symptom burden from cancer or chronic illness are most often treated as inpatients in the hospital setting. Physical symptoms such as pain, confusion, and shortness of breath may exacerbate symptoms related to trauma and may also blur the patient's and provider's ability to differentiate between symptoms that drive the treatment plan. Trauma-informed care is significantly more challenging to operationalize in a hospital setting and requires more broad culture change, including thoughtful shifting of priorities from cost efficiency to patient-centered care.

Social workers, orienting from a biopsychosocial and system perspective, have the training and skills to model elements of trauma-informed care for their multidisciplinary colleagues as they implement them into daily practice in the hospital. In addition to modeling co-creation of care plans with patients that aim to maximize stress management, social workers can demonstrate the self-reflection and self-awareness that is necessary to do this work. Providers and clinicians working with patients with chronic and serious illness must understand their own sense of self in practice, including their own trauma history, coping strategies, and positions of power within sociopolitical systems. When there is a shared traumatogenic environment, such as during the COVID-19 pandemic, providers' personal exposure to illness and threat occurs in parallel with those of their patients (Tosone et al., 2012). Cultivating an appreciation of how stress manifests in our own bodies; our own narratives around illness, death, and dying; and supported self-care strategies in professional and personal life increase our ability to connect authentically with the experience of our patients. This is essential across environments where patients are seen for primary, specialty, or acute care for chronic and serious illness.

Telemedicine, vastly more common since the COVID-19 pandemic, has created another healthcare environment where trauma-informed practices should be considered and applied. Gerber et al. (2020) consider ways to promote an environment of

Table 13.1 Trauma-informed interventions and approaches

	Acute care social worker	Suggested language with patients	Advocacy for change within healthcare system
Addressing power	Co-create treatment plans Assess for experiences of racism, misogyny, homophobia, ageism, and other forms of oppression in psychosocial assessments	*"What would you like us to focus on in our work together?"* *"We know that racism exists in healthcare. How has this affected you (and your family)?"*	Encourage the use of language that humanizes the individuals receiving care Facilitate a learning environment where implicit biases are identified and challenged Encourage open dialogue among teams about healthcare disparities (nationally, locally) and name inequities when appropriate Remind teams of the inherent power differential within the healthcare system Consider your own feelings of power/powerlessness in your work environment
Fostering curiosity and illness narratives	Consider framing health issues and associated health behaviors as ways that patients have organized cognitively, emotionally, and relationally around trauma Assess communication preferences and include others with patient's permission Explore their thoughts and feelings about their health Actively listen for patient/family/community narratives around illness, death, and dying	*"What helps the most when you're in the hospital?"* *"What do I need to know about you as a person to take the best care of you that I can?"* *"If we talk about test results or changes to your plan, is there anyone you'd like with you for support?"* *"What are you hoping for during this hospital stay? What worries you?"* *"Can you tell me more about your brother's illness and how it affected you?"*	Reframe patients' disruptive behavior as coping strategies activated under stress Encourage curiosity during interactions with patients and their support systems Encourage a strength-based, rather than deficit-focused, approach Educate the team and staff on the impact of these narratives on the individual's healthcare decision-making

(continued)

Table 13.1 (continued)

	Acute care social worker	Suggested language with patients	Advocacy for change within healthcare system
Increasing sense of control	Use invitations in conversation to allow patients/families the opportunities to take a break Ask for names and pronouns Orient and reorient, repeating information as needed Consider breaking up decisions or goals into small tasks Offer opportunities to have control over daily routine Allow the patient/support system to name what is important Prepare for care transitions	*"The doctors have recommended that you continue physical therapy in a facility. Would it be okay to talk about what this would look like?"* *"Is it okay to keep going?"* *"Would it be okay to leave you a list of facilities to look over today, and we can make some choices tomorrow?"* *"What's a good time for me to return tomorrow to follow up?"* *"What else haven't I asked that is important for me and your team to know to take the best care of you?"* *"I'd like us to talk about what you can expect when you return home, and how you might reach out for help if you're having a difficult time."*	Encourage teams to identify when choices may exist and offer these to patients Assess the learning style of the patient/support system and tailor informational materials appropriately; encourage the hospital to have a range of resources easily accessible to staff Anticipate barriers as patients transition from settings of care (hospital to home; hospital to skilled nursing facility)
Attunement	Remain calm and consistent; utilize transparency in communication Explore with the patient how to prepare for moments when they may become activated by reminders of trauma or experience heightened fear response Establish and maintain therapeutic boundaries and utilize transparency when reinforcing the boundaries Elicit feedback	*"How will you know if you're feeling unsafe in this visit?"* *"How can you let me know to slow down, or that you need to take a break?"* *"How can I help support you right now?"* *"Is there anything I (or we) missed?"*	It is not expected or acceptable for providers to tolerate emotional or physical abuse from patients/caregivers. Reinforcing boundaries helps us all feel safe.

(continued)

Table 13.1 (continued)

	Acute care social worker	Suggested language with patients	Advocacy for change within healthcare system
Flexibility	Encourage a nuanced care plan, individualizing as much as can be accommodated Obtain information about the patient's daily routine and advocate for the care plan to orient around it as much as possible		Encourage the team to consider timing of blood draws/vital signs to minimize sleep disruption

SAMHSA (2014), Levenson (2020), Ortiz (2017), and Chochinov (2007)

safety during the virtual visit, including a pre-appointment screen to explore possible barriers such as an unsafe home environment, lack of privacy, or availability of necessary technology. It is helpful for a team member, one whom the patient is familiar with, to provide information about the telemedicine visit, orient them to technology and security, and explore any questions or concerns in advance. The provider should choose an environment that is quiet and private and has a neutral backdrop and not sit too close to the camera. The authors also suggest that during the visit, the provider orient the patient to unusual sounds that may occur during the visit, such as nearby construction or interruptions by team members.

As in a traditional face-to-face encounter, it is beneficial for the provider and patient to collaboratively set an agenda for the visit. The provider can consider utilizing more verbal expressions of curiosity and empathy than in a traditional face-to-face encounter where it is easier to observe nonverbal communication. The provider must have a greater awareness of their vocal intonation, facial expression, and gestures while also attuning more closely to that of their patients. The exchange of nonverbal communication, relatively spontaneous and fluid in a face-to-face encounter, is now more strained through technology. For those whose home environment does not feel secure, the structure provided by the traditional in-person clinic appointment may have provided a greater sense of safety. Some patients may find that they disconnect or dissociate more readily in remote visits than when in person. Additionally, many patients may feel embarrassed by their home environment. Waiting for patients to invite conversation with the provider about their surroundings may increase feelings of control and privacy. Frequent check-ins ensure effective communication in the event that the Internet is unstable.

For many patients, engaging in online healthcare is a new experience of technology, which has been primarily used for entertainment and as a supplemental form for socialization (Porges, 2020). Repurposing technology for medical care during the pandemic has served as a necessary lifeline, but it is important to be aware of the ways in which providers, clinicians, and patients are all working harder to facilitate connection. At the same time, we should understand that telemedicine allows for a greater sense of safety for certain patients. The ability to engage from a familiar setting can feel stabilizing and allow for self-regulation. Many patients are benefiting from the fact that telemedicine eliminates the cost and time of traveling to the clinic and allows for participation in care by family and friends. This conservation of resources may be essential depending on the patient's needs.

If possible, allowing choice of an in-person or virtual visit, or even a hybrid model over the course of treatment, allows for variation. Regardless of the modality, however, the provider or clinician should consider their work to be highly relational and plan collaboratively with their patient on how to safely connect in their care. This requires education on ways to enhance safety during virtual visits.

During a single encounter or over the course of the relationship with a trauma survivor, they may offer details about their trauma history. It is important for health professionals to know how to respond appropriately and have mental health resources on hand for referral (Raja et al., 2015). Traditionally, mental health and trauma screens are not conducted in medical settings. Any kind of trauma screening should be conducted by a trained mental health provider who explores gently and with the patient's explicit and unpressured permission and with the shared expectation that the information is to enhance the medical treatment plan and not for the purpose of engaging in trauma treatment during the visit (Raja et al., 2015; Reeves, 2015). These questions may feel unexpected and intrusive if not asked thoughtfully in a trauma-informed care setting, where staff are prepared to provide psychoeducation around the connection between the trauma history and illness and offer support, such as a grounding exercise that helps facilitate reorientation, should the patient become dysregulated.

While information about past trauma may be relevant for both providers and patients and inform an individualized treatment plan, universal trauma-informed approaches ensure that the care the patient receives is responsive to their needs regardless of the assessment and may even be more effective to help soothe and regulate in the moment (Raja et al., 2015; SAMHSA, 2014).

The trust that builds from the assessment of traumatic responses and standardized trauma-informed interventions may lead the patient and provider to consider a referral for a formal mental health assessment. This assessment can be conducted in a trauma-informed manner, at the patient's pace, and with the consideration that there may be limited qualified providers and clinicians who can conduct longer-term trauma-specific therapy (Levenson, 2020; Raja et al., 2015).

Psychosocial Interventions

As the "patient" identity edges to the fore, individuals with serious illness often grapple with their understanding of self and of their roles within relationships, community, and greater society. They may experience a deep sense of loss and instability as they grieve these aspects of their identity that have helped to ground and orient them over the course of their lives. Narrative interventions can be utilized by clinical social workers to help the patient reflect and integrate this new identity with others that have been more prominent or meaningful (Glick et al., 2018). Exploring a broader view of the self that is rooted in individual values may allow for greater flexibility in how the patient perceives themselves as they adjust to life with serious illness. An example of this is Dignity Therapy, or Dignity Model interventions that coach the patient through assessment of their personal narrative in the context of serious illness (Chochinov, 2007). The primary question asked, "What do I need to know about you as a person to take the best possible care of you?" (Dignity Toolkit, n.d.), while based on existential theories, is also trauma-informed. The structured questions that may follow can be a helpful starting place for social workers looking to integrate narrative interventions in their care for patients with serious illness.

Aligning with family or community narratives around health and illness can also help the patient see themselves reflected in the stories of others whom they identify with. In this way, they may experience a renewed strength by becoming grounded in a collective narrative and be able to access this as a type of guide for being present with illness in the here-and-now or as a path forward as they envision their future. Considering the community or collective narrative as a resource may be unfamiliar to those who trained and are practicing in the United States, where individualism is a dominant ideology. However, storytelling during illness and bereavement is universal (Neimeyer, 2005). It involves the recounting of challenging experiences in the medical setting, which in turn influences the dominant narrative about medical care at the end of life between families, communities, and across generations.

Polyvagal Theory and Interventions

Polyvagal theory offers a view on how the autonomic nervous system operates when under stress or threat and also when being soothed and in a restorative state. This theory suggests how to work with patients to interpret their stress response and work toward self- and co-regulation. Porges and Dana (2018) describe the two branches of the autonomic nervous system, the sympathetic and parasympathetic nervous systems, which respond to stressful or harmful stimuli with the goal of keeping us safe and alive. When activated by a perceived threat, the sympathetic nervous system prepares the body to engage and fight or flee from the dangerous stimulus. The parasympathetic nervous system prepares the body to freeze or shut down. Each works through a complex neurobiological process that initiates the release of stress hormones that work to rev up or power down the biological functions to seek safety. The parasympathetic nervous system, through the vagus nerve, is split into the dorsal vagal and ventral vagal systems. The dorsal vagal system helps to control and slow breathing, heart rate, and digestion, and the ventral vagal system facilitates social engagement for connection and safety, which is also critical to survival (Porges & Dana, 2018). Chronic stress, or an ongoing perception of threat, may keep the sympathetic nervous system activated more often than not, leading to long-term health effects such as high blood pressure and high cortisol levels.

In order for restoration, health, and growth to occur, Porges and Dana (2018) note that the nervous system cannot be activated or in a state of defense. The ventral vagal system needs to be engaged for social engagement and for regulation and maintenance of the dorsal vagal and sympathetic nervous systems. This allows the ability to be open to and attend to social cues that signal safety in relationship with others, such as facial expressions, tone of voice, and body language. As healthcare professionals, this can help us assess, with our patients, when they are hyper-aroused (hypervigilance, racing thoughts, anxiety) or hypo-aroused (moving slowly, numb, speaking rationally about difficult topics with no apparent emotion) and out of tune with their environment and how to help them move into a more balanced state where their bodies can feel safe. This balanced state is what Porges and Dana (2018) refer to as the window of tolerance, where a person can engage critical thinking, orient to and attune to the environment, and relate to others calmly without feeling overwhelmed or experiencing the urge to pull away. For some patients, the window of tolerance is quite large, where they can accommodate a wide range of daily stressful stimuli while remaining engaged with others and retaining access to their critical thinking. For others, such as survivors of trauma, the window of tolerance is much narrower; these individuals can tolerate a lesser amount of stress before hyper- or hypo-arousal is triggered.

Grounding techniques can be helpful interventions, easily utilized in medical settings to help reorient a patient who is hyper- or hypo-aroused, whose nervous system might be perceiving and responding to a life-threatening stimulus. Bringing them to a quiet location and facilitating their orientation to the room, the environment, and attendant physical sensations (feet on the floor, back on the chair or bed) can help shift toward homeostasis. Drinking cold water and moving the body or parts of the body can help shift from hypo-arousal to a more comfortable baseline while simply noticing one's breath can help shift from hyper-arousal to a more balanced state. Psychoeducation that encourages patients to scan and attend to their body's sensations, both the purely physical and in terms of noticing how/where emotions are experienced in their body, can help support a growing sense of awareness and agency over emotional and physical responses that may typically feel overwhelming (Feldman, 2017). The process of a provider noticing and caring about a patient's physiological responses, and having some expertise in helping guide patients through managing their responses, can provide a form of relational attunement and grounding.

Conclusion

Compared to other members of the medical team, social workers are uniquely trained to understand the impact of trauma experienced by individuals as a result of childhood and adult adversity and systemic discrimination. We are educated in a person-in-environment perspective and consider a holistic view of a patient when they present to a healthcare setting (Feldman, 2017). In these settings, we observe the ways in which trauma can influence the patient's experience of serious illness, beginning with their engagement with preventative care, to their response to changes in their body, to coping with rigorous treatment schedules and medical follow-up. By better recognizing traumatic responses, more than focusing on labeling experiences as "Trauma," we can help patients navigate their healthcare experience in a more grounded, healing-oriented, and less damaging way.

It is essential that we begin to shift the culture of the healthcare system to one that is holistically healing-centered. Social workers can champion these efforts through implementation of trauma-informed care, supporting policies and practices that are more responsive to a range of patient experiences. This can be done through their interactions within their teams, such as with modeling of self-reflection and psychoeducation about the impact of trauma and reframing of patient and caregiver responses under a trauma-informed lens. This can also be done in their clinical work with patients across medical settings, as they work collaboratively to consider the patient's dynamic responses to illness with curiosity and humility and co-create treatment plans that help them feel more safe within their bodies and when navigating their care. In this way, trauma-informed care can be healing for those receiving care and empowering for providers in their work of healing others.

Author's Reflection

Trauma is a tricky subject in healthcare. With death on the not-too-distant horizon and fears of powerlessness abound, everyone is in survival mode, after all, providers and patients alike. For many years, I was blind to how little I really knew about trauma and assumed my MSW training and clinical exposure to intense situations was education enough. My professional understanding of trauma went from being "something that happened to soldiers and survivors of assault" (big T Traumas) to eventually including things like the interpersonal and developmental traumas that come from inconsistently getting your socio-emotional needs for safety, attunement, and proximity met, too (little t traumas), among others. It was an awakening to learn that those things weren't just unpleasant – depending on how and when they were experienced, they can literally change the nervous system!

I received my formal somatic trauma therapy training after 15 years of working in palliative care. It was a series of lightbulb moments and realizing how much this information could have better informed my work when I was on the front lines in the hospital. When we screen for trauma history in healthcare now, we're mostly asking people to self-identify with big T Traumas only, for the most part, and we are missing a lot. So many of our patients are having trauma reactions like prolonged hyper-arousal and dissociation, or intense mistrust and hypervigilance, and they may not even realize it. They may think they are just sensitive, anxious, or depressed or feel they are constantly being abandoned or misled (our healthcare system does just that, frequently, and not evenly across all social groups). They are not able to consciously connect with their body's learned response to overwhelm and fear. Illness becomes another trauma, and as clinicians, we end up either dismissing the patient for being "dramatic" or feeling powerless to help. On a personal level, I've found neither of those stances particularly gratifying.

As someone who has been both a hospital patient and a hospital clinician, I have a profound appreciation for what healthcare does to the nervous system as it seeks to heal the body. Learning about trauma is really hard; it makes us rethink our own narratives and work and exposes us to the vulnerability of being human and the limits of our control. Our hope in writing this chapter was to help social workers better understand what they're seeing in patients who are exhibiting signs of trauma and, perhaps, better understand some of their own responses, too. With better understanding comes the opportunity to provide better care to people whose resources are depleted by the experience of illness and for healthcare providers to better connect to their own sense of efficacy in easing suffering and healing.

After all, for all of us, in consciousness, there is healing. – A.N.

Reflection Questions

1. What did you learn about trauma in this chapter that you did not know before?
2. How might the trauma of systemic oppression impact an individual's experience of healthcare?
3. How might you intervene with a patient who is displaying signs of a trauma history? What would you look for and what would you do?

References

American Psychiatric Association. (2013). *Diagnostic and statistical manual of mental disorders* (5th ed.).

Bosco, M. A., Gallinati, J. L., & Clark, M. E. (2013). *Conceptualizing and treating comorbid chronic pain and PTSD*. Pain Research and Treatment.

Brady, K. T., & Back, S. E. (2012). Childhood trauma, posttraumatic stress disorder, and alcohol dependence. *Alcohol Research, 34*(4), 408–413.

Chochinov, H. M. (2007). Dignity and the essence of medicine: The A, B, C, and D of dignity conserving care. *BMJ, 335*(7612), 184–187.

Clark, D. (1999). 'Total pain', disciplinary power and the body in the work of Cicely Saunders, 1958–1967. *Social Science & Medicine, 49*(6), 727–736.

Cloitre, M., Hyland, P., Bisson, J. I., Brewin, C. R., Roberts, N. P., Karatzias, T., & Shevlin, M. (2019). ICD-11 posttraumatic stress disorder and complex posttraumatic stress disorder in the United States: A population-based study. *Journal of Traumatic Stress, 32*(6), 833–842.

Davidson, J. E., Jones, C., & Bienvenu, O. J. (2012). Family response to critical illness: Postintensive care syndrome–family. *Critical Care Medicine, 40*(2), 618–624.

de Saxe Zerden, L., Cadet, T. J., Galambos, C., & Jones, B. (2020). Social work's commitment and leadership to address social determinants of health and integrate social care into health care. *Journal of Health & Human Services Administration, 43*(3).

Diamond, L. C., Wilson-Stronks, A., & Jacobs, E. A. (2010). Do hospitals measure up to the national culturally and linguistically appropriate services standards? *Medical Care*, 1080–1087.

Dignity Toolkit. (n.d.). https://www.dignityincare.ca/en/toolkit.html

Diop, M. S., Taylor, C. N., Murillo, S. N., Zeidman, J. A., James, A. K., & Burnett-Bowie, S. A. M. (2021). This is our lane: Talking with patients about racism. *Women's Midlife Health, 7*(1), 1–8.

Dubus, N., & Howard, H. (2016). Current realities and future vision: Developing an interprofessional, integrated health care workforce. *Social Work in Health Care, 55*(9), 766–778.
Feldman, D. B. (2017). Stepwise psychosocial palliative care: A new approach to the treatment of posttraumatic stress disorder at the end of life. *Journal of Social Work in End-of-Life & Palliative Care, 13*(2–3), 113–133.
Felitti, V. J., Anda, R. F., Nordenberg, D., Williamson, D. F., Spitz, A. M., Edwards, V., Koss, M. P., & Marks, J. S. (1998). Relationship of childhood abuse and household dysfunction to many of the leading causes of death in adults: The adverse childhood experiences (ACE) study. *American Journal of Preventive Medicine, 14*, 245–258.
Ganzel, B. (2018). Trauma-informed hospice and palliative care. *The Gerontologist, 58*(3), 409–419.
Gerber, M. R., Elisseou, S., Sager, Z. S., & Keith, J. A. (2020). Trauma-informed telehealth in the COVID-19 era and beyond. *Federal Practitioner, 37*(7), 302–308.
Glick, D. M., Cook, J. M., Moye, J., & Kaiser, A. P. (2018). Assessment and treatment considerations for post traumatic stress disorder at end of life. *American Journal of Hospice and Palliative Medicine, 35*(8), 1133–1139.
Hamberger, L. K., Barry, C., & Franco, Z. (2019). Implementing trauma-informed care in primary medical settings: Evidence-based rationale and approaches. *Journal of Aggression, Maltreatment & Trauma, 28*(4), 425–444.
Herman, J. L. (1992). Complex PTSD: A syndrome in survivors of prolonged and repeated trauma. *Journal of Traumatic Stress, 5*, 377–391.
Jones, K. F., Ho, J. J., Sager, Z., Childers, J., & Merlin, J. (2022). Adapting palliative care skills to provide substance use disorder treatment to patients with serious illness. *American Journal of Hospice & Palliative Medicine, 39*(1), 101–107.
Kelly-Irving, M., & Delpierre, C. (2019). A critique of the adverse childhood experiences framework in epidemiology and public health: Uses and misuses. *Social Policy and Society, 18*(3), 445–456.
Knight, C. (2015). Trauma-informed social work practice: Practice considerations and challenges. *Clinical Social Work Journal, 43*(1), 25–37.
Larkin, H., Felitti, V. J., & Anda, R. F. (2014). Social work and adverse childhood experiences research: Implications for practice and health policy. *Social Work in Public Health, 29*(1), 1–16.
Levenson, J. (2017). Trauma-informed social work practice. *Social Work, 62*(2), 105–113.
Levenson, J. (2020). Translating trauma-informed principles into social work practice. *Social Work, 65*(3), 288–298.
Neimeyer, R. (2005). Grief, loss, and the quest for meaning: Narrative contributions to bereavement care. *Bereavement Care, 24*(2), 27–30.
Ortiz, A. (2017). *Liberation in the exam room.* Southern Jamaica Plain Medical Center.
Peikes, D. N., Reid, R. J., Day, T. J., Cornwell, D. D., Dale, S. B., Baron, R. J., Brown, R. S., & Shapiro, R. J. (2014). Staffing patterns of primary care practices in the comprehensive primary care initiative. *The Annals of Family Medicine, 12*(2), 142–149.
Porcelli, P., Guidi, J., Sirri, L., Grandi, S., Grassi, L., Ottolini, F., Pasquini, P., Picardi, A., Rafanelli, C., Rigatelli, M., Sonino, N., & Fava, G. A. (2013). Alexithymia in the medically ill. Analysis of 1190 patients in gastroenterology, cardiology, oncology and dermatology. *General Hospital Psychiatry, 35*(5), 521–527.
Porges, S. W. (2020). The COVID-19 pandemic is a paradoxical challenge to our nervous system: A polyvagal perspective. *Clinical Neuropsychiatry, 17*(2), 135–138.
Porges, S. W., & Dana, D. (2018). *Clinical applications of the polyvagal theory: The emergence of polyvagal-informed therapies.* (Norton series on interpersonal neurobiology). WW Norton & Company.
Prigerson, H. G., Kakarala, S., Gang, J., & Maciejewski, P. K. (2021). History and status of prolonged grief disorder as a psychiatric diagnosis. *Annual Review of Clinical Psychology, 17*, 109–126.

Raja, S., Hasnain, M., Hoersch, M., Gove-Yin, S., & Rajagopalan, C. (2015). Trauma informed care in medicine: Current knowledge and future research directions. *Family & Community Health, 38*(3), 216–226.

Ramanuj, P., Ferenchik, E., Docherty, M., Spaeth-Rublee, B., & Pincus, H. (2019). Evolving models of integrated behavioral health and primary care. *Current Psychiatry Reports, 21*(1), 1–12.

Reeves, E. (2015). A synthesis of the literature on trauma-informed care. *Issues in Mental Health Nursing, 36*(9), 698–709.

Rowe, J. M., Rizzo, V. M., Vail, M. R., Kang, S. Y., & Golden, R. (2017). The role of social workers in addressing nonmedical needs in primary health care. *Social Work in Health Care, 56*(6), 435–449.

Sirri, L., Fava, G. A., & Sonino, N. (2013). The unifying concept of illness behavior. *Psychotherapy and Psychosomatics, 82*(2), 74–81.

Substance Abuse and Mental Health Services Administration. (2014). *SAMHSA's concept of trauma and guidance for a trauma-informed approach. HHS Publication No. (SMA) 14-4884.* Substance Abuse and Mental Health Services Administration.

Tosone, C., Nuttman-Shwartz, O., & Stephens, T. (2012). Shared trauma: When the professional is personal. *Clinical Social Work Journal, 40*, 231–239.

Vanderlip, E. R., Rundell, J., Avery, M., Alter, C., Engel, C., Fortney, J., & Williams, M. (2016). *Dissemination of integrated care within adult primary care settings: The collaborative care model.* American Psychiatric Association and Academy of Psychosomatic Medicine.

Wilson, D. M., Underwood, L., & Errasti-Ibarrondo, B. (2021). A scoping research literature review to map the evidence on grief triggers. *Social Science & Medicine, 282*, 114109.

Chapter 14
Contemporary Issues in Healthcare

Meredith Hemphill and Alicia Tennenbaum

Introduction

This chapter examines the face of healthcare today and the impact its features have on the overall well-being of people who are chronically and seriously ill. This topic arises in recognition of how the processes we refer to as *getting better* or *managing illness* are shaped in dialogue with systems of care and those governing bodies, laws, and regulations that define their scope. Today, healthcare systems are managing more demand as the numbers of adults with chronic conditions increase. To prevent such illnesses from worsening, resources and programs are being expanded to prevent crises and manage such illnesses better from a preventative, long-term viewpoint.

Initially linked to casework for maternal health, venereal diseases, and crisis intervention in epidemics such as influenza, social work presence in healthcare spaces and impact is far greater today (Ruth & Marshall, 2017). Today, social workers are involved in case management, discharge planning and short-term counseling, and interdisciplinary case review and more. They also have the potential to become involved and collaborate with other disciplines on those programs and initiatives focused on positive change in health and healthcare. This chapter suggests that the inclusion of their voices and values can greatly benefit patients and address some of the largest issues in medical care today.

M. Hemphill (✉)
City Center Psychotherapy, New York, NY, USA
e-mail: drhemphill@citycenterpsychotherapy.com

A. Tennenbaum
Mount Sinai Hospital, New York, NY, USA
e-mail: Alicia.tennenbaum@mountsinai.org

M. Hemphill, A. Nathanson (eds.), *The Practice of Clinical Social Work in Healthcare*, Essential Clinical Social Work Series,
https://doi.org/10.1007/978-3-031-31650-0_14

Healthcare Today

Healthcare is challenged by increasing demand for complex care. The United States has a higher proportion of older adults (65 years or above) in its population than ever before (16% in 2018), and this is expected to continue to increase to 23% – 95 million older individuals – by 2060 (Population Reference Bureau, 2019). In parallel, the United States is seeing higher numbers of age-related illnesses and diseases. Six in ten (or 60%) of all Americans now live with at least one chronic disease (Centers for Disease Control and Prevention [CDC], 2019). Chronic diseases that appear more commonly in older age, such as heart disease and cancer, account for the greatest numbers of deaths in the United States (National Center for Health Statistics [NCHS], 2021).

Such illnesses and conditions often need complex and/or long-term care management to prevent dire health outcomes. As demonstrated in this book's chapters on cancer, a common care path for people with cancer involves repeated and ongoing testing and monitoring, arduous treatment, multiple teams and specialists, transitions in care from inpatient to outpatient and from active treatment to remission, palliative care, and, possibly, more. Similarly, the management of heart disease can be complex for the patient and their care team, committed to delaying or preventing disease progression and health crisis. In recognition of the potential for better health outcomes through good complex care (which includes consistent engagement with healthcare teams when disease impact and symptoms are minimal), care management of chronic diseases such as cardiovascular disease, chronic obstructive pulmonary disease (COPD), and diabetes is closely monitored and used to rank "high performance" within hospitals (NYC Health and Hospitals, 2022).

How can healthcare systems keep pace with rising care needs? Alongside some expansion of services and resources, there is an effort toward improving the productivity and efficiency of healthcare providers and the "proper" utilization of services by patients. For this reason, a heavy task list is common to clinical and administrative professions in healthcare facilities. For example, an average physician's assistant's (PA's) tasks to complete – with around 19 patients a day (Florence Health, 2019) – include medical information gathering, physical exams and diagnosing and/or review of diagnosis list, treatment plan reviews, medication list review and management, note-taking and collaboration, and consultation with other members of the medical team (Indeed, 2021). These tasks and processes are intended to promote the "accurate" utilization of services – i.e., to help medical appointments proceed better and more quickly, with relevant data already collected and in-hand.

Cost-saving initiatives are also common in healthcare facilities as they strive to meet demand. An estimated $760 billion is "wasted" in American health spending per year (Frakt, 2019, para. 6). To reduce this number, healthcare facilities monitor trends in usage and have developed analytics to identify patients at high risk for readmission to hospitals (Lexis Nexis, n.d.) based on social determinants such as housing insecurity, history of substance abuse, etc. They then develop programs that aim to reduce unnecessary administration of costly services and care. An example of such a program is the Hospital Readmission Reduction Program, which has been created to reduce reimbursement costs associated with avoidable hospital readmissions by penalizing those facilities whose readmission numbers are 3% or above the expected rate. As the following section shows, many programs have also been developed to target the core social issues related to readmission risk. By helping patients overcome barriers to initiating or continuing needed care, the likelihood of bigger and costlier interventions is reduced.

The trend toward improving healthcare system efficiency may also explain an increased focus on communication between providers, especially during a transition in care or when multiple care settings are involved. Transitions from one setting to another (for instance, from an inpatient floor to home) are proven to increase risk of adverse health events and slow rates of recovery (Agency for Healthcare Research and Quality, 2018). Detailed discharge notes and increased case management presence are two examples of many best practices that can mitigate adverse effects of transitions. Many of these beneficial practices are executed by social workers.

Alongside the rising need for complex symptom management, palliative care utilization has increased. People diagnosed with chronic conditions involving complex symptoms often find those symptoms distressing, disruptive, and overwhelming, making the need for the expertise of palliative care teams apparent, and such teams or departments are increasingly commonplace in major hospitals today.

Health Insurance

The opportunity to receive care, get healthier, and have the associated psychosocial burden of illness lightened is partially determined by a patient's health insurance coverage. With insurance that offers adequate coverage, patients are spared the burden of paying for the majority of their medical care and treatment. Yet out-of-pocket costs for treatments and services, deductibles, and exhaustion of coverage for certain types of services damage the financial well-being of many – especially those who are very ill and are receiving extensive treatments and/or those who were financially struggling pre-illness (Chi, 2019).

The proportion of uninsured people was 10.9% in 2019, a rate that has steadily increased since 2016 "amid efforts to alter the availability and affordability of coverage" (Tolbert, 2020, para. 4). This refers to some states' refusal to take up the Affordable Care Act (ACA) marketplaces, which make health insurance coverage more affordable. The Supreme Court heard and ruled against Texas and 17 other GOP states who argued that the ACA was unconstitutional and who sought to repeal it in Texas v. United States/Azar (Hagen, 2021). Despite this upholding, the strength of the ACA safety net remains uneven. State policymakers decide if the marketplace is made available (and to what extent) or allow other short-term plans that are not ACA compliant to be offered, with the effect of destabilizing ACA marketplaces and raising ACA plan premiums (Norris, n.d.). This is concerning for those individuals who might not otherwise be able to afford insurance, those who are vulnerable to job loss and underemployment, or whose incomes rest just above pre-ACA Medicaid thresholds. Yet, ACA markets are unlikely to close soon. The COVID Relief Bill passed in March 2021 bolstered it with a government subsidy aimed at easing the strain of an increasing "sick pool" and economic downturn caused by COVID-19 shutdowns. Supporters of the ACA point to both the necessity of the emergency aid provided by the COVID-19 Relief Bill and its long-term problems. Levey (2021), for example, suggests that the increasing reliance on federal subsidies to cover premiums for private commercial health plans leaves those who have enrolled in marketplace insurance plans vulnerable anew if either changes or ends.

The likelihood of being uninsured is greater for undocumented individuals, for whom Emergency Medicaid continues to be the only insurance option available. Inadequate on many counts, it requires that individuals meet Medicaid eligibility and offers only receiving emergency care (for an illness or disease that has not been identified previously); preventive care and care for a chronic condition that is not "emergent" or acute will not be covered. This has not changed with COVID-19's devastating effects. Because of these long-standing limitations of eligibility and coverage, undocumented individuals are less likely to receive timely, comprehensive, and uninterrupted care. The fear of mounting bills that could be left unpaid can keep individuals who are undocumented from going to a doctor to address physical symptoms or to follow through with recommended care.

The psychosocial impact of being seriously ill and having no insurance can be easily imagined. It can lead to avoidance of costly diagnosis and care; it can force the seriously ill individual to make choices between multiple challenges to survival. Should that person choose health or work/rent/food/caregiving of others? Is that person presented with a choice at all, or does life maintenance require that health needs are not met?

Even the person who *is* insured may suffer great financial hardship when in need of long-term care or intensive treatment and procedures. Chi (2019) shows how financial hardship (caused by paying insurance premiums, co-pays, or uncovered procedures or services) seriously impedes a person's ability to cope with illness and exacerbates anxiety, depression, and a sense of helplessness. Additionally, it is likely to delay detection, start of care, and compliance (i.e., likelihood of completing treatment uninterrupted). This suggests that the person with financial stress is likely to have treatment and care experiences that are more fraught and fragmented than the person without it; it also suggests that the person with financial stress has more of a mental and emotional load to bear than the person who is less affected by high care costs or has fewer of them. The noxious effects of financial burden are well captured by the term "financial toxicity" (FT) (Chi, 2019).

Research suggests that FT is experienced by many Americans: one in five report having financial problems because of increased medical expenses (Institute of Medicine, 2008). The number affected and depth of impact increases alongside the length and complexity of care received. Delago-Guay et al. (2015) studied the financial distress of 149 adults with advanced cancer, noting that over 305 of these patients rated this type of distress as more intense than that brought on by physical, familial, or emotional difficulties. Chi (2019) notes that these financial distress levels remain constant regardless of insurance status, the implication being that having health insurance does not tend to plug the drain of healthcare costs enough to lessen distress. Rather, these findings suggest that length and complexity of treatment is the primary determinant of a patient's sense of financial burden.

Health Disparity

The continued existence of substantial health disparities between race, ethnicity, income level, and geography has been described in each Social Justice section in this book. They speak to another trend in illness and disease today: The incidence and impact of many serious illnesses are felt disproportionately among certain demographic groups. These Social Justice sections outline research and literature demonstrating that serious, life-threatening consequences of illness are more common for people of color and/or people with fewer resources (i.e., less income, greater distance to top healthcare facilities, fewer social supports) across many diagnoses. As discussed throughout, these poorer health outcomes are partially due to reluctance to engage with medical professionals due to distrust of medical establishments that have, historically, been responsible for harming and/or delivering subpar care delivered to people of certain racial or ethnic groups, gender identities, and socioeconomic statuses. This book's authors have also argued repeatedly that healthcare professionals, and the infrastructure of institutional care, in many cases do not display the cultural congruence and humility that could make a meaningful difference in the care of disadvantaged groups. Many of our authors have highlighted how ongoing bias and racism affect the delivery of care within various illness groups and called for overhauls of systems of care that extend beyond more comprehensive training of medical professionals. For example, in the chapter on organ transplant, there is a call for more culturally informed assessments of transplant candidates and a greater awareness of larger societal disenfranchisement that impacts transplant eligibility and discussion of candidacy, in order to protect individual patients from being denied needed transplants unfairly as a result of implicit bias.

The costs of care can also account for disparities in care, leading to interruptions in care, narrowing of care choices, and to less than full engagement in treatment and monitoring of illnesses. Chi (2019) speaks of the prevalence of and multifaceted effect of financial toxicity – that is, the negative psychosocial and life consequences of high care costs. The author argues that, when such care costs are levied onto a person who is already financially struggling, the impact turns from unpleasant and anxiety-provoking to a serious barrier to ongoing treatment and care (Chi, 2019).

To address suspected causes of health disparities, governing bodies in healthcare are focused on prevention, early detection, and care delivery issues. Hospitals have outreach and population health departments, programming, and reports dedicated to identifying and addressing significant and concerning health issues in their surrounding communities, particularly those that affect racial or cultural groups disproportionately (Dennelly, 2019). For example, the American College of Surgeons (ACS, 2020), which sets standards for cancer care, has multiple requirements for accreditation-seeking cancer centers to more proactively reach out to neighboring community members and support them through early detection of cancers and possible subsequent treatment. These requirements recognize the harm of late detection, the need for and responsibility of facilities to overcome barriers to accessing care, the preventable factors in interrupted treatment and lack of follow-up in survivorship care, and the life-saving value of addressing those factors (ACS, 2020). Benefits such as extended at-home monitoring and long-term care are also offered for Medicaid and Medicare recipients who are especially challenged by management of low-grade illness and at higher risk for health decline (e.g., low-income senior citizens and people with one or more physical, intellectual, developmental disabilities) (National Council on Disability, n.d.).

It is difficult to determine to what extent these initiatives and programs do, in fact, prevent or reduce the severity of illness for targeted groups. Institutional and government research relies on comparisons between current incidence and mortality rates and projected ones and between current and past utilization of healthcare services, and of course, such comparisons leave room for other explanations of findings. If mortality rates caused by complications from diabetes are below expectations in 2060, they could indicate a reverse in trend *or* indicate an inaccurate prediction. Lower-than-expected rates could be caused, in some part, by prevention and early detection efforts *or* by other factors entirely.

Programs also aim to make quality-of-life improvements for people who are ill, including augmenting ability to carry out their activities in daily living (ADLs); physical therapy at home targets improvement in strength, flexibility, and mobility to promote recovery and prevent illness recurrence. Some other programs focus on the management of mental health issues, supporting mental health alongside physical health needs (Prince et al., 2007); still others provide companion services. It is commonly understood that home health aide services have multiple complementary benefits: physical assistance, enhanced sense of connection, and prevention of low mood that may, in turn, impact physical (as well as mental) health (Chi & Hemphill Ruden, 2019).

Healthcare facilities also work to maintain and enhance *continuity of care*. Goodwin (2021) portrays continuity of care (the transition of care plans and health information from one care team or facility to another) as critically important to a person's health and difficult to secure in today's healthcare landscape, defined as it is by specialization, insurance and financial problems, and other obstacles to accessing timely and effective care. Today, a patient may not have one physician or medical team who can be trusted to act as gatekeeper and point person in the management and oversight of their health problems, and they may frequently move between healthcare settings (i.e., community-based programs, outpatient facilities, and/or various inpatient departments or floors). To improve continuity, hospitals require thorough communication between healthcare professionals during known transitions of care and review documents used in transition of care (such as discharge plans), evaluating their comprehensiveness. In another effort to ensure uninterrupted care, administrators may also work closely with medical teams and their patients to schedule appointments that maintain the care plan while also accounting for individual needs and preferences. For instance, the person who needs early morning appointments so that she can get to work later in the day may be given such time slots consistently for this reason.

Guiding Principles in Healthcare

There are several conceptual and organizational frameworks that guide service and service delivery in healthcare systems today and will drive the future development of healthcare systems.

The "triple aim" of healthcare – "better care, better cost, and better health" (Dennelly, 2019, p. 276) – directs healthcare toward care experience, improving health outcomes and reducing per capita costs (Berwick et al., 2008). This three-pronged approach can be found between the lines of hospital administration operations, oversight, and data review. For example, patient advocate roles are created within hospitals as part of an aim toward delivering "better care" and patient advocates are tasked with receiving patient complaints and intervening toward resolution of care issues identified through them (Health Net Federal Services, n.d.). "Better costs" efforts are evident in the stated aim of hospitals to reduce the number of non-urgent, unnecessary emergency room visits that currently account for billions of dollars annually (Garber, 2019). "Better health" efforts by healthcare facilities are those research and programmatic initiatives within them that identify and improve health outcomes and reduce mortality rates.

Another concept is "patient-centered care." This is a framework for guiding goals of care discussions, care, and treatment plans with the patient's preferences, values, and priorities to the fore. Although this perspective might appear obvious and commonsensical to the social worker who is committed to a holistic view of an individual's experience, it is a departure from the traditional medical approach. The latter focuses on a person's physical health alone, sometimes at the expense of the person's well-being overall. What are examples of a shift of perspective in medicine toward patient-centered care? The patient satisfaction rating within hospitals is one; it prioritizes the patient's experience of care delivery. It is one of several metrics used to determine a hospital's provision of *excellence in care*. The Medicare Hospice Benefit and Medicare policy in palliative care for cancer patients is another example. It is a federal policy that recognizes the need to elevate physical, emotional, and spiritual suffering common to life-threatening illnesses with preventive and symptom-focused care alongside other holistic services (Marmo & Lane, 2020). The policy's extension of benefit to Medicare patients is supported by research that shows that the utilization of comfort care is a positive medical and patient-centered move. Such research shows that comfort care delays death, increases quality of life, *and* maintains the seriously ill person's sense of wholeness (Marmo & Lane, 2020).

This *integrated healthcare model* is a guiding principle for many healthcare facilities now, too. It is both a structure for care and a method of addressing multiple psychosocial and health needs simultaneously (Dennelly, 2019). Integrated healthcare systems consolidate care so that interconnected, consequential issues are addressed. It is designed to better ensure that mental health issues that would be otherwise unknown and/or unattended are addressed and alleviated. Dennelly (2019) highlights its importance in behavioral health, suggesting that it can overcome the stigma attached to receiving related services and reach people whose presence at a clinic or primary care facility may partially result from mental health disorders (depression, anxiety, substance misuse, or somatic symptoms) or psychosocial problems (i.e., elder abuse, intimate partner violence, homelessness, child abuse).

COVID-19

The COVID-19 pandemic is now widely acknowledged as a collective trauma that has threatened individuals, communities, and infrastructures of support and care. COVID-19 has brought the threat of severe illness and death to us all and has involved the witnessing of both. People we care for, worked with, or were intimately involved with have died or been severely ill. Beyond our personal circles, the sheer volume of cases and deaths we have learned about can be overwhelming as well.

It is important to recognize that crises in healthcare preceded COVID-19 in the form of preexisting understaffing and capacity issues. The COVID-19 crisis was not introduced to infrastructures that were thoroughly prepared and well-equipped for large surges in care needs. Rather, the hospitalizations and long-term care needs of some COVID-19 patients, and the new expectation that healthcare facilities *surge up* to meet these needs, landed on an already taxed healthcare system – one with shortages of healthcare staff, beds, and equipment preceding this pandemic. Thus, at the height of COVID-19-related surges, patients who needed intensive care may have had to wait longer than usual for intensive care unit intervention or inpatient hospital beds. The pandemic has exacerbated preexisting problems in healthcare and news coverage of COVID-19 incidence and mortality rates has put a powerful spotlight on them (Brody, 2021). However, while the need for a wider pool of healthcare workers (as well as other resources) has been made evident, the issue of recruitment and retention of onsite healthcare workers remains. In fact, the World Health Organization predicts that there will be a shortfall of 14.5 million healthcare workers globally by 2030 (2022).

Hospital and healthcare settings have also offered enhanced support services for patients and their workers in response to this crisis, which have included extended counseling benefits to service providers like social workers. The management of supporting self, coworkers and staff, patients, care teams, and institutions has been described by social workers in healthcare settings as overwhelming, frightening, anxiety producing, and depressing and as mentally, physically, and emotionally exhausting (Tosone, 2021). Piccolino (2021) discusses how social workers have walked in parallel with their patients, witnessing and supporting patients as their own health, security, and safety are at risk and as they face and cope with the same reality and fears.

Social Work's Presence in Healthcare

Social work's presence in healthcare facilities depends on institutional and departmental advocacy and support. Some departments or offices have onsite social workers; others have "offsite" social work assistance (i.e., social workers who follow patients from elsewhere); still others do not have social workers available to them. Similarly, while the benefit of social workers being part of goals of care and advance care conversations has been suggested in social work literature (e.g., Berzoff & Silverman, 2004), social workers can often be left out of such conversations. Because most hospitals with a limited social work headcount rely on referral systems to identify patients who receive psychosocial support and assistance, not all patients are seen or supported by healthcare social workers. Only those patients who refer themselves or who are referred by their medical team as needing social work assessment and intervention receive it. As a result, a patient and their support network may face the distress of health issues without social work intervention.

What a social worker does and how that person approaches the overarching goal of psychosocial support can vary, too. The inpatient social worker's tasks and focus are often primarily focused on hospital discharge, the project of ensuring that a person continues to heal at home or in another facility (partially to reduce costs to hospitals and patients for longer-than-medically needed inpatient stays). Berkman and Rehr (1972) identify the goal of the inpatient social worker as attending to the patient's immediate needs and facilitating a "socially oriented discharge plan" (p. 577) that supports their "recovery needs" (p. 567). In descriptions of inpatient social work (e.g., Renata, 2019), this orientation that focuses on immediate, short-term physical and psychosocial needs continues to be widely supported and heavily defines the role and tasks of inpatient social workers. Some commentators on inpatient social work push for comprehensive assessment and intervention of common mental health issues, including post-traumatic stress disorder (PTSD) (Jasphy, 2018). They call for expanding the parameters of "successful" discharge, prioritizing and adding a person's psychosocial health to the list of considerations for ensuring a "good" discharge out of the hospital.

Social workers in outpatient roles may be expected to engage more in the kind of work that is traditionally considered therapeutic. They are more likely to conduct short-term counseling focused on the psychological and emotional impact of illness; even if they do not engage in sessions devoted to a person's coping, they may use therapeutic approaches and concepts, and psychoeducation, during nontherapeutic interventions (such as case management, resource acquisition, or advocacy). In this way, a social worker who is working to secure transportation assistance for a client might engage in a therapeutic dialogue with that person about the feelings surrounding the stress of getting to/from appointments. Another social worker intervention that can have dual benefits is that of facilitator. When the social worker facilitates an open dialogue between medical team and patient about goals of care, for instance, that person utilizes therapeutic skills of assessment, creates a safe space for exploration of what's important to the patient, and better ensures mutual understanding between parties. This has therapeutic, as well as practical, impact – helping all parties get closer to an agreed-upon care plan.

Depending on the setting within healthcare (as well as the culture of the institution and team), social workers may be expected to have certain training and competencies. Palliative care social workers must learn and possess the "values and attitudes that allow them to engage therapeutically with those experiencing loss, death, and suffering" (Berzoff & Silverman, 2004, xxv), as well as working knowledge of relevant resources. Social workers who work within emergency rooms must work well in crisis, rapidly identifying what they can offer to ameliorate immediate issues and manifesting calm and reassurance in presenting such offerings.

With the rise of new programming outlined in the Health Disparity section, there is also a new opportunity for social workers to step into new roles and duties. Social workers may also step into leadership roles to create and implement behavioral health initiatives or weigh in on programs with behavioral health components aimed at improving physical health and care usage.

Social Work's Prerogative in Healthcare

Social work recognizes that work toward a person's betterment is a multifaceted endeavor rooted in a belief in their inherent dignity and worth and equal rights (Berzoff & Silverman, 2004). It is marked by its attunement to and active involvement in the systematic and contextual issues that impact individuals' and groups' agency and by its recognition of these issues as potential barriers to identifying and voicing patient care preferences and to processing and recovering from health-related experiences.

In healthcare, this social work purview can manifest at each level of patient engagement and advocacy. At the micro level, it can appear as active listening to the patient as they share their illness experience, as conceptualizing the patient's experience as an individual and nuanced one, and as responding to the patient empathetically from that understanding and awareness. It can look like advocacy for those who are – or have the potential to be – inequitably treated or disenfranchised due to race, culture, religion, socioeconomic status, sexual orientation, gender identity, disability, and/or age. It can appear as resource allocation and referrals to and coordination of care with outside service providers for patients with limited resources. It involves sensitivity to variations in ability or capacity to navigate complex systems in healthcare and care management (including work, state, and federal benefits). At the mezzo level, it can appear as active involvement with medical teams, health groups, leadership of healthcare institutions, and organizations. By being present at such tables, the social worker has greater opportunity to assess gaps of care across patient groups and to give voice to the patients' common experiences and perspective of them. At the macro level, it encourages the social worker to incorporate Rawls' (1971) theoretical approach of individual justice (entitlement to individual rights) and distributive justice (equitable distribution of resources) into their practice. In other words, the social worker in healthcare should examine the systems of care that affect patients from a social justice lens and speak up when they are found to be unjust or unequitable. When patients' rights are protected in some cases only, when resources (like preventive services) are disproportionately given and/or given to *some* only, the social worker looks for avenues of change.

To support the healthcare social worker's effort toward this end, education, training, and supervisory support related to affecting change within highly politicized organizations is relevant and valuable. Heifetz et al. (2009) offer a diagnostic tool for professionals at any level of seniority within such organizations who are interested in spearheading improvement. It begins with: What is the challenge and what does resolution look like? It continues by questioning institutional values and reasons for maintaining the status quo (risks of changing, competing values, loyalties, and alliances, etc.) (Heifetz et al., 2009). This tool may be helpful to social workers wondering where to begin such processes of change. To effectively advocate, social workers in healthcare would also be well advised to develop a working knowledge of laws and regulations, along with team/department/agency composition and dynamics, and to apply this knowledge in the formulation and presentation of recommendations for change for individual patients and patient groups. This is likely to be helpful as they navigate barriers to change, such as institutional constraints and restrictions, and seek to anchor discourse with other professional groups (such as hospital administrators or medical teams) in mutually agreed-upon values, objectives, and goals. Risks, competing values, and conflicting alliances often become less significant considerations when parties are reminded of a shared core value, such as optimal care of the person who is ill.

References

Agency for Healthcare Research and Quality. (2018, June). Chartbook on care coordination. *Transitions of care*. https://www.ahrq.gov/research/findings/nhqrdr/chartbooks/carecoordination/measure1.html

American College of Surgeons. (2020). *Optimal resources for cancer care*. https://www.facs.org/-/media/files/quality-programs/cancer/coc/optimal_resources_for_cancer_care_2020_standards.ashx

Berkman, B. G., & Rehr, H. (1972). The "sick-role" cycle and the timing of social work intervention. *Social Service Review, 46*(4).

Berwick, D. M., Nolan, T. W., & Whittington, J. (2008). The triple aim: Care, health, and cost. *Health Affairs, 27*(3).

Berzoff, J., & Silverman, P. (2004). *Living with dying: Handbook for end-of-life healthcare practitioners*. Columbia University Press.

Brody, J. E. (2021, February 8). Pandemic lessons in improving the medical system. *The New York Times*. https://www.nytimes.com/2021/02/08/well/live/medical-system-improvements.html
Centers for Disease Control and Prevention. (2019). *About chronic diseases*. https://www.cdc.gov/chronicdisease/about/index.htm
Chi, M. (2019, September). The hidden cost of cancer: Helping clients cope with financial toxicity. Special issue on healthcare. *Clinical Social Work Journal, 47*(3), 249–257.
Chi, M., & Hemphill Ruden, M. (2019, September). Introduction to "best practice in psychosocial healthcare: Complexity, compromise, and innovation". Special issue on healthcare. *Clinical Social Work Journal, 47*(3), 233–235.
Delgao-Guay, M., Ferrer, J., Rieber, A. G., Rhondai, W., Tayjasanant, S., Ochoa, J., et al. (2015). Financial distress and its associations with physical and emotional symptoms and quality of life among advanced cancer patients. *The Oncologist, 20*(9), 1092–1098.
Dennelly, L. (2019). Navigating psychosocial challenges in primary care with an integrated behavioral health model. *Clinical Social Work Journal, 3*, 276–283. https://doi.org/10.1007/s10615-019-00708-0
Florence Health. (2019, October 2). *PAs and NPs spend much less time with patients than they want – here's why*. https://huddle.florence-health.com/discover/content/article/how-much-time-pas-nps-wish-they-spend-with-patients-vs-do/
Frakt, A. (2019, October 7). The huge waste in the U.S. health system. *The New York Times*. https://www.nytimes.com/2019/10/07/upshot/health-care-waste-study.html
Garber, J. (2019, November 11). Are we ignoring the systemic factors behind "inappropriate" use of emergency care? *Lown Institute*. https://lowninstitute.org/are-we-ignoring-the-systemic-factors-behind-inappropriate-use-of-emergency-care/rgencycare?
Goodwin, J. S. (2021). Continuity of care matters in all health care settings. *JAMA Network*. https://www.Users/meredith/Downloads/goodwin_2021_ic_210044_1616042424.75384%20(1).pdf
Hagen, L. (2021, June 17). Supreme court dismisses red state challenge to Obamacare. *US News*. https://www.usnews.com/news/national-news/articles/2021-06-17/supreme-court-dismisses-red-state-challenge-to-obamacare
Health Net Federal Services. (n.d.). *Hospital patient advocates*. https://www.hnfs.com/content/hnfs/home/tw/bene/res/hospital-stay/patient_advocates.html
Heifetz, R.A., Linsky, M., & Grashow, A. (2009). Diagnose the political landscape. Chapter 6. In *The practice of adaptive leadership: Tools and tactics for changing your organization and the world.*
Indeed. (2021). *Physician assistant job description*. https://www.indeed.com/hire/job-description/physician-assistant?gclid=CjwKCAiAs92MBhAXEiwAXTi256yuEMys88XqBHm3vnQqtnoE0x4U4vk8VzvQxumIl2rl9gZdVWCq9RoCj9YQAvD_BwE&aceid=
Jasphy, L. (2018, March 31). The importance of clinical social work in patient care. *The Playbook*. https://www.hss.edu/playbook/the-importance-of-clinical-social-work-in-patient-care/
Levey, N. (2021, March 23). The COVID relief bill expands the affordable care act. It doesn't come cheap. *Policy-ish*. NPR. https://www.npr.org/sections/health-shots/2021/03/23/980364322/the-covid-relief-bill-expanda-the-affordable-care-act-it-doesnt-come-cheap
Lexis Nexis. (n.d.). Studies show that social determinants of health (SDOH) are better indicators of hospital readmission risk than standard EHR care. *White Paper*. https://risk.lexisnexis.com/insights-resources/white-paper/mitigate-hospital-readmission-risk?trmid=HCCRM22.GA.SearchAds.PHGO-568922&gclid=Cj0KCQiA_c-OBhDFARIsAIFg3ez8n_Ei8Wrs8sO3iutViPnybSsTj6LnQjo0G5aQPYH93JKCDWo-nrYaAhh_EALwwcB
Marmo, S., & Lane, S. R. (2020, May 13). Social justice and advanced cancer patients: An analysis of key policies. *Journal of Policy Practice and Research, 1*, 37–54.
National Center for Health Statistics. (2021, December). *NCHS data brief, 427*. https://www.cdc.gov/nchs/data/databriefs/db427.pdf

National Council on Disability. (n.d.). *Appendix F. Disability-related Medicaid service coverages.* https://ncd.gov/publications/2013/20130315/20130513_AppendixF
Norris, L. (n.d.). States vary considerably in terms of how they manage their insurance markets and health insurance exchanges. *Healthinsurance.org*. https://www.healthinsurance.org/health-insurance-marketplaces/
NYC Health and Hospitals. (2022). *U.S. news and world report recognizes seven NYC health and hospitals facilities as "high performing" across specialties.* nychealthandhospitals.org/pressrelease/u-s-news-recognizes-nyc-health-hospitals-facilities-as-high-performing/
Piccolino, S. (2021). On the front lines of the fight against the COVID-19 pandemic: Meaning-making and shared trauma. In *Shared trauma, shared resilience during a pandemic*. Springer.
Population Reference Bureau. (2019). *Fact sheet: Aging in America*. https://www.prb.org/resources/fact-sheet-aging-in-the-united-states/
Prince, M., Patel, V., Saxena, S., Maj, M., Maselko, J., Philips, M. R., & Rahman, A. (2007). No health without mental health. *Lancet, 370*, 859–877.
Rawls, J. (1971). *A theory of social justice*. Cambridge.
Renata, R. (2019, March 4). *What are the duties of a social worker in the hospital?* https://careertrend.com/about-6327303-job-description-patient-coordinator.html
Ruth, B. J., & Marshall, J. W. (2017). A history of social work in public health. *American Journal of Public Health, 107*(3 Suppl), S236–S242.
Tolbert, J. (2020, November 6). *Key fact about the uninsured population*. https://www.kff.org/uninsured/issue-brief/key-facts-about-the-uninsured-population/
Tosone, C. (2021). Introduction. In *Shared trauma, shared resilience during a pandemic.*
World Health Organization. (2022). *Health workforce requirements for universal health coverage and the sustainable development goals.* https://apps.who.int/iris/bitstream/handle/10665/250330/9789241511407-?sequence=1

Epilogue

Meredith Hemphill

With 75% of social workers expected to be working in healthcare by 2027 (Ruth & Marshall, 2017), the demand for our specialized skill sets is increasingly imperative. We, social workers in the healthcare field, have more than a list of concrete tasks and responsibilities; we have a working paradigm of psychosocial care – a way of understanding the experiences of people who are ill and their families – that can drive how care is provided to them, and this can elevate the overall quality of care.

When we better understand what we bring to the table, we may also critically engage more with our role, particularly in interdisciplinary settings. This may manifest as a heightened curiosity when receiving referrals: *Why am I really being asked to see this person? What is this person going through that lies beyond their medical symptoms, and how does that impact their physical health?* Or it could result in advocating for different tasks to be included in their day-to-day work, which focus more on a patient's overall well-being: *Can I be involved in more interdisciplinary meetings for patient groups or institutional initiatives? How should I suggest something new?*

It is important for social workers to approach their work from their professionally based viewpoint and, when they do so, they are bound to see themselves differently in the execution of their work.

When we, as healthcare social workers, are in touch with what we can bring to the healthcare systems we serve, we recognize ourselves as a necessary and important part of the provision of care and can intervene skillfully, and positively impact the care for our patients so that they can navigate physical illness and the journey to physical wellness as completely and smoothly as possible.

M. Hemphill
City Center Psychotherapy, New York, NY, USA
e-mail: drhemphill@citycenterpsychotherapy.com

M. Hemphill, A. Nathanson (eds.), *The Practice of Clinical Social Work in Healthcare*, Essential Clinical Social Work Series,
https://doi.org/10.1007/978-3-031-31650-0

Reference

Ruth, B. J., & Marshall, J. W. (2017). A history of social work in public health. *American Journal of Public Health, 107*(3, Suppl), S236–S242.

Index

M. Hemphill, A. Nathanson (eds.), *The Practice of Clinical Social Work in Healthcare*, Essential Clinical Social Work Series,
https://doi.org/10.1007/978-3-031-31650-0

Printed in the USA
CPSIA information can be obtained
at www.ICGtesting.com
LVHW011555300723
753856LV00001B/2

9 783031 316494